Reproduction in Domestic Ruminants VII

Society of Reproduction and Fertility Volume 67

Proceedings of the Eighth International Symposium on Reproduction in Domestic Ruminants

Anchorage, Alaska
September 2010

Edited by:
MC Lucy, JL Pate, MF Smith and TE Spencer

Nottingham
University Press

Nottingham University Press
Manor Farm, Church Lane, Thrumpton
Nottingham NG11 0AX, United Kingdom
www.nup.com

NOTTINGHAM

First published 2010

British Library Cataloguing in Publication Data
Reproduction in Domestic Ruminants VII
I. Lucy, M.C. II. Pate, J.L. III. Smith, M.F. IV. Spencer, T.E.

ISBN: 978-1-907284-14-4
ISSN: 2045-872X

Disclaimer

Every reasonable effort has been made to ensure that the material in this book is true, correct, complete and appropriate at the time of writing. Nevertheless, the publishers and authors do not accept responsibility for any omission or error, or for any injury, damage, loss or financial consequences arising from the use of the book.

Typeset by Nottingham University Press, Nottingham
Printed and bound by H. Charlesworth and Co Ltd, UK

Contents

SPERM IN THE REPRODUCTIVE TRACT

Chairperson: Zvi Roth

THE RUMINANT CORPUS LUTEUM

Chairperson: Joy Pate

CRITICAL ISSUES FACING GLOBAL RUMINANT PRODUCTION

Chairperson: Reinaldo Cooke

MANAGING FERTILITY IN DOMESTIC RUMINANTS

Chairperson: George Perry

UNIQUE ASPECTS OF REPRODUCTION IN DIVERSE RUMINANT SPECIES

Chairperson: Tom Geary

Preface

The Eighth International Ruminant Reproduction Symposium was held at the Hilton Hotel in Anchorage, Alaska, USA on September 3-7, 2010. There were 209 delegates from 32 countries including participants from Mexico and South America, USA and Canada, Europe, the Middle East and Asia, and Australia and New Zealand. The only continents without representation were Africa and Antarctica. The delegates received tremendous hospitality during the conference thanks in part to the hard work of Scott Doonan of the Hilton Anchorage.

This volume contains the proceedings of 32 scientific presentations that were made over 12 conference sessions. The task of nominating plenary speakers fell upon the North American Scientific Organizing Committee with subcommittee chairs representing the diverse aspects of ruminant reproductive biology (Fuller Bazer, Marc-André Sirard, Larry Reynolds, Milan Shipka, Carlos Gutiérrez, Keith Inskeep, Susan Suarez, Jose Santos, and Terry Nett). These chairs recruited additional international members in their efforts to create a balanced program with global representation. The final program included sessions on: The Ruminant Genome; Developmental Processes in Ruminants; The Ruminant Transcriptome; Assessing Gene Function in Ruminants; Pluripotency in Ruminant Stem Cells; Ruminant Neuroendocrinology; The Eric Lamming Memorial Lecture on Ovulation; Oocyte and Follicular Development in Ruminants; Sperm in the Reproductive Tract; The Ruminant Corpus Luteum; Critical Issues Facing Global Ruminant Production; Managing Fertility in Domestic Ruminants; and Unique Aspects of Reproduction in Diverse Ruminant Species. Invited speakers received a bottle of "Epididymal Reserve" cabernet sauvignon from Phil Senger of Current Conceptions, Inc.

A conference dinner was held at the Sheraton with memorable views of Mt. McKinley (the highest mountain in North America and approximately 200 km from Anchorage). Pioneer Awards were made to Drs. Fuller Bazer (Texas A&M University) and Gordon Niswender (Colorado State University) for their significant contributions to science through the development of novel technologies, the creation of new knowledge, and the mentoring of the next generation of ruminant reproductive biologists. Drs. William Thatcher and Jenny Juengel kindly agreed to make award presentations. Special thanks to Professor Keith Inskeep (West Virginia University) for agreeing to present the conference summary and Professor Robert Webb (Nottingham) for acting as master of ceremonies for the evening.

We gratefully acknowledge the financial support of Arm & Hammer Animal Nutrition, the College of Agriculture, Food, and Natural Resources, the Division of Animal Sciences, and the Mizzou Advantage Program at the University of Missouri, Pfizer Animal Health, the Beef Reproduction Task Force, Current Conceptions Inc., the Society for Reproduction and Fertility, Elanco Animal Health, IMV Technologies, and Intervet Schering-Plough Animal Health.

The local organizing committee (LOC) that consisted of Matt Lucy and Mike Smith from the University of Missouri, Joy Pate from Pennsylvania State University, and Tom Spencer from Texas A&M University acted as scientific editors for this volume. Their task would have been far more difficult without the help of fellow scientists who reviewed invited papers and abstracts. This volume could not have been competed without the work Sarah Keeling (Nottingham University Press) who assembled and typeset these proceedings. Special thanks go to Cinda

Hudlow, Emily Newsom, Ky Pohler, and Emma Jinks from the University of Missouri for their significant participation in various aspects of the book project. The beautiful photographs on the cover of this book were submitted by Marc-André Sirard and Alex Evans. Many thanks to all who submitted entries to the cover photo contest.

A final and most-important thank you goes to Christine Pickett, Sharon Rhodes and Margaret Arredondo of the University of Missouri Conference Office. These individuals, with little or no connection to our field of science, demonstrated unparalleled and tireless dedication to the success of the 2010 Ruminant Reproduction Symposium. This symposium would have not been possible without them. We will be forever grateful for their efforts on our behalf.

Matt Lucy
Chairman, LOC

Pioneer Awards

It has become a tradition at recent Ruminant Reproduction Symposia (Colorado Springs, 1998; Crieff, 2002; and Wellington, 2006) to recognize the outstanding contributions of a select group of individuals to our understanding of ruminant reproduction. Therefore, the local organizing committee decided to acknowledge the lifetime achievements of two highly distinguished North American scientists. The criteria which formed the basis of the Pioneer Award included the following: 1) Development of new knowledge that opened areas of research in ruminant reproduction, 2) Development of new technologies that have enabled other investigators to make important contributions to ruminant reproductive biology, 3) A person who is recognized as an international scholar, 4) Known for his/her contributions toward mentoring younger scientists, and 5) An individual with a record of contributing and participating in the Ruminant Reproduction Symposium over the years. Although the committee recognized the important contributions of several North American researchers, we are pleased to recognize both Fuller W. Bazer (Texas A&M University) and Gordon D. Niswender (Colorado State University) with the Pioneer Award at the 2010 Ruminant Reproduction Symposium.

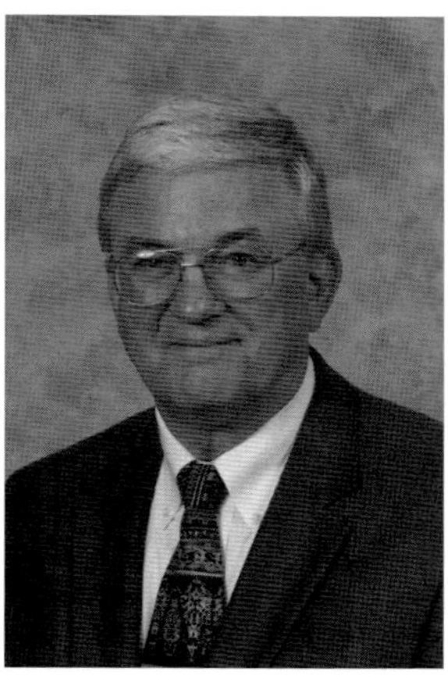

Fuller W. Bazer

Regents Fellow, Distinguished Professor and O.D. Butler Chair Texas A&M University

Fuller Bazer received a Bachelor's degree in biology from the Centenary College of Louisiana in 1960 and Master of Science degree from Louisiana State University in 1963. From 1963 to 1965, he served as a Lieutenant in the U.S. Army. In 1965, he decided to continue his graduate training at North Carolina State University, where he earned his Doctor of Philosophy degree with Drs. L.C. Ulberg and A.J. Clawson in 1969. While pursuing his graduate degrees, he developed an interest in early pregnancy biology that became a passion and theme of his distinguished research career. In 1968, Fuller joined the Department of Animal Science at the University of Florida as an Assistant Professor and rose through the ranks to Graduate Research Professor in 1988. In 1992, he moved to Texas A&M University where he was named the O.D. Butler Chair in Animal Science and served in a number of administrative roles including Director of the Institute for Biosciences and Technology, Associate Dean of the College of Agriculture and Life Sciences, and Associate Vice President for Research. He was named a Regent's Fellow in 1999 and a Distinguished Professor in 2004.

Dr. Fuller Bazer is known worldwide for his research in the area of conceptus-maternal interactions that span the gamut of domestic animals from ruminants to pigs and horses. The biology of how the conceptus (embryo and its associated placental membranes) communicates with the mother to establish and maintain pregnancy has been the focus of Dr. Bazer's research career and his collaborations with Drs. Bill Thatcher and Mike Roberts at the University of Florida and with Drs. Bob Burghardt, Greg Johnson, Tom Spencer and Guoyao Wu at Texas A&M University have been particularly productive in this regard. Earlier in his career he examined how ovarian hormones and the uterus regulate growth and development of the conceptus of domestic animals. He and his colleagues made significant contributions to our understanding of pregnancy recognition signaling in both pigs and sheep. In 1977, he and Bill Thatcher published the endocrine-exocrine theory of pregnancy recognition in pigs. While at the University of Florida, he, Mike Roberts and Bill Thatcher published a series of papers that established interferon tau (IFNT) as the pregnancy recognition signal in ruminants that had direct paracrine actions on the uterus to inhibit endometrial production of luteolytic pulses of $PGF_{2\alpha}$, thereby preventing regression of the corpus luteum and maintaining progesterone that is necessary for pregnancy. Those studies required the development of unique models including the catheterization of the uterus and unilateral pregnancy. Always a proponent of how agricultural research can benefit human medicine, Fuller and his colleagues established that IFNT was useful as a therapy for the treatment of autoimmune diseases such as rheumatoid arthritis and multiple sclerosis. His research studies have resulted in over 400 scientific articles, reviews and book chapters during his career.

Fuller has a comprehensive knowledge and passion for Reproductive Biology and its implications in the broader world of scientific research which has been acknowledged by his receipt of numerous awards including the: Alexander von Humboldt Research Award in Agriculture; American Society of Animal Science Physiology and Endocrinology Award; Society for the Study of Reproduction Research Award, Distinguished Service Award, Carl G. Hartman Award, and Trainee Mentor Award; Texas A&M University and the Association of Former Students Distinguished Achievement Awards in Research; Wolf Prize in Agriculture; and most recently the Society for Reproduction and Fertility Distinguished Research Award.

He has had a lifelong commitment to graduate education and training postdoctoral fellows, and his research has involved partnerships with over 90 trainees (graduate students and postdoctoral fellows). One of the unique qualities of Dr. Bazer is his selflessness and service as a teacher and trusted mentor to trainees in reproductive biology as well as faculty members at Texas A&M and abroad. His service to the scientific community is too extensive to review here but includes providing recombinant proteins to investigators worldwide, serving as President and Director of the Society for the Study of Reproduction, Editor of Biology of Reproduction, co-founder of the Reproductive Tract Biology Gordon Research Conference, review panels for the USDA, BARD and NIH, and as a reviewer for countless scientific journals and granting agencies.

In summary, Fuller W. Bazer is an outstanding scientist, educator, and mentor who has made enormous contributions to our understanding of pregnancy biology in domestic ruminants.

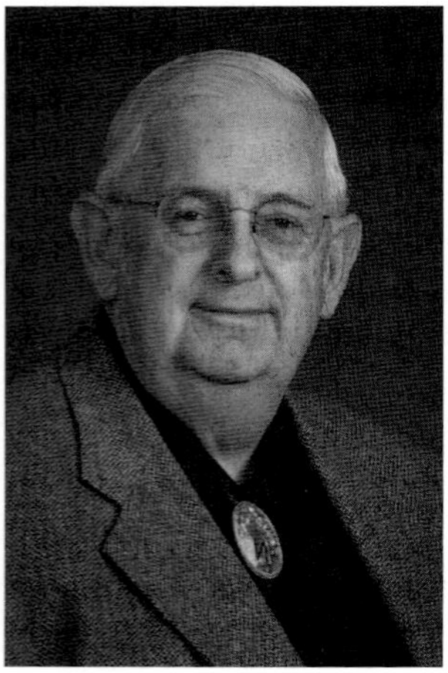

Gordon D. Niswender

University Distinguished Professor
Colorado State University

Gordon Niswender received a degree in agricultural education from the University of Wyoming. Shortly before graduation he attended a seminar by Dr James N. Wiltbank and decided to join Dr. Wiltbank's research and graduate training program at the University of Nebraska to pursue a Master of Science degree. While working with Dr. Wiltbank he developed an interest in regulation of the corpus luteum, which would become a consistent theme throughout his distinguished research career. In 1964 he joined Dr. Phillip Dzuik (Animal Genetics Laboratory) at the

University of Illinois and received the PhD degree (1967) in Animal Sciences and Physiology. Gordon joined the laboratory of Dr. Rees Midgley as a postdoctoral fellow and later became an assistant professor at the University of Michigan. While at Michigan he developed radioimmunoassays for FSH, LH, progesterone, and testosterone and the preceding assays have been used for reliable measurement of the preceding hormones in a variety of species including domestic ruminants. He is known worldwide for the generation of an antiserum to LH (GDN #15) that has been used to measure circulating concentrations of LH in numerous species. His original publication in 1969 entitled "Radioimmunoassay for bovine and ovine luteinizing hormone (Endocrinology 84:1166-1173) has been designated a Citation Classic. In 1972, Gordon joined the Department of Biomedical Sciences at Colorado State University (CSU) where he rose through the ranks and was named a University Distinguished Professor in 1987.

Regulation of the corpus luteum has been the focus of Dr. Niswender's research career and his long-term collaborations with Drs. Terry Nett and Heywood Sawyer have been particularly fruitful in this regard. Earlier in his career he examined the relationship among changes in circulating concentrations of progesterone, luteal blood flow, and both occupied and unoccupied LH receptors. He and his colleagues made significant contributions to our understanding of the mechanism of action of LH through his studies on LH receptor binding, receptor internalization, and signal transduction in luteal cells. He also developed receptor assays for $PGF_{2\alpha}$ and PGE_2 and investigated the role of these prostaglandins in luteolysis and maternal recognition of pregnancy in ruminants. The preceding studies led to characterization of the morphological, biochemical, and physiological differences between small and large steroidogenic luteal cells. He and his colleagues demonstrated that small luteal cells have a relatively low basal secretion of progesterone but are highly responsive to LH. Alternatively, large luteal cells have a high basal secretion of progesterone and are not responsive to LH. Gordon and his colleagues have focused on the cellular interactions between small and large steroidogenic luteal cells during luteolysis and developed a model for the regulation of luteal function based on the interaction of these two cell types. His research studies have been published in 214 refereed journal articles and 41 book chapters.

Gordon has been the recipient of numerous prestigious awards including the Animal Physiology and Endocrinology Award by the American Society of Animal Science, Research Award from the Society for the Study of Reproduction, Endocrine Society Ayerst Award, Merit Award from the National Institutes of Health, Distinguished Service Award from the Society for the Study of Reproduction, and the Carl G. Hartman Award from the Society for the Study of Reproduction.

He has had a life-long commitment to graduate education and training postdoctoral fellows. He has served as the mentor for 6 MS students, 20 PhD students and 32 postdoctoral fellows and he is well known as a mentor who is both tough and committed to the professional development of his mentees. His service to the scientific community is too extensive to review here but includes providing antisera for radioimmunoassays to investigators worldwide, serving as Treasurer and President of the Society for the Study of Reproduction, serving on the Board of Directors for the Ovarian Workshop, over ten years of service to the National Institutes of Health in various capacities, and helping to organize the first International Ruminant Reproduction Symposium.

In summary, Gordon Niswender is an outstanding scientist, educator, and mentor who has made enormous contributions to our understanding of corpus luteum physiology in domestic ruminants.

Ruminant reproduction: recent findings and future challenges, a summary

EK Inskeep

Division of Animal and Nutritional Sciences, West Virginia University, Morgantown, WV 26506-6108

Introduction

This conference has provided a valuable update on knowledge of reproductive physiology, and its genetic and environmental regulation, in a variety of domesticated and wild ruminants. Researchers have begun to examine genetic factors in model systems such as maturation and capacitation of sperm, follicular selection, maturation and ovulation, and luteal function in pregnant and non-pregnant females, as well as placental development and function. New knowledge of details of these processes reinforces basic concepts of the importance of neuroendocrine regulation of testicular and ovarian function, particularly in regard to roles of steroid hormones in determining fertility. One is struck by the multiplicity of effects of key hormones and the precision of timing of their secretion required for maximum reproductive performance, especially in the lactating female.

Greater understanding of genomic, proteomic and metabolomic factors is being obtained and interpretations of "omics" data are improving. A greater number of papers included data from use of new genetic and associated "omics" technologies than ever before. The elucidation of roles of non-coding RNAs, especially micro-RNAs, is revealing detailed knowledge of regulatory steps in oocyte maturation and early embryogenesis. Despite numerous steps forward, many mysteries of mechanisms of action in both the male and the female are yet to be solved.

We've seen and heard reviews of a series of careful step-by-step analyses of significant questions in reproductive physiology and endocrinology. Sometimes the work has been done by the reviewers and their colleagues. In other cases, more extensive networks of researchers were involved, either as collaborators, building on others' work, or working independently.

Biotechnology

The initial paper by Taylor *et al.* highlighted the economy of new technologies and rapid progress in understanding the ruminant genome, with predictions of how these methods will allow manipulation in the future. The power of newer methods was emphasized further by Sinclair *et al.* and Anthony *et al.* One statement by Taylor *et al.* was that "genetic progress in milk production is expected to double due to the decrease in generation interval ... achieved by a reduced need to progeny test young bulls..." There is a danger that this prediction might portend a further decrease in reproductive fitness of lactating dairy cows unless selection programs consider reproductive traits. However, the authors optimistically concluded that such information will "guide the engineering of transgenic animals with increased adaptation to changing production environments, disease resistance, reproductive and productive capabilities."

Bauersachs *et al.* evaluated and illustrated techniques for analyses of genomic, transcriptomic, and proteomic databases. These analyses provide opportunities for linking quantitative and

Corresponding author E-mail: einskeep@wvu.edu

molecular genetics to expand knowledge of genetic regulation of reproductive traits. Although these databases have revealed antagonistic relationships between production and fertility at the molecular level, some alleles were found that had favorable effects on yield traits and a fertility trait.

A wide variety of actions has been ascribed to non-coding RNAs in the mouse (Tesfaye *et al.*), but relatively little is known in ruminants. This is certainly an area of fertile ground for ruminant studies. The micro RNAs are particularly exciting, as it appears that they play major roles in regulating activation of the embryonic genome (Sirard) and are altered in oocytes derived from persistent follicles (Lingenfelter *et al.* 2007), which in preliminary work (Taft, Jr. 1999) appeared to have progressed in meiosis to nuclear stage II. Current knowledge of the timing and factors involved in the maternal:embryo transition of genomic control was reviewed in detail by Sirard, who pointed to the 8-cell stage as a major point of transition. He noted that transcription factors decrease through the 8-cell stage, then increase again at the blastocyst, but some transcription factors that are only maternal in origin, do not show that recovery. Tesfaye *et al.* predicted that micro RNAs will be considerably involved in post-transcriptional gene regulation and be regulated epigenetically.

Another component of the genome recently described in more detail is endogenous retroviruses. As discussed by Spencer *et al.*, these beta retroviruses began to enter the genome millions of years ago or entered thousands of years ago, but may still be invading. Although many are non-functional, others play important biological roles. They can prevent entry of other retroviruses by receptor interference. Some are expressed specifically in uterine luminal and glandular epithelia and in trophectoderm of the conceptus. These play essential roles in elongation of the conceptus and in growth and development of trophectoderm and could possibly predict the type of implantation in these species. Two questions come to mind: (1) Is there any potential for contraceptive effects in animal populations by blocking those retrovirus components that are essential to placentation? (2) Could any of these retroviruses qualify for use as vectors for gene insertion?

Comparative data have been a prominent feature of this symposium

Comparisons across species can be very valuable in stimulating our thinking. Data reported here provide great encouragement relative to the breadth of studies involved and the variety of species being studied. However, the multitude of data on mice give cause for concern that rodents may be substituted for food animals in too many cases for the long term good of animal agriculture. While reduced funding for food animal research has caused a search for funding from biomedical sources (Ireland *et al.* 2008), it appears to have caused a shift to use of research animals from which data may or may not be extrapolated readily to food animals.

On the other hand, much of what has been learned in food animals has derived from clues gleaned from studies of lower mammals. Clarke & Smith credited the basis for their work with gonadotropin inhibitory hormone to its discovery in the hypothalamus of an even more remote species, the quail. It will be important in the future to maintain an appropriate balance and the ruminant-oriented scientist will necessarily read and study a wide selection of non-ruminant literature in the search for clues to mechanisms.

Given the increased presentation of comparative data at this venue than at previous symposia in the series, a naive science writer in attendance might conclude that there has been great success in transgenics that led to ruminant rats, ruminant mice and ruminant pigs. I am reminded of the time when my younger son was raising cattle as a 4-H youth project. Tom reasoned that winter feeding costs (and his labor) could be reduced by transferring a gene for hibernation into the beef cow. My own dream was that isolation of the factor that caused identical quadruplets in the armadillo might allow similar division of early zygotes in food animals if that factor were injected into the oviduct. Subsequent separation of the divided embryos should facilitate an increase in genetic efficiency of embryo transfer. Might such a gene exist in dams of identical twins?

These science fiction-type ideas might not be as farfetched as one would think when considered in light of successes in rodents with transplantation of testicular stem cells. The most exciting new finding in that area is that germ cell clumps were formed in THY1-enriched spermatogonial stem cells from the bull cultured with growth factors and bovine embryonic fibroblasts as feeder cells (Oatley). Successful transplantation of spermatogonial stem cells from superior bulls into testes of average bulls would be an alternative to AI for the beef industry, in which AI is limited by extensive conditions. Of course, such a procedure also would contribute to a loss of heterozygosity in the population.

Studies of embryonic and fetal mortality are revealing species differences in types and patterns of loss, and genetic, environmental and epigenetic factors involved in those losses. Analyses of genomic, proteomic and metabolomic information may identify opportunities for interventions to prevent these losses or overcome detrimental characteristics.

Another positive feature of this symposium is the increase in number of submitted papers. Particularly noticeable to this reviewer is a greater emphasis on male reproduction among those submitted papers. The male has been neglected in some quarters in recent years. At this meeting, several submitted papers provided detailed elaboration of concepts discussed in the review papers.

Characterization of the ruminant genome and its components in reproductive tissues, including placenta

Productive efforts to characterize ruminant genomes have been reported in the whole animal, ovary and oocyte, testis and spermatozoa, oviduct, uterus, and placenta. Developmental programming by dietary manipulation is receiving increasing emphasis. Fowden *et al.* characterized environmental effects on several placental functions and effects on fetal or birth weights. Nutrition at critical times during prenatal development is clearly a major factor and produces epigenetic effects that carry over into adulthood. They described a variety of roles of the placenta and the importance of imprinted genes and IGF2 in placental development and adaptation. In reading their report, the widely used ratio of fetal weight to placental weight seems a crude measure of placental efficiency. It would appear that more precise data are obtained in studies using catheterization of fetal and maternal vessels to collect sequential samples for analyses. Would some measures of placental function lend themselves to evaluation in a manner that would yield a relative value, similar to residual feed intake?

The importance of DNA methylation in gene expression and epigenetic effects, and effects of diet on DNA methylation were emphasized by both Fowden *et al.* and Sinclair *et al.* The latter authors delineated knowledge of DNA methylation in the germline in mice and how little is known in ruminants. They introduced the term "methylome" in regard to methylation status of genes. They presented evidence of dietary regulation, effects of environmental chemicals, and epigenetic changes and raised an important question, Why are "effects of peri-conceptional nutrient restriction manifest more in male than female offspring" in both rats and sheep? They further noted a neglect of research into effects of paternal nutrition on epigenetic programming through the germline. Germane to current concerns in the human population, they showed that dietary limits to methylation in the ewe led to adult obesity in the offspring.

"Knockdown" of gene expression was used by Anthony *et al.* to assess gene function in sheep placenta. With a short-hairpin RNA targeting sheep proline-rich protein 15, a nuclear protein expressed during elongation of the conceptus, introduced into the trophoblast, the conceptus died or failed to develop by day 15 postcoitum. Mechanism of action of the gene is not known. They also discussed development and use of cultures of cattle or sheep trophoblast cell lines in assessing gene function and regulation, and limitations to *in vitro* techniques.

Seasonal and neuroendocrine studies

In conjunction with the symposium in Crieff, Scotland 8 years ago, I had the great privilege of visiting with Gerald Lincoln and seeing his highly seasonal Soay sheep. The work since that time (Lincoln & Hazlerigg) has been very productive and led to a concept that annual transitions are generated by birth and death of cells and tissue regeneration throughout the life cycle, which Lincoln & Hazlerigg referred to as "the histogenesis hypothesis". In Soay sheep, these annual transitions in response to photoperiod occur in tissues of the pars tuberalis of the anterior pituitary gland and in the sub-ventricular zone of the mediobasal hypothalamus. Although they illustrated annual changes regulated by the pars tuberalis with prolactin, they pointed out that in the past, too much emphasis was placed on products without realizing the changes occurring in sources of those products.

Clarke & Smith described the roles and regulation of two relatively recently discovered products, kisspeptin and gonadotropin inhibitory hormone and showed associated histological changes. In 2004, when Bob Goodman and I were preparing the revised chapter on the estrous cycle of the ewe for the Knobil and Neill book (Goodman & Inskeep, 2006), we resisted the suggestion by Associate Editor Tony Plant, that perhaps we should include some mention of kisspeptin, arguing that it had hardly been examined in the sheep. How wrong we were to ignore it! That became clear as Clarke & Smith described how kisspeptin functions in two different hypothalamic areas to regulate GnRH secretion. Particularly striking is the fact that a single cell type contains kisspeptin, neurokinin B and dynorphin, thus mediating both positive and negative feedback of sex steroids. Gonadotropin inhibitory hormone has direct inhibitory effects on GnRH neurons and changes seasonally, both in number of cells producing it (fitting with the histogenesis hypothesis) and in number of GnRH cells contacted by terminals of GnIH cells. The authors noted that seasonal changes require 6 to 9 weeks. Yet seasonal anoestrus can be abrogated by introduction of the male (as discussed in earlier symposia in this series, Walkden-Brown *et al.* 1999). Genetic selection for fertility in May (northern hemisphere) in response to only the male, led to some animals cycling throughout the seasonal period of expected anoestrus (Vincent *et al.* 2000). The mechanism of action of male introduction represents an opportunity for further neuroendocrine studies.

Sperm quality, storage and function

Sutovsky & Lovercamp reviewed new approaches using biomarkers to assess sperm quality and characterization of the proteome of sperm. Prediction of fertility from examination of semen has long been elusive. A combination of techniques was used to identify ubiquitin, 15-lipoxygenase, thioredoxin SPTRX3/TXNDC8, platelet activating factor-receptor, arylsulfatase A, glycan-specific lectins and acrosome-binding lectins as potentially valuable markers of sperm defects. These molecules show promise for greater accuracy in assessing semen samples using flow cytometry and imaging methodologies.

Sperm storage and movement in the oviduct were discussed by Hung & Suarez, who used a comparative approach and noted that most ruminant work had been done in *Bos taurus*. They identified the uterotubal junction as a key site regulating passage of sperm into the oviduct and discussed how genetic defects, expressed in the proteome of sperm, can prevent that passage. In mice, microscopic observation of the behavior of sperm in the oviduct was a useful technique. Prolonged motile life of sperm is facilitated by binding to cilia of the oviductal epithelium and by delayed capacitation. Capacitation and hyperactivation allow sperm to be released from the oviductal epithelium and move toward the site of fertilization in the ampulla. Each of these processes and whether sperm are guided toward eggs by chemotaxis are not fully understood.

Gadella provided a very extensive review of the fertilization process, including attachment of sperm to the zona pellucida, hypermotility, zona drilling, blocks to polyspermy and sperm-oocyte fusion. His paper was one of the most thorough in the entire conference in citation of the pertinent literature and in analyzing dogma versus knowledge. To one who recalls when Dan Szollosi & Hans Ris (1961) first described the process of fusion of sperm and oocyte membranes to engulf the sperm into the ooplasm in the rat, it seems that knowledge has come a very long way. Gadella, too, provided a new "omics" term, suggesting the need for studies of "glycomics" to further understand the fertilization process.

Follicles and oocytes

Studies of follicular development and selection have led to interesting progress in understanding that process during the last two decades. One concept detailed here (Smith *et al.*) is that selection of a single ovulatory follicle in the cow may be predicated upon negative regulation of the action of FSH and IGF1 on granulosa cells in follicles destined to become subordinate and atretic. This step occurs after the negative regulatory factor has been down regulated in the lead (dominant, selected) follicle by IGF1 and FSH. The concept arose from characterization of the transcriptome of bovine oocytes. The presence of five expressed sequence tags of mRNA for a neuropeptide, cocaine and amphetamine-regulated transcript (CARTPT), known to have pleiotropic effects, led the Michigan State group to explore its role in the ovary, and ultimately to this concept.

In their paper on the extracellular matrix in the ovary, Rodgers & Irving-Rodgers discussed how focal intra-epithelial matrix (focimatrix), a novel type of basal lamina, may be involved in maturation of granulosa cells. Focimatrix appears before selection of the dominant follicle and increases thereafter. It will be interesting to see if these changes are related to the destruction of CARTPT in the dominant follicle. These authors identified three other roles of extracellular matrix and described variation in its composition in the ovary. They made a case for the bovine ovary as a model for human polycystic ovarian syndrome (known as PCOS), because of its content of fibrillins and their binding to TGFβ binding proteins. They identified a relationship of oocyte quality to ultrastructure of the follicular basal lamina. And finally, they provided evidence that hyaluronan and versican, matrices produced by granulosa cells, contributed to increases in follicular fluid due to their osmotic potential.

Just as Smith's group has patiently dissected the role of CART in follicular selection in the cow, Murdoch and his colleagues have step-by-step tested components of the mechanism of ovulation in the ewe. They started earlier and with less sophisticated genetic data, but have achieved a similar end. Many of the steps in the ovulatory process fit with the hypotheses in Espey's classic review (1980, updated in 1994). However, Murdoch's work has delineated in the ewe the important role of the ovarian surface epithelium. From that knowledge, they have developed hypotheses for a mechanism by which ovulatory damage to the ovarian surface epithelium can lead to ovarian cancer.

Evans *et al.* have identified greater pregnancy success in animals with greater numbers of antral follicles in the ovary, a trait that is repeatable from cycle to cycle within an animal, and is associated with variations in hormonal concentrations. However, early data indicate that number of antral follicles may be subject to prenatal programming and reduced dramatically by nutritional restriction in the dam during gestation. While ovulation rate in sheep is associated with specific genes, a specific genetic relationship for antral follicle count in cattle appears to be indicated only by breed differences at this time. Daughters of restricted animals did have increased blood pressure and circumference of the aorta at slaughter (a surprising combination) in addition to the effect on follicle number.

Corpus Luteum

Miyamoto *et al.* found over 4200 papers on corpora lutea in domestic ruminants. They approached luteal development and function as a continuum from formation through gaining function to luteolysis. They especially assessed potential luteotropic roles of growth factors (VEGF, FGF2 and IGFs) and studies of differing sensitivity to $PGF_{2\alpha}$ of the early versus mid-cycle corpus luteum. They embraced the concept that life of the corpus luteum depends on the balance of luteotropic and luteolytic factors and hypothesized that $PGF_{2\alpha}$, well known as a luteolysin, acts as a luteotropin in the early corpus luteum. That postulate is in contrast to the work by Sayre *et al.* (2000) in which repeated injection of $PGF_{2\alpha}$ at 8-h intervals up-regulated luteolysis early in the estrous cycle, and it must be evaluated in relation to other data. Consider the early demonstrations by Milvae *et al.* (1986) that other arachidonic acid derivatives have luteotropic or steroidogenic effects early in the cycle. Consider also the enzymatic complement of the corpus luteum as delineated in numerous papers by Michel Fortier, Joe Arosh and their colleagues (e.g., Arosh *et al.* 2004a,b). The enzymatic complement of the ovary includes 9-keto-reductase, which interconverts $PGF_{2\alpha}$ and PGE_2, the direction depending upon substrate concentration. Numerous studies have established luteotropic effects of PGEs on maintenance of corpora lutea in cattle and sheep (see Weems *et al.* 2006, for review).

The review by Skarzynski & Okuda provided a concept and model of luteolysis in the cow that differs somewhat from the models proposed by McCracken *et al.* (1999), by Niswender *et al.* (2007) in the sheep, by Ginther *et al.* (2010) for natural lutolysis in the cow, or by Weems *et al.* (2006) in their comprehensive review. The current reviewers placed greater emphasis on luteal blood flow and resultant hypoxia. However, they agree that luteal oxytocin is not the only regulator of uterine secretion of $PGF_{2\alpha}$ in the cow and is probably not required for that secretion (see Inskeep, 2004 or 2010 for a thorough discussion of timing of luteolysis by progesterone).

Many of the ideas in these papers on corpora lutea must be re-evaluated in relation to the differences in changes during natural (or simulated natural) luteolysis and changes in response to bolus injections of $PGF_{2\alpha}$, as recently documented in a series of papers by Ginther and his colleagues (e.g., 2010).

Hansen and coworkers thoroughly detailed the changes in dogma necessary to accommodate the important new findings (1) that interferon tau is secreted into the uterine vein and that (2) interferon tau has actions in the corpus luteum to support its maintenance during maternal recognition of pregnancy in sheep. This major change needs to be translated rapidly and effectively into the reproductive physiology classroom and textbooks. The linkage of these effects of interferon tau to the anti-luteolytic effects of the E prostaglandins deserves further examination and clarification in future research (Pratt *et al.* 1977, 1979; Silvia *et al.* 1984; Weems *et al.* 2006; Lee *et al.* 2010; McCracken *et al.* 2010; Stephen *et al.* 2010). Hansen *et al.* also discussed the induction of interferon stimulated glycoproteins in blood cells, which parallels secretion of interferon tau and provides a diagnostic test for pregnancy.

The camelid placenta does not produce progesterone, so all camelid species are dependent on the corpus luteum throughout pregnancy. In dromedary camels, Skidmore *et al.* found that progesterone-treated recipients that had not ovulated could get pregnant from transferred embryos. To avoid continued daily injections, they induced new corpora lutea later by treatment with eCG and GnRH. Interestingly, 50% remained pregnant after withdrawal of exogenous progesterone, a proportion equal to that observed in cattle in which a new corpus luteum was induced during days 28 to 36 of pregnancy (Bridges *et al.* 2000), after previous maintenance by exogenous progestogen during absence of a corpus luteum.

The lactating dairy cow

Despite the variety of assigned subjects, 7 of the speakers centered some or all of their concerns on the lowered fertility rates of the high producing, lactating dairy cow (Santos *et al.*, Evans *et al.*, Lonergan, Sartori *et al.*, Burke & Verkerk, Wiltbank *et al.*, and Smith *et al.*) and an 8th (Zicarelli) addressed similar problems in dairy buffalo, a species that is gaining in numbers more rapidly than cattle. Numerous factors have been identified as contributing to success or failure of pregnancy in these animals. These factors include concentrations of estradiol or progesterone at critical periods, antral follicle counts in the ovaries, temperature stress, concentrations of non-esterified fatty acids during negative energy balance in the early postpartum period, timing of hormonal treatments and management factors.

As an example of the factors listed above, low progesterone during (1) the cycle before breeding, (2) the first few days after breeding, (3) maternal recognition of pregnancy, or (4) placentation, has major negative impacts on pregnancy success (Inskeep & Dailey, 2005). However, various attempts to overcome low progesterone at these times have met with limited or sporadic success.

Similarly, inadequate exposure to estradiol during the immediate preovulatory period can interfere with oocyte maturation and luteal function or lifespan. Wiltbank *et al.* discussed the metabolism of steroids in high producing cows and Day *et al.*, from work in beef cattle, pointed out that treatment with estradiol in regimens for synchronization of oestrus can be beneficial. In cows in which duration of proestrus was shortened by treatment with GnRH, life span of the corpus luteum in beef cows was less than 12 days in 74% of 38 animals in which duration of proestrus averaged only 1.3 days before induced ovulation, compared with only 30% of 40 animals in which duration of proestrus averaged 2.3 days (Mussard *et al.* 2007; Bridges *et al.* 2010). Cordoba & Fricke (2002) found short cycles in 51% of 49 lactating dairy cows that returned to service after timed insemination on an OvSynch program.

Prevention of early secretion of $PGF_{2\alpha}$ (which causes a short luteal phase; reviewed by Inskeep, 2004 and Inskeep & Dailey, 2005) in response to the post-ovulatory rise in progesterone required a sequence of pre-ovulatory exposure to progesterone and estrogen (Kieborz-Loos *et al.* 2003). That sequence has not occurred at the first ovulation at puberty or after parturition, and can be lacking if follicles are ovulated prematurely in other situations. Thus, if follicular maturation, and hence exposure of the reproductive tract to estrogen, was inadequate, premature secretion of $PGF_{2\alpha}$ could be the reason for occurrence of short luteal phases after GnRH. Conversely, excessive estradiol can damage the oocyte (as in the case of persistent follicles; Cooperative Regional Research Project NE 161, 1996), interfere with maternal recognition of pregnancy (Breuel *et al.* 1993), or disrupt placentation (Bridges *et al.* 2000).

Particularly valuable in understanding limitations to fertility in the early postpartum period has been the innovative work by Leroy *et al.* (2008a,b), discussed in the review by Lonergan.

They showed that increased non-esterified fatty acids in follicular fluid during negative energy balance compromised oocyte and embryo quality.

Are there solutions for management of the lactating dairy cow?

A particularly challenging dilemma is the continued decrease in reproductive performance of high-yielding, lactating dairy cows. There is a clear need for further research into the basic mechanisms of reproductive performance in the dairy cow, as discussed thoroughly by Lonergan. He pointed to follicular development, poor exhibition of oestrus, lowered oocyte quality, altered sperm transport, suboptimal reproductive tract environment and embryonic and fetal losses as contributors and the need to determine the relative contributions of each to lowered fertility rates within a given situation.

There is an eminent need for innovative thinking about the utilization of what is already known. The insistence that breeding in large herds must be tied to timed ovulation, without estrous detection, has been shown to be helpful in pregnancy rate in some herds (Wiltbank *et al.*, Santos *et al.*). In others, it may contribute to the problem, rather than the solution. Particularly, it may promote selection against expression of oestrus. Treatments to control variables and avoid heat detection have become ever more complicated as illustrated by Wiltbank *et al.* for the dairy cow and Day *et al.* for the beef cow. Variations in these methods have been necessary in Zebu cattle (Sartori *et al.*) and water buffaloes (Zicarelli). Water buffaloes are especially compromised by seasonality and by the nearly complete lack of homosexual behavior in the female (Usmani *et al.* 1983). Like the dairy cow, buffaloes are encumbered by high late embryonic mortality. Sartori *et al.* noted the smaller antral follicles and corpora lutea in *Bos indicus* compared with *Bos taurus* and the lowered dosages of hormones needed because of greater feedback sensitivity. Burke & Verkerk discussed how the increased constraints of both larger herd size and external influences of consumers, environmental issues and animal welfare concerns affect the more extensive production system in New Zealand. New Zealand dairying is seasonal and supports the largest sector of agricultural exports. They reviewed practices developed, including effectiveness, shortcomings and side effects, and supported a need for simpler schemes of treatment for reproductive management.

R. A. Dailey has proposed a simpler scheme of synchronization that would not use timed breeding, but require observation for oestrus just 3 days in each three-week period (presented in detail in Inskeep & Dailey 2010). However, when that scheme was submitted to use in two herds, analyses of the data collected revealed only 54% complete compliance with even that simple scheme (RA Dailey, unpublished); non-compliant inseminations have been reported as a problem with more involved schemes (Stevenson & Phatak 2005).

Rodriguez-Martinez *et al.* (2008) compiled data showing that duration of oestrus had changed over time, especially in American Holsteins. Although Rottensten & Touchberry (1957) reported a heritability of 21%, duration of oestrus has not been considered in selection programs. Exhibition of a detectable oestrus allows proper timing of insemination, and is indicative of appropriate maturation of the oocyte and readiness of the reproductive tract to establish pregnancy. Sartori *et al.* noted that when groups of synchronized Holstein and Nelore cows were run together, approximately 90% of mounts were within breed.

In early studies (Inskeep *et al.* 1961), conception was defined as birth of a live calf and inheritance of conception rate at first service was examined in Holsteins bred to high fertility AI sires (60- to 90-day non-return rate in the upper two-thirds of the bulls in the stud). Heritability of conception rate to first service, estimated from intra-sire correlations of paternal half-sib groups, was approximately 8.5%. Based upon that estimate, if one were to select daughters of bulls in the upper 25% of sires for daughter's conception rate, based upon 20 previous daughters, the expected advantage would be 4.7% in the next generation. Selection based upon conception rate to first service has not been implemented, but some schemes now utilize daughter pregnancy rate. More recently, Bamber *et al.* (2009) estimated the heritability of pregnancy loss after 30 days as 49%, which should make that trait a more effective tool for selection.

In a different approach, Khatib *et al.* (2008) found that the gene, signal transducer and activator of transcription 5A (*STAT5A*), was associated with sperm factors that caused low fertilization rate *in vitro*, with death rates of *in vitro* fertilized embryos, and with milk composition in Holstein cows. It appeared that selection for heterozygotic females could promote both successful pregnancy and increased production.

Lonergan illustrated changing attitudes in selection programs to put less emphasis on production and more emphasis on reproduction and health. Selection for strength and duration of expression of oestrus and for conception to first AI, against pregnancy loss, or for specific genes that regulate components of the reproductive process seem appropriate to recommend. These approaches may prove far more valuable to sustainability of dairy production than the extensive efforts at minor modifications in hormonal treatments designed to facilitate timed breeding. Santos *et al.* illustrated successes on farms that have adopted integrated approaches, including consideration of cow comfort, transition cow management, aggressive postpartum health monitoring and manipulation of the ovarian cycle to increase insemination rate, as well as introduction of selection for fertility.

Other new findings

This reviewer was surprised to learn that the family Camelidae originated in North America (Skidmore *et al.*); they seem more plentiful on other continents. Progress in facilitating AI and embryo transfer was achieved in dromedary camels by synchronizing follicular waves using GnRH and prostaglandin analogues.

Preservation of endangered wild species is an increasing concern in studies in zoos throughout the world and has received increasing emphasis. Just last week, expectation of birth of a Sumatran rhinoceros from AI was announced at the Cincinnati Zoo. Santiago-Moreno *et al.* shared their experience in sperm collection and preservation in the Spanish ibex. Males with larger, more symmetrical horns had better semen quality, thus aiding selection of candidate males. They have developed a captive breeding program, synchronized ovulation using a method that was effective in dairy goats and obtained fertility rates of 25 to 63%. Interestingly, only dominant females became pregnant. In addition, they have produced live hybrids with domestic goats. As in other wild ruminants in the Mediterranean region, seasonal reproductive activity began earlier in males than in females.

In Alaska, reindeer and caribou, members of the same species, are of great interest. Reindeer are the only cervids indigenous to the arctic environment (Shipka & Rowell) and the only deer in which male and female both grow antlers. The females do not show homosexual behaviour. Their gestation length has been the subject of great variation in fragmentary reports. The data showed that they are seasonal breeders with an estrous cycle of 18 to 29 days, mean 24 days. Gestation length was quite variable, from 198 to 229 days and depended on when in the season the female was bred. The variability makes them somewhat comparable to the horse, but the effect of season on timing makes one wonder what mechanism is operating that contributes to such wide variability. Progesterone in blood rose more rapidly in animals bred later, which could be a clue to that mechanism.

Final remarks

Drs. Michael Smith and Matthew Lucy asked me to predict where we are headed in studies of reproduction in ruminants; what is not known and needs to be learned. I have interspersed some suggestions derived from the reviews presented by the 31 speakers at the symposium. It is clear that such thoughtful reviews can help to make planning research more efficient, that tomorrow's researchers will need to be more widely read and that more cost effective methodologies will help with the research task. Even so, funding will be a limiting factor. I believe we should be thinking more and publishing less.

New methods for genetic studies will enable more readily identified genes for study. That will provide opportunities for programmatic, sequential studies that lead from discovery of a gene to understanding the role of its product. There will still be a need for basic physiological studies of that product (example CART) and its actions and for application of knowledge in applied research.

Finally, there is a great need for unbiased dialogue among workers who are operating with different models of their understanding of a process or system. *Dogma needs to be challenged!* That is the road to greater understanding and challenging it together should help to fulfill Carl Hartman's statement in the early days of our discipline, "Science should be fun!"

Acknowledgements

I thank the organizers, Drs. Mike Smith, Matt Lucy, Joy Pate and Tom Spencer for the invitation to prepare and present this summary and their support of my attendance at the symposium in addition to funds from West Virginia University. The opportunity to read 30 papers in advance of the meeting allowed me to learn more than from any other scientific meeting I have ever attended. To the writers and presenters, I express my congratulations on excellent reviews and my hope for forgiveness if I have misinterpreted your data or conclusions.

References

Arosh JA, Banu SK, Chapdelaine P, Madore E & Fortier MA 2004a Prostaglandin biosynthesis, transport and signaling in corpus luteum: a basis for autoregulation of luteal function. *Endocrinology* **145** 2551-2560.

Arosh JA, Banu SK, Kimmins S, Chapdelaine P, MacLaren LA & Fortier MA 2004b Effect of interferon tau on prostaglandin biosynthesis, transport and signaling during maternal recognition of pregnancy in cattle: Evidence of polycrine action of PGE_2. *Endocrinology* **145** 5280-5293.

Bamber RL, Shook GE, Wiltbank MC, Santos JEP & Fricke PM 2009 Genetic parameters for anovulation and pregnancy loss in cattle. *J Dairy Sci* **92** 5739–5753.

Breuel KF, Lewis PE, Schrick FN, Lishman AW, Inskeep EK & RL Butcher 1993 Factors affecting fertility in the postpartum cow: role of the oocyte and follicle in conception rate. *Biol Reprod* **48** 655–661.

Bridges GA, Mussard ML, Burke CR & Day ML 2010 Influence of the length of proestrus on fertility and endocrine function in female cattle. *Anim Reprod Sci* **117** 208-215.

Bridges PJ, Wright DJ, Buford WI, Ahmad N, Hernandez-Fonseca H, McCormick ML, Schrick FN, Dailey RA, Lewis PE & Inskeep EK. 2000 Ability of induced corpora lutea to maintain pregnancy in beef cows. *J Anim Sci* **78** 2942-2949.

Cooperative Regional Research Project, NE-161 1996 Relationship of fertility to patterns of ovarian follicular development and associated hormonal profiles in dairy cows and heifers. *J Anim Sci* **74** 1943–1952.

Cordoba MC & Fricke PM 2002 Initiation of the breeding season in a grazing-based dairy by synchronization of ovulation. *J Dairy Sci* **85** 5739-5753.

Espey LL 1980 Ovulation as an inflammatory reaction – a hypothesis. *Biol Reprod* **22** 73-106.

Espey LL 1994 Current status of the hypothesis that mammalian ovulation is comparable to an inflammatory reaction. *Biol Reprod* **50** 233-238.

Ginther OJ, Shrestha HK, Fuenzalida MJ, Shahiduzzaman, AKM, Hannan MA & Beg MA 2010 Intrapulse temporality between pulses of a metabolite of prostaglandin F2α and circulating concentrations of progesterone before, during, and after spontaneous luteolysis in heifers. *Theriogenology* (In press).

Goodman RL & Inskeep EK 2006 Neuroendocrine control of the ovarian cycle of the sheep. In *Knobil and Neill's Physiology of Reproduction*, 3rd Ed pp 2389-2447. Ed JD Neill. Amsterdam: Elsevier.

Inskeep EK 2004 Preovulatory, postovulatory, and post-maternal recognition effects of concentrations of progesterone on embryonic survival in the cow. *J Anim Sci* **82** (E. Suppl.) E24-E39.

Inskeep EK 2010 Time-dependent embryotoxicity of the endogenous luteolysin prostaglandin $F_2\alpha$ in ruminants. In Endocrine Toxicology pp 240-255. Eds C. Eldridge and J.T. Stevens. Informa Healthcare: London.

Inskeep EK & Dailey RA 2005 Embryonic death in cattle. *Vet Clin Food Anim* **21** 437-461.

Inskeep EK & Dailey RA 2010. Maximizing embryonic and early fetal survival in dairy cattle. In *WCDS Advances in Dairy Technology* **22** 51-69. Lorraine Doepel, Editor.

Inskeep EK, Tyler WJ & Casida LE 1961 Hereditary variation in conception rate of HolsteinFriesian cattle. *J Dairy Sci* **44** 1857-1862.

Ireland JJ, Roberts RM, Palmer GH, Bauman DE & Bazer FW 2008 A commentary on domestic animals as dual-purpose models that benefit agricultural and biomedical research. *J Anim Sci* **86** 2797-2805.

Khatib H, Monson RL, Schutzkus V, Kohl DM, Rosa GJM, & Rutledge JJ 2008 Mutations in the *STAT5A* gene are associated with embryonic survival and milk composition in cattle. *J Dairy Sci* **91** 784–793.

Kieborz-Loos KR, Garverick HA, Keisler DH, Hamilton SA, Salfen BE, Youngquist RS & Smith MF 2003 Oxytocin-induced secretion of prostaglandin $F_2\alpha$ in postpartum beef cows: Effects of progesterone and estradiol-17β treatment. *J Anim Sci* **81** 1830–1836.

Lee J, Stephen SD, McCracken JA, Banu S, Nithy TK & Arosh JA 2010 Selective increased luteal prostaglandin E2 compared to F2alpha biosynthesis and signaling are critical for luteal protection and resistance during establishment of pregnancy in sheep. Society for the Study of Reproduction, 43rd Annual Meeting, Milwaukee WI Abst 231.

Leroy JL, Opsomer G, Van Soom A, Goovaerts IG & Bols PE 2008a Reduced fertility in high-yielding dairy cows: are the oocyte and embryo in danger? Part I. The importance of negative energy balance and altered corpus luteum function to the reduction of oocyte and embryo quality in high-yielding dairy cows. *Reprod Domest Anim* **43** 612-622.

Leroy JL, Van Soom A, Opsomer G, Goovaerts IG & Bols PE 2008b Reduced fertility in high-yielding dairy cows: are the oocyte and embryo in danger? Part II. Mechanisms linking nutrition and reduced oocyte and embryo quality in high-yielding dairy cows. *Reprod Domest Anim* **43** 623-632.

Lingenfelter BM, Dailey RA, Inskeep EK, Vernon MW, Poole DH, Rhinehart JD & Yao J 2007 Changes of maternal transcripts in oocytes from persistent follicles in cattle. *Molec Reprod Devel* **74** 265-272.

McCracken JA, Custer EE & Lamsa JC 1999 Luteolysis: A neuroendocrine-mediated event. *Physiological Reviews* **79** 263-324.

McCracken JA, Lee J, Stephen SD, Banu S, Nithy TK & Arosh JA 2010 Selective transport of PGF2a and PGE2 from uterus to ovary during luteolysis and during the establishment of pregnancy in sheep. Society for the Study of Reproduction, 43rd Annual Meeting, Milwaukee WI Abst 233.

Milvae RA, Alila HW & Hansel W 1986 Involvement of lipoxygenase products of arachidonic acid metabolism in bovine luteal function. *Biol Reprod* **35** 1210-1215.

Mussard ML, Burke CR, Behlke EJ, Gasser CL & Day ML 2007 Influence of premature induction of a luteinizing hormone surge with gonadotropin-releasing hormone on ovulation, luteal function and fertility in cattle. *J Anim Sci* **85** 937–943.

Niswender GD, Davis TL, Griffith RH, Bogan RL, Monser K, Bott RC, Bruemmer JE, & Nett TM 2007 Judge, jury, and executioner: the auto-regulation of luteal function. *Society of Reproduction and Fertility Supplement* **64** 191-206.

Pratt BR, Butcher RL & Inskeep EK 1977 Antiluteolytic effect of the conceptus and PGE_2 in ewes. *J Anim Sci* **45** 784791.

Pratt BR, Butcher RL & Inskeep EK 1979 Effect of continuous intrauterine administration of prostaglandin E_2 on lifespan of corpora lutea of nonpregnant ewes. *J Anim Sci* **48** 14411446.

Rodriguez-Martinez H, Hultgren J, Båge R, Bergqvist A-S, Svensson C, Bergsten C, Lidfors L, Gunnarsson S, Algers B, Emanuelson U, Berglund B, Andersson G, Håård M, Lindhé B, Stålhammar H, & Gustafsson H 2008 Reproductive performance in high-producing dairy cows: Can we sustain it under current practice? In: *IVIS Reviews in Veterinary Medicine*, I.V.I.S. (Ed.). International Veterinary Information Service, Ithaca NY (www.ivis.org), Updated: 12-Dec-2008; R0108.1208 (Open Journal).

Rottensten K & Touchberry RW 1957 Observations on the degree of expression of estrus in cattle. *J Dairy Sci* **40** 1457-1465.

Sayre BL, Taft R, Inskeep EK & Killefer J 2000 Increased expression of insulin-like growth factor binding protein-1 during induced regression of bovine corpora lutea. *Biol Reprod* **63** 21–29.

Silvia WJ, Ottobre JS & Inskeep EK 1984 Concentrations of prostaglandins E_2, $F_{2\alpha}$, and 6-keto-prostaglandin $F_{1\alpha}$ in the utero-ovarian venous plasma of nonpregnant and early pregnant ewes. *Biol Reprod* **30** 936944.

Stephen SD, Lee J, Banu S, McCracken JA, Nithy TK & Arosh JA 2010 Effects of early pregnancy and estrous cycle on survival and apoptotic pathways lead to endurance or death of corpus luteum in sheep. Society for the Study of Reproduction, 43rd Annual Meeting, Milwaukee WI Abst 232.

Stevenson JS and Phatak AP 2005 Inseminations at estrus induced by resynchronization before application of synchronized estrus and ovulation. *J Dairy Sci* **88** 399-405.

Szollosi, DG & Ris H 1961 Observations on sperm penetration in the rat. *J Biophys Biochem Cytology* **10** 275-283.

Taft RA Jr 1999 Oocyte morphology and estrogen concentration following a reduction in progesterone in beef cattle. Ph.D. Dissertation West Virginia University 72 pp.

Usmani RH, Iqbal J, Lewis GS & Inskeep EK 1983 Reproduction in female dairy buffalo. West Virginia University, Div. of Int. Agr. For. Pub. **95**, 35 pp.

Vincent JN, McQuown EC & Notter DR 2000 Duration of the seasonal anestrus in sheep selected for fertility in a fall-lambing system. *J Anim Sci* **78** 1149–1154.

Walkden-Brown SW, Martin GB & Restall BJ 1999 Role of male-female interaction in regulating reproduction in sheep and goats. *J Reprod Fertil (Suppl* **54***)* 243-257.

Weems CW, Weems YS & Randel RD 2006 Prostaglandins and reproduction in female farm animals. *Vet J* **171** 206–228.

Genomic tools for characterizing monogenic and polygenic traits in ruminants - using the bovine as an example

JF Taylor, RH Chapple, JE Decker, SJ Gregg, JW Kim, SD McKay, HR Ramey, MM Rolf, TM Taxis and RD Schnabel

S135B Animal Sciences Research Center, University of Missouri, Columbia, USA 65211

Next generation sequencing platforms have democratized genome sequencing. Large genome centers are no longer required to produce genome sequences costing millions. A few lanes of paired-end sequence on an Illumina Genome Analyzer, costing <$10,000, will produce more sequence than generated only a few years ago to produce the human and cow assemblies. The *de novo* assembly of large numbers of short reads into a high-quality whole-genome sequence is now technically feasible and will allow the whole genome sequencing and assembly of a broad spectrum of ruminant species. Next-generation sequencing instruments are also proving very useful for transcriptome or resequencing projects in which the entire RNA population produced by a tissue, or the entire genomes of individual animals are sequenced, and the produced reads are aligned to a reference assembly. We have used this strategy to examine gene expression differences in tissues from cattle differing in feed efficiency, to perform genome-wide single nucleotide polymorphism discovery for the construction of ultrahigh-density genotyping assays, and in combination with genome-wide association analysis, for the identification of mutations responsible for Mendelian diseases. The new 800K SNP bovine genotyping assays possess the resolution to map trait associations to the locations of individual genes and the 45 million polymorphisms identified in >180X genome sequence coverage on over 200 animals can be queried to identify the polymorphisms present within positional candidate genes. These new tools should rapidly allow the identification of genes and mutations underlying variation in cattle production and reproductive traits.

Introduction

The higher ruminants are believed to have rapidly speciated in the Mid-Eocene, resulting in five distinct extant families: Antilocapridae, Giraffidae, Moschidae, Cervidae, and Bovidae. While there are about 200 species of ruminants (Hackmann & Spain 2010), few have been domesticated (cattle, goats, sheep, bison, yaks, buffalo, deer, etc) and the phylogeny describing the evolutionary relationships among species has yet to be fully resolved (Decker *et al*. 2009). Similarly, the history of domestication and breed formation within a species such as cattle is

Corresponding author E-mail: taylorjerr@missouri.edu

poorly understood. In fact, the number and location of prehistoric domestication events for the extinct aurochs (*Bos primigenius*) has been controversial, and the ancestry of many of the modern breeds of cattle is unknown (Decker *et al.* 2009). Knowledge of these relationships is of more than academic and conservation interest since the evolutionary history of breeds and species will shed insight into the genes and pathways which control phenotypes which are either shared or diverged among species or breeds. For example, Angus and Shorthorn cattle both accumulate large amounts of intramuscular fat (marbling) and their close genetic relationship as breeds suggests that the genetic mechanisms underlying marbling (loci at which naturally occurring variants induce phenotypic effects and allele frequencies at these loci) are quite similar. On the other hand, Angus and Wagyu cattle are both black-hided and marble highly but are distantly related (Decker *et al.* 2009). Since the cattle phylogeny contains few black-hided breeds and the propensity to marble varies dramatically among the more recently formed breeds, there are two possible explanations for these phenomena. In the case of coat color, either independent mutations have occurred at a single gene (e.g., Melanocortin 1 receptor, *MC1R*) leading to black coat color (Klungland *et al.* 1995), or mutations in two independent genes within the same (melanocortin) pathway have occurred (Candille *et al.* 2007). On the other hand, marbling is inherited as a quantitative trait and for the breeds to have similar high means, either the same genes control variation in both breeds (with allele frequency distributions that generate similar means), or the breeds share a core of identical genes and also breed specific genes for which variation contributes to within breed variation, and the similarity of breed means. These hypotheses are testable by a number of different approaches. However, the point to be made here is that the superimposition of phenotypes on phylogenies (species or breed trees) allows the identification of experimental models which can contribute to the eludication of the genes and pathways responsible for variation within populations and the evolution of population specific phenotypes.

Genetic analysis within a species

Monogenic phenotypes

Hypotheses concerning the mode of inheritance and allelism (whether or not a mutation within the same gene is responsible for a phenotype) can be determined by pedigree analysis and by making experimental crosses. For example, we characterized a fatal movement disorder of Chinese Crested dogs that was clinically and pathologically indistinguishable from a condition known as canine multiple system degeneration that had previously been recognized in Kerry Blue Terriers (O'Brien *et al.* 2005). We showed that the disease segregated as an autosomal recessive and by making crosses between Chinese Crested and Kerry Blue Terrier carriers of the disease allele, we were able to show that mutations within the same gene were responsible for the disease in both breeds. Since both diseases are recessive and are likely due to the loss of gene function, this result also strongly suggests that the disease is identical in both breeds and not simply that the disorder was clinically and pathologically indistinguishable between the breeds. Because microsatellite loci (primarily dinucleotide repeat polymorphisms which could be amplified by PCR and scored on a fragment size analyzer) were plentifully available in dog, we were able to perform a linkage analysis within an extended family and localize the disease locus to a 15 Mb region of dog chromosome 1. This region was subsequently fine-mapped using additional markers and more distantly related affected dogs to reduce the size of the interval harboring the disease locus to less than 1 Mb. Because the sequence assembly for the dog genome (a Boxer) had just become available, we were able to identify and then sequence exons from candidate genes (e.g., *PARK2*) within this region; however, we are yet to identify the causal mutation underlying this disease. The reasons for this are that: 1) The region contains 27 genes and a number of these could be viable candidates, 2) Although we targeted exons for sequence analysis, we really have no idea what kind of mutation we are looking for – it could certainly be noncoding or a duplication of a coding region – neither of which would be detected by our exon sequencing strategy, and 3) the region is large and until very recently there have been no straightforward or cost-effective methods for sequencing large targeted regions of DNA from individuals.

When individuals belong to extended nuclear families, linkage analysis tests the concordance between phenotype and genotype to establish linkage of the disease locus to a specific chromosomal region. For example, if the disease is known to be inherited as a fully penetrant autosomal recessive we would expect all affected progeny within a family to have inherited the same combination of chromosomal fragments from each of their parents in the region of the disease locus and all unaffected progeny to have inherited different chromosomal combinations. Because only a single meiosis separates parents and progeny there is only a very limited opportunity for recombination to rearrange the parental chromosomal haplotypes (combination of alleles present on a single chromosome or region of a chromosome) present in the progeny and the size of the chromosomal region harboring the disease locus is determined by the number of affected progeny included in the mapping population. Additionally, the resolution of detection of recombination breakpoints is determined by the resolution of the marker map used to perform the linkage analysis. Until very recently, microsatellites were used for almost all linkage analyses and these markers could only be multiplexed in groups of 6-8, meaning that 40-50 separate PCR reactions had to be performed on each individual's DNA to achieve a genome-wide marker map density of one marker per 10 Mb. Not only is microsatellite genotyping slow and tedious, but it is expensive at a cost of $0.25-$1 per produced genotype.

The evolutionary history of the majority of domesticated livestock species differs dramatically from that of human. Modern humans arose from a small effective population size some 100,000 years ago and the population has recently been rapidly expanding, leading to a relatively large current effective population size ($N_e \approx 7{,}000$, Tenesa *et al.* 2007). On the other hand, the domestication of all livestock species occurred within the last 10,000 years (Loftus *et al.* 1994, Giuffra *et al.* 2000), breed societies were formed only within the last 200 years, and the population bottlenecks created by these events have led to relatively small current effective population sizes in cattle ($N_e \approx$ 100-200, Bovine HapMap Consortium 2009). As a consequence, many monogenic traits, such as disease are caused by novel rare mutations within human populations, but within a domesticated ruminant species, the majority are caused by a single founder event and all copies of the disease allele within a population are identical by descent to the allele present in the founder individual. Since the original mutation occurred on a single chromosome (with a specific haplotype surrounding the disease allele) which has subsequently been rearranged by recombination within descendants, we expect that all individuals with a fully penetrant autosomal recessive disease are actually homozygous for a small core haplotype that is identical to that present in the founder individual. The size of this haplotype can be quite small if the mutation is old and many generations of recombination have occurred since the occurrence of the original mutation and microsatellite mapping usually does not possess the resolution to detect these core haplotypes.

Recently, high density single nucleotide polymorphism (SNP) genotyping assays have been developed for several ruminant species including cattle (Matukumalli *et al.* 2009) and sheep (Magee *et al.* 2010). While these first generation assays allow the detection of genotypes at ~50,000 loci, second generation assays allowing the detection of ~777,000 SNPs now available for cattle (http://www.illumina.com/documents/%5Cproducts%5Cdatasheets%5Cdatasheet_bovineHD.pdf). These assays allow a completely different approach to the mapping of genes influencing monogenic and polygenic loci within species based upon the linkage disequilibrium (LD) between loci that are physically close together on a chromosome. LD is usually measured as the squared correlation coefficient between alleles that are present at two different loci, and the extent of this correlation is influenced by the age of the two mutations and the evolutionary history of the population. In populations such as human, which have large effective population sizes, the correlation between two loci that are old and have moderately high allele frequencies is quite low, whereas in domesticated ruminant populations, these correlations are much larger (Bovine HapMap Consortium 2009). Thus, we would expect that the core haplotypes harboring a disease mutation in, e.g., cattle populations would be quite large and that the resolution of the BovineSNP50 assay (Matukumalli *et al.* 2009) would be sufficient to detect regions of homozygosity in affected animals that might be only quite distantly related. This is, in fact, exactly the case, and the assay allows the rapid localization of recessive disease mutations by case control genome-wide association (GWA) analysis which seeks to identify genomic regions in which all affected individuals are homozygous for a core haplotype, and unaffected individuals are not homozygous for this haplotype (Charlier *et al.* 2008, Meyers *et al.* 2010).

The approach can be modified in a rather interesting way to detect regions of the genome that have undergone recent selective sweeps within a population. Strong selection for a phenotype determined by genotype at a single locus will result in the rapid fixation of a single allele at the causal locus. However, because only relatively few generations of selection (from an evolutionary perspective) are required to drive the selected allele to fixation, we expect LD to drag relatively large flanking chromosomal regions to fixation in the process. Thus, the signature of a selective sweep is the loss of variability within the genome in a region flanking a strongly selected allele in all individuals within a population (Nielsen *et al.* 2005). As time passes following the selective sweep new mutations or migration into the population will allow the accumulation of variation in the region, however, variation will remain reduced within the selected region for a very large number of generations. For example, the locus responsible for the presence or absence of horns in cattle (the polled locus) was first mapped to the centromeric end of chromosome 1 (BTA1) by Georges *et al.* (1993) and was subsequently fine mapped to a 1 Mb region of this chromosome (Drögemüller *et al.* 2005, Wunderlich *et al.* 2006). Horns are inherited as a recessive with the horned phenotype being ancestral and the polled allele being derived. Strong selection within a breed to produce only polled cattle should have produced a selective sweep for the polled allele leaving a strong signature of selection detectable as loss of polymorphism within the region of the genome harboring this gene. To test this, we examined the minor allele frequencies (MAF, frequency of the rarer of the two alleles present at each SNP) of 54,442 SNPs scored in 3,668 registered Angus bulls to identify genomic regions in which losses of diversity suggested the presence of strong selective sweeps. Strong evidence of a selective sweep was found between 1.71-2.01 Mb (UMD3.0 assembly) on BTA1 where 11 consecutive SNP spanning 301 kb had MAF <0.005 (Figure 1). While 7,964 of the 54,442 tested SNP (14.6%) had MAF < 0.005, the probability that 11 consecutive SNP would have small MAF is vanishingly small (despite the fact that they are not inherited independently) and this suggests that a strong recent selective sweep was focused on this region of the Angus genome. Not coincidentally, this region is located within the 1 Mb region identified as harboring the polled locus by Drögemüller *et al.* (2005).

The largest region of the Angus genome (555 kb) in which 10 consecutive SNPs possessed MAF<0.008 was on BTA12 from 25.88-26.43 Mb and contains 8 annotated genes which clearly warrant further investigation as to their involvement in the determination of various

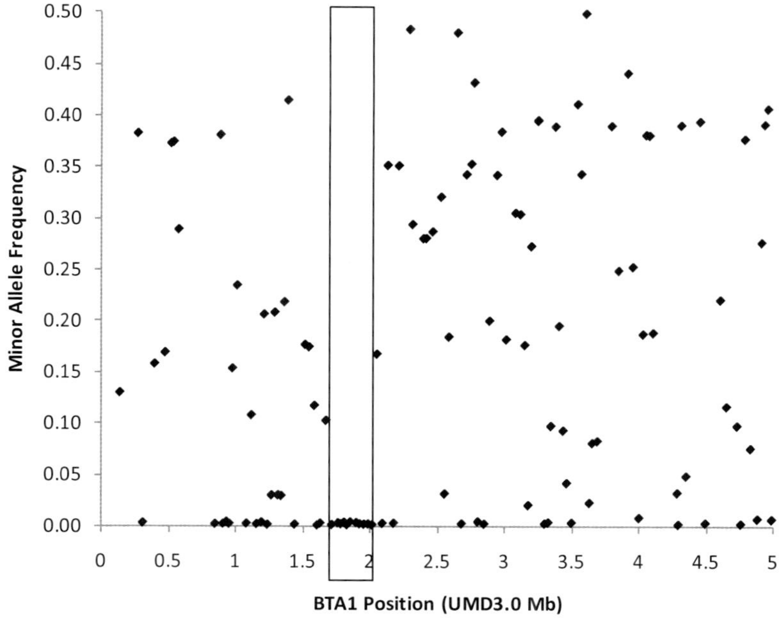

Fig. 1. Minor allele frequency for 116 BovineSNP50 SNP loci mapped to the first 5 Mb of bovine chromosome 1 in the UMD3.0 sequence assembly scored in 3,668 registered Angus bulls. The plot reveals a region of 11 consecutive SNPs spanning 301 kb with minor allele frequency less than 0.005 within the 1 Mb region previously shown to harbor the horn/poll locus (Drögemüller *et al.* 2005).

phenotypes. At the center of this interval is *CNGB1* in which mutations have been found to be responsible for an autosomal recessive form of retinitis pigmentosis in human (Bareil *et al.* 2001). Interestingly, the region harboring the *MC1R* locus on BTA18 which is responsible for black/non-black coat color possessed 5 consecutive SNP with MAF < 0.008 and spanned 320 kb suggesting that selective sweeps of similar intensity occurred for black coat color and polled in Angus cattle. The fact that MAF $\neq 0$ in these intervals is most likely due to genotyping error which is similar in magnitude to these allele frequencies; however, it could also be due to the incomplete elimination of the recessive alleles at these loci, the accumulation of new mutations or the introgression of new haplotypes – all of which are testable hypotheses.

Polygenic phenotypes

There have been many linkage and LD mapping experiments performed in cattle to identify loci that contribute to variation in quantitative (polygenic) traits such as growth, carcass quality, feed efficiency and fertility using families produced either within breeds (McClure *et al.* 2010), by crosses between breeds (Kim *et al.* 2003) or by the analysis of populations of individuals in the absence of pedigree information (Barendse *et al.* 2007). Linkage analysis to detect quantitative trait loci (QTLs) requires the assembly of families of individuals in which the phenotypes of progeny which inherited differing combinations of parental alleles are statistically contrasted to detect the presence of nearby genes of large effect on the phenotype. As with linkage analysis to detect monogenic trait loci, the resolution of the chromosomal intervals detected to harbor QTL is usually quite poor with confidence intervals often spanning 50% or more of a chromosome due to limits to the numbers of progeny produced within families (Kim *et al.* 2002). However, linkage analysis of QTLs suffers from two additional shortfalls (Sellner *et al.* 2007). First, the only loci that can be detected are those for which the parents happen to be heterozygous, which means that many QTL will go undetected within any one experiment simply due to lack of parental heterozygosity. Second, the magnitude of QTLs that can be detected (statistical power of the experiment) is also limited by family size. The majority of early linkage analyses which employed microsatellite genotyping of half-sib, back cross or F_2 families used only a few hundred progeny and typically detected no more than 3-5 QTLs per analyzed trait. The largest such analysis was performed by McClure *et al.* (2010) who scored 402 marker loci (predominantly microsatellites) in 38 Angus half-sib families comprising 1,622 steers and an extended pedigree of 1,769 Angus sires and detected an average of 48.1 QTL per analyzed trait. This result is in remarkable agreement with the estimate of 50-100 genes predicted to underlie variation in quantitative traits in dairy populations assuming that the polymorphisms in these genes were neutral with respect to fitness (Hayes & Goddard 2001).

GWA analysis utilizes SNPs evenly spaced throughout the genome to detect the presence of nearby QTLs. In its simplest form, the analysis is performed one SNP at a time by performing an F-test to establish if the mean phenotype differs among individuals with different SNP genotypes. Because the presence of LD requires that alleles at the QTL and SNP locus be correlated, the distribution of QTL genotypes present within each of the SNP genotype classes differs (Figure 2). Consequently, even though the flanking SNP locus itself generally has no effect on phenotype, a test to determine whether the phenotypic mean differs among individuals with different SNP genotypes will be significant if there is a large effect QTL nearby that is in strong LD with the tested SNP. This turns out to be a rather important assumption because manipulation of the formulae in Figure 2C shows that for two loci to be in very strong LD it is necessary (but not sufficient) that they have very similar allele frequencies. However, the vast majority of genotyping assays are designed to include only SNPs that have high MAF in the populations in which the assay is intended to be used. Therefore, by definition, these assays are designed to detect only those common variants that underlie phenotype within any genotyped population. This, at least in part, explains the missing heritability in human GWA studies (Maher 2008) where common SNP variants are used to detect rare causal variants (and they don't!). Similarly, the extent of LD estimated within the genomes of species using these assays (e.g., BovineHap Project 2009) is misleading because what is actually being estimated is the linkage disequilibrium between common variants separated by specific physical distances. While the true distributions of QTL effects that underlie quantitative traits in livestock are unknown, in all likelihood they are biased towards common variants. Hayes & Goddard (2001) empirically estimated that 17 and 35% of the largest effect QTL explained 90% of the genetic variance in dairy and swine, respectively. Thus, 50K common SNPs appear to be sufficient to perform GWA studies within breeds of ruminants for the purpose of identifying the genes of large effect which explain the majority of genetic variation within quantitative traits.

We used the BovineSNP50 assay to genotype 3,240 animals from 5 beef breeds (Table 1) with Warner-Bratzler shear force (WBSF) measures of beef tenderness. We also genotyped 7 SNPs in a 150 kb region spanning calpastatin (*CAST*) on BTA7 and 43 SNPs in a 208 kb region spanning calpain (*CAPN1*) on BTA29. Both genes have previously been shown to be associated with WBSF in several beef breeds. Because pedigree relationships within populations can result in the stratification of samples into families that result in spurious associations in GWA (MacLeod *et al.* 2010), we performed a more sophisticated analysis in which a genomic relationship matrix was estimated for each breed group using the animal's genotypes and all SNP effects were simultaneously estimated by best linear unbiased prediction (VanRaden 2008). Figure 3 shows the standardized estimated SNP allele substitution effects in the 4 breeds with

A)

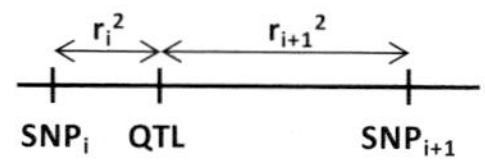

B)

QTL genotype	QQ	Qq	qq
Genotypic Mean	a	d	-a

C)

Allele frequency		P_i	$1-P_i$
	Alleles	A_i	B_i
P_Q	Q	$P_QP_i + D$	$P_Q(1-P_i) - D$
$1-P_Q$	q	$(1-P_Q)P_i - D$	$(1-P_Q)(1-P_i) + D$

$D = Cov(SNP_i, QTL)$

$r_i^2 = D^2/[P_Q(1-P_Q)P_i(1-P_i)]$

D)

SNP Genotype		A_iA_i		...		B_iB_i	
QTL Genotype	QQ	Qq	qq	...	QQ	Qq	qq
Frequency	$(P_QP_i+D)^2$	$2(P_QP_i+D)[(1-P_Q)P_i-D]$	$[(1-P_Q)P_i-D]^2$	...	$[P_Q(1-P_i)-D]^2$	$2[P_Q(1-P_i)-D]\times[(1-P_Q)(1-P_i)+D]$	$[(1-P_Q)(1-P_i)+D]^2$

Fig. 2. Affect of LD between loci on multilocus genotype frequencies. A) Representation of a chromosomal architecture with two SNPs flanking a QTL with LD r_i^2 and r_{i+1}^2 between each SNP and the QTL, respectively, B) QTL is defined such that genotypes have different mean phenotypes (genotypic values), C) Manifestation of LD is the overrepresentation of two haplotype classes and underrepresentation of the remaining two haplotype classes by an amount D (the covariance between alleles at the two loci) relative to the expectation under independence of alleles at the two loci, and D) Effect of LD on QTL genotype frequencies within each of the SNP genotype classes.

Table 1. Estimates of genetic parameters for Warner Bratzler Shear Force in 5 beef breeds. Each breed was separately analyzed using an animal model incorporating a gender × herd-of-origin × slaughter contemporary group and using a genomic relationship matrix estimated from 40,645 SNPs.

	Warner-Bratzler Shear Force (kg)			
Breed	N	σ_A^2	σ_E^2	h^2
Angus	651	0.2184	0.2036	0.52
Charolais	695	0.2275	0.2664	0.46
Hereford	1,095	0.1500	0.7325	0.17
Limousin	283	0.0723	0.7227	0.09
Simmental	516	0.0580	0.6917	0.08
Total	3,240			

largest sample sizes. Remarkably, these plots show little concordance between the regions harboring WBSF quantitative trait loci (QTL) across breeds with the exception of the effect of *CAPN1* which is large in all breeds. Similar results have been seen when performing GWA for milk traits in Jersey and Holstein populations (Dorian Garrick, *pers. comm.*) and suggest either that different QTL are responsible for trait variation in different breeds, or that the resolution of

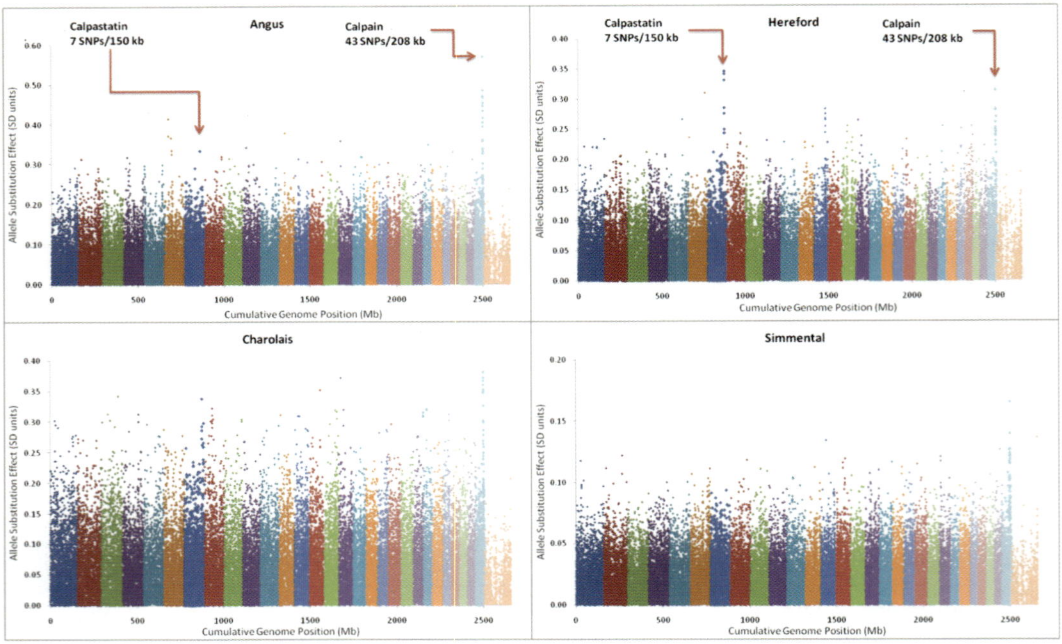

Fig. 3. Manhattan plots of SNP allele substitution effects for WBSF for 40,645 SNPs in 4 breeds. Genomic locations of CAST (BTA7) and CAPN1 (BTA29) are indicated by red arrows.

the BovineSNP50 assay is not sufficient to detect the QTLs which are for the most part identical across breeds, but differ in LD with nearby SNPs due to breed specific differences in MAF. We believe the latter explanation to be the most likely, since the average genome-wide SNP spacing in this study was 65 kb except for the region on BTA29 harboring *CAPN1* which had an average SNP spacing of 4.8 kb and produced one strongly associated SNP in all 5 breeds with the same allele being desirable across all breeds. Nevertheless, this is a very important issue which must be resolved before significant further efforts are made to identify the genes that underlie quantitative traits in domesticated ruminant species.

Gene hunting

The process of identifying the genes and mutations that underlie QTL has been hampered by the lack of genome sequences from which to identify suitable candidate genes, the large size of the QTL regions identified by linkage analysis and the inability to sequence large regions of genomic DNA to hunt for polymorphisms which may be responsible for trait variation (Sellner *et al.* 2007). Following 20 years of QTL mapping in cattle, very few genes and mutations underlying QTL have been identified – *DGAT1* and *ABCG2* with effects on milk traits in dairy cattle and perhaps *CAST* and *CAPN1* with effects on beef tenderness, although the causal mutations within these genes do not appear to have been identified. This situation appears to be about to quickly change. Genome sequences assembled from long-read Sanger sequencing have been produced for the cow (Bovine Genome Sequencing and Analysis Consortium 2009; Zimin *et al.* 2009) and genome projects are underway in buffalo, sheep and deer. High-density genotyping assays have been developed for sheep and cattle which allow large numbers of samples to be rapidly genotyped for large numbers of SNPs. These assays allow the localization of QTL by LD analysis which generally results in far smaller QTL regions than are produced in linkage analyses. Finally, next-generation sequencing technologies are revolutionizing many aspects of biological and genomic research, and in particular, make it possible to very simply sequence large chromosomal intervals to seek polymorphisms which may underlie monogenic or polygenetic traits. By simply resequencing the entire genome of a disease-affected individual and focusing only on the sequences that align to the region harboring the disease locus, all mutations present within the region (relative to the reference sequence) can be identified. While this approach may sound wasteful, it is a very effective way to rapidly identify candidate mutations and allows the examination of the candidate region for duplications and deletions. To identify candidate mutations underlying an autosomal recessive neurological disease in dogs, we first mapped the disease locus by GWA to a small region of canine chromosome 4 and then produced a 9X average depth sequence coverage of the entire genome of an affected dog using just four lanes of a single Illumina Genome Analyzer IIx (GA IIx) flow cell at a total cost of under $10,000. The dog was homozygous by descent for the disease causing region of chromosome 4 and Figure 4 shows a view of the sequence pile up for the *LOC489223* gene from this dog when aligned by NextGENe (http://www.softgenetics.com/NextGENe.html) to the CanFam2 Boxer dog assembly. This figure shows two mutations leading to amino acid substitutions within this gene which become candidates for the disease-causing mutation. The final step to this analysis is to genotype mutations detected within the candidate region to establish (by concordance with disease phenotype) which of the detected polymorphisms is causal. If the candidate region is large, there may be many hundreds or even thousands of detected polymorphisms and currently, there is no inexpensive genotyping platform which allows simultaneously assaying this number of polymorphisms in a few hundred individuals to establish the identity of the causal polymorphism. This appears to be the single remaining limitation to the detection of the genes and polymorphisms which underlie disease and quantitative trait variation.

Genomic selection

Fortunately, for the purpose of implementing marker-assisted selection of livestock for almost any trait (including fertility) it is not necessary to identify the genes which underlie genetic variation in the trait. Probably the most important breakthrough in genetic improvement in the last 25 years has been the recent demonstration that Genomic Selection (GS) first proposed by Meuwissen *et al.* (2001) can be effectively implemented within breeds of cattle using the BovineSNP50 assay. GS is a methodology to predict animals' breeding values from high-density SNP panels which utilizes a two-stage approach in which animals with phenotypes and genotypes are first used in a training analysis to establish relationships between individual SNPs and trait variation (the normalized values of these SNP effects are shown in Figure 3) and then the inferred breeding value prediction equations are validated in independent populations. In subsequent generations, the breeding values of animals may be estimated at birth from their BovineSNP50 genotypes and the prediction equations. This technology has revolutionized dairy cattle breeding worldwide and genetic progress in milk production is expected to double due to the decrease in generation interval that has been achieved by a reduced need to progeny test young bulls and the high accuracies of the molecular estimates of breeding value (Hayes *et al.* 2009, VanRaden *et al.* 2009).

The technology is also being deployed within the US beef industry, however, the much lower use of artificial insemination (AI) within the industry and the broader composition of

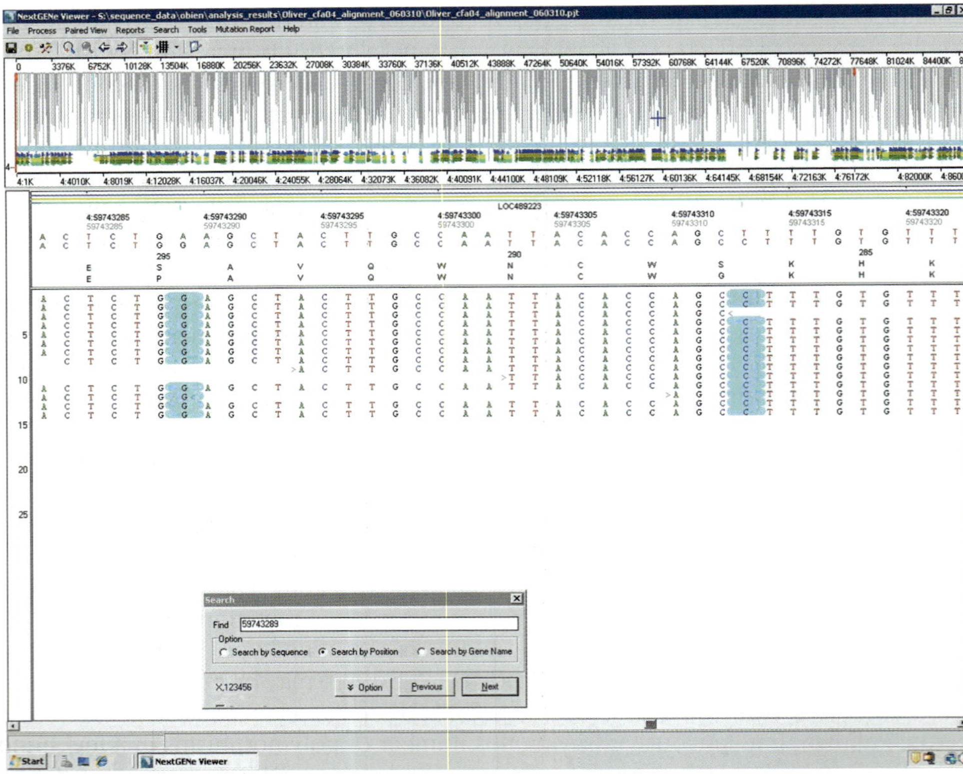

Fig. 4. Screenshot of a NextGENe browser view showing a 14X depth of coverage of sequence produced from a dog homozygous for genomic region on canine chromosome 4 harboring an allele causal for an autosomal recessive neurological disease reveals two charged amino acid substitutions in *LOC489223*. The dog was whole genome sequenced to an average depth of 9X and the only sequence used for mutation discovery was that which aligned to the region of the Boxer reference sequence which was established by LD analysis as harboring the disease causing allele.

breeds employed for U.S. beef production have slowed adoption relative to the dairy industry. First, it has been very difficult to assemble the large training populations needed to develop models with high predictive power. In Angus, the numerically most important beef breed in the US, we have now genotyped only 3,668 registered bulls – far less than the 8,000 Holsteins genotyped when GS was deployed within the dairy industry. Second, the majority of commercial beef animals are bred by natural service and the cost of genotyping young bulls must be amortized over a much smaller number of progeny that are produced by AI sires. It has been vital in the beef industry to reduce the cost of DNA testing to enable GS to be deployed broadly within the industry. When we first developed molecular breeding value prediction equations using genetic evaluations provided by the American Angus Association (AAA) and 41,028 BovineSNP50 SNPs genotyped in 1,710 registered Angus bulls, we developed a reduced set of 384 SNPs which were predictive of breeding values for marbling, ribeye muscle area, backfat thickness and yearling weight to reduce the cost of DNA testing. Validation was performed by genotyping an independent set of 285 bulls and estimating genetic correlations between molecular estimates of breeding value and estimates produced in a multivariate mixed linear model analysis using progeny data (MacNeil *et al.* 2010). Despite the small numbers of tested SNPs, these correlations were 0.65, 0.58, 0.50 and 0.54, respectively. Based upon these results, the AAA now delivers "combined" estimates of genetic merit based upon all sources of available data (molecular, pedigree and phenotype) to the US beef industry. GS has swept through the US beef and dairy industries within less than three years of the development of the BovineSNP50 assay and the technology has been seamlessly adopted by both industries. However, the Angus national genetic evaluation system is now run weekly rather than bi-annually to allow rapid delivery of DNA test results to producers. This rate of technology adoption is almost unprecedented within animal agriculture and is driven by two factors: 1) the technology has been demonstrated to work in dairy cattle, and 2) it provides information that producers desire and for which they are willing to pay.

Genetic analysis across species

Because we cannot make viable crosses between the majority of ruminant species, we cannot use traditional mapping approaches to identify the genes responsible for the phenotypic differences that have evolved following speciation events. In fact, until recently it has been difficult to even reconstruct the evolutionary history of species such as the ruminants which rapidly radiated. Decker *et al.* (2009) have shown that tools developed to detect variation within a species such as the BovineSNP50 assay can be accurately applied as tools to explore orthologous single nucleotide sequences among closely related species. While SNPs remain variable within a species for no more than 1-2 million years with one allele becoming fixed either due to drift or selection, it appears that recurrent mutations occur at the same loci within different species and that different alleles become fixed within different lineages. Thus, genotyping tools such as the BovineSNP50 assay are capable of detecting the nucleotide that is present at the position in an outgroup species' genome that is orthologous to each SNP within the bovine genome. Remarkably, as genetic distance from cow increases, these nucleotides are not all identical (representing the nucleotide present in the genome of the common ancestor of all advanced ruminants). Of the 40,843 bovine SNP used to study the evolution of 61 higher ruminant species, Decker *et al.* (2009) found that 21,019 were phylogenetically informative among the non-cattle species. This result suggests that there are likely to be a very large number of differences between the genome sequences of ruminants and even if whole genome sequences existed for every ruminant species, sequence-based GWA which attempted to identify mutations concordant with species' phenotypes are likely to reveal large numbers of loci consistent with the phenotype differences among species. Despite this, many causal mutations responsible for the differences among species (along with many false positives) will be among the set of congruent genotypes and may point to gene targets for study within hybridized species (e.g., Bison × Cattle) or for mutation studies within transgenic models.

The more usual form of analysis will be to compare gene content between species to identify othologs shared between all ruminants *versus* those that are lineage specific (including duplicated genes) and to identify genes putatively under selection as manifested by differing rates of synonymous and non synonymous substitutions. This approach was employed to identify innate immunity genes specific to the cattle lineage, some of which appear to be under strong selection within the species (Bovine Genome Sequencing and Analysis Consortium 2009). However, there are a number of problems inherent to this form of analysis. The divergence between species can make it difficult to establish gene orthology (same gene descended from a common ancestor) – although this is not likely to be an issue for the higher ruminants which are diverged by about 29 million years. A more important problem is that the majority of ruminant genes can only be identified by prediction programs or through their similarity to better studied human genes. Naturally, this means that lineage specific genes are those that are most likely to be missed in this form of analysis. Finally, with only a single representative sequenced within each species, we have no idea about which sites are variable within a species and this makes it difficult to estimate the synonymous *versus* nonsynonymous substitution rates within genes. However, the next few years are likely to result in the generation of enormous amounts of genome and transcriptome sequence within entire clades of species which will change the way that we study biology.

Tools and reagents

SNPs and SNP chips

The identification of SNPs within species for which very little genomic information is available is now relatively straight forward. By the next-generation sequencing of reduced representation libraries produced either by restriction digestion of genomic DNA and fragment size selection (Van Tassell *et al.* 2008) or tissue transcript libraries from individual animals or pools of animals, it is now possible to rapidly identify hundreds of thousands of SNPs and simultaneously estimate MAF. More recently, to generate SNPs for the design of 800K SNP Illumina and Affymetrix assays, we used an Illumina GA IIx to sequence 5 mate-pair and 5 paired-end genomic DNA libraries for each of: 1) a pool of 10 Brahman (*Bos taurus indicus*), 2) a pool of 15 Hanwoo (Korean *Bos taurus taurus*), and 3) 3 individual high-impact Angus bulls (Table 2). Sequence data were trimmed, filtered and aligned to the UMD3.0 sequence assembly for polymorphism discovery using NextGENe and resulted in the discovery of more than 20 million putative SNPs (Table 2). Other public efforts led to the identification of over 45 million polymorphisms in 200 individuals or pools of individuals sequenced to varying depths. The identification of the same SNPs within different individuals or breeds testifies to the validity of these loci and avoids the problem of sequencing errors being identified as SNPs. Such SNPs provide the foundation for the design of high density genotyping assays which are straightforward but very expensive to develop using Illumina Infinium or Affymetrix Axiom chemistry due to the high cost of oligonucleotide synthesis. Thus, it remains to be seen whether these assays will have broad species utilization in the future, or if the cost of genotyping will decrease to the point that genome-wide genotypes will be produced by sequencing.

Table 2. Generation of whole genome sequence data from 3 cattle breeds within the authors' laboratory at the University of Missouri.

Library	GAIIx Lanes	Post-Filter Reads (million)	Total Bases (billion)	Genome Coverage (2.685Gb = 1X)	Average Read Length (bp)	Unfiltered SNPs and Indels (million)
Brahman (N = 10)	13	454.4	32.942	12.27	72.12	19.9[a]
Hanwoo (N = 15)	16	497.5	35.221	13.11	70.97	18.7[a]
Angus (N = 3)	34	1,179.3	97.304	36.23	78.92	14.8[a]
B/R New Design 036	9	310.0	23.565	8.77	75.18	
GDAR SVF Traveler 234D	17	591.0	52.813	19.66	87.50	7.2[b]
N Bar Emulation EXT	9	278.3	20.926	7.79	74.08	
All Libraries	98	2,131.2	165.467	61.61	75.97	

[a]Delivered to Affymetrix and/or Illumina based upon 47X total genome coverage
[b]Based upon the current 19.66X coverage for this animal

Also of importance is the fact that these SNPs and sequences will nearly all be placed within the public domain over the coming 12 months which will produce a public resource of very considerable value. Researchers interested in the diversity within specific genes can query these data to extract the information they need without the need for expensive and costly resequencing projects.

De novo genome sequences and sequence annotation

The current sequence assemblies for agricultural species are all in early iterations and contain significant errors including contigs assembled to the wrong chromosomes, inverted scaffolds and rudimentary annotations. Currently, the animal used to produce the bovine genome sequence assembly (Hereford, L1 Dominette 01449) is being sequenced to a much greater depth on an Illumina GA IIx using mate-pair and paired-end libraries to provide a much greater depth of sequence coverage which will be reassembled along with the existing Sanger reads by the Salzberg group at the University of Maryland. However, the annotation of the assembly requires a great deal of work and transcript libraries produced from a large number of tissues at different stages of development need to be sequenced in RNA-seq experiments to identify the genes and splice variants present within the genome (Mortazavi *et al.* 2008).

It now appears to be feasible to generate *de novo* genome sequence assemblies from short-read sequencing technologies (Ruiqiang *et al.* 2010) and the increasing read-lengths and decreasing costs per Gb of sequence will undoubtedly lead to a rapid increase in the number of *de novo* sequence assemblies produced for ruminants. Furthermore, we will also begin to see many more 100 genome or 1,000 genome projects for individual species which will assist us to identify important functional variants and genomic regions that are under strong selection. Knowledge of the regions within a genome that are variable will also greatly assist in the comparison of genomes between species.

Other applications of next-generation sequencers

Next-generation sequencing instruments are powerful tools for examining genome-wide phenomena. In addition to sequencing DNA and RNA populations, methodologies have been developed which allow the capture (and identification by sequencing) of genomic regions to which proteins such as transcription factors bind (CHIP-seq, Johnson *et al.* 2007), which are methylated (e.g., reduced representation bisulphate sequencing, Meissner *et al.* 2007), or which are physically close together within cells derived from specific tissue types (Hi-C, Lieberman-Aiden *et al.* 2009). These tools will revolutionize our understanding of genome organization and function.

Conclusions

Next-generation sequencing technologies are having enormous impacts in fundamental biology and applied animal agriculture. As competing technologies emerge and the cost of sequencing decreases, we will begin to see the genomes and transcriptomes of closely related- ruminants sequenced, and comparative analyses will point to the genes, structural differences and polymorphisms responsible for the evolution of phenotypic differences between species. Furthermore, many representatives from different breeds and species will be sequenced, which will lead to a much better understanding of the fundamental causes of genetic variation within a species.

While this information will enable genetic improvement within species utilizing existing genetic variation, it will also guide the engineering of transgenic animals with increased adaptation to changing production environments, disease resistance, reproductive and productive capabilities (Fahrenkrug *et al.* 2010). Both approaches to animal improvement will be needed to meet the world's human dietary needs in the very near future.

Acknowledgements

We thank the Circle A Ranch and the MFA, Inc. for providing samples and data, and the American Angus Association for providing pedigree data and expected progeny differences for Angus sires. JFT is supported by National Research Initiative Grant no. 2008-35205-04687 from the USDA Cooperative State Research, Education, and Extension Service, Agriculture and Food Research Initiative grant number 2009-65205-05635 from the USDA National Institute of Food and Agriculture and grant 13321 from the Missouri Life Science Research Board.

References

Bareil C, Hamel CP, Delague V, Arnaud B, Demaille J & Claustres M 2001 Segregation of a mutation in CNGB1 encoding the beta-subunit of the rod cGMP-gated channel in a family with autosomal recessive retinitis pigmentosa. *Human Genetics* **108** 328-334.

Barendse W, Reverter A, Bunch RJ, Harrison BE, Barris W & Thomas MB 2007 A validated whole-genome association study of efficient food conversion in cattle. *Genetics* **176** 1893-1905.

Bovine Genome Sequencing and Analysis Consortium 2009 The genome sequence of taurine cattle: a window to ruminant biology and evolution. *Science* **324** 522-528.

Bovine HapMap Consortium 2009 Genome Wide Survey of SNP Variation Uncovers the Genetic Structure of Cattle Breeds. *Science* **324** 528-532.

Candille SI, Kaelin CB, Cattanach BM, Yu B, Thompson DA, Nix MA, Kerns JA, Schmutz SM, Millhauser GL & Barsh GS 2007 A -defensin mutation causes black coat color in domestic dogs. *Science* **318** 1418-1423.

Charlier C, Coppieters W, Rollin F, Desmecht D, Agerholm JS, Cambisano N, Carta E, Dardano S, Dive M, Fasquelle C, Frennet JC, Hanset R, Hubin X, Jorgensen C, Karim L, Kent M, Harvey K, Pearce BR, Simon P, Tama N, Nie H, Vandeputte S, Lien S, Longeri M, Fredholm M, Harvey RJ & Georges M 2008 Highly effective SNP-based association mapping and management of recessive defects in livestock. *Nature Genetics* **40** 449-454.

Decker JE, Pires JC, Conant GC, McKay SD, Heaton MP, Chen K, Cooper A, Vilkki J, Seabury CM, Caetano AR, Johnson GS, Brenneman RA, Hanotte O, Eggert LS, Wiener P, Kim JJ, Kim KS, Sonstegard TS, Van Tassell CP, Neibergs HL, McEwan JC, Brauning R, Coutinho LL, Babar ME, Wilson GA, McClure MC, Rolf MM, Kim J, Schnabel RD & Taylor JF 2009 Resolving the evolution of extant and extinct ruminants with high-throughput phylogenomics. *Proceedings of the National Academy of Science U S A.* **106** 18644-18649.

Drögemüller C, Wöhlke A, Mömke S & Distl O 2005 Fine mapping of the polled locus to a 1-Mb region on bovine chromosome 1q12. *Mammalian Genome* 16 613-620.

Fahrenkrug SC, Carlson DF, Doran T, Van Eenennaam A, Galli C, Hackett PB, Li N, Maga EA, Murray JD, Taylor JF, Wheeler M, Whitelaw B & Glenn B 2010 Precision genetics for complex objectives in animal agriculture. *Journal of Animal Science* doi:10.2527/jas.2010-2847.

Georges M, Drinkwater R, King T, Mishra A, Moore SS, Nielsen D, Sargeant LS, Sorensen A, Steele MR, Zhao X, Womack JE & Hetzel J 1993 Microsatellite mapping of a gene affecting horn development in Bos taurus. *Nature Genetics* **4** 206-210.

Giuffra E, Kijas JM, Amarger V, Carlborg O, Jeon JT & Andersson L 2000 The origin of the domestic pig: independent domestication and subsequent introgression. *Genetics* **154** 1785-1791.

Hackmann TJ & Spain JN 2010 Invited review: Ruminant ecology and evolution: Perspectives useful to ruminant livestock research and production. *Journal of Dairy Science* **93** 1320-1334.

Hayes B & Goddard ME 2001 The distribution of the effects of genes affecting quantitative traits in livestock. *Genetics Selection Evolution* **33** 209-229.

Hayes BJ, Bowman PJ, Chamberlain AJ & Goddard ME 2009 Invited review: Genomic selection in dairy cattle: progress and challenges. *Journal of Dairy Science* **92** 433-443.

Johnson DS, Mortazavi A, Myers RM & Wold B 2007 Genome-Wide Mapping of *in vivo* protein-DNA interactions. *Science* **316** 1497-1502.

Kim J-J, Davis SK & Taylor JF 2002 Application of non-parametric bootstrap methods to estimate confidence intervals for QTL location in a beef cattle QTL experimental population. *Genetics Research* **79** 259-263.

Kim J-J, Farnir F, Savell J & Taylor JF 2003. Detection of QTL for growth and beef carcass fatness traits in a cross between *Bos taurus* (Angus) and *Bos indicus* (Brahman) cattle. *Journal of Animal Science* **81** 1933-1942.

Klungland H, Våge DI, Gomez-Raya L, Adalsteinsson S & Lien S 1995 The role of melanocyte-stimulating hormone (MSH) receptor in bovine coat color determination. *Mammalian Genome* **6** 636-639.

Lieberman-Aiden E, van Berkum NL, Williams L, Imakaev M, Ragoczy T, Telling A, Amit I, Lajoie BR, Sabo PJ, Dorschner MO, Sandstrom R, Bernstein B, Bender MA, Groudine M, Gnirke A, Stamatoyannopoulos J, Mirny LA, Lander ES & Dekker J 2009 Comprehensive mapping of long-range interactions reveals folding principles of the human genome. Science **326** 289-293.

Loftus RT, MacHugh DE, Bradley DG, Sharp PM & Cunningham P 1994 Evidence for two independent domestications of cattle. *Proceedings of the National Academy of Science U S A.* **91** 2757–2761.

MacLeod IM, Hayes BJ, Savin KW, Chamberlain AJ, McPartlan HC & Goddard ME 2010 Power of a genome scan to detect and locate quantitative trait loci in cattle using dense single nucleotide polymorphisms. *Journal of Animal Breeding and Genetics* **127** 133-142.

MacNeil MD, Northcutt SL, Schnabel RD, Garrick DJ & Taylor JF 2010 Genetic correlations between carcass traits and molecular breeding values in Angus cattle. *Proceedings of the 9th World Congress on Genetics Applied to Livestock Production*. August 1-6, Leipzig, Germany.

Magee DA, Park SDE, Scraggs E, Murphy AM, Doherty ML, Kijas JW, International Sheep Genomics Consortium & MacHugh DE 2010 Technical note: High fidelity of whole-genome amplified sheep (Ovis aries) DNA using a high-density single nucleotide polymorphism array-based genotyping platform. *Journal of Animal Science* published online Jun 18, 2010.

Maher B 2008 Personal genomes: The case of the missing heritability. *Nature* **456** 18-21.

Matukumalli LK, Lawley CT, Schnabel RD, Taylor JF, Allan MF, Heaton MP, O'Connell J, Moore SS, Smith TP, Sonstegard TS & Van Tassell CP 2009 Development and characterization of a high density SNP genotyping assay for cattle. *PLoS One* **4** e5350.

McClure MC, Morsci NS, Schnabel RD, Kim JW, Yao P, Rolf MM, McKay SD, Gregg SJ, Chapple RH, Northcutt SL & Taylor JF 2010 A genome scan for quantitative trait loci influencing carcass, post-natal growth and reproductive traits in commercial Angus cattle. *Animal Genetics* May 10. [Epub ahead of print].

Meissner A, Mikkelsen TS, Gu H, Wernig M, Hanna J, Sivachenko A, Zhang X, Bernstein BE, Nusbaum C, Jaffe DB, Gnirke A, Jaenisch R & Lander ES 2007 Genome-scale DNA methylation maps of pluripotent and differentiated cells. *Nature* **454** 766-771.

Meuwissen TH, Hayes BJ & Goddard ME 2001 Prediction of total genetic value using genome-wide dense marker maps. *Genetics* **157** 1819-1829.

Meyers SN, McDaneld TG, Swist SL, Marron BM, Steffen DJ, O'Toole D, O'Connell JR, Beever JE, Sonstegard TS & Smith TP 2010 A deletion mutation in bovine SLC4A2 is associated with osteopetrosis in Red Angus cattle. *BMC Genomics* **11** 337.

Mortazavi A, Williams BA, McCue K, Schaeffer L & Wold B 2008 Mapping and quantifying mammalian transcriptomes by RNA-Seq. *Nature Methods* **5** 621-628.

Nielsen R, Williamson S, Kim Y, Hubisz MJ, Clark AG & Bustamante C 2005 Genomic scans for selective sweeps using SNP data. *Genome Research* **15** 1566-1575.

O'Brien DP, Johnson GS, Schnabel RD, Khan S, Coates JR, Johnson GC & Taylor JF 2005 Genetic mapping of canine multiple system degeneration and ectodermal dysplasia loci. *Journal of Heredity* **96** 727-734.

Ruiqiang L, Fan W, Tian G, Zhu H, He L, Cai J, Huang Q, Cai Q, Li B, Bai Y, Zhang Z, Zhang Y, Wang W, Li J, Wei F, Li H, Jian M, Li J, Zhang Z, Nielsen R, Li D, Gu W, Yang Z, Xuan Z, Ryder OA, Leung FC, Zhou Y, Cao J, Sun X, Fu Y, Fang X, Guo X, Wang B, Hou R, Shen F, Mu B, Ni P, Lin R, Qian W, Wang G, Yu C, Nie W, Wang J, Wu Z, Liang H, Min J, Wu Q, Cheng S, Ruan J, Wang M, Shi Z, Wen M, Liu B, Ren X, Zheng H, Dong D, Cook K, Shan G, Zhang H, Kosiol C, Xie X, Lu Z, Zheng H, Li Y, Steiner CC, Lam TT, Lin S, Zhang Q, Li G, Tian J, Gong T, Liu H, Zhang D, Fang L, Ye C, Zhang J, Hu W, Xu A, Ren Y, Zhang G, Bruford MW, Li Q, Ma L, Guo Y, An N, Hu Y, Zheng Y, Shi Y, Li Z, Liu Q, Chen Y, Zhao J, Qu N, Zhao S, Tian F, Wang X, Wang H, Xu L, Liu X, Vinar T, Wang Y, Lam T, Yiu S, Liu S, Zhang H, Li D, Huang Y, Wang X, Yang G, Jiang Z, Wang J, Qin N, Li L, Li J, Bolund L, Kristiansen K, Wong GK, Olson M, Zhang X, Li S, Yang H, Wang J & Wang J 2010 The sequence and de novo assembly of the giant panda genome. *Nature* **463** 311-317.

Sellner EM, Kim JW, McClure MC, Taylor KH, Schnabel RD & Taylor JF 2007 Applications of Genomic Information in Livestock. *Journal of Animal Science* **85** 3148-3158.

Tenesa A, Navarro P, Hayes BJ, Duffy DL, Clarke GM, Goddard ME & Visscher PM 2007 Recent human effective population size estimated from linkage disequilibrium. *Genome Research* **17** 520–526.

VanRaden PM 2008 Efficient Methods to Compute Genomic Predictions. *Journal of Dairy Science* **91** 4414–4423.

VanRaden PM, Van Tassell CP, Wiggans GR, Sonstegard TS, Schnabel RD, Taylor JF & Schenkel FS 2009 Invited review: reliability of genomic predictions for North American Holstein bulls. *Journal of Dairy Science* **92** 16-24.

Van Tassell CP, Smith TPL, Matukumalli LK, Taylor JF, Schnabel RD, Lawley CT, Haudenschild CD, Moore SS, Warren WC & Sonstegard TS 2008 Simultaneous SNP discovery and allele frequency estimation by high throughput sequencing of reduced representation genomic libraries. *Nature Methods* **5** 247-252.

Wunderlich KR, Abbey CA, Clayton DR, Song Y, Schein JE, Georges M, Coppieters W, Adelson DL, Taylor JF, Davis SL & Gill CA 2006 A 2.5-Mb contig constructed from Angus, Longhorn and horned Hereford DNA spanning the polled interval on bovine chromosome 1. *Animal Genetics* 37 592-594.

Zimin AV, Delcher AL, Florea L, Kelley DR, Schatz MC, Puiu D, Hanrahan F, Pertea G, Van Tassell CP, Sonstegard TS, Marçais G, Roberts M, Subramanian P, Yorke JA & Salzberg SL 2009 A whole-genome assembly of the domestic cow, Bos taurus. Genome Biology **10** R42.

Creating new knowledge for ruminant reproduction from rapidly expanding and evolving scientific databases

S Bauersachs, H Blum, S Krebs, T Fröhlich, GJ Arnold and E Wolf

Laboratory for Functional Genome Analysis (LAFUGA), Gene Center, Ludwig-Maximilians-Universität München, Feodor-Lynen-Str. 25, D-81377 Munich, Germany

Declining fertility is a major problem for the dairy industry. Recent developments of Omics-technologies facilitate a comprehensive analysis of molecular patters in gametes, embryos and tissues of the reproductive tract which may help to identify the reasons for impaired fertility. Large Omics-datasets require appropriate bioinformatics analysis in the context of rapidly expanding and evolving scientific databases. This overview summarizes the current status of ruminant genome projects, describes currently existing resources for ruminant genomics, transcriptomics and proteomics as well as databases and tools for the interpretation and exploitation of transcriptomics and proteomics datasets. Gene set enrichment analysis (GSEA) and transcription factor binding site (TFBS) analyses are strategies for the identification of regulatory genes. In general, the comprehensive analysis of molecular traits by Omics-technologies can enhance the interpretation of genome-wide association studies, providing insights into the biological pathways linking genotype and phenotype, and their modulation by endogenous and environmental factors.

Introduction

Reproductive success is a key component of economic production with ruminants, affecting both productivity and genetic progress. The decrease in dairy cattle fertility is a worldwide problem and a major cause of cow culling and economic losses. It is widely accepted that there is a strong association between high milk production and low fertility in dairy herds; however the reasons for the negative relationship between these traits remain to be resolved. On the one hand, metabolic problems that may be associated with high yield can influence molecular pathways controlling fertility at different levels and in various organs of the reproductive tract. On the other hand, preferential selection for production traits in the past may have led to genotypes in dairy cattle that are suboptimal for reproductive competence (Lucy 2001).

Reproductive success is determined by a cascade of biological processes: maturation and selection of gametes, fertilization, pre- and post-implantation embryonic development, fetal growth regulation, birth and early postnatal development of offspring. Among those, a reduction in fertilization and embryonic survival rates has been suggested as the most important component for decreasing reproductive efficiency in dairy cattle (Santos et al. 2004). Holistic and sensitive Omics-technologies characterizing the transcriptome, proteome, metabolome etc. of cells or tissues facilitate a comprehensive description of molecular patterns of gametes, embryos and

Corresponding author E-mail: ewolf@lmb.uni-muenchen.de

their maternal environment. For instance, our previous studies of bovine endometrium revealed characteristic transcriptome changes during the estrous cycle (Bauersachs et al. 2005; Mitko et al. 2008) and during early pregnancy (Bauersachs et al. 2006; Klein et al. 2006). Interestingly, we and others observed a different response of the endometrium to cloned vs. fertilized embryos (Bauersachs et al. 2009; Mansouri-Attia et al. 2009), suggesting the endometrium as a sensor for embryo quality and disturbed embryo-maternal communication in the peri-implantation period as a reason for structural and functional alterations of the placenta in clone pregnancies. Thus, changes of molecular patterns during development may point to genes or pathways that have an effect on reproductive success. Consequently, molecular patterns identified by Omics-technologies in organs and tissues that are relevant for reproduction can be viewed as "intermediate phenotypes" (Schadt 2009) of fertility, whose comprehensive description, interpretation and modeling may help to understand the genetic basis of cellular functions that are important for fertility (Figure 1).

This article provides an overview of the currently existing databases and bioinformatics tools that can be used to interpret Omics-data in the context of reproduction and other traits of ruminants.

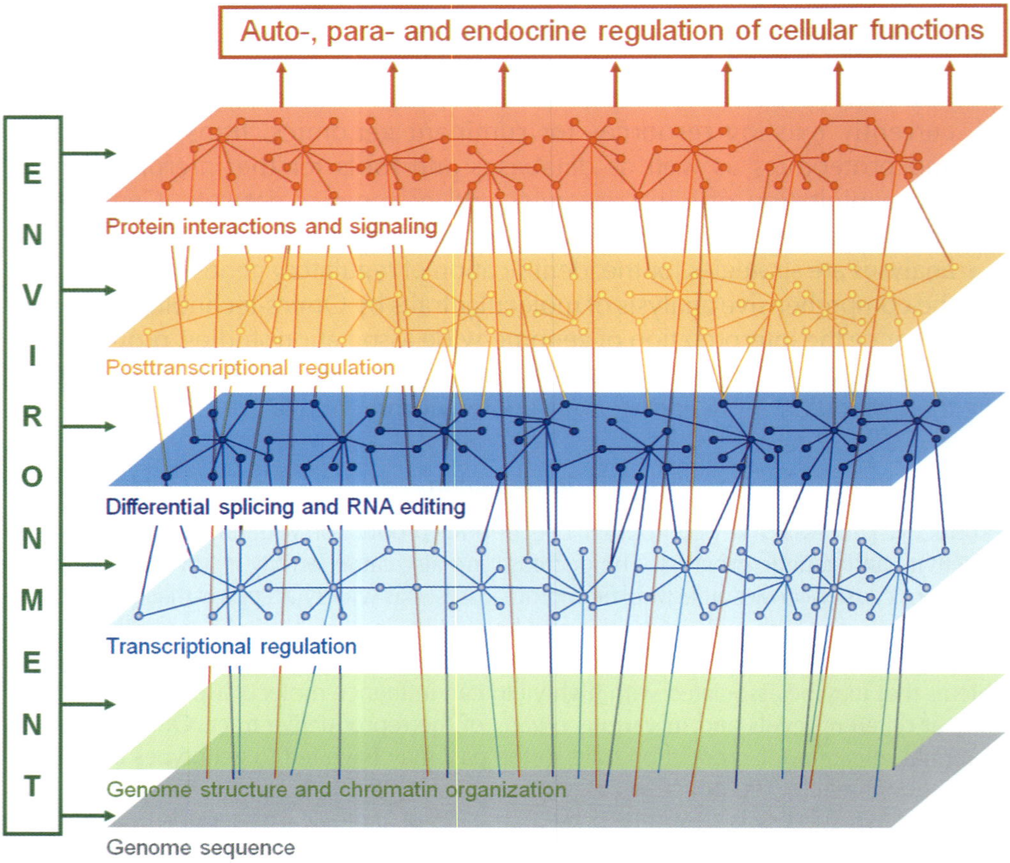

Fig. 1. Flow of genetic information via different classes of molecules producing molecular patterns and networks which affect cellular and organ functions. Integrating large-scale, high-dimensional molecular and physiological data holds promise for defining the molecular networks that respond to genetic and environmental perturbations of the physiological functions. The different layers of information provide a hierarchy of intermediate phenotypes, RNA being the most proximal non-DNA species of all molecular entities in the cell. Complex epigenomic mechanisms and interactions between the different classes of molecules modulate the flow of genetic information into biological functions.

Current status of ruminant genome projects

The largest current publicly available sequence database is GenBank located at the NCBI and contains nucleotide sequences of more than 300,000 organisms (Benson et al. 2009). GenBank is a collaborative effort between the International Nucleotide Sequence Database Collaboration (INSDC) of the NCBI, the DNA Data Bank of Japan (DDBJ) and the European Molecular Biology Laboratory (EMBL) Nucleotide Sequence Database (EMBL-Bank) at the European Bioinformatics Institute (EBI). Within this collaboration databases are synchronized by exchange and update of data. Founded in 1982, the content of GenBank has been growing exponentially, doubling approximately every 18 months (Figure 2). It currently comprises nearly $120*10^9$ nucleotides (GenBank release 177, April 2010). The generation of nucleotide sequence data was significantly accelerated by the development of powerful strategies for whole genome shotgun sequencing (WGS). The content of the WGS database grew faster than that of GenBank and exceeded it within two years (Figure 2). Among the twenty most sequenced organisms in GenBank Release 177 *Bos taurus* is the only ruminant species with a finished genome sequence, listed with roughly 5 gigabases of DNA/RNA sequences (Table 1) and 1.56 millions of expressed sequence tag (EST) records. The current assembly of the *Bos taurus* genome, Btau_4.0, is based on whole genome shotgun sequencing with 7× sequence coverage and comprises the sequence of all chromosomes except for the Y chromosome. The current release of GenBank contains no annotated genomes of other ruminants and only relatively small numbers of mRNA sequence data of other ruminants (e.g. mRNA entries: sheep: 3055, water buffalo: 695). This situation might be improved by the efforts of International Sequencing Consortia to sequence the Y chromosome of *Bos taurus* and the ovine genome (http://www.intlgenome.org/viewDatabase.cfm; Table 2).

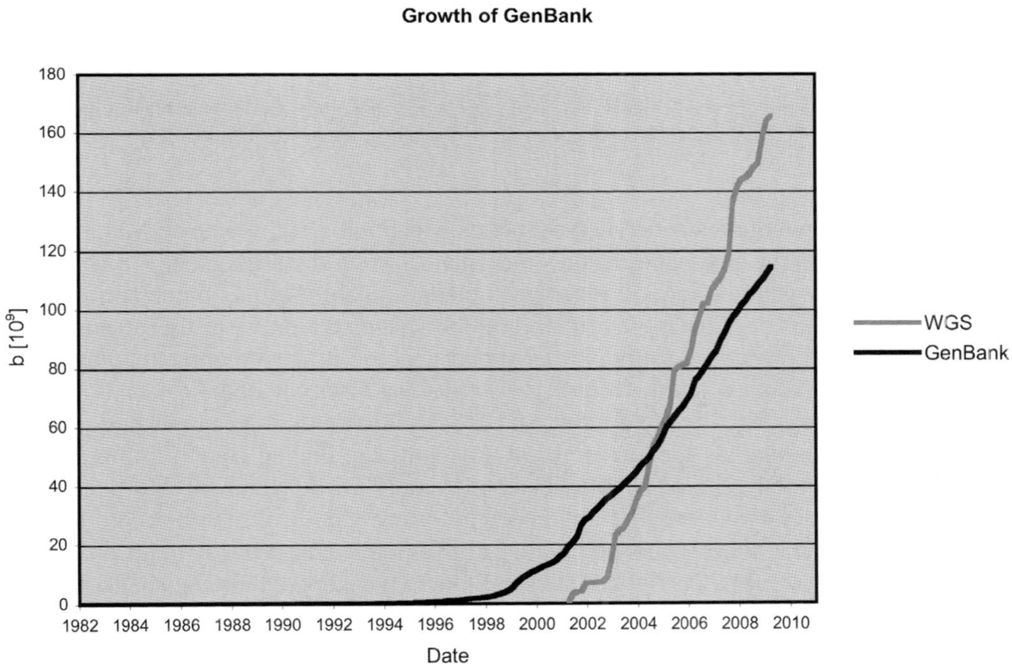

Fig. 2. Growth of GenBank. The number of bases in GenBank between 1982 and 2010 is blotted as black line, whereas the gray line displays the number of bases from whole genome shot gun sequencing projects. The data are derived from the distribution release note of GenBank release 177.

Table 1. Twenty most sequenced organisms in GenBank Release 177 (April 2010)

Entries	Bases*	Species
14661813	14675829480	*Homo sapiens*
7864719	8850187116	*Mus musculus*
2000118	6283974613	*Rattus norvegicus*
2179964	5355764557	*Bos taurus*
3890820	5034163602	*Zea mays*
3217695	4778268370	*Sus scrofa*
1697206	3052524947	*Danio rerio*
228209	1352880670	*Strongylocentrotus purpuratus*
1241806	1195864179	*Oryza sativa Japonica Group*
1753889	1185779622	*Nicotiana tabacum*
1423873	1146958794	*Xenopus (Silurana) tropicalis*
1205719	1043367600	*Drosophila melanogaster*
213748	999755722	*Pan troglodytes*
2286014	993961755	*Arabidopsis thaliana*
1435337	932443900	*Canis lupus familiaris*
655957	911105678	*Vitis vinifera*
808694	889675519	*Gallus gallus*
1840687	864995575	*Glycine max*
79871	816072773	*Macaca mulatta*
1216189	748184685	*Ciona intestinalis*

*: DNA/RNA, excluding chloroplast and mitochondrial sequences, metagenomic sequences, Whole Genome Shotgun sequences, and 'constructed' CON-division sequences. Ovine sequences are not included.

With the development of next-generation sequencing technologies the time-consuming process of generation of genome sequences has been dramatically shortened. Recently, a first draft sequence of the ovine genome sequence has been made available with a limited annotation that was produced by 454 sequencing and mapping the sheep sequences to the bovine genome sequence reordered according to the virtual sheep genome (www.sheephapmap.org/, www.livestockgenomics.csiro.au/). Furthermore, a low-coverage assembly of the alpaca (*Vicugna pacos*) is available that is actually not a ruminant but is similar to ruminants in its physiology and is thus generally classified as pseudo-ruminant. Recently, the Beijing Genomics Institute (BGI) has announced, that the genome of the Tibetan Antelope, a wild ruminant, has been finished (http://www.genomics.cn/en/search_show.php?type=show&id=530). Furthermore additional ruminant genomes might be sequenced within the Genome 10K project which plans whole-genome sequencing of 10.000 vertebrate species (http://www.genome10k.org/) (Genome 2009).

Current resources for ruminant genomics, transcriptomics and proteomics

The bovine reference genome is the first finished and fully annotated ruminant genome sequence (Elsik et al. 2009). Data from the bovine genome sequencing project as well as other genome sequencing projects are available through a number of genome browsers (e.g. Ensembl and UCSC genome browser) and genome project databases (Table 2). Comparative genome alignments with other vertebrate genomes are available through these genome browsers, providing a source for comparative genome annotation. A specialized tool for visualizing the results of the mammalian genome comparative analysis is Evolution Highway that was used to decode the bovine genome evolutionary history (Elsik et al. 2009). In the context of genetic studies comparative genome annotation is of great value for positional cloning of bovine QTL. The Bovine Genome Database (http://bovinegenome.org) provides - in addition to the bovine genome sequence - up to date gene models and annotations and integration of physical and linkage maps with sequence, QTL, and SNP data. The investigation of variations in the genome is of major importance for animal breeding. For cattle and sheep there are large-scale ongoing SNP genotyping projects for genomic selection and HapMap development (bovinehapmap.org, sheephapmap.org). Publically available data in the context of QTL and GWAS analysis can be obtained for example from the Animal QTL database, the Bovine QTL viewer, and the USDA MARC website (see Table 2). Data derived from gene expression analyses can be found in public functional genomics data repositories such as Gene Expression Omnibus (GEO) and ArrayExpress (Table 2).

An important point for transcriptome and proteome analyses is a comprehensive gene annotation. Annotation data for protein-coding and non-coding transcripts and protein sequences can be downloaded, e.g. via Ensembl's BioMart. Genome annotation pipelines are using different strategies for gene annotation based on the alignment of sequences from public sequence databases, comparative alignment of Ensembl human and mouse proteins, and *ab initio* gene predictions. Another strategy to obtain full-length transcript and protein sequences is the generation of clusters of ESTs and full-length mRNA sequences derived from the same gene locus (UniGene, see Table 2). There are also attempts to find orthologous genes of several completely sequenced eukaryotic genomes (HomoloGene, see Table 2). In order to provide a defined functional description and classification of genes the Gene Ontology (GO) project has developed three structured controlled vocabularies (ontologies) that describe gene products in terms of their associated biological processes, cellular components and molecular functions in a species-independent manner. Genes are assigned based on data from the literature, on belonging to a known protein family, but also merely based on the presence of conserved protein domains. For ruminants only bovine genes are included in the GO classification. Likewise, only bovine genes are assigned to Kyoto Encyclopedia of Genes and Genomes (KEGG) metabolic, signaling and disease pathways.

With the discovery of small regulatory RNAs or so-called microRNAs (miRNAs) a database containing all known miRNA sequences was developed (mirBase, Table 2). In the current release (mirBase 15) there are 665 bovine and 4 ovine miRNAs. However, as many miRNAs are highly conserved between species annotations from other mammals can be used for ruminants where no annotation is available.

In addition to the information based on nucleic acid sequences and abundance, availability of data generated on the protein level is indispensable, since in all biological systems a broad spectrum of regulation phenomena occur on the protein level (e.g., secretion, activation of protein precursors by protein cleavage or phosphorylation, feedback inhibition, translational regulation, etc.). These crucial events are not mirrored by mRNA abundances, and their analysis is therefore addressable exclusively on the protein level. Moreover, the existence of mRNA in a tissue or cell type does not provide unequivocal evidence for the presence of the corresponding protein. As a consequence of substantial efforts in high resolution mass spectrometry (MS) of proteins and peptides, identification and quantification of thousands of proteins has become feasible and affordable during the last decade (for review, see Frohlich & Arnold 2006).

Table 2. Genomic resources for ruminant research

Resource	Content	Web site/Source
NCBI Genomic Biology	Links to genomic biology tools and resources for Bos taurus, Bubalus bubalis, Capra hircus, Ovis aries	www.ncbi.nlm.nih.gov/Genomes/
NCBI Entrez Genome Project database	Collection of complete and incomplete (in-progress) large-scale sequencing, assembly, annotation, and mapping projects for cellular organisms	www.ncbi.nlm.nih.gov/sites/entrez?db=genomeprj
Ensembl Genome Browser	Genome annotation for Bos taurus and Vicugna pacos	www.ensembl.org/Bos_taurus/Info/Index
UCSC Genome Browser	Genome annotation for Bos taurus	genome.ucsc.edu/cgi-bin/hgGateway?hgsid=158064562&clade=mammal&org=Cow&db=0
BioMart	Annotation tool	www.ensembl.org/biomart/martview
Entrez Gene	Searchable database of genes, from RefSeq genomes, and defined by sequence and/or located in the NCBI Map Viewer	www.ncbi.nlm.nih.gov/gene
HomoloGene	System for automated detection of homologs among the annotated genes of several completely sequenced eukaryotic genomes	www.ncbi.nlm.nih.gov/homologene
UniGene	UniGene entries are sets of transcript sequences that appear to come from the same transcription locus (gene or expressed pseudogene), together with information on protein similarities, gene expression, cDNA clone reagents, and genomic location	www.ncbi.nlm.nih.gov/sites/entrez?db=unigene
miRBase	Bovine and ovine micro RNAs	www.mirbase.org/cgi-bin/mirna_summary.pl?org=bta
Gene Expression Omnibus	Database for curated gene expression datasets	www.ncbi.nlm.nih.gov/geo
ArrayExpress Archive	Database of functional genomics experiments including gene expression	www.ebi.ac.uk/microarray-as/ae
Bos taurus genome project	Bovine Genome Database project	http://bovinegenome.org
Bovine HapMap project	Large-scale bovine single nucleotide polymorphism (SNP) genotyping for genomic selection and HapMap development	http://bovinehapmap.org
Animal Quantitative Trait Locus (QTL) database	Houses all publicly available QTL data on livestock animal species for easily locating and making comparisons within and between species	www.genome.iastate.edu/cgi-bin/QTLdb/index
Bovine QTL viewer	Contains all available public domain bovine QTL data for both dairy and beef traits	genomes.sapac.edu.au/bovineqtl
USDA MARC	Cattle and sheep genome maps	www.ars.usda.gov/main/docs.htm?docid=2340
Evolution Highway	Collaborative project designed to provide a visual means for simultaneously comparing genomes of multiple amniote species	http://evolutionhighway.ncsa.uiuc.edu
Ovis aries genome project	Home page of the International Sheep Genomics Consortium	www.sheephapmap.org
CSIRO livestock genomics web site	Access to data generated by genomics projects for major livestock species, major focus on the cattle and sheep genome mapping and sequencing projects, provides access to interactive genome maps of cattle and sheep and to the results of the Bacterial Artificial Chromosome (BAC) library contiging project for cattle	www.livestockgenomics.csiro.au

Due to the bioinformatics algorithms used for MS-based protein identification, comprehensive genomic databases of the organisms analyzed (or at least a closely related species) are indispensable prerequisites for protein identification. Hence, the availability of the bovine genome database (http://www.ncbi.nlm.nih.gov, Elsik et al. 2009) represents a milestone with respect to protein identifications in ruminants. Whole genome sequencing and annotation of sheep and other ruminants are currently in progress and will further stimulate the generation of data on the protein level.

Through various proteomic approaches performed during the last years, a tremendous amount of data has been generated, giving rise to the generation of databases focused on protein data. The most prominent of these is the "UniProt" database (***uni***versal ***prot***ein; www.uniprot.org), representing the largest collection of protein information from a broad variety of organisms and viruses. Uniprot combines data from Swiss-Prot, TrEMBL (Translated EMBL Nucleotide Sequence Data Library) (Boeckmann et al. 2003) and PIR (**P**rotein **I**nformation **R**esource, Wu et al. 2006) and is updated frequently.

Besides pure sequence data, UniProt provides information about post-translational modifications and functional aspects as well as relevant links to structural and gene ontology databases. A special feature of the Swiss-Prot part of UniProt is the manual annotation and review process performed by experts in the field, thereby providing a superior level of data reliability and relevance as compared to datasets automatically generated by unsupervised, computer based data mining.

To facilitate public access to the huge number of datasets generated in proteomic approaches, several databases are currently established containing raw data from mass spectrometry based protein identifications (peak lists, intensities, identified peptides etc.). Two prominent examples are the PRIDE database (**PR**oteomics **IDE**ntifications, Vizcaino et al. 2009) managed by the EBI at the EMBL and the "Peptide Atlas" (Deutsch et al. 2008) managed by the Seattle Proteome Center, containing data from 60 and 12 species (releases May 2010), respectively. Data from ruminants are contained only in PRIDE, currently comprising 66 different proteins from *Bos taurus* (PRIDE core version 2.8.0).

The benefit of these databases lies in the possibility to quickly gain information about the level of expression of proteins in individual cells, tissues or body fluids. Moreover, post-translational modifications identified by mass spectrometry can frequently be assigned to distinct amino acid positions of the protein. As a special advantage, the public availability of mass spectrometry raw data facilitates their re-analysis using rapidly evolving new algorithms.

The low number of ruminant data so far contained in PRIDE reflects both the lack of obligation to deposit raw data of proteomic experiments in public databases along with publication in scientific journals as well as the rather initial status of proteome research in farm animals. Along with ongoing new guidelines for proteomic data publication and exciting developments in protein analysis, e.g., mass spectrometry based quantification of proteins using SRM (**S**elected **R**eaction **M**onitoring) technology (Lange et al. 2008; Picotti et al. 2010), protein databases will provide a widely applicable source of information in the fields of basic research as well as veterinary medicine and animal reproduction.

Databases and tools to exploit transcriptomics and proteomics datasets for ruminants

As already mentioned the GO database provides a defined description of genes regarding the categories "Biological Process", "Molecular Function", and "Cellular Component". There are numerous tools for the analysis of GO terms associated with a list of differentially expressed transcripts or proteins (see Table 3). Many of these tools provide quantitatively enriched GO terms associated with a gene list, i.e. GO terms for which significantly more associated genes were found than expected by chance. The processing of the results of such analyses can be very laborious due to the redundant structure of the GO categories. The "Functional Annotation Clustering" tool of the Database for Annotation, Visualization and Integrated Discovery (DAVID) (Dennis et al. 2003) reduces this problem by clustering enriched functional categories (from GO and other databases) that have overlapping gene contents.

Table 3. Tools for the bioinformatics analysis of Omics-data

Tool	Function	Web site/Source
Gene Ontology	provides a controlled vocabulary of terms for describing gene product characteristics and gene product annotation data	geneontology.org/
GO tools for analysis of gene expression/microarray datasets	overview of tools for Gene Ontology analysis of lists of differentially expressed genes/mRNAs or proteins	geneontology.org/GO.tools.microarray.shtml#goarray
Gene Set Enrichment Analysis (GSEA)	computational method that determines whether an a priori defined set of genes shows statistically significant, concordant differences between two biological states (e.g. phenotypes)	www.broadinstitute.org/gsea/
Database for Annotation, Visualization and Integrated Discovery (DAVID)	functional annotation, functional classification, gene ID conversion, gene name batch viewer	david.abcc.ncifcrf.gov/
CoPub text mining tool	text mining tool for detection of co-occuring biomedical concepts in abstracts from the Medline literature database significantly linked to a differential gene set	services.nbic.nl/cgi-bin/copub3/CoPub.pl
oPOSSUM	detection of over-represented transcription factor binding sites in the promoters of sets of genes	www.cisreg.ca/oPOSSUM/
KEGG pathway database	collection of manually drawn pathway maps	www.genome.jp/kegg/pathway.html
NCI/Nature Pathway Interaction Database	biomolecular interactions and cellular processes assembled into authoritative human signaling pathways	pid.nci.nih.gov/index.shtml
STRING	database and analysis tool for known and predicted protein-protein interactions	string.embl.de/newstring_cgi/show_input_page.pl?UserId=JE8TU8ELDuNa&sessionId=I1hDAbLNVFLZ
Cytoscape	open source bioinformatics software platform for visualizing molecular interaction networks and integrating these interactions with gene expression profiles and other state data	www.cytoscape.org/

A different strategy for the analysis of lists of differentially expressed genes or proteins is text-mining of PubMed abstracts with CoPub to analyze gene-gene co-citation and co-citation of genes with keywords (Table 3). This analysis identifies biological or disease-related keywords overrepresented within the differentially expressed genes.

Microarray datasets can also be characterized by comparison with gene sets derived from other gene expression studies or from defined functional categories by the use of "Gene set enrichment analysis" (GSEA) (Subramanian et al. 2005). GSEA compares a gene expression dataset with different collections of gene sets: positional gene sets, curated gene sets, motif gene sets, computational gene sets, and GO gene sets (for detailed explanation see www.broadinstitute.org/gsea/msigdb/index.jsp). The genes of an expression dataset are ranked according to differential expression with the most significantly up-regulated genes at the top and the most significantly down-regulated genes at the bottom. Based on the positions of the genes of the gene sets in the ranked gene expression dataset enrichment towards an end of the ranked list is calculated that indicates concordance of the gene set with the gene expression dataset. User-provided gene sets can also be used for comparison with the expression dataset. GSEA results can be helpful for example in concluding from regulatory mechanisms that are known for a given gene set or from gene sets which belong to defined functional categories or cellular pathways (Figure 3).

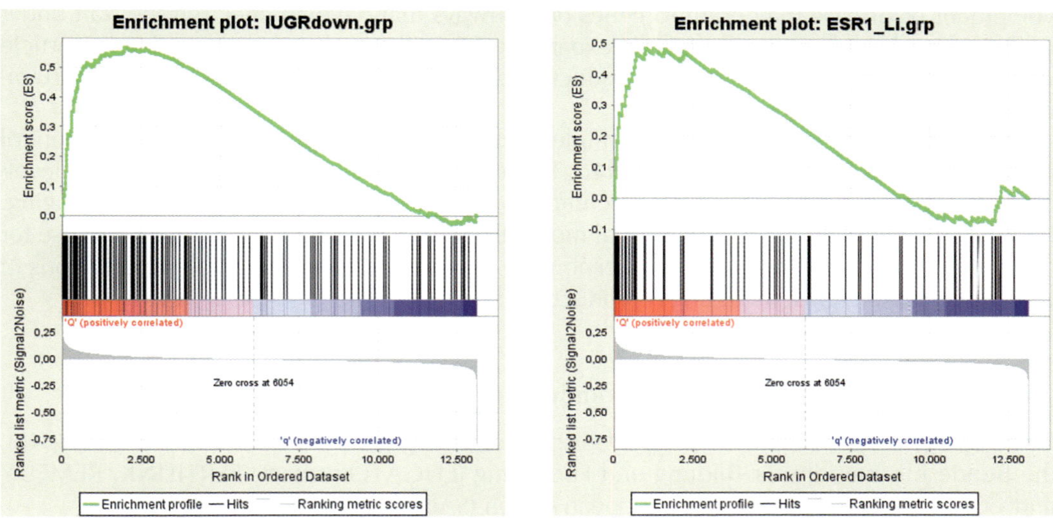

Fig. 3. Gene Set Enrichment Analysis. A set of 161 genes associated with human intrauterine growth retardation was tested for enrichment in a dataset of gene expression linked to the presence of a QTL haplotype for stillbirth risk (due to fetal overgrowth) in cattle (left). The enrichment result confirms that the differentially expressed QTL-associated genes are functionally linked to fetal growth. The same dataset was tested with a set of 67 genes reported to be estrogen-responsive in cattle (right). The enrichment result suggests involvement of estrogen-regulated genes and thus confirms *ESR1* as a functional candidate gene for the stillbirth QTL.

A further strategy to identify regulatory mechanisms underlying the observed gene expression changes is the identification of potential transcription factors by the analysis of regulatory motifs in the promoter regions of the differentially expressed genes, e.g. using oPOSSUM (Ho Sui et al. 2007). Unfortunately, this tool is available only for human, mouse and rat, i.e. the analysis in other species assumes conserved regulatory elements in the corresponding promoter regions.

Nevertheless, a comparative study of human and bovine transcription factor binding sites (TFBS) (Zadissa et al. 2007) encourages the use of human promoter databases for the inference of bovine gene regulation. In our recent study on local and systemic responses of the bovine mammary gland to experimental infection with a pathogenic *Escherichia coli* strain, TFBS analysis suggested NFkB and STAT1 as regulators of genes involved in immune response, inflammation, acute phase response and chemokine/cytokine signaling, which were differentially expressed locally in the infected quarter of the mammary gland (Mitterhuemer et al. 2010).

Finally, the potential interactions of the identified differentially expressed genes or proteins among themselves and with other genes or proteins could be of interest. There are also a number of different databases and tools for interaction analyses, for example STRING, a searchable database for known and predicted protein-protein interactions (Jensen et al. 2009).

Conclusions and perspectives

Holistic and sensitive Omics-technologies characterizing the transcriptome, proteome, metabolome and other molecular characteristics of cells or tissues facilitate the comprehensive description of molecular patterns of tissues that are associated with particular physiological or pathophysiological conditions. Importantly, dynamic changes of these patterns during development or disease may point to genes or pathways that have an effect on the trait under investigation. It is clear that the rapidly expanding scientific databases described in this article will help to dissect mechanisms of reproductive physiology and other important traits of ruminants at the molecular level.

In addition to the development and implementation of Omics-phenotypes, a refinement of physiological readouts is urgently required. Those can be obtained, for example, by the development of non-invasive longitudinal techniques such as remote/indirect sensing or imaging. Integrating large-scale, high-dimensional molecular and physiological data holds promise for defining the molecular networks that respond to genetic and environmental perturbations of physiological functions, including reproduction.

Acknowledgments

Our studies were/are supported by the Deutsche Forschungsgemeinschaft (FOR478, FOR1041), the Bundesministerium für Bildung und Forschung (FUGATO-projects FERTILINK, REMEDY and COMPENDIUM), and by the European Union (SABRE, ERIN, PluriSys).

References

Bauersachs S, Ulbrich SE, Gross K, Schmidt SEM, Meyer HHD, Einspanier R, Wenigerkind H, Vermehren M, Blum H, Sinowatz F & Wolf E 2005 Gene expression profiling of bovine endometrium during the oestrous cycle: detection of molecular pathways involved in functional changes. *Journal of Molecular Endocrinology* **34** 889-908.

Bauersachs S, Ulbrich SE, Gross K, Schmidt SEM, Meyer HHD, Wenigerkind H, Vermehren M, Sinowatz F, Blum H & Wolf E 2006 Embryo-induced transcriptome changes in bovine endometrium reveal species-specific and common molecular markers of uterine receptivity. *Reproduction* **132** 319-331.

Bauersachs S, Ulbrich SE, Zakhartchenko V, Minten M, Reichenbach M, Reichenbach H-D, Blum H, Spencer TE & Wolf E 2009 The endometrium responds differently to cloned versus fertilized embryos. *Proceedings of the National Academy of Sciences of the United States of America* **106** 5681-5686.

Benson DA, Karsch-Mizrachi I, Lipman DJ, Ostell J & Sayers EW 2009 GenBank. *Nucleic Acids Research* **38** D46-51.

Boeckmann B, Bairoch A, Apweiler R, Blatter MC, Estreicher A, Gasteiger E, Martin MJ, Michoud K, O'Donovan C, Phan I, Pilbout S & Schneider M 2003

The SWISS-PROT protein knowledgebase and its supplement TrEMBL in 2003. *Nucleic Acids Research* **31** 365-370.

Dennis G, Jr., Sherman BT, Hosack DA, Yang J, Gao W, Lane HC & Lempicki RA 2003 DAVID: Database for Annotation, Visualization, and Integrated Discovery. *Genome Biology* **4** P3.

Deutsch EW, Lam H & Aebersold R 2008 PeptideAtlas: a resource for target selection for emerging targeted proteomics workflows. *EMBO Reports* **9** 429-434.

Elsik CG, Tellam RL, Worley KC, Gibbs RA, Muzny DM, Weinstock GM, Adelson DL, Eichler EE, Elnitski L, Guigo R, Hamernik DL, Kappes SM, Lewin HA, Lynn DJ, Nicholas FW, Reymond A, Rijnkels M, Skow LC, Zdobnov EM, Schook L, Womack J, Alioto T, Antonarakis SE, Astashyn A, Chapple CE, Chen HC, Chrast J, Camara F, Ermolaeva O, Henrichsen CN, Hlavina W, Kapustin Y, Kiryutin B, Kitts P, Kokocinski F, Landrum M, Maglott D, Pruitt K, Sapojnikov V, Searle SM, Solovyev V, Souvorov A, Ucla C, Wyss C, Anzola JM, Gerlach D, Elhaik E, Graur D, Reese JT, Edgar RC, McEwan JC, Payne GM, Raison JM, Junier T, Kriventseva EV, Eyras E, Plass M, Donthu R, Larkin DM, Reecy J, Yang MQ, Chen L, Cheng Z, Chitko-McKown CG, Liu GE, Matukumalli LK, Song J, Zhu B, Bradley DG, Brinkman FS, Lau LP, Whiteside MD, Walker A, Wheeler TT, Casey T, German JB, Lemay DG, Maqbool NJ, Molenaar AJ, Seo S, Stothard P, Baldwin CL, Baxter R, Brinkmeyer-Langford CL, Brown WC, Childers CP, Connelley T, Ellis SA, Fritz K, Glass EJ, Herzig CT, Iivanainen A, Lahmers KK, Bennett AK, Dickens CM, Gilbert JG, Hagen DE, Salih H, Aerts J, Caetano AR, Dalrymple B, Garcia JF, Gill CA, Hiendleder SG, Memili E, Spurlock D, Williams JL, Alexander L, Brownstein MJ, Guan L, Holt RA, Jones SJ, Marra MA, Moore R, Moore SS, Roberts A, Taniguchi M, Waterman RC, Chacko J, Chandrabose MM, Cree A, Dao MD, Dinh HH, Gabisi RA, Hines S, Hume J, Jhangiani SN, Joshi V, Kovar CL, Lewis LR, Liu YS, Lopez J, Morgan MB, Nguyen NB, Okwuonu GO, Ruiz SJ, Santibanez J, Wright RA, Buhay C, Ding Y, Dugan-Rocha S, Herdandez J, Holder M, Sabo A, Egan A, Goodell J, Wilczek-Boney K, Fowler GR, Hitchens ME, Lozado RJ, Moen C, Steffen D, Warren JT, Zhang J, Chiu R, Schein JE, Durbin KJ, Havlak P, Jiang H, Liu Y, Qin X, Ren Y, Shen Y, Song H, Bell SN, Davis C, Johnson AJ, Lee S, Nazareth LV, Patel BM, Pu LL, Vattathil S, Williams RL, Jr., Curry S, Hamilton C, Sodergren E, Wheeler DA, Barris W, Bennett GL, Eggen A, Green RD, Harhay GP, Hobbs M, Jann O, Keele JW, Kent MP, Lien S, McKay SD, McWilliam S, Ratnakumar A, Schnabel RD, Smith T, Snelling WM, Sonstegard TS, Stone RT, Sugimoto Y, Takasuga A, Taylor JF, Van Tassell CP, Macneil MD, Abatepaulo AR, Abbey CA, Ahola V, Almeida IG, Amadio AF, Anatriello E, Bahadue SM, Biase FH, Boldt CR, Carroll JA, Carvalho WA, Cervelatti EP, Chacko E, Chapin JE, Cheng Y, Choi J, Colley AJ, de Campos TA, De Donato M, Santos IK, de Oliveira CJ, Deobald H, Devinoy E, Donohue KE, Dovc P, Eberlein A, Fitzsimmons CJ, Franzin AM, Garcia GR, Genini S, Gladney CJ, Grant JR, Greaser ML, Green JA, Hadsell DL, Hakimov HA, Halgren R, Harrow JL, Hart EA, Hastings N, Hernandez M, Hu ZL, Ingham A, Iso-Touru T, Jamis C, Jensen K, Kapetis D, Kerr T, Khalil SS, Khatib H, Kolbehdari D, Kumar CG, Kumar D, Leach R, Lee JC, Li C, Logan KM, Malinverni R, Marques E, Martin WF, Martins NF, Maruyama SR, Mazza R, McLean KL, Medrano JF, Moreno BT, More DD, Muntean CT, Nandakumar HP, Nogueira MF, Olsaker I, Pant SD, Panzitta F, Pastor RC, Poli MA, Poslusny N, Rachagani S, Ranganathan S, Razpet A, Riggs PK, Rincon G, Rodriguez-Osorio N, Rodriguez-Zas SL, Romero NE, Rosenwald A, Sando L, Schmutz SM, Shen L, Sherman L, Southey BR, Lutzow YS, Sweedler JV, Tammen I, Telugu BP, Urbanski JM, Utsunomiya YT, Verschoor CP, Waardenberg AJ, Wang Z, Ward R, Weikard R, Welsh TH, Jr., White SN, Wilming LG, Wunderlich KR, Yang J & Zhao FQ 2009 The genome sequence of taurine cattle: a window to ruminant biology and evolution. *Science* **324** 522-528.

Frohlich T & Arnold GJ 2006 Proteome research based on modern liquid chromatography-tandem mass spectrometry: separation, identification and quantification. *Journal of Neural Transmission* **113** 973-994.

Genome KCoS 2009 Genome 10K: a proposal to obtain whole-genome sequence for 10,000 vertebrate species. *Journal of Heredity* **100** 659-674.

Ho Sui SJ, Fulton DL, Arenillas DJ, Kwon AT & Wasserman WW 2007 oPOSSUM: integrated tools for analysis of regulatory motif over-representation. *Nucleic Acids Research* **35** W245-252.

Jensen LJ, Kuhn M, Stark M, Chaffron S, Creevey C, Muller J, Doerks T, Julien P, Roth A, Simonovic M, Bork P & von Mering C 2009 STRING 8--a global view on proteins and their functional interactions in 630 organisms. *Nucleic Acids Research* **37** D412-416.

Klein C, Bauersachs S, Ulbrich SE, Einspanier R, Meyer HHD, Schmidt SEM, Reichenbach H-D, Vermehren M, Sinowatz F, Blum H & Wolf E 2006 Monozygotic twin model reveals novel embryo-induced transcriptome changes of bovine endometrium in the preattachment period. *Biology of Reproduction* **74** 253-264.

Lange V, Picotti P, Domon B & Aebersold R 2008 Selected reaction monitoring for quantitative proteomics: a tutorial. *Molecular Systems Biology* **4** 222.

Lucy MC 2001 Reproductive loss in high-producing dairy cattle: where will it end? *Journal of Dairy Science* **84** 1277-1293.

Mansouri-Attia N, Sandra O, Aubert J, Degrelle S, Everts RE, Giraud-Delville C, Heyman Y, Galio L, Hue I, Yang X, Tian XC, Lewin HA & Renard JP 2009 Endometrium as an early sensor of in vitro embryo manipulation technologies. *Proceedings of the National Academy of Sciences of the United States of America* **106** 5687-5692.

Mitko K, Ulbrich SE, Wenigerkind H, Sinowatz F, Blum H, Wolf E & Bauersachs S 2008 Dynamic changes in messenger RNA profiles of bovine endometrium during the oestrous cycle. *Reproduction* **135** 225-240.

Mitterhuemer S, Petzl W, Krebs S, Mehne D, Klanner A, Wolf E, Zerbe H & Blum H 2010 Escherichia coli infection induces distinct local and systemic transcriptome responses in the mammary gland. *BMC Genomics* **11** 138.

Picotti P, Rinner O, Stallmach R, Dautel F, Farrah T, Domon B, Wenschuh H & Aebersold R 2010 High-throughput generation of selected reaction-monitoring assays for proteins and proteomes. *Nature Methods* **7** 43-46.

Santos JEP, Thatcher WW, Chebel RC, Cerri RLA & Galvao KN 2004 The effect of embryonic death rates in cattle on the efficacy of estrus synchronization programs. *Animal Reproduction Science* **82-83** 513-535.

Schadt EE 2009 Molecular networks as sensors and drivers of common human diseases. *Nature* **461** 218-223.

Subramanian A, Tamayo P, Mootha VK, Mukherjee S, Ebert BL, Gillette MA, Paulovich A, Pomeroy SL, Golub TR, Lander ES & Mesirov JP 2005 Gene set enrichment analysis: a knowledge-based approach for interpreting genome-wide expression profiles. *Proceedings of the National Academy of Sciences of the United States of America* **102** 15545-15550.

Vizcaino JA, Cote R, Reisinger F, Foster JM, Mueller M, Rameseder J, Hermjakob H & Martens L 2009 A guide to the Proteomics Identifications Database proteomics data repository. *Proteomics* **9** 4276-4283.

Wu CH, Apweiler R, Bairoch A, Natale DA, Barker WC, Boeckmann B, Ferro S, Gasteiger E, Huang H, Lopez R, Magrane M, Martin MJ, Mazumder R, O'Donovan C, Redaschi N & Suzek B 2006 The Universal Protein Resource (UniProt): an expanding universe of protein information. *Nucleic Acids Research* **34** D187-191.

Zadissa A, McEwan JC & Brown CM 2007 Inference of transcriptional regulation using gene expression data from the bovine and human genomes. *BMC Genomics* **8** 265.

Developmental programming of the ovine placenta

AL Fowden, JW Ward, FBP Wooding and AJ Forhead

Department of Physiology, Development & Neuroscience, University of Cambridge, Downing Street, Cambridge, CB2 3EG, UK

The pattern of intrauterine growth and size at birth, in particular, programmes the structure and function of tissues later in life in many species, which has important implications for the incidence of adult-onset generative diseases in human populations. In mammals, the main determinant of intrauterine growth is the placental supply of nutrients which, in turn, depends on the size, morphology, transport characteristics and endocrine function of the placenta. However, compared to somatic tissues, little is known about the developmental programming of the placenta. This review examines the epigenetic regulation of placental phenotype with particular emphasis on the nutrient transfer capacity of the ovine placenta and environmental factors shown to cause developmental programming of other tissues. Overall, the placenta is responsive to environmental factors and uses a number of different strategies to adapt its phenotype to help support fetal growth during adverse intrauterine conditions. It is, therefore, not just a passive conduit for nutrient transfer to the fetus but alters its nutrient supply capacity dynamically to optimise fetal nutrient acquisition. Thus, the placental epigenome provides both a memory of environmental conditions experienced during development and an index of the future well being of the offspring.

Introduction

Size at birth is critical in determining life expectancy. In human populations, the smaller the neonate the less likely it is to survive at birth and more likely it is to develop adult onset, life threatening diseases, such as hypertension, coronary heart disease and Type 2 diabetes (Barker, 1994). Similarly, in domesticated species including ruminants, natural and experimental restriction of fetal growth leads to poor neonatal viability and a failure to thrive postnatally (Greenwood & Bell 2003). Low birth weight in these animals is also associated with abnormalities in metabolic, endocrine, reproductive and cardiovascular function in later life (McMillen & Robinson 2005). Together, the epidemiological and experimental observations have led to the concept that conditions experienced *in utero* lead to a specific epigenotype with phenotypic consequences long after birth. The process by which environmental conditions during early life permanently alter tissue structure and function is known as developmental programming.

In mammals, the main determinant of size at birth is the placental supply of nutrients for fetal growth. In turn, this depends on the size, morphology, transport characteristics and

Corresponding author E-mail: alf1000@cam.ac.uk

endocrine function of the placenta (Sibley *et al.* 2005; Fowden *et al.* 2006b). Experimental manipulation of placental growth in sheep and other species leads to altered fetal growth and postnatal physiological abnormalities, consistent with the human epidemiological findings (Fowden *et al.*, 2008). Epigenetic regulation of placental phenotype may, therefore, be an important mechanism by which environmental conditions programme intrauterine development. Indeed, recent human studies have shown that the adverse cardiovascular consequences of low birth weight are related to the shape and size of the placenta at birth (Barker *et al.* 2010). However, compared to somatic tissues (McMillen & Robinson 2005; Gluckman *et al.* 2009), little is known about the programming of the placenta *per se*. This review examines epigenetic regulation of placental phenotype with particular emphasis on the nutrient transfer capacity of the ovine placenta and environmental factors shown experimentally to cause developmental programming of other tissues.

Placental size and morphology

Placental size directly affects the capacity for nutrient transfer via changes in the trophoblast surface area for transport and, when measured as placental weight, is directly related to fetal body weight at term in many species including ruminants (Baur 1977; Mellor 1983). In sheep, direct experimental restriction of placental growth by removal of implantation sites, multiple pregnancy or by embryo transfer between breeds of different sizes reduces fetal weight (Owens *et al.* 1987; Dwyer *et al.* 2005; Reynolds *et al.* 2005). Placental weight and, hence, birth weight is also determined by parity of the ewe (Dwyer *et al.* 2005). In addition, placental weight at term is affected by a wide range of environmental factors, although their specific effects depend on the severity, duration and gestational age at the onset of the perturbation (Table 1).

Both under- and over-nutrition affect placental weight at term (Table 1). Periconceptual undernutrition from 60 days before conception up to implantation at ≈ 30 days of pregnancy appears to have little effect on placental growth but, when the period of undernutrition occurs during the main period of placental growth from 40-75 days, placental weight is often increased at term (Table 1). If the period of nutrient deprivation extends into mid to late gestation, placental weight is generally lower than normal at term but not if undernutrition is confined solely to late gestation (Table 1). In addition, the body condition score of the ewe at conception, an index of pre-pregnancy nutritional state, and genetic adaptation to poor nutritional conditions can alter the placental response to subsequent undernutrition, particularly during mid gestation (Kelly 1992; Osgerby *et al.* 2003; Vonnahme *et al.* 2006). In contrast, over-nutrition for most of gestation leads to placental growth restriction at term (Table 1), especially in growing adolescents (Redmer *et al.* 2004).

Ovine placental weight appears less sensitive to changes in fetal and maternal hormone concentrations. Variations in maternal growth hormone (GH), IGF-1 and insulin levels during mid or late gestation appear to have little effect on the weight of the total placenta or of individual placentomes (DiGiacomo & Hay 1989; Harding *et al.* 1997; Wallace *et al.* 2006; Wright *et al.* 2008). Similarly, manipulating fetal hormone concentrations by exogenous infusion or endocrine gland ablation has shown that fetal pituitary, thyroid and adrenal hormones have little effect on total placental weight at term, although they influence fetal growth (see Fowden & Forhead, 2009). Placental weight near term is also unaffected by fetal administration of leptin and IGF-1 for 5-10 days during late gestation (Bloomfield *et al.* 2002; Forhead *et al.* 2008). However, maternal administration of natural or synthetic glucocorticoids during late gestation reduces placental weight in association with fetal growth restriction (Jensen *et al.* 2002; Braun *et al.* 2007). Since glucocorticoid concentrations are altered by conditions, such as hyperthermia, undernutrition and hypoxaemia (see Fowden & Forhead 2009), these hormones may mediate, in part, the effects of environmental stimuli on the placenta. Indeed, in natural conditions, the placental effects of many of these environmental factors are likely to be multi-factorial as conditions such hypoxaemia and hyperthermia reduce food intake in pregnant ewes (Alexander & Williams 1977; Jacobs *et al.* 1988; Regnault *et al.* 2005).

Even during adverse conditions, fetal weight is still directly related to placental weight (Wallace *et al.* 2005; Quigley *et al.* 2008). However, often, the effects of these conditions are more pronounced on the placenta than fetus (Table 1). When placental growth is restricted, placental efficiency increases as more grams of fetus are produced per gram of placenta than in normal conditions (see Fowden *et al* 2009). Greater placental efficiency is also seen with maternal glucocorticoid treatment, multiple pregnancy and increasing parity of the ewe (Jensen *et al.* 2002; Dwyer *et al.* 2005). Hardier breeds of sheep also tend to have higher placental efficiencies than breeds evolutionarily adapted to better nutritional conditions (Dwyer *et al.*, 2005). These observations suggest that the placenta can adapt to the fetal nutrient demands for growth and help maintain normal fetal growth when its own growth is compromised. These adaptations may have a morphological or functional origin.

Ovine placentomes can be classified into 4 types, A to D, using their gross morphological appearance (Vatnick *et al.* 1991). The smaller, rounder A and B type placentomes predominate throughout gestation and, on average, account for about 60% or more of the total number under normal conditions. The larger, flatter C and D type placentomes are less common but increase in frequency during late gestation, although their numbers appear to decrease again close to term (see Fowden *et al.* 2006b). In general, adverse environmental conditions during the period of maximal placental growth lead to a shift from A-type placentomes to the more everted types later in gestation (Table 1). While this shift is often associated with placental growth restriction, changes in placentome frequency distribution have been observed without any change in total placental weight in response to both environmental and hormonal stimuli (Penninga & Longo 1998; Bloomfield *et al.* 2002). This has lead to the suggestion that the presence of more C and D-type placentomes is an adaptation to increase placental efficiency and the transfer of nutrients to the fetus (Heasman *et al.* 1998; Steyn *et al.* 2001; Vonnahme *et al.* 2006). Certainly, in carunclectomized ewes with small placentas composed solely of large D-type placentomes, the rate of glucose transfer to the fetus per gram of placenta is enhanced relative to controls (Owens *et al.* 1987; 1989). However, in normal conditions during late gestation, there is little, if any, evidence for changes in placental weight, efficiency or glucose transfer with the frequency of C/D type placentomes (Figure 1A-C).

In late gestation, adverse conditions either have little effect on placentome distribution or reduce the incidence of C/D placentome types (Table 1). This may be the consequence of elevated cortisol concentrations as both maternal and fetal glucocorticoid treatment in late gestation increases the frequency of A/B type placentomes (Jensen *et al.* 2002; 2005; Ward *et al.* 2006). By tagging individual placentomes before fetal treatment, cortisol was shown to decrease, or even reverse, the normal rate of placentome eversion with increasing gestational age, consistent with the prepartum decline in C/D placentome frequency seen during the natural fetal cortisol surge (Ward *et al.* 2006; Fowden *et al.* 2006b). Since placental glucose delivery to cortisol infused fetuses per gram of placenta is higher in animals with proportionately more A/B type placentomes (Figure 1D), the cortisol-induced slowing of the progressive ontogenic shift towards more everted placentomes may be an adaptive response to help maintain the fetal nutrient supply during late gestation (Ward *et al.* 2006). Thus, the gross morphology of the ovine placenta may be functionally significant in nutrient transport when cortisol concentrations are high.

Table 1. Effects of environmental cues during pregnancy on feto-placental growth and placental morphology in sheep near term (>130 days).

		% Control Weight			
Treatment	Period of Treatment	Placenta	Fetus	Morphological Changes	Reference
Nutrition					
Overnutrition	-89-133	87%	100%	Less C/D type placetomes	Quigley et al. 2008
	0-128	49%	63%	Reduced mean placetome weight Decreased capillary surface density	Wallace et al. 2000 Redmer et al. 2004
Hyperglycaemia	115-135	86%	98%		Aldoretta et al. 1994
Undernutrition	-89-133	73%	82%	More C/D type placetomes	Quigley et al. 2008
	-60 -30	97%	107-93%	More D type placetomes	Oliver et al. 2005; Rumball et al. 2008
	-14-70	120%	97%	Less A more D placentomes	Steyn et al. 2001
	0-90 0-130	98% 93%	90% 83%	Normal placetomes distribution Reduced caruncle capillary area density	Luther et al. 2007
	28-80	160-120%	107-100%	Less A more B type placentomes Smaller placetomes across all types Increased fetal compared to placetome	Heasman et al. 1998 Dandrea et al. 2001 Gnanalingham et al. 2007
	30-96	130%	100%		McCrabb at al. 1991
	22-135	81%	88%	Less B more C&D placetomes	McMullen et al. 2004; Osgerby et al. 2002
	50-145	77%	67%	Less fetal tissue in placetomes	Alexander & Williams 1971
	91-135	100%	100%		McMullen et al. 2004
	115-144	100%	100%		Edwards & McMillen 2001
Hypoglycaemia	70-135	68%	71%		Carver & Hay 1995
	100-135	69%	72%		Aldoretta et al. 1994
	115-135	100%	100%		DiGiacomo & Hay 1989

Table 1. Contd.

Restrict placental blood flow					
Uterine	115-138	73-66%	85-68%		Lang et al. 2000
Cord constriction	125-128	80%	100%	Less D type placetomes	Gardner et al. 2002
Embolization	125-135	78%	87%		Gangon et al. 1996
Hypoxia					
High Altitude	0 –110	100%	100%	Less A more B ,C, & D placetomes	Penninga & Longo 1998;
	30- term	108%	71%	Increased capillary area	Parraquez et al. 2006
	49 -140	100%	100%	Increased vascular area Decreased number of vessels Increased coiling	Krebs et al. 1997
Hypoxic chamber	30-135	77%	79%		Jacobs et al. 1988
	120-141	89%	83%		
Hyperthermia	40 -120	49%	58%	Increased number of fetal vessels Decreased number of maternal vessels Increased coiling of fetal vessels	Regnault et al. 2002; 2003
	50-100	68%	76%		Alexander & Williams 1971
	50-145	31%	49%		
	64-138	42%	73%	Decreased protein content	Early et al. 1991
	100-145	59%	71%		Alexander & Williams 1971
Glucocorticoid Treatment					
Mother	104, 111, 118	100%	87%	Fewer BNC	Braun et al. 2007
	115 -125	100%	110%	More B type placetomes	Jensen et al. 2005
	118 -128	75%	93%	Less A type placetomes	Jensen et al. 2002
Fetus	125 -130	100%	100%	More A and less D type placetomes Lower BNC numbers	Ward et al. 2002; 2006

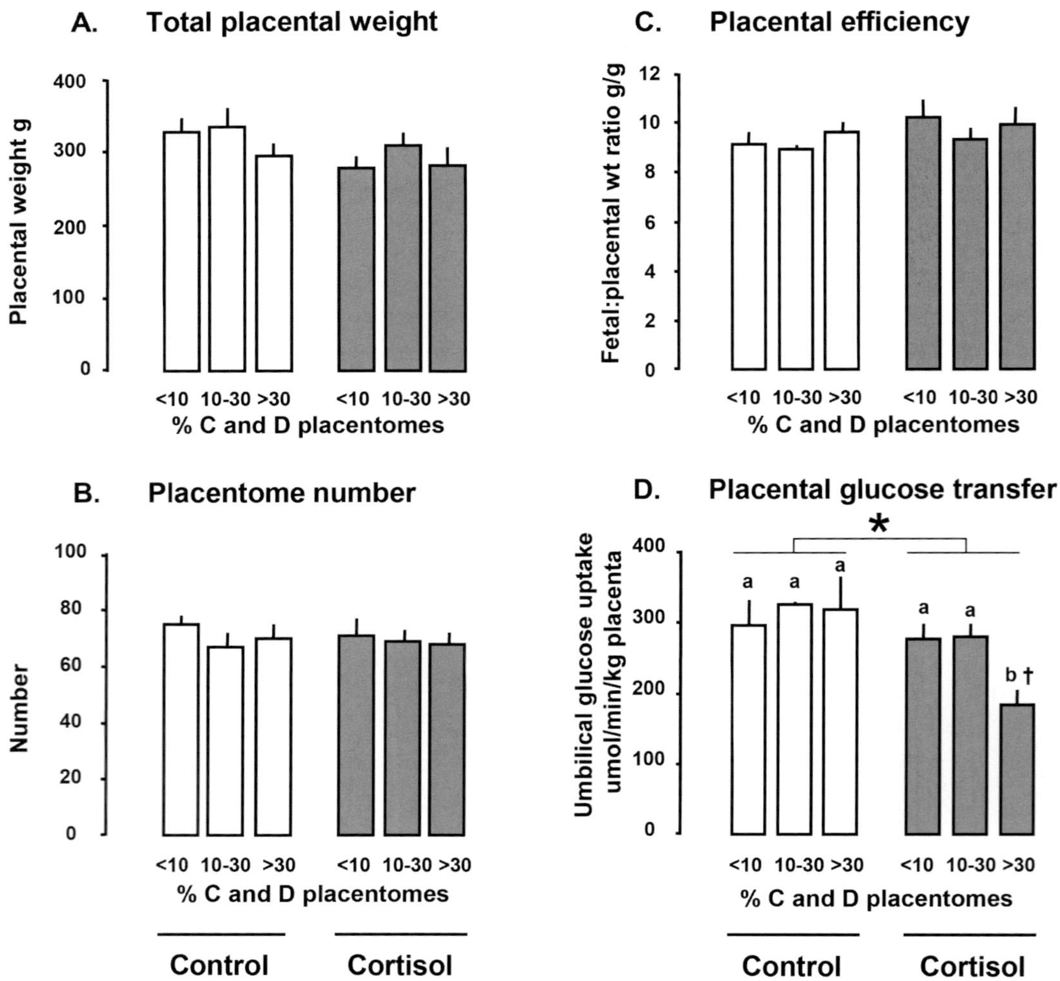

Fig. 1. Mean (±SE) values of A) total placental weight, B) placentome number, C) placental efficiency measured as gram fetus per gram placenta and D) placental glucose transfer calculated as umbilical uptake per gram placenta at the prevailing glucose concentration gradient in single sheep fetuses either infused with cortisol (1-2mg/kg fetus/day, shaded columns) or in the control state (saline infused or untreated, open columns) before delivery at 127-131 days with respect to the frequency distribution of more everted C and D type placentomes expressed as a percentage of the total placentome number (<10%, 10-30%, >30%). * significant effect of treatment $P<0.02$ two-way ANOVA. In D) within treatments, columns with different letters as superscripts are significantly different from each other $P<0.05$ (two-way ANOVA). † significantly different from respective saline infused placentome type ($P<0.05$, t-test). Number of fetuses in A), B) and C) are Controls; <10% n = 18, 10-30%, n = 8; >30%, n= 11: Cortisol; <10% n = 7, 10-30% n = 11, >30% n = 6. In D) numbers are Controls; <10% n = 6, 10-30% n = 3, >30% n =5: Cortisol; 10% n = 5, 10-30% n = 4, >30% n = 6. Data from Gardner *et al.* 2002; Ward 2002; Ward *et al.* 2002; 2006 and Fowden, Forhead and Wooding, unpublished observations).

Much less is known about environmental influences on ovine placental ultra-structure. Glucocorticoid administration to either the ewe or fetus in late gestation prematurely decreases the number of binucleate cells (BNC) in the fetal trophectoderm (Ward *et al.* 2002; Braun *et al.* 2007), consistent with the prepartum decline in BNC numbers as fetal cortisol levels rise towards term (Wooding & Burton 2008). These cells produce placental lactogen (PL) and migrate across the maternal-fetal interface throughout pregnancy to form a syncytium by fusion with the maternal epithelium. They are, therefore, involved in placental remodelling and maternal PL delivery, both of which may influence placental efficiency (Fowden *et al.* 2009). Reduced PL concentrations have been observed in hyperthermic and overnourished ewes, although these changes probably reflect the reduced placental mass rather than decreased BNC numbers or PL content per cell (Regnault *et al.* 2005; Lea *et al.* 2007). In contrast, periconceptional undernutrition leads to raised maternal and fetal PL levels in late gestation despite normal placental weight, which suggests that BNCs can be regulated nutritionally (Oliver *et al.* 2005).

Between 50 days and term, the surface area for nutrient exchange increases in the ovine placenta along with increases in the number and/or area of the capillaries in the caruncular (maternal) and cotyledonary (fetal) portions of the placentomes (Stegmann 1975; Reynolds *et al.* 2005). The cotyledonary increments are greater due to branching angiogenesis and an increase in capillary density (Reynolds *et al.* 2010). In part, the vascular changes are driven by the fetal nutrient demands as between breed embryo transfer has shown that constraining fetal growth below its genetic potential increases placental vascularity in several species including sheep (Biensen *et al.* 1999; Allen *et al.* 2002; Reynolds *et al.* 2005). Placental vascularity also changes in response to environmental stressors (Table 1) and with gross placentome type, although not consistently across the A to D spectrum (Vonnahme *et al.* 2008). Consequently, increasing placental vascularity may explain, in part, the increased efficiency of the small placenta but does not provide a functional rationale for the shift towards more everted placentome types after adverse conditions early in development.

Both increases and decreases in the number, area and density of the placental capillaries have been observed during poor intrauterine conditions with differential responses in the cotyledonary and caruncular vasculature in some instances (Krebs *et al.* 1997; Regnault *et al.* 2002; Luther *et al.* 2007; Redmer *et al.* 2009). At high altitude, placental capillaries become more branched and looped, and their average luminal area increases in both the cotyledonary and caruncular regions (Krebs *et al.* 1997). Similar increases in vessel tortuosity have been observed in placentomes from hyperthermic ewes, in association with an increase in cotyledonary capillary number (Regnault *et al.* 2002). In addition, both over- and under-nutrition during the period of maximal placental growth affects angiogenesis with regional alterations in capillary area and/or number density, which become less pronounced with increasing gestational age (Redmer *et al.* 2004; Luther *et al.* 2007; Zhu *et al.* 2009). In many of these conditions, the changes in placental vascularity are accompanied by alterations in placental expression of various angiogenic factors (Reynolds *et al.* 2005). These include the vascular endothelial growth factor (VEGF), angiopoietin and fibroblast growth factor protein families as well as their respective receptors, all of which have several isoforms (Reynolds *et al.* 2010). By altering blood flow and surface area for exchange, these environmentally-induced changes in placental vascularity and morphology will modify nutrient transfer, particularly of lipophilic molecules, like oxygen, which cross the placenta by simple diffusion. However, to date, little is known about the epigenetic regulation of the thickness and morphology of the interhemal membrane also important in determining the passive diffusional characteristics of the placenta.

Placental transport characteristics

For facilitated diffusion and active transport, placental nutrient transport capacity depends not only on trophoblast surface area but also on expression of nutrient transporters per unit area. Transplacental diffusion of nutrients into the fetal circulation is also determined by the transplacental concentration gradient and the rate of nutrient utilisation by the utero-placental tissues themselves (Hay 2006; Fowden *et al.* 2009). All of these factors change with gestational age and during adverse intrauterine conditions (Regnault *et al.* 2005; Fowden *et al.* 2008). For example, between mid and late gestation, there are increases in the placental abundance of glucose transporter-3 (GLUT3), the transplacental glucose concentration gradient and in the relative proportion of uterine glucose uptake transfered to the sheep fetus (Fowden 1997; Hay 2006). Since some of the glucose carbon used *in utero* is passed onto the fetus as lactate (Hay 2006), changes in placental lactate production towards term and during adverse conditions will also influence the apparent glucose transfer capacity of the ovine placenta (Fowden 1997).

In late gestation, transplacental glucose transfer is altered by a range of nutritional and other perturbations, although the extent to which these changes are due to genuine alterations in the placental glucose transport capacity appears to depend on the specific insult (Table 2). For instance, the small placenta of hyperthermic ewes transports more glucose per kg placenta than controls, primarily as a result of an increased transplacental glucose concentration gradient caused by fetal hypoglycaemia (Table 2). At the normal glucose concentration gradient, the capacity for glucose transport per kg of hyperthermic placenta is actually 20-30% lower than control due to reduced placental expression of the glucose transporters (GLUT), GLUT1 and GLUT8 (Thureen *et al.* 1992, Regnault *et al.* 2003: Limesand *et al.* 2005). Conversely, the weight specific glucose transfer capacity is increased in the small placenta of carunclectomised ewes (Table 2). Similarly, 25-50% increases in placental glucose transfer capacity have been observed with prolonged maternal hypoglycaemia or restricted dietary intake when the reduced transplacental concentration gradient is taken into account (Table 2). These changes in glucose transport are accompanied by altered patterns of placental GLUT1 and GLUT3 expression, which are isoform specific and temporally distinct depending on the insult (Das *et al.* 1998; 2000; Bell *et al.* 1999; Dandrea *et al.* 2001). In contrast, when placental growth is restricted by over-nutrition of young animals, there is no change in glucose transport capacity or GLUT expression per gram placenta, despite the reductions in placental and fetal mass (Wallace *et al*, 2005). Fetal glucocorticoid over-exposure also has no effect on the weight specific capacity for placental glucose transport or on placental GLUT1 and GLUT3 expression, although umbilical glucose uptake per gram placenta is reduced as a result of increased uteroplacental glucose consumption (Table 2). The ovine feto-placental unit, therefore, adopts different strategies to help maintain a fetal glucose supply during adverse conditions depending on the specific insult. This may relate, in part, to the degree of placental growth restriction and/or to the maternal and fetal endocrine mileux.

Compared to the GLUTs, less is known about the regulation of amino acid transporters in the ovine placenta during adverse conditions. There are at least nine different amino acid transporter systems with distinct functional characteristics yet overlapping specificities that function to actively accumulate amino acids in the placenta and, then, facilitate their passive transfer into the fetal circulation (Regnault *et al.* 2005). Transplacental amino acid flux varies with the specific amino acid and the maternal concentration. It is also affected by catabolism and transamination of amino acids within the placenta itself (Regnault *et al.* 2005). In sheep, changes in the transplacental amino acid transport have been observed in response to hyperthermia, undernutrition and maternal administration of GH, IGF-I and glucocorticoids (Liechty *et al.* 1991; Liu *et al.* 1994; Ross *et al.* 1996; Harding *et al.* 1997; Timmerman *et al.* 2000). In

Table 2. Effects of environmental conditions on the characteristics of transplacental glucose transport in sheep fetuses near term (>130 days) expressed as percentage change from control values. (↑ = increase. ↓= decrease.)

Treatment	Glucose transport per kg placenta†	Transplacental glucose gradient	Uteroplacental glucose consumption per kg placenta	Glucose transport capacity per kg placenta‡	Glucose transporters	References
Nutrition						
Overnutrition	No Δ	No Δ	No Δ	No Δ	No ΔGLUT 1 & 3	Wallace et al.2002;2004
Hyperglycaemia	No Δ - ↑10%	↑ 55%	↑ 120%	?	↓GLUT1 & 3	Aldoretta et al. 1994 Das et al. 1998; 2000
Undernutrition	↓ 60%	↓ 40%	↓ 43%	↑ 50%	↑GLUT1 & 3	Leury et al. 1990 Bell et al. 1999 Dandrea et al. 1998
Hypoglycaemia	↓ 45-80%	↓ 48%	↓ 16-30%	No Δ to ↑25%	↓GLUT1 No Δ GLUT3	Aldoretta et al. 1994 Carver & Hay 1995 Das et al. 1998; 2000
Hyperthermia	↑ 25%	↑ 10%-15%	No Δ	↓ 20-30%	↓GLUT1 & 8	Thureen et al. 1992 Wallace et al. 2005 Limesand et al. 2004
Glucocorticoid treatment	↓ 20%	No Δ	↑ 70%	No Δ	No Δ GLUT1 & 3	Ward, 2002 Ward et al. 2004
Placental growth restriction††	↑ 37%	↑ 37%	No Δ	↑ 55%	?	Owens et al. 1987; 1989

† = measured as umbilical glucose uptake per kg placenta at the prevailing transplacental glucose concentration gradient. ‡ = measured either as clearance of non-metabolisable glucose analogue or as umbilical uptake per kg placenta at the normal glucose concentration gradient. †† = ewes carunclectomised before pregnancy. ? = unknown. Δ = change.

particular, there are reductions in the placental delivery of leucine, threonine, glutamate and alanine to the fetus. There are also changes in uteroplacental handling and inter-organ shuttling of essential and gluconeogenic amino acids in response to heat stress and undernutition (Liechty *et al.* 1991; Ross *et al.* 1996; Timmerman *et al.* 2000). In rodents, environmental stimuli, such as undernutrition and dietary composition, alter placental expression of the accumulative System A amino acid transporters (Jansson *et al.* 2006; Jones *et al.* 2009; Coan *et al.* 2010) but little is known about the epigenetic regulation of amino acid transporters in ovine placenta.

Placental endocrine function

The placenta produces a number of hormones including steroids, peptides, cytokines, glycoproteins and eicosanoids, which are released into both the fetal and maternal circulation (see Fowden *et al.* 2008; Fowden & Forhead 2009). Some of these hormones, such as progesterone, placental lactogen, the cytokines and placental variants of GH and prolactin have metabolic actions in the mother that favour nutrient delivery to the fetus (Gootwine 2004). In sheep, maternal concentrations of placentally derived hormones, such as progesterone and placental lactogen, are lower than normal during adverse conditions, such as hyperthermia, overfeeding, undernutrition and glucocorticoid overexposure (Regnault *et al.* 2002; Wallace *et al.* 2004; 2005; Braun *et al.* 2007). This is due, in part, to the reduced placental mass but may also reflect cyto-architectural changes in the placenta caused, for instance, by altered BNC dynamics (Table 1). Receptors for these hormones are present in the ovine placenta and binding of ligands, such as IGF-I, to their receptors has been shown to alter placental clearance of non-metabolisable glucose and amino acid analogues *in vivo* (Harding *et al.* 1994; Gootwine 2004).

Other placental hormones, such as the prostaglandins (PG)E_2 and $F_{2\alpha,}$ also affect the fetal supply of nutrients and oxygen but more indirectly by actions on fetal endocrine function, regional blood flow and myometrial contractility (see Fowden & Forhead 2009). In sheep, undernutrition during late gestation increases uteroplacental activity of PGH synthase and the production of $PGF_{2\alpha}$ and PGE_2 (Whittle *et al.* 2001). These increments in PG synthesis are directly related to the degree of maternal hypoglycaemia and the fall in uteroplacental glucose consumption and can be reversed by restoring normoglycaemia by re-feeding or glucose infusion into the fasted animal (Fowden *et al.* 1994). The ovine placenta has also been shown to contain PG dehydrogenase (PGDH), an enzyme which converts biologically active PGs into their inactive keto metabolites (Whittle *et al.* 2001). Uteroplacental output of these metabolites rises towards term and in response to undernutrition during late gestation (Fowden *et al.* 1994). In part, the nutritionally induced changes in PG production and metabolism may be due to the concomitant rise in glucocorticoid concentrations as cortisol has been shown to increase production of $PGF_{2\alpha}$ and PGE_2 by enhancing PGH synthase activity and decreasing PGDH activity in ovine placenta (Whittle *et al.* 2001). Sensitivity of placental PGDH and PGH synthase to nutritional and endocrine stimuli increases with increasing gestational age in parallel with the rise in fetal cortisol concentrations and the onset of myometrial contractile activity towards term (Fowden *et al.* 1994).

The ovine placenta also inactivates a range of hormones, including glucocorticoids, catecholamines, IGFs, thyroxine (T_4) and tri-iodothyronine (T_3), which limits their effectiveness in the fetus (Fowden & Forhead 2004). For example, placental type III deiodinase converts T_4 to biologically inactive reverse-T_3 and maintains a high fetal clearance rate of T_3, the most biologically active thyroid hormone (Forhead *et al.*, 2006). Similarly, the placental enzyme, 11ß-hydroxysteroid dehydrogenase type 2 (11ßHSD2), converts active glucocorticoids to their inactive metabolites, which reduces placental and fetal exposure to the higher cortisol concentrations found in the maternal circulation (Seckl 2004). Its placental activity is down regulated by undernutrition and both maternal and fetal administration of glucocorticoids in sheep (Whorwood *et al.* 2001; Clarke *et al.* 2002; Kerzner *et al.* 2002; McMullen *et al.* 2004; Gnanalingham *et al.* 2007). In turn, by altering placental cortisol bioavailability, these environmentally-induced changes in 11ßHSD2 activity influence placental production and metabolism of other glucocorticoid sensitive hormones, such as the PGs, progesterone, oestrogens, placental lactogen and active thyroid hormones (see Fowden & Forhead 2004; 2009). Furthermore, there are changes in the placental abundance of glucocorticoid and other hormone receptors in response to maternal undernutrition, which will affect hormone bioavailability within the placental tissues (Whorwood *et al.* 2001; Gnalingham *et al.* 2007; Yiallourides *et al.* 2009). Epigenetic changes in placental hormone production may, therefore, alter placental delivery of nutrients to the fetus either by paracrine actions on placental transport characteristics or by endocrine actions on maternal metabolism that alter nutrient allocation between the maternal and uteroplacental tissues (Fowden *et al.* 2006b). These programmed endocrine changes may also determine the length of gestation and the development of maternal tissues, such as the mammary glands, with implications for nutrition and growth after birth.

Molecular mechanisms of placental programming

Compared to the mouse placenta (Fowden *et al.* 2006a), relatively little is known about the molecular mechanisms by which environmental factors alter the morphological and functional development of the ovine placenta. Using microarrays, recent studies have shown that hypoxia and dietary protein deprivation alter expression of over 200 genes in the mouse placenta with specific up-regulation of genes involved in apoptosis and inhibition of cell growth (Gheorghe *et al.* 2010). Gene deletion studies have demonstrated that imprinted genes, which are expressed monoallelically in a parent-of-origin manner, have a disproportionately important role in placental development (Reik *et al.* 2003; Fowden *et al.* 2006b). In particular, the imprinted *Igf2-H19* gene locus has been shown to affect both trophoblast morphology and nutrient transfer (Reik *et al.* 2003; Coan *et al.* 2008b). Deletion of the placental specific P0 transcript of the *Igf2* gene causes placental growth retardation but increases placental efficiency in association with up-regulation of placental glucose and amino acid transfer and of placental expression of *Slc2a3*/GLUT3 and *Slc38a4*, an isoform of the System A amino acid transporters (Constancia *et al.* 2002; 2005). During late gestation, expression of this *Igf2P0* transcript is altered in conjunction with changes in nutrient transfer by maternal dietary manipulations and when placental growth is restricted naturally (Coan *et al.* 2008a&b; 2010). Collectively, these studies suggest that placental *Igf2* has a major role as an environmental sensor and adapts placental phenotype to help support fetal growth in mice.

Both IGF-II and IGF-I are expressed in ruminant placenta, particularly early in gestation, as is the primary IGF receptor, IGF1R (Wooding & Burton 2008). In ovine placentomes, expression of the IGFs, IGF1R and their binding proteins is altered in a regional and temporally specific manner by environmental factors including hyperthermia, maternal GH administration, overnutrition and both acute and chronic under-nutrition at various stages of pregnancy (Osgerby *et al.* 2004; McMullen *et al.* 2005; de Vrijer *et al.* 2006; Gnanalingham *et al.* 2007; Wright *et al.* 2008; Yiallourides *et al.* 2009). Indeed, the smaller the placenta the higher the IGF-II abundance in moderately nourished ewes (Osgerby *et al.* 2003), which suggests that placental IGF-II may act to enhance growth of the compromised placenta, as occurs in mice (Coan *et al.* 2008b). In addition, both under and over-nutrition alter the intracellular signalling pathways downstream of IGF1R in ovine placentas (Zhu *et al.* 2007; 2009), which has implications for placental protein synthesis, cell proliferation and expression of nutrient transporters, independently of IGF concentrations (Jansson & Powell 2007).

At the chromatin level, epigenetic regulation of gene expression can occur by changes in DNA methylation, histone modifications and/or siRNA abundance (Gluckman *et al.* 2009). In somatic tissues, changes in DNA methylation and histone modifications have been observed in the promoters of key metabolic genes in the adult offspring of rats malnourished or glucocorticoid treated during pregnancy, which parallel alterations in gene expression and enzyme activity (see Burdge *et al.* 2007). Changes in hepatic DNA methylation have also been observed in rat and sheep fetuses of mothers fed methyl deficient diets (Rees *et al.* 2000; Sinclair *et al.* 2007). In part, this may be due to reduced hepatic activity of DNA methytranferase responsible for maintaining DNA methylation during cell replication (Lillycrop *et al.* 2007). Even less is known about these processes in the placenta. When histone H3 trimethylation is prevented in mice by deletion of a specific histone methytransferase, vascular development of the definitive hemochorial placenta is impaired as embryonic blood vessels fail to invade the labyrinthine layer, resulting in embryonic lethality at 11.5 days (Hu *et al.* 2010). Similarly, inhibition of DNA methylation by 5-azacytidine administration to pregnant rats, leads to a small placenta at term with impaired development of the labyrinthine trophoblast (Šerman *et al.* 2007). Hypomethylation and biallelic expression of the *H19* gene locus is also seen in the overgrown placenta of cloned cattle (Curchoe *et al.* 2009). In addition, hypomethylation of the imprinting control region of the *IGF2/H19* domain, or of the domain itself, has been observed in placentas of growth restricted human infants in some but not all studies (Tabano *et al.* 2010; Bourque *et al*, 2010). Genes involved in DNA methylation and histone modifications are down-regulated in mouse placenta after maternal hypoxia and protein deprivation during the second half of pregnancy but whether this alters the methylation status of any of the other affected placental genes remains unknown (Gheorghe *et al.* 2010). Maternal undernutrition was not associated with altered methylation of the promoter regions of the *Igf2* or *Slc38a4* genes in the mouse placenta, despite changes in their expression in late gestation (Coan *et al.* 2010).

Conclusions

Environmental factors have an important role in programming the placental phenotype (Figure 2). They may act, directly, on placental development or, indirectly, through changes in the maternal endocrine environment (Figure 2). Together, they programme the nutrient transfer capacity of the placenta by altering its size and morphology, its transport characteristics and its endocrine function. In turn, these placental adaptations affect the fetal endocrine environment and the absolute and relative quantities of nutrients supplied to the fetus with consequences for intrauterine development and offspring phenotype (Figure 2). They also alter maternal adaptation to pregnancy and the allocation of maternal resources to feto-placental development. The memory of early environmental events can, therefore, be transmitted to the fetus long after the original insult through the placental epigenome. Thus, the placenta is not just a passive conduit for nutrients but adapts its nutrient transfer capacity dynamically during environmental challenges to optimise fetal acquisition of nutrients for growth given the prevailing nutrient availability.

Acknowledgements

We would like to thank all the members of the Department of Physiology, Development and Neuroscience who have helped with these studies over the years. We are also indebted to the

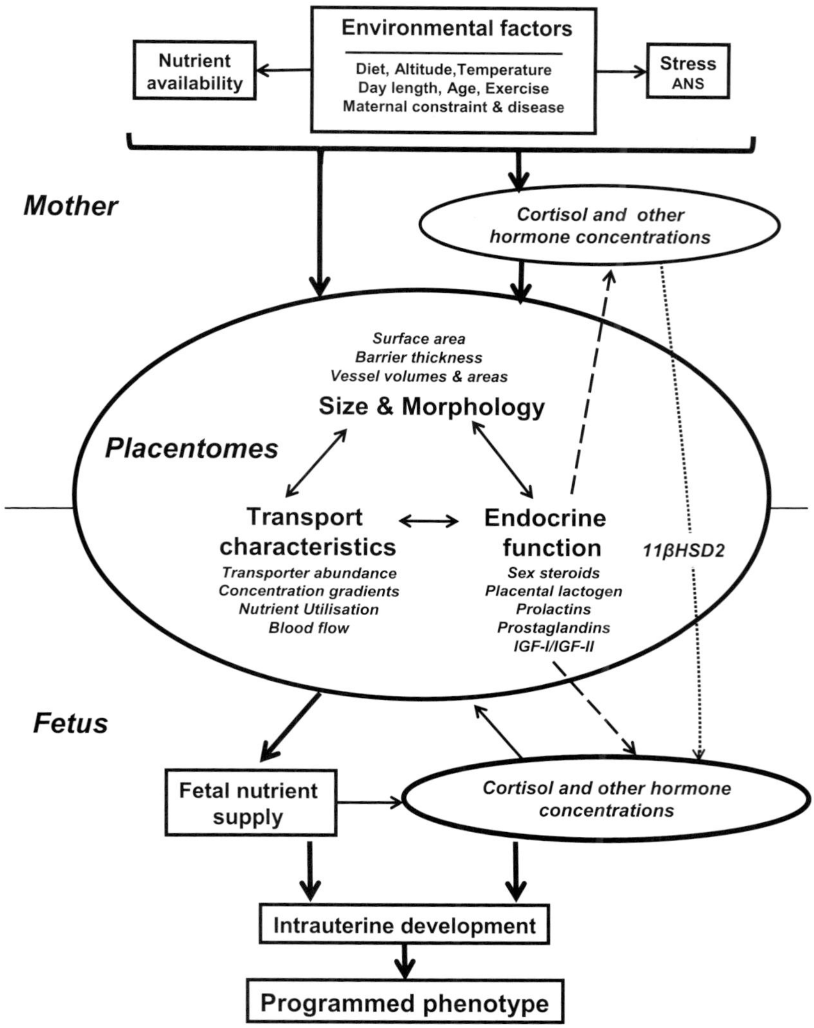

Fig. 2. Schematic diagram showing the role of environmental factors in controlling placental phenotype and the consequences of these regulatory actions for intrauterine development and developmental programming of the offspring. ANS, Autonomic Nervous System. 11ßHSD2, 11ß-hydroxysteroid dehydrogenase type 2. IGFI/IGFII, Insulin-like growth factors I and II.

BBSRC, the Royal Society, the Wellcome Trust and the Centre for Trophoblast Research for their funding of the research.

References

Aldoretta PW, Carver TD & Hay WW 1994 Ovine utero-placental glucose and oxygen metabolism in relation to chronic changes in maternal and fetal glucose concentrations. *Placenta* **15** 753-764.

Alexander G & Williams D 1971 Heat stress and development of the conceptus in domestic sheep. *J Agric Sci* **76** 53-72.

Allen WR, Wilsher S, Turnbull C, Stewart F, Ousey J, Rossdale PD & Fowden AL 2002 Influence of maternal size on placental, fetal and postnatal growth in the horse: I Development in utero. *Reproduction* **123**, 454-465.

Barker DJP 1994 Mothers, Babies and Disease. BMJ Publishing Group, London.

Barker DJP, Thornburg KL, Osmond C, Kajantie E & Eriksson JG 2010 The surface area of the placenta and hypertension in the offspring in later life. *Int J Dev Biol* **54** 525-530.

Baur R 1977 Morphometry of the placental exchange area. *Adv Anat Emb Cell Bio* **5**, 1-63.

Bell AW, Hay WW & Ehrhardt RA 1999 Placental transport of nutrients and its implications for fetal growth. *J Reprod Fert Suppl* **54**, 401-410.

Biensen NJ, Wilson ME, Ford SP 1999 The impacts of uterine environment and fetal genotype as conceptus size and placental vascularity during late gestation in pigs. *J Anim Sci* **77**, 954-959.

Bloomfield FH, van Zijl PL, Bauer MK & Harding JE 2002 A chronic low dose infusion of insulin-like growth factor I alters placental function but does not affect fetal growth. *Reprod Fert Dev* **14** 393-400.

Bourgue DK, Avila L, Peñaherrera M, von Dadelszen P, Robinson WP 2010 Decreased placental methylation at the *H19/IGF2* imprinting control region is associated with normotensive intrauterine growth restriction but not preeclampsia. *Placenta* **31** 197-202.

Braun T, Li S, Moss TJM, Newnham JP, Challis JRG, Gluckman PD & Sloboda DM 2007. Maternal betamethasone administration reduces binucleate cell number and placental lactogen in sheep. *J Endocrinol* **194** 337-347.

Burdge GC Hanson MA, Slater-Jefferies JL & Lillycrop KA 2007 Epigenetic regulation of transcription: a mechanism for inducing variations in phenotype (fetal programming) by differences in nutrition during early life? Brit J Nutr 97 1036-1046.

Carver TD & Hay WW 1995 Uteroplacental carbon substrate metabolism and oxygen consumption after long term hypoglycaemia in pregnant sheep. *Am J Physiol* **269**, E299-E308.

Clarke K, Ward JW, Forhead AJ, Giussani DA & Fowden AL 2002 Regulation of 11□-hydroxysteroid dehydrogenase type 2 activity in ovine placenta by fetal cortisol. *J Endocrinol* **172**, 527-534.

Coan PM, Angiolini E, Sandovici I, Burton GJ, Constancia M & Fowden AL 2008a Adaptations in placental nutrient transfer capacity to meet fetal growth demands depend on placental size in mice. *J. Physiol.* **586** 4567-4576.

Coan PM, Fowden AL, Constancia, M, Ferguson-Smith AC, Burton GJ & Sibley CP 2008b Disproportionate effects of *Igf2* gene knockout on placental morphology and diffusional exchange characteristics in the mouse. *J. Physiol.* 586 5023-5032.

Coan PM, Vaughan OR, Sekita Y, Finn SL, Burton GJ, Constancia M & Fowden, AL 2010 Adaptations in placental phenotype support fetal growth during undernutrition of pregnant mice. *J. Physiol* **588** 527-538.

Constancia M, Angiolini E, Sandovic I, Smith P, Smith R, Kelsey G, Dean W, Ferguson-Smith A, Sibley C, Reik W, Fowden AL 2005 Adaptation of nutrient supply to fetal demand in the mouse involves interaction between the *Igf2* gene and placental transporter systems. *PNAS* **102** 19219-19224.

Constancia M, Hemburger M, Hughes J, Dean W, Ferguson-Smith A, Fundele R, Stewart F, Kelsey G, Fowden A, Sibley C & Reik W 2002 Placental-specific IGF2 is a major modulator of placental and fetal growth. *Nature* **417** 945-948.

Curchoe CL, Zhang S, Yang L, Page R & Tian XC 2009 Hypomethylation trends in the intergenic region of the imprinted IGF2 and H19 genes in cloned cattle. *Anim Reprod Sci* **116** 213-225.

Dandrea J, Wilson ME, Gopalakrishna G, Heasman L, Budpa H, Stephenson T & Symonds ME 2001 Maternal nutritional manipulation of placental growth and glucose transporter 1 (GLUT1) abundance in sheep. *Reproduction* **122** 793-800.

Das UG, Farouk Sadiq H, Soares MJ, Hay WW & Devaskar SU 1998 Time dependent physiological regulation of rodent and ovine glucose transporter (GLUT-1) protein. *Am J Physiol* **274** R339-R347.

Das UG, He J, Ehrhardt RA, Hay WW, Devaskar SU 2000 Time dependent physiological regulation of ovine placental Glut-3 transporter protein. *Am J Physiol* **279** R2252-R2261.

DiGiacomo JE, Hay WW 1989 Regulation of placental glucose transfer and consumption by fetal glucose production. *Ped Res* **25** 429-434.

Dwyer CM, Calvert SK, Farish M, Donbavand J & Pickup HE 2005 Breed, litter and parity effects on placental weight and placentome number , and consequences for neonatal behaviour of the lamb. *Theriogenology* **63** 1092-1110.

Early RJ, McBride BW, Vatnick I & Bell AW 1991 Chronic heat stress and perinatal development in sheep. II Placental cellularity and metabolism. *J. Anim Sci.* **69** 3610-3616.

Edwards LJ & McMillen IC 2001 Maternal undernutrition increases arterial blood pressure in the sheep fetus during late gestation. *J Physiol* **533** 561-570.

Forhead AJ, Curtis K, Kapstein E, Visser TJ & Fowden AL. 2006 Developmental control of iodothyronine deiodinases by cortisol in the ovine fetus and placenta near term. *Endocrinol* **147**, 5988-5994.

Forhead AJ, Lamb CA, Franko KL, O'Connor DM, Wooding FBP, Cripps RL, Ozanne SE, Blanche D, Shen QW, Du M & Fowden AL (2008). Role of leptin in the regulation of growth and carbohydrate metabolism in the ovine fetus during late gestation. *J. Physiol* **586** 2393-2403.

Fowden AL 1997 Comparative aspects of fetal carbohydrate metabolism. *Equine Vet J* **24** (Suppl.), 19-25.

Fowden AL & Forhead AJ 2004 Endocrine mechanisms of intrauterine programming. *Reproduction* **127**, 515-526.

Fowden AL & Forhead AJ 2009 Hormones as epigenetic signals in developmental programming. *Exp Physiol* **94** 607-625.

Fowden AL, Forhead AJ, Coan PM & Burton GJ 2008 The placenta and intrauterine programming. *J. Neuroendocrinol.* 20 439-450.

Fowden AL, Ralph M, Silver M 1994 Nutritional regulation of uteroplacental prostraglandin production and metabolism in pregnant ewes and mares during late gestation. *Exp Clin Endo* **102** 212-221.

Fowden AL, Sferruzzi-Perri AN, Coan PM, Constancia M & Burton GJ 2009 Placental efficiency and adaptation: Endocrine regulation. *J. Physiol.* **587** 3459-3472.

Fowden AL, Sibley C, Reik W & Constancia M 2006a Imprinted genes, placental development and fetal growth. *Hormone Res* **65** Suppl 3, 49-57.

Fowden AL, Ward JW, Wooding FPB, Forhead AJ & Constancia M 2006b Programming placental nutrient transport capacity. *J Physiol* **572** 5-15.

Gangon R, Johnston L & Murotsuki M 1996 Fetalplacental embolization in late gestation ovine fetus: alterations in umbilical blood flow and fetal heart rate pattern. *Am J Obstet Gynec* **175** 63-72.

Gardner DS, Ward JW, Giussani DA, Fowden AL 2002 The effects of a reversible period of adverse intrauterine conditions during late gestation on fetal and placental weight and placetome distribution in sheep. *Placenta* **23** 459-466.

Gheorghe CP, Goyal R, Mittal A & Longo LD 2010 Gene expression in the placenta: maternal stress and epigenetic responses. *Int J Dev Biol* **54** 507-523.

Gnanalingham MG, Williams P, Wilson V, Bisphan J, Hyatt MA, Pellicano A, Budge H, Stephenson T, Symonds ME 2007 Nutritional manipulation between early to mid gestation: effects on uncoupling protein-2, glucocorticoid sensitivity, IGF-I receptor and cell proliferation but not apoptosis in the ovine placenta. *Reproduction* **134** 615-623.

Gootwine E 2004 Placental hormones and fetal-placental development. *Anim Reprod Sci* **82** 551-566

Greenwood PL & Bell AW 2003 Consequences of intrauterine growth retardation for postnatal growth, metabolism and pathophysiology. Reproduction Suppl **61** 195-206.

Gluckman PD, Hanson MA, Buklijas T, Low FM & Beedle AS 2009 Epigenetic mechanisms that underpin metabolic and cardiovascular diseases. *Nat Rev Endocrinol* **5** 401-408

Harding JE, Evans PC & Gluckman PD 1997 Maternal growth hormone treatment increases placental diffusion capacity but not fetal or placental growth in sheep. *Endo*crinol **138** 5352-5358.

Harding JE, Liu L, Evans PC & Gluckman PD 1994 Insulin-like growth factor I alters feto-placental protein and carbohydrate metabolism in fetal sheep. *Endocrinol* **134** 1509-1514.

Hay WW. 2006 Placental-fetal glucose exchange and fetal glucose metabolism. *Trans Am Clin Climatol Assoc* **117** 321-339.

Heasman L, Clarke L, Stephenson TJ & Symonds ME 1998 Influence of maternal nutrient restriction in early to mid-gestation on placental and fetal development at term in sheep. *Pediatr Res* **44** 546-551.

Hu M, Sun X-J, Zhang Y-L, Kuang Y, Hu C-Q, wu W-L, Shen S-H, Du T-T, Li H, He F, Xiao H-S, Wang Z-G, Liu T-X, Hu H, Huang Q-H, Chen S-J, Chen Z 2010 Hsitone H3 lysine 36 methyltansferase *Hypb/Setd2* is required for embryonic vascular remodeling. *PNAS* **107** 2956-2961.

Jacobs R, Robinson JS, Owens JA, Falconer J & Webster MED 1988 The effect of prolonged hypobaric hypoxia on growth of fetal sheep. *J. Develop. Physiol.* **19** 97-112.

Jansson N, Pettersson J, Haafiz A, Ericsson A, Palmberg I, Tranberg M, Ganapathy V, Powell TH, Jansson T 2006 Downregulation of placental transport of amino acids precedes the development of intrauterine growth restriction in rats fed a low protein diet. *J Physiol* **576** 935-945.

Jansson T & Powell TL 2007 Role of the placenta in fetal programming: underlying mechanisms and potential intervention approaches. *Clin Sci* **113** 1-13.

Jensen EG, Gallaher BW, Breier BH & Harding JE 2002 The effect of chronic maternal cortisol infusion on the late-gestation fetal sheep. *J Endo*crinol **174** 27-36.

Jensen E, Wood CE & Keller-Wood M 2005 Chronic alterations in ovine corticosteroid levels influence uterine blood flow and placental and fetal growth. *Am J Physiol Regul Integr Comp Physiol* **288** R54-R61.

Jones HN, Woollett LA, Barour N, Prasad PD, Powell TL & Jansson T 2009 High-fat diet before and during pregnancy causes marked up-regulation of placental nutrient transport and fetal overgrowth in C57/BL6 mice. *FASEB J* **23** 271-278.

Kelly RW 1992 Nutrition and placental development. *Proc Nutr Soc Aust* **17** 203-211.

Kerzner LS, Stonesweet BS, Wu K-Y, Sadowska G & Malee MP 2002 Antenatal dexamethasone: Effect on ovine placental 11□ hydroxysteroid dehydrogenase Type 2 expression and fetal growth. *Ped Res* **52** 706-712.

Krebs C, Longo LD & Leiser R 1997 Term ovine placental vasculature: comparison of sea level and high altitude conditions by corrosion cast and histomorphometry. *Placenta* **18** 43-51.

Lang U, Baker RS, Khoury J & Clark KE 2000 Effects of chronic reduction in uterine blood flow on fetal and placental growth in the sheep. *Am J Physiol Regulatory Integrative Comp Physiol* **279** R53-R59.

Lea RG, Wooding P, Stewart I, Hannah LT, Morton S, Wallace K, Aitken RP, Milne JS, Regnault TR, Anthony RV & Wallace JM 2007 The expression of ovine placental lactogen, StAR and progesterone-associated steroidogenic enzymes in placentae of overnourished adolescent ewes. *Reproduction* **133** 785-796.

Leury BJ, Bird AR, Chandler KD & Bell AW 1990 Glucose partitioning in the pregnant ewe: effects of undenutrition and exercise. *Brit J Nutr* **64** 449-462.

Liechty EA, Kelley J & Lemons JA 1991 Effect of fasting on uteroplacental amino acid metabolism in the pregnant sheep. *Biol Neonate* **60** 207-214.

Lillycrop KA, Slater-Jefferies JL, Hanson MA, Godfrey KM, Jackson AA & Burdge GC 2007 Induction of altered epigenetic regulation of the hepatic glucocorticoid recpetor in the offspring of rats fed a protein-restricted diet during pregnancy suggests that reduced DNA methyltransferase expression is involved in impaired DNA methylation and changes in histone modifications. Brit. J. Nutr. 97 1064-1073

Limesand SW, Regnault TRH & Hay WW. Characterisation of glucose transporter 8 (GLUT8) in the ovine placenta of normal and growth restricted fetuses. *Placenta* **25** 70-77.

Liu L, Harding JE, Evans PC & Gluckman PD 1994 Maternal insulin-like growth factor-I infusion alters feto-placental carbohydrate and protein metabolism in pregnant sheep. *Endocrinol* **135** 895-900.

Luther J, Milne J, Aitkin R, Matsuzaki M, Reynolds L, Redmer D & Wallace J 2007 Placental growth, angiogenic gene expression, and vascular development in undernourished adolescent sheep. *Biol Reprod* **77** 351-357.

McCrabb GJ, Egan AR & Hosking BJ 1991 Maternal undernutrition during mid-gestation in sheep. Placental size and its relationship to calcium transfer during late gestation. *Brit. J Nutr.* **65** 157-168.

McMillen IC & Robinson JS 2005 Developmental origins of metabolic syndrome: prediction, plasticity and programming. *Physiol Rev* **85** 571-633.

McMullen S, Ogersby JC, Thurston LM, Gadd TS, Wood PJ, Wathes DC & Michael AE 2004 Alterations in placental 11 □-hydroxysteroid dehydrogenase (11□HSD) activity and fetal cortisol: cortisone ratios induced by nutritional restriction prior to conception and as defined stages of gestation in ewes. *Reproduction* **127** 717-725.

McMullen S, Ogersby JC, Milne JS Wallace JM & Wathes DC 2005 The effects of acute nutrient restriction in the mid-gestaional ewe on maternal and fetal nutrient status, the expression of placental growth factors and fetal growth. *Placenta* **26** 25-33.

Mellor DJ. 1983 Nutritional and placental determinants of foetal growth rate in sheep and consequences for the newborn lamb. *Br Vet J* **139** 307-324.

Oliver MH, Hawkins P & Harding JE 2005 Periconceptual undernutrition alters growth trajectory and metabolic and endocrine response to fasting in late gestation fetal sheep. *Ped Res* **57** 591-598.

Osgerby JC, Wathes DC, Howard D & Gadd TS 2002 The effect of maternal undernutrition on ovine fetal growth. *J Endocrinol* **173** 131-141.

Osgerby JC, Gadd TS & Wathes DC 2003 Effect of maternal body condition on placental and fetal growth and the insulin-like growth factor axis in Dorset ewes. *Reproduction* **125** 717-731

Osgerby JC, Wathes DC, Howard D & Gadd TS 2004 The effect of maternal undernutrition on the placental growth trajectory and the uterine insulin-like growth factor axis in the pregnant ewe. *J Endocrinol* **182** 89-103.

Owens JA, Falconer J & Robinson JS 1989 Glucose metabolism in pregnant sheep when placental growth is restricted. *Am J Physiol* **257** R350-R357.

Owens JA, Falconer J, Robinson JS 1987 Restriction of placental size in the sheep enhances the efficiency of placental transfer of antipyrine, 3-O-methyl-D-glucose but not of urea. *J Dev Physiol* **9** 457-464.

Parraquez VH, Atlagich M, Diaz, R, Cepeda R, Gonzalez C Delos Reyes M, Bruzzone ME, Behn C & Raggi LA 2006 Ovine placenta at high altidue: comparison of animals with different times of adaptation to hypoxic environment *J. Anim. Sci.* **95** 151-157.

Penninga L & Longo LD 1998 Ovine placentome morphology: effect of high altitude, long-term hypoxia. *Placenta* **19** 187-193.

Sibley CP, Turner MA, Cetin I, Ayuk P, Boyd CAR, D'Souza SW, Glazier JD, Greenwood SL, Jansson T & Powell T 2005 Placental phenotypes of intrauterine growth. *Ped Res* **58**, 827-832.

Quigley SP, Kleeman DO, Walker SA, Speck PA, Rudiger SR, Nattrass GS, DeBlasio MJ & Owens JA 2008 Effect of variable long term maternal feed allowance on the development of the ovine placenta and fetus. *Placenta* **29** 539-548.

Redmer DA, Wallace JM & Reynolds LP. 2004 Effect of nutrient intake during pregnancy on fetal and placental growth and vascular development. *Dom Anim Endo* **27** 199-217.

Redmer DA, Luther JS, Milne JS, Aitkin RP, Johnson ML, Borowicz PP, Borowicz MA, Reynolds LP & Wallace JM 2009 Fetoplacental growth and vascular development in overnourished sheep at day 50, 90 and 130 of gestation. *Reproduction* **137** 749-757.

Rees WD, Hay SM, Brown DS, Antipatis C & Palmer RM 2000. Maternal protein deficiency causes hypermethylation of DNA in the livers of rat fetuses. *J Nutr* **130** 1821-1826.

Regnault TRH, Galan HL, Parker TA & Anthony RV 2002 Placental development in normal and compromised pregnancies- a review. *Placenta* **23** Suppl A Trophoblast Research **16** S119-S129.

Regnault TRH, Friedman JE, Wilkening RB, Anthony RV & Hay WW 2005 Fetoplacental transport and utilization of amino acids in IUGR. A Review. *Placenta* **26** Suppl 1, S52-S62.

Regnault TRH, de VRijer B, Galan HL, Davidsen ML, Trembler KA, Battaglia FC, Wilening RB & Anthony RV 2003 The relationship between transplacental O_2 diffusion and placental expression of PIGF, FEGF and their eceptors in the placental insufficiency model of fetal growth restriction. *J. Physiol* **550** 641-656.

Reik W, Constancia M, Fowden AL, Anderson N, Dean W, Ferguson-Smith AC, Tycko B & Sibley C 2003 Regulation of supply and demand for maternal nutrients in mammals by imprinted genes. *J. Physiol* **547** 35-44.

Reynolds LP, Borowicz PP, Vonnahme KA, Johnson ML, Grazul-Bilska AT, Wallace JM, Caton JS & Redmer DA 2005 Animal models of placental angiogenesis. *Placenta* **26** 689-708.

Reynolds LP, Borowicz PP, Caton JS, Vonnahme KA, Luther JS Buchanan DS, Hafez SA, Grazul-Bilska AT & Redmer DA 2010 Uteroplacental vascular development and placental function: an update. *Int J Dev Biol* **54** 355-365.

Ross JC, Fennessey PV, Wilkening RP, Battaglia FC & Meschia G 1996 Placental transport and fetal utilization of leucine in a model of fetal growth retardation. *Am J Physiol* **270** E491-E503.

Rumball CWH, Harding JE, Oliver MH & Bloomfield FH 2008 Effects of twin pregnancy and periconceptual undernutrition on maternal metabolism, fetal growth and glucose-insulin axis function in ovine pregnancy. *J. Physiol* **586** 1399-1411.

Seckl JC 2004 Prenatal glucocorticoids and long term programming. *Eur J Endocrinol* Suppl. **3**, U49-62.

Šerman L, Vlahović M, Šijan M, Bulić-Jakuš, Šerman A, Sinčić N, Matijević R, Jurić-Lekić & Katušić A 2007 The impact of 5-azacytidine on placental weight, glycoprotein pattern and proliferating cell nuclear antigen expression in rat placenta. *Placenta* **28** 803-811.

Sibley CP, Turner MA, Cetin I, Ayuk P, Boyd CA, D'Souza SW, Glazier JD, Greenwood SL, Jansson T & Powell T 2005. Placental phenotypes of intrauterine growth. *Pediatr. Res.* **58**: 827-832.

Sinclair KD, Allegrucci C, Singh R, Gardner DS, Sebastian S, Bispham J, Thurston A, Huntley JF, Rees WD, Maloney CA, Lea RG, Craigon J, McEvoy TG & Young LE 2007 DNA mehylation, insulin resistance and blood pressure in offspring determined by maternal periconceptional B vitamin and methonine status. PNAS 104 19351-19356.

Stegeman HJ 1975 Placental development in the sheep and its relation to fetal development. *Bijdragen to V de Dierkunde* **44**, 3-73.

Steyn C, Hawkins P, Saito T, Noakes DE, Kingdom JCP, & Hanson MA 2001 Undernutrition during the first half of gestation increases the predominance of fetal tissue in late gestation ovine placentomes. *Eur J Obstet Gynec Reprod Biol* **98**, 165-170.

Tabano S, Colpietro P, Cetin I, Grati FR, Zanutto S, Mandò C, Antonazzo P, Pileri P, Rossella F, Larizza L, Sirchia SM, Miozzo M 2010 Epigenetic modulation of the *IGF2/H19* imprinted domain in human embryonic and extra-embrynic compartments and its possible role in fetal growth restriction. *Epigenetics* **5** 313-321.

Thureen PJ, Trembler KA, Meschia G, Makowski EL, Wilkening RB. 1992 Placental glucose transport in heat-induced fetal growth retardation. *Am J Physiol* **263** R578-R585.

Timmerman M, Teng C, Wilkening RP, Fennessey P, Battaglia FC, Meschia G. 2000 Effect of dexamethasone on fetal hepatic glutamine-glutanate exchange. *Am J Physiol* **278** E839-E845.

Vatnick I, Schoknect IPA, Danigrad R & Bell AW 1991 Growth and metabolism of the placenta after unilateral fetectomy in twin pregnant ewes. *J Dev Physiol* **15**, 351-356.

Vonnahme KA, Arndt WJ, Johnson ML, Borowicz PP & Reynolds LP 2008 Effect of morphology on placentome size, vascularity and vasoreactivity in late pregnant sheep. *Biol Reprod* **79** 976-982.

Vonnahme KA, Hess BW, Nijland MJ, Nathanielsz PW & Ford SP 2006 Placentomal differentiation may compensate for maternal nutrient restriction in ewes adapted to harsh range conditions. *J Anim Sci* **84** 3451-3459.

de Vrijer B, Davidsen ML, Wilkening RB, Anthony RV & Regnault, TRH 2006 Altered placental and fetal expression of IGFs and IGF-binding proteins associated with intrauterine growth restriction in fetal sheep during early to mid-pregnancy. *Pediatr Res* **60** 507-512.

Wallace JM, Aiken RP, Milne JS & Hay WW 2004 Nutritionally mediated placental growth restriction in the growing adolescent: consequences for the fetus. *Biol Reprod* **71** 1055-1062.

Wallace JM, Bourke DA, Aitken RP, Milne JS & Hay WW 2002 Placental glucose transport in growth restricted pregnancies induced by overnourishing adolescent sheep. *J Physiol* **547** 85-94.

Wallace JM, Matsuzaki M, Milne J & Aiken R 2006 Late but not early gestational maternal growth hormone treatment increases fetal adiposity in overnourished adolescent sheep. *Biol Reprod* **75** 231-239.

Wallace JM, Regnault TRH, Limesand SW, Hay WW & Anthony RV 2005 Investigating the causes of low birth weight in contrasting ovine paradigms. *J Physiol* **565** 19-26.

Ward JW 2002 Feto-placental metabolism: Regulation by cortisol. PhD Thesis. University of Cambridge.

Ward JW, Forhead AJ, Wooding FBP & Fowden AL 2006 Functional significance and cortisol dependence of the gross morphology of ovine placetome during late gestation. *Biol Reprod* **74** 137-145.

Ward JW, Wooding FBP & Fowden AL 2002 The effect of cortisol on the binucleate cell population in the ovine placenta during late gestation. *Placenta* **23** 451-458.

Ward JW, Wooding FPB & Fowden AL 2004 Ovine feto-placental metabolism. *J Physiol.* **554**, 529-541.

Whittle WL, Patel FA, Alfaidy N, Holloway AC, Fraser M, Gyomovey S, Lye SJ, Gibb W, Challis JRG 2001 Glucocorticoid regulation of human and ovine parturition: the relationship between fetal hypothalamic-pituitary-adrenal axis activation and intrauterine prostagladin production. *Biol Reprod* **64** 1019-1032.

Whorwood CB, Firth KM, Budge H & Symonds ME 2001 Maternal undernutrition during early to mid gestation programs tissue-specific alterations in the expression of the glucocorticoid receptor, 11□hydroxsterond dehydrogenase isoforms, and type I angiotensin II receptor in neonatal sheep. *Endocrinol* **142** 2854-2864.

Wooding FBP & Burton GJ 2008 Comparative Placentation. Springer

Wright CD, Orbus RJ, Regnault TRH & Anthony RV 2008 Effects of early gestation GH administration on placental and fetal development in sheep. *J. Endocrinol* **198** 91-99.

Yiallourides M, Sebert SP, Wilson V, Sharkey D, Rhind SM, Symonds ME & Budge H 2009 The differential effects of the timing of maternal nutrient restriction in the ovine placenta on glucocorticoid sensitivity, uncoupling protein 2, peroxisome prolifertor-activated receptor-γ and cell proliferation. *Reproduction* **138** 601-608.

Zhu MJ, Du M, Hess BW, Nathanielsz PW & Ford SP 2007 Periconceptional nutrient restriction in the ewe alters MAPK/ERK1/2 and PI3K/Akt growth signaling pathways and vascularity in the placentome . Placenta **28** 1192-1199.

Zhu MJ, Du M, Nijland MJ, Nathanielsz PW, Hess BW, Moss GE & Ford SP 2009 Down-regulation of growth signalling pathways linked to a reduced cotyledonary vascularity in placentomes of over-nourished obese pregnant ewes. Placenta **30** 405-410.

Dietary regulation of developmental programming in ruminants: epigenetic modifications in the germline

KD Sinclair, A Karamitri and DS Gardner

Schools of Biosciences and Veterinary Medicine and Science, University of Nottingham, Sutton Bonington, Leicestershire, LE12 5RD, UK

Ruminants have been utilised extensively to investigate the developmental origins of health and disease, with the sheep serving as the model species of choice to complement dietary studies in the rat and mouse. Surprisingly few studies, however, have investigated delayed effects of maternal undernutrition during pregnancy on adult offspring health and a consistent phenotype, together with underlying mechanistic pathways, has not emerged. Nevertheless, when broad consideration is given to all studies with ruminants it is apparent that interventions that are initiated very early in gestation, and/or prior to conception, lead to greater effects on adult physiology than those that are specifically targeted to late gestation. Effects induced following dietary interventions at the earliest stages of mammalian development have been shown to arise as a consequence of alterations to key epigenetic processes that occur in germ cells and pluripotent embryonic cells. Currently, our understanding of epigenetic programming in the germline is greatest for the mouse, and is considered in detail in this article together with what is known in ruminants. This species imbalance, however, looks set to change as fully annotated genomic maps are developed for domesticated large animal species, and with the advent of 'next-generation' DNA sequencing technologies that have the power to globally map the epigenome at single-base-pair resolution. These developments would help to address such issues as sexually dimorphic epigenetic alterations to DNA methylation that have been found to arise following dietary restrictions during the peri-conceptional period, the effects of paternal nutritional status on epigenetic programming through the germline, and transgenerational studies where, in future, greater emphasis in domesticated ruminants should be placed on traits of agricultural importance.

Introduction

Ruminant species (predominantly sheep) have been used in what we now term a 'developmental programming' context since early in the 20th century. Indeed, in the first issue of The Proceedings of the Nutrition Society a paper was presented on 'The Influence of Diet on Pregnancy and Lactation in the Mother, the Growth and Viability of the Foetus, and Post-Natal Development'

Corresponding author E-mail: Kevin.Sinclair@nottingham.ac.uk

(Garry, 1944). At that time, the emphasis was on productive traits as influenced by maternal diet; that is, how to maximise the efficiency of meat production before, during and after the Great Wars. Slightly earlier, Joseph Barcroft was interested in how organs metabolised and handled gases in solution, particularly oxygen, and this led him to utilise pregnant ruminants, first the goat (Barcroft *et al.* 1934) and then the sheep (Barcroft & Barron 1936) to investigate aspects of fetal physiology; being a unique gaseous (hypoxic) environment. Since that time, thanks largely to the collective efforts of scientists such J Hammond, LR Wallace, R McCance & E Widdowson and, more recently, JJ Robinson, the pregnant ruminant has been extensively utilised as a model to investigate fetal physiology and responses to a variety of nutritional and non-nutritional stimuli.

Maternal diet and developmental programming in ruminants

Central to the current thesis are the ewe's predicted responses to a change in the supply of a variety of dietary micro- and macro-nutrients, which can influence maternal body composition at the onset of pregnancy, nutrient partitioning (e.g. amino acids and polyamines; Kwon *et al.*, 2004) and fetal development during pregnancy, and the ewe's subsequent lactational ability and lamb performance. Surprisingly, the first studies in sheep to truly embrace the concept originally proposed by Barker & Osmond (1986), that maternal nutrition during pregnancy could impinge on the long-term well being of offspring, didn't materialise until 11-12 years later, and these studies only considered the impact of variations in maternal diet on aspects of fetal growth and development (Trahair *et al.* 1997; Clarke *et al.* 1998; Gallaher *et al.* 1998; Warnes *et al.* 1998). A PubMed search (accessed May 21st 2010) for the MESH term "maternal nutritional physiological phenomena and sheep" returned 121 papers of which 87 were original contributions (not reviews). Of these, 35 were original research articles which investigated the delayed effects of maternal undernutrition on adult offspring. For example, Bloomfield *et al* (2003) described an association between 10 days severe undernutrition close to term in sheep and a greater pituitary (but not adrenal) response to stress in their offspring at 30 months of age.

After excluding descriptive reports of tissue and sex-specific molecular changes in offspring due to variations in maternal nutrition, there are approximately 17 papers that reported a characterised phenotype in adult offspring (Table 1). The physiological outcomes described within these papers are variable, reflecting (1) the different breeds of sheep used, (2) different nutritional interventions at (3) different gestational time-points and (4) different post-natal ages. Thus, we know that reduced nutrient intake by pregnant dams can influence appetite and tissue energy oxidative capacity (Sebert *et al.* 2009; Jorgensen *et al.* 2009), glucose-insulin metabolism (Gardner *et al.* 2005; Burt *et al.* 2007; Ford *et al.* 2007; Poore *et al.* 2007; Todd *et al.* 2009; Rhodes *et al.* 2009), hypothalamic-pituitary-adrenal axis function (Bloomfield *et al.* 2003; Gardner *et al.* 2006; Chadio *et al.* 2007), cardiovascular and renal function (Gardner *et al.* 2004; Williams *et al.* 2007; Chan *et al.* 2009; Cleal *et al.* 2007; Gopalakrishnan *et al.* 2005), behavioural responses (Dwyer *et al.* 2003; Erhard *et al.* 2004; Hernandez *et al.* 2009) and immune function (Sinclair *et al.* 2007; Eckersall *et al.* 2008). In summarising these studies it is clear that variations in maternal nutrition interact with maternal body composition to alter cellular function within the organs of offspring; for example, corticotrophin/adrenocorticotrophin sensitivity within the pituitary/adrenal with respect to programming of the HPA axis or the density/activity of insulin signalling proteins in peripheral tissues with respect to programming of glucose-insulin dynamics. However, a consistent phenotype has not emerged and whilst the other 18 papers demonstrating descriptive effects invariably infer mechanistic insights to one or other of the physiological systems programmed, a clear mechanistic pathway remains elusive.

Table 1. Studies investigating the effect of maternal nutrient restriction on adult offspring physiological function in sheep

Dietary paradigm	Period of nutrient restriction before or during gestation (days): -60 0 30 80 147	Observed physiological phenotype	Reference
10-15% wt loss (-61 to 30 days)		↓ (10%) glucose tolerance (10mth)	Todd *et al* 2009
10-15% wt loss (-61 to 30 days)		altered behavioural responses	Hernandez *et al* 2009
30% ME (-60 to 7 days)		↑ fetal BP (3-8±2.5 mmHg)	Edwards & McMillen 2002
MD diet (-56 to 6 days)		↓ insulin sensitivity (males) at 2yr ↑ BP (11 ± 2 mmHg)	Sinclair *et al* 2007
30% ME (0 to 30 days)		↑ HPA axis in female *vs.* male	Chadio *et al* 2007
50% ME (1 to 30 days)		↑ adult PP at 1 yr (5 ± 1 mmHg)	Gardner *et al* 2004
50% ME (1 to 30 days)		↓ baroreflex sensitivity to AII	Gardner *et al* 2006
50% ME (1 to 95 days)		↑ adult BP at 3 yr (10 ± 2 mmHg)	Gopalakrishnan *et al* 2004
50% ME (1 to 95 days)		altered behavioural responses	Erhard *et al* 2004
50% ME (28 to 78 days)		↓ (~ 15%) glucose tolerance at 8 mth	Burt *et al* 2007
50% ME (28 to 78 days)		↓ (~ 15%) glucose tolerance at 8 mth	Ford *et al* 2008
50% ME (28 to 80 days)		↓ BP (6 mth , 8 ± 3 mmHg). ↓ (40 ± 12 %) nephron number	Gopalakrishnan *et al* 2005
30% ME (31 to 100 days)		little to no effect	Chadio *et al* 2007
35% ME (28 to 147 days)		↓ ewe-lamb bonding behaviour at birth	Dwyer *et al* 2003
30% ME (65 to 125 days)		↓ immune response to vaccination	Eckersall *et al* 2008
50% ME (110 to 147 days)		↓ (first phase) insulin sensitivity at 1 yr	Gardner *et al* 2005

Key: % ME, percentage reduction in metabolisable energy intake fed to ewes; MD diet, a methyl deficient diet; mth, months; Day 0, conception (147 days in the sheep); BP, blood pressure; PP, pulse pressure; HPA, hypothalamic-pituitary-adrenal axis; yr, year; RAAS, renin-angiotensin-aldosterone axis; GTT, glucose tolerance test; p24, postnatal age in months.

In recent years, a few studies with sheep have experimentally tested the developmental programming hypothesis by combining a post-natal nutritional challenge after exposure to a pre-natal nutritional insult (Table 2). We asked the question whether moderate adult obesity would exacerbate the effects on the offspring of maternal global energy restriction, and tested the hypothesis by longitudinally sampling the offspring in a lean and then obese condition (Rhodes *et al.* 2009). We found little evidence of programming by maternal global energy restriction *per se*, but some support for the hypothesis that development of obesity would reveal a deleterious phenotype (altered glucose-insulin handling), albeit very mild. The only other studies to have used a similar approach, but with an entirely different experimental paradigm (i.e. 2x2 factorial arrangement; prenatal undernutrition [1-31 days gestation] x postnatal undernutrition [pair-fed to achieve 85% growth of control sheep]) found that post-natal intervention had the greater effect on adult physiology (e.g. a 5-6 mm Hg greater increase in mean arterial pressure to Angiotensin II) (Cleal *et al.* 2007)) and a ~30% increase in insulin appearance after a glucose tolerance test in male offspring only (Poore *et al.* 2007).

Peri-conceptional diet and developmental programming in ruminants

Taken together, *a priori* assumptions about the expected adult phenotype when utilising either postnatal overnutrition (greater deterioration of metabolic control) or postnatal undernutrition (improvement of metabolic control) are not clear cut and further work in this area is warranted. Nevertheless, when broad consideration is given to all studies conducted in ruminants it is apparent that interventions that are initiated very early in gestation (and/or prior to conception) lead to greater effects on adult physiology than those that are specifically targeted to late gestation. This is most evident in the study of Sinclair *et al* (2007) in which dietary methyl group deficiency for 8 weeks before and 6 days into gestation (i.e. embracing the periods of oocyte growth and maturation, and pre-implantation embryo development) revealed a 11 mm Hg increase in mean arterial pressure and a 30% increase in the pressor response to infused angiotensin II in two-year-old male offspring. Responses such as this at the earliest stages of mammalian development hint at the importance of key epigenetic processes that occur in germ cells and pluripotent embryonic cells, and that subsequently determine offspring health.

The present article, therefore, will provide a contemporary overview of these molecular processes drawing, where necessary, on information acquired from mice and other mammalian species, before reviewing our current state of knowledge with respect to ruminants. Finally, current limitations and outstanding issues are indentified, and consideration given to future priorities for research funding.

DNA methylation programming in the germline

The aforementioned processes of development are regulated in a temporal and spatial manner by a series of carefully orchestrated alterations to the transcriptome which arise as a consequence of covalent modifications to DNA and associated histone proteins that act in concert with chromatin structure in a cell-lineage specific manner. Over the last 20 years there has been an exponential increase in activity in the field of epigenetics and mammalian development with more than 7000 research articles and 2000 reviews dedicated to the topic. For a contemporary overview of some of the broader aspects of this area the reader is directed elsewhere (Reik, 2007; Petronis, 2010). Instead, attention in the current article is directed towards epigenetic programming in the germline, with consideration given to covalent modifications to components of the nucleosome (the functional subunit of chromatin) and, in particular, to DNA.

Table 2. Studies investigating variations in dam and lamb nutrition on adult offspring physiological function in sheep.

Dietary paradigm	Period of nutrient restriction during or after gestation (months) 0 1 T P3 P6 P12 P18 P24		Reference
Dam: 50% ME (0-1 mth) Lamb: 85% growth (3-6mth)		↓ (30%) insulin sensitivity	Poore *et al* 2007
Dam: 50% ME (0-1 mth) Lamb: 85% growth (3-6mth)		↑ RAAS response (5-8mmHg) to furosemide at 2.5yr	Cleal *et al* 2007
Dam: 50% ME (1-2.5 mth) Lamb: Ad lib (3-12 mth)		↓ renal function at 1 yr	Williams *et al* 2007
Dam: 50% ME (1-2.5 mth) Lam: Ad lib (3-12 mth)		↑ BP (10 $\pm$ 2 mmHg) at 1 yr	Chan *et al* 2009
Dam: 50% ME (1-2.5 mth) Lamb: Ad lib (3-12 mth)		Subtle effects on energy balance	Sebert *et al* 2009
Dam: 30% ME (2-4.3 mth) Lamb: 1.5M (18-24 mth)		↑ peak insulin to GTT at 1.5yr	Rhodes *et al* 2009
Dam: 50% ME (0-1 mth) Lamb: high-fat (0-6mth)		↓ (40%) mitochondrial activity & VO_{2max}	Jorgensen *et al* 2009

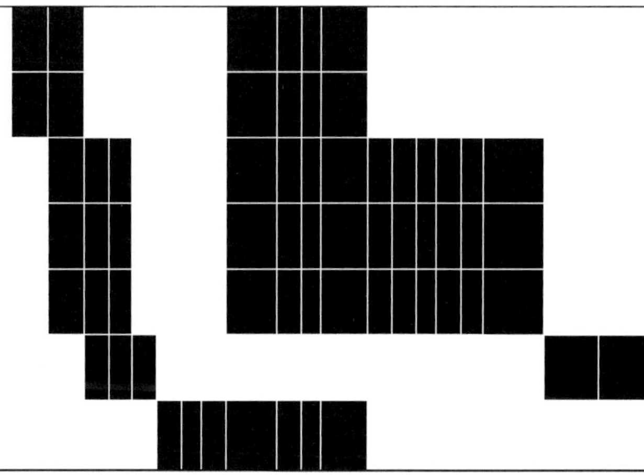

Key: % ME, percentage reduction in metabolisable energy intake fed to ewes; MD diet, a methyl deficient diet; mth, months; T, term (147 days in the sheep); BP, blood pressure; PP, pulse pressure; HPA, hypothalamic-pituitary-adrenal axis; yr, year; RAAS, renin-angiotensin-aldosterone axis; GTT, glucose tolerance test; p24, postnatal age in months.

DNA methylation

DNA methylation involves the covalent addition of a methyl group to the number 5 carbon atom of the cytosine pyrimidine ring and is targeted to CpG dinucleotides which are recognised by DNA methyltransferases (DNMTs) (Goll & Bestor, 2005). Unlike single-copy genes, repeat sequences in the genome are CpG rich and are usually highly methylated. This is thought to confer chromosomal stability and to regulate the extent of recombination, but it also serves to silence transposable elements which constitute around 45% of the human genome (Lander *et al.*, 2001). In contrast, single-copy genes are usually deficient in CpGs, which tend to cluster as 'CpG islands', and co-localise with the promoters of most constitutively expressed genes (Illingworth & Bird, 2009). Around 40% of mammalian genes contain CpG islands in or close to their promoters. Whilst the majority of these are hypomethylated, tissue-specific differences in the extent of CpG island methylation exist. Indeed, it has been estimated that tissue-specific differentially methylated sequences constitute at least 5% of total CpG islands in the genome (Song *et al.*, 2005), and these serve to regulate gene expression, lineage specification and differentiation during development. In the case of imprinted genes CpG islands can, in addition, reside distally to the promoter at so-called differentially methylated (DMR) or imprint control (ICR) regions. However, non-CpG island methylation and indeed non-CpG methylation are known to exist in the mouse and human. Emerging data, using 'next generation' deep sequencing and array based technologies, indicate that the former may represent a more important determinant of tissue-specific gene expression, whereas the latter appears to be specific to embryonic stem cells (Lister *et al.*, 2009). Using comprehensive high-throughput array-based relative methylation (CHARM) analysis, Irizarry *et al.* (2009) found that tissue differentially methylated regions (t-DMR), which are functionally related to gene expression, do not occur in promoters or in CpG islands but in adjacent (i.e. within 2kb) lower density sequences which they termed "CpG island shores". Other recent studies (e.g. Ball *et al.*, 2009; Maunakea *et al.*, 2010) support the notion that t-DMR at non-CpG islands within gene bodies may be more important in regulating highly expressed genes than DNA methylation in 5′ CpG island promoters, where covalent modifications to histones may have a more prominent role.

The mouse germline

Much of what we know about changes to DNA methylation in the germline pertains to studies conducted in the mouse (Lees-Murdock and Walsh, 2008; Sanz *et al.*, 2010) with only limited data available for ruminants and other species (discussed later). Briefly, between days 11.5 and 12.5 *post coitum* in the mouse, single copy imprinted and non-imprinted genes, together with repeat sequences, are synchronously demethylated in both male and female genomes. However, in contrast to imprinted and single-copy genes, repeat sequences are only partially demethylated, a process hypothesised to minimise transposition and stabilise chromosome integrity (Hajkova *et al.*, 2002). At the same time X-chromosome reactivation is initiated. This involves a loss of methylation at the DMR regulating X-inactive specific transcript (*Tsix*) and X (inactive)-specific transcript, antisense (*Xist*) expression (Boumil *et al.*, 2006). *De novo* methylation occurs later during gametogenesis and, in contrast to demethylation, occurs asynchronously, both between and within various sequence classes and between male and female genomes. The timing of methylation acquisition in the female gamete coincides with the stage of oocyte growth leading up to the re-initiation of meiosis and is associated with increased expression of genes (i.e. *Dnmt3a, Dnmt3b* and *Dnmt3L*) involved in *de novo* methylation (Lucifero *et al.*, 2007).

Epigenetic events during syngamy are again best studied in the mouse where the paternally derived genome is actively (in the absence of DNA replication) demethylated during the first cell cycle. The identification of a putative demethylase, however, had remained elusive for many years (Ooi & Bestor, 2008). Recently, however, key roles for Activation-Induced cytidine Deaminase (AID) (Popp *et al.*, 2010; Bhutani *et al.*, 2010) and components of the elongator complex (Okada *et al.*, 2010) in paternal DNA demethylation have been demonstrated in mouse primordial germ cells and zygotes, although the precise mechanisms of their action remain to be determined. The maternal pronucleus and paternal ICRs are able to maintain their hypermethylated state during this period due, in part, to the actions of PGC7/Stella (Nakamura *et al.*, 2007), a maternal factor essential for early development, which can protect these regions from demethylation although, once again, the precise mechanism of protection has not been established. The protected state of the maternal genome at syngamy may also be related to the methylation status of lysine residues K9 and K27 on histone H3 which are thought to guard against active demethylation (Santos *et al.*, 2005). In contrast to the paternal genome, the maternal genome is passively demethylated with each cell cycle and round of DNA replication during early pre-implantation development. DNA methylation imprints, however, are maintained. Recent evidence indicates that this is largely achieved through the actions of maternally and zygotically derived Dnmt1, which are speculated to specifically target DMRs by some unknown mechanism (Hirasawa *et al.*, 2008).

By the blastocyst stage global differences in DNA methylation are evident between the extraembryonic and embryonic lineages in the mouse (Morgan *et al.*, 2005). In contrast to the trophectoderm (TE), there is clear evidence of extensive *de novo* methylation within the inner cell mass (ICM). The *de novo* methylase Dnmt3b is known to preferentially localise to the ICM in mouse blastocysts (Watanabe *et al.*, 2002). Also, specific histone modifications such as the aforementioned trimethylation of K9 and K27 on histone H3 are enriched in the ICM relative to the TE (Erhardt *et al.*, 2003). Over-expression of the histone methyltransferase (RMT4/CARM1), that methylates arginine 26 of Histone H3, has been shown to upregulate Nanog and Sox2 expression in individual blastomeres of 4-cell embryos. The expression of these factors is believed to ultimately lead to the preferential allocation of blastomeres to the ICM (Torres-Padilla *et al.*, 2007). Although somewhat controversial, these observations indicate that epigenetic modifications can influence cell fate determination and lineage commitment during the earliest stages of mammalian development.

The ruminant germline

In contrast to the mouse strikingly little is known about epigenetic modifications to DNA and associated proteins during gametogenesis in ruminants. However, broadly in keeping with the mouse, global DNA methylation (determined using a 5-methylcytosine antibody and quantified by fluorescence microscopy) has been shown to increase in growing oocytes from the late pre-antral through to the large-antral stage of follicle development (Russo *et al.*, 2007). As yet, nothing is known about how acquisition of DNA methylation may differ between the various sequence classes.

The process of active demethylation during syngamy, described earlier for the paternal genome in the mouse, appears to differ between species (Fulka *et al.*, 2008). Similar to the mouse, a dramatic loss of cytosine methylation from the male pronucleus is observed in the rat, human and cow, but not in the rabbit and sheep. Through the use of interspecies intracytoplasmic sperm injection, Beaujean *et al.* (2004a) were able to demonstrate that the more extreme loss of paternal DNA methylation in the mouse compared to the sheep pronucleus arises as a consequence of the enhanced resistance of sheep sperm to demethylation and the greater demethylating capacity of the mouse ooplasm. The molecular basis for these differences is currently not known. In the mouse, histone H3K9 acetylation and methylation status is mechanistically linked to DNA methylation but, although a similar configuration for this histone exists in the sheep zygote, it is not related to the level of DNA methylation in the male pronucleus (Hou *et al.*, 2008). The functional significance of these species differences in demethylation following fertilisation is also unclear. They may merely reflect pre-existing levels of methylation in the male pronucleus at the time of syngamy, which are comparatively low in sheep (Beaujean *et al.*, 2004b).

The subsequent loss of DNA methylation during the early pre-implantation period is also more extreme in the mouse than either the cow or sheep genomes. Indeed, only at the blastocyst stage is demethylation apparent in the sheep TE, whereas cells of the ICM remain methylated (Beaujean *et al.*, 2004b). Therefore, whilst the outcome of methylation differences at the blastocyst stage is similar for the mouse and sheep (hypermethylated ICM and hypomethylated TE), the manner in which these comparable states are reached differs between the species. This may reflect differences in the timing of key developmental stages, such as embryonic transcription activation which, in ruminant species, occurs later than in the mouse at around the 8 to 16-cell stage. Nevertheless, despite these species differences it is evident that sweeping epigenetic changes to both DNA and associated proteins occur through the germline, rendering germ cells and pluripotent embryonic cells vulnerable to environmentally induced epigenetic dysregulation.

Dietary manipulation of epigenetic programming in the germline

With the foregoing discussion in mind it is surprising to note that there has been little attempt to investigate nutritional induced epigenetic programming in the germline. Most studies with ruminants and other species have tended to focus on the epigenetic consequences of procedures used in assisted reproduction, such as ovarian stimulation, intra-cytoplasmic sperm injection and embryo culture (Grace and Sinclair, 2009), or reprogramming during somatic cell nuclear transfer (Niemann *et al.*, 2008). These studies clearly highlight the vulnerability of gametes and pluripotent embryonic cells to environmentally-induced epigenetic dysregulation. Those investigators that have assessed aspects of dietary induced epigenetic programming have tended to focus on the regulation of specific metabolic pathways in rodents exposed to some form of global nutrient restriction throughout *in utero* development (Burdge and Lillycrop, 2010).

Some of our early investigations into the mechanistic basis of the 'Large Offspring Syndrome' (LOS; Sinclair *et al.*, 2000a), however, suggested that the composition of the diet of embryo donor ewes could influence both the incidence and severity of the observed LOS phenotypes. At least in the sheep, the aberrant fetal phenotype is associated with a loss of imprinting and expression of the gene encoding the type 2 insulin-like growth factor receptor (*IGF2R*) which, in turn, arises as a consequence of a loss of methylation on the second intron DMR of the gene (Young *et al.*, 2001). Elevated plasma urea concentrations in zygote-donor ewes in subsequent studies were induced by feeding high-nitrogen diets from the onset of oestrous synchronisation and ovarian stimulation, two weeks prior to AI and zygote recovery. Plasma urea concentrations were negatively correlated to *IGF2R* expression in the fetal heart and kidney which, together with the positive correlation between plasma urea and conceptus mass, confirmed an involvement of nitrogen/urea metabolism in the aetiology of the LOS (Powell *et al.*, 2006).

In cattle we have shown that the feeding of specially formulated diets that lead to elevated plasma ammonium and urea concentrations can impair post-fertilisation development of oocytes (Sinclair *et al.*, 2000b). Related studies in the mouse revealed that elevated ammonium concentrations during culture can alter the expression of the imprinted gene *H19* and impair fetal development (Lane and Gardner, 2003); although similar levels of ammonium during oocyte growth in a long-term follicle culture system did not alter the methylation status of DMRs in three imprinted genes (*Snrpn*, *Igf2r* and *H19*) in MII oocytes (Anckaert *et al.*, 2009). In the rat, the feeding of a LPD for just the first 4 days of gestation led to post-natal hypertension in male offspring (Kwong *et al.*, 2000), and a reduction in *H19* and *Igf2* transcript expression in fetal male, but not female, livers (Kwong *et al.*, 2006). However, *H19* transcript expression was not associated with altered methylation at its DMR in that study.

Sticking with the theme of imprinting, human subjects who were prenatally exposed to famine during the Dutch Hunger Winter in 1944-45 had, as aged adults, reduced *IGF2* DMR methylation compared with their unexposed, same-sex siblings (Heijmans *et al.*, 2008). Significantly, this only applied to those subjects who were exposed during the peri-conceptional period and not during late gestation. Whilst this epigenetic modification in DNA methylation was not related to transcript expression, these data provide the first evidence in a human population for the epigenetic basis of the developmental origins of adult disease. More recently, peri-conceptional folic acid use was shown to increase the level of *IGF2* DMR methylation of DNA extracted from whole blood of infant children (Steegers-Theunissen *et al.*, 2009). Interestingly, *IGF2R* DMR methylation in that study was correlated with the concentration of S-adenosyl methionine (SAM) in maternal blood.

As an initial step to provide a link between maternal diet and epigenetic alterations to DNA methylation we investigated aspects of the linked methionine-folate cycles in human embryonic stem cells (Steele *et al.*, 2005), somatic cells and oocytes from the bovine ovary, and bovine pre-implantation embryos (Kwong *et al.*, 2010). Analyses revealed that transcripts for most of the enzymes and transporters involved in these cycles were present in all cell types from both species. There were, however, some noticeable similarities and differences both between the two species and between cell types within species. For example, in contrast to cells of the spleen, transcripts for the folate receptor *FOLR2* were absent in human and bovine embryonic cells, and were also not present in oocytes and somatic cells within the bovine ovarian follicle. Methionine-adenosyl transferase (MAT) (EC 2.5.1.6) is an enzyme that catalyses the activation of methionine by ATP to form SAM. The isoenzyme encoded by *MAT1A* exists as two proteins with moderate to high K_m values for methionine, but transcripts for *MAT1A* were either absent or very poorly expressed in both human and bovine embryonic cells, and all cells within the bovine ovary, indicating that these different cell types are not accustomed to metabolising high concentrations of methionine so typical of contemporary cell and embryo culture media. Most strikingly in the cow was the absence of transcripts for the enzyme betaine-homocysteine methyltransferase (EC 2.1.1.5) in all somatic cells of the bovine ovary, as well as in the bovine oocyte and pre-implantation embryo. This may reflect species-specific differences in the importance of this enzyme for these cell types. It certainly indicates that these cycles function differently between species, and also between cell type within a species.

With the foregoing characterisations in mind we sought to assess if restricting the dietary supply of specific methyl-cycle metabolites (i.e. vitamin B_{12}, methionine and folate) in the diet of embryo donor ewes could lead to epigenetic modifications to DNA methylation in offspring with long-term implications for animal health. Methyl deficient or control diets were offered from 8 weeks before, until 6 days after, conception by AI. This duration of exposure ensured that the critical periods of DNA methylation programming in the germline of sheep (Beaujean *et al.*, 2004b; Russo *et al.*, 2007) were incorporated. Embryos were recovered and transferred singly to normally fed surrogates. Neither pregnancy rate nor birth weight was affected in this study but adult offspring were heavier and fatter, elicited altered immune responses to antigenic challenge, were insulin resistant and had high blood pressure (Sinclair *et al.*, 2007). In keeping with studies in the rat (Kwong *et al.*, 2000; Kwong *et al.*, 2006) these effects were most evident in male offspring. The altered methylation status of 4% of 1,400 CpG islands examined by restriction landmark genome scanning (RLGS) in the fetal liver revealed compelling evidence of a widespread epigenetic mechanism associated with this nutritionally programmed effect. Furthermore, more than half of the affected loci were specific to males. These intriguing observations point to sexually dimorphic epigenetic programming during early pre-implantation development and merits further investigation.

Current limitations, outstanding issues and future priorities

Genome maps in ruminants have been under development for the last decade. Whilst the bovine genome has been fully sequenced and is largely annotated (Elsik *et al.*, 2009), sheep and goat maps are still under construction. The lack of genomic sequence information in the sheep has proved a significant barrier to progress and required us to use RLGS as a non-selective screening technique for the methylome to define the proportion of genes affected by peri-conceptional maternal nutrition (Sinclair *et al.*, 2007). In contrast, the power of 'next-generation' DNA sequencing technologies to globally map the epigenome was recently demonstrated in human pluripotent embryonic stem cells and terminally differentiated fetal fibroblasts. Lister *et al.* (2009) published the first complete DNA-methylation map of the human genome at single-base-pair resolution and their analyses challenges a number of existing theories in the field. For example, as eluded to earlier, whereas in fetal fibroblasts almost all DNA methylation occurs at CpG dinucleotides, around 25% of methylation sites in pluripotent stem cells do not occur at CpGs but on cytosines that neighbour other bases, in particular adenosine. The function, significance and enzymes involved in non-CpG methylation, however, remain to be identified. Nevertheless, large-scale analysis of genome-wide DNA methylation by deep sequencing of bisulphite-treated DNA represents a future advancement to current RLGS protocols and methods that array immunoprecipitated methylated DNA; the former is limited by methylation sensitive restriction endonucleases available, and uses radiolabelled phosphorus, whilst the latter is biased towards CpG-rich sequences and exhibits poor sensitivity for low CpG dense regions (i.e. those outside CpG islands) (Beck & Rakyan, 2008; Thu *et al.*, 2009).

Several outstanding issues emerge from the studies cited earlier in this article. For example, the fact that the effects of peri-conceptional nutrient restriction manifest more in male than female offspring in contrasting species (i.e. rat and sheep), and that this is consistent with sexually dimorphic epigenetic alterations to DNA methylation (at least in the sheep), is of profound importance. Sexual dimorphism in the development and metabolism of pre-implantation embryos is well established in ruminants and other mammalian species (Gutiérrez-Adán *et al.*, 2006). Epigenetic differences between male and female bovine blastocysts have also recently been reported (Bermejo-Álvarex *et al.*, 2008). Using a methylation-sensitive PCR technique, these authors assessed the methylation status of 6 genomic regions in male and female bovine blastocysts and found one region, close to a variable number tandem repeat sequence, to be differentially methylated. The authors concluded that there may be genomic region-specific differences in epigenetic status between male and female bovine blastocysts which may apply to other single-copy genes involved in regulating full-term development. Although this remains to be determined, the potential exists to identify loci in the pre-implantation embryo that, in terms of epigenetic programming, are altered by maternal diet in a sexually dimorphic manner.

A neglected area of research concerns the effect of paternal nutritional status on epigenetic programming through the germline and the consequences for offspring health and well being. Indirect evidence that environmentally induced defects programmed into the male gamete can alter offspring health and fertility come from transgenerational studies in the rat investigating the effects of maternal protein restriction during pregnancy (Harrison & Langley-Evans, 2008) and pregnant rats exposed to the agricultural fungicide vinclozolin (Guerrero-Bosagnna & Skinner, 2009). In both cases phenotypic defects were transmitted via the male germline, at least to the F2 generation, indicating that defects programmed into the male gamete can alter offspring health. Furthermore, the studies with vinclozolin were extended to demonstrate epigenetic alterations to DNA methylation in epididymal sperm which persisted to F3 offspring.

There also needs to be greater emphasis in the future on assessing the effects of specific components of the maternal diet during clearly defined periods of gestation. To that end due care and consideration should be given to the processes of nutrient storage, transport and function in the pregnant animal offered a nutrient deficient diet, as this will lead to the onset of body tissue depletion followed by deficiency, dysfunction and ultimately disease (Sinclair and Singh, 2007). In the past the timing and extent of nutrient restriction has frequently been inadequately monitored, greatly hindering data interpretation. Finally, and returning to the interests of the pioneering scientists listed at the beginning of this article, greater consideration should be made in future towards understanding the programming of traits of agricultural importance.

Conclusions

The foregoing discussion highlights the need to fully sequence and annotate the genomes of domesticated animal species, in particular the sheep, so that full advantage can be made of the contemporary molecular tools available to provide the mechanistic insights required in the field of developmental programming of health and disease. This is best exemplified by the extent of knowledge in epigenetic programming through the germline in the mouse compared to other mammalian species. Large animals, such as the sheep, represent a more appropriate model to study the developmental origins of health and disease because their mature size, and associated reproductive rate, metabolism and physiology are more similar to that of humans. Domestic ruminants are also species of commercial interest, so that in the future perhaps more emphasis should be placed on studying traits of economic importance where animals are offered more thoughtfully formulated diets that facilitate the study of specific micro-and macro-nutrients.

Acknowledgements

AK is supported by a grant from the British Heart Foundation (PG/08/124/26414)

References

Anckaert E, Adriaenssens T, Romero S & Smitz J 2009 Ammonium accumulation and use of mineral oil overlay do not alter imprinting establishment at three key imprinted genes in mouse oocytes grown and matured in a long-term follicle culture. *Biol Reprod* **81** 666-73.

Ball MP, Li JB, Gao Y, Lee JH, LeProust EM, Park IH, Xie B, Daley GQ & Church GM 2009 Targeted and genome-scale strategies reveal gene-body methylation signatures in human cells. *Nat. Biotechnol.* **27** 361-368.

Barcroft J, Flexner LB & McClurkin T 1934 The output of the foetal heart in the goat. *J Physiol* **82** 498-508.

Barcroft J & Barron DH 1936 The genesis of respiratory movements in the foetus of the sheep. *J Physiol* **88** 56-61.

Barker DJ & Osmond C 1986 Infant mortality, childhood nutrition, and ischaemic heart disease in England and Wales. *Lancet* **1** 1077-81.

Beaujean N, Hartshorne G, Cavilla J, Taylor JE, Gardner J, Wilmut I, Meehan R & Young L 2004b Non-conservation of mammalian preimplantation methylation dynamics *Curr Biol* **14** R266-7.

Beaujean N, Taylor JE, McGarry M, Gardner J, Wilmut I, Loi P, Ptak G, Galli C, Lazzari G, Bird A, Young LE & Meehan RR 2004a The effect of interspecific oocytes on demethylation of sperm DNA. *Proc Natl Acad Sci U S A* **101** 7636-40.

Beck S & Rakyan VK 2008 The methylome: approaches for global DNA methylation profiling. *Trends in Genetics* **24** 231-7

Bermejo-Álvarex P, Rizos D, Rath D, Lonergan P & Gutierrez-Adan A 2008 Epigenetic differences between male and female bovine blastocysts produced in vitro. *Physiol Genomics* **32** 264-272.

Bhutani N, Brady JJ, Damian M, Sacco A, Corbel SY & Blau HM 2010 Reprogramming towards pluripotency requires AID-dependent DNA demethylation. *Nature* **463** 1042-7.

Bloomfield FH, Oliver MH, Giannoulias CD, Gluckman PD, Harding JE & Challis JR 2003 Brief undernutrition in late-gestation sheep programs the hypothalamic-pituitary-adrenal axis in adult offspring. *Endocrinology* **144** 2933-2940.

Boumil RM, Ogawa Y, Sun BK, Huynh KD & Lee JT 2006 Differential methylation of Xite and CTCF sites in Tsix mirrors the pattern of X-inactivation choice in mice. *Mol Cell Biol* **26** 2109-17.

Burdge GC & Lillycrop KA 2010 Nutrition, Epigenetics, and Developmental Plasticity: Implications for Understanding Human Diseas. *Annu Rev Nutr* Apr 20 (Electronic publication ahead of print).

Burt BE, Hess BW, Nathanielsz PW & Ford SP 2007 Flock differences in the impact of maternal dietary restriction on offspring growth and glucose tolerance in female offspring. *Soc Reprod Fertil Suppl* **64** 411-24.

Chadio SE, Kotsampasi B, Papadomichelakis G, Deligeorgis S, Kalogiannis D, Menegatos I & Zervas G 2007 Impact of maternal undernutrition on the hypothalamic-pituitary-adrenal axis responsiveness in sheep at different ages postnatal. *J Endocrinol* **192** 495-503.

Chan LL, Sebert SP, Hyatt MA, Stephenson T, Budge H, Symonds ME & Gardner DS 2009 Effect of maternal nutrient restriction from early to midgestation on cardiac function and metabolism after adolescent-onset obesity. *Am J Physiol Regul Integr Comp Physiol* **296** R1455-63.

Clarke L, Heasman L, Juniper DT & Symonds ME 1998 Maternal nutrition in early-mid gestation and placental size in sheep. *Br.J Nutr.* **79** 359-364.

Cleal JK, Poore KR, Boullin JP, Khan O, Chau R, Hambidge O, Torrens C, Newman JP, Poston L, Noakes DE, Hanson MA & Green LR 2007 Mismatched pre- and postnatal nutrition leads to cardiovascular dysfunction and altered renal function in adulthood. *Proc Natl Acad Sci U.S.A* **104** 9529-33.

Dwyer CM, Lawrence AB, Bishop SC & Lewis M 2003 Ewe-lamb bonding behaviours at birth are affected by maternal undernutrition in pregnancy. *Br J Nutr* **89** 123-36.

Eckersall PD, Lawson FP, Kyle CE, Waterston M, Bence L, Stear MJ & Rhind SM 2008 Maternal undernutrition and the ovine acute phase response to vaccination. *BMC Vet Res* **4** 1.

Edwards LJ & McMillen IC 2002 Impact of maternal undernutrition during the periconceptional period, fetal number, and fetal sex on the development of the hypothalamo-pituitary adrenal axis in sheep during late gestation. *Biol Reprod* **66** 1562-9.

Elsik CG, Tellam RL, Worley KC *et al*. 2009 The genome sequence of taurine cattle: a window to ruminant biology and evolution. *Science* **324** 522-8.

Erhardt S, Su IH, Schneider R, Barton S,Bannister AJ, Perez-Burgos L, Jenuwein T, Kouzarides T,Tarakhovsky A & Surani MA 2003 Consequences of the depletion of zygotic and embryonic enhancer of zeste 2 during preimplantation mouse development. *Development* **130** 4235-48.

Erhard HW, Boissy A, Rae MT & Rhind SM 2004 Effects of prenatal undernutrition on emotional reactivity and cognitive flexibility in adult sheep. *Behav Brain Res* **151** 25-35.

Ford SP, Hess BW, Schwope MM, Nijland MJ, Gilbert JS, Vonnahme KA, Means WJ, Han H & Nathanielsz PW 2007 Maternal undernutrition during early to mid-gestation in the ewe results in altered growth, adiposity, and glucose tolerance in male offspring. *J Anim Sci* **85** 1285-94.

Fulka H, St John JC, Fulka J & Hozak P 2008 Chromatin in early mammalian embryos: achieving the pluripotent state. *Differentiation* **76** 3-14.

Gallaher BW, Breier BH, Keven CL, Harding JE & Gluckman PD 1998 Fetal programming of insulin-like growth factor (IGF)-I and IGF-binding protein-3: evidence for an altered response to undernutrition in late gestation following exposure to periconceptual undernutrition in the sheep. *J Endocrinol.* **159** 501-8.

Gardner DS, Pearce S, Dandrea J, Walker R, Ramsay MM, Stephenson T & Symonds ME 2004 Peri-implantation undernutrition programs blunted angiotensin II evoked baroreflex responses in young adult sheep. *Hypertension* **43** 1290-6.

Gardner DS, Tingey K, Van Bon BW, Ozanne SE, Wilson V, Dandrea J, Keisler DH, Stephenson T & Symonds ME 2005 Programming of glucose-insulin metabolism in adult sheep after maternal undernutrition. *Am J Physiol Regul Integr Comp Physiol* **289** R947-54.

Gardner DS, Van Bon BW, Dandrea J, Goddard PJ, May SF, Wilson V, Stephenson T & Symonds ME 2006 Effect of periconceptional undernutrition and gender on hypothalamic-pituitary-adrenal axis function in young adult sheep *J Endocrinol* **190** 203-12.

Garry RC 1944 The Influence of Diet on Pregnancy and Lactation in the Mother, the Growth and Viability of the Foetus, and Post-Natal Development. Part 1. Pregnancy. *Proceedings of the Nutrition Society* 1 226-48.

Goll MG & Bestor TH 2005 Eukaryotic cytosine methyltransferases. *Annu Rev Biochem* **74** 481-514.

Gopalakrishnan GS, Gardner DS, Rhind SM, Rae MT, Kyle CE, Brooks AN, Walker RM, Ramsay MM, Keisler DH, Stephenson T & Symonds ME 2004 Programming of adult cardiovascular function after early maternal undernutrition in sheep. *Am J Physiol Regul Integr Comp Physiol* **287** R12-20.

Gopalakrishnan GS, Gardner DS, Dandrea J, Langley-Evans SC, Pearce S, Kurlak LO, Walker RM, Seetho IW, Keisler DH, Ramsay MM, Stephenson T & Symonds ME 2005 Influence of maternal pre-pregnancy body composition and diet during early-mid pregnancy on cardiovascular function and nephron number in juvenile sheep. *Br J Nutr* **94** 938-47.

Grace KS & Sinclair KD 2009 Assisted reproductive technology, epigenetics, and long-term health: a developmental time bomb still ticking. *Semin Reprod Med* **27** 409-16.

Guerrero-Bosagna CM & Skinner MK 2009 Epigenetic transgenerational effects of endocrine disruptors on male reproduction. *Semin Reprod Med* **27** 403-408.

Gutiérrez-Adán A, Perez-Crespo M, Fernandex-Gonzalez R, Ramirez MA, Moreira P, Pintado B, Lonergan P & Rizos D 2006 Developmental consequences of sexual dimorphism during pre-implantation embryonic development. *Reprod Domest Anim* **41** Suppl 2 54-62.

Hajkova P, Erhardt S, Lane N, Haaf T, El-Maarri O, Reik W, Walter J & Surani MA 2002 Epigenetic reprogramming in mouse primordial germ cells. *Mech Dev* **117** 15-23.

Harrison M & Langley-Evans SC 2008 Intergenerational programming of impaired nephrogenesis and hypertension in rats following maternal protein restriction during pregnancy. *Br J Nutr* **101** 1020-1030.

Heijmans BT, Tobi EW, Stein AD, Putter H, Blauw GJ, Susser ES, Slagboom PE &Lumey, LH 2008 Persistent epigenetic differences associated with prenatal exposure to famine in humans. *Proc Natl Acad Sci U S A* **105** 17046-9.

Hernandez CE, Harding JE, Oliver MH, Bloomfield FH, Held SD & Matthews LR 2009 Effects of litter size, sex and periconceptional ewe nutrition on side preference and cognitive flexibility in the offspring. *Behav Brain Res* **204** 82-7.

Hirasawa R, Chiba H, Kaneda M, Tajima S, Li E, Jaenisch R & Sasaki H 2008 Maternal and zygotic Dnmt1 are necessary and sufficient for the maintenance of DNA methylation imprints during preimplantation development. *Genes Dev* **22** 1607-16.

Hou J, Liu L, Zhang J, Cui XH, Yan FX, Guan H, Chen YF & An XR 2008 Epigenetic modification of histone 3 at lysine 9 in sheep zygotes and its relationship with DNA methylation. *BMC Dev Biol* **8** 60.

Illingworth RS & Bird AP 2009 CpG islands--'a rough guide'. *FEBS Lett* **583** 1713-20.

Irizarry RA, Ladd-Acosta C, Wen B, Wu Z, Montano C, Onyango P, Cui H, Gabo K, Rongione M, Webster M, Ji H, Potash JB, Sabunciyan S, Feinberg AP. 2009 The human colon cancer methylome shows similar hypo- and hypermethylation at conserved tissue-specific CpG island shores. *Nat Genet.* **41** 178-186.

Jorgensen W, Gam C, Andersen JL, Schjerling P, Scheibye-Knudsen M, Mortensen OH, Grunnet N, Nielsen MO & Quistorff B 2009 Changed mitochondrial function by pre- and/or postpartum di *et al*terations in sheep. *Am J Physiol Endocrinol Metab* **297** E1349-57.

Kwon H, Ford SP, Bazer FW, Spencer TE, Nathanielsz PW, Nijland MJ, Hess BW &Wu G 2004 Maternal nutrient restriction reduces concentrations of amino acids and polyamines in ovine maternal and fetal plasma and fetal fluids. *Biology of Reproduction* **71** 901-908.

Kwong WY, Wild AE, Roberts P, Willis AC & Fleming TP 2000 Maternal undernutrition during the preimplantation period of rat development causes blastocyst abnormalities and programming of postnatal hypertension. *Development* **127** 4195-202.

Kwong W Y, Miller DJ, Ursell E, Wild AE, Wilkins AP, Osmond C, Anthony FW & Fleming TP 2006 Imprinted gene expression in the rat embryo-fetal axis is altered in response to periconceptional maternal low protein diet. *Reproduction* **132** 265-77.

Kwong WY, Adamiak SJ, Gwynn A, Singh R & Sinclair KD 2010 Endogenous folates and single-carbon metabolism in the ovarian follicle, oocyte and preimplantation embryo *Reproduction* **139** 705-15.

Lander ES, Linton LM, Birren B *et al.* 2001 Initial sequencing and analysis of the human genome. *Nature* **409** 860-921.

Lane M & Gardner DK 2003 Ammonium induces aberrant blastocyst differentiation, metabolism, pH regulation, gene expression and subsequently alters fetal development in the mouse. *Biol Reprod* **69** 1109-17.

Lees-Murdock DJ & Walsh CP 2008 DNA methylation reprogramming in the germline. *Adv Exp Med Biol* **626** 1-15.

Lister R, Pelizzola M, Dowen RH et al. 2009 Human DNA methylomes at base resolution show widespread epigenomic differences *Nature* **462** 315-322

Lucifero D, La Salle S, Bourc'his D, Martel J, Bestor TH & Trasler JM 2007 Coordinate regulation of DNA methyltransferase expression during oogenesis. *BMC Dev Biol* **7** 36.

Maunakea AK, Nagarajan RP, Bilenky M, Ballinger TJ, D'Souza C, Fouse SD, Johnson BE, Hong C, Nielsen C, Zhao Y, Turecki G, Delaney A, Varhol R, Thiessen N, Shchors K, Heine VM, Rowitch DH, Xing X, Fiore C, Schillebeeckx M, Jones SJ, Haussler D, Marra MA, Hirst M, Wang T & Costello JF 2010 Conserved role of intragenic DNA methylation in regulating alternative promoters. *Nat. 466* 253-257.

Morgan HD, Santos F, Green K, Dean W & Reik W 2005 Epigenetic reprogramming in mammals. *Hum Mol Genet* **14** R47-58.

Nakamura T, Arai Y, Umehara H, Masuhara M,Kimura T, Taniguchi H, Sekimoto T, Ikawa M, Yoneda Y, Okabe M, Tanaka S, Shiota K & Nakano T 2007 PGC7/Stella protects against DNA demethylation in early embryogenesis. *Nat Cell Biol* **9** 64-71.

Niemann H, Tian XC, King WA & Lee RS 2008 Epigenetic reprogramming in embryonic and foetal development upon somatic cell nuclear transfer cloning. *Reproduction* **135** 151-63.

Okada Y, Yamagata K, Hong K, Wakayama, T & Zhang Y 2010 A role for the elongator complex in zygotic paternal genome demethylation. *Nature* **463** 554-8.

Ooi SK & Bestor TH 2008 The colorful history of active DNA demethylation. *Cell* **133** 1145-8.

Petronis A 2010 Epigenetics as a unifying principle in the aetiology of complex traits and diseases. *Nature* **465** 721-727.

Poore KR, Cleal JK, Newman JP, Boullin JP, Noakes DE, Hanson MA & Green LR 2007 Nutritional challenges during development induce sex-specific changes in glucose homeostasis in the adult sheep. *Am J Physiol Endocrinol Metab* **292** E32-9.

Popp C, Dean W, Feng S, Cokus SJ, Andrews S, Pellegrini M, Jacobsen SE & Reik W 2010 Genome-wide erasure of DNA methylation in mouse primordial germ cells is affected by AID deficiency. *Nature* **463** 1101-5.

Powell K, Rooke JA, McEvoy TG Ashworth CJ, Robinson JJ, Wilmut I, Young LE, Sinclair KD 2006 Zygote donor nitrogen metabolism and in vitro embryo culture perturbs in utero development and IGF2R expression in ovine fetal tissues. *Theriogenology* **66** 1901-12.

Reik, W. 2007 Stability and flexibility of epigenetic gene regulation in mammalian development. *Nature* **447** 425-32,

Rhodes P, Craigon J, Gray C, Rhind SM, Loughna PT & Gardner DS 2009 Adult-onset obesity reveals prenatal programming of glucose-insulin sensitivity in male sheep nutrient restricted during late gestation. *PLoS One* **4** e7393.

Russo V, Martelli A, Berardinelli P, Di Giacinto O, Bernabo N, Fantasia D, Mattioli M & Barboni B 2007 Modifications in chromatin morphology and organization during sheep oogenesis. *Microsc Res Tech* **70** 733-44.

Santos F, Peters AH, Otte AP, Reik W & Dean W 2005 Dynamic chromatin modifications characterise the first cell cycle in mouse embryos. *Dev Biol* **280** 225-36.

Sanz LA, Kota SK & Feil R 2010 Genome-wide DNA demethylation in mammals. *Genome Biol* **11** 110.

Sebert SP, Hyatt MA, Chan LLY, Patel N, Bell RC, Keisler D, Stephenson T, Budge H, Symonds ME & Gardner DS 2009 Maternal Nutrient Restriction between Early and Midgestation and Its Impact Upon Appetite Regulation after Juvenile Obesity. *Endocrinology* **150** 634-41.

Sinclair KD, Young LE, Wilmut I & McEvoy TG 2000a In-utero overgrowth in ruminants following embryo culture: lessons from mice and a warning to men. *Hum Reprod* 15(Suppl 5) 68–86

Sinclair KD, Kuran M, Gebbie FE, Webb, R & McEvoy TG 2000b Nitrogen metabolism and fertility in cattle: II. Development of oocytes recovered from heifers offered diets differing in their rate of nitrogen release in the rumen. *J. Anim Sci* **78** 2670-2680.

Sinclair KD, Allegrucci C, Singh R, Gardner DS, Sebastian S, Bispham J, Thurston A, Huntley JF, Rees WD, Maloney CA, Lea RG, Craigon J, McEvoy TG & Young LE 2007 DNA methylation, insulin resistance, and blood pressure in offspring determined by maternal periconceptional B vitamin and methionine status. *Proc Natl Acad Sci U S A* **104** 19351-6.

Sinclair KD & Singh R 2007 Modelling the developmental origins of health and disease in the early embryo. *Theriogenology* **67** 43-53.

Song F, Smith JF, Kimura MT, Morrow AD, Matsuyama T. Nagase H & Held WA 2005 Association of tissue-specific differentially methylated regions (TDMs) with differential gene expression. *Proc Natl Acad Sci U S A* **102** 3336-41.

Steegers-Theunissen RP, Obermann-Borst SA, Kremer D, Lindemans J, Siebel C, Steegers EA, Slagboom PE & Heijmans BT 2009 Periconceptional maternal folic acid use of 400 microg per day is related to increased methylation of the IGF2 gene in the very young child *PLoS One* **4** e7845.

Steele W, Allegrucci C, Singh R, Lucas E, Priddle H, Denning C, Sinclair K & Young L 2005 Human embryonic stem cell methyl cycle enzyme expression: modelling epigenetic programming in assisted reproduction? *Reprod Biomed Online* **10** 755-66.

Thu KL, Pikor LA, Kennett, JY, Alvarez CE & Lam WL 2009 Methylation analysis by DNA immunoprecipitation *J Cell Physiol* **222** 522-531.

Todd SE, Oliver MH, Jaquiery AL, Bloomfield FH & Harding JE 2009 Periconceptional undernutrition of ewes impairs glucose tolerance in their adult offspring. *Pediatr Res* **65** 409-13.

Torres-Padilla ME, Parfitt DE, Kouzarides T & Zernicka-Goetz M 2007 Histone arginine methylation regulates pluripotency in the early mouse embryo. *Nature* **445** 214-8.

Trahair JF, DeBarro TM, Robinson JS & Owens JA 1997 Restriction of nutrition in utero selectively inhibits gastrointestinal growth in fetal sheep. *J Nutr* **127** 637-41.

Warnes KE, Morris MJ, Symonds ME, Phillips ID, Clarke IJ, Owens JA & McMillen IC 1998 Effects of increasing gestation, cortisol and maternal undernutrition on hypothalamic neuropeptide Y expression in the sheep fetus. *J Neuroendocrinol* **10** 51-7.

Watanabe D, Suetake I, Tada T & Tajima S 2002 Stage- and cell-specific expression of Dnmt3a and Dnmt3b during embryogenesis. *Mech Dev* **118** 187-90.

Williams PJ, Kurlak LO, Perkins AC, Budge H, Stephenson T, Keisler D, Symonds ME & Gardner DS 2007 Hypertension and impaired renal function accompany juvenile obesity: The effect of prenatal diet. *Kidney Int* **73** 279-89.

Young LE, Fernandes K, McEvoy TG, Butterwith SC, Gutierrez CG, Carolan C, Broadbent PJ, Robinson JJ, Wilmut I & Sinclair KD 2001 Epigenetic change in IGF2R is associated with fetal overgrowth after sheep embryo culture. *Nat Genet* **27** 153-4.

The noncoding genome: implications for ruminant reproductive biology

D Tesfaye[1], MM Hossain[2] and K Schellander[1]

[1] *Institute of Animal Science, University of Bonn, Endenicher Allee 15, 53115 Bonn, Germany;* [2] *Dept. of Animal Breeding and Genetics, Bangladesh Agricultural University, Mymensingh-2202, Bangladesh*

Advances in the analyses of human and other higher eukaryotic genomes have disclosed a large fraction of the genetic material (ca 98%) which does not code for proteins. Major portion of this non-coding genome is in fact transcribed into an enormous repertoire of functional non coding RNA molecules (ncRNAs) rather than encoding any proteins. Recent fascinating and fast progress in bioinformatic, high-throughput sequencing and other biochemical approaches have fuelled rapid growth in our appreciation of the tremendous number, diversity and biological importance of these ncRNAs in the hidden layer of gene regulation both at transcriptional and post-transcriptional level. Broadly ncRNAs fall into three size classes namely, ~20 nucleotides for the large family of microRNAs (miRNAs), to 25-200 nucleotides for other different families of small RNAs and finally to over thousands of nucleotides for macro ncRNAs involved in eukaryotic gene regulation. Among the ncRNAs that have revolutionized our understanding of eukaryotic gene expression, microRNAs (miRNAs) have recently been emphasized extensively with enormous potential for playing a pivotal role in disease, fertility and development. They are found to be potentially involved in various aspects of physiological regulation of reproductive tissues (testis, ovary, endometrium and oviduct), cells (sperm and oocytes) and embryonic development in addition to other body systems. Here, we review the recent work on miRNAs in details and some other small ncRNAs briefly in animal models focusing on their diverse roles in the physiology of reproductive cells and tissues together with their implications for ruminant reproductive biology.

Introduction

Proteomic analysis of genome sequences in the past highlighted only mRNA-coding genes and non-protein-coding transcripts were often overlooked. Genomic analysis in the last decade however revealed that with an increase in genome complexity, the protein coding fractions of genome is much fewer compared to non-coding portion. It is estimated, that around 98% of the transcriptional outputs of eukaryotic genomes consist of large proportion of RNAs, which do not encode proteins (Adams *et al.* 2000). This vast untranslated fraction of the genome harbors thousands of genes which lead to transcription of a remarkable number of functional non-coding RNAs (Mattick & Makunin 2006). Beside the initial discovery of the ribosomal

Corresponding author E-mail: tesfaye@itw.uni-bonn.de

RNAs, small nuclear RNAs and transfer RNAs that are involved in mRNA splicing and translation, many more classes and types of recently discovered ncRNAs are also known to be involved in the regulatory functions namely, but not limited to, transcriptional and post transcriptional gene regulation, chromosome replication, RNA processing, site-specific RNA modification, DNA methylation, telomere synthesis and length differentiation, protein degradation and protein translocation (Storz 2002, Hannon *et al.* 2006). Ongoing identification of new classes of non-coding RNAs (ncRNAs) and new member of existing classes presently underscores the paramount importance of ncRNAs function at many levels essential for gene expression and genome stability.

Types of ncRNAs are emerging from occasional discoveries with varying in size, mechanisms of biosynthesis and their regulatory mechanisms. However, their list is continuously and tremendously increasing and getting appreciation for their functional importance. Broadly, ncRNAs could be differentiated into three classes according to their range in size. Among them, the tiny one known as miRNAs which ranges in size about 20-24 nucleotides (nt) and have been found to modulate development of mammals and engaged in disease development as well as contributing to the fertility of different species through post transcriptional gene regulation. The group of ncRNAs ranging in size 100-200 nt are designated as small RNAs commonly found as translational regulators in bacteria and some other species as well. Lastly, the ncRNAs comprising the majority of longer transcripts to over 10000 nt in size are called macro ncRNAs involved in epigenetic regulation of gene expression in eukaryotes (Hutvagner & Zamore 2002, Storz 2002). In contrast to the uncertainty surrounding the function of most mammalian macro ncRNAs, imprinted macro ncRNAs have clearly been identified as regulator of flanking genes by DNA methylation (Koerner *et al.* 2009). Small non coding RNAs such as miRNAs, short interfering RNAs, piwi-interacting RNAs and short nucleolar RNAs are associated with trans-acting functions, whereas macro ncRNAs are so far only associated to cis-acting functions.

However, as knowledge on the types and the members of each type are still limited, most of these biochemically abundant species of ncRNAs are yet to be discovered. It is likely that there are many more ncRNAs than was ever suspected. Here we review the recent reports on the small non-coding RNAs with particular emphasis on miRNAs in details and some other selected small ncRNAs briefly in animal models focusing on their diverse roles in the physiology of reproductive cells (germ cells) and tissues (testis, ovary, endometrium, oviduct and embryo) together with their implications for ruminant reproductive biology.

Small non-coding RNAs and gene regulation

The notion of the sncRNAs is not new - for example 5S rRNAs, U6 RNA, snoRNAs, BC200 RNA, etc. were discovered long before, but they are only recently highlighted because of growing list of classes and members of sncRNAs which are found to be physiologically important as riboregulators. A short list of several classes of sncRNAs in different species with their potential functions are presented but not limited to Table 1. Among these all ncRNAs, miRNAs and some other small ncRNAs have revolutionized our understanding of a hidden layer of new gene regulation now-a-days. MiRNAs are the well characterized ones getting more attention to the scientific community due to their high level of importance. Diverse expression pattern of miRNAs and high number of their potential target mRNAs suggest their involvement in the regulation of various developmentally related genes at post-transcriptional level (Lau *et al.* 2001, Lai 2003, Ambros 2004, Bartel 2004, Alvarez-Garcia & Miska 2005, Plasterk 2006, Chen & Rajewsky 2007). The tiny (18-24 nt in length) and single-stranded, derived from primary transcripts termed as "pri-miRNAs", having an RNA hairpin structure of 60-120 nt with a mature

Table 1. Classes of small ncRNAs (≤ 200 nt) in different species with their functions

Class of sncRNA	Length (nt)	Potential/probable function	Example species	Reference
Small interfering RNA (siRNA)	19–21	Target mRNA cleavage	Reported in many species	(Fire *et al.* 1998), Reviewed in (Rana 2007)
Trans-acting siRNA (tasiRNA)	21–22	mRNA cleavage	Arabidopsis	(Peragine *et al.* 2004, Vazquez *et al.* 2004)
MicroRNA (miRNA)	19–25	Translational repression	Mammals, Birds, flies, Nematodes, etc. (conserved)	(Lee *et al.* 1993, Bagga *et al.* 2005)
Repeat-associated siRNA (rasiRNA)	24–27	Transposon control, transcriptional silencing	Yeast, plants & flies	(Aravin *et al.* 2001, Reinhart & Bartel 2002, Volpe *et al.* 2002, Grewal & Moazed 2003, Carrington 2005)
Piwi-interacting RNA (piRNA)	26–31	Transposon control in germ cells	Mammals	(O'Donnell & Boeke 2007)
Small-scan RNA (scnRNA)	~ 28	Histone methylation, DNA elimination	Tetrahymena	(Mochizuki *et al.* 2002)
gCYb gRNA	68	Directs insertion & excision of uridines	*T. brucei*	(Kable *et al.* 1997, Souza *et al.* 1997, Simpson *et al.* 2000)
RyhB sRNA	80	Targets mRNAs for degradation	*E. coli*	(Masse & Gottesman 2002)
DsrA sRNA	87	Preventing formation of an inhibitory mRNA structure	*E. coli*	(Wassarman *et al.* 1999, Altuvia & Wagner 2000)
U18 C/D snoRNA	102	Directs 29-0-ribose methylation of target rRNA	*S. cerevisiae*	(Samarsky & Fournier 1999, Kiss 2001)
OxyS	109	Represses ranslation by occluding ribosome binding	*E. coli*	(Wassarman *et al.* 1999, Altuvia & Wagner 2000)
4.5S RNA	114	Protein translocation	*E. coli*	(Wassarman *et al.* 1999, Keenan *et al.* 2001)
6S RNA	184	Transcription: Modulates promoter use	*E. coli*	(Wassarman *et al.* 1999, Wassarman & Storz 2000)
U2 snRNA	186	RNA processing: Core of spliceosome	Human	(Gu *et al.* 1998, Will & Luhrmann 2001)
BC1 RNA	142–165	Amplification of short interspersed elements	Rodents	(Shen *et al.* 1997)
snR8 H/ACA snoRNA	189	Directs pseudouridylation of target rRNA	*S. cerevisiae*	(Samarsky & Fournier 1999, Kiss 2001)
BC200 RNA	195–205	Encodes a neural small cytoplasmic RNA	Primates, human	(Martignetti & Brosius 1993)

miRNA in one of the two strands (Fig. 1). This hairpin in turn is cleaved from the pri-miRNA in the nucleus by the double-strand-specific ribonuclease, Drosha (Lee *et al.* 2002). The resulting precursor miRNA (pre-miRNA) is transported to the cytoplasm via a process that involves Exportin-5 (Yi *et al.* 2003) and subsequently cleaved by Dicer (Lee *et al.* 2003) to generate a short, double-stranded RNA duplex. One of the strands of the miRNA duplex is incorporated into a protein complex termed RNA induced silencing complex (RISC). RISC is guided by the incorporated miRNA strand to mRNAs containing complementary sequences in 3´ untranslated region to 7- to 8-nt region of 5´ end of miRNA called seed sequence, which primarily results in inhibition of mRNA translation (Pillai *et al.* 2005) (Fig. 1). Blocking the translation of mRNAs occurs through interaction of RISC with eukaryotic translation initiation factor 6, which prevents assembly of 80S ribosomes (Chendrimada *et al.* 2007), or through inhibition of translation after initiation (Jackson & Standart 2007). Recent reports have also indicated that miRNA, with or without perfect sequence complementarity, can cause an increase in mRNA degradation by endonucleolytic cleavage or deadenylation, respectively (Jackson & Standart 2007) or changes in proteins associated with RISC can cause a shift from translational inhibition to translational enhancement (Vasudevan *et al.* 2007, Orom *et al.* 2008). Those mRNAs which are repressed by miRNAs are further stored in the cytoplasmic foci called P-bodies (Liu *et al.* 2005a, Liu *et al.* 2005b, Rehwinkel *et al.* 2005). MiRNAs have found to play an integral part of animal gene regulatory networks as one of the most abundant classes of gene regulators.

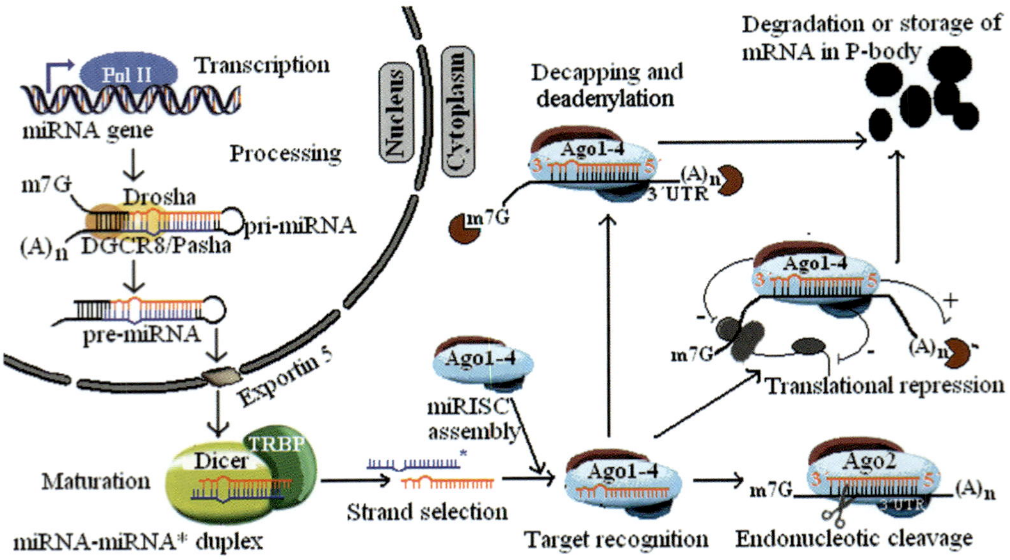

Fig. 1. Biogenesis of miRNAs and their mechanism of gene regulation.
Pri-miRNAs, which are generally synthesized by RNA polymerase II, are trimmed in the nucleus by Drosha to generate a ~60-nt pre-miRNA which is exported to the cytoplasm, where it is further processed by Dicer, in association with one of the four mammalian Argonaute proteins (Ago) and TBRP. Target mRNAs are recognized by miRNAs in the form of ribonucleoprotein complexes (miRNPs) through sequence complementarity, usually between the miRNA and sequences in the 3´-UTR of the mRNA. The miRNP complex which is loaded onto the target mRNA exhibits direct or indirect effect in translational repression. Direct effects occur either through inhibition of initiation (-) of translation through binding Ago2 to m^7G (7-methyl-G cap) results in prevention of ribosome association with the target mRNA, or through inhibition of translation post-initiation, which includes premature ribosome drop off, slowed or stalled elongation, and co-translational protein. In addition to direct effects on translation (or protein accumulation), miRNPs can have other effects on targeted mRNAs, including promoting deadenylation (+), which might result in degradation (increased turnover) (Nilsen 2007). Translational repression and/or deadenylation occurs followed by decapping and exonuclease-mediated degradation if base-pairing is partially complementary or, in the case of perfect complementarity and provided the miRNP contains specifically Ago2, may result in endonucleolytic cleavage of the mRNA at the site where the miRNA is annealed (Standart & Jackson 2007).

Despite the fact that animal miRNAs, which are the focus of this review, have a significant importance in the reproductive process, the other types of small noncoding RNA with distinct properties also deserve more attention. Small interfering RNAs (siRNAs) differ from miRNAs mainly in their Origin. They are the products of long, Dicer-processed, double-stranded (ds) RNAs that silence genes by cleaving their target mRNAs (Fig. 2A) [reviewed in Reference (Chu & Rana 2007)]. The RNAi was first discovered by introduction of long ds RNAs into C. elegans (Fire *et al.* 1998). Like endogenous miRNAs, long dsRNAs are processed by the Dicer-TRBP-PACT complex [reviewed in Reference (Chu & Rana 2007, Rana 2007)]. This dsRNA-processing step creates RNA with 2-nt overhangs at their 3´ ends and phosphate groups at their 5´ termini. The anti-sense strand of siRNA, known as the guide strand serves as the template for sequence-specific gene silencing by the RNAi machinery (Fig. 2A). The sense strand is known as the passenger strand. Subsequent to Dicer processing, the 21–23 nt guide strand of duplex siRNA is loaded into Ago2 to form the effector siRISC. Ago2 is the endonuclease responsible for the cleavage activity of siRISC. With perfect base pairing and formation of an A-form helix structure between the siRNA guide strand and its target mRNA, siRISC cleaves its target 10–11 nt from the 5´ end of the guide siRNA strand, and the complex is recycled for the next round of target mRNA cleavage. mRNAs cleaved by siRISC are subsequently degraded by cellular exonucleases, resulting in robust depletion of target genes [reviewed in (Chu & Rana 2007, Rana 2007)].

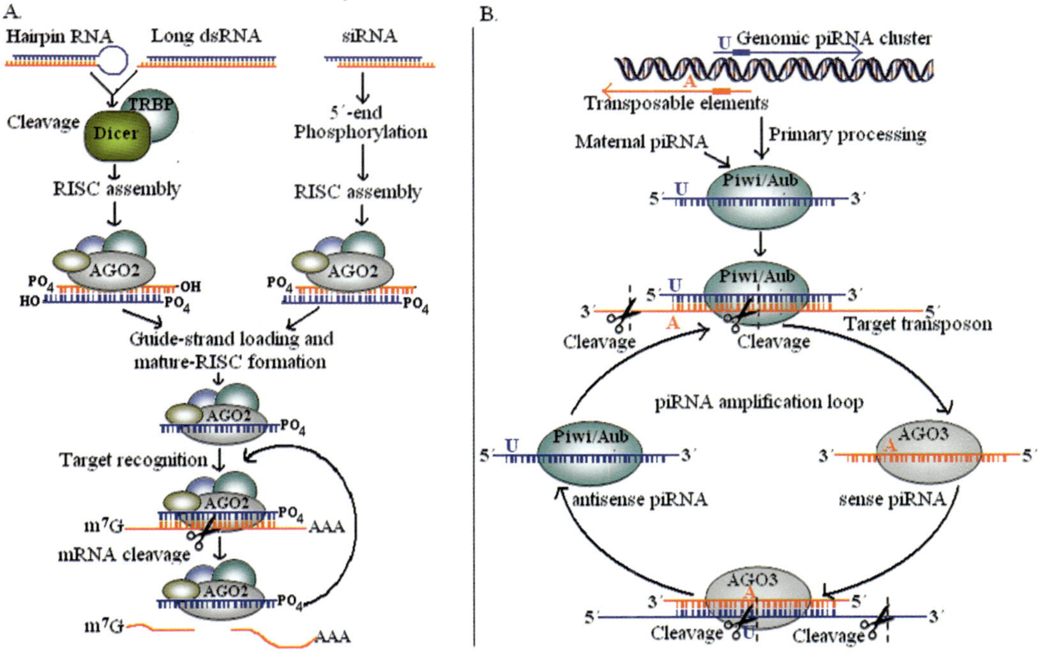

Fig. 2. Gene silencing by siRNAs (A) and biogenesis of piRNAs (B).

Piwi-interacting RNAs (piRNAs) are a third group of small RNAs (24- to 30-nt) generated by a Dicer-independent mechanism and are associated with members of the Piwi family, a subtype of Argonaute proteins with MIWI, MILI, and MIWI2 orthologs (Kuramochi-Miyagawa *et al.* 2001, Aravin *et al.* 2006, Lau *et al.* 2006, Watanabe *et al.* 2006). PiRNAs can be derived from either transposons and other repeated sequence elements or complex DNA sequence elements (Aravin *et al.* 2007, Brennecke *et al.* 2007, Houwing *et al.* 2007). Those piRNAs which are derived from repeated sequence elements are specifically designated as repeat-associated small interfering RNAs (rasiRNAs). Based on the studies in Drosophila and mouse, piRNA has been found to be produced like ping-pong manner, in which Ago3 bound to sense-strand piRNAs catalyzes antisense-strand cleavage at an A:U base-pair that generates the 5´ end of antisense piRNAs (Fig. 2B) (Aravin *et al.* 2007, Brennecke *et al.* 2007, Gunawardane *et al.* 2007). The 5´ ends of the resulting cleavage products are proposed to be associated with Aub or Piwi, with nucleolytic processing of the 3´ overhangs generating mature 23- to 30-nt antisense piRNAs (Fig. 2B). The mature antisense piRNA Argonaute complexes are then proposed to bind and cleave sense strand RNAs, silencing gene expression and generating the 5´ end of sense-strand piRNA precursors that will be associated with Ago3. Processing of the 3´ overhang produces mature sense-strand piRNAs, completing the cycle (Fig. 2B) reviewed by (Klattenhoff & Theurkauf 2008). Genetic studies in mice, *Drosophila* and zebrafish showed that piRNAs are crucial to germline development (Kuramochi-Miyagawa *et al.* 2004, Carmell *et al.* 2007, Houwing *et al.* 2007) and proteins involved in piRNA production have also been implicated in the control of gene expression in somatic cells (Pal-Bhadra *et al.* 2004, Grimaud *et al.* 2006).

Function of miRNAs in reproduction

miRNAs are estimated to comprise 1–5% of animal genes (Bartel 2004, Bentwich *et al.* 2005, Berezikov *et al.* 2005) or a given genome could encode nearly thousands of miRNAs (Bentwich *et al.* 2005). Moreover, a typical miRNA regulates hundreds of target genes (Brennecke *et al.* 2005, Krek *et al.* 2005, Lewis *et al.* 2005, Xie *et al.* 2005) and altogether they could target a large proportion of genes up to 30% of the genome (Lim *et al.* 2005). Changes in the expression of even a single miRNA found to have a significant impact on the outcome of diverse cellular activities. Inhibition of miRNA biogenesis has been found to be resulted in developmental arrest in mouse and fish (Bernstein *et al.* 2003, Wienholds *et al.* 2003, Giraldez *et al.* 2005) and female infertility in mouse (Otsuka *et al.* 2007, Otsuka *et al.* 2008). Investigation on the potential role of miRNA in reproduction up-to-date has been accomplished by the different approach. First, by identifying the population of miRNAs in the germ cells and reproductive tissues through cloning method. Second, by investigating the expression of candidate miRNA or group of miRNAs using microarray platform or RT-PCR approach. Third, by localizing candidate miRNA in the tissue or cell using in-situ hybridization approach. Forth, by knocking down global miRNA expression by creating Dicer1 knockout mice. Finally, by investigating specific miRNA function through using the oligonucleotide inhibitors and/or miRNA mimics or precursors. Accounting the studies and approaches published so far, the following sub-sections describe the role of miRNAs with respect to reproductive biology.

Function of miRNAs in the female reproduction

Expression and regulation of miRNAs in the mammalian ovarian cells and their function

Dynamically regulated, complex and coordinated ovarian functions include sequential recruitment, selection and growth of the follicles, atresia, ovulation and luteolysis are under control of closely coordinated endocrine and paracrine factors. All these factors are controlled by tightly regulated expression and interaction of a multitude of genes in different compartments of the ovary (Bonnet *et al.* 2008). As one of the major classes of gene regulators, miRNAs are considered to be involved in the regulation of ovarian genes (Ro *et al.* 2007a, Hossain *et al.* 2009). Several studies expanding from identification and expression profiling to functional involvement of miRNAs in the ovary have been carried out in different animal species. Four attempts have led to identify the distinct and major population of miRNAs in 2 weeks old and adult mouse ovary (Ro *et al.* 2007b), adult mouse ovary and testis (Mishima *et al.* 2008), adult bovine ovary (Hossain *et al.* 2009) and new born mouse ovary (Ahn *et al.* 2010) through small RNA library construction and sequencing. Regardless of species these studies showed that let-7 family, miR-21, miR-99a, miR-125b, miR-126, miR-143, miR-145 and miR-199b to be most commonly abundant miRNAs in the ovary. The presence of miRNAs and their differential expression can give the primary clue for their potential role in ovarian function. However, further functional characterization of these miRNAs in different cell types of ovary (oocyte, granulosa, theca cells and ovarian stroma) at different follicular stage or at different estrus cycle remains to be elucidated. Although bioinformatic prediction and analysis of ovary specific mRNAs targets for these enriched miRNAs revealed several molecular and cellular pathways and physiological functions important for ovarian follicular development (Hossain *et al.* 2009), atresia, ovulation as well as ovarian dysfunction, the identification of functional target mRNAs remains to be validated by appropriate wet lab experiment.

Several studies highlighted the expression and regulation of some individual miRNAs in different ovarian cells especially in oocyte and granulosa cells. After disclosing the absence or less role of sperm born miRNAs in mammalian fertilization (Amanai *et al.* 2006), further studies were directed towards these two cell types (oocyte and granulosa). For example, the first attempt was made in 2006 and the study identified small number of miRNAs as well as some other small noncoding RNAs (rasiRNAs, gsRNAs) in mouse oocyte (Watanabe *et al.* 2006). However, further identification of miRNAs in oocytes through direct cloning method is still missing rather more initiative has been taken for microarray or RT-PCR based miRNAs detection through homologous or heterologous approach. For example, the differential expression of miRNAs has been identified during bovine oocyte maturation and preimplantation embryo development in-vitro using the heterologous approach (Tesfaye *et al.* 2009).

The Microarray experiments show that Dicer1 is highly expressed and functionally important in the oocytes during folliculogenesis as well as in the mature oocytes (Su *et al.* 2002, Choi *et al.* 2007, Murchison *et al.* 2007). Conditional knockout of Dicer1 in growing oocytes revealed unaffected oocyte growth and folliculogenesis during the early stage but meiosis I has been found to be arrested with defective spindle organization in oocytes lacking Dicer1 (Murchison *et al.* 2007). Moreover, transcriptional analysis through microarray experiments has identified the major portion of the transcripts as misregulated in Dicer1-deficient oocytes. These efforts not only provide initial evidence for the role of miRNAs in the oocyte but also suggested that a large proportion of the maternal genes are directly or indirectly under the control of miRNAs (Murchison *et al.* 2007, Tang *et al.* 2007). However, Suh *et al.* studied the effect of deletion of another miRNAs processing molecules called Dgcr8 and revealed contrasting conclusion that the effects on the phenotypes in Dicer deficient oocytes are rather due to endogenous siRNAs (Suh *et al.* 2010). Moreover, the expression level of miRNAs in Dgcr8 deficient oocyte found to be reduced as similar to the Dicer deficient oocyte. In addition, there was no effect due to deletion of Dgcr8 allele even from maternal and zygotic genome on the phenotype as well as mRNA profile which were very unlikely for Dicer deficient oocytes. These findings show that miRNA function is globally suppressed during oocyte maturation and preimplantation development.

The progress of the study on miRNAs is higher in case of granulosa cells compared to oocyte and other ovarian cell types. For example, study of expression of miRNAs by Fiedler et al. (2008) in mouse mural granulosa cells collected before and after an ovulatory dose of hCG identified miR-132 and miR-212 as highly upregulated following LH/hCG induction.

Further analysis of these two miRNAs in cultured granulosa cells revealed the roles in the post-transcriptional regulation of CtBP1 gene which is known to be interacting with steroidogenic factor-1 and acts as a co-repressor of nuclear receptor target genes. Recently, studies have been conducted to know the role of miRNAs in human granulosa cells (GC) by transfecting 187 individual synthetic miRNA precursors that mimic endogenous precursor miRNAs representing the majority of human miRNAs (Sirotkin *et al.* 2009a). Interestingly, they have screened 80 miRNAs which control both proliferation and apoptosis in ovarian granulosa cells, as well as they have identified miRNAs which promote and suppress these processes utilizing a genome-wide miRNA screen. Transfection of cultured human granulosa cells with 11 out of 80 tested miRNA constructs resulted in significant increase in percentage of cells containing PCNA a cell proliferation marker. These were mir-108, mir-7, mir-9, mir-105, mir-128, mir-132, mir-141, mir-142, mir-152, mir-188 and mir-191. Eleven out of the 80 miRNAs tested in the same experiment (mir-15a, mir-96, mir-92, mir-124, mir-18, mir-29a, mir-125a, mir-136, mir-147, mir-183 and mir-32) found to promote up to 2-fold accumulation of Bax - proapoptic marker in human primary granulosa cells. However, the detailed regulatory mechanism for regulating such two processes through targeting which mRNAs by the individual miRNAs are unknown and remains to be disclosed in future investigation.

The most recent work highlighted one miRNA (miR-224) in detail for regulation of granulosa cell proliferation and thereafter has shown to affect ovarian estrogen release in mouse (Yao *et al.* 2010). In that experiment miR-224 expression was found to be regulated by TGF-ß/Smads pathway through inhibiting TGF-ß superfamily type I receptors (SB431542) which leads to blockage of phosphorylation of the downstream effectors Smad2/3 in vitro in granulosa cells. The ectopic expression of miR-224 was suggested to enhance TGF- ß 1-induced granulosa cell proliferation through targeting Smad4. This was a good demonstration for the notion that miRNAs could control or promote TGF- ß 1-induced GC proliferation and ovarian estrogen release. However, there are many more miRNAs and their mechanism involved in the function of granulosa cells is still remaining to be elucidated. So, to further clarify the role of miRNAs in oogenesis and folliculogenesis, generation of knockouts or knocking down the individual miRNAs could help to understand their critical roles in ovarian development as well as ovarian cellular functions. Information on the regulatory role of miRNAs in the ovarian cells of ruminants compared to human and mouse are so limited and these are the open field for the researcher working on ruminant reproductive biology. Currently, the expression and functional evidence of miRNAs in the follicular theca cells in any physiological states of any species remains to be elucidated.

Ovarian steroidogenesis and miRNAs

Recent studies revealed interesting relationship between ovarian steroids and miRNAs. Several studies suggested ovarian steroid dependent biogenesis & maturation of miRNAs and reversely some set of miRNAs could regulate the secretion of ovarian steroid. It has been first demonstrated that ovarian steroids influence the expression of some miRNAs (hsa-miR20a, hsa-miR21 and hsa-miR26a) in endometrial stromal cell and glandular epithelial cell in human (Pan *et al.* 2007). The molecular mechanism by which ovarian steroids regulate the expression of miRNAs was unclear but such regulatory function has been suggested to alter the expression of their target genes and cellular activities manifested by their products thereby (Pan *et al.* 2007). It has been also shown that LH/hCG regulates the expression of selected miRNAs, which affect posttranscriptional gene regulation in mouse within ovarian granulosa cells (Fiedler *et al.* 2008). Estrogen was found to suppress the levels of a set of miRNAs in mice and human cultured cells through estrogen receptor α (ERα) by associating with the Drosha complex and preventing the conversion of pri-miRNAs into pre-miRNAs (Yamagata *et al.* 2009). As down-regulation of miRNAs appeared to stabilize human VEGF mRNA, the posttranscriptional control by estrogen appears to mediate the half-life of estrogen target genes via regulated miRNA maturation (Yamagata *et al.* 2009). In addition, upregulation of subset of miRNAs in female mice lacking estrogen receptor α and down regulation of some miRNAs in the estrogen target organ (Uterus) was observed following estradiol (E2) treatment in ovariectomized female mice (Macias *et al.* 2009). Altogether these studies suggested that ERα bound to E2 inhibits the production of a subset of miRNAs by a mechanism whereby ERα blocks Drosha-mediated processing of a subset of miRNAs by binding to Drosha in a p68/p72-dependent manner and inducing the dissociation of the microprocessor complex from the pri-miRNA (Macias *et al.* 2009).

In contrast, some miRNAs are also found to play important role in the ovarian steroidogenesis (Sirotkin *et al.* 2009b). Genome-wide screening of miRNAs revealed the involvement of miRNAs in control of release of the ovarian steroid hormones progesterone, androgen and estrogen in human ovarian cells (Sirotkin *et al.* 2009b). They have evaluated the effect of transfection of cultured primary ovarian granulosa cells with gene constructs encoding the majority of identified human pre-miRNAs on release of progesterone, testosterone and estradiol was also evaluated. These results revealed thirty-six out of 80 tested miRNA constructs inhibiting the progesterone release in granulosa cells and 10 miRNAs have been found to promote progesterone release. Subsequent transfection of cells with antisense constructs to two selected miRNAs (mir-15a and mir-188) revealed induction of progesterone output due to lack of blockage of progesterone release. While fifty-seven tested miRNAs were found to inhibit testosterone release, only one miRNA (mir-107) enhanced testosterone output. Fifty-one miRNAs suppressed estradiol release, while none of the 80 miRNAs tested were found to stimulate it (Sirotkin *et al.* 2009b). However, the complex regulatory mechanisms for controlling miRNAs biogenesis by the steroids or vice versa are still unclear. The involvement of miRNAs for such mechanisms as regulator of several hundreds of genes as potential target could be much higher than ever speculated.

Role of miRNAs in other female reproductive tissues and disease conditions

Both physical and functional integrity of the oviduct is responsible for the transport and protection of the oocyte during fertilization and early embryo development through shuttle the oocyte/embryo toward the uterus and secreting necessary proteins. As the activity of this organ largely depends on the level of estrogen and progesterone, it is likely that transcriptional regulation for the cyclic phenotypic changes of the oviduct and uterus could be under control of miRNAs as evidenced in the ovary. But, the expression and regulatory network of miRNAs for the physiology of oviduct is still an open field for investigation. The loss- or gain-of-function studies of Dicer have evidenced primarily the importance of miRNAs for oviductal functions. Conditional inactivation of *Dicer* in the mesenchyme of the developing Müllerian ducts, in ovarian granulosa cells and mesenchyme-derived cells of the oviducts and uterus revealed female sterility in mouse. Several other reproductive defects including decreased ovulation rates, compromised oocyte and embryo integrity, prominent bilateral paratubal (oviductal) cysts, adenomyosis, shorter and hypotrophic oviduct and uterus have been reported in mouse (Hong *et al.* 2008, Nagaraja *et al.* 2008, Gonzalez & Behringer 2009). Thus, findings revealed diverse and critical roles of Dicer and its miRNA products for postnatal differentiation, development and function of the female reproductive tract as well as female fertility. However, expression and functional characterization of individual miRNAs for the physical and functional integrity of oviduct is yet to be investigated.

The uterus, which undergoes cyclic changes throughout the menstrual or estrous cycle during embryo implantation, is also largely dependent on ovarian steriod. The receptivity of uterus during blastocyst implantation is achieved through transition from elevated estrogen dependent highly proliferative state to progesterone dependent highly secretory state. MiRNAs could also be involved in this uterine change through regulating or interfering the post transcriptional and translational activity of vast number of genes which are supported by the initial conditional inactivation of Dicer studies. In addition, several studies have reported the regulation of miRNAs in the endometrium by the ovarian steroid (Pan *et al.* 2007, Toloubeydokhti *et al.* 2008, Macias *et al.* 2009). Differential expression of miRNAs in endometrial carcinogenesis and between uterine leiomyoma versus normal myometrium has been studied (Boren *et al.* 2008, Marsh *et al.* 2008). Differential expression of miRNAs in endometrium of women with and without endometriosis has been evidenced and revealed importance of miRNAs in normal endometrial cellular activities, pathogenesis of endometriosis and associated reproductive condition (Pan *et al.* 2007, Teague *et al.* 2009). Additionally, a reduced expression of miR-199a and miR-16 may work synergistically to promote an inflammatory environment by up-regulating COX-2 protein levels, thereby promoting prostaglandin production, neoangiogenesis and estradiol mediated cellular proliferation in endometriotic tissues (Teague *et al.* 2009). So, in addition to the study of conditional inactivation of Dicer, studies on the identification of miRNA expression in the normal & diseased uterus and the characterization of some individual miRNA in the uterus (normal & endometriotic) as well as in the uterine implantation site (discussed in previous section) has shade initial light onto the importance of miRNAs regulating physiological changes of the uterus in response to steroids and pregnancy as well as in pathogenic condition.

In addition to their importance in the regulation of normal ovarian physiology as described in the previous section, recently it has become evident that miRNAs play a major role in ovarian tumorigenesis. Several miRNA expression profiling studies have identified changes in miRNA patterns that take place during ovarian cancer development (Iorio *et al.* 2007, Dahiya *et al.* 2008, Giannakakis *et al.* 2008, Laios *et al.* 2008, Nam *et al.* 2008, Yang *et al.* 2008a, Zhang *et al.* 2008, Wyman *et al.* 2009, Bendoraite *et al.* 2010). Candidate miRNAs which were found to be most commonly altered in ovarian carcinoma compared to normal tissue from different study (observed at least in three experiments) are let-7 family, miR-100, miR-106b, miR-10b, miR-125b, miR-143, miR-145, miR-155, miR-15a, miR-199b, miR-200a, miR-200b, miR-200c, miR-21, miR-22, miR-222, miR-368, miR-424 and miR-99a. The majority of these deregulated miRNAs including miR-15a, miR-34a, miR-34b ; miR-210 and let-7 family were found to be down-regulated in human ovarian cancer, hence suggested to act as tumor suppressor and thereby represent potential targets for therapy (Johnson *et al.* 2005, Giannakakis *et al.* 2008, Kumar *et al.* 2008, Zhang *et al.* 2008). The downregulation of major miRNAs in the epithelial ovarian cancer has been found due to both genomic losses and epigenetic alterations (Zhang *et al.* 2008). Further understanding the underlying mechanisms of how miRNAs are regulated in normal or disease condition together with identification of their specific target genes and their functions might lead to increase reproductive efficiency and the development of preventive or therapeutic strategies by regulating specific target genes associated with such reproductive disorders.

MiRNAs in the male reproduction

Importance of miRNAs in male reproduction has been shown by analyzing the expression and regulation of miRNAs in the testicular cells with their putative functions. MiRNAs were first detected from the testis during establishing the techniques reliable for genome-wide miRNA profiling (Barad *et al.* 2004, Liu *et al.* 2004). A number of miRNAs differentially expressed during testicular development and bioinformatic identification of several possible male germ cell target mRNAs has been reported (Yu *et al.* 2005). Further analysis revealed mir-122a targeting transition protein 2 (Tnp2) mRNA, a testis-specific and post-transcriptionally regulated mRNA in postmeiotic germ cells first suggested the miRNAs mediated posttranscriptional regulation in the mammalian testis. Small RNAs cDNA library constructed and identified 52 distinct miRNAs as well as other small noncoding RNAs (rasiRNAs and gsRNAs) in the testis (Watanabe *et al.* 2006). The evidence for the potential involvement of the miRNA pathway in the regulation of male germ cell (GC) development were reported by localizing testis-expressed miRNAs (miR-21, let-7a, miR-122a), in the chromatoid body of male GCs and expected to have control in post-meiotic GC differentiation (Kotaja *et al.* 2006). In 2007 Novotny and his coworkers lay out the potential involvement of miRNAs in post-transcriptional regulation in the testis by the miR-17-92 cluster during meiotic recombination (Novotny *et al.* 2007). In the same year several individual efforts were made to clone miRNAs from the testes in a large scale. Through small RNA cloning method Ro et al. (2007a) identified 141 miRNAs from the mouse testis including 29 novel miRNAs and from the pattern of expression they have suggested twenty eight candidate miRNAs which are preferentially (22) or exclusively (6) expressed in the mouse testis for further functional studies. Comparison of miRNAs pattern between immature and mature mouse testes through miRNA microarray (with 892 miRNA probes) identified 19 significantly different miRNAs expression (Yan *et al.* 2007). Future studies ablating specific miRNAs using transgenic technologies or by other suitable approach will help us better understand the role of individual miRNAs in gonadal development. The expression patterns of several members of the miRNA pathway in the testis namely Dicer (Dcr), Drosha, Ago1, Ago2, Ago3 and Ago4 are identified to express in pachytene spermatocytes, round and elongated spermatids and Sertoli cells (Gonzalez-Gonzalez *et al.* 2008). Moreover, miRNAs were found to be localized to XY body of spermatocytes including the nucleolus of Sertoli cells (Marcon *et al.* 2008). The transgenic male mouse lacking Dcr in germ cells were found to be subfertile both due to the defect in the transition from round to elongating spermatids and production of sperm with abnormal motility (Maatouk *et al.* 2008). Recent study has identified that about 86% of X-linked miRNAs actually escape meiotic sex chromosome inactivation (MSCI) during spermatogenesis and transcriptional silencing of genes on X & Y chromosomes was found to occur in mid-to-late pachytene spermatocytes (Song *et al.* 2009). Further more, selective ablation of Dcr in Sertoli cells has led to infertility due to complete absence of spermatozoa and progressive testicular degeneration (Papaioannou *et al.* 2009). In the same study altered expression of several key genes such as Gdnf, Kitl, Man2a2, and Serpina5 which are essential for spermatogenesis, was revealed as a result of the miRNA mediated post-transcriptional control in the Sertoli cells leading to abnormal spermatogenesis. The existence, preferential and temporal differential expression of miRNAs and the involvement of their machinery genes especially Dcr in the mature and immature testis as well as in different testicular cells has evidenced the functional role of miRNAs in the physiology of testis. Despite various studies carried out on comparative expression analysis of hundreds of testicular miRNAs, there is a tremendous research gap in the investigation of exact functional role of specific miRNAs in the development and proliferation of germ cells in testis.

miRNAs regulation of embryonic development process and stem cells maintenance

The well-orchestrated expression of genes that are derived from the maternal and/or embryonic genome is required for the onset and maintenance of distinct morphological changes during the embryonic development. Optimum regulation of genes or critical gene regulatory event in favor of early embryonic development have been shown to be directly (individual miRNAs study) or indirectly (disrupting miRNAs biogenesis) under the control of miRNAs. Disruption of Dicer1 - an enzyme important for biogenesis of miRNAs and RNA interference related pathways in mammals was first demonstrated and shown that loss of Dicer1 lead to lethality early in development, where Dicer1-null embryos were found to be depleted of stem cells in mouse (Bernstein *et al.* 2003). Another report has been published in the same year to show the importance of Dicer1 in vertebrate development through inactivation of the Dicer1 gene in zebrafish and subsequently observed the early developmental arrest (Wienholds *et al.* 2003). While defective generation of miRNAs was observed in Dicer-null mouse embryonic stem cells with severe defects in differentiation both in vitro and in vivo, the re-expression of Dicer in the knockout cells has been found to rescue these defective phenotypes (Kanellopoulou *et al.* 2005). Additionally, maternal miRNAs have been shown to be essential for the earliest stages of mouse embryonic development through the loss of maternal inheritance of miRNAs following specific deletion of Dicer from growing oocytes (Tang *et al.* 2007). So, these initial reports suggested that miRNAs are essential for embryonic development as the effect of loss of Dicer1 could primarily arise from an inability to process endogenous miRNAs which later on functioning in gene regulation. While critical roles for miRNAs biogenesis in the early embryonic development are well established, roles for individual miRNAs have only recently been investigated mostly in the mouse.

The role of miRNAs has been suggested first for differentiation or maintenance of tissue identity during early embryonic development in zebrafish (Wienholds *et al.* 2005). Several attempts were made to clone miRNAs from the embryo or embryonic tissues to understand the miRNA-mediated regulation of embryonic development. A significant number of miRNAs has been identified at specific stages of mouse embryonic development through massively parallel signature sequencing technology (Mineno *et al.* 2006) and in bovine embryo through small RNAs library construction (Coutinho *et al.* 2007). The coexistence of dynamic synthesis and degradation of miRNAs has been shown but overall quantity and stage-dependent miRNAs increases as the embryos develop during mouse preimplantation stage embryonic development (Yang *et al.* 2008b). Even, during the preimplantation stage miRNAs are shown to participate in directing the highly regulated spatiotemporally expressed genetic network as well. In vitro gain- and loss-of-function experiments showed that the expression of cyclooxygenase-2, a gene critical for implantation, is post-transcriptionally regulated by two miRNAs namely: mmu-miR-101a and mmu-miR-199a* (Chakrabarty *et al.* 2007). Another study has identified higher expression of miR-21 in the subluminal stromal cells at implantation sites on day 5 of pregnancy but not detected during pseudo-pregnancy or even under delayed implantation (Hu *et al.* 2008). This revealed that the expression of mmu-miR-21 in the implantation sites regulated by the active blastocysts. Moreover, in the same study, the role of miR-21 in embryo implantation has been suggested due to targeted regulation of the Reck gene (Hu *et al.* 2008). Recent microarray based miRNAs expression profiling in elongated cloned and in vitro-fertilized bovine embryos has suggested that the reprogramming of miRNAs occurred in cloned bovine elongated embryos (Castro *et al.* 2010). However, status of reprogramming error in the extra embryonic tissues (or placenta) has not yet been separated which could be the main reason for the cloned pregnancy loss during the first trimester.

Recent studies identified a unique set of miRNAs expressed and its functional importance in embryonic stem cells (ES cells). Initial effort has identified that miR-290 through miR-295 (miR-290 cluster) are ES cell-specific and there after suggested that they could potentially participate in early embryonic processes such as the maintenance of pluripotency in mouse

(Houbaviy *et al.* 2003). Similar study in human has also identified some clustered miRNAs (miR-296, miR-301 and miR-302: homologous to the miRNAs reported by Houbaviy *et al.* in mouse) specifically expressed in human ES cells and not in differentiated embryonic cells or adult tissues (Suh *et al.* 2004). These clustered miRNA organization is presumably effective for coordinated regulation of their expression and regulation of common targets because a common seed is shared between some miR-290 cluster miRNAs, miR-302a-d and miR-93 (Houbaviy *et al.* 2003, Houbaviy *et al.* 2005). The role of miR-290 cluster in embryogenesis has been evidenced in a study, in which the generation of a mouse mutant with a homozygous deletion of the miR-290 cluster resulted in the death of embryos (Ambros & Chen 2007). By the loss- or gain-of-function studies of Dicer, DGCR8 and ES-related miRNA genes such as miR-290-295 cluster have strongly suggested that miRNAs play an important role in ES cell maintenance, differentiation (Benetti *et al.* 2008, Sinkkonen *et al.* 2008) and lineage determination (Kanellopoulou *et al.* 2005, Wang *et al.* 2007, Ivey *et al.* 2008, Tay *et al.* 2008). Despite the fact that knowledge on the role of miRNAs in the embryonic development and stem cell maintenance, differentiation and lineage in mouse and human is increasingly building, it is yet to be elucidated for ruminants.

miRNAs regulation of epigenetics in reproduction and early development

The term epigenetics refers to all heritable changes in gene expression that are not associated with concomitant alterations in the DNA sequence. Reversible DNA methylation and histone modifications are known to have profound effects on controlling gene expression. Correct DNA methylation patterns are paramount for the generation of functional gametes with pluripotency states, embryo development, placental function and the maintenance of genome architecture and expression in somatic cells. Aberrancies in both the epigenetic and in the miRNA regulation of genes have been documented to be important in diseases and early development. Very little is known about the miRNAs mediated epigenetic processes or epigenetic control of miRNAs expression, which are potentially involved in regulating reproduction and early development. The potential role of Dicer has been postulated in heterochromatin formation (Fukagawa *et al.* 2004). In addition, Dicer-deficient mutants are shown to reduce epigenetic silencing of expression from centromeric repeat sequences as a result of alterations in DNA methylation and histone modifications (Kanellopoulou *et al.* 2005). As contradictory to this, no apparent changes were observed in the centromeric heterochromatin later on (Murchison *et al.* 2005). However, controversial result were reported by recent studies, where the Dicer deficient stem cells were found to have reduced levels of both de novo DNA methylation and DNA methyltransferases (Dnmts) (Benetti *et al.* 2008, Sinkkonen *et al.* 2008) as well as increased telomere recombination and elongation (Benetti *et al.* 2008). These results supported a model in which the miR-290 cluster maintains ES cells by controlling de novo DNA methylation via Rbl2 and indirectly telomere homeostasis and by repressing the self-renewal program through modulating the epigenetic status of pluripotency genes upon differentiation [reviewed in (Wang *et al.* 2009)].

Epigenetic regulation by the miRNAs has opened up a new dimension of mode of regulation from translational suppression and classic RNAi degradation. In addition to regulation of gene expression at the posttranscriptional level in the cytoplasm, recent findings suggest additional roles for miRNAs in the nucleus. MiRNAs which are encoded within the promoter region of genes could be involved in silencing such genes at transcription level epigenetically. Such cis-regulatory roles of miRNAs have been observed in transcriptional silencing of POLR3D expression and endothelial nitric oxide synthase (eNOS) promoter activity (Zhang *et al.* 2005,

Kim *et al.* 2008). Moreover, miR-122 has been shown to facilate replication of hepatitis C viral RNAs without affecting mRNAs translation or RNA stability (Jopling *et al.* 2005).

Recently, aberrant epigenetic reprogramming of imprinted miR-127 in cloned murine embryos has been reported in relation to the aberrant epigenetic reprogramming of the mouse retrotransposon-like gene Rtl1 (Cui *et al.* 2009). MiRNA-mediated switching of chromatin remodeling complexes in neural development by repression of BAF53a has been observed in mouse (Yoo *et al.* 2009). This repression is accomplished through the 3´ UTR of BAF53a and mediated by the simultaneous activities of miR-9* and miR-124. Repressor-element-1-silencing transcription factor participates in this switch by repressing miR-9* and miR-124, thereby permitting BAF53a expression in neural progenitors. Interestingly, the aberrant DNA methylation and histone modifications could simultaneously induce silencing of miRNAs in colorectal cancer (Bandres *et al.* 2009). The relation of miRNA and epigenetics is presently being elucidated. So, much less is known about the specific miRNA and their targets to regulate epigenetic machinery or epigenetic regulation of specific miRNAs that are required for normal physiological condition or for any phenotypic effects, but this area of research is rapidly moving forward.

Implication of sncRNAs for ruminant reproductive biology and challenges

Non-coding RNAs comprise the major part of the mammalian transcriptome and have been suggested to play an important role in the regulation of gene expression. They are important in most epigenetic mechanisms as is exemplified by the role of small RNAs in silencing of transposable elements, miRNAs in gene expression control, large RNAs in X-chromosome inactivation and DNA imprinting and "heritable" RNAs in non-mendelian epigenetic inheritance. Moreover, DNA methylation and histone modifications can be directed by different types of ncRNAs. Among the sncRNAs, miRNAs seem well suited to maintain the delicate balance between normal reproductive biology, system development and tissue maintenance versus deregulated growth and tumor formation. These small non-coding RNAs have been found to play a central role in various cellular activities, including developmental processes, cell growth, differentiation and apoptosis, cell–cell communication, inflammatory and immune responses through gene expression stability. As many of these processes are an integrated part of gonadal functions, germ cell formation, differentiation, uterine and oviductal cellular activities during different stage of reproduction and steroid synthesis, it is possible to postulate the potential role of miRNAs in regulation of reproductive processes along with other physiological functions. Alteration of the expression of miRNAs in any of these processes could lead to subsequent infertility, reproductive and other steroid-dependent disorders with ultimate failure in reproduction.

Being an important gene regulator, miRNAs could be an interesting avenue to resolve lot of questions on different regulatory mechanisms of ruminant's reproductive process. Posttranscriptional gene regulation by miRNAs during the periods of ovarian follicular development, atresia and luteolysis could be an interesting field of investigation in ruminants. This is particularly interesting since the ovarian follicle is a complex structure composed of different types of cells that are functionally related and constantly changing and differentiating. Investigations are required but remains to be elucidated for the role of miRNAs in the interaction between granulosa and theca cells which are essential for biosynthesis estrogen. In vitro culture models for a single cell type (primary granulosa), co-cultures of theca and granulosa cells or whole follicle cultures could be utilized for elucidating such miRNAs mediated regulation to overcome the technical difficulties in in-vivo experiment. Identification of the whole set of miRNAs in different ovarian cells in ruminants is paramount important for any functional study. To accomplish this, miRNAs microarray could be a useful approach either by using arrays from ruminants or by heterologous approaches by using platform from other species like mouse or human. A direct identification through construction of ovarian cell specific small RNAs library can also be an option. In addition to identification, miRNA microarray could be also useful to describe dynamic changes in miRNA transcript levels in closely related to regulatory events of gene expression for successful follicular development to explain how this is all managed by the different ovarian cell types. Although hundreds of genes, which are important for ovarian physiology, are predicted to be potential target of miRNAs (Hossain *et al.* 2009), all these targets should be validated to elucidate key points of such regulation. Thereafter, it might be possible to draw a fine description of the role of miRNAs in the molecular mechanisms of the dynamic processes occurring in these different compartments of ovary during follicular development and might provide insight into how we might be able to enhance reproductive efficiencies.

In the absence of transcription, synthesis of hundreds of new products and disappearance of many proteins during oocyte maturation after germinal vesicle breakdown and early embryogenesis indicating fine regulation of hundreds of transcripts by a mechanism other than transcription. These changes could possibly largely rely on and controlled by miRNAs, but it is still remains to be elucidated. In addition, it has been evidenced that the bidirectional interactions between oocyte and somatic cells control folliculogenesis. In this communication oocyte secretes soluble paracrine factors that act on its adjacent granulosa cells, which in turn regulate oocyte development in bi-directional communication axis (Gilchrist *et al.* 2004). Further investigations are required to know the role of miRNAs in paracrine signaling and gapjuntional exchange and control of regulatory molecules through intercellular communication between oocytes and granulosa cells.

A large number of target genes for a single miRNA and multiple miRNAs targeting the expression of one gene have been recognized as a major challenge in the assessment of the role of specific miRNAs and establishing precise miRNA-target networks. Moreover, the identification of functional targets represents a major hurdle in our understanding of miRNA function for complex phenomena of reproduction in different ruminant species due to lack of complete genomic information, suitable bio-informatic tools and difficulty to carry out in-vivo functional studies. A few number of knockout studies in mice have been carried out to show the involvement of regulatory miRNAs in mammalian reproduction. However, the knowledge on the functions of specific miRNAs from mouse knockout models cannot be systematically applied to ruminants. So, for large ruminant, the production of transgenic animals could help to elucidate miRNAs mediated regulation of reproductive process in vivo. However, the success of such approaches is limited due to technical difficulty, cost of making null miRNA transgenics and extended time frame required to observe the effect in reproductive processes in ruminants.

Presently, our understanding of non-coding RNAs specially miRNAs function in reproductive biology is very limited and much remains to be uncovered in this exciting field of investigation. Better understanding of small non-coding RNAs, especially miRNA-mediated regulatory effects could be potentially used for regulation of ruminant reproductive processes including fertility and for treatment of reproductive and other steroid-dependent disorders in near future and results can be applied in other species due to high level of conservation of miRNAs between species.

Conclusion

Non-coding RNAs comprise the majority of the mammalian transcriptome and have been suggested to play an important role in the regulation of gene expression. In contrast to the uncertainty surrounding the function of most mammalian ncRNAs, imprinted macro ncRNAs have clearly been shown to regulate flanking genes epigenetically and small non-coding RNAs have been shown to have tremendous transcriptional regulation for normal physiology or disease condition of different types of tissues and cells. Among the sncRNAs, miRNAs are the well characterized one which could maintain the delicate balance between normal reproductive biology, system development and tissue maintenance versus deregulated growth and tumor formation. The studies on the role miRNAs in disease development are much extensive than on reproductive biology and furthermore very limited in ruminant species compared to human and mouse. Conditional Dicer1 knockout mice have been used to show the consequences that the lack of miRNA have on ovarian, testicular, oviductal, uterine, oocyte, and embryonic function and development. To date, much of the work on miRNAs has focused on expression profiling rather than their regulation and functional characterization within specific tissues and cells or during the reproductive process. However, this area of research is rapidly moving forward and it is expected that a lot of information regarding miRNA-mediated posttranscriptional gene regulation and their epigenetic regulation in ruminant reproduction biology will be known within the next several years. Studies to identify the specific miRNAs, their target genes and post transcriptional regulatory network will further shed light on the importance of specific miRNA both for the development and function of reproductive tissues as well as disease condition. Once relevant miRNAs and functional targets are identified, possible clinical use for these molecules will represent the next front line and may lead to novel strategies for better enhancing or manipulating reproductive efficiency.

References

Adams MD, Celniker SE, Holt RA, Evans CA, Gocayne JD, Amanatides PG, Scherer SE, Li PW, Hoskins RA, Galle RF, George RA, Lewis SE, Richards S, Ashburner M, Henderson SN, Sutton GG, Wortman JR, Yandell MD, Zhang Q, Chen LX, Brandon RC, Rogers YH, Blazej RG, Champe M, Pfeiffer BD, Wan KH, Doyle C, Baxter EG, Helt G, Nelson CR, Gabor GL, Abril JF, Agbayani A, An HJ, Andrews-Pfannkoch C, Baldwin D, Ballew RM, Basu A, Baxendale J, Bayraktaroglu L, Beasley EM, Beeson KY, Benos PV, Berman BP, Bhandari D, Bolshakov S, Borkova D, Botchan MR, Bouck J, Brokstein P, Brottier P, Burtis KC, Busam DA, Butler H, Cadieu E, Center A, Chandra I, Cherry JM, Cawley S, Dahlke C, Davenport LB, Davies P, de Pablos B, Delcher A, Deng Z, Mays AD, Dew I, Dietz SM, Dodson K, Doup LE, Downes M, Dugan-Rocha S, Dunkov BC, Dunn P, Durbin KJ, Evangelista CC, Ferraz C, Ferriera S, Fleischmann W, Fosler C, Gabrielian AE, Garg NS, Gelbart WM, Glasser K, Glodek A, Gong F, Gorrell JH, Gu Z, Guan P, Harris M, Harris NL, Harvey D, Heiman TJ, Hernandez JR, Houck J, Hostin D, Houston KA, Howland TJ, Wei MH, Ibegwam C, Jalali M, Kalush F, Karpen GH, Ke Z, Kennison JA, Ketchum KA, Kimmel BE, Kodira CD, Kraft C, Kravitz S, Kulp D, Lai Z, Lasko P, Lei Y, Levitsky AA, Li J, Li Z, Liang Y, Lin X, Liu X, Mattei B, McIntosh TC, McLeod MP, McPherson D, Merkulov G, Milshina NV, Mobarry C, Morris J, Moshrefi A, Mount SM, Moy M, Murphy B, Murphy L, Muzny DM, Nelson DL, Nelson DR, Nelson KA, Nixon K, Nusskern DR, Pacleb JM, Palazzolo M, Pittman GS, Pan S, Pollard J, Puri V, Reese MG, Reinert K, Remington K, Saunders RD, Scheeler F, Shen H, Shue BC, Siden-Kiamos I, Simpson M, Skupski MP, Smith T, Spier E, Spradling AC, Stapleton M, Strong R, Sun E, Svirskas R, Tector C, Turner R, Venter E, Wang AH, Wang X, Wang ZY, Wassarman DA, Weinstock GM, Weissenbach J, Williams SM, WoodageT, Worley KC, Wu D, Yang S, Yao QA, Ye J, Yeh RF, Zaveri JS, Zhan M, Zhang G, Zhao Q, Zheng L, Zheng XH, Zhong FN, Zhong W, Zhou X, Zhu S, Zhu X, Smith HO, Gibbs RA, Myers EW, Rubin GM & Venter JC 2000 The genome sequence of Drosophila melanogaster. *Science* **287** 2185-2195.

Ahn HW, Morin RD, Zhao H, Harris RA, Coarfa C, Chen ZJ, Milosavljevic A, Marra MA & Rajkovic A 2010 MicroRNA transcriptome in the newborn mouse ovaries determined by massive parallel sequencing. *Mol Hum Reprod* **(In press)**.

Altuvia S & Wagner EG 2000 Switching on and off with RNA. *Proc Natl Acad Sci U S A* **97** 9824-9826.

Alvarez-Garcia I & Miska EA 2005 MicroRNA functions in animal development and human disease. *Development* **132** 4653-4662.

Amanai M, Brahmajosyula M & Perry AC 2006 A restricted role for sperm-borne microRNAs in mammalian fertilization. *Biol Reprod* **75** 877-884.

Ambros V 2004 The functions of animal microRNAs. *Nature* **431** 350-355.

Ambros V & Chen X 2007 The regulation of genes

and genomes by small RNAs. *Development* **134** 1635-1641.

Aravin A, Gaidatzis D, Pfeffer S, Lagos-Quintana M, Landgraf P, Iovino N, Morris P, Brownstein MJ, Kuramochi-Miyagawa S, Nakano T, Chien M, Russo JJ, Ju J, Sheridan R, Sander C, Zavolan M & Tuschl T 2006 A novel class of small RNAs bind to MILI protein in mouse testes. *Nature* **442** 203-207.

Aravin AA, Naumova NM, Tulin AV, Vagin VV, Rozovsky YM & Gvozdev VA 2001 Double-stranded RNA-mediated silencing of genomic tandem repeats and transposable elements in the D. melanogaster germline. *Curr Biol* **11** 1017-1027.

Aravin AA, Sachidanandam R, Girard A, Fejes-Toth K & Hannon GJ 2007 Developmentally regulated piRNA clusters implicate MILI in transposon control. *Science* **316** 744-747.

Bagga S, Bracht J, Hunter S, Massirer K, Holtz J, Eachus R & Pasquinelli AE 2005 Regulation by let-7 and lin-4 miRNAs results in target mRNA degradation. *Cell* **122** 553-563.

Bandres E, Agirre X, Bitarte N, Ramirez N, Zarate R, Roman-Gomez J, Prosper F & Garcia-Foncillas J 2009 Epigenetic regulation of microRNA expression in colorectal cancer. *Int J Cancer* **125** 2737-2743.

Barad O, Meiri E, Avniel A, Aharonov R, Barzilai A, Bentwich I, Einav U, Gilad S, Hurban P, Karov Y, Lobenhofer EK, Sharon E, Shiboleth YM, Shtutman M, Bentwich Z & Einat P 2004 MicroRNA expression detected by oligonucleotide microarrays: system establishment and expression profiling in human tissues. *Genome Res* **14** 2486-2494.

Bartel DP 2004 MicroRNAs: genomics, biogenesis, mechanism, and function. *Cell* **116** 281-297.

Bendoraite A, Knouf EC, Garg KS, Parkin RK, Kroh EM, O'Briant KC, Ventura AP, Godwin AK, Karlan BY, Drescher CW, Urban N, Knudsen BS & Tewari M 2010 Regulation of miR-200 family microRNAs and ZEB transcription factors in ovarian cancer: evidence supporting a mesothelial-to-epithelial transition. *Gynecol Oncol* **116** 117-125.

Benetti R, Gonzalo S, Jaco I, Munoz P, Gonzalez S, Schoeftner S, Murchison E, Andl T, Chen T, Klatt P, Li E, Serrano M, Millar S, Hannon G & Blasco MA 2008 A mammalian microRNA cluster controls DNA methylation and telomere recombination via Rbl2-dependent regulation of DNA methyltransferases. *Nat Struct Mol Biol* **15** 268-279.

Bentwich I, Avniel A, Karov Y, Aharonov R, Gilad S, Barad O, Barzilai A, Einat P, Einav U, Meiri E, Sharon E, Spector Y & Bentwich Z 2005 Identification of hundreds of conserved and nonconserved human microRNAs. *Nat Genet* **37** 766-770.

Berezikov E, Guryev V, van de Belt J, Wienholds E, Plasterk RH & Cuppen E 2005 Phylogenetic shadowing and computational identification of human microRNA genes. *Cell* **120** 21-24.

Bernstein E, Kim SY, Carmell MA, Murchison EP, Alcorn H, Li MZ, Mills AA, Elledge SJ, Anderson KV & Hannon GJ 2003 Dicer is essential for mouse development. *Nat Genet* **35** 215-217.

Bonnet A, Dalbies-Tran R & Sirard MA 2008 Opportunities and challenges in applying genomics to the study of oogenesis and folliculogenesis in farm animals. *Reproduction* **135** 119-128.

Boren T, Xiong Y, Hakam A, Wenham R, Apte S, Wei Z, Kamath S, Chen DT, Dressman H & Lancaster JM 2008 MicroRNAs and their target messenger RNAs associated with endometrial carcinogenesis. *Gynecol Oncol* **110** 206-215.

Brennecke J, Aravin AA, Stark A, Dus M, Kellis M, Sachidanandam R & Hannon GJ 2007 Discrete small RNA-generating loci as master regulators of transposon activity in Drosophila. *Cell* **128** 1089-1103.

Brennecke J, Stark A, Russell RB & Cohen SM 2005 Principles of microRNA-target recognition. *PLoS Biol* **3** e85.

Carmell MA, Girard A, van de Kant HJ, Bourc'his D, Bestor TH, de Rooij DG & Hannon GJ 2007 MIWI2 is essential for spermatogenesis and repression of transposons in the mouse male germline. *Dev Cell* **12** 503-514.

Carrington JC 2005 Small RNAs and Arabidopsis. A fast forward look. *Plant Physiol* **138** 565-566.

Castro FO, Sharbati S, Rodriguez-Alvarez LL, Cox JF, Hultschig C & Einspanier R 2010 MicroRNA expression profiling of elongated cloned and in vitro-fertilized bovine embryos. *Theriogenology* **73** 71-85.

Chakrabarty A, Tranguch S, Daikoku T, Jensen K, Furneaux H & Dey SK 2007 MicroRNA regulation of cyclooxygenase-2 during embryo implantation. *Proc Natl Acad Sci U S A* **104** 15144-15149.

Chen K & Rajewsky N 2007 The evolution of gene regulation by transcription factors and microRNAs. *Nat Rev Genet* **8** 93-103.

Chendrimada TP, Finn KJ, Ji X, Baillat D, Gregory RI, Liebhaber SA, Pasquinelli AE & Shiekhattar R 2007 MicroRNA silencing through RISC recruitment of eIF6. *Nature* **447** 823-828.

Choi Y, Qin Y, Berger MF, Ballow DJ, Bulyk ML & Rajkovic A 2007 Microarray analyses of newborn mouse ovaries lacking Nobox. *Biol Reprod* **77** 312-319.

Chu CY & Rana TM 2007 Small RNAs: regulators and guardians of the genome. *J Cell Physiol* **213** 412-419.

Coutinho LL, Matukumalli LK, Sonstegard TS, Van Tassell CP, Gasbarre LC, Capuco AV & Smith TP 2007 Discovery and profiling of bovine microRNAs from immune-related and embryonic tissues. *Physiol Genomics* **29** 35-43.

Cui XS, Zhang DX, Ko YG & Kim NH 2009 Aberrant epigenetic reprogramming of imprinted microRNA-127 and Rtl1 in cloned mouse embryos. *Biochem Biophys Res Commun* **379** 390-394.

Dahiya N, Sherman-Baust CA, Wang TL, Davidson B, Shih Ie M, Zhang Y, Wood W, 3rd, Becker KG & Morin PJ 2008 MicroRNA expression and identification of putative miRNA targets in ovarian cancer. *PLoS One* **3** e2436.

Fiedler SD, Carletti MZ, Hong X & Christenson LK

2008 Hormonal regulation of MicroRNA expression in periovulatory mouse mural granulosa cells. *Biol Reprod* **79** 1030-1037.

Fire A, Xu S, Montgomery MK, Kostas SA, Driver SE & Mello CC 1998 Potent and specific genetic interference by double-stranded RNA in Caenorhabditis elegans. *Nature* **391** 806-811.

Fukagawa T, Nogami M, Yoshikawa M, Ikeno M, Okazaki T, Takami Y, Nakayama T & Oshimura M 2004 Dicer is essential for formation of the heterochromatin structure in vertebrate cells. *Nat Cell Biol* **6** 784-791.

Giannakakis A, Sandaltzopoulos R, Greshock J, Liang S, Huang J, Hasegawa K, Li C, O'Brien-Jenkins A, Katsaros D, Weber BL, Simon C, Coukos G & Zhang L 2008 miR-210 links hypoxia with cell cycle regulation and is deleted in human epithelial ovarian cancer. *Cancer Biol Ther* **7** 255-264.

Gilchrist RB, Ritter LJ & Armstrong DT 2004 Oocyte-somatic cell interactions during follicle development in mammals. *Anim Reprod Sci* **82-83** 431-446.

Giraldez AJ, Cinalli RM, Glasner ME, Enright AJ, Thomson JM, Baskerville S, Hammond SM, Bartel DP & Schier AF 2005 MicroRNAs regulate brain morphogenesis in zebrafish. *Science* **308** 833-838.

Gonzalez-Gonzalez E, Lopez-Casas PP & del Mazo J 2008 The expression patterns of genes involved in the RNAi pathways are tissue-dependent and differ in the germ and somatic cells of mouse testis. *Biochim Biophys Acta* **1779** 306-311.

Gonzalez G & Behringer RR 2009 Dicer is required for female reproductive tract development and fertility in the mouse. *Mol Reprod Dev* **76** 678-688.

Grewal SI & Moazed D 2003 Heterochromatin and epigenetic control of gene expression. *Science* **301** 798-802.

Grimaud C, Bantignies F, Pal-Bhadra M, Ghana P, Bhadra U & Cavalli G 2006 RNAi components are required for nuclear clustering of Polycomb group response elements. *Cell* **124** 957-971.

Gu J, Chen Y & Reddy R 1998 Small RNA database. *Nucleic Acids Res* **26** 160-162.

Gunawardane LS, Saito K, Nishida KM, Miyoshi K, Kawamura Y, Nagami T, Siomi H & Siomi MC 2007 A slicer-mediated mechanism for repeat-associated siRNA 5′ end formation in Drosophila. *Science* **315** 1587-1590.

Hannon GJ, Rivas FV, Murchison EP & Steitz JA 2006 The expanding universe of noncoding RNAs. *Cold Spring Harb Symp Quant Biol* **71** 551-564.

Hong X, Luense LJ, McGinnis LK, Nothnick WB & Christenson LK 2008 Dicer1 is essential for female fertility and normal development of the female reproductive system. *Endocrinology* **149** 6207-6212.

Hossain MM, Ghanem N, Hoelker M, Rings F, Phatsara C, Tholen E, Schellander K & Tesfaye D 2009 Identification and characterization of miRNAs expressed in the bovine ovary. *BMC Genomics* **10** 443.

Houbaviy HB, Dennis L, Jaenisch R & Sharp PA 2005 Characterization of a highly variable eutherian microRNA gene. *RNA* **11** 1245-1257.

Houbaviy HB, Murray MF & Sharp PA 2003 Embryonic stem cell-specific MicroRNAs. *Dev Cell* **5** 351-358.

Houwing S, Kamminga LM, Berezikov E, Cronembold D, Girard A, van den Elst H, Filippov DV, Blaser H, Raz E, Moens CB, Plasterk RH, Hannon GJ, Draper BW & Ketting RF 2007 A role for Piwi and piRNAs in germ cell maintenance and transposon silencing in Zebrafish. *Cell* **129** 69-82.

Hu SJ, Ren G, Liu JL, Zhao ZA, Yu YS, Su RW, Ma XH, Ni H, Lei W & Yang ZM 2008 MicroRNA expression and regulation in mouse uterus during embryo implantation. *J Biol Chem* **283** 23473-23484.

Hutvagner G & Zamore PD 2002 RNAi: nature abhors a double-strand. *Curr Opin Genet Dev* **12** 225-232.

Iorio MV, Visone R, Di Leva G, Donati V, Petrocca F, Casalini P, Taccioli C, Volinia S, Liu CG, Alder H, Calin GA, Menard S & Croce CM 2007 MicroRNA signatures in human ovarian cancer. *Cancer Res* **67** 8699-8707.

Ivey KN, Muth A, Arnold J, King FW, Yeh RF, Fish JE, Hsiao EC, Schwartz RJ, Conklin BR, Bernstein HS & Srivastava D 2008 MicroRNA regulation of cell lineages in mouse and human embryonic stem cells. *Cell Stem Cell* **2** 219-229.

Jackson RJ & Standart N 2007 How do microRNAs regulate gene expression? *Sci STKE* **2007** re1.

Johnson SM, Grosshans H, Shingara J, Byrom M, Jarvis R, Cheng A, Labourier E, Reinert KL, Brown D & Slack FJ 2005 RAS is regulated by the let-7 microRNA family. *Cell* **120** 635-647.

Jopling CL, Yi M, Lancaster AM, Lemon SM & Sarnow P 2005 Modulation of hepatitis C virus RNA abundance by a liver-specific MicroRNA. *Science* **309** 1577-1581.

Kable ML, Heidmann S & Stuart KD 1997 RNA editing: getting U into RNA. *Trends Biochem Sci* **22** 162-166.

Kanellopoulou C, Muljo SA, Kung AL, Ganesan S, Drapkin R, Jenuwein T, Livingston DM & Rajewsky K 2005 Dicer-deficient mouse embryonic stem cells are defective in differentiation and centromeric silencing. *Genes Dev* **19** 489-501.

Keenan RJ, Freymann DM, Stroud RM & Walter P 2001 The signal recognition particle. *Annu Rev Biochem* **70** 755-775.

Kim DH, Saetrom P, Snove O, Jr. & Rossi JJ 2008 MicroRNA-directed transcriptional gene silencing in mammalian cells. *Proc Natl Acad Sci U S A* **105** 16230-16235.

Kiss T 2001 Small nucleolar RNA-guided post-transcriptional modification of cellular RNAs. *EMBO J* **20** 3617-3622.

Klattenhoff C & Theurkauf W 2008 Biogenesis and germline functions of piRNAs. *Development* **135** 3-9.

Koerner MV, Pauler FM, Huang R & Barlow DP 2009 The function of non-coding RNAs in genomic imprinting. *Development* **136** 1771-1783.

Kotaja N, Bhattacharyya SN, Jaskiewicz L, Kimmins S, Parvinen M, Filipowicz W & Sassone-Corsi P 2006 The chromatoid body of male germ cells: similarity with processing bodies and presence of Dicer and microRNA pathway components. *Proc Natl Acad Sci U S A* **103** 2647-2652.

Krek A, Grun D, Poy MN, Wolf R, Rosenberg L, Epstein EJ, MacMenamin P, da Piedade I, Gunsalus KC, Stoffel M & Rajewsky N 2005 Combinatorial microRNA target predictions. *Nat Genet* **37** 495-500.

Kumar MS, Erkeland SJ, Pester RE, Chen CY, Ebert MS, Sharp PA & Jacks T 2008 Suppression of non-small cell lung tumor development by the let-7 microRNA family. *Proc Natl Acad Sci U S A* **105** 3903-3908.

Kuramochi-Miyagawa S, Kimura T, Ijiri TW, Isobe T, Asada N, Fujita Y, Ikawa M, Iwai N, Okabe M, Deng W, Lin H, Matsuda Y & Nakano T 2004 Mili, a mammalian member of piwi family gene, is essential for spermatogenesis. *Development* **131** 839-849.

Kuramochi-Miyagawa S, Kimura T, Yomogida K, Kuroiwa A, Tadokoro Y, Fujita Y, Sato M, Matsuda Y & Nakano T 2001 Two mouse piwi-related genes: miwi and mili. *Mech Dev* **108** 121-133.

Lai EC 2003 microRNAs: Runts of the Genome Assert Themselves. *Current Biology* **13** R925-R936.

Laios A, O'Toole S, Flavin R, Martin C, Kelly L, Ring M, Finn SP, Barrett C, Loda M, Gleeson N, D'Arcy T, McGuinness E, Sheils O, Sheppard B & J OL 2008 Potential role of miR-9 and miR-223 in recurrent ovarian cancer. *Mol Cancer* **7** 35.

Lau NC, Lim LP, Weinstein EG & Bartel DP 2001 An abundant class of tiny RNAs with probable regulatory roles in Caenorhabditis elegans. *Science* **294** 858-862.

Lau NC, Seto AG, Kim J, Kuramochi-Miyagawa S, Nakano T, Bartel DP & Kingston RE 2006 Characterization of the piRNA complex from rat testes. *Science* **313** 363-367.

Lee RC, Feinbaum RL & Ambros V 1993 The C. elegans heterochronic gene lin-4 encodes small RNAs with antisense complementarity to lin-14. *Cell* **75** 843-854.

Lee Y, Ahn C, Han J, Choi H, Kim J, Yim J, Lee J, Provost P, Radmark O, Kim S & Kim VN 2003 The nuclear RNase III Drosha initiates microRNA processing. *Nature* **425** 415-419.

Lee Y, Jeon K, Lee JT, Kim S & Kim VN 2002 MicroRNA maturation: stepwise processing and subcellular localization. *EMBO J* **21** 4663-4670.

Lewis BP, Burge CB & Bartel DP 2005 Conserved seed pairing, often flanked by adenosines, indicates that thousands of human genes are microRNA targets. *Cell* **120** 15-20.

Lim LP, Lau NC, Garrett-Engele P, Grimson A, Schelter JM, Castle J, Bartel DP, Linsley PS & Johnson JM 2005 Microarray analysis shows that some microRNAs downregulate large numbers of target mRNAs. *Nature* **433** 769-773.

Liu CG, Calin GA, Meloon B, Gamliel N, Sevignani C, Ferracin M, Dumitru CD, Shimizu M, Zupo S, Dono M, Alder H, Bullrich F, Negrini M & Croce CM 2004 An oligonucleotide microchip for genome-wide microRNA profiling in human and mouse tissues. *Proc Natl Acad Sci U S A* **101** 9740-9744.

Liu J, Rivas FV, Wohlschlegel J, Yates JR, 3rd, Parker R & Hannon GJ 2005a A role for the P-body component GW182 in microRNA function. *Nat Cell Biol* **7** 1261-1266.

Liu J, Valencia-Sanchez MA, Hannon GJ & Parker R 2005b MicroRNA-dependent localization of targeted mRNAs to mammalian P-bodies. *Nat Cell Biol* **7** 719-723.

Maatouk DM, Loveland KL, McManus MT, Moore K & Harfe BD 2008 Dicer1 is required for differentiation of the mouse male germline. *Biol Reprod* **79** 696-703.

Macias S, Michlewski G & Caceres JF 2009 Hormonal regulation of microRNA biogenesis. *Mol Cell* **36** 172-173.

Marcon E, Babak T, Chua G, Hughes T & Moens PB 2008 miRNA and piRNA localization in the male mammalian meiotic nucleus. *Chromosome Res* **16** 243-260.

Marsh EE, Lin Z, Yin P, Milad M, Chakravarti D & Bulun SE 2008 Differential expression of microRNA species in human uterine leiomyoma versus normal myometrium. *Fertil Steril* **89** 1771-1776.

Martignetti JA & Brosius J 1993 BC200 RNA: a neural RNA polymerase III product encoded by a monomeric Alu element. *Proc Natl Acad Sci U S A* **90** 11563-11567.

Masse E & Gottesman S 2002 A small RNA regulates the expression of genes involved in iron metabolism in Escherichia coli. *Proc Natl Acad Sci U S A* **99** 4620-4625.

Mattick JS & Makunin IV 2006 Non-coding RNA. *Hum Mol Genet* **15 Spec No 1** R17-29.

Mineno J, Okamoto S, Ando T, Sato M, Chono H, Izu H, Takayama M, Asada K, Mirochnitchenko O, Inouye M & Kato I 2006 The expression profile of microRNAs in mouse embryos. *Nucleic Acids Res* **34** 1765-1771.

Mishima T, Takizawa T, Luo SS, Ishibashi O, Kawahigashi Y, Mizuguchi Y, Ishikawa T, Mori M, Kanda T & Goto T 2008 MicroRNA (miRNA) cloning analysis reveals sex differences in miRNA expression profiles between adult mouse testis and ovary. *Reproduction* **136** 811-822.

Mochizuki K, Fine NA, Fujisawa T & Gorovsky MA 2002 Analysis of a piwi-related gene implicates small RNAs in genome rearrangement in tetrahymena. *Cell* **110** 689-699.

Murchison EP, Partridge JF, Tam OH, Cheloufi S & Hannon GJ 2005 Characterization of Dicer-deficient murine embryonic stem cells. *Proc Natl Acad Sci U S A* **102** 12135-12140.

Murchison EP, Stein P, Xuan Z, Pan H, Zhang MQ, Schultz RM & Hannon GJ 2007 Critical roles for Dicer in the female germline. *Genes Dev* **21** 682-693.

Nagaraja AK, Andreu-Vieyra C, Franco HL, Ma L, Chen R, Han DY, Zhu H, Agno JE, Gunaratne PH, DeMayo FJ & Matzuk MM 2008 Deletion of Dicer in somatic cells of the female reproductive tract causes sterility. *Mol Endocrinol* **22** 2336-2352.

Nam EJ, Yoon H, Kim SW, Kim H, Kim YT, Kim JH, Kim JW & Kim S 2008 MicroRNA expression profiles in serous ovarian carcinoma. *Clin Cancer Res* **14**

2690-2695.

Nilsen TW 2007 Mechanisms of microRNA-mediated gene regulation in animal cells. *Trends Genet* **23** 243-249.

Novotny GW, Sonne SB, Nielsen JE, Jonstrup SP, Hansen MA, Skakkebaek NE, Rajpert-De Meyts E, Kjems J & Leffers H 2007 Translational repression of E2F1 mRNA in carcinoma in situ and normal testis correlates with expression of the miR-17-92 cluster. *Cell Death Differ* **14** 879-882.

O'Donnell KA & Boeke JD 2007 Mighty Piwis defend the germline against genome intruders. *Cell* **129** 37-44.

Orom UA, Nielsen FC & Lund AH 2008 MicroRNA-10a binds the 5'UTR of ribosomal protein mRNAs and enhances their translation. *Mol Cell* **30** 460-471.

Otsuka M, Jing Q, Georgel P, New L, Chen J, Mols J, Kang Young J, Jiang Z, Du X, Cook R, Das SC, Pattnaik AK, Beutler B & Han J 2007 Hypersusceptibility to Vesicular Stomatitis Virus Infection in Dicer1-Deficient Mice Is Due to Impaired miR24 and miR93 Expression. *Immunity* **27** 123-134.

Otsuka M, Zheng M, Hayashi M, Lee JD, Yoshino O, Lin S & Han J 2008 Impaired microRNA processing causes corpus luteum insufficiency and infertility in mice. *J Clin Invest* **118** 1944-1954.

Pal-Bhadra M, Leibovitch BA, Gandhi SG, Rao M, Bhadra U, Birchler JA & Elgin SC 2004 Heterochromatic silencing and HP1 localization in Drosophila are dependent on the RNAi machinery. *Science* **303** 669-672.

Pan Q, Luo X, Toloubeydokhti T & Chegini N 2007 The expression profile of micro-RNA in endometrium and endometriosis and the influence of ovarian steroids on their expression. *Mol Hum Reprod* **13** 797-806.

Papaioannou MD, Pitetti JL, Ro S, Park C, Aubry F, Schaad O, Vejnar CE, Kuhne F, Descombes P, Zdobnov EM, McManus MT, Guillou F, Harfe BD, Yan W, Jegou B & Nef S 2009 Sertoli cell Dicer is essential for spermatogenesis in mice. *Dev Biol* **326** 250-259.

Peragine A, Yoshikawa M, Wu G, Albrecht HL & Poethig RS 2004 SGS3 and SGS2/SDE1/RDR6 are required for juvenile development and the production of trans-acting siRNAs in Arabidopsis. *Genes Dev* **18** 2368-2379.

Pillai RS, Bhattacharyya SN, Artus CG, Zoller T, Cougot N, Basyuk E, Bertrand E & Filipowicz W 2005 Inhibition of translational initiation by Let-7 MicroRNA in human cells. *Science* **309** 1573-1576.

Plasterk RH 2006 Micro RNAs in animal development. *Cell* **124** 877-881.

Rana TM 2007 Illuminating the silence: understanding the structure and function of small RNAs. *Nat Rev Mol Cell Biol* **8** 23-36.

Rehwinkel J, Behm-Ansmant I, Gatfield D & Izaurralde E 2005 A crucial role for GW182 and the DCP1:DCP2 decapping complex in miRNA-mediated gene silencing. *RNA* **11** 1640-1647.

Reinhart BJ & Bartel DP 2002 Small RNAs correspond to centromere heterochromatic repeats. *Science* **297** 1831.

Ro S, Park C, Sanders KM, McCarrey JR & Yan W 2007a Cloning and expression profiling of testis-expressed microRNAs. *Dev Biol* **311** 592-602.

Ro S, Song R, Park C, Zheng H, Sanders KM & Yan W 2007b Cloning and expression profiling of small RNAs expressed in the mouse ovary. *RNA* **13** 2366-2380.

Samarsky DA & Fournier MJ 1999 A comprehensive database for the small nucleolar RNAs from Saccharomyces cerevisiae. *Nucleic Acids Res* **27** 161-164.

Shen MR, Brosius J & Deininger PL 1997 BC1 RNA, the transcript from a master gene for ID element amplification, is able to prime its own reverse transcription. *Nucleic Acids Res* **25** 1641-1648.

Simpson L, Thiemann OH, Savill NJ, Alfonzo JD & Maslov DA 2000 Evolution of RNA editing in trypanosome mitochondria. *Proc Natl Acad Sci U S A* **97** 6986-6993.

Sinkkonen L, Hugenschmidt T, Berninger P, Gaidatzis D, Mohn F, Artus-Revel CG, Zavolan M, Svoboda P & Filipowicz W 2008 MicroRNAs control de novo DNA methylation through regulation of transcriptional repressors in mouse embryonic stem cells. *Nat Struct Mol Biol* **15** 259-267.

Sirotkin AV, Laukova M, Ovcharenko D, Brenaut P & Mlyncek M 2009a Identification of microRNAs controlling human ovarian cell proliferation and apoptosis. *J Cell Physiol* **223** 49-56.

Sirotkin AV, Ovcharenko D, Grossmann R, Laukova M & Mlyncek M 2009b Identification of microRNAs controlling human ovarian cell steroidogenesis via a genome-scale screen. *J Cell Physiol* **219** 415-420.

Song R, Ro S, Michaels JD, Park C, McCarrey JR & Yan W 2009 Many X-linked microRNAs escape meiotic sex chromosome inactivation. *Nat Genet* **41** 488-493.

Souza AE, Hermann T & Goringer HU 1997 The guide RNA database. *Nucleic Acids Res* **25** 104-106.

Standart N & Jackson RJ 2007 MicroRNAs repress translation of m7Gppp-capped target mRNAs in vitro by inhibiting initiation and promoting deadenylation. *Genes Dev* **21** 1975-1982.

Storz G 2002 An expanding universe of noncoding RNAs. *Science* **296** 1260-1263.

Su AI, Cooke MP, Ching KA, Hakak Y, Walker JR, Wiltshire T, Orth AP, Vega RG, Sapinoso LM, Moqrich A, Patapoutian A, Hampton GM, Schultz PG & Hogenesch JB 2002 Large-scale analysis of the human and mouse transcriptomes. *Proc Natl Acad Sci U S A* **99** 4465-4470.

Suh MR, Lee Y, Kim JY, Kim SK, Moon SH, Lee JY, Cha KY, Chung HM, Yoon HS, Moon SY, Kim VN & Kim KS 2004 Human embryonic stem cells express a unique set of microRNAs. *Dev Biol* **270** 488-498.

Suh N, Baehner L, Moltzahn F, Melton C, Shenoy A, Chen J & Blelloch R 2010 MicroRNA function is globally suppressed in mouse oocytes and early embryos. *Curr Biol* **20** 271-277.

Tang F, Kaneda M, O'Carroll D, Hajkova P, Barton SC, Sun YA, Lee C, Tarakhovsky A, Lao K & Surani MA 2007 Maternal microRNAs are essential for mouse zygotic development. *Genes Dev* **21** 644-648.

Tay YM, Tam WL, Ang YS, Gaughwin PM, Yang H, Wang W, Liu R, George J, Ng HH, Perera RJ, Lufkin T, Rigoutsos I, Thomson AM & Lim B 2008 MicroRNA-134 modulates the differentiation of mouse embryonic stem cells, where it causes post-transcriptional attenuation of Nanog and LRH1. *Stem Cells* **26** 17-29.

Teague EM, Print CG & Hull ML 2009 The role of microRNAs in endometriosis and associated reproductive conditions. *Hum Reprod Update* **16** 142-165.

Tesfaye D, Worku D, Rings F, Phatsara C, Tholen E, Schellander K & Hoelker M 2009 Identification and expression profiling of microRNAs during bovine oocyte maturation using heterologous approach. *Mol Reprod Dev* **76** 665-677.

Toloubeydokhti T, Pan Q, Luo X, Bukulmez O & Chegini N 2008 The expression and ovarian steroid regulation of endometrial micro-RNAs. *Reprod Sci* **15** 993-1001.

Vasudevan S, Tong Y & Steitz JA 2007 Switching from repression to activation: microRNAs can up-regulate translation. *Science* **318** 1931-1934.

Vazquez F, Vaucheret H, Rajagopalan R, Lepers C, Gasciolli V, Mallory AC, Hilbert JL, Bartel DP & Crete P 2004 Endogenous trans-acting siRNAs regulate the accumulation of Arabidopsis mRNAs. *Mol Cell* **16** 69-79.

Volpe TA, Kidner C, Hall IM, Teng G, Grewal SI & Martienssen RA 2002 Regulation of heterochromatic silencing and histone H3 lysine-9 methylation by RNAi. *Science* **297** 1833-1837.

Wang Y, Keys DN, Au-Young JK & Chen C 2009 MicroRNAs in embryonic stem cells. *J Cell Physiol* **218** 251-255.

Wang Y, Medvid R, Melton C, Jaenisch R & Blelloch R 2007 DGCR8 is essential for microRNA biogenesis and silencing of embryonic stem cell self-renewal. *Nat Genet* **39** 380-385.

Wassarman KM & Storz G 2000 6S RNA regulates E. coli RNA polymerase activity. *Cell* **101** 613-623.

Wassarman KM, Zhang A & Storz G 1999 Small RNAs in Escherichia coli. *Trends Microbiol* **7** 37-45.

Watanabe T, Takeda A, Tsukiyama T, Mise K, Okuno T, Sasaki H, Minami N & Imai H 2006 Identification and characterization of two novel classes of small RNAs in the mouse germline: retrotransposon-derived siRNAs in oocytes and germline small RNAs in testes. *Genes Dev* **20** 1732-1743.

Wienholds E, Kloosterman WP, Miska E, Alvarez-Saavedra E, Berezikov E, de Bruijn E, Horvitz HR, Kauppinen S & Plasterk RH 2005 MicroRNA expression in zebrafish embryonic development. *Science* **309** 310-311.

Wienholds E, Koudijs MJ, van Eeden FJ, Cuppen E & Plasterk RH 2003 The microRNA-producing enzyme Dicer1 is essential for zebrafish development. *Nat Genet* **35** 217-218.

Will CL & Luhrmann R 2001 Spliceosomal UsnRNP biogenesis, structure and function. *Curr Opin Cell Biol* **13** 290-301.

Wyman SK, Parkin RK, Mitchell PS, Fritz BR, O'Briant K, Godwin AK, Urban N, Drescher CW, Knudsen BS & Tewari M 2009 Repertoire of microRNAs in epithelial ovarian cancer as determined by next generation sequencing of small RNA cDNA libraries. *PLoS One* **4** e5311.

Xie X, Lu J, Kulbokas EJ, Golub TR, Mootha V, Lindblad-Toh K, Lander ES & Kellis M 2005 Systematic discovery of regulatory motifs in human promoters and 3′ UTRs by comparison of several mammals. *Nature* **434** 338-345.

Yamagata K, Fujiyama S, Ito S, Ueda T, Murata T, Naitou M, Takeyama K, Minami Y, O'Malley BW & Kato S 2009 Maturation of microRNA is hormonally regulated by a nuclear receptor. *Mol Cell* **36** 340-347.

Yan N, Lu Y, Sun H, Tao D, Zhang S, Liu W & Ma Y 2007 A microarray for microRNA profiling in mouse testis tissues. *Reproduction* **134** 73-79.

Yang H, Kong W, He L, Zhao JJ, O'Donnell JD, Wang J, Wenham RM, Coppola D, Kruk PA, Nicosia SV & Cheng JQ 2008a MicroRNA expression profiling in human ovarian cancer: miR-214 induces cell survival and cisplatin resistance by targeting PTEN. *Cancer Res* **68** 425-433.

Yang Y, Bai W, Zhang L, Yin G, Wang X, Wang J, Zhao H, Han Y & Yao YQ 2008b Determination of microRNAs in mouse preimplantation embryos by microarray. *Dev Dyn* **237** 2315-2327.

Yao G, Yin M, Lian J, Tian H, Liu L, Li X & Sun F 2010 MicroRNA-224 is involved in transforming growth factor-beta-mediated mouse granulosa cell proliferation and granulosa cell function by targeting Smad4. *Mol Endocrinol* **24** 540-551.

Yi R, Qin Y, Macara IG & Cullen BR 2003 Exportin-5 mediates the nuclear export of pre-microRNAs and short hairpin RNAs. *Genes Dev* **17** 3011-3016.

Yoo AS, Staahl BT, Chen L & Crabtree GR 2009 MicroRNA-mediated switching of chromatin-remodelling complexes in neural development. *Nature* **460** 642-646.

Yu Z, Raabe T & Hecht NB 2005 MicroRNA Mirn122a reduces expression of the posttranscriptionally regulated germ cell transition protein 2 (Tnp2) messenger RNA (mRNA) by mRNA cleavage. *Biol Reprod* **73** 427-433.

Zhang L, Volinia S, Bonome T, Calin GA, Greshock J, Yang N, Liu CG, Giannakakis A, Alexiou P, Hasegawa K, Johnstone CN, Megraw MS, Adams S, Lassus H, Huang J, Kaur S, Liang S, Sethupathy P, Leminen A, Simossis VA, Sandaltzopoulos R, Naomoto Y, Katsaros D, Gimotty PA, DeMichele A, Huang Q, Butzow R, Rustgi AK, Weber BL, Birrer MJ, Hatzigeorgiou AG, Croce CM & Coukos G 2008 Genomic and epigenetic alterations deregulate microRNA expression in human epithelial ovarian cancer. *Proc Natl Acad Sci U S A* **105** 7004-7009.

Zhang MX, Ou H, Shen YH, Wang J, Coselli J & Wang XL 2005 Regulation of endothelial nitric oxide synthase by small RNA. *Proc Natl Acad Sci U S A* **102** 16967-16972.

Endogenous retroviruses of sheep: a model system for understanding physiological adaptation to an evolving ruminant genome

TE Spencer[1], SG Black[1], F Arnaud[2,3] and M Palmarini[2]

[1]Center for Animal Biotechnology and Genomics, Department of Animal Science, Texas A&M University, College Station, TX, USA; [2]Institute of Comparative Medicine, University of Glasgow Veterinary School, Glasgow, Scotland, UK; [3]Present address: UMR754, EPHE, Université de Lyon 1, INRA, Ecole Nationale Vétérinaire de Lyon, IFR 128, Lyon, France

Endogenous retroviruses (ERVs) are present in the genome of all vertebrates and are remnants of ancient exogenous retroviral infections of the host germline transmitted vertically from generation to generation. Sheep betaretroviruses offer a unique model system to study the complex interaction between retroviruses and their host. The sheep genome contains 27 endogenous betaretroviruses (enJSRVs) related to the exogenous and pathogenic Jaagsiekte sheep retrovirus (JSRV), the causative agent of a transmissible lung cancer in sheep. The enJSRVs can protect their host against JSRV infection by blocking early and late steps of the JSRV replication cycle. In the female reproductive tract, enJSRVs are specifically expressed in the uterine luminal and glandular epithelia as well as in the conceptus (embryo and associated extraembryonic membranes) trophectoderm and *in utero* loss-of-function experiments found the enJSRVs envelope (env) to be essential for conceptus elongation and trophectoderm growth and development. Collectively, available evidence in sheep and other mammals indicate that ERVs coevolved with their hosts for millions of years and were positively selected for biological roles in genome plasticity and evolution, protection of the host against infection of related pathogenic and exogenous retroviruses, and placental development.

Introduction

Endogenous retroviruses (ERVs) are present in the genome of all vertebrates and are vertically transmitted as stable, inherited Mendelian genes (Boeke & Stoye 1997). ERVs are thought to arise from ancient infections of the germline of the host by exogenous retroviruses, and they have heavily colonized the genome of all animal species. The obligatory integration step of the retroviral replication cycle allowed, during evolution, the incorporation of the viral genome (provirus) into the host genome (**Fig. 1**). In fact, more that 40% of the human genome is comprised by transposable elements, and ERVs account for approximately 8% of the human

Corresponding author E-mail: tspencer@tamu.edu

genome (Kurth & Bannert 2010) (**Fig. 2**). Retrotransposition or re-infection of the germline can generate further insertions augmenting the number of ERVs loci in the genome (Gifford & Tristem 2003). A complete ERV "provirus", i.e. the retroviral genome integrated into the host cell genome, shares the same genomic structure of an exogenous retrovirus, which is four viral genes (*gag, pro, pol*, and *env*) flanked by two long terminal repeats (LTRs) (**Fig. 3**). The *gag* gene encodes for the major viral structural protein, while *pro* and *pol* encode for the viral enzymatic machinery necessary for the viral replication cycle. The *env* gene encodes for the envelope glycoprotein (Env) that is inserted in the lipid bilayer of the exterior membrane to form the viral envelope and mediates entry of the virus into susceptible cells via a receptor. The LTRs contain enhancer and promoter elements that direct expression of the viral genes.

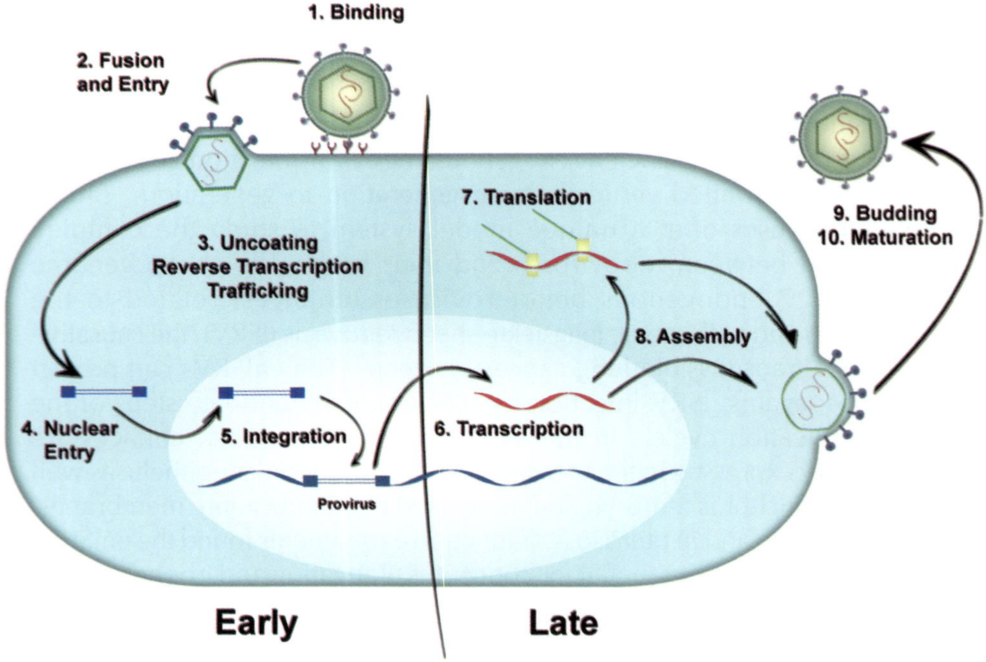

Fig. 1. Life cycle of retroviruses. The retroviral life cycle is arbitrarily divided into two phases, early and late. The stages in each phase are shown above. Interactions between viral and host cell restriction factors occur at every stage of the viral life cycle. The infecting virus attaches to a specific receptor on the cellular plasma membrane with the SU portion of the viral Env protein leading to fusion and entry. Reverse transcription then generates a double-stranded DNA copy of the RNA genome. The provirus is transported into the nucleus and integrated into chromosomal DNA. Transcription by the cellular machinery generates RNA copies that are then translated in the cytoplasm. Virion proteins and progeny RNA assemble at the cell boundary and the plasma membrane, and progeny virus is released into a mature viral particle.

ERVs are widespread throughout vertebrate genomes (Herniou *et al.* 1998). Some ERVs are highly related to exogenous retroviruses, including Jaagsiekte sheep retrovirus (JSRV), mouse mammary tumor virus (MMTV), feline leukemia virus (FeLV), and avian leukemia virus (ALV), which are currently active and infect sheep, mice, cats and chickens, respectively (Boeke & Stoye 1997). These ERVs are generally referred to as "modern" ERVs, because they integrated

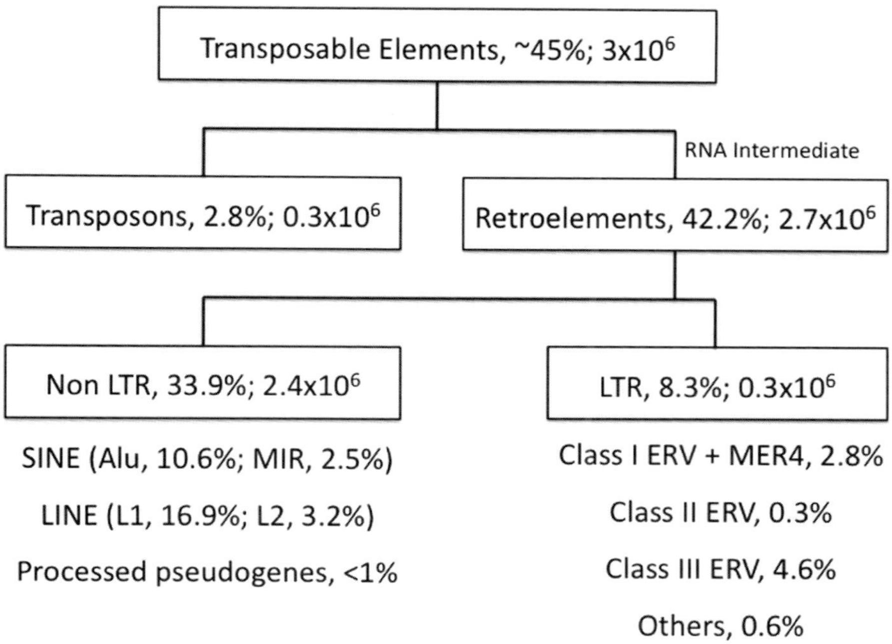

Fig. 2. Endogenous retroviruses are transposable elements. Transposable elements are stretches of DNA that cut and splice themselves out of the genome into another region, contributing to genetic diversity in a variety of organisms (Bannert & Kurth 2004, Biemont & Vieira 2006). Approximately 45% of the human genome is composed of transposable elements. Transposable elements can be divided into DNA transposons, which act *via* a DNA intermediate, and retrotransposons that use a RNA intermediate. DNA transposons comprise 2.8% of the transposable elements of the human genome, while the remaining 42.2% are retrotransposons. Retrotransposons can be further divided into non LTR elements (33.9%), comprising the long and short interspersed elements (LINEs and SINEs respectively), and LTR elements (8.3%) that are endogenous retroviruses (ERVs). Figure adapted from Bannert & Kurth (Bannert & Kurth 2004).

into the host genome after speciation and are closely related to exogenous viruses that are still infectious. Indeed, most ERVs do not have an exogenous counterpart. Some modern ERVs are still able to produce infectious virus due to the lack of inactivating mutations. Modern ERVs can also have insertionally polymorphic loci, since they are not completely fixed in a particular population and are still undergoing endogenization. In contrast, "ancient" ERVs invaded the genomes before speciation and, consequently, are present in every individual at the same genomic location of phylogenetically related species (Coffin 2004). Over time, ERV accumulate mutations, insertions, and recombinations, particularly if their expression brings deleterious consequences for the host (Boeke & Stoye 1997). Consequently, the majority of integrated retroviral sequences are non-functional remnants ("fossils") of exogenous related sequences.

The biological significance of ERVs has been debated for several decades and in the past they were generally thought to be "junk DNA" (Bock & Stoye 2000), but mounting evidence reveals that selected ERVs have a variety of beneficial roles to their host (Jern & Coffin 2008, Varela *et al.* 2009, Kurth & Bannert 2010). The presence of transcriptionally active ERVs with intact open reading frames conserved million of years after integration support the idea that some

ERVs were selected and co-opted by the host for specific biological roles until they became true essential genes (de Parseval & Heidmann 2005). In this review, we will focus on the biological roles of sheep JSRV-related endogenous betaretroviruses (enJSRVs) in genome plasticity and evolution, protection from exogenous and pathogenic JSRV, and placental development.

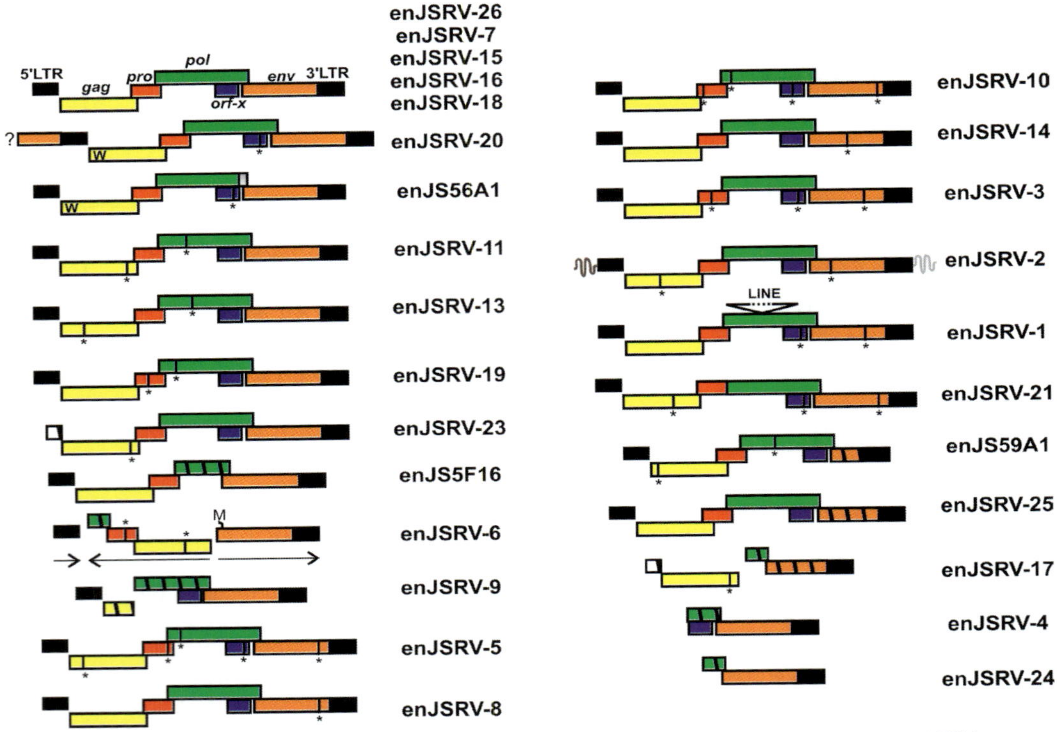

Fig. 3. Representative enJSRVs proviruses present within the sheep genome. Five enJSRVs display an intact genomic organization typical of replication competent proviruses (top). The "W" present in the Gag protein of enJS56A1 and enJSRV-20 indicates the R21W substitution that confers transdominant properties to these two proviruses. The 5′ flanking region of enJSRV-20 contains an *env* gene indicated by a box and a question mark (?). Vertical lines with an asterisk (*) represent stop codons, while hatched boxes indicate deletions. enJSRV-6 harbours a recombined structure with internal sequence in the opposite direction compared to the 5′ and 3′ LTRs of the provirus. The first methionine (indicated by the letter M) of the *env* gene of enJSRV-6 is present after the usual start codon. Figure reproduced from Arnaud and coworkers (Arnaud *et al.* 2007a).

Endogenous and exogenous betaretroviruses of domestic sheep: enJSRVs/JSRV

Domestic sheep harbor at least 27 copies of ERVs in their genome, termed enJSRVs (**Fig. 3**), because they are highly related to the exogenous and pathogenic Jaagsiekte sheep retrovirus (JSRV) (Arnaud *et al.* 2007a). JSRV is the causative agent of ovine pulmonary adenocarcinoma, a transmissible lung cancer of sheep (Palmarini *et al.* 1999). A unique feature of JSRV among oncogenic retroviruses is that its Env glycoprotein is the main determinant of cell transformation both *in vitro* and *in vivo* (Maeda *et al.* 2001, Wootton *et al.* 2005, Caporale *et al.* 2006). The JSRV Env is able to induce lung adenocarcinomas in immunocompetent sheep when expressed by a JSRV-based vector under the control of the JSRV LTR (Caporale *et al.* 2006). Although the mitogen activated protein kinase (Ras-MEK-MAPK), Rac1, and phosphoinositide 3-kinase (PI3K-AKT-mTOR) pathways are implicated in JSRV-induced cell transformation, it still remains to be determined how the viral Env engages the cell signaling network to activate these pathways (Palmarini *et al.* 2001b, Maeda *et al.* 2005, De Las Heras *et al.* 2006, Varela *et al.* 2006, Maeda & Fan 2008).

The majority of the 27 enJSRV proviruses in sheep are defective as a result of deletions, nonsense mutations, and recombinations; however, five enJSRV proviruses contain intact genomes with uninterrupted open reading frames for all retroviral genes (**Fig. 3**) (Arnaud *et al.* 2007a). These enJSRV loci are insertionally polymorphic in the domestic sheep population. JSRV and enJSRVs have a high degree of similarity (~85-89% identity at the nucleotide level). enJSRVs are present in sheep and goats, but not cattle or other species. Integration of enJSRVs began before the split between the genus Ovis and the genus Capra, approximately 5 to 7 million years ago, and continued after sheep domestication (~ 10,000 years ago) (Arnaud *et al.* 2007a, Chessa *et al.* 2009) (**Fig. 4**). Interestingly, a particular enJSRV provirus, enJSRV-26, is thought to have integrated in the host less than 200 years ago and may be a unique integration event occurred in a single animal (Arnaud *et al.* 2007a). Thus, the enJSRVs are most likely still invading the sheep genome.

enJSRVs viral interference

enJSRVs can block JSRV replication at both early and late stages of the retroviral cycle (**Fig. 1**). Both JSRV and enJSRVs use the same cellular receptor for entry called HYAL2 (hyaluronidase 2), a glycosylphosphatidylinositol (GPI)-anchored protein (Rai *et al.* 2001, Arnaud *et al.* 2007a). As described for other viruses, enJSRVs Env can prevent JSRV entry by a classic mechanism of receptor interference (Spencer *et al.* 2003). In addition, two enJSRV loci (enJS56A1 and enJSRV-20) can block JSRV replication at a late stage of the retroviral replication cycle by a block referred to as JSRV late restriction (Mura *et al.* 2004, Arnaud *et al.* 2007a, Murcia *et al.* 2007). These two transdominant proviruses entered the host genome 3 million years ago before and during speciation within the genus *Ovis* (Arnaud *et al.* 2007a) (**Fig. 4**). They subsequently acquired in two temporally distinct events a defective Gag polyprotein *via* a substitution of an arginine at the position 21 (typical of a replication competent virus) to a tryptophan residue. JSRV late restriction likely occurs *via* the production of defective Gag protein by the transdominant proviruses that form viral particles and/or multimers with the functional Gag proteins, which then accumulate in the cytoplasm as pre-aggresome structures that are subsequently degraded by the proteasome. Therefore, the transdominant proviruses prevent Gag proteins of the competent virus to interact with the trafficking cellular machinery and ultimately the release of viral particles (Arnaud *et al.* 2007b, Murcia *et al.* 2007).

Available evidence strongly supports the hypothesis that selection of transdominant enJSRV loci protected sheep against infection with related exogenous retroviruses, including JSRV and perhaps enzootic nasal tumor virus or ENTV. Both proviruses with transdominant (protective) genotype/phenotypes became fixed in the host genome of the domestic sheep (*Ovis aries*), supporting the idea of their positive selection during or immediately before sheep domestication (9,000 years ago) (**Fig. 4**). These data support the hypothesis that ERVs could help the host to fight retroviral infections (Palmarini *et al.* 2004).

ERVs and placental development

ERVs have been speculated to play a physiological role in placenta morphogenesis for almost three decades considering that retroviral particles have been frequently observed in the reproductive tract (Kalter *et al.* 1975, Smith & Moore 1988, Harris 1991). In fact, ERVs are

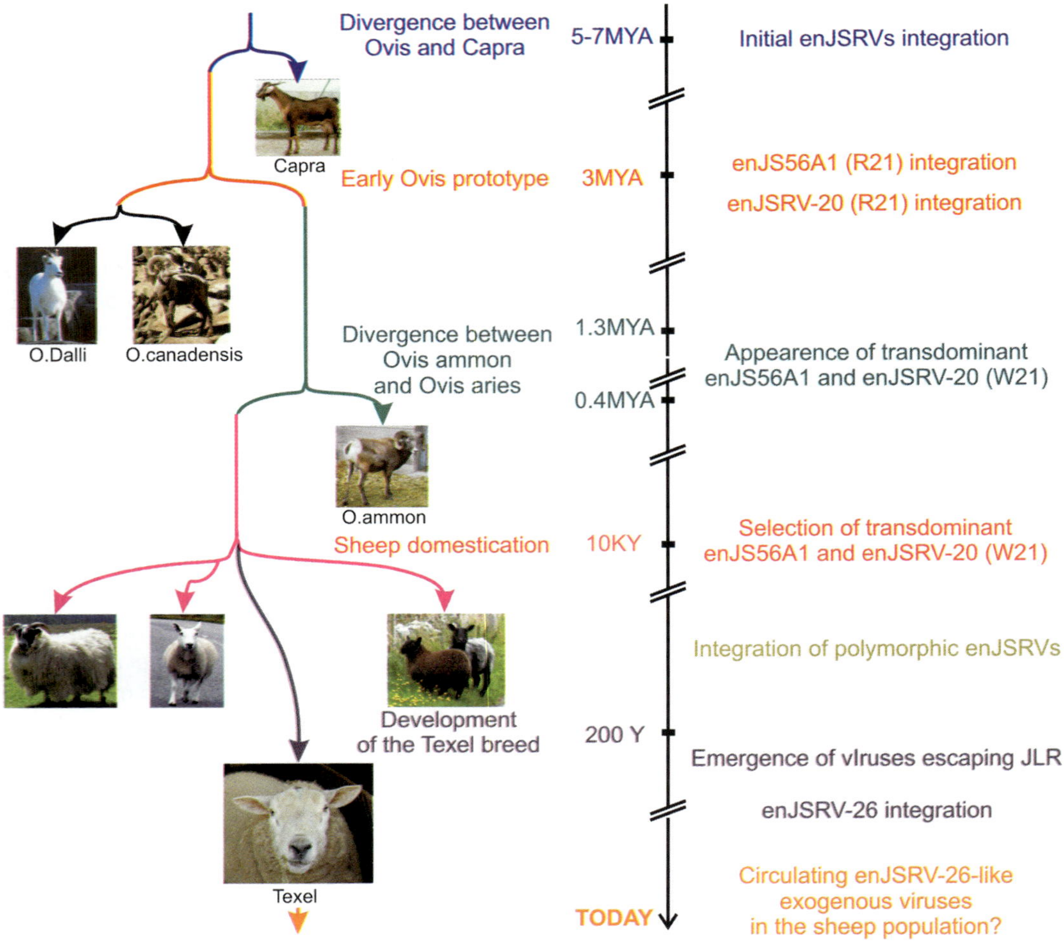

Fig. 4. Dates and events associating the evolutionary history of enJSRVs and their host**.** Schematic diagram illustrating key events of the evolutionary history of enJSRVs with estimated dates during the evolution of the domestic sheep and the Caprinae. Figure reproduced from Arnaud and coworkers (Arnaud *et al.* 2008).

abundant in the genital tract and placenta of various animal species (Harris 1991, Harris 1998). Indeed, a number of intact ERV *env* genes have been identified in primates (syncytin-1 and -2) (Venables *et al.* 1995, Blond *et al.* 2000, de Parseval *et al.* 2003), Muridae (syncytin-A and -B in mouse, rat, gerbil, vole, and hamster) (Dupressoir *et al.* 2005), and rabbits (syncytin-Ory1) (Heidmann *et al.* 2009). In each case, the protein products of the nonorthologous ERV *env* genes, termed syncytins, are highly fusogenic in transfection assays and preferentially expressed in the syncytiotrophoblast. The syncytiotrophoblast is a multinucleated cell that lines the outer surface of the placenta, derived by intercellular fusion of mononuclear cytotrophoblast cells, and responsible for the transport of oxygen, nutrients and waste products, production of hormones, and immune tolerance (Watson & Cross 2005). In both humans and mice, one of the two syncytins (human syncytin-2 and mouse syncytin-B) is immunosuppressive and, rather unexpectedly, the other (human syncytin 1 and mouse syncytin-A) is not, although both are able to induce cell-cell fusion (Mangeney *et al.* 2007). Syncytin-A plays an important biological role in syncytiotrophoblast development, because *syncytin-A* null mice die *in utero* due to failure of trophoblast cells to fuse and form one of the two syncytiotrophoblast layers present in the mouse placenta (Dupressoir *et al.* 2009). Given that some syncytins are immunosuppressive, they may play a role in fetomaternal tolerance, although this concept has not been mechanistically tested *in vivo* (Mangeney *et al.* 2007). The presence of intact env genes that are expressed in the multinucleated syncytiotrophoblasts of the placenta and preserved over thousands of years, together with the observation that they elicit fusion of cells in vitro, led to the speculation that ERVs play an essential role in placental development and were positively selected for a convergent fundamental role in the evolution of placental mammals and development of viviparity (Villarreal 1997, Mi *et al.* 2000, Dupressoir *et al.* 2005, Heidmann *et al.* 2009).

In sheep, enJSRVs are abundantly expressed in the epithelia lining the different tissues of the female reproductive tract (vagina, cervix, uterus and oviduct) (Palmarini *et al.* 2000, Dunlap *et al.* 2005). In the uterus, both enJSRVs RNA and protein are detected specifically in the endometrial luminal epithelium (LE) and in the glandular epithelia (GE) (Spencer *et al.* 1999, Palmarini *et al.* 2000, Palmarini *et al.* 2001a). In addition, the enJSRVs *env* are expressed in the trophectoderm cells of the placenta in a temporal fashion that is coincident with key events in conceptus elongation and onset of trophoblast giant binucleate cell (BNC) differentiation (Dunlap *et al.* 2005). Within the placenta, enJSRVs are most abundant in the trophoblast giant BNC and multinucleated synytial plaques within the placentomes throughout pregnancy. The RNA of enJSRVs is first detected in the conceptus on day 12 (Dunlap *et al.* 2005). Interestingly, hyaluronoglucosaminidase 2 (HYAL2), a cellular receptor for both JSRV and enJSRVs Env (Rai *et al.* 2001, Arnaud *et al.* 2007a), is detected exclusively in the BNC and the multinucleated syncytial plaques of the placenta (Dunlap *et al.* 2005). These observations led to the hypothesis that enJSRVs and HYAL2 are important for placental growth and differentiation in sheep (Spencer *et al.* 2007). Indeed, injection of morpholinos that inhibit enJSRV Env production into the uteri of pregnant sheep on day 8 of pregnancy compromised conceptus elongation, resulting in reduced mononuclear trophoblast cell outgrowth and loss of trophoblast giant BNC differentiation (Dunlap *et al.* 2006). The biological role of HYAL2 in sheep conceptus development and differentiation has not been determined. **Figure 5** presents a current hypothesis on the biological roles of enJSRVs Env and HYAL2 in trophoblast development and differentiation in the sheep conceptus during early pregnancy.

Interestingly, the enJSRVs Env have a high degree of similarity with the oncogenic exogenous JSRV Env; thus, it is tempting to speculate that both endogenous and exogenous JSRV Env share similar mechanisms to induce trophoblast proliferation/differentiation and cell transformation, respectively, since placental morphogenesis has features similar to tumorigenesis and metastasis (Soundararajan & Rao 2004, Ferretti *et al.* 2007). Indeed, the Ras-MEK-MAPK, Rac1, and PI3K-AKT-mTOR signalling pathways involved in JSRV-induced cell transformation are important regulators of trophoblast growth and differentiation in human and rodent placentae (Pollheimer & Knofler 2005).

Conclusions

ERVs are present in the genomes of all vertebrates (Gifford & Tristem 2003) and can be used as DNA fossils to unravel virus-host coevolution over millions of years (Coffin 2004, Chessa *et al.* 2009). The domestic sheep constitutes a powerful model to study the biological significance

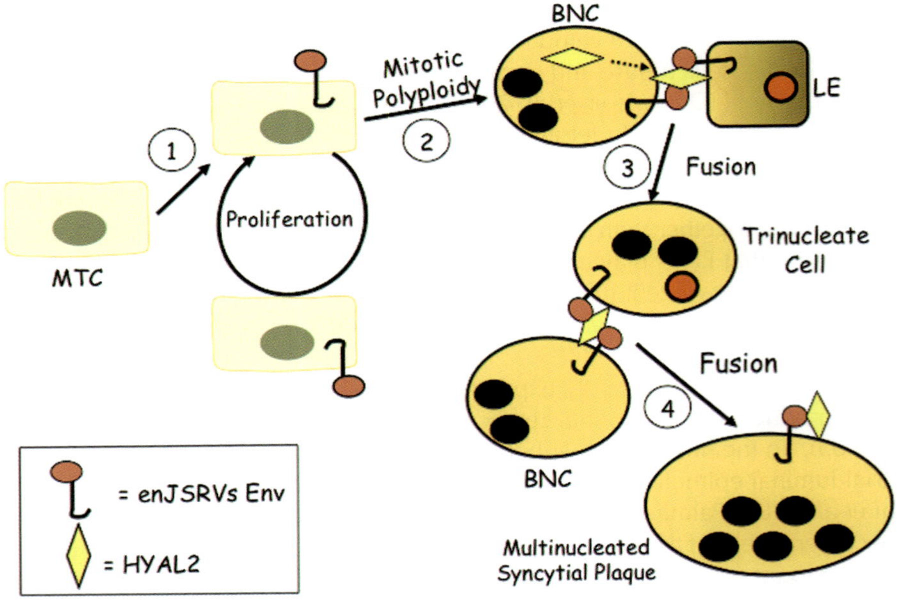

Fig. 5. Hypothesis on the biological role of enJSRVs Env and HYAL2 in trophoblast differentiation in sheep. During pregnancy, trophoblast giant binucleate cells (BNC) begin to differentiate from mononuclear trophoblast cells (MTC) on day 14. First, MTC begin to express enJSRVs envelope (Env) in the conceptus on day 12 (Step 1). Second, results from microscopy studies support the idea that binucleated trophectoderm cells or trophoblast giant BNC are derived from karyokinesis without cytokinesis (endoreduplication) or mitotic polyploidy (Step 2). Next, the newly formed BNC that are co-expressing enJSRVs *env* and *HYAL2* initially fuse with enJSRVs *env*-expressing endometrial luminal epithelial (LE) cells, forming a trinucleated fetomaternal hybrid cell (Step 3). During this period, the BNC and LE cells express enJSRV *env* RNA, whereas only the BNC express *HYAL2*. In fact, *HYAL2* mRNA is not detectable in uterine cells. By days 20 to 25, virtually all of the endometrial LE cells are fused with the BNC. Fourth, other newly formed BNC fuse with trinucleate cells to form a multinucleated syncytial plaque (Step 4). During most of gestation, the BNC continue to differentiate from the MTC and then fuse with each other and existing multinucleated syncytia to form multinucleated syncytial plaques with 20-25 nuclei. The multinucleated syncytial plaques and BNC form the basis of the cotyledons of the placenta that interdigitate with caruncles of the endometrium to develop and form placentomes.

of ERVs given the contemporary presence in this animal species of a pathogenic exogenous retrovirus (JSRV) and the biologically active enJSRVs (Arnaud *et al.* 2007a, Arnaud *et al.* 2008). During evolution, the first driving force that positively selected and fixed enJSRVs in sheep population was their ability to protect their host against infection by related pathogenic retroviruses (Palmarini *et al.* 2004, Arnaud *et al.* 2008). However, the enJSRVs Env are also essential for placental development in sheep (Dunlap *et al.* 2006). Collective evidence from studies of primates, rodents, rabbits and sheep supports the idea that independently acquired, nonorthologous ERVs were positively selected for a convergent physiological role in evolution and development of the placenta. Studies with enJSRVs and JSRV as well as other ERVs expressed in the placenta help us understand how ERVs evolved from infectious elements to essential genes (de Parseval & Heidmann 2005).

Acknowledgements

We are grateful to the members of the Laboratory for Uterine Biology and Pregnancy of Texas A&M University and the Laboratory of Viral Pathogenesis of the University of Glasgow Faculty of Veterinary Medicine for stimulating discussions. Work in the laboratory of the authors is supported by NIH grant HD052745, a program grant of the Wellcome Trust and by a Strategic Research Developmental Grant by the Scottish Funding Council.

References

Arnaud F, Caporale M, Varela M, Biek R, Chessa B, Alberti A, Golder M, Mura M, Zhang YP, Yu L, Pereira F, Demartini JC, Leymaster K, Spencer TE & Palmarini M 2007a A paradigm for virus-host coevolution: sequential counter-adaptations between endogenous and exogenous retroviruses. *PLoS Pathog* **3** e170.

Arnaud F, Murcia PR & Palmarini M 2007b Mechanisms of late restriction induced by an endogenous retrovirus. *J Virol* **81** 11441-11451.

Arnaud F, Varela M, Spencer TE & Palmarini M 2008 Coevolution of endogenous betaretroviruses of sheep and their host. *Cell Mol Life Sci* **65** 3422-3432.

Bannert N & Kurth R 2004 Retroelements and the human genome: new perspectives on an old relation. *Proc Natl Acad Sci U S A* **101 Suppl 2** 14572-14579.

Biemont C & Vieira C 2006 Genetics: junk DNA as an evolutionary force. *Nature* **443** 521-524.

Blond JL, Lavillette D, Cheynet V, Bouton O, Oriol G, Chapel-Fernandes S, Mandrand B, Mallet F & Cosset FL 2000 An envelope glycoprotein of the human endogenous retrovirus HERV-W is expressed in the human placenta and fuses cells expressing the type D mammalian retrovirus receptor. *J Virol* **74** 3321-3329.

Bock M & Stoye JP 2000 Endogenous retroviruses and the human germline. *Curr Opin Genet Dev* **10** 651-655.

Boeke JD & Stoye JP 1997 Retrotransposons , endogenous retroviruses and the evolution of retroelements. In *Retroviruses*, pp. 343-436.

Caporale M, Cousens C, Centorame P, Pinoni C, De Las Heras M & Palmarini M 2006 Expression of the jaagsiekte sheep retrovirus envelope glycoprotein is sufficient to induce lung tumors in sheep. *J Virol* **80** 8030-8037.

Chessa B, Pereira F, Arnaud F, Amorim A, Goyache F, Mainland I, Kao RR, Pemberton JM, Beraldi D, Stear MJ, Alberti A, Pittau M, Iannuzzi L, Banabazi MH, Kazwala RR, Zhang YP, Arranz JJ, Ali BA, Wang Z, Uzun M, Dione MM, Olsaker I, Holm LE, Saarma U, Ahmad S, Marzanov N, Eythorsdottir E, Holland MJ, Ajmone-Marsan P, Bruford MW, Kantanen J, Spencer TE & Palmarini M 2009 Revealing the history of sheep domestication using retrovirus integrations. *Science* **324** 532-536.

Coffin JM 2004 Evolution of retroviruses: fossils in our DNA. *Proc Am Philos Soc* **148** 264-280.

De Las Heras M, Ortin A, Benito A, Summers C, Ferrer LM & Sharp JM 2006 In-situ demonstration of mitogen-activated protein kinase Erk 1/2 signalling pathway in contagious respiratory tumours of sheep and goats. *J Comp Pathol* **135** 1-10.

de Parseval N & Heidmann T 2005 Human endogenous retroviruses: from infectious elements to human genes. *Cytogenet Genome Res* **110** 318-332.

de Parseval N, Lazar V, Casella JF, Benit L & Heidmann T 2003 Survey of human genes of retroviral origin: identification and transcriptome of the genes with coding capacity for complete envelope proteins. *J Virol* **77** 10414-10422.

Dunlap KA, Palmarini M, Adelson DL & Spencer TE 2005 Sheep endogenous betaretroviruses (enJSRVs) and the hyaluronidase 2 (HYAL2) receptor in the ovine uterus and conceptus. *Biol Reprod* **73** 271-279.

Dunlap KA, Palmarini M, Varela M, Burghardt RC, Hayashi K, Farmer JL & Spencer TE 2006 Endogenous retroviruses regulate periimplantation placental growth and differentiation. *Proc Natl Acad Sci U S A* **103** 14390-14395.

Dupressoir A, Marceau G, Vernochet C, Benit L, Kanellopoulos C, Sapin V & Heidmann T 2005 Syncytin-A and syncytin-B, two fusogenic placenta-specific murine envelope genes of retroviral origin conserved in Muridae. *Proc Natl Acad Sci U S A* **102** 725-730.

Dupressoir A, Vernochet C, Bawa O, Harper F, Pierron G, Opolon P & Heidmann T 2009 Syncytin-A knockout mice demonstrate the critical role in placentation of a fusogenic, endogenous retrovirus-derived, envelope gene. *Proc Natl Acad Sci U S A* **106** 12127-12132.

Ferretti C, Bruni L, Dangles-Marie V, Pecking AP & Bellet D 2007 Molecular circuits shared by placental and cancer cells, and their implications in the proliferative, invasive and migratory capacities of trophoblasts. *Hum Reprod Update* **13** 121-141.

Gifford R & Tristem M 2003 The evolution, distribution and diversity of endogenous retroviruses. *Virus Genes* **26** 291-315.

Harris JR 1991 The evolution of placental mammals. *FEBS Lett* **295** 3-4.

Harris JR 1998 Placental endogenous retrovirus (ERV): structural, functional, and evolutionary significance. *Bioessays* **20** 307-316.

Heidmann O, Vernochet C, Dupressoir A & Heidmann T 2009 Identification of an endogenous retroviral envelope gene with fusogenic activity and placenta-specific expression in the rabbit: a new "syncytin" in a third order of mammals. *Retrovirology* **6** 107.

Herniou E, Martin J, Miller K, Cook J, Wilkinson M &

Tristem M 1998 Retroviral diversity and distribution in vertebrates. *J Virol* **72** 5955-5966.

Jern P & Coffin JM 2008 Effects of retroviruses on host genome function. *Annu Rev Genet* **42** 709-732.

Kalter SS, Heberling RL, Helmke RJ, Panigel M, Smith GC, Kraemer DC, Hellman A, Fowler AK & Strickland JE 1975 A comparative study on the presence of C-type viral particles in placentas from primates and other animals. *Bibl Haematol* **40** 391-401.

Kurth R & Bannert N 2010 Beneficial and detrimental effects of human endogenous retroviruses. *Int J Cancer* **126** 306-314.

Maeda N & Fan H 2008 Signal transduction pathways utilized by enzootic nasal tumor virus (ENTV-1) envelope protein in transformation of rat epithelial cells resemble those used by jaagsiekte sheep retrovirus. *Virus Genes* **36** 147-155.

Maeda N, Fu W, Ortin A, de las Heras M & Fan H 2005 Roles of the Ras-MEK-mitogen-activated protein kinase and phosphatidylinositol 3-kinase-Akt-mTOR pathways in Jaagsiekte sheep retrovirus-induced transformation of rodent fibroblast and epithelial cell lines. *J Virol* **79** 4440-4450.

Maeda N, Palmarini M, Murgia C & Fan H 2001 Direct transformation of rodent fibroblasts by jaagsiekte sheep retrovirus DNA. *Proc Natl Acad Sci U S A* **98** 4449-4454.

Mangeney M, Renard M, Schlecht-Louf G, Bouallaga I, Heidmann O, Letzelter C, Richaud A, Ducos B & Heidmann T 2007 Placental syncytins: Genetic disjunction between the fusogenic and immunosuppressive activity of retroviral envelope proteins. *Proc Natl Acad Sci U S A* **104** 20534-20539.

Mi S, Lee X, Li X, Veldman GM, Finnerty H, Racie L, LaVallie E, Tang XY, Edouard P, Howes S, Keith JC, Jr. & McCoy JM 2000 Syncytin is a captive retroviral envelope protein involved in human placental morphogenesis. *Nature* **403** 785-789.

Mura M, Murcia P, Caporale M, Spencer TE, Nagashima K, Rein A & Palmarini M 2004 Late viral interference induced by transdominant Gag of an endogenous retrovirus. *Proc Natl Acad Sci U S A* **101** 11117-11122.

Murcia PR, Arnaud F & Palmarini M 2007 The transdominant endogenous retrovirus enJS56A1 associates with and blocks intracellular trafficking of Jaagsiekte sheep retrovirus Gag. *J Virol* **81** 1762-1772.

Palmarini M, Gray CA, Carpenter K, Fan H, Bazer FW & Spencer T 2001a Expression of endogenous betaretroviruses in the ovine uterus: effects of neonatal age, estrous cycle, pregnancy and progesterone. *J Virol* **75** 11319-11327.

Palmarini M, Hallwirth C, York D, Murgia C, de Oliveira T, Spencer T & Fan H 2000 Molecular cloning and functional analysis of three type D endogenous retroviruses of sheep reveals a different cell tropism from that of the highly related exogenous jaagsiekte sheep retrovirus. *Journal of Virology* **74** 8065-8076.

Palmarini M, Maeda N, Murgia C, De-Fraja C, Hofacre A & Fan H 2001b A phosphatidylinositol-3-kinase (PI-3K) docking site in the cytoplasmic tail of the Jaagsiekte sheep retrovirus transmembrane protein is essential for envelope-induced transformation of NIH3T3 cells. *Journal of Virology* **75** 11002-11009.

Palmarini M, Mura M & Spencer TE 2004 Endogenous betaretroviruses of sheep: teaching new lessons in retroviral interference and adaptation. *J Gen Virol* **85** 1-13.

Palmarini M, Sharp JM, De las Heras M & Fan H 1999 Jaagsiekte sheep retrovirus is necessary and sufficient to induce a contagious lung cancer in sheep. *Journal of Virology* **73** 6964-6972.

Pollheimer J & Knofler M 2005 Signalling pathways regulating the invasive differentiation of human trophoblasts: a review. *Placenta* **26 Suppl A** S21-30.

Rai SK, Duh FM, Vigdorovich V, Danilkovitch-Miagkova A, Lerman MI & Miller AD 2001 Candidate tumor suppressor HYAL2 is a glycosylphosphatidylinositol (GPI)-anchored cell-surface receptor for jaagsiekte sheep retrovirus, the envelope protein of which mediates oncogenic transformation. *Proc Natl Acad Sci U S A* **98** 4443-4448.

Smith CA & Moore HD 1988 Expression of C-type viral particles at implantation in the marmoset monkey. *Hum Reprod* **3** 395-398.

Soundararajan R & Rao AJ 2004 Trophoblast 'pseudo-tumorigenesis': significance and contributory factors. *Reprod Biol Endocrinol* **2** 15.

Spencer TE, Johnson GA, Bazer FW, Burghardt RC & Palmarini M 2007 Pregnancy recognition and conceptus implantation in domestic ruminants: roles of progesterone, interferons and endogenous retroviruses. *Reprod Fertil Dev* **19** 65-78.

Spencer TE, Mura M, Gray CA, Griebel PJ & Palmarini M 2003 Receptor usage and fetal expression of ovine endogenous betaretroviruses: implications for coevolution of endogenous and exogenous retroviruses. *J Virol* **77** 749-753.

Spencer TE, Stagg AG, Joyce MM, Jenster G, Wood CG, Bazer FW, Wiley AA & Bartol FF 1999 Discovery and characterization of endometrial epithelial messenger ribonucleic acids using the ovine uterine gland knockout model. *Endocrinology* **140** 4070-4080.

Varela M, Chow YH, Sturkie C, Murcia P & Palmarini M 2006 Association of RON tyrosine kinase with the Jaagsiekte sheep retrovirus envelope glycoprotein. *Virology* **350** 347-357.

Varela M, Spencer TE, Palmarini M & Arnaud F 2009 Friendly viruses: the special relationship between endogenous retroviruses and their host. *Ann N Y Acad Sci* **1178** 157-172.

Venables PJ, Brookes SM, Griffiths D, Weiss RA & Boyd MT 1995 Abundance of an endogenous retroviral envelope protein in placental trophoblasts suggests a biological function. *Virology* **211** 589-592.

Villarreal LP 1997 On viruses, sex, and motherhood. *J Virol* **71** 859-865.

Watson ED & Cross JC 2005 Development of structures and transport functions in the mouse placenta. *Physiology (Bethesda)* **20** 180-193.

Wootton SK, Halbert CL & Miller AD 2005 Sheep retrovirus structural protein induces lung tumours. *Nature* **434** 904-907.

Putative role of cocaine- and amphetamine-regulated transcript (*CARTPT*) in dominant follicle selection in cattle

GW Smith[1,2,3], A Sen[1,2], JK Folger[1,2] and JJ Ireland [2,3]

Laboratory of Mammalian Reproductive Biology and Genomics[1], Departments of Animal Science[2] and Physiology[3], Michigan State University, East Lansing, MI 48824-1225

The mechanisms regulating development of a single (dominant) follicle capable of ovulation during each follicular wave in cattle and atresia of remaining follicles (dominant follicle selection) are not well understood. FSH and IGF1 are known regulators of follicle growth and granulosa cell estradiol production during follicular waves. Recent evidence indicates cocaine and amphetamine regulated transcript (*CARTPT*), with intraovarian expression only in single-ovulating species, is a novel regulator of follicular development. The mature CARTPT peptide (CART) is a potent negative regulator of FSH and IGF1 action on granulosa cells in vitro and can inhibit follicular estradiol production in vivo. Follicular fluid CART concentrations in healthy follicles decrease after dominant follicle selection and *CARTPT* mRNA is lower in healthy versus atretic follicles collected prior to and early after initiation of follicle dominance, suggestive of a regulatory role in the selection process. The inhibitory actions of CART on FSH signaling and estradiol production are dependent on the $G_{o/i}$-subclass of inhibitory G proteins and linked to multiple components of the FSH signal transduction pathway resulting in reduced *CYP19A1* mRNA and estradiol production. Evidence to date supports a potential important functional role for CART in regulation of dominant follicle selection and the species-specific ovulatory quota in monotocous species.

Introduction

The ovarian cycle is central to the reproductive process, because only mature ovarian follicles release oocytes to be fertilized. However, > 99.9% of follicles die via atresia at various stages of folliculogenesis and never ovulate. Antral follicle development occurs in a characteristic wave like pattern in monotocous species including cattle and humans (Fortune 1994, Ginther *et al.* 2001, Baerwald *et al.* 2003). A transient increase in serum FSH precedes the onset of a follicular wave and stimulates emergence of a cohort of small antral follicles. Typically, in the face of declining FSH concentrations, a single dominant follicle out of this cohort is selected to continue to grow to ovulatory size (Fortune *et al.* 2004), and produces increased amounts of estradiol. The remaining smaller "subordinate" follicles rapidly lose their capacity to produce estradiol and die via atresia (Richards & Hedin 1988, Sunderland *et al.* 1994, Mihm *et al.* 1997, Baerwald *et al.* 2003). The process whereby development of a single (dominant) follicle capable of ovulation during each

---

Corresponding author E-mail: smithge7@msu.edu

follicular wave and atresia of remaining follicles occurs is referred to as dominant follicle selection. Selection of a single dominant follicle is an evolutionarily conserved mechanism critical to control of number of offspring per pregnancy in monotocous species. Production of estradiol by the dominant follicle is essential for follicular growth and triggers the preovulatory gonadotropin surge to promote resumption of meiosis and ovulation (Fortune 1994, Greenwald & Roy 1994, Vander *et al.* 1994). Estradiol producing capacity is lost in ovarian follicles before apoptosis and morphological signs of atresia (Sunderland *et al.* 1994, Austin *et al.* 2001). While the key role of pituitary gonadotropins in mediating the wave like pattern of follicular development is well established, the intrafollicular mechanisms and regulatory molecules that are obligatory for selection of a single dominant follicle during each follicular wave have not been fully established.

Differences in the milieu of intrafollicular factors between the future dominant and subordinate follicles are believed to have a role in selection (Beg *et al.* 2002, Beg & Ginther 2006). A prominent local role for multiple growth factor systems, including the IGFs, in selection has been proposed (Fortune *et al.* 2001, Knight & Glister 2003, Webb *et al.* 2003, Fortune *et al.* 2004). The IGFs increase granulosa cell proliferation, synergize with gonadotropins to promote granulosa cell differentiation (Spicer & Echternkamp 1995), stimulate estradiol production (Spicer *et al.* 1993, Gutierrez *et al.* 1997) and enhance sensitivity to FSH (Monget & Monniaux 1995). Concentrations of free IGF1 diverge in the largest versus second largest follicle within a cohort of growing follicles during follicular waves (Beg *et al.* 2002, Rivera & Fortune 2003b). These results support a functional role for increased IGF1 bioavailability in future dominant follicles during selection. Intrafollicular IGF1 bioavailability is regulated by the low molecular weight IGF binding proteins (IGFBP) and IGFBP4 and IGFBP5 levels are regulated by IGFBP proteases (Rivera & Fortune 2003a). Follicular fluid IGFBP levels are greater in atretic versus healthy follicles (Echternkamp *et al.* 1994, de la Sota *et al.* 1996, Stewart *et al.* 1996, Mihm *et al.* 1997). Lower levels of IGFBP4 and IGFBP5 are present in the largest growing follicles during selection and in the dominant follicle compared with smaller (subordinate) follicles (Rivera & Fortune 2003a). Follicles with reduced IGFBP4 and IGFBP5 also displayed higher levels of proteolytic activity for IGFBP4 and IGFBP5 (Rivera & Fortune 2003a), activity attributed to PAPPA (Mazerbourg *et al.* 2001, Rivera & Fortune 2003b, Spicer 2004). Furthermore, studies have shown that the follicle with the lowest follicular fluid IGFBP4 levels in a cohort prior to selection is destined to become the dominant follicle (Mihm *et al.* 2000).

A combination of FSH and IGF1 is well established to regulate estradiol production and growth of follicles during follicular waves in cattle (Beg & Ginther 2006). While the role of FSH in initiating emergence of a follicular wave is well established, dominant follicle selection occurs as FSH concentrations are declining (Adams *et al.* 1992, Sunderland *et al.* 1994). A combination of follicle ablations and experimental suppression of FSH concentrations below normal levels at onset of diameter deviation has been used to functionally demonstrate greater FSH responsiveness of the future dominant follicle versus future subordinate follicles in cattle (Ginther *et al.* 2003). However, *FSHR* mRNA (Xu *et al.* 1995, Bao *et al.* 1997, Evans & Fortune 1997) and FSHR binding (Ireland & Roche 1982, Ireland & Roche 1983a, Ireland & Roche 1983b, Braden *et al.* 1986) do not increase coincident with selection. Hence, rather than enhanced FSH action, it is plausible that local (intrafollicular) inhibition of FSH action could be functionally linked to selection. Observed temporal regulation of cocaine- and amphetamine– regulated transcript (*CARTPT*) expression during a follicular wave and observed negative effects of mature form of the CARTPT peptide (CART) on FSH and IGF1 action, also suggest a potential functional role for *CARTPT* as a mediator of dominant follicle selection. The focus of this review is on intrafollicular expression, actions and mechanism of action of *CARTPT*; evidence supportive of a functional role for *CARTPT* in regulation of dominant follicle selection.

Discovery and intrafollicular expression of *CARTPT*

The dawning of the genomics and genome sequencing era in livestock has provided tremendous potential for advancement in understanding of the molecular mechanisms involved in regulation of ovarian follicular development. During experiments reported in 2004 designed to characterize the transcriptome of bovine oocytes and generate an oocyte cDNA microarray for physiological studies (Yao *et al.* 2004), we identified five expressed sequence tags with similarity to *CARTPT*. Expression of *CARTPT* mRNA in the mammalian ovary had not been reported previously. The presence of *CARTPT* mRNA in the bovine oocyte was of considerable interest because CART is a well characterized neuropeptide with documented biological activity. Numerous pleiotropic actions of CART, including anorexigenic (Kristensen *et al.* 1998, Lambert *et al.* 1998, Vrang *et al.* 1999, Hunter *et al.* 2004), neuroendocrine (Vrang *et al.* 2000, Baranowska *et al.* 2003, Kuriyama *et al.* 2004, Raptis *et al.* 2004, Smith *et al.* 2004) and anti-psychostimulant effects (Jaworski *et al.* 2003, Kim *et al.* 2003, Kuhar *et al.* 2005) have been described in the brain. To date, the gastrointestinal tract (Ekblad *et al.* 2003), pancreatic cells (Wierup *et al.* 2005, Wierup *et al.* 2006) and ovarian granulosa cells (Sen *et al.* 2007, Sen *et al.* 2008, Lv *et al.* 2009) are the prominent non-neural sites of *CARTPT* action described. Furthermore, *in vitro* model systems for investigation of *CARTPT* mechanism of action linked to a downstream physiological response had not been described at the time of the serendipitous discovery of *CARTPT* expression in the bovine ovary. Thus, CART met initial criteria for a potential novel intrafollicular regulatory molecule of interest and further experiments were conducted to characterize bovine ovarian *CARTPT* expression and investigate its intrafollicular localization and potential regulatory role.

While intraovarian *CARTPT* expression was initially documented in the oocyte, the granulosa cell layer is the prominent source of *CARTPT* expression in the bovine ovary. To date, the function of CART of oocyte origin is unclear. In initial studies, *CARTPT* mRNA and peptide localization was observed specifically in the granulosa cell layer of some but not all antral follicles and not in preantral follicles (Kobayashi *et al.* 2004). The temporal expression of *CARTPT* mRNA in granulosa cells of antral, but not preantral follicles suggests that local CART action is presumably restricted to follicles that have undergone advanced stages of differentiation.

To further define the window of follicular development when biological actions of CART are most likely manifest, temporal changes in granulosa cell *CARTPT* mRNA and follicular fluid CART concentrations were determined in bovine follicles collected at the following specific stages of the first follicular wave: 1) predeviation (d 1.5 after emergence of the first follicular wave), 2) early dominance (first day in wave when one follicle in cohort is 2 mm larger than others), 3) mid dominance (second day in wave that dominant follicle does not increase in size), 4) loss of dominance (first day that a new cohort in second follicular wave appears) and 5) preovulatory (1 d after $PGF_{2\alpha}$ injection on d 7 post estrus). Health status of each follicle was determined by calculating follicular fluid estradiol: progesterone ratios. Follicles with an estradiol: progesterone ratio ≥ 1 are estrogen-active and healthy and follicles with an estradiol: progesterone ratio < 1 are estrogen-inactive and atretic (Ireland & Roche 1982, Ireland & Roche 1983a, Sunderland *et al.* 1994). Results revealed granulosa cell *CARTPT* mRNA and follicular fluid CART concentrations are higher in estrogen inactive atretic follicles versus estrogen active healthy follicles collected during (predeviation stage) and immediately after selection (early dominance stage) and relatively low in follicles collected at remaining stages of a follicular wave (Lv *et al.* 2009). Furthermore, follicular fluid CART levels are decreased in estrogen-active healthy follicles coincident with dominant follicle selection (Lv *et al.* 2009). Observed elevated granulosa cell *CARTPT* mRNA and follicular fluid CART concentrations in estrogen-inactive subordinate compared with estrogen-active potential dominant follicles, coupled with the higher follicular fluid CART concentrations in healthy follicles collected before versus immediately after selection (Lv *et al.* 2009) support a potential functional role for *CARTPT* in the process of dominant follicle selection.

CARTPT regulation of estradiol production and mechanism of action

The observed negative relationship of *CARTPT* expression with follicle health status and temporal regulation of granulosa cell *CARTPT* expression during follicular waves in cattle is suggestive of a functional role in dominant follicle selection. Hence the ability of CART to inhibit granulosa cell estradiol production in vitro was investigated using a long term culture system where cells gain significant estradiol producing capacity with time in culture and respond in a dose-dependent fashion to FSH (Sen *et al.* 2007) and IGF1 (Gutierrez *et al.* 1997) with an increase in estradiol production. Treatment with CART inhibits (in a dose-dependent fashion) FSH-stimulated estradiol production and *CYP19A1* mRNA expression by bovine granulosa cells (Sen *et al.* 2007). Treatment with CART also suppresses IGF1-stimulated estradiol production in this culture system (Fig. 1). Collectively, results demonstrate potent inhibitory effects of CART on actions of two of the major tropic hormones for estradiol production during the selection process. Furthermore, CART treatment can also reduce LH-induced production of androstenedione, the androgen precursor for estradiol synthesis, by theca tissue collected prior to (pre deviation stage) and early post selection (early dominance stage), but not at later stages of a follicular wave (Lv *et al.* 2009). Thus, the inhibitory effects of CART on estradiol production in vivo during selection could be mediated indirectly by inhibition of production of theca cell androgen precursor for estradiol biosynthesis and well as directly through actions on FSH- and IGF1-stimulated granulosa cell estradiol production.

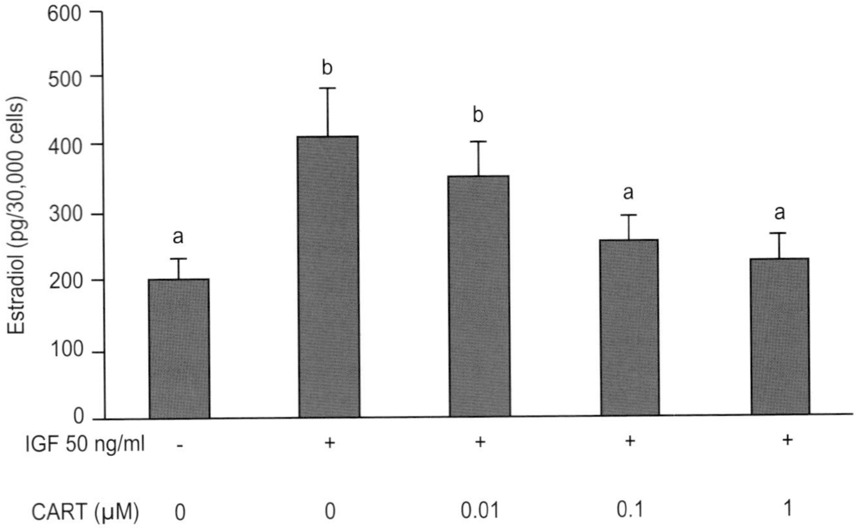

Fig. 1. Dose dependent inhibitory effect of CART on IGF1-induced granulosa cell estradiol production in vitro. Serum-free long-term granulosa cell culture was performed using previously described procedures (Sen *et al.* 2007, Sen *et al.* 2008). Cells were cultured for 7 d in the presence or absence of 50 ng/ml LR3 IGF1. Every 48 h, 75% of media was replaced with fresh medium containing appropriate treatments. CART treatments (0, 0.01, 0.1 and 1 μM) were initiated on d 6 of culture and continued for 24 h. On d 7, media was removed for estradiol assay and the cells were washed 2X, trypsinized and cell number determined. Data (pg estradiol) were normalized to 30,000 cells and bars (mean +/- SEM of four replicate experiments) with different superscripts denote significant differences across treatments ($P < 0.05$). Note dose dependent (> 90%) inhibition of IGF1-induced estradiol production in response to CART treatment.

To confirm physiological relevance of inhibitory effects of CART on estradiol production obtained in vitro, the effects of intrafollicular injection of CART (into early dominant follicles) on follicular estradiol production and granulosa cell *CYP19A1* mRNA in vivo was performed (Lv *et al.* 2009) using our previously validated ultrasound mediated intrafollicular injection procedures (Peters *et al.* 2004, Li *et al.* 2006, Li *et al.* 2007). Ultrasound mediated intrafollicular injection provides a powerful tool for administration of ligands, antagonists, inhibitors etc into follicles at specific stages of a wave to test gene function/contribution to mechanisms associated with selection.

In above described studies, elevation of concentrations of CART in follicular fluid approximately 3-fold resulted in a 54% reduction in follicular fluid estradiol and a 96% decrease in granulosa cell *CYP19A1* mRNA 24 h post injection, with no effect on follicle size (Lv *et al.* 2009). Concentrations of androstenedione were not affected, but this was not unexpected as injection of CART occurred after the selection process was complete. Thus, CART can negatively regulate follicular estradiol production and *CYP19A1* mRNA in vivo supporting a potential physiological role for CART in negative regulation of granulosa cell estradiol production during selection of the dominant follicle.

To further dissect the mechanisms involved in *CARTPT* regulation of granulosa cell estradiol production, effects of CART treatment on specific components of the FSH signal transduction cascade were determined using a combination of pharmacological inhibitors, siRNA mediated gene knockdown strategies and biochemical assays. FSH-induced granulosa cell cAMP accumulation and estradiol production is Ca^{2+} dependent and CART can inhibit FSH-stimulated Ca^{2+} influx (Sen *et al.* 2007). Furthermore, it is well known that FSH activates the cAMP-protein kinase A pathway leading to *CYP19A1* expression and estradiol production (Richards 2001, Richards *et al.* 2002). Treatment with CART induces a dose dependent decrease in cAMP accumulation in bovine granulosa cells in response to FSH or forskolin treatment (Sen *et al.* 2007). However, inhibitory effects of CART on FSH-stimulated estradiol production are not mediated solely by inhibition of cAMP accumulation, as CART also inhibits estradiol production in response to treatment of granulosa cells with 8-Br-cAMP (Sen *et al.* 2007). The ability of CART to inhibit 8-Br-cAMP-induced estradiol production clearly indicates that cAMP is not the sole limiting factor involved in the negative effects of CART on FSH signaling. Thus, CART likely regulates other FSH-induced signaling proteins obligatory for estradiol production that are downstream of cAMP.

Bovine granulosa cell estradiol production in response to FSH is also Erk 1/2 (MAPK 3/1) and Akt (AKT1) dependent (Sen *et al.* 2007) and a growing body of evidence supports a prominent role for regulation of MAPK3/1 and AKT1 pathways in the selection process. Subordinate follicles collected near the time of selection of the dominant follicle had reduced levels of phosphorylated AKT1 in granulosa cells and phosphorylated MAPK3/1 and AKT1 in theca cells when compared to bovine dominant follicles (Ryan *et al.* 2007). In addition, intrafollicular administration of MAPK3/1 and AKT1 inhibitors into growing sheep follicles disrupted growth and estradiol production (Ryan *et al.* 2008). Evidence suggests that CART may function as an endogenous negative regulator of MAPK3/1 and AKT1 signaling associated with dominant follicle selection. Transient CART stimulation of bovine granulosa cells shortens the duration of FSH-induced MAPK3/1 and AKT1 signaling while a prolonged CART treatment completely blocks FSH-induced MAPK3/1 and AKT1 activation (Sen *et al.* 2008). The CART-induced accelerated termination of MAPK3/1 and AKT1 signaling is mediated both by induced expression and impaired ubiquitin-mediated proteasome degradation of the mitogen-activated protein kinase (MAPK) phosphatases dual specific phosphatase 5 (DUSP5) and protein phosphatase 2A (PP2A). Stimulation of granulosa cells with CART alone induces MAPK3/1 activation and CART-induced expression of DUSP5 is MAPK3/1 dependent. Ablation (using siRNA) of DUSP5 and (or) PP2A in cultured granulosa prevents the CART-induced early termination of MAPK3/1 and AKT1 signaling (Sen *et al.* 2008). Results support CART-induced suppression of MAPK3/1 and AKT1 signaling as an important component of its inhibitory actions on FSH-stimulated estradiol production.

Despite pleiotropic actions of CART on bovine granulosa cells and described anorexigenic (Kristensen *et al.* 1998, Lambert *et al.* 1998, Vrang *et al.* 1999, Hunter *et al.* 2004), neuroendocrine (Vrang *et al.* 2000, Baranowska *et al.* 2003, Kuriyama *et al.* 2004, Raptis *et al.* 2004, Smith *et al.* 2004) and anti-psychostimulant (Jaworski *et al.* 2003, Kim *et al.* 2003, Kuhar *et al.* 2005) effects of CART in the brain, the molecular identity of the receptor mediating biological actions of CART remains undetermined. Binding studies using the AtT20 cell line (Vicentic *et al.* 2005), PC12 cells (Maletinska *et al.* 2007) and primary neural cell cultures (Jones & Kuhar 2008) provide direct evidence for existence of a putative CART receptor. Specific, saturable, high affinity binding (kD 0.468 nM) of CART to bovine granulosa cells has been detected and granulosa cell CART binding is increased in response to FSH treatment in vitro (Folger *et al.* 2009), suggesting that the transient increase in FSH preceding initiation of each follicular wave may be important for conferring granulosa cell CART responsiveness to the recruited cohort of follicles. Furthermore, previously described actions of CART on bovine granulosa cells are dependent on activity of the o/i subclass ($G_{o/i}$) of inhibitory G proteins and blocked by pretreatment with a $G_{o/i}$ inhibitor. Thus, results suggest that CART actions are presumably mediated by binding to a G-protein ($G_{o/i}$) coupled receptor of unknown identity.

Collectively, results of above described studies support the following model (Fig. 2) depicting the intracellular mechanism of action of CART in inhibition of FSH-induced MAPK3/1 and AKT1 signaling in bovine granulosa cells associated with dominant follicle selection. Upon binding to its receptor ($G_{o/i}$ linked), CART inhibits FSH-stimulated Ca^{2+} influx, cAMP accumulation and MAPK3/1 (Erk 1/2) and AKT1 (Akt) signaling resulting in reduced *CYP19A1* mRNA and estradiol production. Inhibitory effects of CART on MAPK3/1 and AKT1 signaling are mediated by accelerated dephosphorylation of phosphorylated MAPK3/1 (pErk1/2) and AKT1 (pAkt). CART-induced early termination of the FSH-induced MAPK3/1 and AKT1 signaling pathways are mediated via induced expression and decreased proteasome degradation of DUSP5 and PP2A. CART-induced expression of DUSP5 is dependent on MAPK3/1 thereby exhibiting a negative feedback loop where activated MAPK3/1 induces DUSP5 expression which in turn terminates MAPK3/1 activation.

Proposed functional role for *CARTPT* in dominant follicle selection

Follicular waves in cattle can be divided chronologically into two distinct phases, the predominance phase and the dominance phase. Events occurring during the predominance phase are obligatory for selection of a single dominant follicle and culminate with dominant follicle development during the dominance phase. A transient increase in FSH at the beginning of the predominance phase triggers emergence of each follicular wave (Fortune 1994, Ireland *et al.* 2000, Fortune *et al.* 2001). After emergence, follicles in the cohort initially grow at a similar rate (common growth phase) (Beg & Ginther 2006). Molecular determinants predictive of the future subordinate follicles, such as high IGFBP4 concentrations, have been identified as early as the predeviation stage (Mihm *et al.* 2000), but follicle ablation studies have demonstrated that all follicles in the cohort retain the capacity to become the dominant follicle during this common growth phase (Beg & Ginther 2006). Diameter deviation is defined as the divergence in growth rates between the two largest follicles in a follicular wave, during which time the

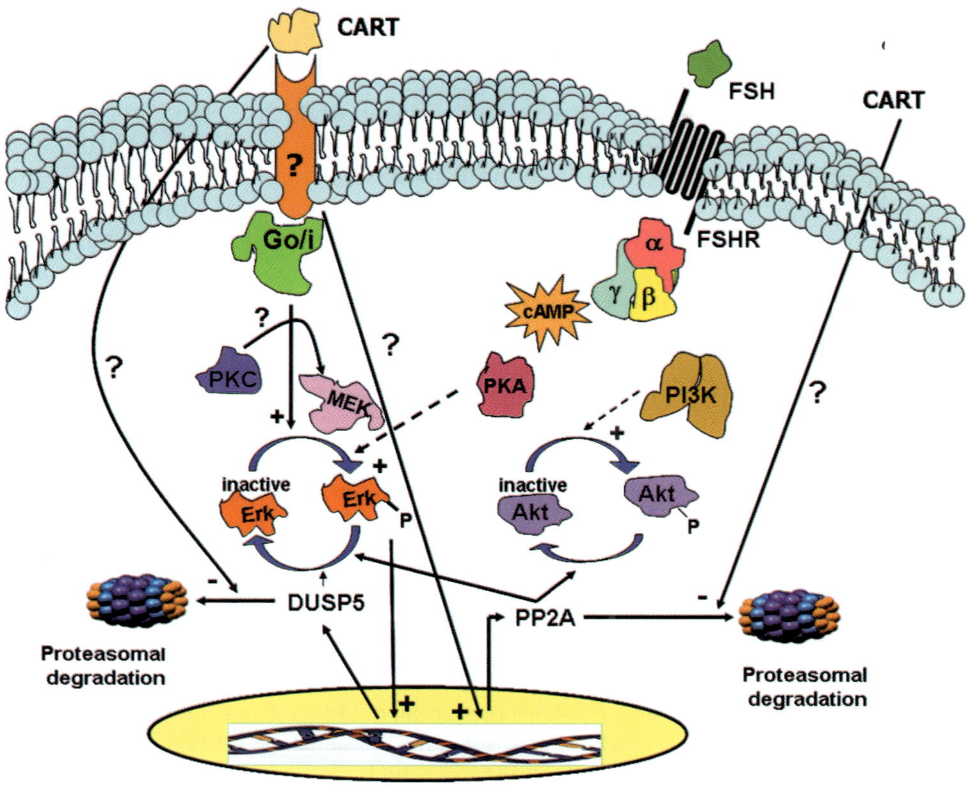

Fig. 2. Proposed model for the intracellular mechanism of CART action in inhibition of FSH stimulated MAPK 3/1 and AKT1 signaling in bovine granulosa cells. FSH stimulates MAPK3/1 (Erk1/2) and AKT1 (Akt) activation while CART treatment accelerates the termination of FSH-induced Erk1/2 and Akt signaling. CART stimulation alone also induces Erk1/2 activation in bovine granulosa cells. Expression of DUSP5 is dependent on Erk1/2 thereby exhibiting a negative feedback loop where activated Erk1/2 induces DUSP5 expression which in turn terminates Erk1/2 activation. CART-induced DUSP5 expression is functionally required for CART-induced termination of Erk 1/2 signaling and is mediated by Erk1/2 and transcription dependent mechanisms. CART increases PP2A expression which is also functionally required for CART-induced termination of Erk 1/2 and Akt activation and CART regulation of PP2A expression is mediated by transcription dependent and independent mechanisms. CART treatment also impairs the proteasomal degradation of both DUSP5 and PP2A resulting in their accumulation (Reprinted from Sen *et al.* 2008).

largest (future dominant follicle) continues to grow and the future subordinate follicle experiences a reduced growth rate and diminished estradiol production (Beg & Ginther 2006). The onset of diameter deviation occurs when the largest follicle reaches 8.5 mm in dairy cattle (Ginther *et al.* 2001, Beg *et al.* 2002) and marks initiation of divergence in growth rate and estradiol producing capacity between the F1 or largest (future dominant) and F2 or second largest (future subordinate) growing follicles resulting in acquisition of dominance and completion of the predominance phase and selection. While the role of FSH in initiating emergence of a follicular wave is well established, dominant follicle selection occurs as FSH concentrations are declining (Adams *et al.* 1992, Sunderland *et al.* 1994).

Greater FSH responsiveness of the future dominant follicle versus future subordinate follicles in cattle has been demonstrated previously (Ginther *et al.* 2003), but is not likely linked to differences in *FSHR* expression as *FSHR* mRNA (Xu *et al.* 1995, Bao *et al.* 1997, Evans & Fortune 1997) and FSHR binding (Ireland & Roche 1982, Ireland & Roche 1983a, Ireland & Roche 1983b, Braden *et al.* 1986) do not increase coincident with selection. Thus, local (intrafollicular) inhibition of FSH action in the future subordinate follicle could help mediate selection. A reduction in follicular fluid CART concentrations in the future dominant follicle occurs within this key time period (Lv *et al.* 2009). Therefore, it is plausible that CART functionally mediates reduced FSH responsiveness of future subordinate follicles during selection. CART is a potent inhibitor of multiple components of the granulosa cell FSH signaling pathway culminating in reduced estradiol production and *CYP19A1* mRNA (Sen *et al.* 2007, Sen *et al.* 2008). Greater intrafollicular CART concentrations and potentially greater CART responsiveness (granulosa cell CART binding sites) may target negative actions of CART specifically to the future subordinate follicles during selection.

Given the proposed role of CART in inhibition of FSH action in future subordinate follicles, what are the mechanisms that allow escape from such inhibitory effects in cases of co-dominant follicles or allow a future subordinate follicle (F2) to become dominant if the future dominant follicle (F1) is destroyed? Ultrasound mediated follicle ablation at the beginning of deviation has been utilized to gain further insight into the mechanisms associated with dominant follicle selection (Beg & Ginther 2006). Ablation of the largest follicle at the onset of deviation allows the second largest follicle to become dominant (Ko *et al.* 1991, Adams *et al.* 1993) and results in a transient increase in FSH (Ginther *et al.* 2002) which presumably helps promote continued growth of the second largest follicle. Furthermore, greater FSH concentrations prior to deviation (Kulick *et al.* 2001, Lopez *et al.* 2005) and a delay in the nadir of FSH concentrations (Lopez *et al.* 2005) are characteristic of follicular waves in which cattle display co-dominant follicles versus those in which a single dominant follicle develops. Our results indicate that granulosa cell *CARTPT* mRNA is reduced in vitro in response to FSH treatment (Lv *et al.* 2009). Hence it is possible that the higher FSH accompanying ablation of the largest follicle at deviation, or in waves in which co-dominant follicles develop, is sufficient to overcome the inhibitory effects of CART on FSH action and (or) to reduce *CARTPT* expression allowing the follicle in question to become dominant.

In addition to the regulatory role of FSH, differences in the milieu of intrafollicular factors between the future dominant and subordinate follicles are believed to have a role in selection (Beg *et al.* 2002, Beg & Ginther 2006). Concentrations of free IGF1 diverge in the largest (F1) versus second largest (F2) follicles within a cohort of growing follicles during follicular waves (Beg *et al.* 2002, Rivera & Fortune 2003b). Granulosa cell *CARTPT* mRNA is reduced in response to IGF1 treatment in vitro (Lv *et al.* 2009). Thus, it is possible that the enhanced IGF1 bioavailability in the future dominant follicle is responsible for observed reduction in follicular CART concentrations during dominant follicle selection. Furthermore, CART is a potent inhibitor of IGF1-stimulated estradiol production by bovine granulosa cells (Fig. 1). Thus, CART-induced inhibition of IGF1 action in future subordinate follicles may help promote dominant follicle selection. However, it is not yet known whether inhibitory effects of CART on IGF1 action are also mediated by stimulation of IGFBP expression.

Based on results described herein, the following model (Fig. 3) is proposed to explain the potential role of *CARTPT* in dominant follicle selection. This model is focused on the time period (onset of diameter deviation) where divergence in growth rate and steroidogenic capacity of the largest (F1; future dominant follicle) and second largest growing follicle (F2; future subordinate follicle) occurs during the first follicular wave, resulting in acquisition of dominance by the F1 follicle. Actions of FSH and IGF1 in the F1 follicle promote sustained growth and estradiol production resulting in selection as the dominant follicle and such actions are mediated in part by enhanced FSH- and IGF1-stimulated MAPK3/1 and AKT1 signaling. Enhanced CART signaling in the F2 (future subordinate follicle), but not the F1 follicle, causes inhibition of FSH and IGF1 action resulting in inhibition of MAPK3/1 and AKT1 signaling, reduced estradiol production and *CYP19A1* mRNA, cessation of growth, and development as a subordinate follicle. It is also proposed that elevated CART and perhaps CART receptor expression in subordinate follicles, potentially due to negative regulation of *CARTPT* and CART receptor expression by IGF1 specifically in the F1 follicle, targets CART actions specifically to the F1 (subordinate follicle) at this key time point during follicular development.

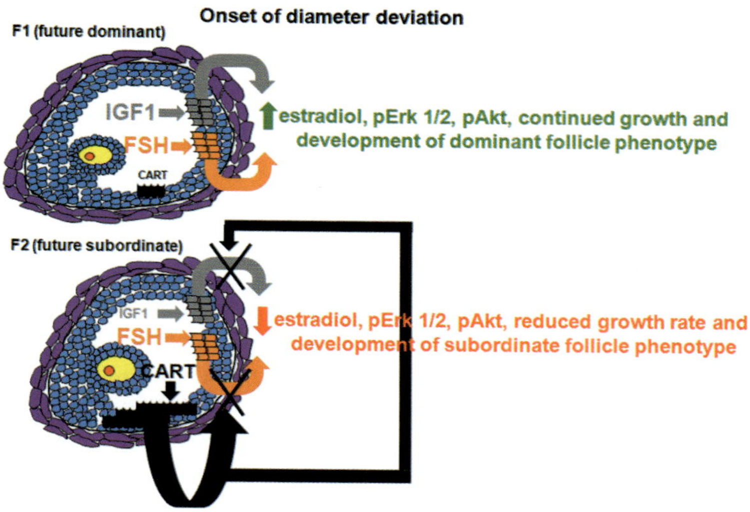

Fig. 3. Proposed model depicting differential actions of CART in F1 (future dominant) versus F2 (future subordinate) follicles at time of diameter deviation culminating in completion of dominant follicle selection. Actions of FSH (orange) and IGF1 (gray) in the F1 follicle promote activation of MAPK3/1 (Erk 1/2) and AKT1 (Akt) signaling (denoted by increased phosphorylated (p) Erk 1/2 and pAkt) and continued growth and estradiol production culminating in acquisition of dominant follicle phenotype. Enhanced CART signaling (black) in the F2 (future subordinate) but not the F1 follicle causes inhibition (X) of FSH (orange) and IGF1 action (gray) resulting in suppression of Erk 1/2 and Akt signaling, reduced estradiol production, cessation of follicular growth, and development of subordinate follicle phenotype. Elevated CART and perhaps CART receptor (■) expression in the F2 follicle, potentially due to negative regulation by IGF1 specifically in the F1 follicle, targets CART's actions specifically to the F2 (subordinate follicle) at this key time point during follicular development.

Conclusions

Collectively, results described above support a novel local role for CART in regulation of follicular development in cattle. Expression of *CARTPT* is temporally regulated at specific stages of a follicular wave with greater *CARTPT* expression in atretic versus healthy follicles early in a wave and a pronounced decrease in intrafollicular CART concentrations in healthy follicles accompanying selection of the dominant follicle (Lv *et al.* 2009). Expression of *CARTPT* mRNA is negatively regulated by FSH and IGF1 (Lv *et al.* 2009), factors stimulatory to follicular growth and granulosa cell estradiol production. Results of in vitro culture experiments established CART as a potent negative regulator of IGF1-stimulated bovine granulosa cell estradiol production (Fig. 1) and of multiple components of the FSH signal transduction cascade resulting in reduced estradiol production and *CYP19A1* mRNA (Sen *et al.* 2007, Sen *et al.* 2008). Similar effects of CART on estradiol production and *CYP19A1* mRNA were observed in vivo following ultrasound mediated intrafollicular injection of CART (Lv *et al.* 2009). Collectively, results presented support the proposed role for CART as a functional mediator of selection of a single dominant follicle during each follicular wave in cattle and perhaps in other mono-ovulatory species. In contrast, CART is not present in the ovaries of rats (Murphy *et al.* 2000) and *CARTPT* mutant mice are fertile (Asnicar *et al.* 2001). Furthermore, *CARTPT* expression is undetectable in ovaries of polytocous farm species such as the pig (Lv and Smith, unpublished observations) or in ovaries of sexually mature mice (Sen and Smith, unpublished observations). These observations suggest that poly-ovulatory species such as rodents may require a less stringent selection mechanism to ovulate multiple follicles thus providing an evolutionary explanation for the absence of *CARTPT* expression in the ovary of polytocous species. Hence, we hypothesize that *CARTPT* functions as a "gatekeeper" of the species-specific ovulatory quota in monotocous species such as cattle.

Acknowledgements

Described studies of *CARTPT* expression and regulation and CART actions in the bovine ovary were supported by National Research Initiative Competitive Grant no. 2005-35203-16011 from the USDA National Institute of Food and Agriculture, Agriculture and Food Research Initiative Competitive Grant no. 2009-65203-05700 from the USDA National Institute of Food and Agriculture, and the Michigan Agricultural Experiment Station.

References

Adams GP, Matteri RL, Kastelic JP, Ko JC & Ginther OJ 1992 Association between surges of follicle-stimulating hormone and the emergence of follicular waves in heifers. *J Reprod Fertil* **94** 177-188.

Adams GP, Kot K, Smith CA & Ginther OJ 1993 Effect of a dominant follicle on regression of its subordinates in heifers. *Can J Anim Sci* **73** 267-275.

Asnicar MA, Smith DP, Yang DD, Heiman ML, Fox N, Chen YF, Hsiung HM & Koster A 2001 Absence of cocaine- and amphetamine-regulated transcript results in obesity in mice fed a high caloric diet. *Endocrinology* **142** 4394-4400.

Austin EJ, Mihm M, Evans AC, Knight PG, Ireland JL, Ireland JJ & Roche JF 2001 Alterations in intrafollicular regulatory factors and apoptosis during selection of follicles in the first follicular wave of the bovine estrous cycle. *Biol Reprod* **64** 839-848.

Baerwald AR, Adams GP & Pierson RA 2003 Characterization of ovarian follicular wave dynamics in women. *Biol Reprod* **69** 1023-1031.

Bao B, Garverick HA, Smith GW, Smith MF, Salfen BE & Youngquist RS 1997 Changes in messenger ribonucleic acid encoding luteinizing hormone receptor, cytochrome P450-side chain cleavage, and aromatase are associated with recruitment and selection of bovine ovarian follicles. *Biol Reprod* **56** 1158-1168.

Baranowska B, Wolinska Witort E, Chmielowska M, Martynska L & Baranowska Bik A 2003 Direct effects of cocaine-amphetamine-regulated transcript (CART) on pituitary hormone release in pituitary cell culture. *Neuroendocrinol Lett* **24** 224-226.

Beg MA, Bergfelt DR, Kot K & Ginther OJ 2002 Follicle selection in cattle: dynamics of follicular fluid factors during development of follicle dominance. *Biol Reprod* **66** 120-126.

Beg MA & Ginther OJ 2006 Follicle selection in cattle and horses: role of intrafollicular factors. *Reproduction* **132** 365-377.

Braden TD, Manns JG, Cermak DL, Nett TM & Niswender GD 1986 Follicular development following parturition and during the estrous cycle in beef cows. *Theriogenology* **25** 833-843.

de la Sota RL, Simmen FA, Diaz T & Thatcher WW 1996 Insulin-like growth factor system in bovine first-wave dominant and subordinate follicles. *Biol Reprod* **55** 803-812.

Echternkamp SE, Howard HJ, Roberts AJ, Grizzle J & Wise T 1994 Relationships among concentrations of steroids, insulin-like growth factor-I, and insulin-like growth factor binding proteins in ovarian follicular fluid of beef cattle. *Biol Reprod* **51** 971-981.

Ekblad E, Kuhar M, Wierup N & Sundler F 2003 Cocaine- and amphetamine-regulated transcript: distribution and function in rat gastrointestinal tract. *Neurogas-*

troenterol Motil **15** 545-557.

Evans AC & Fortune JE 1997 Selection of the dominant follicle in cattle occurs in the absence of differences in the expression of messenger ribonucleic acid for gonadotropin receptors. *Endocrinology* **138** 2963-2971.

Folger JK, Jimenez Krassel F, Ireland JJ & Smith GW 2009 Role of cocaine and amphetamine regulated transcript (CART) in regulation of antral follicle development in cattle: Demonstration of inhibitory effects of the CART peptide on follicular estradiol production and granulosa cell aromatase mRNA in vivo and potential FSH regulation of CART receptor binding. *Biol Reprod* **Supplement 1** 156.

Fortune JE 1994 Ovarian follicular growth and development in mammals. *Biol Reprod* **50** 225-232.

Fortune JE, Rivera GM, Evans AC & Turzillo AM 2001 Differentiation of dominant versus subordinate follicles in cattle. *Biol Reprod* **65** 648-654.

Fortune JE, Rivera GM & Yang MY 2004 Follicular development: the role of the follicular microenvironment in selection of the dominant follicle. *Anim Reprod Sci* **82-83** 109-126.

Ginther OJ, Beg MA, Bergfelt DR, Donadeu FX & Kot K 2001 Follicle selection in monovular species. *Biol Reprod* **65** 638-647.

Ginther OJ, Beg MA, Bergfelt DR & Kot K 2002 Activin A, estradiol, and free insulin-like growth factor I in follicular fluid preceding the experimental assumption of follicle dominance in cattle. *Biol Reprod* **67** 14-19.

Ginther OJ, Beg MA, Donadeu FX & Bergfelt DR 2003 Mechanism of follicle deviation in monovular farm species. *Anim Reprod Sci* **78** 239-257.

Greenwald GS & Roy SK 1994. Follicular development and its control. In *The Physiology of Reproduction*, pp. 629-724. Eds E Knobil & JD Neil. New York: Raven Press.

Gutierrez CG, Campbell BK & Webb R 1997 Development of a long-term bovine granulosa cell culture system: induction and maintenance of estradiol production, response to follicle-stimulating hormone, and morphological characteristics. *Biol Reprod* **56** 608-616.

Hunter RG, Philpot K, Vicentic A, Dominguez G, Hubert GW & Kuhar MJ 2004 CART in feeding and obesity. *Trends Endocrinol Metab* **15** 454-459.

Ireland JJ & Roche JF 1982 Development of antral follicles in cattle after prostaglandin-induced luteolysis: changes in serum hormones, steroids in follicular fluid, and gonadotropin receptors. *Endocrinology* **111** 2077-2086.

Ireland JJ & Roche JF 1983a Development of nonovulatory antral follicles in heifers: changes in steroids in follicular fluid and receptors for gonadotropins. *Endocrinology* **112** 150-156.

Ireland JJ & Roche JF 1983b Growth and differentiation of large antral follicles after spontaneous luteolysis in heifers: changes in concentration of hormones in follicular fluid and specific binding of gonadotropins to follicles. *J Anim Sci* **57** 157-167.

Ireland JJ, Mihm M, Austin E, Diskin MG & Roche JF 2000 Historical perspective of turnover of dominant follicles during the bovine estrous cycle: key concepts, studies, advancements, and terms. *J Dairy Sci* **83** 1648-1658.

Jaworski JN, Vicentic A, Hunter RG, Kimmel HL & Kuhar MJ 2003 CART peptides are modulators of mesolimbic dopamine and psychostimulants. *Life Sci* **73** 741-747.

Jones DC & Kuhar MJ 2008 CART receptor binding in primary cell cultures of the rat nucleus accumbens. *Synapse* **62** 122-127.

Kim JH, Creekmore E & Vezina P 2003 Microinjection of CART peptide 55-102 into the nucleus accumbens blocks amphetamine-induced locomotion. *Neuropeptides* **37** 369-373.

Knight PG & Glister C 2003 Local roles of TGF-beta superfamily members in the control of ovarian follicle development. *Anim Reprod Sci* **78** 165-183.

Ko JC, Kastelic JP, Del Campo MR & Ginther OJ 1991 Effects of a dominant follicle on ovarian follicular dynamics during the oestrous cycle in heifers. *J Reprod Fertil* **91** 511-519.

Kobayashi Y, Jimenez Krassel F, Li Q, Yao J, Huang R, Ireland JJ, Coussens PM & Smith GW 2004 Evidence that cocaine- and amphetamine-regulated transcript is a novel intraovarian regulator of follicular atresia. *Endocrinology* **145** 5373-5383.

Kristensen P, Judge ME, Thim L, Ribel U, Christjansen KN, Wulff BS, Clausen JT, Jensen PB, Madsen OD, Vrang N, Larsen PJ & Hastrup S 1998 Hypothalamic CART is a new anorectic peptide regulated by leptin. *Nature* **393** 72-76.

Kuhar MJ, Jaworski JN, Hubert GW, Philpot KB & Dominguez G 2005 Cocaine- and amphetamine-regulated transcript peptides play a role in drug abuse and are potential therapeutic targets. *AAPS J* **7** E259-265.

Kulick LJ, Bergfelt DR, Kot K & Ginther OJ 2001 Follicle selection in cattle: follicle deviation and codominance within sequential waves. *Biol Reprod* **65** 839-846.

Kuriyama G, Takekoshi S, Tojo K, Nakai Y, Kuhar MJ & Osamura RY 2004 Cocaine- and amphetamine-regulated transcript peptide in the rat anterior pituitary gland is localized in gonadotrophs and suppresses prolactin secretion. *Endocrinology* **145** 2542-2550.

Lambert PD, Couceyro PR, McGirr KM, Dall Vechia SE, Smith Y & Kuhar MJ 1998 CART peptides in the central control of feeding and interactions with neuropeptide Y. *Synapse* **29** 293-298.

Li Q, Jimenez-Krassel F, Kobayashi Y, Ireland JJ & Smith GW 2006 Effect of intrafollicular indomethacin injection on gonadotropin surge-induced expression of select extracellular matrix degrading enzymes and their inhibitors in bovine preovulatory follicles. *Reproduction* **131** 533-543.

Li Q, Jimenez-Krassel F, Bettegowda A, Ireland JJ & Smith GW 2007 Evidence that the preovulatory rise in intrafollicular progesterone may not be required for ovulation in cattle. *J Endocrinol* **192** 473-483.

Lopez H, Sartori R & Wiltbank MC 2005 Reproductive

hormones and follicular growth during development of one or multiple dominant follicles in cattle. *Biol Reprod* **72** 788-795.

Lv L, Jimenez-Krassel F, Sen A, Bettegowda A, Mondal M, Folger JK, Lee KB, Ireland JJ & Smith GW 2009 Evidence supporting a role for cocaine- and amphetamine-regulated transcript (CARTPT) in control of granulosa cell estradiol production associated with dominant follicle selection in cattle. *Biol Reprod* **81** 580-586.

Maletinska L, Maixnerova J, Matyskova R, Haugvicova R, Sloncova E, Elbert T, Slaninova J & Zelezna B 2007 Cocaine- and amphetamine-regulated transcript (CART) peptide specific binding in pheochromocytoma cells PC12. *Eur J Pharmacol* **559** 109-114.

Mazerbourg S, Overgaard MT, Oxvig C, Christiansen M, Conover CA, Laurendeau I, Vidaud M, Tosser Klopp G, Zapf J & Monget P 2001 Pregnancy-associated plasma protein-A (PAPP-A) in ovine, bovine, porcine, and equine ovarian follicles: involvement in IGF binding protein-4 proteolytic degradation and mRNA expression during follicular development. *Endocrinology* **142** 5243-5253.

Mihm M, Good TE, Ireland JL, Ireland JJ, Knight PG & Roche JF 1997 Decline in serum follicle-stimulating hormone concentrations alters key intrafollicular growth factors involved in selection of the dominant follicle in heifers. *Biol Reprod* **57** 1328-1337.

Mihm M, Austin EJ, Good TE, Ireland JL, Knight PG, Roche JF & Ireland JJ 2000 Identification of potential intrafollicular factors involved in selection of dominant follicles in heifers. *Biol Reprod* **63** 811-819.

Monget P & Monniaux D 1995 Growth factors and the control of folliculogenesis. *J Reprod Fertil Suppl* **49** 321-333.

Murphy KG, Abbott CR, Mahmoudi M, Hunter R, Gardiner JV, Rossi M, Stanley SA, Ghatei MA, Kuhar MJ & Bloom SR 2000 Quantification and synthesis of cocaine- and amphetamine-regulated transcript peptide (79-102)-like immunoreactivity and mRNA in rat tissues. *J Endocrinol* **166** 659-668.

Peters MW, Pursley JR & Smith GW 2004 Inhibition of intrafollicular PGE2 synthesis and ovulation following ultrasound-mediated intrafollicular injection of the selective cyclooxygenase-2 inhibitor NS-398 in cattle. *J Anim Sci* **82** 1656-1662.

Raptis S, Fekete C, Sarkar S, Rand WM, Emerson CH, Nagy GM & Lechan RM 2004 Cocaine- and amphetamine-regulated transcript co-contained in thyrotropin-releasing hormone (TRH) neurons of the hypothalamic paraventricular nucleus modulates TRH-induced prolactin secretion. *Endocrinology* **145** 1695-1699.

Richards JS & Hedin L 1988 Molecular aspects of hormone action in ovarian follicular development, ovulation, and luteinization. *Annu Rev Physiol* **50** 441-463.

Richards JS 2001 Perspective: the ovarian follicle--a perspective in 2001. *Endocrinology* **142** 2184-2193.

Richards JS, Russell DL, Ochsner S, Hsieh M, Doyle KH, Falender AE, Lo YK & Sharma SC 2002 Novel signaling pathways that control ovarian follicular development, ovulation, and luteinization. *Recent Prog Horm Res* **57** 195-220.

Rivera GM & Fortune JE 2003a Proteolysis of insulin-like growth factor binding proteins -4 and -5 in bovine follicular fluid: implications for ovarian follicular selection and dominance. *Endocrinology* **144** 2977-2987.

Rivera GM & Fortune JE 2003b Selection of the dominant follicle and insulin-like growth factor (IGF)-binding proteins: evidence that pregnancy-associated plasma protein A contributes to proteolysis of IGF-binding protein 5 in bovine follicular fluid. *Endocrinology* **144** 437-446.

Ryan KE, Casey SM, Canty MJ, Crowe MA, Martin F & Evans AC 2007 Akt and Erk signal transduction pathways are early markers of differentiation in dominant and subordinate ovarian follicles in cattle. *Reproduction* **133** 617-626.

Ryan KE, Glister C, Lonergan P, Martin F, Knight PG & Evans AC 2008 Functional significance of the signal transduction pathways Akt and Erk in ovarian follicles: In vitro and in vivo studies in cattle and sheep. *J Ovarian Res* **1** 2.

Sen A, Bettegowda A, Jimenez-Krassel F, Ireland JJ & Smith GW 2007 Cocaine- and amphetamine-regulated transcript regulation of follicle-stimulating hormone signal transduction in bovine granulosa cells. *Endocrinology* **148** 4400-4410.

Sen A, Lv L, Bello N, Ireland JJ & Smith GW 2008 Cocaine- and amphetamine-regulated transcript accelerates termination of follicle-stimulating hormone-induced extracellularly regulated kinase 1/2 and Akt activation by regulating the expression and degradation of specific mitogen-activated protein kinase phosphatases in bovine granulosa cells. *Mol Endocrinol* **22** 2655-2676.

Smith SM, Vaughan JM, Donaldson CJ, Rivier J, Li C, Chen A & Vale WW 2004 Cocaine- and amphetamine-regulated transcript activates the hypothalamic-pituitary-adrenal axis through a corticotropin-releasing factor receptor-dependent mechanism. *Endocrinology* **145** 5202-5209.

Spicer LJ, Alpizar E & Echternkamp SE 1993 Effects of insulin, insulin-like growth factor I, and gonadotropins on bovine granulosa cell proliferation, progesterone production, estradiol production, and (or) insulin-like growth factor I production in vitro. *J Anim Sci* **71** 1232-1241.

Spicer LJ & Echternkamp SE 1995 The ovarian insulin and insulin-like growth factor system with an emphasis on domestic animals. *Domest Anim Endocrinol* **12** 223-245.

Spicer LJ 2004 Proteolytic degradation of insulin-like growth factor binding proteins by ovarian follicles: a control mechanism for selection of dominant follicles. *Biol Reprod* **70** 1223-1230.

Stewart RE, Spicer LJ, Hamilton TD, Keefer BE, Daw-

son LJ, Morgan GL & Echternkamp SE 1996 Levels of insulin-like growth factor (IGF) binding proteins, luteinizing hormone and IGF-I receptors, and steroids in dominant follicles during the first follicular wave in cattle exhibiting regular estrous cycles. *Endocrinology* **137** 2842-2850.

Sunderland SJ, Crowe MA, Boland MP, Roche JF & Ireland JJ 1994 Selection, dominance and atresia of follicles during the oestrous cycle of heifers. *J Reprod Fertil* **101** 547-555.

Vander AJ, Sherman JH & Luciano DS 1994. Reproduction. In *Human physiology: The mechanisms of body function*, pp. 661-692. Eds KM Prancan & JW Bradley. New York: McGraw-Hill.

Vicentic A, Lakatos A & Kuhar MJ 2005 CART (cocaine- and amphetamine-regulated transcript) peptide receptors: Specific binding in AtT20 cells. *Eur J Pharmacol* **528** 188-189.

Vrang N, Tang Christensen M, Larsen PJ & Kristensen P 1999 Recombinant CART peptide induces c-Fos expression in central areas involved in control of feeding behaviour. *Brain Res* **818** 499-509.

Vrang N, Larsen PJ, Kristensen P & Tang Christensen M 2000 Central administration of cocaine-amphetamine-regulated transcript activates hypothalamic neuroendocrine neurons in the rat. *Endocrinology* **141** 794-801.

Webb R, Nicholas B, Gong JG, Campbell BK, Gutierrez CG, Garverick HA & Armstrong DG 2003 Mechanisms regulating follicular development and selection of the dominant follicle. *Reprod Suppl* **61** 71-90.

Wierup N, Richards WG, Bannon AW, Kuhar MJ, Ahren B & Sundler F 2005 CART knock out mice have impaired insulin secretion and glucose intolerance, altered beta cell morphology and increased body weight. *Regul Pept* **129** 203-211.

Wierup N, Bjorkqvist M, Kuhar MJ, Mulder H & Sundler F 2006 CART regulates islet hormone secretion and is expressed in the beta-cells of type 2 diabetic rats. *Diabetes* **55** 305-311.

Xu Z, Garverick HA, Smith GW, Smith MF, Hamilton SA & Youngquist RS 1995 Expression of follicle-stimulating hormone and luteinizing hormone receptor messenger ribonucleic acids in bovine follicles during the first follicular wave. *Biol Reprod* **53** 951-957.

Yao J, Ren X, Ireland JJ, Coussens PM, Smith TP & Smith GW 2004 Generation of a bovine oocyte cDNA library and microarray: resources for identification of genes important for follicular development and early embryogenesis. *Physiol Genomics* **19** 84-92.

Assessing gene function in the ruminant placenta

RV Anthony, JD Cantlon, KC Gates, SH Purcell and CM Clay

Animal Reproduction and Biotechnology Laboratory, Department of Biomedical Sciences, College of Veterinary Medicine and Biomedical Sciences, Colorado State University, Fort Collins, CO 80523

The placenta provides the means for nutrient transfer from the mother to the fetus, waste transfer from the fetus to the mother, protection of the fetus from the maternal immune system, and is an active endocrine organ. While many placental functions have been defined and investigated, assessing the function of specific genes expressed by the placenta has been problematic, since classical ablation-replacement methods are not feasible with the placenta. The pregnant sheep has been a long-standing animal model for assessing *in vivo* physiology during pregnancy, since surgical placement of indwelling catheters into both maternal and fetal vasculature has allowed the assessment of placental nutrient transfer and utilization, as well as placental hormone secretion, under unanesthetized-unstressed steady state sampling conditions. However, in ruminants the lack of well-characterized trophoblast cell lines and the inefficiency of creating transgenic pregnancies in ruminants have inhibited our ability to assess specific gene function. Recently, sheep and cattle primary trophoblast cell lines have been reported, and may further our ability to investigate trophoblast function and transcriptional regulation of genes expressed by the placenta. Furthermore, viral infection of the trophoectoderm layer of hatched blastocysts, as a means for placenta-specific transgenesis, holds considerable potential to assess gene function in the ruminant placenta. This approach has been used successfully to "knockdown" gene expression in the developing sheep conceptus, and has the potential for gain-of-function experiments as well. While this technology is still being developed, it may provide an efficient approach to assess specific gene function in the ruminant placenta.

Introduction

The placenta is a multifaceted organ that plays critical roles in maintaining and protecting the developing fetus. These roles include transferring nutrients from the mother to the fetus and waste secretion from the fetus to the mother, acting as a barrier for the fetus against pathogens and the maternal immune system, and serving as an active endocrine organ. As the "vehicle" for amino acid, fatty acid, glucose and oxygen transfer to the fetus, the placenta utilizes a variety of transport mechanisms (Regnault *et al.* 2005; Jones *et al.* 2007). Nutrient supply to the fetus is not only dependent on available transport mechanisms, but also on the amount of placental substrate and hormone metabolism. At mid-gestation, the majority of substrate taken up by the gravid uterus is consumed by the placenta (Bell *et al.* 1986) but the proportion of

Corresponding author E-mail: Russ.Anthony@Colostate.edu

substrate utilized by the placenta declines as gestation advances, with more transferred to the fetus. A portion of the nutrients utilized by the placenta serves to fuel the placenta as an active endocrine organ. The placenta is capable of secreting a plethora of hormones, growth factors and cytokines, many of which are also produced by other endocrine or non-endocrine organs (Talamantes & Ogren 1988). Some of these are true placental hormones since they are not produced by other organs and have known or inferred functions during pregnancy. Included in this category are the conceptus interferons, chorionic gonadotropins, and members of the growth hormone (GH)/prolactin (PRL) gene family (Roberts & Anthony 1994). While we know a great deal about the function of the placenta, we still know little about the specific function of individual genes expressed within the placenta.

Assessing specific gene function in the placenta has been difficult, since classical ablation-replacement strategies are not feasible with the placenta. The ability to surgically place and maintain catheters in both the maternal and fetal circulation of pregnant sheep (Meschia *et al.* 1965; Battaglia *et al.* 1968), allowing non-stressed repetitive sampling, has provided considerable insight into placental function in ruminants. However, the lack of ruminant-specific trophoblast cell lines or efficient means to alter specific gene expression within the placenta has often precluded the direct testing of gene function. Non-ruminant trophoblast-derived cell lines have been useful when examining ruminant gene regulation, but the recent availability of cattle (Talbot *et al.* 2000; Shimada *et al.* 2001) and sheep (Farmer *et al.* 2008) cell lines may allow a more robust assessment of ruminant gene regulation and function *in vitro*. Furthermore, recent *in vivo* loss-of-function experiments have been reported in sheep, where either antisense morpholino oligonucleotides were introduced into the uterine lumen (Dunlap *et al.* 2006), or blastocysts were infected with lentivirus expressing a short-hairpin RNA construct before embryo transfer (Purcell *et al.* 2009). Use of these newer experimental approaches may well provide the mechanism by which to directly assess placental gene function in ruminants.

Formation and structure of the ruminant placenta

In contrast to primates and rodents, the ruminant conceptus does not undergo invasive implantation. Rather the blastocyst, comprised of the inner cell mass (ICM) and the blastocoele cavity surrounded by a single layer of trophectoderm, elongates into a filamentous conceptus (Guillomot 1995). Extraembryonic primitive endoderm develops from the ICM and migrates beneath the trophectoderm, differentiating into visceral endoderm (beneath the ICM) and parietal endoderm (PE) beneath the trophectoderm (Flechon *et al.* 2007). As the conceptus elongates, the PE elongates with the trophectoderm (Flechon *et al.* 2007), taking on a multinucleated syncytial morphology but retaining the characteristics of polarized epithelium. By 15 days post coitus (dpc) in sheep, and 19-20 dpc in cattle, formal apposition occurs between the trophectoderm and uterine luminal epithelium (Guillomot 1995), followed a day later by adhesion along the feto-maternal interface. The process of apposition and adhesion coincides with expansion of the allantois from the hind-gut, providing fusion with the chorion and vascularization in the areas of maternal caruncle projections (Stegeman 1974). Interdigitation of the chorionic epithelium with the uterine epithelium located in the non-glandular caruncles provides for the initial formation of individual placentomes (Boshier 1969), comprised of the fetal cotyledon and maternal caruncle. As pregnancy progresses, growth of the fetomaternal interface leads to an apposing network of fetal and maternal villi. The fetal cotyledonary villous tree, when mature, is comprised of stem, intermediate and terminal villi (Leiser *et al.* 1997), within which are stem arteries and veins, intermediate arterioles and venules, and terminal capillaries, respectively.

Coincident with the time of conceptus apposition is the appearance of chorionic binucleate cells (BNC; Guillomot *et al.* 1981) within the trophectoderm layer. The BNC result from consecutive nuclear divisions of trophectoderm uninucleate cells (UNC), without cytokinesis following the second division (Wooding 1992), and comprise 15-20% of the trophectoderm. Essentially throughout gestation, 15-20% of the BNC are migrating through the tight junctions formed by the UNC (Wooding 1983). Fusion of the BNC with uterine epithelial cells form trinucleate cells, and continued fusion of BNC with the initial trinucleate cells result in the formation of syncytial plaques, comprised of 20-25 nuclei, linked by tight junctions (Wooding 1984; Wooding 1992). At mid-gestation in sheep and goats the fetomaternal interface is totally comprised of syncytium (Wooding 1984; Wooding 1992). By contrast, in cattle and deer, the uterine epithelium is reestablished, such that continued BNC migration and fusion results in transient trinucleate cells (Wooding & Wathes 1980). The formation, migration and fusion of BNC not only serves in the development and formation of the expanding fetal villi and the fetomaternal interface, but they also serve in the synthesis and delivery of placental hormones, such as placental lactogen (PL; Milosavljevic *et al.* 1989; Kappes *et al.* 1992) to the maternal circulation.

This brief description of ruminant placenta development and structure is meant to provide an appreciation of the complexity of the ruminant placenta. If one just considers the villous tree of the fetal cotyledon, it is comprised of UNC, BNC, villous mesenchyme, vascular endothelial and smooth muscle cells, and the proportion of each within a single cotyledon changes as pregnancy progresses (Kappes *et al.* 1992). Furthermore, there is the fetomaternal syncytium, and when separating the placentome into its cotyledon and caruncle components, residual tissue from either the maternal or fetal components contaminate the other (Bridger *et al.* 2007). Consequently, the recent use of microarray-based gene profiling methods to assess placental gene expression (Everts *et al.* 2008) in cattle may be confounded by the multiple cell types present in the ruminant placenta. Subsequent quantitative reverse transcriptase-polymerase chain reaction (qRT-PCR) can be used to validate the changes in mRNA concentration (Aston *et al.* 2009), but the combination of subsequent qRT-PCR and *in situ* hybridization (Ushizawa *et al.* 2007) likely gives a clearer interpretation of the microarray results. However, important changes in mRNA concentrations of "lowly"-expressed genes might be overlooked or muted by the relative composition of the tissue used for RNA isolation. Use of laser-capture microdissection to harvest the cell population of interest (e.g., trophoblast layer) may enhance the validity of the results obtained from gene profiling experiments.

In vitro assessment of placental gene function

For years, *in vitro* investigation into ruminant placental gene regulation and function was hampered by the lack of ruminant-specific cell lines. Often human or rat choriocarinoma cell lines were used to investigate the transcriptitional regulation of sheep and cattle genes expressed in the placenta (e.g., Liang *et al.* 1999; Ezashi *et al.* 2001; Limesand *et al.* 2004). To provide relevance to the ruminant, we also utilized nuclear extracts from isolated sheep BNC in DNase footprinting (Liang *et al.* 1999), electrophoretic mobility shift assays (Limesand *et al.* 2004) and Southwestern analysis (Jeckel *et al.* 2009), to verify the results obtained with choriocarcinoma cell lines. In our experience (Liang *et al.* 1999; Limesand *et al.* 2004; Jeckel *et al.* 2009) BeWo cells (human choriocarcinoma cell line) have served as a useful model system for studying the transcriptional regulation of sheep PL. Recently, Bridger *et al.* (2007) reported the establishment of trophoblast cultures from cattle placentomes, and subsequently they reported the culture of BNCs for 90 days in culture (Landim *et al.* 2007) and proliferation of bovine trophoblast cell line F3 in response to epidermal growth factor (Hambruch *et al.* 2010). During early passages (P2) of the F3 cells, the BNC expressed PL, but in later passages (P18) PL was no longer detectable (Hambruch *et al.* 2010). As yet, there are no reports of successful transfection or other genetic manipulations of these cells. With the ovine trophoblast cells that we harvested to isolate nuclear protein (Liang *et al.* 1999; Limesand *et al.* 2004), part of these cells were placed in culture and passaged, and attempts were made to transfect these cells by a variety of techniques (e.g., lipid-mediated transfection, electroporation, $CaPO_4$ precipitation) without success. Our only success in transforming these cells was when we infected them with an adenoviral construct (Figure 1) or lentiviral construct, both of which expressed enhanced green fluorescent protein (EGFP) under the control of the cytomegalovirus promoter. This approach was successful in obtaining EGFP expression in BNCs (Figure 1), but since the number of BNC diminished considerably with each successive passage, we have not pursued this approach further. It may however, be a useful approach to examine transcriptional regulation of genes expressed by BNC.

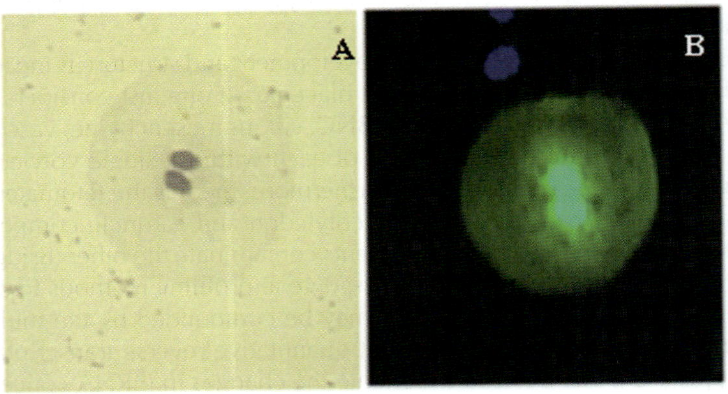

Fig. 1. Binucleate cell (BNC) expression of enhanced green fluorescent protein (EGFP). BNC were isolated from 100 dpc sheep placenta, placed in culture and infected with an adenovirus vector expressing EGFP. Panel A: Hemotoxylin stained BNC. Panel B: Direct fluorescence microscopy of BNC expressing EGFP. Nuclei were stained with DAPI. 400X magnification.

As noted in the introduction, the methods used to generate two trophoblast cell lines from cattle blastocysts have been described. One cell line (CT-1 cells; Talbot *et al.* 2000) was generated by plating 10-11 dpc hatched blastocysts on a feeder layer of STO mouse fibroblast cells. The second cell line (BT-1 cells; Shimada *et al.* 2001) was generated by culturing blastocysts on collagen-coated dishes, in the absence of a feeder cell, but cell growth was accelerated when cultured in the presence of bovine endometrial fibroblast-conditioned medium. Both cell lines express interferon-τ, but the BT-1 cells have been shown to generate BNC (Nakano *et al.* 2002), and express PL and pregnancy-associated glycoproteins (Ushizawa *et al.* 2005). It was demonstrated that the expression of metalloproteinases and tissue inhibitors of metalloproteinases by BT-1 cells could be regulated by exposure to several cytokines, including tumor necrosis factor-α and interleukin-1α, demonstrating the responsiveness of BT-1 cells to exogenous stimuli (Hirata *et al.* 2003). In a similar fashion, exposure of CT-1 cells to granulocyte-macrophage colony-stimulating-factor resulted in increased interferon-τ expression (Michael *et al.* 2006). Furthermore, Ezashi *et al.* (2008) demonstrated that both Distal-less 3 (DLX3) and ETS2 are expressed by CT-1 cells and that transfection of CT-1 cells with small interfering RNA designed to target DLX3 resulted in reduced interferon-τ production. The summation of the various studies reported with either BT-1 or CT-1 cells suggest that these cell lines may be quite useful in examining ruminant trophoblast gene regulation and function. It has yet to be clearly demonstrated how efficiently these cells can be transfected for transcriptional regulation studies and/or genetic manipulation of function.

In contrast to the BT-1 and CT-1 cell lines, which were derived from outgrowths of hatched blastocyts, Farmer *et al.* (2008) reported the generation of oTr-1 and oTr-F cell lines from 15 dpc sheep conceptuses. The elongated conceptuses were minced, and cultured either on plastic (oTr-1) or on collagen coated dishes (oTr-F). These cell lines were established and used to investigate the function of galectin 15 (LGALS15) in trophectoderm migration and attachment (Farmer *et al.* 2008). LGALS15 promoted oTr proliferation and migration, and the effect of LGALS15 on migration could be inhibited with a c-Jun N-terminal kinase inhibitor, but not with a Rho-kinase inhibitor. Seeking an *in vitro* cell culture system to investigate regulation and function of proline-rich 15 (PRR15), a nuclear protein with peak expression at 15-16 dpc in sheep conceptuses (Purcell et al. 2009), we obtained oTr-1 cells developed in Dr. R.C. Burghardt's laboratory (Texas A&M University) from Dr. T.E. Spencer (Texas A&M University). Analysis of PRR15 and interferon-τ mRNA isolated from the oTr-1 cells by qRT-PCR indicated that the expression of these two genes was considerably lower in oTr-1 cells, when compared to 15 dpc conceptus mRNA. Subsequently, we generated a series of oTR cell lines (oTR-17, -18, -19, -23 and -25) from 15 dpc sheep conceptuses using the methods of Farmer *et al.* (2008), and found that when these cells are cultured on plastic, PRR15 and interferon-τ mRNA concentrations were quite low. Consequently, we compared the expression of PRR15 by oTR cells when cultured on plastic or various concentrations of Matrigel® for 48 hours. As evidenced in Figure 2, PRR15 mRNA concentration increased significantly when oTR cells were plated on a 1 mm cushion of Matrigel®, at a concentration of 6 mg/ml. There is a notable phenotypic change in the oTR cells following plating on Matrigel®, as evidenced in Figure 3. During the first hour of culture on Matrigel® the cells begin to migrate and by 3 hours have formed clusters of cells (Figure 3), which continue to condense and invade into the matrix. Expression of PRR15 mRNA increases in a time-dependent manner when oTR cells are cultured on Matrigel®, until 36 hours, at which time its mRNA concentration plateaus. The phenotypic behavior of the oTR cells cultured on Matrigel® is similar to what we observe with human ACH-3P cells (Hiden *et al.* 2007), and what has been reported for first trimester human cytotrophoblast cells (Librach *et al.* 1991) and mouse trophoblast stem cells (Lei *et al.* 2007), suggesting greater inter-species trophoblast cell similarity than might be anticipated.

From this discussion, it is obvious that there are a number of ruminant-specific trophoblast cell isolation and culture systems now available for use in assessing placental gene function *in vitro*. There are differences in gestational age at isolation, subsequent culture conditions, and possibly in responsiveness. All of these approaches utilize continual culture and passage of primary cells, which opens the door for passage related changes in cell phenotype, responsiveness, and usefulness. While a number of "markers" have been used to assess human cytotrophoblast cells and the various cell lines available (Hiden *et al.* 2007; Hannan *et al.* 2010), as yet a similar strategy has not been fully developed for assessing ruminant trophoblast cell lines. This will require investigators reaching consensus as to which markers should be used, and the sharing of reagents. Regardless, the availability of these ruminant trophoblast cell lines should be quite useful in assessing placental gene function in ruminants, but the results from such studies should always be put in context with what we know about *in vivo* function.

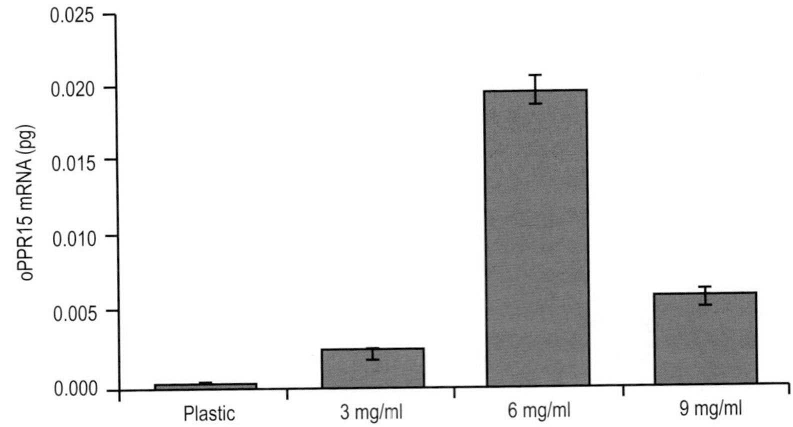

Fig. 2. PRR15 mRNA concentration in oTR cells cultured on Matrigel®. oTR-17 cells were plated on plastic culture dishes, or on dishes coated with 3, 6 or 9 mg/ml of Matigel® for 48 hours. PRR15 mRNA concentration was assessed by qRT-PCR as described in Purcell *et al.* (2009).

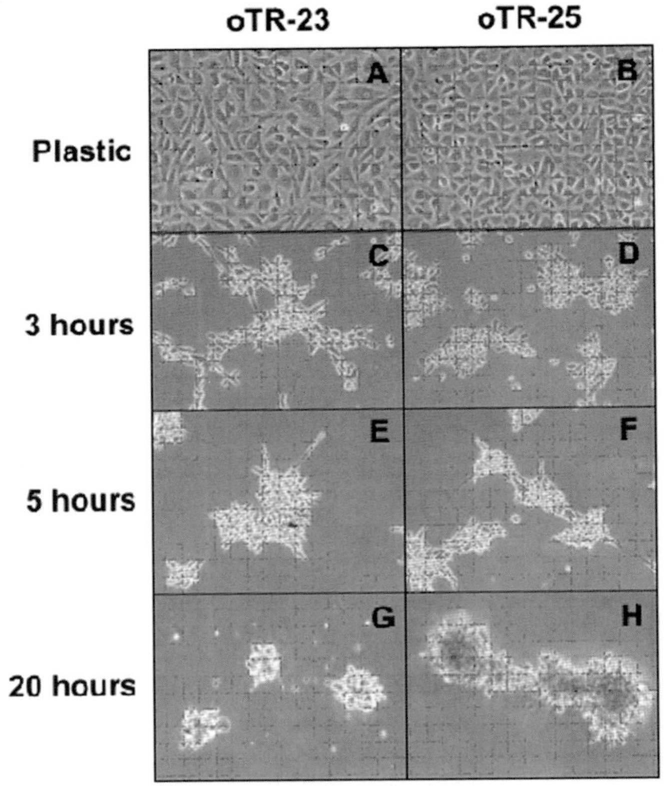

Fig. 3. Phenotypic change in oTR cells cultured on Matrigel®. oTR-23 and oTR-25 cells were cultured on plastic culture dishes, or on dishes coated with 6 mg/ml of Matrigel®. Panels A & B: oTR-23 and -25 cells grown on plastic. Picture was taken just before harvesting the cells for plating onto Matrigel®. Panels C & D: oTR-23 and -25 cells following 3 hours of culture on Matrigel®. Panels E & F: oTR-23 and -25 cells following 5 hours of culture on Matrigel®. Panels G & H: oTR-23 and -25 cells following 20 hours of culture on Matrigel®. 100X magnification.

In vivo assessment of placental gene function

In vivo assessment of placental function

While our understanding of the function of specific genes expressed within the ruminant placenta may lag behind other species, especially rodents, we do have a better understanding of actual placental function in ruminants than we do in other species. This results from the ability to surgically place and maintain catheters in both the maternal and fetal vasculature in sheep (Meschia *et al.* 1965; Battaglia *et al.* 1968), allowing repetitive sampling of both maternal and fetal blood under non-stressed conditions. Placement of catheters in both maternal and fetal vessels (Figure 4) not only allows for infusion of substrate, but also simultaneous sampling of arterial-venous concentration differences on both sides of the placenta, allowing application of the Fick principle (Meschia *et al.* 1980). Simultaneous sampling of arterial-venous differences, along with measures of blood flow in uterine and umbilical vessels, provides for the determination of uteroplacental utilization and or metabolism (Hay 1991). This approach has been applied extensively to placental uptake and utilization of O_2, glucose and amino acids, but as inferred in Figure 4, it can also be applied to other tissues (e.g., hind limb skeletal muscle, liver, etc.) within the fetus (Anderson *et al.* 2001; Teng *et al.* 2002). At mid gestation, uteroplacental O_2 consumption by the placenta accounts for approximately 80% of total O_2 uptake by the uterus (Bell *et al.* 1986), and during late gestation, uteroplacental O_2 consumption is essentially equivalent to O_2 consumption by the fetus (Meschia *et al.* 1980). Of the oxygen consumed by the placenta, 90% can be accounted for by oxidative phosphorylation of glucose (Meschia *et al.* 1980), as 80% of the glucose taken up by the uteroplacental unit is consumed (Hay 1991). These data demonstrate how metabolically active the placenta is, and can only be determined under steady state conditions. Simultaneous collection of maternal and fetal arterial and venous blood samples can be collected in ruminants, an experimental approach that is not permissible in humans or feasible in rodents. This experimental approach can also be applied to placental hormone production and secretion in ruminants, as Schoknecht *et al.* (1992) demonstrated that the PL entry rate into fetal sheep circulation increases with increasing gestational age even though fetal concentrations of PL plateau by 90 days of gestation (Kappes *et al.* 1992).

As methods develop to alter specific gene expression in the ruminant placenta (see below), the utility of being able to assess placental function *in vivo* will become advantageous. For example, it has been demonstrated *in vivo*, using two distinct sheep models of intrauterine growth restriction (Wallace *et al.* 2005), that placental delivery of O_2, glucose and amino acids to the umbilical circulation is impaired. The ability to ablate the expression of specific nutrient transporters within the placenta, incorporating steady-state *in vivo* transfer studies into the experimental paradigm, would provide considerable insight into the role of individual placental transport mechanisms. Additionally, the ability to enhance or ablate the expression of specific placental hormones, followed by *in vivo* assessment of the physiological impact using the approaches outlined above, could finally provide a direct assessment of the physiological role and necessity of these hormones.

In vivo assessment of gene function

Transgenesis in mice has been used for approximately 30 years to examine the effect of "adding" genes. Similarly, homologous recombination in mouse embryonic stem cells as a means of functionally deleting genes has been used to study specific gene function for over 20 years. Unfortunately, comparable efficient methods have not been forthcoming for ruminants, especially

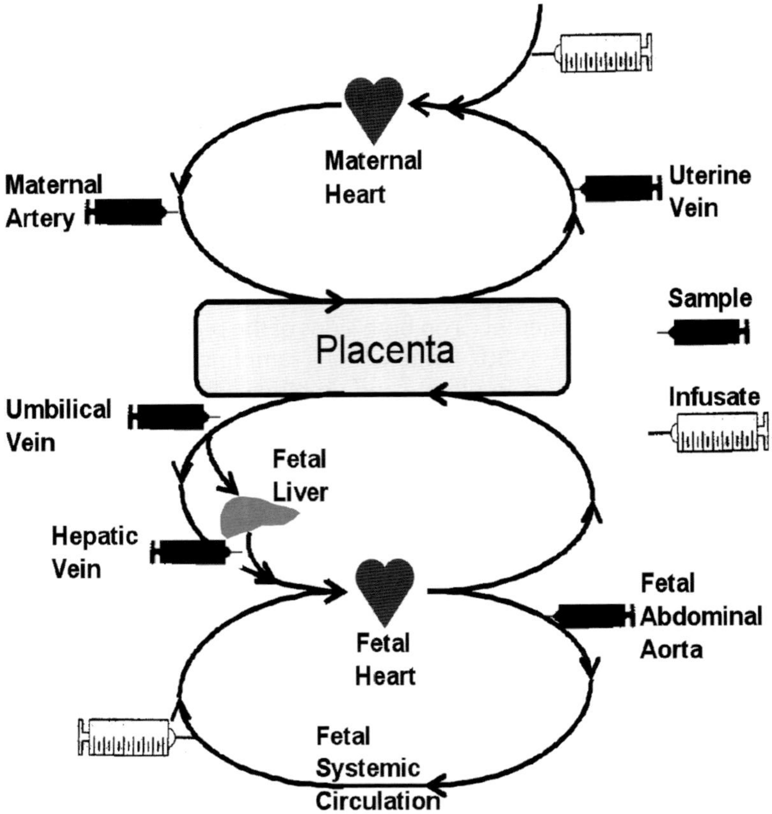

Fig. 4. Schematic representation of *in vivo* preparation of pregnant sheep used to measure utero-placental and fetal uptake and metabolism of O_2 and nutrients. Infusate can be administered to either maternal or fetal circulation, and blood samples drawn simultaneously from either circulation.

for genes expressed by the placenta. Consequently, until recently, there have not been viable approaches available to directly assess the function of genes expressed in the ruminant placenta. Dunlap *et al.* (2006) reported the successful use of morpholino oligonucleotides, infused into the uterine lumen on 8 dpc, to examine the impact of inhibiting the expression of the endogenous retrovirus enJSRV *env* within sheep conceptuses. Antisense morpholiono oligonucleotides utilize morpholine rings in their structure in place of deoxyribose, and are designed to hybridize with RNA sequences encompassing the translational start site, or an exon/intron splice-acceptor site (Summerton 1999). Hybridization at these sites provides steric blocking of translation and or pre-mRNA splicing in an RNase H independent fashion (Summerton 1999). By infusing antisense morpholino oligonucletides designed against enJSRV *env*, Dunlap *et al.* (2006) demonstrated that enJSRV *env* plays an important role in trophectoderm growth and differentiation in elongating sheep conceptuses. This is a useful approach to study early events in conceptus growth and placentation. However, since the approach relies on transient transfection, efficacy of morpholino oligonucleotide mediated gene "knockdown" is lost as the conceptus/placenta proliferates.

Steric blocking of translation or pre-mRNA splicing interferes with production of the gene product of interest, but does not target the mRNA for destruction. Naturally occurring micro RNA (miRNA) provide a mechanism of defense against virus infection and or endogenous gene regulation (He and Hannon 2004), through RNA interference (RNAi). As depicted in Figure 5, primary miRNA transcripts are processed in the nucleus by the RNase III activity of Drosha, yielding pre-miRNA with a characteristic hairpin-loop structure, that are exported out of the nucleus. The pre-miRNA are further processed in the cytoplasm by the RNase III activity of Dicer, yielding a 22-base pair duplex, or mature miRNA. The miRNA serves as the "guide" sequence incorporated into the RNA-induced silencing complex (RISC). When RISC complexes with the target transcript, Argonaute, a component of RISC that possesses RNase H activity, cleaves the mRNA thus targeting it for nuclease-mediated degradation. If there is imperfect complementarity between the "guide" sequence and the target, Argonaute may not cleave the target, but rather recruit additional proteins that ultimately inhibit translation of the target (Figure 5). Furthermore, many endogenous miRNA target the 3′-untranslated regions of mRNA, such that the miRNA-RISC complex represses translation, rather than initiating mRNA degradation.

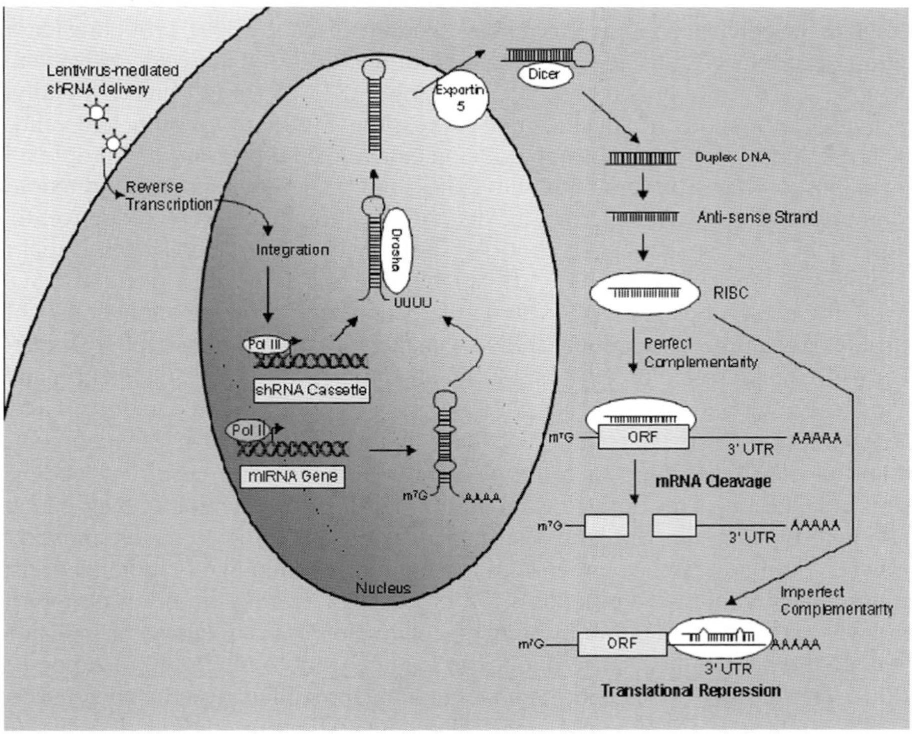

Fig. 5. Schematic representation of the generation, processing and function of miRNA or shRNA. Both miRNA and shRNA are processed in the nucleus by Drosha, and further processed in the cytoplasm by Dicer, yielding a 22 base pair duplex. The antisense strand of the duplex complexes with RISC, acting as a "guide" sequence for hybridization with the "target" transcript. If there is perfect complementarity between the "guide" and "target sequences, the "target" sequence undergoes cleavage and degradation. With incomplete complementarity, translation of the "target" sequence is inhibited by the RISC complex.

Based on our knowledge of how endogenous miRNA are generated, processed and function (He and Hannon 2004), this information has been used to develop and use exogenous RNAi to modify gene expression. Short-hairpin RNA (shRNA) introduced into cells (Paddison *et al.* 2002) are processed in the same fashion as endogenous miRNA. Cassettes encoding a shRNA often consist of inverted repeats separated by a loop sequence and followed by a short poly(T) track to terminate transcription (Paddison *et al.* 2002). Typically, the shRNA-encoding cassette is inserted downstream of a RNA polymerase III promoter (Paddison *et al.* 2004), within the targeting vector of choice. The targeting vector can be a simple plasmid used for transfection of cells *in vitro*, or it can be a viral vector, such as adenovirus or lentivirus. Adenoviral vectors have numerous advantages, primarily the ease in obtaining high titer stocks of virus and the infectivity of the virus, but suffer from the fact that they only provide for transient expression, such that the "effect" may be washed out over time in a rapidly proliferating tissue such as the ruminant placenta. By contrast, lentiviral vectors provide for stable integration into the host genome making them ideal for "long-term" transgenesis. Lentiviral constructs are often easier to generate than adenoviral constructs, but it is more difficult to generate high-titer stocks of lentivirus.

As noted above, when shRNA are introduced into cells, either *in vitro* or *in vivo*, the shRNA is processed in the cell like endogenous miRNA (Paddinson *et al.* 2002), providing for targeted-degradation of mRNA or translational repression of that mRNA (Figure 5). However, not all shRNAs work, and it is not uncommon to design and test 3 to 5 shRNA before identifying one that effectively "knocks down" specific-gene expression. Furthermore, sufficient validation of a shRNA is needed to verify that it is not inducing generalized repression of multiple mRNA or off-target effects, or that its introduction into cells is not triggering interferon induction and an innate immune response. Often, investigators will scramble the shRNA sequence, to render it non-functional, and use that as the control. The drawback of that approach is that it is difficult to know that the scrambled shRNA is capable of interacting with Dicer and RISC, which would yield the most robust control. Alternatively, one can introduce a functional shRNA as the control. For example, a functional shRNA that targets a mRNA transcript not expressed by the cell or tissue of interest. Purcell *et al.* (2009) utilized a shRNA that targeted human PRR15, but due to three nucleotide mismatches with the sheep mRNA sequence, it did not alter sheep PRR15 expression, providing a robust control for their subsequent *in vivo* experiments.

Hofmann *et al.* (2004) infected cattle oocytes with a lentiviral construct leading to the expression of EGFP in calves derived from *in vitro* fertilization. Similarly, they infected fetal fibroblasts with the recombinant lentivirus and used these as donor cells for somatic cell nuclear transfer. Both approaches underscore the potential for lentiviral-mediated transgenesis in ruminants. Lentiviral-mediated expression of shRNA targeting the prion protein in goats and cattle was accomplished either by somatic cell nuclear transfer (goats) or injection of the lentivirus into the perivitelline space of oocytes (cattle), prior to *in vitro* fertilization (Golding *et al.* 2006). These two reports confirmed the potential for lentiviral-mediated transgenesis, as well as shRNA-mediated RNAi in ruminants. Recently, we reported (Purcell *et al.* 2009) the infection of day 8 sheep blastocysts with a lentiviral construct designed to target the mRNA encoding PRR15, a nuclear protein expressed by the elongating ruminant conceptus. We utilized a replication-deficient lentiviral construct generated by Rubinson *et al.* (2003), such that when hatched blastocysts were exposed to the virus, only the outer trophectoderm would be infected. Exposing three blastocysts to 300,000 transforming units of the virus in 100μl drops for 4 to 6 hours resulted in uniform infection of the trophectoderm. Infected blastocysts were then surgically transferred to synchronized recipient ewes. The lentivirus construct used (LL3.7; Rubinson *et al.* 2003) contains an EGFP expression cassette driven by the cytomegalovirus promoter, and an insertion site for the shRNA cassette downstream of the mouse U6 promoter, a RNA polymerase III promoter. As reported in Purcell *et al.* (2009), infection of blastocysts with a lentivirus that did not contain a shRNA cassette, or with one containing a shRNA cassette that targets human PRR15 mRNA (discussed earlier), did not impact conceptus development by 15 dpc, and there was uniform expression of EGFP in the conceptus trophectoderm. In contrast, infecting blastocysts with the lentivirus expressing the shRNA targeting sheep PRR15 mRNA resulted in conceptus demise or a failure to develop by 15 dpc. While we continue to investigate the exact function of PRR15, our results demonstrate the utility of lentiviral-mediated transgenesis in the ruminant placenta. Furthermore, while our efforts were ongoing, Georgiades *et al.* (2007) and Okada *et al.* (2007) reported trophoblast-specific lentiviral-mediated gene transfer in mice, again by infecting the hatched blastocysts. These three reports (Geogiades *et al.* 2007; Okada *et al.* 2007; Purcell *et al.* 2009) provide the "proof of concept" that lentiviral-mediated transgenesis can be directed to the placenta specifically. Since lentiviral constructs are stably integrated into the host genome, any derivative of the trophectoderm should express the "transgene" throughout the remainder of gestation, providing the opportunity to directly assess the function of genes expressed by the ruminant placenta. Furthermore, this approach could be expanded to "gain of function" experiments, where a transgene would be expressed under the control of a tissue-specific promoter, or under the control of a "regulated" promoter that could be "turned on or off" at various times during gestation.

Conclusions

Historically we have gained considerable insight into the physiological function and processes of the placenta from studies using ruminants. This is especially true for sheep which have been used extensively for *in vivo* studies assessing placental functions affecting fetal-placental development. However, it has been difficult to directly assess specific gene function in the ruminant placenta. The generation of cattle or sheep trophoblast cell lines is providing ruminant-specific assessment of gene function and regulation *in vitro*. Furthermore, reports of lentiviral-mediated transgenesis specifically in the trophoblast lineage provide the potential to expand assessment of gene function in the placenta *in vivo*. The use of RNAi *in vivo* is a powerful tool in determining the importance of specific genes expressed in the placenta, and when coupled with maternal and fetal catheterization, the impact on placental and fetal physiology can be assessed simultaneously. Results from these *in vivo* approaches coupled with *in vitro* investigations using the appropriate ruminant trophoblast cell line could yield powerful strategies for uncovering new biological functions and underlying molecular mechanisms. With these new approaches in hand, the future for assessing gene function in the ruminant placenta is bright.

References

Anderson MS, He J, Flowers-Ziegler J, Devaskar SU & Hay WW 2001 Effects of selective hyperglycemia and hyperinsulinemia on glucose transporters in fetal ovine skeletal muscle. *American Journal of Physiology* **281** R1256-1263.

Aston KI, Li GP, Hicks BA, Sessions BR, Davis AP, Winger QA, Rickords LF, Stevens JR & White KL 2009 Global gene expression analysis of bovine somatic cell nuclear transfer blastocysts and cotyledons. *Molecular Reproduction and Development* **76** 471-482.

Battaglia FC, Meschia G, Makowski EL & Bowes W 1968 The effect of maternal oxygen inhalation upon fetal oxygenation. *Journal of Clinical Investigation* **47** 548-555.

Bell AW, Kennaugh JM, Battaglia FC, Makowski EL & Meshcia G 1986 Metabolic and circulatory studies of fetal Lamb at midgestation. *American Journal of Physiology* **250** E538-544.

Boshier DP 1969 A histological and histochemical examination of implantation and early placentome formation in sheep. *Journal of Reproduction and Fertility* **19** 51–61.

Bridger PS, Haupt S, Klisch K, Leiser R, Tinneberg HR & Pfarrer C 2007 Validation of primary epitheloid cell cultures isolated from bovine placental caruncles and cotyledons. *Theriogenology* **68** 592-603.

Dunlap KA, Palmarini M, Varela M, Burghardt RC, Hayashi K, Farmer JL & Spencer TE 2006 Endogenous retroviruses regulate periimplantation placental growth and differentiation. *Proceedings of the National Academy of Sciences* **103** 14390-14395.

Everts RE, Chavatte-Palmer P, Razzak A, Hue I, Green CA, Oliveira R, Vignon X, Rodriguez-Zas SL, Tian XC, Yang X, Renard J-P & Lewin HA 2008 Aberrant gene expression patterns in placentomes are associated with phenotypically normal and abnormal cattle cloned by somatic cell nuclear transfer. *Physiological Genomics* **33** 65-77.

Ezashi T, Das P, Gupta R, Walker A & Roberts RM 2008 The role of homeobox protein distal-less 3 and its interaction with ETS2 in regulating bovine interferon-tau gene expression-synergistic transcriptional activation with ETS2. *Biology of Reproduction* **79** 115-124.

Ezashi T, Ghosh D & Roberts RM 2001 Repression of Ets-2-induced transactivation of the τ-interferon promoter by oct-4. *Molecular and Cellular Biology* **21** 7883-7891.

Farmer JL, Burghardt RC, Jousan FD, Hansen PJ, Bazer FW & Spencer TE 2008 Galectin 15 (LGALS15) functions in trophectoderm migration and attachment. *FASEB Journal* **22** 548-560.

Flechon JE, Flechon B, Degrouard J & Guillomot M 2007 Cellular features of the extra-embryonic endoderm during elongation in the ovine conceptus. *Genesis* **45** 709-715.

Georgiades P, Cox B, Gertsenstein M, Chawengsaksophak K & Rossant J 2007 Trophoblast specific gene manipulation using lentivirus-based vectors. *Biotechniques* **42** 317-324.

Golding MC, Long CR, Carmell MA, Hannon GJ & Westhusin ME 2006 Suppression of prion protein in livestock by RNA interference. *Proceedings of the National Academy of Science* **103** 5285-5290.

Guillomot M 1995 Cellular interactions during implantation in domestic ruminants. *Journal of Reproduction and Fertility Supplement* **49** 39-51.

Guillomot M, Flechon JE & Wintenberger-Torres S 1981 Conceptus attachment in the ewe: an ultrastructural study. *Placenta* **2** 169-182.

Hambruch N, Haeger J-D, Dilly M & Pfarrer 2010 EGF stimulates proliferation in the bovine placental trophoblast cell line F3 via RAS and MAPK. *Placenta* **31** 67-74.

Hannan NJ, Paiva P, Dimitriadis E & Salamonsen LA 2010 Models for study of human embyro implantation: choice of cell lines. *Biology of Reproduction* **82** 235-245.

Hay Jr WW 1991 In vivo measurements of placental transport and metabolism. *Proceedings of the Nutrition Society* **50** 355-362.

He L & Hannon GJ 2004 MicroRNAs: Small RNAs with a big role in gene regulation. *Nature Reviews Genetics* **5** 522-531.

Hiden U, Wadsack C, Prutsch N, Gauster M, Weiss U, Frank H-G, Schmitz U, Fast-Hirsch C, Hengstschlager M, Potgens A, Ruben A, Knofler M, Haslinger P, Huppertz B, Bilban M, Kaufmann P & Desoye G. 2007 The first trimester human trophoblast cell line ACH-3P: A novel tool to study autocrine/paracrine regulatory loops of human trophoblast subpopulations – TNF-α stimulates MMP15 expression. *BMC Developmental Biology* **7** 137.

Hirata, M, Sato T, Tsumagari M, Shimada A, Nakano H, Hashizume K & Ito A 2003 Differential regulation of the expression of matrix metalloproteinase's and tissue inhibitors of metalloproteinase's by cytokines and growth factors in bovine endometrial stromal cells and trophoblast cell line BT-1 in vitro. *Biology of Reproduction* **68** 1276-1281.

Hofmann A, Zakhartchenko V, Weppert M, Sebald H, Wenigerkind H, Brem G, Wolf E & Pfeifer A 2004 Generation of transgenic cattle by lentiviral gene transfer into oocytes. *Biology of Reproduction* **71** 405-409.

Jeckel KM, Limesand SW & Anthony RV 2009 Specificity protein-1 and -3 trans-activate the ovine placental lactogen gene promoter. *Molecular and Cellular Endocrinology* **307** 118-124.

Jones HN, Powell TL & Jannson T 2007 Regulation of placental nutrient transport – a review. *Placenta* **28** 763-774.

Kappes SM, Warren WC, Pratt SL, Liang R & Anthony RV 1992 Quantification and cellular localization of ovine placental lactogen messenger ribonucleic acid expression during mid- and late gestation. *Endocrinology* **131** 2829-2838.

Landim LP, Miglino MA, Pfarrer C, Ambrosio CE & Garcia JM 2007 Culture of mature trophoblastic giant cells from bovine placentomes. *Animal Reproduction Science* **98** 357-364.

Lei T, Hohn H-P, Behr & Denker H-W 2007 Influences of extracellular matrix and of conditioned media on differentiation and invasiveness of trophoblast stem cells. *Placenta* **28** 14-21.

Leiser R, Krebs C, Ebert B & Dantzer V 1997 Placental vascular corrosion cast studies: A comparison between ruminants and humans. *Microscopy Research and Technique* **38** 76–87.

Liang R, Limesand SW & Anthony RV 1999 Structure and transcriptional regulation of the ovine placental lactogen gene. *European Journal of Biochemistry* **265** 883-895.

Librach CL, Werb Z, Fitzgerald ML, Chiu K, Corwin NM, Esteves RA, Grobelny D, Galardy R, Damsky CH & Fisher SJ 1991 92-kD type IV collagenase mediates invasion of human cytotrophoblasts. *Journal of Cell Biology* **113** 437-449.

Limesand SW, Jeckel KM & Anthony RV 2004 Purα, a single-stranded DNA binding protein, augments placental lactogen gene transcription. *Molecular Endocrinology* **18** 447-457.

Meschia G, Battaglia FC, Hay WW & Sparks JW 1980 Utilization of substrates by the ovine placenta in vivo. *Federation Proceedings* **39** 245-249.

Meschia G, Cotter JR, Breathnach CS & Barron DH 1965 The diffusibility of oxygen across the sheep placenta. *Quarterly Journal of Experimental Physiology and Cognate Medical Sciences* **50** 466-480.

Michael DD, Wagner SK, Ocon OM, Talbot NC, Rooke JA & Ealy AD 2006 Granulocyte-macrophage colony-stimulating-factor increases interferon-τ protein secretion in bovine trophectoderm cells. *American Journal of Reproductive Immunology* **56** 63-67.

Milosavljevic M, Duello TM & Schuler LA 1989 In situ localisation of two prolactin related mRNAs to binucleate cells of bovine placentomes. *Endocrinology* **125** 883-889.

Nakano H, Shimada A, Imai K, Takezawa T, Takahashi T & Hashizume K 2002 Bovine trophoblastic cell differentiation on collagen substrata: formation of binucleate cells expressing placental lactogen. *Cell and Tissue Research* **307** 225-235.

Okada Y, Ueshin Y, Isotani A, Saito-Fujita T, Nakashima H, Kimura K, Mizoguchi A, Oh-hora M, Mori Y, Ogata M, Oshima RG, Okabe M & Ikawa M 2007 Complementation of placental defects and embryonic lethality by trophoblast-specific lentiviral gene transfer. *Nature Biotechnology* **25** 233-237.

Paddison PJ, Caudy AA, Bernstein E, Hannon GJ & Conklin DS 2002 Short hairpin RNAs (shRNAs) induce sequence-specific silencing in mammalian cells. *Genes and Development* **16** 948-958.

Paddison PJ, Caudy AA, Sachidanandam R & Hannon GJ 2004 Short hairpin activated gene silencing in mammalian cells. *Methods in Molecular Biology* **265** 85-100.

Purcell SH, Cantlon JD, Wright CD, Henkes LE, Seidel GE & Anthony RV 2009 The involvement of proline-rich 15 in early conceptus development in sheep. *Biology of Reproduction* **81** 1112-1121.

Regnault TRH, Friedman JE, Wilkening RB, Anthony RV & Hay WW 2005 Fetoplacental transport and utilization of amino acids in IUGR – a review. *Placenta* **26** S52-62.

Roberts RM & Anthony RV 1994 Molecular biology of the trophectoderm and placental hormones. In *Molecular Biology of the Female Reproductive System,* pp 395-440. Ed JK Findlay. San Diego: Academic Press.

Rubinson DA, Dillon CP, Kwiatkowski AV, Sievers C, Yang L, Kopinja J, Zhang M, McManus MT, Gertler FB, Scott ML & Van Parijs L 2003 A lentivirus-based system to functionally silence genes in primary mammalian cells, stem cells and transgenic mice by RNA interference. *Nature Genetics* **33** 401-406.

Schoknecht PA, Currie WB & Bell AW 1992 Kinetics of placental lactogen in mid- and late-gestation ovine fetuses. *Journal of Endocrinology* **133** 95-100.

Shimada A, Nakano H, Takahashi T, Imai K & Hashizume K 2001 Isolation and characterization of a bovine blastocyst-derived trophoblastic cell line, BT-1: development of a culture system in the absence of feeder cell. *Placenta* **22** 652-662.

Stegeman JHJ 1974 Placental development in the sheep and its relation to fetal development. A qualitative and quantitative anatomic and histologic study. *Bijdragen Tot De Dierkunde* **44** 3-72.

Summerton J 1999 Morpholino antisense oligomers: the case for an RNase H-independent structural type. *Biochimica et Biophysica Acta* **1489** 141-158.

Talamantes F & Ogren L 1988 The placenta as an endocrine organ: polypeptides. In *The Physiology of Reproduction,* pp 2093-2144. Eds E Knobil & J Neill. New York: Raven Press.

Talbot NC, Caperna TJ, Edwards JL, Garrett W, Wells KD & Ealy AD 2000 Bovine blastocyst-derived trophectoderm and endoderm cell cultures: interferon-τ and transferrin expression as respective in vitro markers. *Biology of Reproduction* **62** 235-247.

Teng C, Battaglia FC, Meschia G, Narkewicz MR & Wilkening RB 2002 Fetal hepatic and umbilical uptakes of glucogenic substrates during a glucagon-somatostatin infusion. *American Journal of Physiology* **282** E542-550.

Ushizawa K, Takahashi T, Hosoe M, Ishiwata H, Kaneyama K, Kizaki K & Hashizume K 2007 Global gene expression analysis and regulation of the principal genes expressed in bovine placenta in relation to the transcription factor AP-2 family. *Reproductive Biology and Endocrinology* **5** 17.

Ushizawa K, Takahashi T, Kaneyama K, Tokunaga, Tsunoda Y & Hashizume K 2005 Gene expression profiles of bovine trophoblastic cell line (BT-1) analyzed by a custom cDNA microarray. *Journal of Reproduction and Development* **51** 211-220.

Wallace JM, Regnault TRH, Limesand SW, Hay Jr WW & Anthony RV 2005 Investigating the causes of low birth weight in contrasting ovine paradigms. *Journal of Physiology* **565** 19-26.

Wooding FBP 1983 Frequency and localization of binucleate cells in the placentomes of ruminants. *Placenta* **4** 527-540.

Wooding FBP 1984 Role of binucleate cells in fetomaternal cell fusion at implantation in sheep. *American Journal of Anatomy* **170** 233-250.

Wooding FBP 1992 Current topic: The synepitheliochorial placenta of ruminants: binucelate cell fusions and hormone production. *Placenta* **13** 101-113.

Wooding FBP & Wathes 1980 Binucleate cell migration in the bovine placentome. *Journal of Reproduction and Fertility* **59** 425-430.

Spermatogonial stem cell biology in the bull: development of isolation, culture, and transplantation methodologies and their potential impacts on cattle production

JM Oatley

Center for Reproductive Biology and Health, Department of Dairy and Animal Science, The Pennsylvania State University, University Park, PA 16802

Widespread adoption of artificial insemination as a breeding practice has allowed for expanded use of desirable genetics from specific sires and greatly influenced production traits in dairy cattle populations worldwide. In fact, the average dairy cow in the US in 2009 produced 4.5 times more milk than in 1940 when commercialization of artificial insemination began. While many factors have contributed to this rapid increase in levels of milk production, genetic gain through expanded utilization of germlines from specific sires has been a major contribution. In comparison, use of artificial insemination in beef cattle populations has been limited due to challenges with implementing intensive management strategies required for success. Thus, there is need for alternative reproductive tools to expand use of desirable male genetics in the beef cattle industry. The process of sperm production, termed spermatogenesis, is supported by a tissue-specific stem cell population referred to as spermatogonial stem cells (SSCs). These unique cells have the capacity for infinite self-renewal and long-term regeneration of spermatogenesis following transplantation. In rodents, methods for isolating, culturing, and transplanting SSCs have been devised. For beef cattle, transplanting SSCs isolated from a donor male into the testes of recipient males in which donor-derived spermatogenesis occurs and offspring with donor genetics are produced from natural breeding has great potential as an alternative to artificial insemination. This potential reproductive strategy would allow for expansive use of genetics from desirable sires that overcomes the logistical challenges of artificial insemination. Translation of the methods devised for rodents to cattle is at the forefront of development. Devising means for isolating an SSC-enriched cell fraction from donor testes and identifying conditions that support long-term maintenance and proliferation of bovine SSCs in vitro are two tools that would greatly accelerate the pace at which transplantation will become a commercially viable option for cattle industries. Recent studies showed that expression of THY1 by SSCs is a conserved phenotype between rodents and cattle, and selection of the THY1+ fraction from

Corresponding author E-mail: jmo15@psu.edu

donor testes can be used for isolating an SSC-enriched germ cell population. In addition, the conditions devised for expanding the number of rodent SSCs in vitro continues to serve as the basis for developing conditions that support bovine SSCs. With these tools in hand major advances in developing implementable reproductive tools with SSCs for commercial cattle production will be made in the coming decade.

Introduction

Utilization of desirable genetics is a key aspect of animal agriculture, allowing for rapid expansion of phenotypic improvement in livestock populations. Currently, the most effective means to enhance efficiency of food animal production and improve product quality is through introduction and expansion of specific genetics. In most agriculturally important animal populations the majority of genetic gain is made through the male germline. Thus, male reproductive efficiency is an essential component of livestock production and devising means to expand availability of male genetics can have major economic impacts to the producer and consumer. Spermatozoa are the cell by which genetics of males are passed to the next generation and are a major target for preserving the germline after death and expanding the utilization of superior genetics in cattle populations. One major avenue that sperm have been utilized in cattle production is with artificial insemination (AI). Since its commercialization in the 1940's, AI has had major impacts on cattle production over the last 70 years, especially with genetic improvement of dairy cattle herds (Foote 2002). Widespread adoption of AI in the dairy industry to capitalize on specific genetics has been a main factor for generation of a cattle population in 2009 that produces on average 4.5 times more milk per cow than in 1940 (National Agricultural Statistics Service). It has been estimated thatapproximately 80% of dairy cattle in the US are bred by AI compared to only approximately 5% of beef cattle, resulting in lost opportunities for genetic gains in this industry (Geary et al., 1998; Perry et al. 2002) . Effective implementation of an AI program requires intensive management, posing a practical limitation for beef cattle enterprises in which the majority of animals are typically managed in range conditions where intensive management is challenging. Thus, there is need for devising alternative reproductive strategies that allow for expansion and utilization of the germline from genetically desirable sires in beef cattle populations.

Spermatogenesis and Spermatogonial Stem Cells (SSCs)

Spermatogenesis is the process by which millions of sperm are generated per day in the testis, commencing at puberty and persisting throughout old age in males (Sharpe, 1994). At the foundation of this process are the spermatogonial stem cells (SSCs) which undergo both self-renewal and differentiation. The process of self-renewal maintains a pool of SSCs throughout the life of a male and provides the basis for continual male fertility. Initiation of sperm production occurs when SSC differentiation results in production of daughter progeny, termed A_{paired} (A_{pr}) spermatogonia, which are committed to differentiation rather than self-renewal (de Rooij and Russell, 2000). The A_{pr} spermatogonia then undergo a series of mitotic cell divisions becoming $A_{aligned}$ (A_{al}) spermatogonia and give rise to differentiating type A spermatogonia which undergo another series of amplifying mitotic divisions. These differentiating A spermatogonia mature into intermediate and type B spermatogonia which enter meiosis becoming primary and secondary spermatocytes, and eventually haploid spermatids are produced which undergo a transformation into spermatozoa (Russell et al., 1990). Collectively, the SSCs (also termed A_{single} or A_s), A_{pr}, and A_{al} germ cells are referred to as the undifferentiated spermatogonial population and share many phenotypic and molecular characteristics (Oatley and Brinster 2008). Similar to other tissue-specific stem cell populations SSCs are rare within their residing tissue, constituting an estimated 0.03% of the total testicular cell population in adult mice (Tegelenbosch and de Rooij, 1993). While the SSC population has not been studied in male livestock to any great detail, spermatogenesis is conserved among mammalian species and characteristics defined for SSCs in rodents are likely conserved in higher order mammals such as cattle (Sharpe, 1994). Due to the extreme rarity of SSCs studying and isolating these cells is a major challenge which has hampered the pace at which the biology of these cells has been defined.

Conserved molecular characteristics of SSCs

Currently, molecular markers specific for SSCs that distinguish them from the other undifferentiated spermatogonia (i.e. A_{pr} and A_{al}) have not been described. The only unequivocal measure of SSCs is a functional capacity to regenerate and maintain spermatogenesis. Nonetheless, expression of several molecular markers that distinguish undifferentiated spermatogonia, including SSCs, from differentiating spermatogonia have been identified. Studies in the mouse showed that expression of the transcriptional repressor promyelocytic leukaemia zinc finger (PLZF) is restricted to the undifferentiated spermatogonial population (Buaas et al., 2004; Costoya et al., 2004); whereas, expression of c-KIT is restricted to differentiating spermatogonia (Yoshinaga et al., 1991). Recent studies by Reding et al. (2010) with cattle and Lou et al. (2009) with pigs showed that expression of PLZF is localized to undifferentiated spermatogonia, suggesting at least partial conservation of phenotypic and molecular characteristics of spermatogonia in rodents and livestock. Those same studies showed that expression of ubiquitin carboxyl-terminal esterase L1 (UCHL1) is a general marker of type A spermatogonia in cattle and pigs (Lou et al., 2009; Reding et al., 2010). Currently, localization of c-KIT expression by spermatogonia in livestock has not been reported in detail but will be important to characterize for understanding how the SSC population is defined in agriculturally important animals such as bulls. Overall, use of PLZF, UCHL1, and c-KIT as markers provides a tool to better define different spermatogonial populations including SSCs.

Niche factors regulating SSC fate decisions

Similar to other tissue-specific stem cell populations found in mammals maintenance of a pool of SSCs and regulation of their biological activities is supported by a niche microenvironment (Oatley and Brinster, 2008). This specialized environment is made up of both growth factors and microarchitecture provided by niche support cells. Coordination between the specific growth factors secreted by support cells and expression of receptors by SSCs is essential for maintenance and function of the SSC pool. Thus, defining the support cell populations and their specific contributions to the niche is important given that disruption of these contributions will impair male fertility. The majority of understanding about growth factor components of the SSC niche has been defined using the mouse as a model and conservation of those mechanisms in livestock are only just beginning to be explored (Reding et al., 2010). For mouse SSCs, specific cytokines identified as components of the niche include glilal cell line-derived neurotrophic factor (GDNF), fibroblast growth factor 2 (FGF2), and colony stimulating factor 1 (CSF-1). Reduced expression of GDNF in mice with one null allele results in rapid decline of male fertility following puberty that is attributed to formation of seminiferous tubules devoid of germ cells, a condition referred to as Sertoli-cell-only (Meng et al., 2000). Also, overexpression of GDNF in mice causes accumulation of the undifferentiated spermatogonial population culminating in formation of germ cell tumors (Meng et al., 2000). These in vivo studies suggested that GDNF plays a key role in regulating the fate decisions of SSCs in mammalian testes. Subsequent studies by Kubota et al. (2004a) also utilizing the mouse showed that GDNF could promote long-term survival and expansion of SSC numbers in a serum-free chemically defined environment in vitro, solidifying its role as a key regulator of SSC self-renewal. Because of their intimate association with germ cells and known role as "nurse" cells for spermatogenesis, Sertoli cells have been regarded as the main support cell population for SSC niches. Indeed, Sertoli cells were shown to express GDNF in response to stimulation from follicle stimulating hormone (FSH) which is a key regulator of their functional capacity to support spermatogenesis (Tadokoro et al., 2002). Additional studies by Kubota et al. (2004a) showed that FGF2 supplementation enhances GDNF-induced proliferation of mouse SSCs in vitro but is unable to sustain SSCs as the sole growth factor supplement. Similar to GDNF, production of FGF2 has also been tied to Sertoli cells in the mouse testis (Mullaney and Skinner, 1992). A third factor that contributes to the milieu of extrinsic stimuli that influence SSC self-renewal is CSF-1. In vitro, exposure to soluble CSF-1 enhances GDNF influence on SSC self-renewal specifically and expression of this molecule in vivo is localized to Leydig cells (Oatley et al., 2009). Collectively, these findings implicate both Sertoli and Leydig cells as contributors to the SSC niche in mouse testes. While several key growth factors that regulate SSC self-renewal and survival in vitro have been identified, their rate of proliferation is slow (estimated to be approximately 6 days) and a pure population cannot be maintained suggesting that additional factors affecting their fate decisions have yet to be identified. Unfortunately, expression of GDNF, FGF2, or CSF-1 in the testes of livestock animals has not been reported but will be an area of investigation in the coming decade as more emphasis is placed on translating findings from rodents studies on SSC biology to higher order mammals.

SSC transplantation

A key aspect of SSC biology is their ability for efficient transplantation and regeneration of spermatogenesis. This capability is especially important for altering the genetic makeup of animal populations given that SSCs are the only permanent self-renewing cell type in mammals that contribute genetic information to the next generation. In 1994, Brinster and colleagues reported the regeneration of donor-derived spermatogenesis following microinjection of a single cell suspension of testicular cells isolated from a donor mouse into the testes of recipient mice and offspring containing donor genetics were generated after mating (Brinster and Zimmerman, 1994; Brinster and Avarbock, 1994). These pioneering studies were the first to prove existence of a stem cell population within mammalian testes and opened a new field of study in male reproductive biology. Stem cells are defined by an ability to maintain tissue homeostasis and regenerate long-term tissue function following toxic damage that depletes the tissue of differentiated cells or following transplantation. For the testis, long-term regeneration of spermatogenesis is the defining feature of testicular stem cells. Because the undifferentiated spermatogonial population represents the foundation of spermatogenesis it is believed to contain the testicular stem cells and this regenerating cell population was labeled as spermatogonial stem cells or SSCs. Ever since the first reports of transplantation success, several groups have aimed to extend this methodology to other mammals including humans and livestock.

For cattle, the SSC transplantation method has the potential to provide a novel avenue to (1) immortalize the germline of genetically desirable sires, (2) efficiently expand utilization of desirable male genetics, and (3) provide an efficient means for generation of transgenic cattle. These possibilities are especially applicable to the beef cattle industry where use of AI has historically been limited due to impracticality. One potentially valuable application would be transplantation of SSCs from a desirable donor bull into the testes of a group of recipient bulls in which donor-derived spermatogenesis would occur and the recipients breed by natural service to generate offspring with the donor genetics (Figure 1). This potential reproductive tool would overcome the logistical difficulties associated with implementation of AI, allowing for efficient utilization of desirable male genetics. As a result, genetic gain in beef cattle populations could be enhanced leading to more efficient production of meat and fiber for human consumption. While the potentials are great, translation of SSC transplantation methods devised for mice to cattle has been limited. In mice, isolation of an SSC-enriched fraction from the total testicular cell population for injection into recipient testes has dramatically enhanced the efficiency of SSC transplantation success, and this principal has recently begun to be developed for bulls (Reding et al., 2010).

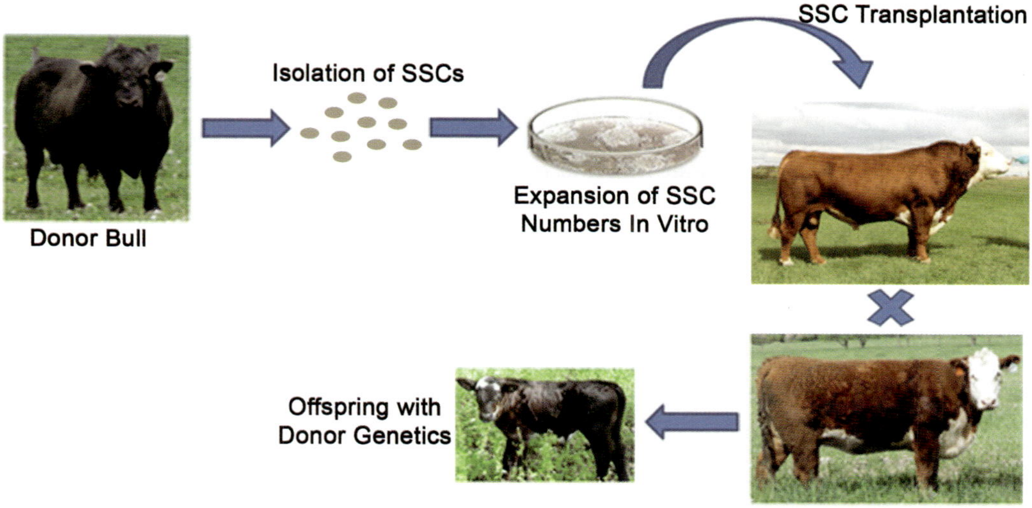

Fig. 1. Scenario for application of SSC transplantation in beef cattle. Isolation of SSCs from the testis of a genetically desirable bull followed by a period of in vitro maintenance that supports their proliferation would provide a source of donor SSCs for transplantation into recipient bulls. Donor-derived spermatogenesis would then occur within recipient testes and these bulls could breed by natural service to generate offspring containing donor genetics. This potential application would provide a novel reproductive tool for expanding the use of desirable male genetics in the beef cattle industry.

Due to rarity of SSCs in mammalian testes extensive regeneration of donor-derived spermatogenesis within recipient testes is limited without enrichment prior to transplantation. This limitation has prompted the search for cell surface markers that could be used with cell sorting technologies such as fluorescent activated cell sorting (FACS) or magnetic activated cell sorting (MACS) to isolate an SSC enriched fraction for transplantation. The mouse has been predominately used as a model to identify cell surface markers of mammalian SSCs. However, recent progress has been made in translating findings in the mouse to bulls (Reding et al., 2010). The first reported markers of mouse SSCs were α6-integrin and β1-integrin which resulted in 8-fold and 4-fold enrichment for SSCs following transplantation, respectively (Shinohara et al., 1999). To date, the greatest enrichment for mouse SSCs based on a single cell surface protein is by selection of the THY1+ cell fraction (Oatley and Brinster, 2008). In adult mouse testes, the THY1+ cell fraction is enriched 30-fold compared to the unselected total testis cell population (Kubota et al., 2004b). Logically, because GDNF is an essential growth factor promoting SSC self-renewal selection of spermatogonia expressing the associated receptors, c-RET and GFRα1, should result in enrichment for SSCs. Unfortunately, both the c-RET+ and GFRα1+ testis cell fractions from adult mice are depleted of SSCs indicating these are not effective markers for isolation of stem cells (Ebata et al., 2005). Other surface proteins identified as markers for rodent SSCs include CD9 (Kanatsu-Shinohara et al., 2004), Ep-CAM (Ryu et al., 2005), and GPR125 (Seandel et al., 2007), but none have shown the level SSC enrichment found with THY1 (Oatley and Brinster 2008).

Conservation of cell surface phenotype for SSCs among mammals is just beginning to be explored. Recent studies by Reding et al. (2010) showed that THY1 is a conserved maker of SSCs in bulls and that selection of the THY1+ cell fraction by MACS results in isolation of an SSC-enriched population from testes of pre-pubertal bulls. The development of SSC transplantation methods in mice was greatly advanced by identification of SSC surface markers that allowed for their isolation (Oatley and Brinster 2006; Oatley and Brinster 2008). With the recent progress in identify markers of SSCs in bulls the pace at which development of SSC transplantation in cattle is sure to increase.

Even without selection of an SSC enriched population for injection several studies have attempted transplantation in bulls utilizing unselected testis cell populations (Izadayar et al., 2003; Herrid et al., 2006; Stockwell et al., 2009;). While none of these studies have provided definitive results of success, important information has been gleaned about feasibility of the testis injection procedure. The greatest challenge for determining success of SSC transplantation in bulls is unequivocal identification of donor-derived spermatogenesis. In rodents, this has been achieved through the use of naturally sterile recipients in which any regeneration of spermatogenesis is donor-derived or with donors that express a marker transgene (e.g. LacZ or GFP) within the germline (Oatley and Brinster 2006). Izadayar et al. (2003) performed homologous and autologous germ cell transplantation with 5 month old Holstein bulls following localized irradiation of recipient testes to deplete endogenous spermatogenesis. At 2.5 months after injection of donor germ cells cross-sections of recipient testes were examined for spermatogenesis histologically and those receiving donor cells contained a greater proportion of seminiferous tubules with both spermatogonia and complete spermatogenesis (Izadayar et al., 2003). Unfortunately, the donor cells were not labeled for detection after transplantation and spermatogenesis within recipient seminiferous tubules could not be unequivocally proven to be donor-derived. Also, by definition transplanted germ cells must support long-term regeneration of spermatogenesis (i.e. several rounds of spermatozoa production) to be considered SSCs but the timeframe of analysis employed by Izadayar et al. (2003) only examined spermatogenesis within recipient bulls after one round of spermatogenesis. Moreover, in mice germ cell development from spermatogonia to spermatozoa occurs over a 35 day period but the first round of spermatogenesis from transplanted SSCs is delayed requiring at least 1.5 cycles or ~52 days (Nagano et al., 1999). In bulls, spermatogenesis is approximately 61 days; thus, identification of donor-derived spermatogenesis after 2.5 months (~75 days) reported by Izadayar et al. (2003) suggests regeneration from transplanted bovine SSCs is accelerated compared to the mouse. Using detectable differences in microsatellite markers Stockwell et al. (2009) detected donor spermatozoa within the ejaculate of recipient bulls 52-98 weeks after injection of germ cells, but their appearance declined over time. These results indicated that the donor-derived spermatozoa were not a result of SSC colonization given that long-term regeneration of spermatogenesis was not achieved. Even with these areas of contention for success of bovine SSC transplantation, previous studies have provided the framework for refinement in the future to develop this technique as a reproductive tool for expanding utilization of the male germline.

Long-term culture of SSCs

In vitro maintenance of SSCs for long periods of time in conditions that support their self-renewal is a key aspect for developing reproductive technologies that utilize these cells to immortalize and expand the use of germlines from desirable males. The rarity of SSCs even if isolated from donor testes is a limiting factor for success of transplantation into recipients and widespread utilization of this technology. The potential for infinite expansion of SSCs in vitro through support of self-renewal would provide millions of these cells for transplantation into hundreds of recipient bulls. Moreover, when combined with cryopreservation methodologies the germline of specific males could be immortalized. These possibilities have advantage over sperm cryopreservation as the standard for germline preservation after death given that sperm are a non renewable resource without the associated SSC population. To date, techniques for long-term maintenance and expansion of SSCs are only available for mice (Kubota et al., 2004a; Oatley and Brinster 2006), rats (Ryu et al., 2005), and hamsters (Kanatsu-Shinohara et al., 2007). Previous studies with cattle have resulted in short-term proliferation of SSCs, but long-term maintenance has not been achieved (Oatley et al., 2004a; Oatley et al., 2004b; Aponte et al., 2005). Additionally, culture of SSCs from other livestock species has not been reported. However, utilizing the mouse system as a basis our lab has made strides in refining culture conditions for maintenance of bovine SSCs (Figure 2).

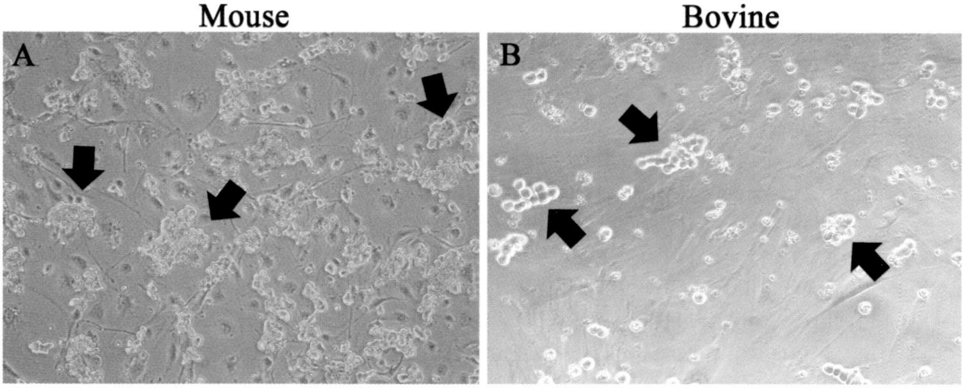

Fig. 2. Formation of germ cell clumps (arrows) in cultures of THY1+ cells isolated from the testes of mice (A) and bulls (B). Cultures were maintained in serum-free chemically defined media with either mouse serum-free nutrient supplement (mSFM, Kubota et al., 2004a) for mouse cells or StemPro® serum-replacement for bovine cells. Also, the media was supplemented with the growth factors GDNF and FGF2. The germ cells loosely attach to an underlying feeder cell monolayer composed of STO cells for mouse cultures and bovine embryonic fibroblasts (BEFs) for bovine cultures. The clumps appear morphologically similar between the two species and mouse cells are proven to contain SSCs. Thus, the formation of these germ cell clumps from bovine testes may contain bona fide SSCs.

For rodents, maintenance and proliferation of SSCs in vitro requires mitotically inactive feeder cell monolayers and optimized serum-free medium with specific nutrient and growth factor supplementations. Feeder cells derived from mouse embryos have proven the most effective at supporting self-renewal of rodent SSCs for several months in vitro (Oatley and Brinster 2006). Immortalized STO (mouse embryonic fibroblast) feeder cell monolayers support expansion of both mouse (Kubota et al., 2004a) and rat (Ryu et al., 2005) SSC numbers for greater than 5 months in culture. In addition, primary mouse embryonic fibroblasts (MEF) support long-term self-renewal of mouse gonocytes (precursors to SSCs) in vitro (Kanatsu-Shinohara et al., 2003). With bulls, primary bovine embryonic fibroblasts (BEF) have been utilized as feeders and support short-term expansion of bovine SSCs (Oatley et al., 2004b). When maintained in complex serum containing medium SSC numbers increased over a 7 day period with BEF feeders, but rapidly declined after 14 days suggesting that long-term self-renewal could not be supported (Oatley et al., 2004b).

In addition to feeder cell monolayers, expansion of rodent SSC numbers in vitro is effectively supported in serum-free medium conditions (Kubota et al., 2004a; Ryu et al., 2005; Kanatsu-Shinohara et al., 2005). In contrast, several cell types, including embryonic stem cells, require the addition of fetal bovine serum (FBS) in basal media to support growth. The complexity of nutrients in FBS preferentially supports proliferation of rapidly dividing cells. Because SSCs divide relatively slowly (Kubota et al., 2004a), other rapidly dividing cell types such as testicular fibroblasts outgrow SSCs when cultured in serum-containing medium resulting in loss of SSCs over time. Also, FBS appears to have toxic effects on mouse and rat SSCs in culture (Kubota et al., 2004a; Ryu et al., 2005). Previous attempts at culturing bovine SSCs have included FBS in basal medium (Dobrinski et al., 2001; Oatley et al., 2002; Oatley et al., 2004a; Oatley et al., 2004b; Aponte et al., 2005). In those studies, short-term expansion of bovine SSCs was observed followed by rapid decline of SSC numbers at which time fibroblast take-over was observed, likely impairing SSC proliferation and survival (Dobrinski et al., 2001; Oately et al., 2002; Oatley et al., 2004b).

For rodent SSCs, a defined serum-free condition composed of Minimal Essential Media Alpha (MEMα) as the base medium with specific nutrient supplementation supports SSC survival and proliferation for extended periods of time (Nagano et al., 2003; Kubota et al., 2004a; Kubota et al., 2004b). Mouse SSC culture conditions developed by Kubota et al. (2004a) utilized a chemically-defined serum-free supplement (mSFM). Extension of this system to support rat SSCs required enrichment of specific components of mSFM leading to creation of a rat serum-free supplement (rSFM; Ryu et al., 2005). In both these supplements each component is added at specific concentrations, providing consistent results because media conditions can be acutely controlled between batches. In less defined conditions, supplementation with commercially produced StemPro® serum-replacement (Invitrogen; Carlsbad, CA) also supports long-term self-renewing expansion of mouse SSCs (Kanatsu-Shinohara et al., 2005). In those conditions, supplement components are proprietary and batch-to-batch variation effects reproducibility of SSC proliferation in vitro. To date, the effects of any basal medium and serum-free condition with nutrient supplementation that supports rodent SSCs in vitro has not been reported with livestock SSCs.

SSC self-renewing proliferation in serum-free conditions is limited without the addition of specific growth factors. Addition of soluble GDNF is essential for expansion of mouse, rat, and hamster SSC numbers when cultured in defined media conditions (Kubota et al., 2004a; Ryu et al., 2005; Kanatsu-Shinohara et al., 2007). Importantly, preliminary studies with bovine germ cells showed that addition of GDNF to complex culture medium enhanced short-term expansion of SSCs over a 14-day period (Oatley et al., 2004b). Studies with the mouse showed that insulin-like growth factor 1 (IGF-1), epidermal growth factor (EGF), FGF2, CSF-1, and leukemia inhibitory factor (LIF) enhance GDNF influence on SSC maintenance and proliferation in serum-free conditions (Kubota et al., 2004a; Kubota et al., 2004b; Kanatsu-Shinohara et al., 2005; Kanatsu-Shinohara et al., 2007). In serum-free medium with specific nutrient (e.g. mSFM, rSFM, or StemPro®) and growth factor supplements SSCs grow as three dimensional clumps of germ cells loosely attached to the feeder cell monolayer (see Figure 2). Similar generation of germ cell clumps in vitro from bovine testis cells has not been reported. Instead, studies by Oatley et al. (2004b) and Aponte et al. (2005 and 2008) have shown maintenance of cells with a fibroblast-like morphology indicating either bovine SSC morphology in vitro is distinctly different from rodents or the cultures did not contain bona fide SSCs.

Translation of conditions that support proliferation of rodent SSCs in vitro to SSCs of other mammals has been challenging and not reported to date in peer reviewed literature. One aid in establishing mouse SSC cultures has been isolation of an SSC-enriched cell fraction from donor testes for initial setup of the culture. Elimination of the non SSC components of a testicular cell population especially the rapidly dividing somatic cells is advantageous for growth of SSCs in vitro. For development of mouse SSC cultures the isolated THY1+ cell fraction was utilized and is commonly used to effectively maintain and expand the number of SSCs in serum-free chemically defined conditions. Recent studies by Reding et al. (2010) showed that the THY1+ cell fraction from bull testes is enriched for SSCs indicating conserved characteristics for these cells among mammalian species. Thus, it is likely that conditions supporting proliferation of mouse SSCs in vitro can serve as a basis for tailoring conditions that support SSCs of other mammals including cattle. In fact, our recent studies have tested the mouse condition of MEMα base medium with StemPro®, GDNF, and FGF2 supplementation with BEF feeders for support of bovine THY1+ SSCs and observed the formation of germ cell clumps resembling those that develop in mouse cultures (Figure 2). For the first time, these cultures may represent maintenance of bovine SSCs in vitro. Future work will involve refining these conditions to support long-term proliferation that can serve as a source of donor SSCs for further development of transplantation methods in bulls.

Conclusions

Major advances in genetic gain of cattle populations can be made with reproductive tools that expand the availability of germlines from desirable males. While AI has been widely used in dairy cattle to achieve this and resulted in major improvements of milk production over the last 70 years, beef cattle populations have lost opportunities for genetic improvement because of the impracticality needed for implementation of AI programs. The unique functions of the SSC population for self-renewal and regeneration of continual spermatogenesis provides a novel alternative to AI for expanding the utilization of desirable male genetics in the beef cattle industry. Reproductive tools based on SSCs such as transplantation are at the forefront of being developed in cattle. In rodents, progression of techniques for isolation, culture, and transplantation of SSCs spanned greater than a decade of research. While several studies have reported limited development of culture conditions for bovine SSCs and transplantation between donor and recipient bulls, none have provided definitive evidence of success that is close to commercialization or useful as a tool in livestock production. One of the major limitations has been lack of methods to isolate an SSC-enriched cell fraction from bull testes. Recently, Reding et al. (2010) reported this capability based on selection of THY1+ cells, adding a key tool for further developing culture and transplantation methods for bulls. Major advances in developing these techniques as usable tools in the cattle industry will be made in the coming decade.

References

Aponte PM, Soda T, Teerds KJ, Mizrak SC, van de Kant HJ & de Rooij DG 2008 Propagation of bovine spermatogonial stem cells in vitro. *Reproduction* **136** 543-557.

Aponte PM, van Bragt MP, de Rooij DG & van Pelt AM 2005 Spermatogonial stem cells: characteristics and experimental possibilities. ***Acta Pathologica, Microbiologica et Immunologica Scandinavica* 113(11-12) 727-742.**

Brinster RL & Avarbock MR 1994 Germline transmission of donor haplotype following spermatogonial transplantation. *Proceedings of the National Academy of Sciences* 91 11303 – 11307.

Brinster RL & Zimmermann JW 1994 Spermatogenesis following male germ-cell transplantation. *Proceedings of the National Academy of Sciences* **91** 11298 – 11302.

Buaas FW, Kirsh AL, Sharma M, McLean DJ, Morris JL, Griswold MD, de Rooij DG & Braun RE 2004 Plzf is required in adult male germ cells for stem cell self-renewal. *Nature Genetics* **36(6)** 647 – 652.

Costoya JA, Hobbs RM, Barna M, Cattoretti G, Manova K, Sukhwani M, Orwig KE, Wolgemuth DJ & Pandolfi PP 2004 Essential role of Plzf in maintenance of spermatogonial stem cells. *Nature Genetics* **36(6)** 653 – 652.

de Rooij DG & Russell LD 2000 All you wanted to know about spermatogonia but were afraid to ask. *Journal of Andrology* **21** 776 – 798.

Dobrinski I, Ogawa T, Avarbock MR & Brinster RL 2001 Effect of the GnRH-agonist leuprolide on colonization of recipient testes by donor spermatogonial stem cells after transplantation in mice. *Tissue and Cell* **33(2)** 200-207.

Ebata KT, Zhang X, Nagano & MC 2005 Expression patterns of cell-surface molecules on male germ line stem cells during postnatal mouse development. *Molecular Reproduction and Development* **72(2)** 171-181.

Foote RH 2002 The history of artificial insemination: Selected notes and notables. *Journal of Animal Science* **80** 1-10.

Geary TW, Whittier JC, Downing ER, LeFever DG, Silcox RW, Holland MD, Nett TM, & Niswender GD 1998 Pregnancy rates of postpartum beef cows that were synchronized using Syncro-Mate-B or the Ovsynch protocol. *Journal of Animal Science* **76** 1523-1527.

Herrid M, Vignarajan S, Davey R, Dobrinski I & Hill JR 2006 Successful transplantation of bovine testicular cells to heterologous recipients. *Reproduction* **132(4)** 617-624.

Izadyar F, Den Ouden K, Stout TA, Stout J, Coret J, Lankveld DP, Spoormakers TJ, Colenbrander B, Oldenbroek JK, Van der Ploeg KD, Woelders H, Kal HB & De Rooij DG 2003 Autologous and homologous transplantation of bovine spermatogonial stem cells. *Reproduction* **126** 765-774.

Kanatsu-Shinohara M, Toyokuni S & Shinohara T 2004 CD9 is a surface marker on mouse and rat male germline stem cells. *Biology of Reproduction* **70** 70 – 75.

Kanatsu-Shinohara M, Muneto T, Lee J, Takenaka M, Chuma S, Nakatsuji N, Horiuchi T & Shinohara T 2007 Long-term culture of male germline stem cells from hamster testes. *Biology of Reproduction* **78(4)** 611-617.

Kanatsu-Shinohara M, Ogonuki N, Inoue K, Miki H, Ogura A, Toyokuni S & Shinohara T 2003 Long-term proliferation in culture and germline transmission of mouse male germline stem cells. *Biology of Reproduction* **69(2)** 612-616.

Kanatsu-Shinohara M, Miki H, Inoue K, Ogonuki N, Toyokuni S, Ogura A & Shinohara T 2005 Long-term culture of mouse male germline stem cells under serum-or feeder-free conditions. *Biology of Reproduction* **72(4)** 985-991.

Kanatsu-Shinohara M, Inoue K, Ogonuki N, Miki H, Yoshida S, Toyokuni S, Lee J, Ogura A & Shinohara T 2007 Leukemia inhibitory factor enhances formation of germ cell colonies in neonatal mouse testis culture. *Biology of Reproduction* **76(1)** 55-62.

Kubota H, Avarbock MR & Brinster RL 2004a Growth factors essential for self renewal and expansion of mouse spermatogonial stem cells. *Proceedings of the National Academy of Sciences* **101** 16489 – 16494.

Kubota H, Avarbock MR & Brinster RL 2004b Culture conditions and single growth factors affect fate determination of mouse spermatogonial stem cells. *Biology of Reproduction* **71** 722 – 731.

Luo J, Megee S & Dobrinski I 2009 Asymmetric distribution of UCH-L1 in spermatogonia is associated with maintenance and differentiation of spermatogonial stem cells. *Journal of Cell Physiology* **220** 460-468.

Meng X, Lindahl M, Hyvönen ME, Parvinen M, de Rooij DG, Hess MW, Raatikainen-Ahokas A, Sainio K, Rauvala H, Lakso M, Pichel JG, Westphal H, Saarma M & Sariola H 2000 Regulation of cell fate decision of undifferentiated spermatogonia by GDNF. *Science* **287** 1489 – 1493.

Mullaney BP & Skinner MK 1992 Basic fibroblast growth factor (bFGF) gene expression and protein production during pubertal development of the seminiferous tubule: follicle-stimulating hormone-induced Sertoli cell bFGF expression. *Endocrinology* **131** 2928-2934.

Nagano M, Avarbock MR & Brinster RL 1999 Pattern and kinetics of mouse donor spermatogonial stem cell colonization in recipient testes. *Biology of Reproduction* **60** 1429-1436.

Nagano M, Ryu BY, Brinster CJ, Avarbock MR, & Brinster RL 2003 Maintenance of mouse male germ line stem cells in vitro. *Biology of Reproduction* **68** 2207-2214.

Oatley JM & Brinster RL 2008 Regulation of spermatogonial stem cells self-renewal in mammals. *Annual Review of Cell Developmental Biology* **24** 263 – 286.

Oatley JM & Brinster RL 2006 Spermatogonial stem cells. *Methods in Enzymology* **419** 259-282.

Oatley JM, Oatley MJ, Avarbock Tobias JW & Brinster RL 2009 Colony stimulating factor 1 is an extrinsic stimulator of mouse spermatogonial stem cell self renewal. *Development* **136(7)** 1191-1199.

Oatley JM, de Avila DM, Reeves JJ & McLean DJ 2004a Testis tissue explant culture supports survival and proliferation of bovine spermatogonial stem cells. *Biology of Reproduction* **70** 625 – 631.

Oatley JM, Reeves JJ & McLean DJ 2004b Biological activity of cryopreserved bovine spermatogonial stem cells during in vitro culture. *Biology of Reproduction* **71** 942-947.

Oatley JM, de Avila DM, McLean DJ, Griswold MD & Reeves JJ 2002 Transplantation of bovine germinal cells into mouse testes. *Journal of Animal Science* **80(7)** 1925-1931.

Perry GA, Smith MF, & Patterson DJ 2002 Evaluation of a fixed-time artificial insemination protocol for postpartum suckled beef cows. *Journal of Animal Science* **80** 3060-4.

Reding SR, Stepnoski AL, Cloninger EW & Oatley JM 2010 THY1 is a Conserved Marker of Undifferentiated Spermatogonia in the Pre-Pubertal Bull Testis. *Reproduction* **139** 893-903.

Russell LD, Ettlin RA, Hikim APS, & Clegg ED 1990 Histological and histocompatability evaluation of the testis. edn1 Clearwater FL, Cache River Press.

Ryu BY, Kubota H, Avarbock MR & Brinster RL 2005 Conservation of spermatogonial stem cell self-renewal signaling between mouse and rat. *Proceedings of the National Academy of Sciences USA* **102(40)** 14302-14307.

Seandel M, James D, Shmelkov SV, Falciatori I, Kim J, Chavala S, Scherr DS, Zhang F, Torres R, Gale NW, Yancopoulos GD, Murphy A, Valenzuela DM, Hobbs RM, Pandolfi PP & Rafii S 2007 Generation of functional multipotent adult stem cells from GPR125+ germline progenitors. *Nature* **449(7160)** 346-350.

Sharpe R 1994 Regulation of spermatogenesis. In *The Physiology of Reproduction*, edn 2, pp 1363 – 1434. Eds E Knobil and JD Neill. New York: Raven Press.

Shinohara T, Avarbock MR & Brinster RL 1999 ß1- and α6-intergrin are surface markers and mouse spermatogonial stem cells. *Proceedings of the National Academy of Sciences* **96** 5505 – 5509.

Stockwell S, Herrid M, Davey R, Brownlee A, Hutton K & Hill JR 2009 Microsatellite detection of donor-derived sperm DNA following germ cell transplantation in cattle. *Reproduction, Fertility and Development* **21(3)** 462-468.

Tegelenbosch RAJ & de Rooij DG 1993 A quantitative study of spermatogonial multiplication and stem cell renewal in the C3H/101 F1 hybrid mouse. *Mutation Research* **290** 193 – 200.

Tadokoro Y, Yomogida K, Ohta H, Tohda A & Nishimune Y 2002 Homeostatic regulation of germinal stem cell proliferation by the GDNF/FSH pathway. *Mechanisms of Development* **113(1)** 29-39.

Yoshinaga K, Nishikawa S, Ogawa M, Hayashi S, Kunisada T, Fujimoto T & Nishikawa S 1991 Role of c-kit in mouse spermatogenesis: identification of spermatogonia as a specific site of c-kit expression and function. *Development* **113(2)** 689-699.

Activation of the embryonic genome

M-A Sirard

Département des Sciences Animales, Centre de Recherche en Biologie de la Reproduction, Université Laval, Sainte-Foy, Québec, Canada, G1K 7P4

Activation of its genome is amongst the essential task the embryo has to undertake following fertilization of the egg. In animal and plants, this activation follows a period of transcriptional silence, which is made necessary by the requirement for an almost complete and functional reprogramming of the DNA coming from both gametes. The process by which DNA is silenced, reprogrammed and reactivated is not fully understood yet but progresses are being made, especially with the help of genomic tools. This review will focus on the recent discoveries made in different animal models and more specifically on the efforts made to further characterize the event of maternal to embryonic transition in bovine embryos.

Introduction

To simplify the reading of this review, a few definitions are required. First the differences between MET: maternal to embryonic transition MZT; maternal to zygotic transition and EGA; embryonic genome activation or ZGA; zygotic genome activation. MET refers mainly to the period during which the source of RNA being used for protein translation transitioned from maternal to embryonic. The term EGA, for "embryonic genome activation", is in fact a sub-event of the MET representing the activation of the embryonic genome required for the initiation of transcription during the MET. In MZT and ZGA, the term embryo is replaced by zygote, but because the term zygote refers to the period where both gametes fuse to form a one cell structure, the term embryo should be used as soon as the cell division occurs. The transition from maternal to embryonic RNA management is a progressive event during which maternal RNAs are depleted by translation and degradation and embryonic RNA gradually increases with the arrival of new ribosomal RNA. This review will focus on the mammalian aspect of the transition and more specifically on the information relevant to the bovine species.

MET: a common feature

The maternal to embryonic transition is not unique to the bovine, or even to animals as plants do experience such a transition between 2 generations (Baroux *et al.*, 2008). The rationale behind such re-organization is the requirement for DNA-chromatin epigenetic reprogramming, which requires a transcriptionally quiet period to ensure a proper selection of the genes to be transcribed (Baroux *et al.*, 2008).. In fact, it is likely that the epigenetic state is a major reason for the transcriptionally silent status of the embryo. This period of transcriptional arrest is often analysed using polymerase II and III inhibitors, such as alpha-amanitin, and its duration is determined by the induced developmental arrest, which varies amongst animals. This arrest can last two hours in Drosophila (Robbins (Robbins, 1980) or as much as 3 days in bovine. In mouse, it lasts one cell cycle but in species like

Corresponding author E-mail: Marc-Andre.Sirard@fsaa.ulaval.ca

Xenopus it last from 15 cell cycles for up to 3000 (Mechali *et al.*, 1990); (Schultz, 2002); (Newport & Kirschner, 1982).

MET: transcriptional silencing in animals

Three main hypotheses are being explored as the source/cause of transcriptional inhibition: 1) The chromatin is not permissive, preventing the polymerase from accessing it 2) The transcriptional machinery is either absent or not functional (ex: requiring specific post-translational modifications such as phosphorylation) and 3) Transcription is aborted by the rapid succession of cell cycles during which the absence of G_0-G_1 prevent normal transcription (Schier, 2007). These hypotheses are still in development and the evidence supporting their existence will be discussed below. To assess transcriptional activity in relation to the first hypothesis, several groups have used the sensitivity to alpha-amanitin, as an indication of requirement for further development (Mechali *et al.*, 1990). Another tool to assess transcriptional activity is the use of reporter genes In Xenopus at the pre-MBT stage (250 cells) (Newport & Kirschner, 1982) and in mouse at the male pronucleus stage (Telford *et al.*, 1990), reporter genes can be expressed and indicate that the embryos retain some capacity to process DNA information, although the structure of the chromatin associated with these vectors remains unknown.

Not only the transcription is controlled or inhibited during the early stages but the destruction of accumulated RNA is also believed to be important for the genomic activation. Recent data indicates that maternal RNA degradation is an important event for embryonic takeover. Genes like *Zelda* in drosophila (Liang *et al.*, 2008) and specific micro-RNA in trout (Ramachandra *et al.*, 2008) are believed to be specifically involved in maternal RNA degradation and indirect inducers of EGA.

MET: the chromatin status

In most mammals, the chromatin status changes through a rapid and active demethylation of the paternal genome and a more passive and progressive demethylation of the maternal genome following fertilization (Santos *et al.*, 2002). During this reprogramming process, the chromatin-induced repressive transcriptional status is believed to ensure embryonic quiescence. The repression is associated with a structural conformation preventing the association of the polymerase with the DNA. For example, the de-acetylation of H3K4 is associated with a repressive status in mouse (Bultman *et al.*, 2006). In Xenopus, the ortholog of Dnmt-1 could have a direct repressive effect on transcription independent of it's DNA methyl transferase catalytic activity that remains to be explained (Dunican *et al.*, 2008). Model animal studies indicate that embryonic genome activation is gradually established from a multi-step progression between a chromatin repressive mechanism and the establishment of the transcription machinery (Baroux *et al.*, 2008).

A recent paper from Koehler (Koehler *et al.*, 2009) illustrates how in the bovine the chromatin high order is modified at the 8 cell stage when compared to earlier stages. They have analysed microscopically the distribution of the eu vs hetero chromatin for different chromosomes (19 and 20) at the 8 cell stage, to show that they are redistributed within the nucleus, potentially to allow transcription to occur. The hypothesis is that transcription occurs mainly out of the chromosomes that are more centrally located in the nuclei.

The modification of the epigenomic marks is recognized to impact gene expression/repression as well. The epigenetic modifications can be observed on the DNA itself and the most accepted process for these type of modifications is methylation of cysteine residues which is associated with repression. Clearly, histones can also be affected by methylation, acetylation, ubiquitination, sumoylation, phospohorylation etc., and each of these modifications may have an enhancer or repressor role depending on the site and on the level of post translational modification. For example, some histone tail sites are double or trimethylated to confer different levels of activity. In oocytes and embryos, the nucleosomes are assembled with histones that sometimes differ from "normal" somatic histones and may play inhibitory roles (McGraw *et al.*, 2006). Indeed in our laboratory, we have explored the role and abundance of bovine H1oo, oocytes-specific linker histones regulating the access of transcription factors to the DNA through nucleosome conformation, and concluded that their presence may affect transcriptional activity (McGraw *et al.*, 2006).

RNA storage

If there is a period without transcription, it almost necessarily requires the accumulation of RNA for protein formation as the proteins have a limited half-life and a cell without instructions cannot adapt to changing environment. In bovine as in other mammals and most animals, the amount of RNA that the oocytes accumulates starts to rise significantly when follicles reach their secondary phase of development (Fair *et al.*, 1997). In somatic cells, the RNA is translated or degraded within hours, therefore, the accumulation of stable in oocyte requires a complete/specific protection mechanism that has evolved in egg producing animals.

Xenopus is the most studied model to assess mRNA fate in animals. The maternal RNA is stored using a specific configuration where the mRNA is de-polyadenylated on the 3′ and capped on the 5′ end. The storage of mRNA is associated with ribonucleoproteins (mRNP), which represses translation. In Xenopus, there is more information about the different proteins involved in the repression of translation, one of which is *maskin*. This protein associates with the cytoplasmic polyadenylation element binding protein (CPEB) located in the 3′ UTR region on mRNA that contains a cytoplasmic polyadenylation *element* (CPE). This association represses translation through the inhibitory action of maskin-eIF4E located at the 5′ end of the RNA (Richter, 2007). The system allows the timed translation of specific mRNA according to a combination of cytoplasmic codes acting on RNA-associated proteins interacting with the 3′UTR sequence of the stored RNAs. The activation of translation seems associated with a longer polyA tail (from 80-150 and higher) while shorted tails (around 20 A) are repressed from translation (Richter 1999). Several regulative motifs and proteins have now been identified as regulators of re-polyadenylation of maternal RNAs (Pique *et al.*, 2008). Maternal RNA must have at least 2 CPE in their 3 'UTR. These sites must be separated by 10-12 nucleotides and if there is a Pumilio-binding element (PBE) upstream of CPE, the repression is even greater. The same author proposes that the maskin protein is recruited by a CPEB dimer, which would explain the importance of the distance between the 2 CPE elements. Progressively, the 3′UTR code is being deciphered allowing our understanding of the precise spatio-temporal regulation of mRNAs during the transition from maternal to embryonic control.

Destruction of targeted maternal RNA

At least 2 degradation pathways are known to influence maternal RNA fate. The first one is controlled by maternally encoded factors and targets the 3′UTR region at specific motifs (Stitzel & Seydoux, 2007), while the second coincides with embryonic genome activation and also uses 3′UTR targets. In Drosophila, sequencing these regions has revealed families of RNA binding proteins associated with RNA fate like SMAUG and Pumilio (De Renzis *et al.*, 2007). In zebra fish, a single miRNA (miR430) drives the repression/destruction of several hundreds of maternal RNAs (Giraldez *et al.*, 2006). A similar observation with Mir-21 has been made more recently in the trout (Ramachandra *et al.*, 2008).

There is a clear demonstration of the importance of RNA degradation in Xenopus, where 2 hrs before the MBT (Mid blastula transition) a new miRNA, miR-427, appears from multimeric genes resulting in the rapid release of millions of copies in the cytoplasm (even the produced RNA is multimeric creating an average target size of 4-8kb on northern blots). The site of action of this miRNA is in the first 60 nucleotides of the 3′UTR of cyclin A1 and B2 but not related to the polyadenylation elements regulating the translation of these cyclins. Since the cyclins are involved in regulating the different phases of the cell cycle including the bypassing of the G1 phase, this help from the embryonic genome ensures the rapid and complete degradation of remaining maternal cyclins within 2 hours and a return to a more somatic cell cycle profile (Lund *et al.*, 2009).

The production of these special miRNA probably requires the activity of some polymerases and therefore requires some transcriptional capacity unless they could be stored as other RNA and release in by a post translational mechanism. Would such transcription would account for the minor genomic activation observed in a few species including the bovine (Memili & First, 1999)?

Transcriptional activation of embryonic genes

Other examples of direct and indirect actions of the embryonic genome on maternal RNA exist. In drosophila, the action of Zelda is associated with a 5′region of targeted genes activated early during embryo formation. According to microarray analyses, at least 279 genes are controlled by Zelda as indicated by their disappearance when Zelda is targeted for destruction by miR309 (Liang *et al.*, 2008). Not surprisingly, Zelda stimulates the expression of miR309, which is responsible for the rapid degradation of specific maternal RNA (Baroux *et al.*, 2008). Unfortunately, the sequence analysis of Zelda did not lead to functional orthologs in mammals. As mentioned above, specific miRNA are produced from the embryonic genome and their role is to destroy maternal RNA. In Xenopus, the transcription of these genes occurs 1-2 hours prior to the main activation of transcription and requires the RNA polymerase, as it can be inhibited by alpha-amanitin (Lund *et al.*, 2009).

If the embryonic genome takes over at the MET, does it mean that all maternal RNA is suddenly useless or destroyed? In mouse, a transcriptomic analysis of late zygotes indicates that around 60 % of de novo transcripts are novel for the embryos while the remaining 40 % was already present in the maternal pool but gets transcribed again in the embryo (Hamatani *et al.*, 2004). We can learn from the same author that a second wave of new transcripts appears between the 4-8 cell stages and the observed new gene products are likely involved in the beginning of the compaction that precedes the differentiation of ICM into trophoblast cells.

Demonstration of transcriptional silence in bovine embryos

Early experiments in the nineties demonstrated that, in the bovine, transcription is activated between the 8 and the 16 cell stage (Barnes & First, 1991). Later on, the possibility of a minor embryonic activation was suggested (Memili & First, 1999), based on the appearance of novel proteins during the 2-4 cell stage. In fact, although evidences have been provided indicating the presence of transcription before the 8 cell stage in the bovine, mainly through alpha-amanitin comparison of proteins gels (Memili & First, 2000), it has not been clearly demonstrated by experiments using specific promoters. However, promising candidates were identified by our lab during transgenic technology development experiments. We found that Beta-galactosidase reporter genes expression occurs only 60 hours post fertilization and does not depend on the number of cell divisions nor possibly fertilization as some 1 cell oocytes turned blue as an indication of transgene transcription at the same time as 8 cell embryos (Gagne *et al.*, 1995). Moreover, several authors have since used reporter genes to identify transgenic embryos using DNA vectors (Murakami *et al.*, 1999) or even artificial chromosomes (Wang *et al.*, 2001) with the same results. Cloning can also be used to evaluate the capabilities of the transcriptional machinery (Bordignon *et al.*, 2003) but it becomes difficult to assess if the transcription observed (often as reported Green fluorescent protein expression) is due to the transfer of some cytoplasmic elements, or to the incomplete reprogramming of the transferred nuclei caused by faulty histones replacement and partial chromatin reconfiguration. Indeed, the transcriptional activity of the fused nucleus as been considered as a negative sign of reprogramming and a bad prognostic of future embryo capacity. Nevertheless, in all these cases, transgene expression is not observed before the 8-16 cell stage or a specific time after activation/fertilization (around 60 hrs). Since bacteria derived transgenes are not associated with histones but rapidly integrate resident cell histones, the chromatin status of the recipient cell is likely to be transmitted to the new DNA quite rapidly. These indirect evidences can be used to support the hypothesis that transgene transcription does not happen in early bovine embryos the same way as in somatic cells.

As mentioned above, the hypothesis of a minor transcriptional activation in bovine embryos has been described (Memili & First, 1999). As a optional explanation for the presence of new "visible RNA" in two to eight cell embryos, the possibility of maternal RNA becoming polyadenylated could be considered. This was addressed by Kanka (Kanka *et al.*, 2009) who validated candidates with specific primers during the reverse transcription to avoid the bias of polyadenylation specific priming. Therefore the question of a minor transcription period before the 8 cell stage remains to be clearly demonstrated in bovine embryos. This could be achieved by using specific promoters for new embryonic genes fused with reporter sequences and injected rapidly post fertilization. It would indicate whether transcription occurs when the right promoter is used, despite the general chromatin configuration. In this case the promoter would have specific characteristics to

Levels of RNA

One of the difficulties in assessing the transcriptional activity through RNA analysis is related to technical aspects such as extraction, reverse transcription and amplification. Because maternal RNA is sometime stored and de-polydeanylated, the length of the polyA tail is an issue. If the tail is short, it requires extraction protocols that do not use the capturing ability of poly T columns or filters. Secondly, if the primers used for the reverse transcription include a polyT sequence, it will exclude an undefined portion of the stored RNA and finally, if a T7 polymerase is used for RNA amplification (as is often the case for microarray experiments), the presence of a polyA tail will likely make a difference since non polyadenylated RNA may not be necessarily amplified. Therefore, much more care should be given to the interpretation of RNA levels prior to the 8 cell stage. These technological considerations have been clearly demonstrated in several papers from our laboratory (Gilbert *et al.*, 2009a; (Gilbert *et al.*, 2009b). In fact, we have seen several examples where the amount of RNA measured with Q-PCR inversely correlated with the protein levels measured by western blots (Vigneault *et al.*, 2009). Therefore, the use of terms like "up regulation" or "down regulation" should be used only from the 8 cell stage onward and in comparison with the proper alpha amanitin controls before the blastocyst stage (Vigneault *et al.*, 2009).

Microarrays analysis of embryonic genome

Although potentially very rich in information as they can probe thousands of gene to assess their level of expression, microarrays data are to be used with caution especially with early embryos. In a recent review by Evsikov (Evsikov & Marin de Evsikova, 2009), several problems are described that users should consider before doing or interpreting microarray data. Firstly, the targets are limited in length and therefore only represent a small portion of the gene they are supposed to indicate. The fact that only 39 % of the changes observed on microarrays are associated with variation of a precise target gene is also somewhat frightening (Kwan *et al.*, 2008). The other 61 % represent initiation and termination sites variants or spliced variants. Secondly, microarrays are not suitable for quantification assays since, in the case of oocytes and embryos, the material needs to be amplified and such amplification creates numerous bias (Gilbert *et al.*, 2009a; Gilbert *et al.*, 2009b). Even in mouse, a 2-cell embryo contains 0.26 pg of RNA, which is four times less than oocytes at 0.95 pg of mRNA (Evsikov & Marin de Evsikova, 2009). The normal methodology promotes the use of equal amounts of mRNA for different biological samples, which is misleading when comparing a comparable number of embryos from different stages unless one can measure very accurately the total amount of each sample and use the exact same. Indeed when we compared ten 8-cells with 10 GV after the same amplification process we have at the end the same amount of aRNA although initially the GV contains several times more RNA than the 8 cells meaning that the genes present in the latter will be over amplified since the process is not linear up to the end, otherwise the end result would be different. Thirdly, due to cross hybridization within gene families, there are several instances when it becomes impossible to assess a specific gene product to a target as the target may hybridize with several genes products from the same family (Kwan *et al.*, 2008). Another problem is the fact that several amplification protocols use the T-7oligo(dT) primer in their first step, indirectly selecting mRNA that have a poly A tail and potentially excluding several of the stored mRNA that are de-polyadenylated, as stated above. Our laboratory has demonstrated such a bias using different primers and real time PCR with pre-MET embryos (Vigneault *et al.*, 2007).

Genes "associated" with the genome activation

It is interesting to look at the functions of genes that are either targeted for destruction or protected from it during the first wave of transcription of the embryonic genome. In drosophila, Gene ontology identified that candidate genes that are destroyed mainly belong to the family of cell cycle proteins, while the conserved ones belong to the transcription factors or RNA transaction processes (binding metabolism, translation) families (Tadros & Lipshitz, 2009). In mouse, unstable mRNA (the ones that disappear) are also associated with the cell cycle but the RNA associated with RNA processing seems to come from the new genome rather than from the protected maternal pool (Hamatani *et al.*, 2004). The mouse maternal to embryonic transition is difficult to analyse, principally due to the rapid activation of the embryonic genome at the end of the first cell cycle when the first division occurs. The microarray information is only partially analysed and it will take further investigations and demonstration to identify the important factors (Li *et al.*; Evsikov & Marin de Evsikova, 2009). Nevertheless, it is clear from the mouse studies that a number of specific factors or transcripts eventually translated into proteins are required for the proper genomic function of the embryo. Factors like Dicer, Ago2 (eukaryotic elongation factor 2c), Atg5 (autophagy related 5) are required to degrade maternal factors (Tsukamoto *et al* 2008). Gene products like *Hr6a* (*Ubiquitin conjugating enzyme E2A*), *Nucleoplasmin 2*, *Tif1a* (*tripartite motif containing 24*) and *Smarca4* are required for chromatin remodelling. Important transcription factor as Oct-4 and Sox 2 influence competence as well as differentiation of blastomeres (Zuccotti *et al.*, 2009). The re-establishment of methylation with Dnmt1 (which also act on chromatin accessibility) and Dnmt3a, involved in de novo methylation, and their impact on the ability of DNA to be transcribed, are to be linked with specific gene activation/inactivation. To this group of better known actors, some new or oocytes specific genes are slowly being added as they are being characterized: Zar-1, *Mater*, Padi6 and Filia as upstream actor of oocyte differentiation (Li *et al.*). The regulation of developmental competence may include the interplay between Oct-4, *Stella* and GCNF (germ cell nuclear factor) during oocyte growth and should be crucial at the end of oocytes maturation (Zuccotti *et al.*, 2009).

Using the rabbit, in which embryonic activation occurs later than the mouse, and is more similar to bovine and human, Léandri made subtractive libraries from early morula and 4 cells embryos (Leandri *et al.*, 2009). The authors used cluster analysis to organize the genes according to their rise or demise from the 4 cell stage to blastocyst. Some of the clustered categories associated with a rise after 4 cells (putatively new embryonic messages, validated by Q-PCR) contain candidates that are common with the bovine. In bovine, the subtraction libraries obtained between the 8 cell plus or minus alpha-amanitin is, like the rabbit, very much enriched with RNA processing elements (Vigneault *et al.*, 2009). Although the list of embryonic early genes is not very long (< 200 genes) several were found in common; *H2Afz* (*histone H 2A*), *SAP18* (*Sin-3 associated proteins*), *SLC family* (*solute carrier family*), *Mthfd1* (*Methylenetetrahydrofolate deshydrogenase*), *ATP 5 b* (*ATP synthase*), *EIF5* (*eukaryotic translation initiation factor 5*) albeit several EIF members are present in both groups, they do not necessarily have the same subtype. Considering that these subtracted libraries are necessarily incomplete and even very partial, the number of similarities is interesting and reassuring for the comparative biology point of view. Not surprisingly, several maternal genes that do decrease during the MET are also common between the rabbit and the bovine studies (Leandri *et al.*, 2009) (Vigneault *et al.*, 2009).

In the pig, embryonic genome activation also occurs later than in the mouse and closer to the rabbit at the 4 cell stage. A recent review from Prather indicates the usefulness of the genomic tools (microarrays and subtractive libraries) to identify the players involved in this process (Prather *et al.*, 2009). In a previous study, they used an array dedicated to this species, even though the genome is incomplete, to profile the transcriptome of the MET period in pig embryos (Whitworth *et al.*, 2005). They have uncovered the importance of several processes such as macroautophagy, which is important for the removal of maternal proteins. This is also being observed in our study in bovine (see below). In the pig, the role of micro RNA also seems important for the degradation of maternal material as loss of function of *EIF2C1* results in the stabilization of specific maternal RNA and development arrest during the MET. *EIF2C1* is part of the RNA-Induced Silencing Complex (RISC) required to process miRNA (Whitworth *et al.*, 2005). However, it is important to note that the role of Dicer and RISC components specifically at the MET are not well understood. The long term effects of disrupting these components are not just important but critical to survival.

Bovine microarrays results

Several recent papers have been published about the MET in bovine and the objective here is not to repeat what has been published but to briefly summarize the pre-and post genomic analysis and then to analyse new results from specific experiments that uncovered genes involved in the bovine MET.

A recent paper from Bettegowda (Bettegowda *et al.*, 2008) has made a list of important genes that are inherited from the maternal pool for continued development or proper embryonic activation. When disrupted, genes like *mater* (Pennetier *et al.*, 2006) *Zar-1*(Pennetier *et al.*, 2004) *NPM2* (Vallee *et al.*, 2008) lead to embryonic arrest phenotypes in the mouse and are present in bovine, but others like *stella*, *HsF1* (*heat shock factor 1*) *RAD* 6 and *basonuclin* have not been identified yet in bovine (Bettegowda *et al.*, 2008). The same group has recently uncovered the importance of a new gene; *importin-alpha 8* or *KPNA7* as a nuclear importer of specific cargo like DNMT1 and HDAC4 and potentially involved in embryonic initiation of transcription (Tejomurtula *et al.*, 2009). Another paper in 2009 (Thelie *et al.*, 2009) confirmed the absence of transcription during the oocyte maturation period and that most (92%) of the maternal transcripts present in oocytes do not re-appear in the blastocyst.

In our laboratory, we have generated a subtractive library to probe the bovine transcriptome in the 8 cell embryo and compare it to 8 cells treated with alpha-amanitin (Vigneault *et al.*, 2009). We found clear evidences that some biological processes are prioritized in the early 8 cell. When the publication of Vigneault et al was submitted 2 years ago, we had limited tools to analyse the system biology value of the data generated. Nonetheless, the lists themselves as organized by functions or GO terms are truly pointing in very specific directions:

- Transcription regulation: 37 transcripts with 50% higher than 5 folds differences
- RNA processing: 40 transcripts with 33% higher than 5 fold differences
- Protein biosynthesis: 38 transcripts with 50 % higher than 5 fold differences
- DNA replication/ nucl. biosynthesis:15 transcripts with 33 % higher than 5 fold
- Protein degradation/modification: 25 transcripts with 50% higher than 5 fold

These 5 GO terms divisions represent the large majority of the known functions associated with the transcript of embryonic origin.

This original bovine data set was then introduced into IPA (Ingenuity pathway analysis). This program uses orthologs for human-mouse or rat to assess links between genes based on the available literature. This program is quite powerful but requires some efforts to ensure a proper analysis with embryonic tissues. Most of the published annotations are associated with the 3 mammalian species above, but since a large portion of transcriptomic studies are derived from cancer analyses, the dataset is enriched with ontogenic relations. Nevertheless, it is quite a powerful tool compared to individual gene search. When the transcriptome is analysed with bovine 8 cells compared to 8 cells with alpha-amanitin, all the differences is on one sided, or "up regulated", in the control without polymerase inhibitor, which makes a lot of sense. Therefore, on the network provided by IPA, all the genes coming from the bovine comparison will be displayed from pink to red depending on the relative intensity of the increased amount of RNA measured. The analysis revealed 11 networks of 15 related molecules or more (table 1). The score indicate an arbitrary value for the Ingenuity analysis which is dependant of the number of molecules involved in a given network (focus molecules)

The functions described in table 1 are in agreement with what is believed to happen at that stage: the resumption of transcription. The visual description of the network is also quite informative. Some example will be given here to highlight particular pathways of interest. The first network is illustrated in figure 1. The first node of interest involves *PSMA, PSMA 2, PSMA3, PSMA6, 20 S proteasome, proteasome 700, immunoproteasome pa28, 26 S proteasome* and *prion protein*. This group fits with the requirement of maternal protein degradation associated with MET in several species (see above). To observe nine interrelated transcripts that are all "upregulated" (see previous comments about the term upregulation) concomitantly is a strong indication that this is not a minor event but an important action in the embryonic program. In addition, the presence of *Snrp*, the transcription elongation factors (TCE family) and the eukaryotic translation elongation factors all indicate the activation of transcription (SKP1 is a kinase involved in transcription regulation), which is even more obvious in network 2.

Table 1. IPA function analysis of the 11 major network at MET in Bovine embryos.

ID	Score	Focus molecules	Top Functions
1	49	28	RNA Post-Transcriptional Modification, Molecular Transport, Nucleic Acid Metabolism
2	42	25	Protein Synthesis, RNA Post-Transcriptional Modification, DNA Replication, Recombination, and Repair
3	41	25	Cancer, Gene Expression, Cell Cycle
4	31	20	RNA Post-Transcriptional Modification, Protein Synthesis, Cellular Assembly and Organization
5	27	19	Protein Synthesis, Cell Death, Gene Expression
6	25	17	Molecular Transport, RNA Trafficking, RNA Post-Transcriptional Mocification
7	23	16	Cell Cycle, Connective Tissue Development and Function, Cancer
8	21	16	Organismal Injury and Abnormalities, Neurological Disease, Behavicr
9	21	15	Cell-To-Cell Signaling and Interaction, Hematological System Development and Function, Immune Cell Trafficking
10	19	14	Cell Signaling, Cellular Assembly and Organization, Cellular Function and Maintenance
11	19	14	Cell Cycle, Cellular Assembly and Organization, Cell Death

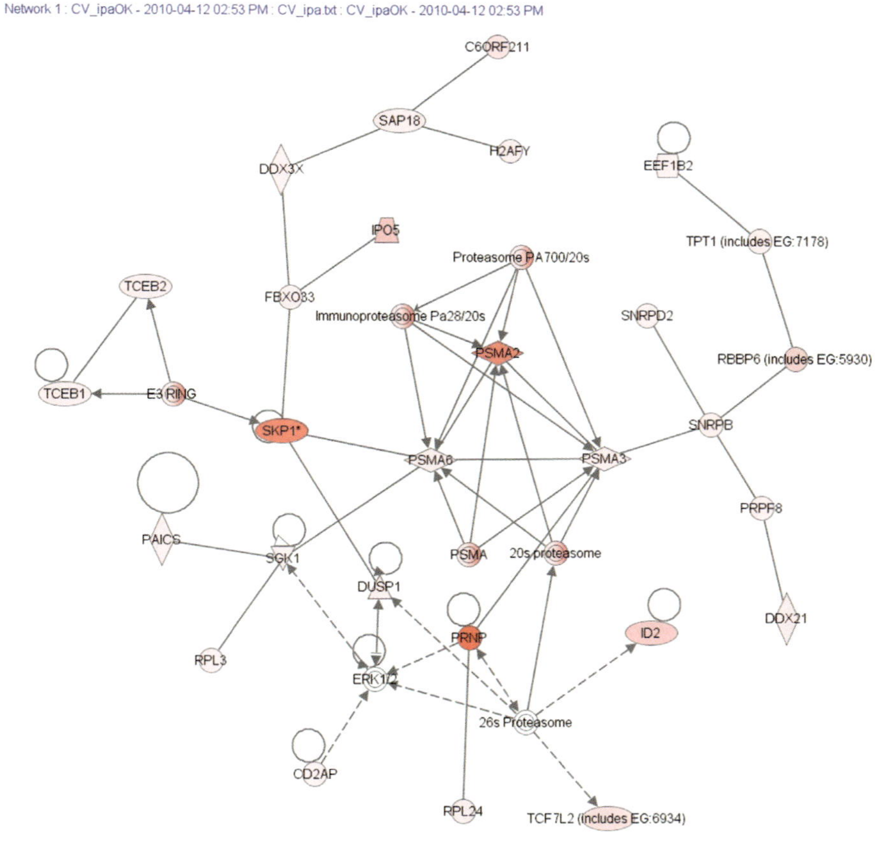

Fig. 1. Illustration of Network 1.

The second network (figure 2) focuses even more on transcriptional activation as several elongation factors are linked together. The concomitant presence of 3 *HNRNP, A2B1* and *A1*, 5 eukaryotic elongation factors *EIF 5, 3A, 3H, 4g, 4G2* and 2 types of *histones H3* associated with active transcription and some importins and transcription regulators such as *ATF1* and *GABPA*, splicing factors as *SF3, B1* and *B3*, indicates that transcriptional activation occurs in the nucleus. The IPA system adds some complementary information to fill the networks and these are not coloured (*Pka, ERK 1-2, Cyclin A*) but indicate potential regulatory mechanisms to investigate.

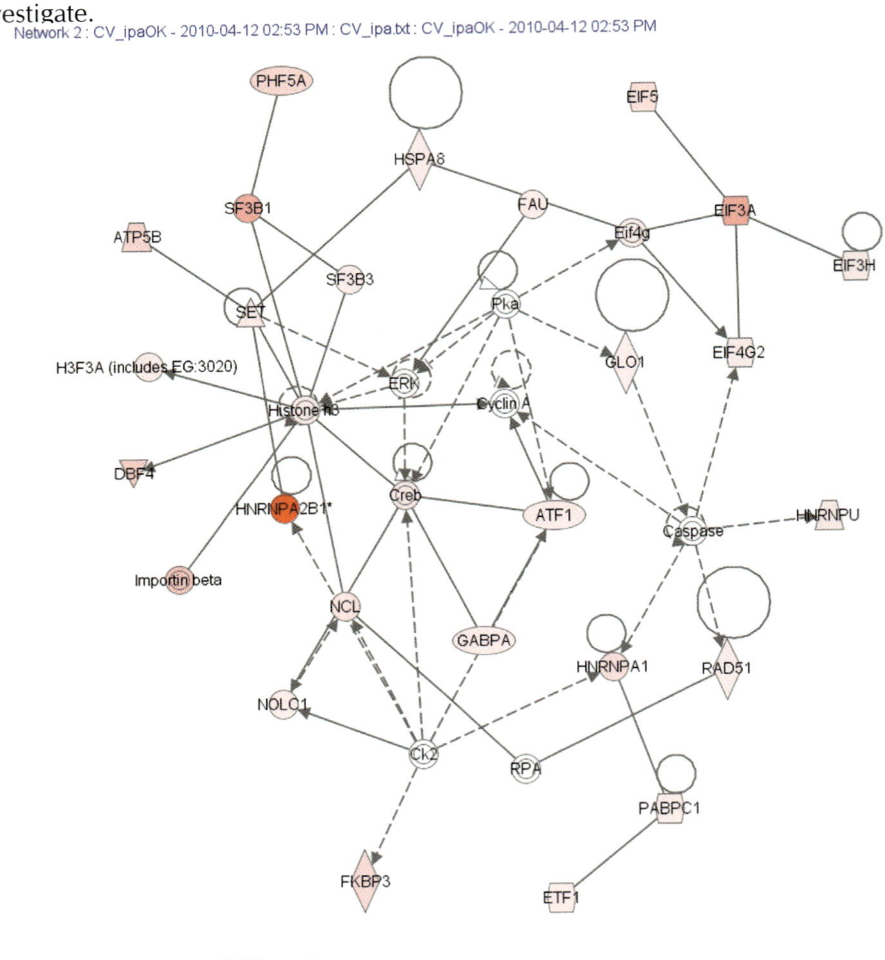

Fig. 2. Illustration of Network 2.

Network 3 (figure 3) also indicates a rise in transcriptional activity as it contains 2 *TBP* (*tata box bonding proteins*), *TAF 7* and *9*, 2 *KLF* genes, *KAT2B, NFYA, YY1* and *REST*, which are all transcriptional regulators. It is interesting to note that the estrogen receptor is linked with 3 of these transcription regulators (*KAT2B, TAF9* and *KLF10*).

The last network to be presented, network 4 (figure 4), is interesting by the finding of a potentially important node in a growth network : *GRB2, growth factor receptor bound protein 2*, which has several molecular functions such as phosphotyrosine binding, SH3/SH2 adaptor activity, epidermal growth factor receptor binding, protein domain specific binding, insulin receptor substrate binding and is involved in the following cellular processes: the MAPKKK

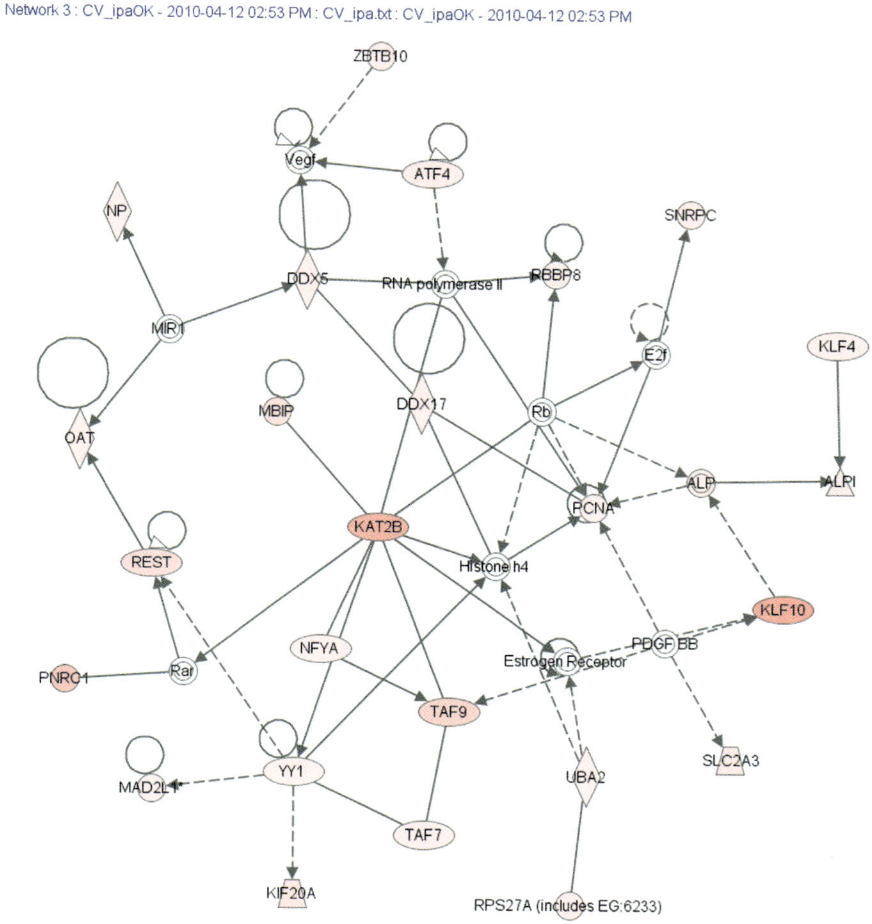

Fig. 3. Illustration of Network 3.

cascade, the epidermal growth factor receptor signalling pathway, Ras protein signal transduction, cell-cell signalling, aging, the insulin receptor signalling pathway, cell differentiation, interspecies interaction between organisms and protein hetero-oligomerization. As it can be observed in figure 4, *GRB2* acts on transcription factors (*MATR3*), on 3 types of ribonucleoproteins (*HNRNP* types *R*, *PF* and *H1*), and on 13 different ribosomal proteins *2,7, 10 A 18, 24, 26, 27, 35 , 37 A, S14, S16, S18* and *S23*. As this *GRB2* was not present in the limited library that was used, it would indicate that we missed it before the use of IPA.

Conclusion

The image behind the puzzle is slowly forming. Looking at the data from other species, particularly the mouse, where single genes can be analyzed using the Knock out approach, the mechanisms of embryonic activation are progressively being revealed. It seems that transcriptional arrest is almost universal in animals although the relationship between the epigenome and transcriptional arrest is still actively investigated and debated. The maternal RNA and

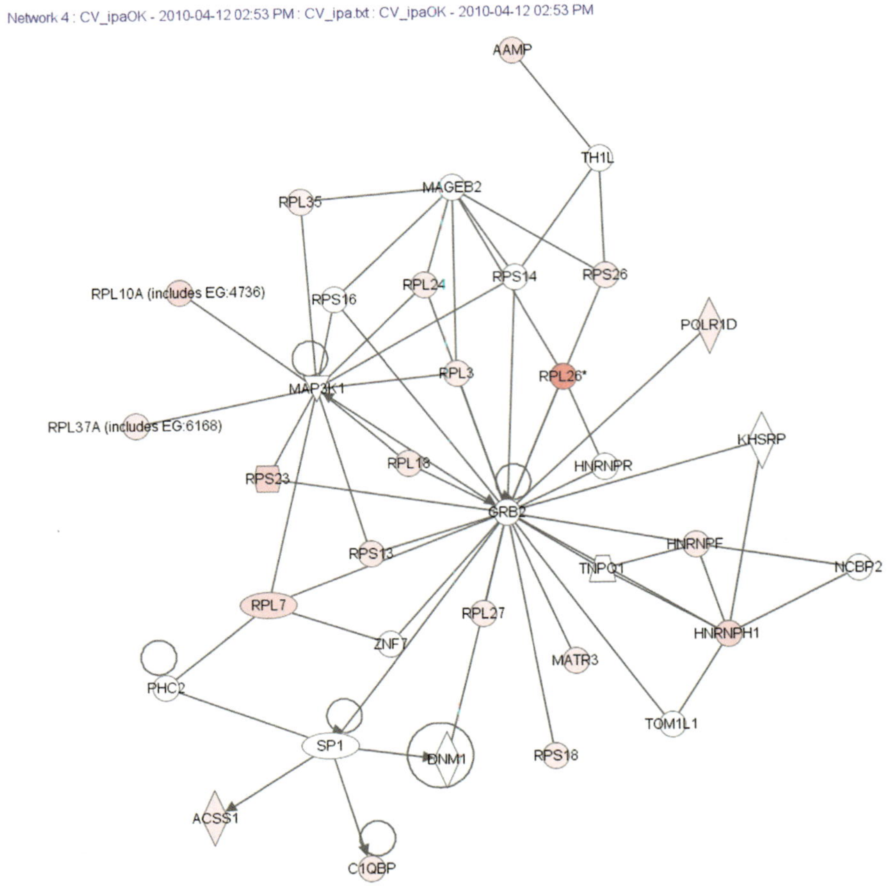

Fig. 4. Illustration of Network 4.

oocyte's proteins are important to trigger embryonic activation as specific products are required for this process, but at the same time the stock pile must be dismantled or destroyed to ensure proper function or activation of the new embryonic genome. The role of miRNAs is confirmed in many vertebrate and invertebrates models but is not defined clearly yet in mammals, albeit the removal of Dicer or other RISC components results in developmental consequences, suggesting an important function of this regulatory mechanism. However, it is important to note that the role of Dicer and RISC components specifically at the MET are not well understood. The long term effects of disrupting these components are not just important but critical to survival. The picture in bovine is getting in line with what has been observed in other mammals and indicates a multistep transcriptional activation around the 8 cell stage. Our findings further suggest that crucial functions are being activated in the early 8 cells, such as protein degradation, ribosome formation and the production of several transcriptional factors and units required for gene expression. These functional analyses are promoting the formulation of new hypotheses for the regulation of this process as new nodes and pathways are being exposed for further testing.

Acknowledgements

The author would like to thank Christian Vigneault for producing the bovine libraries and hybridization results and Julie Nieminen for manuscript revision. Financial support was obtained from NSERC (Natural Sciences and Engineering Research Council of Canada).

References

Barnes F L and First N L. 1991. Embryonic transcription in in vitro cultured bovine embryos. *Mol Reprod Dev*, **29**:117-123.

Baroux C, Autran D, Gillmor C S, Grimanelli D and Grossniklaus U. 2008. The maternal to zygotic transition in animals and plants. *Cold Spring Harb Symp Quant Biol*, **73**:89-100.

Bettegowda A, Lee K B and Smith G W. 2008. Cytoplasmic and nuclear determinants of the maternal-to-embryonic transition. *Reprod Fertil Dev*, **20**:45-53.

Bordignon V, Keyston R, Lazaris A, Bilodeau A S, Pontes J H, Arnold D, Fecteau G, Keefer C and Smith L C. 2003. Transgene expression of green fluorescent protein and germ line transmission in cloned calves derived from in vitro-transfected somatic cells. *Biol Reprod*, **68**:2013-2023.

Bultman S J, Gebuhr T C, Pan H, Svoboda P, Schultz R M and Magnuson T. 2006. Maternal BRG1 regulates zygotic genome activation in the mouse. *Genes Dev*, **20**:1744-1754.

De Renzis S, Elemento O, Tavazoie S and Wieschaus E F. 2007. Unmasking activation of the zygotic genome using chromosomal deletions in the Drosophila embryo. *PLoS Biol*, **5**:e117.

Dunican D S, Ruzov A, Hackett J A and Meehan R R. 2008. xDnmt1 regulates transcriptional silencing in pre-MBT Xenopus embryos independently of its catalytic function. *Development*, **135**:1295-1302.

Evsikov A V and Marin de Evsikova C. 2009. Gene expression during the oocyte-to-embryo transition in mammals. *Mol Reprod Dev*, **76**:805-818.

Fair T, Hulshof S C, Hyttel P, Greve T and Boland M. 1997. Nucleus ultrastructure and transcriptional activity of bovine oocytes in preantral and early antral follicles. *Mol Reprod Dev*, **46**:208-215.

Gagne M, Pothier F and Sirard M A. 1995. Effect of microinjection time during postfertilization S-phase on bovine embryonic development. *Mol Reprod Dev*, **41**:184-194.

Gilbert I, Scantland S, Dufort I, Gordynska O, Labbe A, Sirard M A and Robert C. 2009a. Real-time monitoring of aRNA production during T7 amplification to prevent the loss of sample representation during microarray hybridization sample preparation. *Nucleic Acids Res*, **37**:e65.

Gilbert I, Scantland S, Sylvestre E L, Gravel C, Laflamme I, Sirard M A and Robert C. 2009b. The dynamics of gene products fluctuation during bovine pre-hatching development. *Mol Reprod Dev*, **76**:762-772.

Giraldez A J, Mishima Y, Rihel J, Grocock R J, Van Dongen S, Inoue K, Enright A J and Schier A F. 2006. Zebrafish MiR-430 promotes deadenylation and clearance of maternal mRNAs. *Science*, **312**:75-79.

Hamatani T, Carter M G, Sharov A A and Ko M S. 2004. Dynamics of global gene expression changes during mouse preimplantation development. *Dev Cell*, **6**:117-131.

Kanka J, Kepkova K and Nemcova L. 2009. Gene expression during minor genome activation in preimplantation bovine development. *Theriogenology*, **72**:572-583.

Koehler D, Zakhartchenko V, Froenicke L, Stone G, Stanyon R, Wolf E, Cremer T and Brero A. 2009. Changes of higher order chromatin arrangements during major genome activation in bovine preimplantation embryos. *Exp Cell Res*, **315**:2053-2063.

Kwan T, Benovoy D, Dias C, Gurd S, Provencher C, Beaulieu P, Hudson T J, Sladek R and Majewski J. 2008. Genome-wide analysis of transcript isoform variation in humans. *Nat Genet*, **40**:225-231.

Leandri R D, Archilla C, Bui L C, Peynot N, Liu Z, Cabau C, Chastellier A, Renard J P and Duranthon V. 2009. Revealing the dynamics of gene expression during embryonic genome activation and first differentiation in the rabbit embryo with a dedicated array screening. *Physiol Genomics*, **36**:98-113.

Li L, Zheng P and Dean J. 2010.Maternal control of early mouse development. *Development*, **137**:859-870.

Liang H L, Nien C Y, Liu H Y, Metzstein M M, Kirov N and Rushlow C. 2008. The zinc-finger protein Zelda is a key activator of the early zygotic genome in Drosophila. *Nature*, **456**:400-403.

Lund E, Liu M, Hartley R S, Sheets M D and Dahlberg J E. 2009. Deadenylation of maternal mRNAs mediated by miR-427 in Xenopus laevis embryos. *RNA*, **15**:2351-2363.

McGraw S, Vigneault C, Tremblay K and Sirard M A. 2006. Characterization of linker histone H1FOO during bovine in vitro embryo development. *Mol Reprod Dev*, **73**:692-699.

Mechali M, Almouzni G, Andeol Y, Moreau J, Vriz S, Leibovici M, Hourdry J, Geraudie J, Soussi T and Gusse M. 1990. Genes and mechanisms involved in early embryonic development in Xenopus laevis. *Int J Dev Biol*, **34**:51-59.

Memili E and First N L. 1999. Control of gene expression at the onset of bovine embryonic development. *Biol Reprod*, **61**:1198-1207.

Memili E and First N L. 2000. Zygotic and embryonic gene expression in cow: a review of timing and mechanisms of early gene expression as compared with other species. *Zygote*, **8**:87-96.

Murakami M, Fahrudin M, Varisanga M D and Suzuki T. 1999. Fluorescence expression by bovine embryos after pronuclear microinjection with the EGFP gene. *J Vet Med Sci*, **61**:843-847.

Newport J and Kirschner M. 1982. A major developmental transition in early Xenopus embryos: I. characterization and timing of cellular changes at the midblastula stage. *Cell*, **30**:675-686.

Newport J and Kirschner M. 1982. A major developmental transition in early Xenopus embryos: II. Control of the onset of transcription. *Cell*, **30**:687-696.

Pennetier S, Perreau C, Uzbekova S, Thelie A, Delaleu B, Mermillod P and Dalbies-Tran R. 2006. MATER protein expression and intracellular localization throughout folliculogenesis and preimplantation embryo development in the bovine. *BMC Dev Biol*, **6**:26.

Pennetier S, Uzbekova S, Perreau C, Papillier P, Mermillod P and Dalbies-Tran R. 2004. Spatio-temporal expression of the germ cell marker genes MATER, ZAR1, GDF9, BMP15,andVASA in adult bovine tissues, oocytes, and preimplantation embryos. *Biol Reprod*, **71**:1359-1366.

Pique M, Lopez J M, Foissac S, Guigo R and Mendez R. 2008. A combinatorial code for CPE-mediated translational control. *Cell*, **132**:434-448.

Prather R S, Ross J W, Isom S C and Green J A. 2009. Transcriptional, post-transcriptional and epigenetic control of porcine oocyte maturation and embryogenesis. *Soc Reprod Fertil Suppl*, **66**:165-176.

Ramachandra R K, Salem M, Gahr S, Rexroad C E, 3rd and Yao J. 2008. Cloning and characterization of microRNAs from rainbow trout (Oncorhynchus mykiss): their expression during early embryonic development. *BMC Dev Biol*, **8**:41.

Richter J D. 2007. CPEB: a life in translation. *Trends Biochem Sci*, **32**:279-285.

Robbins L G. 1980. Maternal-zygotic lethal interactions in Drosophila melanogaster: the effects of deficiencies in the zeste-white region of the X chromosome. *Genetics*, **96**:187-200.

Santos F, Hendrich B, Reik W and Dean W. 2002. Dynamic reprogramming of DNA methylation in the early mouse embryo. *Dev Biol*, **241**:172-182.

Schier A F. 2007. The maternal-zygotic transition: death and birth of RNAs. *Science*, **316**:406-407.

Schultz R M. 2002. The molecular foundations of the maternal to zygotic transition in the preimplantation embryo. *Hum Reprod Update*, **8**:323-331.

Stitzel M L and Seydoux G. 2007. Regulation of the oocyte-to-zygote transition. *Science*, **316**:407-408.

Tadros W and Lipshitz H D. 2009. The maternal-to-zygotic transition: a play in two acts. *Development*, **136**:3033-3042.

Tejomurtula J, Lee K B, Tripurani S K, Smith G W and Yao J. 2009. Role of importin alpha8, a new member of the importin alpha family of nuclear transport proteins, in early embryonic development in cattle. *Biol Reprod*, **81**:333-342

Telford N A, Watson A J and Schultz G A. 1990. Transition from maternal to embryonic control in early mammalian development: a comparison of several species. *Mol Reprod Dev*, **26**:90-100.

Thelie A, Papillier P, Perreau C, Uzbekova S, Hennequet-Antier C and Dalbies-Tran R. 2009. Regulation of bovine oocyte-specific transcripts during in vitro oocyte maturation and after maternal-embryonic transition analyzed using a transcriptomic approach. *Mol Reprod Dev*, **76**:773-782.

Tsukamoto S, Kuma A, Murakami M, Kishi C, Yamamoto A, Mizushima N. 2008. Autophagy is essential for preimplantation development of mouse embryos. Science Jul4;321(5885):117-20

Vallee M, Aiba K, Piao Y, Palin M F, Ko M S and Sirard M A. 2008. Comparative analysis of oocyte transcript profiles reveals a high degree of conservation among species. *Reproduction*, **135**:439-448.

Vigneault C, Gilbert I, Sirard M A and Robert C. 2007. Using the histone H2a transcript as an endogenous standard to study relative transcript abundance during bovine early development. *Mol Reprod Dev*, **74**:703-715.

Vigneault C, Gravel C, Vallee M, McGraw S and Sirard M A. 2009. Unveiling the bovine embryo transcriptome during the maternal-to-embryonic transition. *Reproduction*, **137**:245-257.

Vigneault C, McGraw S and Sirard M A. 2009. Spatiotemporal expression of transcriptional regulators in concert with the maternal-to-embryonic transition during bovine in vitro embryogenesis. *Reproduction*, **137**:13-21.

Wang B, Lazaris A, Lindenbaum M, Stewart S, Co D, Perez C, Drayer J and Karatzas C N. 2001. Expression of a reporter gene after microinjection of mammalian artificial chromosomes into pronuclei of bovine zygotes. *Mol Reprod Dev*, **60**:433-438.

Whitworth K M, Agca C, Kim J G, Patel R V, Springer G K, Bivens N J, Forrester L J, Mathialagan N, Green J A and Prather R S. 2005. Transcriptional profiling of pig embryogenesis by using a 15-K member unigene set specific for pig reproductive tissues and embryos. *Biol Reprod*, **72**:1437-1451.

Zuccotti M, Merico V, Redi C A, Bellazzi R, Adjaye J and Garagna S. 2009. Role of Oct-4 during acquisition of developmental competence in mouse oocyte. *Reprod Biomed Online*, **19 Suppl 3**:57-62.

Zuccotti M, Merico V, Sacchi L, Bellone M, Brink T C, Stefanelli M, Redi C A, Bellazzi R, Adjaye J and Garagna S. 2009. Oct-4 regulates the expression of Stella and Foxj2 at the Nanog locus: implications for the developmental competence of mouse oocytes. *Hum Reprod*, **24**:2225-2237.

The role of kisspeptin and gonadotropin inhibitory hormone (GnIH) in the seasonality of reproduction in sheep

IJ Clarke and JT Smith

Dept Physiology, PO Box 13F, Monash University, Clayton, Victoria 3800, Australia

Sheep are seasonal breeders and reproductive status is controlled by photoperiod. Recent recognition of the significant role for kisspeptin and gonadotropin inhibitory hormone (GnIH) in the regulation of gonadotropin releasing hormone (GnRH) cells has provided a new perspective in the seasonal regulation of reproductive activity. Virtually all kisspeptin cells express estrogen receptors and kisspeptin is a potent stimulator of GnRH secretion. Thus, kisspeptin cells provide a conduit by which changes in estrogen feedback effects may be exerted upon GnRH cells. Changes in the activity of kisspeptin cells with season indicate a major role in the seasonal changes in reproductive activity in the ewe. GnIH is an inhibitor of reproductive function and there is mounting evidence that changing activity of this system is also an important determinant of reproductive status. Reciprocal changes in kisspeptin and GnIH activity explain seasonal changes in the function of GnRH cells.

Introduction

Sheep display seasonal patterns of reproduction which is regulated by day length (Robinson 1959). A component of the mechanism that causes a seasonal change in the frequency of luteinizing hormone (LH) pulses was shown in ovariectomised (OVX) ewes, thus being independent of any action of gonadal steroids (Robinson et al. 1985). Earlier work showed that there is an estrogen dependent mechanism that also underlies the transition between breeding and non-breeding seasons (Legan et al. 1977). With development of a model in sheep to measure secretion of gonadotropin releasing hormone (GnRH), it was then possible to attribute the pulses in peripheral plasma levels of LH to pulses of GnRH from the hypothalamus (Clarke and Cummins 1982) Measurements of hypophysial portal plasma concentrations showed that estrogen exerted an enhanced negative feedback effect during the non-breeding season (Karsch et al. 1993).

Gonadal steroid feedback on GnRH secretion governs the reproductive axis (Karsch et al. 1987, Clarke 1993). One of the most fundamental aspects of the operation of the hypothalamo-pituitary gonadal (HPG) axis is the means by which sex steroids act to modulate GnRH secretion and this took some time to resolve. Because GnRH cells do not possess the relevant sex steroid receptors (Herbison 1998), significant efforts were made in various laboratories and species over 3 decades (1970's to 2003) to identify steroid-receptive elements in the brain that relayed feedback information to the GnRH cells. Various cell types were found to express estrogen, pro-

Corresponding author E-mail: iain.clarke@med.monash.edu.au

gesterone and androgen receptors, but evidence of a major conduit remained elusive (Tilbrook et al. 2002). The discovery that kisspeptin and its cognate receptor are essential for normal reproduction (de Roux et al. 2003, Seminara et al. 2006) changed this, as discussed below. These cells provide stimulatory input to the GnRH cells, allowing transmission of sex steroid feedback regulation of reproductive function. Other cells may also participate in sex steroid feedback as well as modulation of GnRH cells by season, stress, immune status, nutritional status etc. Thus, a number of neuronal systems converge on the GnRH cells to determine the output of these cells in terms of GnRH secretion.

Another major advance in our understanding of the secretion and action of GnRH, albeit less well recognized, was the discovery of gonadotrophin inhibitory hormone (GnIH) in the hypothalamus of the quail (Tsutsui et al. 2000). This challenged the concept that gonadotropin secretion was controlled by a singular hypothalamic factor. Evidence that GnIH is important in mammals is now irrefutable. Like kisspeptin, GnIH is an RF-amide peptide but it exerts negative effects on GnRH cells (Ducret et al. 2009) and, at least in some species, the gonadotropes (Clarke et al. 2008). This review will summarise the general properties of these peptides and then evaluate their roles in the regulation of seasonal breeding with special reference to the sheep as a model.

General consideration of the control of GnRH Cells

GnRH neurons exhibit repetitive bursts of action potentials, consistent with phasic secretory activity (Suter et al. 2000). This is translated into the secretory mode as demonstrated by the phasic release of GnRH from cells of the fetal nasal placode of rhesus monkeys studied in culture (Terasawa et al. 1999). In addition, there is communication between GnRH neurons allowing for co-ordinate control (Campbell et al. 2009). If this phasic property of the cells is converted into bursts of secretion of GnRH, then it must be regulated in some fashion, to explain the differences in the patterns of secretion that are seen, for example, during the estrous cycle. The primary means of control is via feedback effects of gonadal steroids.

GnRH cells receive input from brain stem noradrenergic cells (Pompolo et al. 2003a, Rawson et al. 2001), serotoninergic elements of the raphe nucleus (Kiss and Halasz 1985) and a variety of cells of the hypothalamus and the forebrain (Iqbal et al. 2001, Pompolo et al. 2005, Pompolo et al. 2003a, Pompolo et al. 2003b). In addition to direct input to GnRH cells, control may be exerted by systems that form inter-neuronal pathways. Thus, the influence of the estrogen receptive A1 noradrenergic neurons of the brainstem may involve multisynaptic relay via the bed nucleus of the stria terminalis (BNST) or preoptic regions in close vicinity to the GnRH cells (Pereira et al. 2010, Pompolo et al. 2005). Anterograde and retrograde neuronal tracing between the arcuate nucleus of the hypothalamus (ARC) and the preoptic area of the ovine brain indicate that there is very limited direct input to GnRH cells from the former (Backholer et al. 2010, Pompolo et al. 2001). In this regard, even though there is very strong evidence that cells of the ARC play a significant role in the regulation of GnRH cells, there is little evidence of direct neuronal projections that subserve this (Backholer et al. 2010). One caveat on this observation is that ARC cells may project to dendrites of GnRH cells that are not readily seen with standard histolological techniques. The existence of inter-neuronal pathways to GnRH neurons from various regions of the brain would allow complex multifactorial control of the reproductive system, incorporating information in relation to metabolic status, season, stress, immune status, olfactory stimuli etc.

Noradrenergic cells of the brain stem, and forebrain glutamatergic cells and inhibitory cells utilising gamma amino butyric acid (GABA) as a transmitter are important in the regulation of GnRH secretion (Constantin et al. 2010, Kuehl-Kovarik et al. 2002, Pompolo et al. 2003a, Herbison 1997), but these cells do not fulfil all criteria required for mediation of feedback regulators; space does not allow full dissertation on this issue. In 2003, the revelation that kisspeptin cells were essential for reproductive function led to a significant revision in our understanding of how the function of GnRH cells is controlled by 'upstream' elements. This was followed by the gradual acceptance of the role of GnIH, which had been identified 3 years earlier.

Kisspeptin and the control of GnRH cells

There are two major groupings of kisspeptin cells in the mammalian brain, one being in the ARC and the other being in the rostral hypothalamus/POA region. In rodents, the latter group of cells is located in the anteroventral periventricular nucleus (AVPV) and preoptic periventricular nucleus (PeV) (Clarkson et al. 2008, Gottsch et al. 2004, Smith et al. 2005a, Smith et al. 2005b). In the ovine brain, the two synonymous populations of kisspeptin cells are found in the ARC and in the dorsolateral POA (Franceschini et al. 2006). In the ovine brain, kisspeptin cells of the POA provide direct input to GnRH neurons, whereas kisspeptin cells of the ARC may regulate GnRH neurons through an inter-neuronal pathway involving cells of another type (Backholer et al. 2010).

Amongst the neuronal elements that *modulate* GnRH neurons, kisspeptin achieved prominence for a number of reasons. Inactivating mutations in either the gene for kisspeptin (*Kiss1*) or the cognate receptor (GPR54) cause loss of reproductive function (de Roux et al. 2003, Seminara et al. 2003). Supporting the notion that kisspeptin exerts direct action on the GnRH cells, virtually all of these cells express the cognate receptor (GPR54) (Han et al. 2005, Irwig et al. 2004). Indeed, GPR54 is expressed in virtually all GnRH cells in the ewe brain (Smith et al. 2009). Blockade of these receptors with a kisspeptin antagonist, prevents pulsatile LH secretion in a number of species (Roseweir et al. 2009). Other work shows that kisspeptin directly stimulates GnRH secretion (Messager et al. 2005).

In sheep, kisspeptin does not appear to affect LH or FSH release by direct action on pituitary gonadotropes (Smith et al. 2008b). This is in spite of the fact that at least some GPR54 expression can be detected in the pituitary gland by PCR (Smith et al. 2008b). Consistent with this, kisspeptin is not secreted into the hypophysial portal blood in significant amounts (Smith et al. 2008b). Interestingly, however, kisspeptin cells project to the median eminence, where varicose fibres come into close apposition to GnRH fibres (Ramaswamy et al. 2008) and it is possible that there is axo-axonic regulation of GnRH secretion at this level (Keen et al. 2008). Evidence for the action of kisspeptin at the level of the median eminence has been demonstrated in the non-human primate (Keen et al. 2008), based on concordance of pulses of GnRH and kisspeptin in push-pull samples as well as the demonstration that kisspeptin injection to the median eminence stimulated LH secretion. Regarding the latter finding however, it is equivocal as to whether kisspeptin acted on GnRH cell bodies in the mediobasal hypothalamus or whether it acted on secretory terminals.

Kisspeptin cells transmit the negative feedback effect of sex steroids to GnRH cells

GnRH cells do not express estrogen receptor- α (ERα), or androgen receptors (Herbison et al. 1996, Huang and Harlan 1993), but it is clear that sex steroids regulate the secretion of GnRH. In the ovine ARC, virtually all kisspeptin cells express estrogen and progesterone receptors, but only 50% of the kisspeptin population of cells in the lateral POA express ERα (Franceschini et al. 2006). The question arises as to what function is performed by the kisspeptin cells that do not express steroid receptors. As mentioned above, there is good evidence that cells of the ovine ARC do not project directly to GnRH cells, but may exert influence on the latter by an inter-neuronal pathway. On the other hand, kisspeptin cells in the lateral POA of the ovine brain do appear to provide direct neuronal input to GnRH cells (Backholer et al. 2010).

Following ovariectomy, up-regulation of *Kiss1* expression is seen in the ARC kisspeptin cells (Smith et al. 2007) and increased numbers of kisspeptin cells are seen by immunohistochemistry (Pompolo et al. 2006). This shows that chronic effects of gonadal steroids restrain the ARC cells, but not the POA cells, and the effect of ovariectomy is reversed by chronic estrogen treatment (Smith et al. 2009). Virtually all kisspeptin cells in the ARC co-express dynorphin (DYN) and neurokinin B (NKB) (Goodman et al. 2007). This has led to the naming of these cells as K (kisspeptin) N (neurokinin B) Dy (dynorphin) (KNDy) cells (Cheng et al. 2010). The KNDy cells also express both ERα and progesterone receptor at a high level (Franceschini et al. 2006, Foradori et al. 2002), providing the necessary machinery for KNDy cells to mediate both negative and positive feedback effects of sex steroids. There is good evidence that dynorphin plays a role in mediating the negative feedback effect of progesterone (Foradori et al. 2005, Goodman et al. 2004), in addition to the evidence that chronic estrogen treatment down-regulates KNDy cells in OVX ewes (Smith et al. 2009). Further support for the notion that these cells participate in transmitting the negative feedback effect to GnRH cells is the observation that kisspeptin expression in the ARC is reduced in the luteal phase of the estrous cycle (Smith et al. 2009). This does not mean that other cells, such as those that produce enkephalin, may also participate in the negative feedback regulation of GnRH secretion (Walsh et al. 2001), but a major role for the KNDy cells is most likely. As for the involvement of these cells in the negative and positive feedback mechanism, any transmission from the ARC to the GnRH cells of the POA is likely to involve an inter-neuronal pathway. KNDy cells may regulate a subset of GnRH cells in the mediobasal hypothalamus, to exert the negative feedback effect (Goodman et al. 2004).

Kisspeptin and seasonal reproduction

Expression of *Kiss1* in the ARC of ovary-intact ewes is elevated at the onset of the breeding season, as evidenced by manipulations in photoperiod (Wagner et al. 2008). Here, *Kiss1* expression was 3 times higher on a photoperiod of 8 light and 16 dark (8L:16D) than that in animals on longer photoperiods. It is possible this effect could represent the effects of seasonal endogenous steroid production. Importantly, further studies in ewes show even in the absence of gonadal feedback (in OVX ewes with or without chronic estrogen implants) *Kiss1* mRNA and the number of kisspeptin immunoreactive cells is greater in the ARC during the breeding season than in the anestrous season (Smith et al. 2007, Smith et al. 2008a). Moreover, the inhibitory effects of chronic estrogen treatment on *Kiss1* mRNA and kisspeptin expression in the ARC (indicative of negative feedback) are greater during the non-breeding season (Smith et al. 2008a). These data suggest the seasonal change in sensitivity to estrogen, which is a major mechanism for seasonal reproduction, is effected, at least in part, by changing responsiveness of the kisspeptin cells to estrogen. Interestingly, the seasonal effect on *Kiss1* and kisspeptin expression was seen in the ARC, but not the POA. Alternatively, a small, yet significant effect of photoperiod was seen in kisspeptin cells in the POA of ewes transferred to short-day photoperiod (replicating the shift to the breeding season)(Chalivoix et al. 2010). Not surprisingly, a clear increase in kisspeptin cellular expression was also seen in the ARC. The authors suggest that the increase in kisspeptin expression stems from increased kisspeptin synthesis (Chalivoix et al. 2010).

In addition to the seasonal change in *Kiss1* expression and kisspeptin synthesis, the extent to which kisspeptin cells provide input to the GnRH neurons is greater during the breeding season than in the non-breeding season (Smith et al. 2008a). Presumably this input arises from the POA kisspeptin cells although this has not been tested by determining whether the increased input is due to 'recruitment' of cells in the arcuate nucleus. Thus, both the level of kisspeptin expression and the level of kisspeptin input to GnRH neurons are higher during the breeding season, while the negative feedback effects of estrogen on kisspeptin are lower at this time of the year. This is a strong indication that kisspeptin cells play a fundamental role in the seasonal regulation of reproduction.

As the seasonal change in kisspeptin expression in ewes is replicated by manipulation of photoperiod, it appears this may be the primary stimulus governing kisspeptin change. Work in seasonal rodents also provides strong evidence that the seasonal change in kisspeptin levels is due to alterations in photoperiod (Revel et al. 2006, Simonneaux et al. 2008). More importantly, these rodent studies further indicate the photoperiod change in kisspeptin is driven by changes in the pattern of melatonin secretion. Whether this is true in the ovine is not yet determined. Whether melatonin is able to exert its effects directly on kisspeptin cells is not yet known as there are no data to indicate kisspeptin cells possess melatonin receptors.

Role of the A14/A15 dopaminergic nucleus

Dopaminergic neurons located in the A15 region of the hypothalamus are thought to provide considerable input toward the increase in estrogen negative feedback sensitivity during the non-breeding season (for review see (Goodman et al. 2010). These cells are known to hold LH pulse frequency in check during the non-breeding season, but not the breeding season (Havern et al. 1994, Meyer and Goodman 1985). Furthermore, A15 dopaminergic cells are activated by estrogen only during the non-breeding season, but they do not express ERα (Lehman et al. 1996, Lehman and Karsch 1993). Estrogen responsive afferents to these cells may include glutamatergic cells of the POA (Singh et al. 2009).

In spite of the evidence that A14/A15 dopaminergic cells are key players in the seasonal changes in fertility in sheep, these cells do not appear to project directly to GnRH cell bodies (Tillet et al. 1989). Anterograde tracing experiments reveal A15 dopaminergic cells project predominantly to the caudal ARC and the median eminence (Goodman et al. 2010). It is enticing to speculate that the A15 dopaminergic cell projections to the former, communicate directly with kisspeptin cells located in this region, alter their expression and activity, and thereby govern seasonal reproduction.

Gonadotropin inhibitory hormone (GnIH)

GnIH was identified as a hypothalamic factor that inhibits the HPG axis in the quail (Tsutsui et al. 2000) and the role of this peptide is well established for avian species (Tsutsui 2009). It is now clear GnIH also plays an important role in the regulation of reproduction in mammals (Clarke et al. 2009, Smith and Clarke 2010). Mammalian GnIH was first named RF-amide related peptide (RFRP), being a member of the RF-amide family (Hinuma et al. 2000), but it is suggested the original nomenclature (GnIH) should apply to all species (Clarke et al. 2009, Smith and Clarke 2010).

In the sheep brain, *in situ* hybridization identified GnIH-expressing cells in the ventral region of the paraventricular nucleus and the dorsomedial nucleus (Clarke et al. 2008, Dardente et al. 2008, Smith et al. 2008a), with a similar distribution detected using immunohistochemistry, using either a white crowned sparrow GnIH antiserum (Kriegsfeld et al. 2006, Smith et al. 2008a) or an antiserum raised in guinea pigs against human GnIH-3 (Qi et al. 2009). Between 40-80% of GnRH cells show GnIH-immunoreactive varicose fibers in close proximity in the primate, rat, sheep, hamster and mouse brain (Johnson et al. 2007, Kriegsfeld et al. 2006, Qi et al. 2009, Smith et al. 2008a, Wu et al. 2009, Ubuka et al. 2009). This provides a substrate by which GnRH cells may be regulated either directly or indirectly by GnIH. Indeed, GnIH has been shown to directly inhibit the electrical properties of GnRH cells in mice (Wu et al. 2009, Ducret et al. 2009). GnIH-immunoreactive terminals have also been observed in the neurosecretory zone of the median eminence in hamsters, sheep, and primates (Clarke et al. 2008, Dardente et al. 2008, Kriegsfeld et al. 2006, Ubuka et al. 2009). On this basis, a hypophysiotropic role for GnIH is proposed for the sheep (Clarke et al. 2008).

GnIH action on the pituitary gonadotropes

Intravenously (iv) administered GnIH-3 had no effect on basal LH secretion in OVX rats and only minimal (albeit statistically significant) effects on GnRH-stimulated secretion (Rizwan et al. 2009); this was interpreted to mean that GnIH has no major effect on gonadotropes. Others (Murakami et al. 2008) showed a reduction in plasma LH levels in OVX rats 2 h after iv administration, with lack of effect of icv administration. In OVX ewes, systemically administered GnIH-3 reduced pulsatile LH secretion (Clarke et al. 2008), without any effect on the plasma levels of other pituitary hormones, such as growth hormone or prolactin; similar results have also been obtained in the bovine (Kadokawa et al. 2008).
The dose-dependent reduction in GnRH-stimulated LH secretion that is seen in cultures of rat, sheep and bovine pituitary cells, supports the notion of a direct effect of GnIH on gonadotropes (Clarke et al. 2008, Kadokawa et al. 2008, Murakami et al. 2008), although some contrary data have also been reported in studies on rat pituitary cells *in vitro* (Anderson et al. 2009). Such dissimilar results may be due to variable culture conditions or may relate to possible species differences in peripheral GnIH activity. Other lines of evidence also suggest direct pituitary action of GnIH in sheep. Firstly, GnIH-3 eliminates the GnRH-stimulated mobilisation of intracellular calcium in gonadotropes, which is considered mandatory for gonadotropin release (Clarke et al. 2008). Second, GnRH-stimulated up-regulation of *LH*β mRNA levels is also negated by GnIH, which may be due to reduced phosphorylation of extracellular signal-regulated kinase (ERK) (Sari et al. 2009). These data indicate a direct action of GnIH on the pituitary gonadotrope to reduce both synthesis and secretion of LH. *In vitro* treatment of ovine pituitary cell cultures also show an effect of GnIH-3 to reduce FSH secretion in response to GnRH (Clarke et al. 2008) as well as reducing *FSHß* mRNA levels (Sari et al. 2009). Thus, GnIH may inhibit the production/secretion of both gonadotropins.

GnIH and seasonal reproduction

In ewes, a lower number of immunoreactive GnIH cells is detected during the breeding season than in the non-breeding season, but no change was seen in cellular GnIH mRNA expression assessed by *in situ* hybridization (Smith et al. 2008a). Contrary to this, GnIH mRNA expression in Soay ewes (also assessed by *in situ* hybridization) was greater in animals held at a long-day (16L:8D) photoperiod than in those on short day (8L:16D) photoperiod (Dardente et al. 2008). Nevertheless, when these ewes were held on extreme long day photoperiods (22 h light), the effect on GnIH gene expression was lost. It was concluded that GnIH may not play a major role in seasonality (Dardente et al. 2008), but the inhibitory effect may be amplified by an increase in input to GnRH cells during the non-breeding season (see below)(Smith et al. 2008a). Moreover, after transferring ewes to a long-day photoperiod, no effect on GnIH gene expression was apparent in time-points examined before 42 days (Dardente et al. 2008). This lack of a short-term effect is consistent with the notion that the transition between the breeding and non-breeding seasons requires approximately 60 days (Lincoln 1999), and also indicates that the full seasonal transition (and change in GnIH expression) in these ewes may not have occurred.

The lower level of GnIH producing cells that is seen during the breeding season is accompanied by a reduction in the number of GnRH cells contacted by GnIH terminals (Smith et al. 2008a). Given the role of GnIH on the reproductive system, the net effect of these data would indicate the activity of GnIH may be a contributing factor to the inhibition of the reproductive system during the non-breeding season. Further work, including measurement of GnIHR expression in different seasons may be informative.

Kisspeptin and GnIH as key reciprocal regulators in seasonal breeding

Sheep are seasonal breeders, being sexually active in response to short day photoperiod (Karsch et al. 1984, Malpaux et al. 1998). Whereas it has been known for some years that seasonality in sheep is due to alterations in the frequency of generation of GnRH/LH pulses (Robinson et al. 1985), as well as an alteration in the negative feedback effect of ovarian steroids (Legan et al. 1977), there was no identification of a neural substrate that changes with season and controls GnRH secretion accordingly. The A15 dopaminergic nucleus was identified as a key centre in the control of seasonality (Thiery et al. 1995) but as to how this is connected to GnRH secretion is not yet clear. With the revelation of key regulatory function of kisspeptin and GnIH, it is hardly surprising that this has been investigated in relation to seasonal breeding. In the ewe, kisspeptin production (ARC) and input to GnRH cells is reduced in seasonal anestrus and increases at onset of the breeding season (Smith et al. 2008a). Also in the ewe, GnIH protein expression is higher during the non-breeding season than in the breeding season as determined by the number of cells stained with immunohistochemistry (Smith et al. 2008a). Terminal projections from GnIH cells to GnRH neurons are increased during the non-breeding season (Smith et al. 2008a).

Conclusion

Reciprocal changes in kisspeptin and GnIH activity indicate that both RF-amide peptides play a role in seasonal changes in reproductive activity. Kisspeptin treatment of anestrous ewes causes ovulation, offering a potential means by which seasonal acyclicity can be overcome (Caraty et al. 2007). Intervention studies such as reducing GnIH function in the non-breeding season would be instructive.

References

Anderson GM, Relf HL, Rizwan MZ & Evans JJ 2009 Central and peripheral effects of RFamide-related peptide-3 on luteinizing hormone and prolactin secretion in rats. *Endocrinology* **150** 1834-1840.

Backholer K, Smith JT, Rao A, Pereira A, Iqbal J, Ogawa S, Li Q & Clarke IJ 2010 Kisspeptin cells in the ewe brain respond to leptin and communicate with neuropeptide y and proopiomelanocortin cells. *Endocrinology* **151** 2233-2243.

Campbell RE, Gaidamaka G, Han SK & Herbison AE

2009 Dendro-dendritic bundling and shared synapses between gonadotropin-releasing hormone neurons. *Proc Natl Acad Sci U S A* **106** 10835-10840.

Caraty A, Smith JT, Lomet D, Ben Said S, Morrissey A, Cognie J, Doughton B, Baril G, Briant C & Clarke IJ 2007 Kisspeptin synchronizes preovulatory surges in cyclical ewes and causes ovulation in seasonally acyclic ewes. *Endocrinology* **148** 5258-5267.

Chalivoix S, Bagnolini A, Caraty A, Cognie J, Malpaux B & Dufourny L 2010 Effects of photoperiod on kisspeptin neuronal populations of the ewe diencephalon in connection with reproductive function. *J Neuroendocrinol* **22** 110-118.

Cheng G, Coolen LM, Padmanabhan V, Goodman RL & Lehman MN 2010 The kisspeptin/neurokinin B/dynorphin (KNDy) cell population of the arcuate nucleus: sex differences and effects of prenatal testosterone in sheep. *Endocrinology* **151** 301-311.

Clarke IJ 1993 Variable patterns of gonadotropin-releasing hormone secretion during the estrogen-induced luteinizing hormone surge in ovariectomized ewes. *Endocrinology* **133** 1624-1632.

Clarke IJ and Cummins JT 1982 The temporal relationship between gonadotropin releasing hormone (GnRH) and luteinizing hormone (LH) secretion in ovariectomized ewes. *Endocrinology* **111** 1737-1739.

Clarke IJ, Qi Y, Puspita Sari I & Smith JT 2009 Evidence that RF-amide related peptides are inhibitors of reproduction in mammals. *Front Neuroendocrinol* **30** 371-378.

Clarke IJ, Sari IP, Qi Y, Smith JT, Parkington HC, Ubuka T, Iqbal J, Li Q, Tilbrook A, Morgan K, Pawson AJ, Tsutsui K, Millar RP & Bentley GE 2008 Potent Action of RFamide-Related Peptide-3 on Pituitary Gonadotropes Indicative of a Hypophysiotropic Role in the Negative Regulation of Gonadotropin Secretion. *Endocrinology* **149** 5811-5821.

Clarkson J, d'Anglemont de Tassigny X, Moreno AS, Colledge WH & Herbison AE 2008 Kisspeptin-GPR54 signaling is essential for preovulatory gonadotropin-releasing hormone neuron activation and the luteinizing hormone surge. *J Neurosci* **28** 8691-8697.

Constantin S, Jasoni CL, Wadas B & Herbison AE 2010 Gamma-aminobutyric acid and glutamate differentially regulate intracellular calcium concentrations in mouse gonadotropin-releasing hormone neurons. *Endocrinology* **151** 262-270.

Dardente H, Birnie M, Lincoln GA & Hazlerigg DG 2008 RFamide-related peptide and its cognate receptor in the sheep: cDNA cloning, mRNA distribution in the hypothalamus and effect of photoperiod. *J Neuroendocrinol.*

de Roux N, Genin E, Carel JC, Matsuda F, Chaussain JL & Milgrom E 2003 Hypogonadotropic hypogonadism due to loss of function of the KiSS1-derived peptide receptor GPR54. *Proc Natl Acad Sci U S A* **100** 10972-10976.

Ducret E, Anderson GM & Herbison AE 2009 RFamide-related peptide-3, a mammalian gonadotropin-inhibitory hormone ortholog, regulates gonadotropin-releasing hormone neuron firing in the mouse. *Endocrinology* **150** 2799-2804.

Foradori CD, Coolen LM, Fitzgerald ME, Skinner DC, Goodman RL & Lehman MN 2002 Colocalization of progesterone receptors in parvicellular dynorphin neurons of the ovine preoptic area and hypothalamus. *Endocrinology* **143** 4366-4374.

Foradori CD, Goodman RL, Adams VL, Valent M & Lehman MN 2005 Progesterone increases dynorphin a concentrations in cerebrospinal fluid and preprodynorphin messenger ribonucleic Acid levels in a subset of dynorphin neurons in the sheep. *Endocrinology* **146** 1835-1842.

Franceschini I, Lomet D, Cateau M, Delsol G, Tillet Y & Caraty A 2006 Kisspeptin immunoreactive cells of the ovine preoptic area and arcuate nucleus co-express estrogen receptor alpha. *Neurosci Lett* **401** 225-230.

Goodman RL, Coolen LM, Anderson GM, Hardy SL, Valent M, Connors JM, Fitzgerald ME & Lehman MN 2004 Evidence that dynorphin plays a major role in mediating progesterone negative feedback on gonadotropin-releasing hormone neurons in sheep. *Endocrinology* **145** 2959-2967.

Goodman RL, Jansen HT, Billings HJ, Coolen LM & Lehman MN 2010 Neural Systems Mediating Seasonal Breeding in the Ewe. *J Neuroendocrinol.*

Goodman RL, Lehman MN, Smith JT, Coolen LM, de Oliveira CV, Jafarzadehshirazi MR, Pereira A, Iqbal J, Caraty A, Ciofi P & Clarke IJ 2007 Kisspeptin neurons in the arcuate nucleus of the ewe express both dynorphin A and neurokinin B. *Endocrinology* **148** 5752-5760.

Gottsch ML, Cunningham MJ, Smith JT, Popa SM, Acohido BV, Crowley WF, Seminara S, Clifton DK & Steiner RA 2004 A role for kisspeptins in the regulation of gonadotropin secretion in the mouse. *Endocrinology* **145** 4073-4077.

Han SK, Gottsch ML, Lee KJ, Popa SM, Smith JT, Jakawich SK, Clifton DK, Steiner RA & Herbison AE 2005 Activation of gonadotropin-releasing hormone neurons by kisspeptin as a neuroendocrine switch for the onset of puberty. *J Neurosci* **25** 11349-11356.

Havern RL, Whisnant CS & Goodman RL 1994 Dopaminergic structures in the ovine hypothalamus mediating estradiol negative feedback in anestrous ewes. *Endocrinology* **134** 1905-1914.

Herbison AE 1997 Estrogen regulation of GABA transmission in rat preoptic area. *Brain Res Bull* **44** 321-326.

Herbison AE 1998 Multimodal influence of estrogen upon gonadotropin-releasing hormone neurons. *Endocr Rev* **19** 302-330.

Herbison AE, Skinner DC, Robinson JE & King IS 1996 Androgen receptor-immunoreactive cells in ram hypothalamus: distribution and co-localization patterns with gonadotropin-releasing hormone, somatostatin and tyrosine hydroxylase. *Neuroendocrinology* **63** 120-131.

Hinuma S, Shintani Y, Fukusumi S, Iijima N, Matsumoto Y, Hosoya M, Fujii R, Watanabe T, Kikuchi K, Terao Y, Yano T, Yamamoto T, Kawamata Y, Habata Y, Asada

M, Kitada C, Kurokawa T, Onda H, Nishimura O, Tanaka M, Ibata Y & Fujino M 2000 New neuropeptides containing carboxy-terminal RFamide and their receptor in mammals. *Nat Cell Biol* **2** 703-708.

Huang X and Harlan RE 1993 Absence of androgen receptors in LHRH immunoreactive neurons. *Brain Res* **624** 309-311.

Iqbal J, Pompolo S, Sakurai T & Clarke IJ 2001 Evidence that orexin-containing neurones provide direct input to gonadotropin-releasing hormone neurones in the ovine hypothalamus. *J Neuroendocrinol* **13** 1033-1041.

Irwig MS, Fraley GS, Smith JT, Acohido BV, Popa SM, Cunningham MJ, Gottsch ML, Clifton DK & Steiner RA 2004 Kisspeptin activation of gonadotropin releasing hormone neurons and regulation of KiSS-1 mRNA in the male rat. *Neuroendocrinology* **80** 264-272.

Johnson MA, Tsutsui K & Fraley GS 2007 Rat RFamide-related peptide-3 stimulates GH secretion, inhibits LH secretion, and has variable effects on sex behavior in the adult male rat. *Horm Behav* **51** 171-180.

Kadokawa H, Matsui M, Hayashi K, Matsunaga N, Kawashima C, Shimizu T, Kida K & Miyamoto A 2008 Peripheral administration of kisspeptin-10 increases plasma concentrations of GH as well as LH in prepubertal Holstein heifers. *J Endocrinol* **196** 331-334.

Karsch FJ, Bittman EL, Foster DL, Goodman RL, Legan SJ & Robinson JE 1984 Neuroendocrine basis of seasonal reproduction. *Recent Prog Horm Res* **40** 185-232.

Karsch FJ, Cummins JT, Thomas GB & Clarke IJ 1987 Steroid feedback inhibition of pulsatile secretion of gonadotropin-releasing hormone in the ewe. *Biol Reprod* **36** 1207-1218.

Karsch FJ, Dahl GE, Evans NP, Manning JM, Mayfield KP, Moenter SM & Foster DL 1993 Seasonal changes in gonadotropin-releasing hormone secretion in the ewe: alteration in response to the negative feedback action of estradiol. *Biol Reprod* **49** 1377-1383.

Keen KL, Wegner FH, Bloom SR, Ghatei MA & Terasawa E 2008 An increase in kisspeptin-54 release occurs with the pubertal increase in luteinizing hormone-releasing hormone-1 release in the stalk-median eminence of female rhesus monkeys in vivo. *Endocrinology* **149** 4151-4157.

Kiss J and Halasz B 1985 Demonstration of serotoninergic axons terminating on luteinizing hormone-releasing hormone neurons in the preoptic area of the rat using a combination of immunocytochemistry and high resolution autoradiography. *Neuroscience* **14** 69-78.

Kriegsfeld LJ, Mei DF, Bentley GE, Ubuka T, Mason AO, Inoue K, Ukena K, Tsutsui K & Silver R 2006 Identification and characterization of a gonadotropin-inhibitory system in the brains of mammals. *Proc Natl Acad Sci U S A* **103** 2410-2415.

Kuehl-Kovarik MC, Pouliot WA, Halterman GL, Handa RJ, Dudek FE & Partin KM 2002 Episodic bursting activity and response to excitatory amino acids in acutely dissociated gonadotropin-releasing hormone neurons genetically targeted with green fluorescent protein. *J Neurosci* **22** 2313-2322.

Legan SJ, Karsch FJ & Foster DL 1977 The endocrin control of seasonal reproductive function in the ewe: a marked change in response to the negative feedback action of estradiol on luteinizing hormone secretion. *Endocrinology* **101** 818-824.

Lehman MN, Durham DM, Jansen HT, Adrian B & Goodman RL 1996 Dopaminergic A14/A15 neurons are activated during estradiol negative feedback in anestrous, but not breeding season, ewes. *Endocrinology* **137** 4443-4450.

Lehman MN and Karsch FJ 1993 Do gonadotropin-releasing hormone, tyrosine hydroxylase-, and beta-endorphin-immunoreactive neurons contain estrogen receptors? A double-label immunocytochemical study in the Suffolk ewe. *Endocrinology* **133** 887-895.

Lincoln G 1999 Melatonin modulation of prolactin and gonadotrophin secretion. Systems ancient and modern. *Adv Exp Med Biol* **460** 137-153.

Malpaux B, Daveau A, Maurice-Mandon F, Duarte G & Chemineau P 1998 Evidence that melatonin acts in the premammillary hypothalamic area to control reproduction in the ewe: presence of binding sites and stimulation of luteinizing hormone secretion by in situ microimplant delivery. *Endocrinology* **139** 1508-1516.

Messager S, Chatzidaki EE, Ma D, Hendrick AG, Zahn D, Dixon J, Thresher RR, Malinge I, Lomet D, Carlton MB, Colledge WH, Caraty A & Aparicio SA 2005 Kisspeptin directly stimulates gonadotropin-releasing hormone release via G protein-coupled receptor 54. *Proc Natl Acad Sci U S A* **102** 1761-1766.

Meyer SL and Goodman RL 1985 Neurotransmitters involved in mediating the steroid-dependent suppression of pulsatile luteinizing hormone secretion in anestrous ewes: effects of receptor antagonists. *Endocrinology* **116** 2054-2061.

Murakami M, Matsuzaki T, Iwasa T, Yasui T, Irahara M, Osugi T & Tsutsui K 2008 Hypophysiotropic role of RFamide-related peptide-3 (RFRP-3) in the inhibition of LH secretion in female rats. *J Endocrinol* **199** 105-112.

Pereira A, Rawson J, Jakubowska A & Clarke IJ 2010 Estradiol-17beta-responsive A1 and A2 noradrenergic cells of the brain stem project to the bed nucleus of the stria terminalis in the ewe brain: a possible route for regulation of gonadotropin releasing hormone cells. *Neuroscience* **165** 758-773.

Pompolo S, Ischenko O, Pereira A, Iqbal J & Clarke IJ 2005 Evidence that projections from the bed nucleus of the stria terminalis and from the lateral and medial regions of the preoptic area provide input to gonadotropin releasing hormone (GNRH) neurons in the female sheep brain. *Neuroscience* **132** 421-436.

Pompolo S, Pereira A, Estrada KM & Clarke IJ 2006 Colocalization of kisspeptin and gonadotropin-releasing hormone in the ovine brain. *Endocrinology* **147** 804-810.

Pompolo S, Pereira A, Kaneko T & Clarke IJ 2003a Seasonal changes in the inputs to gonadotropin-releasing hormone neurones in the ewe brain: an assessment by conventional fluorescence and confocal microscopy. *J Neuroendocrinol* **15** 538-545.

Pompolo S, Pereira A, Scott CJ, Fujiyma F & Clarke IJ 2003b Evidence for estrogenic regulation of gonadotropin-releasing hormone neurons by glutamatergic neurons in the ewe brain: An immunohistochemical study using an antibody against vesicular glutamate transporter-2. *J Comp Neurol* **465** 136-144.

Pompolo S, Rawson JA & Clarke IJ 2001 Projections from the arcuate/ventromedial region of the hypothalamus to the preoptic area and bed nucleus of stria terminalis in the brain of the ewe; lack of direct input to gonadotropin-releasing hormone neurons. *Brain Res* **904** 1-12.

Qi Y, Oldfield BJ & Clarke IJ 2009 Projections of RFamide-related Peptide-3 Neurons in the Ovine Hypothalamus, with Special Reference to Regions Regulating Energy Balance and Reproduction. *J Neuroendocrinol* In Press.

Ramaswamy S, Guerriero KA, Gibbs RB & Plant TM 2008 Structural interactions between kisspeptin and GnRH neurons in the mediobasal hypothalamus of the male rhesus monkey (Macaca mulatta) as revealed by double immunofluorescence and confocal microscopy. *Endocrinology* **149** 4387-4395.

Rawson JA, Scott CJ, Pereira A, Jakubowska A & Clarke IJ 2001 Noradrenergic projections from the A1 field to the preoptic area in the brain of the ewe and Fos responses to oestrogen in the A1 cells. *J Neuroendocrinol* **13** 129-138.

Revel FG, Saboureau M, Masson-Pevet M, Pevet P, Mikkelsen JD & Simonneaux V 2006 KiSS-1: a likely candidate for the photoperiodic control of reproduction in seasonal breeders. *Chronobiol Int* **23** 277-287.

Rizwan MZ, Porteous R, Herbison AE & Anderson GM 2009 Cells expressing RFamide-related peptide-1/3, the mammalian gonadotropin-inhibitory hormone orthologs, are not hypophysiotropic neuroendocrine neurons in the rat. *Endocrinology* **150** 1413-1420.

Robinson JE, Radford HM & Karsch FJ 1985 Seasonal changes in pulsatile luteinizing hormone (LH) secretion in the ewe: relationship of frequency of LH pulses to day length and response to estradiol negative feedback. *Biol Reprod* **33** 324-334.

Robinson TJ 1959 The estrous cycle of the ewe and doe. *In '(Eds: HH Cole and PT Cupps), Reproduction in Domestic Animals, Academic Press, NY* pp 291-333.

Roseweir AK, Kauffman AS, Smith JT, Guerriero KA, Morgan K, Pielecka-Fortuna J, Pineda R, Gottsch ML, Tena-Sempere M, Moenter SM, Terasawa E, Clarke IJ, Steiner RA & Millar RP 2009 Discovery of potent kisspeptin antagonists delineate physiological mechanisms of gonadotropin regulation. *J Neurosci* **29** 3920-3929.

Sari IP, Rao A, Smith JT, Tilbrook AJ & Clarke IJ 2009 Effect of RF-amide-related peptide-3 on luteinizing hormone and follicle-stimulating hormone synthesis and secretion in ovine pituitary gonadotropes. *Endocrinology* **150** 5549-5556.

Seminara SB, Dipietro MJ, Ramaswamy S, Crowley WF, Jr. & Plant TM 2006 Continuous Human Metastin 45-54 Infusion Desensitizes G Protein-Coupled Receptor 54-Induced Gonadotropin-Releasing Hormone Release Monitored Indirectly in the Juvenile Male Rhesus Monkey (Macaca mulatta): A Finding with Therapeutic Implications. *Endocrinology* **147** 2122-2126.

Seminara SB, Messager S, Chatzidaki EE, Thresher RR, Acierno JS, Jr., Shagoury JK, Bo-Abbas Y, Kuohung W, Schwinof KM, Hendrick AG, Zahn D, Dixon J, Kaiser UB, Slaugenhaupt SA, Gusella JF, O'Rahilly S, Carlton MB, Crowley WF, Jr., Aparicio SA & Colledge WH 2003 The GPR54 gene as a regulator of puberty. *N Engl J Med* **349** 1614-1627.

Simonneaux V, Ansel L, Revel FG, Klosen P, Pevet P & Mikkelsen JD 2008 Kisspeptin and the seasonal control of reproduction in hamsters. *Peptides.*

Singh SR, Hileman SM, Connors JM, McManus CJ, Coolen LM, Lehman MN & Goodman RL 2009 Estradiol negative feedback regulation by glutamatergic afferents to A15 dopaminergic neurons: variation with season. *Endocrinology* **150** 4663-4671.

Smith JT and Clarke IJ 2010 Gonadotropin inhibitory hormone function in mammals. *Trends Endocrinol Metab* **21** 255-260.

Smith JT, Clay CM, Caraty A & Clarke IJ 2007 KiSS-1 messenger ribonucleic acid expression in the hypothalamus of the ewe is regulated by sex steroids and season. *Endocrinology* **148** 1150-1157.

Smith JT, Coolen LM, Kriegsfeld LJ, Sari IP, Jaafarzadehshirazi MR, Maltby M, Bateman K, Goodman RL, Tilbrook AJ, Ubuka T, Bentley GE, Clarke IJ & Lehman MN 2008a Variation in kisspeptin and RFamide-related peptide (RFRP) expression and terminal connections to gonadotropin-releasing hormone neurons in the brain: a novel medium for seasonal breeding in the sheep. *Endocrinology* **149** 5770-5782.

Smith JT, Cunningham MJ, Rissman EF, Clifton DK & Steiner RA 2005a Regulation of Kiss1 gene expression in the brain of the female mouse. *Endocrinology* **146** 3686-3692.

Smith JT, Dungan HM, Stoll EA, Gottsch ML, Braun RE, Eacker SM, Clifton DK & Steiner RA 2005b Differential regulation of KiSS-1 mRNA expression by sex steroids in the brain of the male mouse. *Endocrinology* **146** 2976-2984.

Smith JT, Li Q, Pereira A & Clarke IJ 2009 Kisspeptin neurons in the ovine arcuate nucleus and preoptic area are involved in the preovulatory luteinizing hormone surge. *Endocrinology* **150** 5530-5538.

Smith JT, Rao A, Pereira A, Caraty A, Millar RP & Clarke IJ 2008b Kisspeptin is present in ovine hypophysial portal blood but does not increase during the preovulatory luteinizing hormone surge: evidence that gonadotropes are not direct targets of kisspeptin in vivo. *Endocrinology* **149** 1951-1959.

Suter KJ, Wuarin JP, Smith BN, Dudek FE & Moenter SM 2000 Whole-cell recordings from preoptic/hypothalamic slices reveal burst firing in gonadotropin-releasing hormone neurons identified with green fluorescent protein in transgenic mice. *Endocrinology* **141** 3731-3736.

Terasawa E, Keen KL, Mogi K & Claude P 1999 Pulsatile release of luteinizing hormone-releasing hormone (LHRH) in cultured LHRH neurons derived from the embryonic olfactory placode of the rhesus monkey. *Endocrinology* **140** 1432-1441.

Thiery JC, Gayrard V, Le Corre S, Viguie C, Martin GB, Chemineau P & Malpaux B 1995 Dopaminergic control of LH secretion by the A15 nucleus in anoestrous ewes. *J Reprod Fertil Suppl* **49** 285-296.

Tilbrook AJ, Turner AI & Clarke IJ 2002 Stress and reproduction: central mechanisms and sex differences in non-rodent species. *Stress* **5** 83-100.

Tillet Y, Caldani M & Batailler M 1989 Anatomical relationships of monoaminergic and neuropeptide Y-containing fibres with luteinizing hormone-releasing hormone systems in the preoptic area of the sheep brain: immunohistochemical studies. *J Chem Neuroanat* **2** 319-326.

Tsutsui K 2009 A new key neurohormone controlling reproduction, gonadotropin-inhibitory hormone (GnIH): Biosynthesis, mode of action and functional significance. *Prog Neurobiol* **88** 76-88.

Tsutsui K, Saigoh E, Ukena K, Teranishi H, Fujisawa Y, Kikuchi M, Ishii S & Sharp PJ 2000 A novel avian hypothalamic peptide inhibiting gonadotropin release. *Biochem Biophys Res Commun* **275** 661-667.

Ubuka T, Lai H, Kitani M, Suzuuchi A, Pham V, Cadigan PA, Wang A, Chowdhury VS, Tsutsui K & Bentley GE 2009 Gonadotropin-inhibitory hormone identification, cDNA cloning, and distribution in rhesus macaque brain. *J Comp Neurol* **517** 841-855.

Wagner GC, Johnston JD, Clarke IJ, Lincoln GA & Hazlerigg DG 2008 Redefining the limits of day length responsiveness in a seasonal mammal. *Endocrinology* **149** 32-39.

Walsh JP, Rao A, Thompson RC & Clarke IJ 2001 Proenkephalin and opioid mu-receptor mRNA expression in ovine hypothalamus across the estrous cycle. *Neuroendocrinology* **73** 26-36.

Wu M, Dumalska I, Morozova E, van den Pol AN & Alreja M 2009 Gonadotropin inhibitory hormone inhibits basal forebrain vGluT2-gonadotropin-releasing hormone neurons via a direct postsynaptic mechanism. *J Physiol* **587** 1401-1411.

Mammalian circannual pacemakers

GA Lincoln[1] and DG Hazlerigg[2]

[1]University of Edinburgh, Centre for Reproductive Biology, Queen's Medical Research Institute, Edinburgh EH16 4TJ; [2]University of Aberdeen, School of Biological Sciences, Zoology Building, Aberdeen AB24 2TZ

Circannual clocks drive rhythms in reproduction and many other seasonal characteristics but the underlying control of these long-term oscillators remains a mystery. Now, we propose that circannual timing involves mechanisms that are integral to the ontogenetic life-history programme where annual transitions are generated by cell birth, death and tissue regeneration throughout the life cycle – *the histogenesis hypothesis*. The intrinsic cycle is then timed by cues from the environment. The concept is that in specific sites in the brain, pituitary and peripheral tissues, residual populations of progenitor cells (adult stem cells) synchronously initiate a phase of cell division to begin a cycle. The progeny cells then proliferate, migrate and differentiate, providing the substrate that drives physiological change over long time-spans (e.g. summer/winter); cell death may be required to trigger the next cycle. We have begun to characterise such a tissue-based timer in our Soay sheep model focusing on the pars tuberalis (PT) of the pituitary gland and the sub-ventricular zone of the mediobasal hypothalamus (MBH) as potential circannual pacemakers. The PT is of special interest because it is a melatonin-responsive tissue containing undifferentiated cells, strategically located at the gateway between the brain and pituitary gland. The PT also governs long-photoperiod activation of thyroid hormone dependant processes in the MBH required for neurogenesis. In sheep, exposure to long photoperiod markedly activates BrDU-labelled cell proliferation in the PT and MBH, and acts to entrain the circannual reproductive cycle. Variation in expression and co-ordination of multiple tissue timers may explain species differences in circannual rhythmicity. This paper is dedicated to the memory of Ebo Gwinner[3].

Circannual rhythms and photoperiod time measurement

Organisms utilise two interacting timing mechanisms to regulate long-term cycles in reproduction, hibernation, moult and a plethora of seasonal characteristics (Figure 1). The principle mechanism is circannual rhythm generation where the long-term transitions in physiology are controlled endogenously by some form of interval timer or pacemaker. Circannual rhythms have been characterised in many model species notably hibernating ground squirrels and hamsters (Pengelley & Asmundson, 1974; Mrosovsky, 1978; Zucker, 2001; Concannon et al.,

---

Corresponding author E-mail: gerald.lincoln@ed.ac.uk

[3] This hypothesis was first presented for The Gwinner Lecture at the XI Congress of the European Biological Rhythms Society (EBRS) meeting in Strasbourg, France August 22-28, 2009.

1997; Kondo et al., 2006; Monecke et al., 2009), seasonal breeding deer, sheep and mustellids (Ducker et al., 1973; Goss, 1977, 1984; Herbert et al., 1978; Karsch et al., 1989; Martinet et al., 1992; Gomez-Brunet et al., 2008), seasonal migratory birds (Gwinner, 1986, 1996; Piersma et al., 2008), spawning fish (Dunstan & Bromage, 1988; Randall et al., 1998), and notably in an insect model, the varied carpet beetle *Anthrenus,* that uses a circannual clock to regulate winter diapause and hatching (Nisimura & Numata, 2002; Miyazaki et al., 2005, 2007, 2009). Circannual rhythmicity is also a feature in primates including man (Wickings & Nieschlag, 1980; Wehr, 2001). The intrinsic control is evident by the manner the various physiological rhythms free-run under constant experimental conditions. The endogenous period (circannual tau) is different from the Earth's 12-month year, often closer to 10 months, and synchrony is achieved by entrainment to periodic environmental cues.

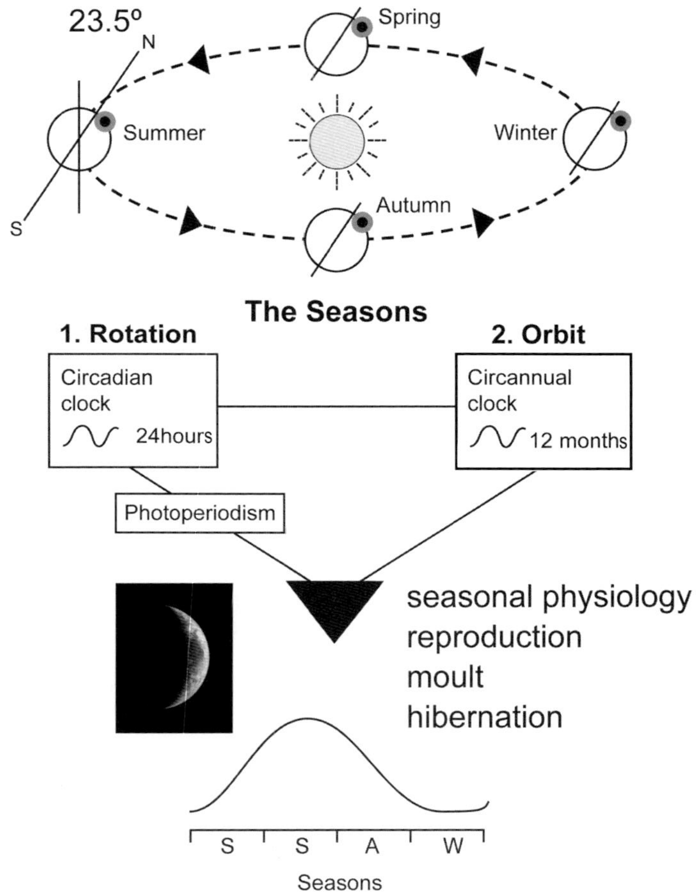

Fig. 1. Endogenous clocks anticipate the Earth's periodicities. Summary of the way the Earth's rotation on its axis every 24h (top panel; line S/N across earth indicates the rotational axis and the filled circle represents point of reference) and orbit around the Sun every 12 months have favoured the evolution of endogenous circadian clocks (based on circadian clock genes) and circannual clocks (based on tissue regeneration – current paper). The ability to respond to the annual cycle in daylength (photoperiod time measurement or photoperiodism) depends on the circadian clock system. Organisms utilise both timing mechanisms to regulate long-term cycles in reproduction, moult, hibernation and other seasonal characteristics.

Circannual rhythmicity is of fundamental importance because it allows complex changes in physiology (e.g. growth of the gonads and secondary sexual characteristics, deposition of fat reserves, growth of the winter coat) to be complete in advance of environmental change as a pre-emptive strategy anticipating the effects of the Earth's orbit (Lincoln, 2006a; Figure 1). It also allows organisms to migrate across time zones while maintaining an intrinsic sense of time, to cope with unpredictable environments such as deserts, and remarkably, to generate synchronous or asynchronous breeding patterns in the tropics according to particular ecological adaptations. Maintaining seasonal animals on a constant photoperiod where the period of the light-dark (LD) cycle differs from 24-h (e.g. 23 or 25-h days) does not affect the period of the free-running circannual rhythm (bird: Gwinner, 1986; Wikelski et al., 2008 - mammal: Carmichael & Zucker, 1986 - insect: Nisimura & Numata, 2002), thus it is unlikely that circannual and circadian timing mechanisms are directly coupled by counting days (so called frequency demultiplication).

The second near universal timing mechanism is photoperiodic time measurement (PTM or photoperiodism). This monitors the annual cycle in daylength, and drives changes in physiology appropriate to the season. Long photoperiods (>12h light/d) activate a summer phenotype and short photoperiods the winter state, with important species-differences in the critical daylength for these responses. This allows animals to vary the breeding season, moult and other characteristics related to latitude of origin. A change in photoperiod can activate or inhibit a seasonal response as a rapid inductive effect commencing within days (Hazlerigg et al., 2004; Nakao et al., 2008), and/or alter the long-term phasing of the endogenous circannual rhythm generators to achieve synchrony with the environment (Woodfill et al., 1994).

In mammals, the mechanism by which photoperiod is decoded is very well characterised (Goldman, 2001; Hazlerigg et al., 2001). This involves the relay of photoperiodic information from the retina to the suprachiasmatic nucleus (SCN) of the rostral hypothalamus. This bilateral tissue acts as the central circadian pacemaker generating a photoperiod-specific signal that governs the 24-h rhythmic pattern of melatonin production by the pineal gland. Melatonin is secreted only at night, and the *duration* of peak production reflects nightlength and thus daylength. The circulating melatonin signal is then interpreted in melatonin target tissues in the brain and pituitary gland that drive seasonal responses. The *pars tuberalis* (PT) of the pituitary gland is the best characterised melatonin target tissue (Hazlerigg et al., 2001; Hazlerigg & Loudon, 2008). It is thought to decode changes in melatonin peak duration through changes in the relative phase of rhythmic *Per* and *Cry* clock gene expression (Lincoln et al., 2002; 2006b) and/or changes in amplitude of *Per* gene expression in the PT (Wagner et al., 2008). Unlike the system generating circannual rhythms, PTM is totally dependant on the endogenous circadian system. This is because circadian clock genes control *both* the pacemaker function of the SCN that shapes the melatonin rhythm, and the decoding mechanisms in the PT that read the melatonin signal (Lincoln, 2006b).

The action of these two basic seasonal timing processes (circannual and PTM) can be dissociated using a constant long photoperiod protocol, as illustrated for sheep (Lincoln et al., 2005). Under the constant photoperiod, the circadian-based melatonin system remains locked to the ambient 24-h photoperiod cycle, while the circannual rhythm generator continues inexorably driving seasonal cycles in physiology (e.g. prolactin secretion). This provides an explanation for the so called 'photorefractory' response (Lincoln et al., 2005). The timing systems can also be dissociated in mammals by pinealectomy (PINX) or pineal denervation by superior cervical ganglionectomy (SCGX), which removes the melatonin signal and blocks photoperiod responsiveness (Woodfill et al., 1993; Lincoln et al., 1989). Such animals continue to express long-term reproductive rhythms albeit more variable than in intact animals. In hibernating ground squirrels, the circannual regulation is so dominant that PINX has only a marginal effect on the timing of seasonal rhythms in body weight and reproduction (Hiebert et al., 2000).

Circannual rhythms throughout life

The long-term study of hibernating chipmunks, *Tamias sibiricus*, by Kondo and colleagues (Kondo et al., 2006) provides the most striking example of biology controlled as an endogenous circannual rhythm. These squirrels were maintained indoors in a simulated winter-like environment of constant dim light and cold temperature, with no daily LD cycle, for up to 11 years (Figure 2). This covered the full lifespan of the animals. Under these static conditions individual animals hibernated periodically expressing phases of hypothermia - each animal showing different circannual timing. The mean circannual tau for the cycle was 10.5 months. This period was significantly shorter than 12 months, thus squirrels must generate a phase-delay in the endogenous rhythm of 1.5 months, using the PTM response, to become stably entrained outdoors.

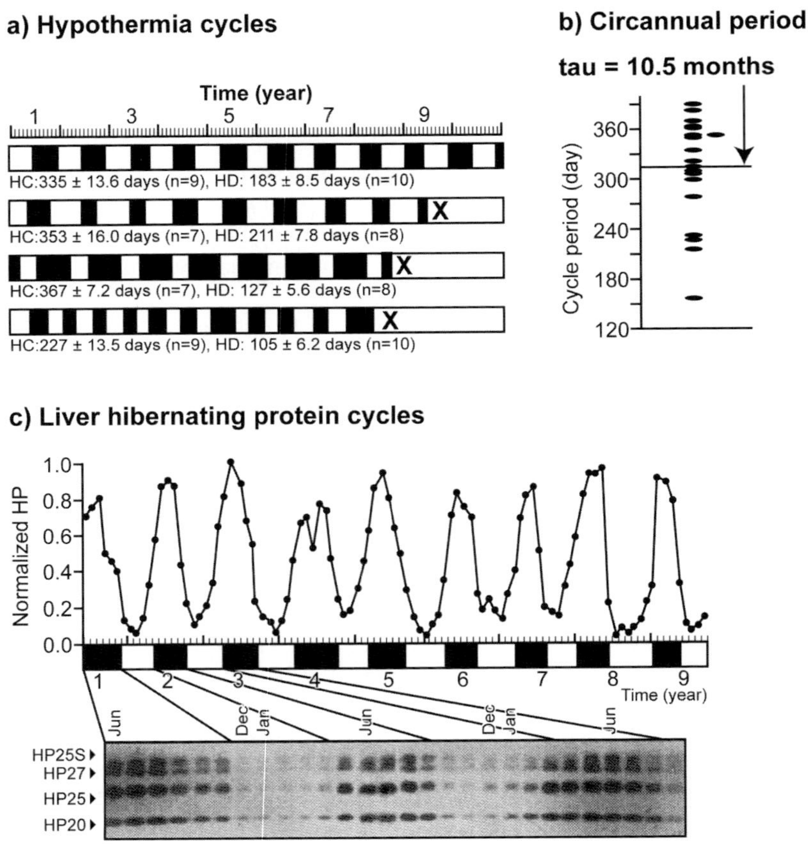

Fig. 2. Kondo's chipmunks. a) Circannual body temperature cycles in individual chipmunks (hibernating squirrels, *Tamias sibiricus*) housed indoors under constant cool temperature (4°C) and dim light for up to 11 years. The filled bars represent the periods of hypothermia associated with hibernation; HC, hibernation cycle (time from onset to next onset of hibernation; HD, hibernation duration; values mean $\pm$ SEM: X animal died). b) Mean period (circannual tau) for the temperature/hibernation rhythm for 16 individual chipmunks under constant conditions (mode: 10.5 months). c) Circannual cycles in the blood concentration of specific liver proteins (called hibernation proteins, HP) in one representative chipmunk related to the temperature/hibernation rhythm (periodic filled bar) and western blots of the concentration of the 3 different HP proteins that form a complex in the blood. The HP 27 protein is shown to dissociate at the choroid plexus entering the CSF, and affects the cold temperature resistance of brain tissue. (Adapted from Kondo et al., 2006).

Closely correlated with the hibernation rhythm were long-term cyclical changes in the blood concentrations of 3 liver proteins (so-called hibernating proteins, HP20, 25, 27) that form complexes in circulating blood. These were shown to dissociate at the level of the brain choroid plexus - with one protein entering the CNS and affecting the low-temperature tolerance of the brain (Kondo et al., 2006). There was no evidence of a progressive decline in the amplitude of the endogenous rhythm through the life history, which is a feature seen in many free-running circannual rhythms (Lincoln et al., 2006).

This remarkable persistence of circannual rhythmicity has also been documented in a passerine bird species, the stonechat *Saxicola torquata*, in a classical study (Gwinner, 2003). A single male bird was kept in the laboratory under an equatorial LD 12:12 lighting regimen for more than 10 years. Testis volume was measured at regular intervals through a minor incision in the abdomen, and the progression of the annual feather moult was scored. The animal expressed a gonadal cycle every 10 months with an associated post-nuptial moult throughout its entire life in captivity, registering 12 complete cycles in 10 years. There was a small change in the relative phasing of the gonadal and pelage rhythms, but they remained closely coupled throughout the life cycle. Parallel studies in other passerine bird species demonstrated that birds hand-reared in captivity, with no contact with their parents and living permanently under constant photoperiod, may express species-specific circannual rhythms in reproduction, moult, body weight and migratory restlessness, thus providing clear evidence for genetic control to a cyclical circannual programme (Gwinner, 1986).

Not all species express 'short-period' circannual rhythms: the great knot, *Calidris tenuirostris,* a long-distance migratory wader, expresses a free-running rhythm >12 months in body mass, moult and feather development under constant LD 12:12 (Piersma et al., 2008). In this case, the body mass and feather growth rhythms in part dissociated, suggesting that they may be regulated by separate oscillatory mechanisms. One specimen of the related red knot, *Calidris canutus,* kept indoors as a pet for 20 years replaced its feathers and changed behaviour circannually throughout life.

Cyclical life histories

The conventional view of the life history in any vertebrate is of a smooth progression from the foetus - to the juvenile - to the adult, and to senescence of old age. In this life history pattern there is a single juvenile to adult transition – we call this the *generic model* (Figure 3, panel A). It represents the sequence of events in short-lived species. The alternative is a *cyclical model* that is potentially more realistic for long-lived species (Figure 3, panel B). In this ontogenetic programme, repeated transitions between active and quiescent occur during adult life, and each represents a circannual cycle. In species adapted to cold and temperate climates, including the chipmunk and migratory birds illustrated above, the cyclic transitions of adulthood are predictably synchronised to the seasons of food plenty and scarcity – with an obvious selective advantage driving the evolution of the circannual clockwork. For species living nearer the equator where conditions are less predictable, expressing a cyclic biology can be equally advantageous, because it can increase an individual's reproductive success. This may involve focusing reproductive effort or avoiding predation, as described for seabird species living near the Equator (Ashmole & Ashmole, 1967; Harris, 1970).

The life cycle pattern in male elephants provides an example of a long-lived, tropical species expressing delayed endogenous circannual rhythmicity and asynchrony (Figure 3C). In both African (*Loxodonta*) and Indian (*Elephas*) elephants, males characteristically express an annual musth cycle regulated by major seasonal swings in testosterone secretion (Cooper et al., 1990; Lincoln & Ratnasooriya, 1996). Elephants reach puberty at 10-15 years of age when still physically immature, and overt behavioural cyclicity only develops in the second half of the life-span from 30-years onwards – by which time the bulls have grown markedly in body size and become socially dominant. The annual patterns of musth behaviour shown by the large bull elephants in the Amboseli National Park in Kenya, close to the Equator, have been recorded over many years (Poole & Moss, 1981; Poole, 1987). These studies demonstrate that mature males have a 2-3 month musth season every year, but each individual develops its own preferred season. This 'personal' timing can be maintained over many years in the mature animals, but can be adjusted by social cues (e.g. death of a dominant male, Poole, 1987). The elephant provides an example of asynchrous cyclicity, similar to that described in tropical axis deer (Loudon & Curlewis, 1988; Lincoln et al., 1994) and fruit bats (O'Brien, 1993; Heideman & Bronson, 1994), although in these smaller species the endogenous cyclicity starts early in the life cycle. One ecological explanation for this phenomenon is that males avoid competition by rutting asynchronously, but as we can now understand, mechanistically they utilise an endogenous circannual clock.

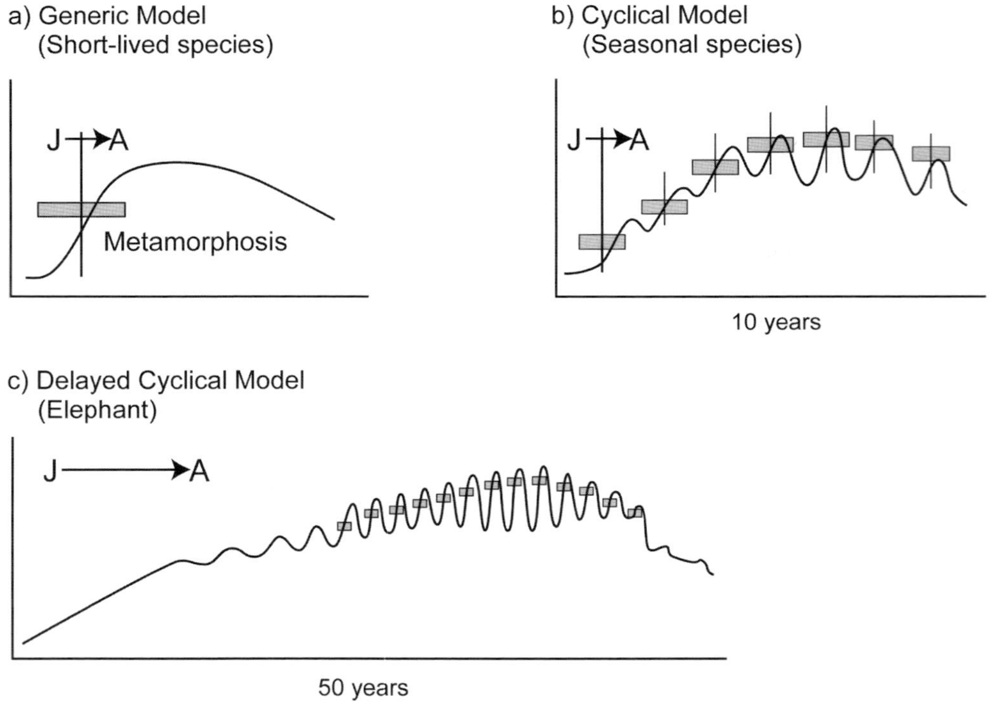

Fig. 3. Vertebrate life-history models illustrating changes in body weight or testis size. a) Generic model depicts a smooth change across the life-history with a single juvenile-adult (J-A) transition (or metamorphosis). This represents a short-lived species. b) Cyclical model with a juvenile-adult (J-A) transition followed by a series of repeated transitions throughout the life-history each representing an endogenous circannual cycle – circannual cycles are an integral part of the life-history programme. This represents a wide spectrum of seasonal species and is regarded as the ancestral pattern for vertebrates. c) Delayed cyclical model where the animal gradually matures and the circannual cyclicity in gonadal activity and sexual behaviour begins in the second half of the life history. This represents the pattern seen in male African (*Loxodonta*) and Indian (*Elephas*) elephants.

The cyclic life-history programme accurately describes a wide spectrum of seasonal species (Figure 3). Because ancestral vertebrates were cold-blooded and most vulnerable to the adverse effects of a seasonal environment, it is logical to expect that endogenous circannual clocks evolved early in vertebrate evolution. This is consistent with the occurrence of circannual rhythmicity in fish (e.g. catfish, Sundararja et al., 1982; trout, Dunstan & Bromage, 1988; Randall et al., 1998; stickleback, Bornestaf & Borg, 2000) and reptiles (e.g. lizard species, Fisher, 1970; Cuellar & Cuellar, 1977; Bertolucci et al., 1999). Moreover, long-lived insects and other invertebrates express circannual rhythms (Miyazaki et a., 2005) – thus circannual timing is likely to be part of ancestral life-history programmes.

Circannual rhythm generators

Ebo Gwinner states in his review of circannual rhythms (Gwinner 1986, p97) 'the most formidable physiological problem in circannual rhythm research arises from the extremely long duration of the process involved. Some of the changes that occur within or between the various fractions of a circannual cycle have time constants that are way beyond the range of time constants known for any neuroendocrine feedback loop and are in many respects reminiscent of developmental processes occurring during ontogeny, e.g. sexual maturation'.

This fits with the concept of the cyclical life history model and supports our new working hypothesis - the *histogenesis hypothesis* (Figure 4). The hypothesis proposes that circannual timing utilizes mechanisms that are an integral part of the ontogenetic life history programme where the intrinsic rhythms depend on cyclical tissue regeneration. Rhythmicity is thought to occur in multiple sites in the brain, pituitary gland and peripheral tissues where populations of progenitor cells/adult stem cells synchronously divide to initiate a new circannual cycle; this is repeated periodically during adulthood. The progeny cells proliferate, migrate and differentiate, similar to the events occurring during embryonic development, providing new tissue in the adult that drives a particular physiological transition. We envisage that some form of feedback signal from the newly differentiated cells acts to terminate the episode of progenitor cell proliferation - thus timing the circannual cycle. The trigger for the next cycle may depend on apoptosis, or some other form of regulated decline in cell function, as part of the timing mechanism.

The very long time constants of the circannual rhythm are presumed to result from the protracted nature of the differentiation process that produce new cell lineages that ultimately take control of a physiological system for many months, combined with the long intrinsic lifespan of these regenerated cells. The novel feature of this hypothesis is not in the idea of regeneration *per se*, since this is a feature in all tissues in the adult, but is in its *synchronous* nature, and in its *hierarchical control* co-ordinated by the brain and pituitary (see below). We propose that there must be mechanisms that govern each step of the cycle of regeneration in a specific tissue. Since 10-monthly circannual rhythms are often reported, this period will be the summation of a series of stages each lasting a few months. The presumption is that a stage is controlled by a set of genes (governing growth factors, neurogenic compounds, etc.) generating the progression of a circannual cycle. This concept of a "sequence of stages" based on tissue regeneration is fundamentally different from that originally proposed by Mrosovsky (Mrosovsky, 1970), where the proposed "stages" were physiological systems, and the cycle was the product of sequentially switching from one physiological state to the next (e.g. growth - reproduction - moult - hibernation). This later model is untenable because circannual rhythms persist after ablating specific physiological systems (Lincoln et al., 2006) and circannual rhythms can dissociate (Gwinner, 1986; Martinet et al., 1992; Piersma et al., 2008).

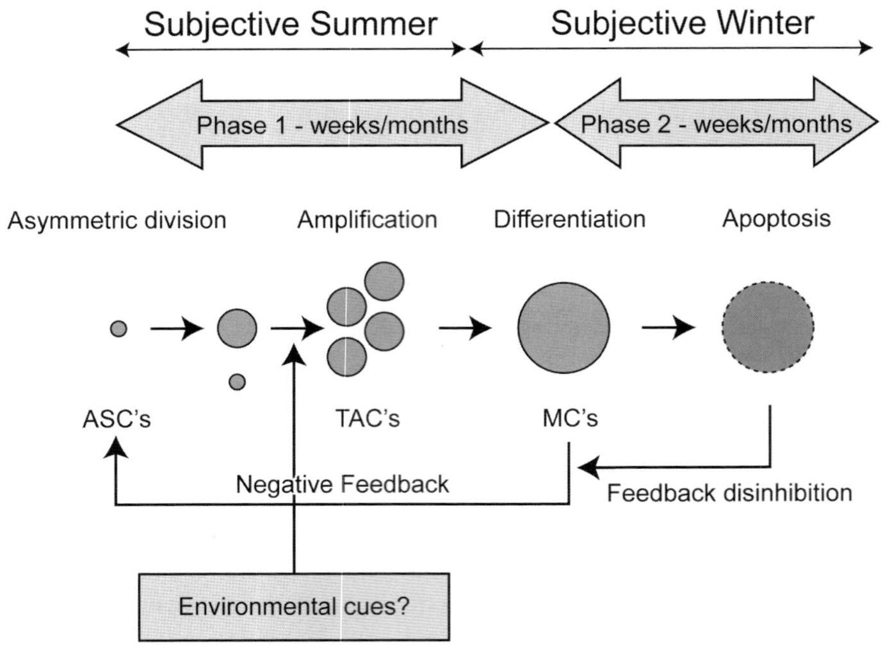

Fig. 4. Working hypothesis for the generation of circannual rhythms by histogenesis. During Phase 1 (subjective summer), adult stem cells (ASCs) divide asymmetrically within a stem cell niche producing transient amplifying cells (TACs) that move out and divide multiple times, before differentiating into mature cells (MCs) that express specific marker genes. We propose that these mature cells produce negative feedback signals that block further ASC and TAC division. This initiates Phase 2 (subjective winter) during which negative inhibition persists until apoptosis of MCs or some other form of spontaneous tissue change causes feedback disinhibition to trigger the next circannual cycle. Environmental cues notably photoperiod, but other factors as well, are thought to be relayed to the sites of tissue regeneration and alter timing. This causes a change in phase (advance or delay according to the stage of the cycle) and permits entrainment to a seasonal environment.

We propose that photoperiod and other environmental cues act at specific stages of the regenerative cycle to alter the period of the circannual rhythm to permit entrainment. This could be during the proliferative phase of the endogenous cycle where the extrinsic signal acts to suppress or prolong the propagation of new cells, thus causing a phase-advance or -delay in the intrinsic cycle generator (Figure 4). This is analogous to the manner daily light signals entrain the circadian clock by affecting the rhythmic expression of specific clock genes (Reppert & Weaver, 2002). A phase-response curve for the effect of long photoperiod has been described in the trout (Dunstan & Bromage, 1988), European hamster (Monecke et al., 2009), and in detail in the carpet beetle, *Anthrenus* (Miyazaki et al., 2007). The circannual clock behaves like a readily entrainable oscillator (Miyazaki et al., 2005; Lincoln et al., 2006). While circannual and circadian rhythms are undoubtedly generated by different genetic mechanisms, their formal entrainment properties are remarkably similar.

Circannual rhythm generators

Histogenesis in the pituitary gland

The pars tuberalis (PT) of the pituitary gland is a very well characterised melatonin target tissue that may act as a specialised circannual timer (Hazlerigg et al., 2001; Lincoln, 2002; Lincoln et al., 2003a & b) (Figure 5). The PT expresses a high density of melatonin mt_1 receptors in the adult in a wide range of seasonal mammals and birds. The tissue is strategically located at the gateway between the brain and pituitary gland, and potentially regulates long-term cycles in several major physiological systems. The main secretory cell-type is the PT thyrotroph - distinct from the thyrotrophs of the pituitary pars distalis (PD) that secrete TSH to control the peripheral thyroid axis (Bockmann et al., 1997; Wittkowski et al., 1999).

The PT cells, by contrast, secrete TSH that acts locally in the mediobasal hypothalamus to regulate thyroid hormone dependant mechanisms and thus drive seasonal biology (Nakao et al., 2008; Hanon et al., 2008; Ono et al., 2009). This involves TSH activation of deiodinase type-2 (DIO_2) in the adjacent tanycytes that line the base of the third ventricle (3V), catalysing the conversion of thyroxin (T4) to its biologically active form tri-iodothyronine (T3). It is the local increase in T3 that activates a cascade of neuroendocrine responses induced by long photoperiod to produce a summer reproductive phenotype (Hazlerigg & Loudon, 2008). The PT cells also secrete other factors that act in a more predictable retrograde manner in the pituitary gland itself. This includes neurokinins that modulate prolactin production by lactotrophs to regulate the seasonal reproductive changes and the pelage moult cycle (Dupre et al., 2010).

Strong evidence that the pituitary gland and particularly the PT acts as a circannual rhythm generator comes from studies using hypothalamo-pituitary disconnected (HPD) Soay sheep (Lincoln et al., 2006). The HPD operation permanently destroys the arcuate nucleus and median eminence and consequently the PT control of the mediobasal hypothalamus, but spares the PT regulation of the lactotrophs (Figure 5). HPD sheep are sexually inactive indicative of the loss of hypothalamic regulation, but continue to express normal cyclical changes in prolactin secretion and the associated moult. Long photoperiod activates, and short photoperiod suppresses, prolactin release (Lincoln & Clarke, 1994; Lincoln, 2002), and exposure to constant long photoperiod produces circannual rhythms in prolactin that persist for at least 4 cycles (Lincoln et al., 2006). Circannual tau is close to 10 months in the HPD sheep. The generation of the circannual rhythm has been mathematically modelled based on the interaction between the melatonin-responsive thyrotroph cells in the PT and the lactotrophs in the PD, and predicts very long feedback delays in the clockwork mechanism (MacGregor & Lincoln, 2008).

The PT may act as a specialised circannual timer because it contains undifferentiated/uncommitted cells that can activate a protracted cycle of cell differentiation and decline (Wittkowski et al., 1999; Hazlerigg, 2001). We have just begun to measure changes in the rate of cell proliferation in the PT and the MBH in Soay sheep using bromodeoxyuridine (BrDU) to label dividing cells (Figure 6). Labelled cell nuclei were counted at 24-hours after BrDU treatment. Proliferation rates in the PT and MBH were maximal at 4 weeks into long photoperiod and decreased spontaneously by 20 weeks long photoperiod associated with the progression of the circannual cycle (photorefractory state). Following a switch in photoperiod, lowest proliferation was at 4 weeks into short photoperiod. This is the beginning of an expansive study to identify the phenotype of the dividing cells and trace their fate after differentiation.

Neurogenesis in the brain

There are multiple sites of neurogenesis in the adult brain that may act as tissue timers and contribute to long-term timing. Of particular interest in relation to thyroid hormone control

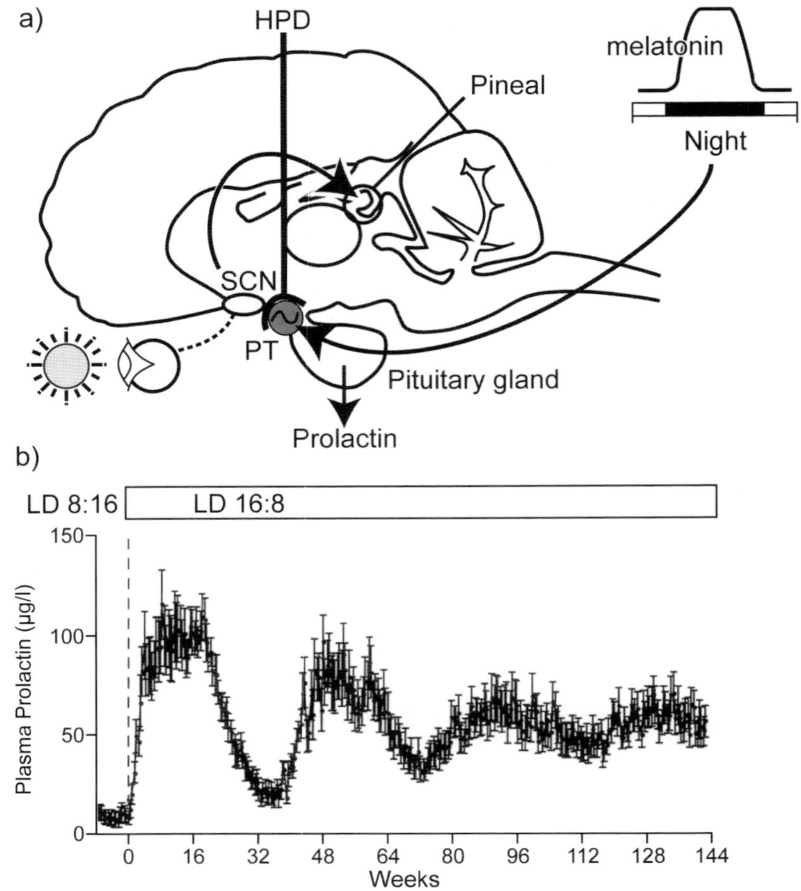

Fig. 5. Hypothalamo-pituitary disconnected (HPD) Soay sheep under constant photoperiod. a) Diagram of the sheep brain illustrating the relay by which light information is transmitted from the retina to the suprachiasmatic nucleus (SCN, central circadian pacemaker) and to the pineal gland that produces a nocturnal melatonin signal that reflects the photoperiod. The melatonin signal acting via the blood is then decoded in the pars tuberalis (PT) of the pituitary gland to affect prolactin secretion from the pituitary lactotrophs. Note, the HPD operation permanently destroys the median eminence and arcuate nucleus isolating the pituitary from direct regulation by the hypothalamus (see HPD, curve line) but maintains the signalling by melatonin. b) Long-term prolactin profiles in HPD Soay transferred from short photoperiod (LD 8:16) to long photoperiod (LD 16:8) and kept under long photoperiod for 144 weeks. A circannual prolactin rhythm was evident in all HPD sheep that persisted for at least 4 cycles becoming asynchronous, and dampening in amplitude with time. The mean circannual tau was 10.2 months. Values are mean ± SEM, n= 10. (Adapted from Lincoln et al., 2006).

by the PT, is the subventricular zone (SZH) surrounding the base of the 3V in the mediobasal hypothalamus. The tanycytes in this region appear to be progenitor cells, whose progeny can migrate into target regions including the lateral hypothalamus and arcuate nuclei to adopt hypothalamic neuronal fates (Xu et al., 2005; Hajihosseini et al., 2008). Changing neurogenesis in the SZH may thus alter the hypothalamic functional set-points, and drive long-term cycles

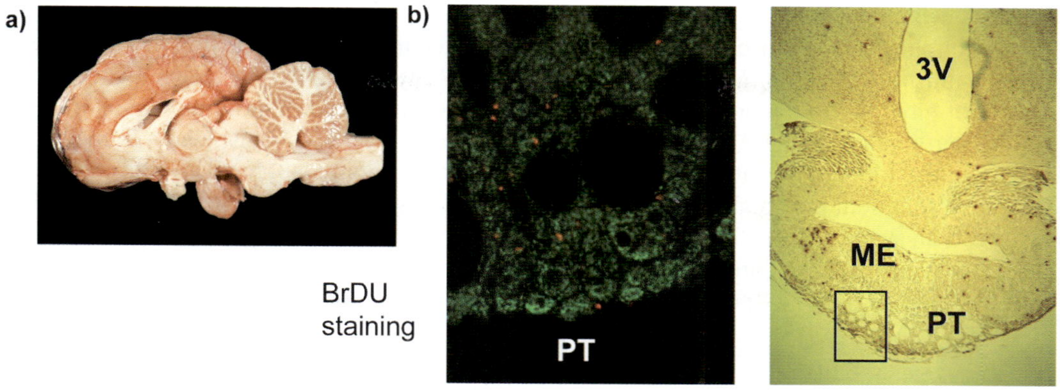

Fig. 6. Photoperiod-induced cell proliferation in the sheep PT and mediobasal hypothalamus. a) Sheep brain cut along the mid-line showing the site of the histological section. b) Coronal section of the sheep pituitary pars tuberalis (PT) and median eminence (ME), immuno-stained to reveal bromo-deoxyuridine (BrDU) labelled cells, indicative of cells that divided within the last 24h. Left panel, PT BrDU positive cells labelled in red; right panel, PT and ME BrDU positive cells labelled in brown. Images from Cathy Wyse.

in physiology and behaviour. This concept is supported by studies of changes in body weight and energy metabolism in laboratory mice induced by the central administration of cilary neurotrophic factor (CNTF) (Kokoeva et al., 2005). This treatment caused cell proliferation in the SZH, migration of progeny cells to the appetite regulatory centres in the paraventricular hypothalamus and differentiation into neurones expressing appetite regulatory peptides. There was a corresponding change in food intake and body weight that lasted several months after the end of treatment. We have recently demonstrated that the *cntf* gene is expressed in the PT and CNTF receptor is expressed in the adjacent mediobasal hypothalamus in our Soay sheep model, consistent with a role in regulating seasonal rhythms (E.Hanon unpublished data).

Cell proliferation also occurs in the adult brain in the subventricular zone of the lateral ventricle (SVZ), producing a rostral stream of progenitor cells that differentiate in the olfactory bulb, and in the subgranular zone (SGZ) of the dentate gyrus of the hippocampus where the new cells become granular cell neurones contributing to learning and spatial memory. Seasonal changes in hippocampal neurogenesis have been well studied in birds related to song control in the breeding season and food caching in winter (Nottebohm, 1989; Barnea & Nottebohm, 1994) and related to repeated long distance migration (Pravosudov et al., 2006). Long-term changes also occur in mammals related to season, photoperiod and/or sex hormonal status (Huang et al., 1998; Galea & McEwen, 1999; Lavenex et al., 2000; Pyter et al., 2005; Xu. et al., 2005). In adult golden hamsters, the number of BrDU positive cells in the dentate gyrus and subependymal zone doubled in animals exposed to short photoperiod (Huang et al., 1998).

Circannual pacemaker shop

The histogenesis hypothesis extends to include regenerative mechanisms in the brain, pituitary and in a range of other peripheral body organs in the control of circannual rhythms. The concept of a circannual pacemaker shop is summarised in Figure 7. In this model, all tissues have a major degree of autonomy in their regeneration and thus can contribute to long-term timing of physiological cycles in the adult. The key feature in animals with a cyclical life history is the degree to which proliferation is synchronised within an organ or physiological system, with the timing entrainable by environmental cues. The evidence for long-term cycling in a peripheral organ is illustrated in chipmunks expressing circannual rhythms in liver proteins related to the control of hibernation (Figure 5). While the cyclicity is intrinsic to different tissues, it may require co-ordination by the PT, mediobasal hypothalamus and possibly elsewhere in the brain, to govern the functional state of the whole body, which requires appropriate phasing of the different circannual pacemakers (Figure 7). This again has parallels with the co-ordination of the circadian system by the SCN. The circannual clockwork is presumed to have much greater inertia because it is based on histogenesis; hence migratory animals (or globe-trotting humans) will not suffer seasonal jet lag!

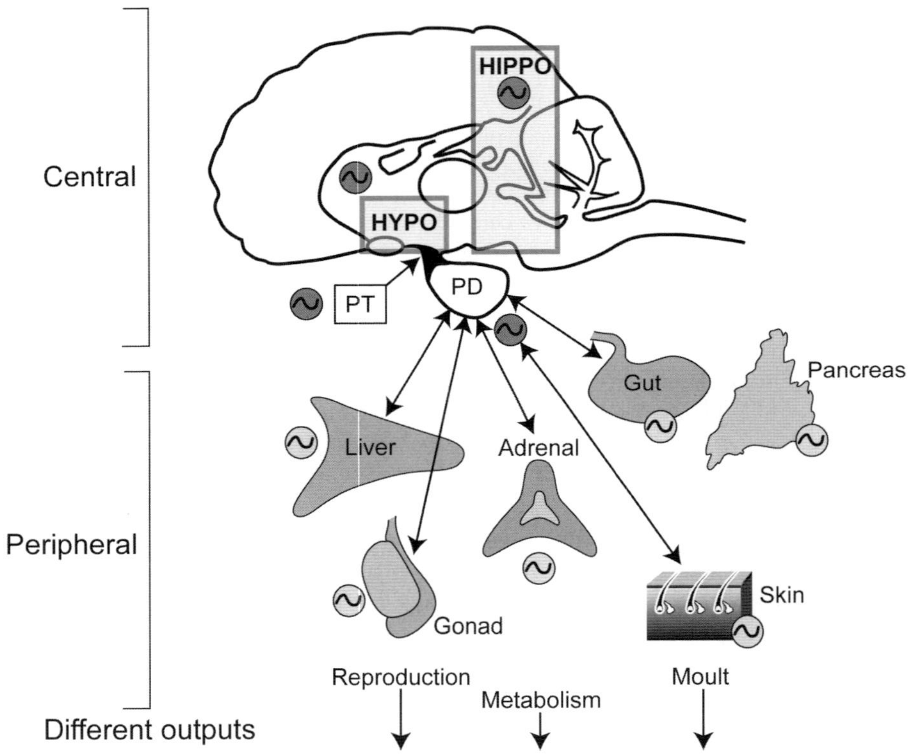

Fig. 7. The Circannual System. The current concept is that there are multiple sites in the brain, pituitary and peripheral organs where cyclical histogenesis contributes to the circannual rhythmicity. Each physiological system (regulating reproduction, metabolism, moult etc) is thought to have its own circannual timer with brain/pituitary sites potentially providing for integration of the multiple systems, and allowing entrainment to environmental cues. Parallels are drawn with the circadian system where the SCN acts as a central pacemaker for peripheral clocks. Autonomy of circannual timers allows for major species differences in the timing of the various physiological rhythms.

The hair follicle provides a model of a tissue-based clock (Schneider et al., 2009). This structure is a mini-organ capable of growing a complete hair over a period of many weeks modulated by hormones and other signals, and the genes controlling the initiation, growth, morphological form, maturation and rest phases are very well characterised based on mutagenesis analysis in mice. Nestin-expressing adult cells localised in the bulb region of the resting hair follicle appear to initiate the next growth cycle, but the intrinsic clock/timer is still a mystery (Schneider et al., 2009). In seasonal animals, the hair follicles alternate between growing short, fine hairs in summer and long, thicker insulating hairs in winter, and the cycle is regulated in part by seasonal changes in prolactin secretion (Choy et al., 1995; Lincoln et al., 2003b). Evidence that this cyclic state is also intrinsically controlled at the level of the skin is provided by a study in red deer (*Cervus elaphus*) in which animals in their winter coat were treated with a subcutaneous implant that infused prolactin locally into the skin over a period of 28 days (Loudon & Jabbour, 1994). This induced the premature growth of a small patch of red summer coat, which subsequently reversed to growing a winter coat, and remained out of synchrony with the hair follicles of the rest of the body for at least 6 months, before realignment. This nicely illustrates a degree of autonomy of timing in a peripheral tissue - fitting into the concept of an integrated timing system (Figure 7).

Regulated regenerative processes are a feature of all tissues and are currently the focus of intensive research effort in liver (Forbes et al., 2002), heart (Anversa et al., 2004), pituitary (Levy 2008; Fauquier et al, 2008; Gleiberman el al., 2008), hair follicles (Schneider et al., 2009) and testis (Davidoff et al., 2004). The aim is to characterise stem cell niches, isolate stem cells and to identify the growth factors and other signals produced by the differentiation of mature cell lineages. In these model systems, synchronous regeneration (as seen in seasonal animals) can be induced by tissue ablation. Resection of a major part of the liver, for example, triggers a synchronous wave of cell division involving multiple progenitor cell types derived from the biliary tree and associated blood vascular structures of the liver. This proliferative process slows once the liver mass recovers to normal indicating the involvement of negative feedback signalling for tissue homeostasis. Similarly, treatment of rats with the toxin ethane dimethanesulphonate (EDS) specifically ablates the Leydig cells in the adult testis removing the source of testosterone, and triggers the synchronous regeneration of a new population of Leydig cells (Davidoff et al., 2004). In this case, stem cells are located in the vascular endothelial tissue of the blood vessels and migrate out into the interstitial tissue and differentiate into new Leydig cells. There is a sequential activation of cell-specific genes over a period of 28 days including the genes regulating testicular steroidogenesis (Davidoff et al., 2004). The local tissue signals that trigger the initial proliferation and later curtail the regeneration response are still to be identified.

Conclusions

We propose that cyclical histogenesis forms the basis of endogenous circannual rhythm generation as an integral part of the life history programme. This is ancestrally cyclical in vertebrates. Regenerative mechanisms persist throughout adulthood driving rhythms of growth and decline across the year. The endogenous timing is adaptive because it allows the organism to profoundly change its physiology and phenotype over long time-scales of many months to anticipate environmental change and thus maximise survival and reproductive success. We present preliminary evidence that cyclical histogenesis occurs in specific sites in the pituitary gland, brain and peripheral tissues that potentially govern circannual rhythms in reproduction, moult and other characteristics. It is likely that each physiological system has its own circannual timer mechanism, integrated centrally to produce the circannual timing system that differs between species. Parallels are drawn with the control of the circadian system where the SCN provides a central pacemaker. At present, the pituitary PT is the best candidate for a central circannual pacemaker. Our current aim is to manipulate cell proliferation mechanisms in the PT and hypothalamus in our Soay sheep model to investigate effects on circannual rhythms, and to characterise the adult stem cell niches in these circannual timing tissues.

Acknowledgements

Our special thanks go to Joan Docherty, Marjorie Thomson, and the staff of the Marshall Building for their dedicated help in running the large animal facility, to Cathy Wyse (University of Aberdeen) and Elodie Hanon (University of Edinburgh) for use of histology images and related data, to Ronnie Grant (University of Edinburgh) for the graphics and to Barbara Helm (University of Konstanz, Germany) for her constructive comments on the manuscript. The work was supported by grants from the MRC and BBSRC, UK

References

Anversa P, Kajstura J, Leri A 2004 Circulating progenitor cells: search for an identity. *Circulation* 110 3158-3160.

Ashmole NP, Ashmole MJ 1967 Comparative feeding ecology of seabirds of a tropicak oceanic island. *Peabody Mus Nat Hist*, Bull 24.

Barnea A, Nottebohm F 1994 Seasonal recruitment of hippocampal neurons in adult free-ranging black-capped chickadees. *Proc Natl Acad Sci* U S A. 91 11217-11221.

Bertolucci C, Leorati M, Innocenti A, Foa A 1999 Circannual variations of lizard circadian activity rhythms in constant darkness. *Behav Ecol Sociobiol* 46 200-209.

Bockmann J, Böckers TM, Winter C, Wittkowski W, Winterhoff H, Deufel T, Kreutz MR 1997 Thyrotropin expression in hypophyseal pars tuberalis-specific cells is 3,5,3′-triiodothyronine, thyrotropin-releasing hormone, and pit-1 independent. *Endocrinology* 138 1019-1928.

Bornestaf C, Borg B 2000 Endogenous breeding cycles in male threespine sticklebacks, *Gasterosteus aculeatus*. *Behaviour* 137 921-932.

Carmichael MS, Zucker I 1986 Circannual rhythms of ground squirrels: a test of the frequency demultiplication hypothesis. *J Biol Rhythms* 1 277-284.

Choy VJ, Nixon AJ, Pearson AJ 1995 Distribution of prolactin receptor immunoreactivity in ovine skin and changes during the wool follicle growth cycle. *J Endocrinol* 155 265-275.

Concannon P, Roberts P, Baldwin B, Tennant B 1997 Long-term entrainment of circannual reproductive and metabolic cycles by Northern and Southern Hemisphere photoperiods in woodchucks (*Marmota monax*). Biol Reprod 57 1008-1015.

Cooper KA Harder JD, Clawson DH, Frederick DL Lodge GA Peachey HC Spellmire TJ Winstel DP 1990 Serum testosterone and musth in captive African and Asian elephants. *Zoo Biol* 9 297-306.

Cuellar HS, Cuellar O 1977 Evidence for endogenous rhythmicity in the reproductive cycle of the parthenogenic lizard *Cnemidophorus uniparens*. Copeia 19 554-557.

Davidoff MS, Middendorff R, Enikolopov G, Riethmacher D, Holstein AF, Müller D 2004 Progenitor cells of the testosterone-producing Leydig cells revealed. *J Cell Biol* 167 935-944.

Ducker MJ, Bowman JC, Temple A 1973 The effect of constant photoperiod on the expression of oestrus in the ewe. *J Reprod Fertil* Suppl 19 143-150.

Dunstan J, Bromage N 1988 The entrainment and gating of the endogenous circannual rhythms of reproduction in the female rainbow trout (*Salmo gairdneri*). *J Comp Physiol* A 164 259-268.

Dupré SM, Miedzinska K, Duval CV, Yu L, Goodman RL, Lincoln GA, Davis JR, McNeilly AS, Burt DD, Loudon AS 2010 Identification of Eya3 and TAC1 as long-day signals in the sheep pituitary. *Curr Biol* 20 829-35.

Fauquier T, Rizzoti K, Dattani M, Lovell-Badge R, Robinson IC 2008 SOX2-expressing progenitor cells generate all of the major cell types in the adult mouse pituitary gland. *Proc Natl Acad Sci* U S A 105 2907-2912.

Fisher K 1970 Untersuchungen zur Jahresperiodik der Fortpflanzung bei mannlichen Ruineneidechsen (*Lacerta sicula campestris* Betta). III. Spontanes Einsetzen und Ausklingen der Gonadenaktivitat; ein Beitrag zur Frage der circannualen Periodik. *Z Vergl Physiol* 66 273-293.

Forbes S, Vig P, Poulsom R, Thomas H, Alison M. 2002 Hepatic stem cells. *J Pathol* 197 510-518. Review.

Galea LA, McEwen BS 1999 Sex and seasonal differences in the rate of cell proliferation in the dentate gyrus of adult wild meadow voles. *Neuroscience* 89 955-964.

Gleiberman AS, Michurina T, Encinas JM, Roig JL, Krasnov P, Balordi F, Fishell G, Rosenfeld MG, Enikolopov G 2008 Genetic approaches identify adult pituitary stem cells. *Proc Natl Acad Sci* U S A 105 6332-6337.

Goldman BD 2001 Mammalian photoperiodic system: formal properties and neuroendocrine mechanisms of photoperiodic time measurement. *J Biol Rhythms* 16 283-301.

Gómez-Brunet A, Santiago-Moreno J, del Campo A, Malpaux B, Chemineau P, Tortonese DJ, Gonzalez-Bulnes A, López-Sebastián A 2008 Endogenous circannual cycles of ovarian activity and changes in prolactin and melatonin secretion in wild and domestic female sheep maintained under a long-day photoperiod. *Biol Reprod* 78 552-62.

Goss RJ 1977 Photoperiodic control of antler cycles in deer. IV Effects of constant light:dark ratios on circannual rhythms. *J Exp Zool* 201 379-382.

Goss RJ 1984 Photoperioduc control of antler cycles in deer. VI Circannual rhythms on altered day lengths. *J Expl Zool* 230 265-272.

Gwinner E 1986 Circannual Rhythms: Endogenous Annual

Clocks in the Organization of Seasonal Processes pp 1-156. Berlin: Springer-Verlag.

Gwinner E 1996 Circadian and circannual programmes in avian migration. *J Exp Biol* 199 39-48.

Gwinner E 2003 Circannual rhythms in birds. *Curr Opin Neurobiol* 13 770-778. Review.

Hajihosseini MK, De Langhe S, Lana-Elola E, Morrison H, Sparshott N, Kelly R, Sharpe J, Rice D, Bellusci S 2008 Localization and fate of Fgf10-expressing cells in the adult mouse brain implicate Fgf10 in control of neurogenesis. *Mol Cell Neurosci* 37 857-868.

Hanon EA, Lincoln GA, Fustin JM, Dardente H, Masson-Pévet M, Morgan PJ, Hazlerigg DG 2008 Ancestral TSH mechanism signals summer in a photoperiodic mammal. *Curr Biol* 18 1147-1152.

Harris MP 1970 Breeding ecology of the swallow-tailed gull, *Creagrus furcatus*. *Auk* 87 215-243.

Hazlerigg DG, Andersson H, Johnston JD, Lincoln G 2004 Molecular characterization of the long-day response in the Soay sheep, a seasonal mammal. *Curr Biol* 14 334-339.

Hazlerigg D, Loudon A 2008 New insights into ancient seasonal life timers. *Curr Biol* 18 R795-R804. Review.

Hazlerigg DG, Morgan PJ, Messager S 2001 Decoding photoperiodic time and melatonin in mammals: what can we learn from the pars tuberalis? *J Biol Rhythms* 2001 16 326-335. Review.

Heideman PD, Bronson FH 1994 An endogenous circannual rhythm of reproduction in a tropical bat, Anoura geoffroyi, is not entrained by photoperiod. *Biol Reprod* 50 607-14.

Herbert J Stracey PM Thorpe DH 1978 Recurrent breeding season in pinealectomized or optic-nerve –sectioned ferrets. *J Endocrinol* 78 389-397.

Hiebert SM, Thomas EM, Lee TM, Pelz KM, Yellon SM, Zucker I 2000 Photic entrainment of circannual rhythms in golden-mantled ground squirrels: role of the pineal gland. *J Biol Rhyth* 15 126-134.

Huang L, DeVries GJ, Bittman EL 1998 Photoperiod regulates neuronal bromodeoxyuridine labeling in the brain of a seasonally breeding mammal. *J Neurobiol* 36 410-420.

Karsch FJ, Robinson JE, Woodfill CJ, Brown MB 1989 Circannual cycles of luteinizing hormone and prolactin secretion in ewes during prolonged exposure to a fixed photoperiod: evidence for an endogenous reproductive rhythm. *Biol Reprod* 41 1034-1046.

Kokoeva MV, Yin H, Flier JS 2005 Neurogenesis in the hypothalamus of adult mice: potential role in energy balance. *Science* 310 679-683.

Kondo N, Sekijima T, Kondo J, Takamatsu N, Tohya K, Ohtsu T 2006 Circannual control of hibernation by HP complex in the brain. *Cell* 125 161-172.

Lavenex P, Steele MA, Jacobs LF 2000 The seasonal pattern of cell proliferation and neuron number in the dentate gyrus of wild adult eastern grey squirrels. *Eur J Neurosci* 12 643-648.

Levy A 2008 Stem cells, hormones and pituitary adenomas. *J Neuroendocrinol* 20 139-140. Review.

Lincoln G, Messager S, Andersson H, Hazlerigg D 2002 Temporal expression of seven clock genes in the suprachiasmatic nucleus and the pars tuberalis of the sheep: evidence for an internal coincidence timer. *Proc Natl Acad Sci* U S A. 99 13890-13895.

Lincoln GA 2002 Neuroendocrine regulation of seasonal gonadotrophin and prolactin rhythms: lessons from the Soay ram model. *Reproduction* Suppl 59:131-147. Review.

Lincoln GA 2006a Melatonin entrainment of circannual rhythms. *Chronobiol Int* 23 301-306.

Lincoln GA 2006b Decoding the nightly melatonin signal through circadian clockwork. *Mol Cell Endocrinol* 252 69-73.

Lincoln GA, Andersson H, Hazlerigg D 2003a Clock genes and the long-term regulation of prolactin secretion: evidence for a photoperiod/circannual timer in the pars tuberalis. *J Neuroendocrinol* 15 390-7. Review.

Lincoln GA, Andersson H, Loudon A 2003b Clock genes in calendar cells as the basis of annual timekeeping in mammals - a unifying hypothesis. *J Endocrinol* 1791-13. Review.

Lincoln GA, Clarke IJ 1994 Photoperiodically-induced cycles in the secretion of prolactin in hypothalamo-pituitary disconnected rams: evidence for translation of the melatonin signal in the pituitary gland. *J Neuroendocrinol* 6 251-60.

Lincoln GA, Clarke IJ, Hut RA, Hazlerigg DG 2006 Characterizing a mammalian circannual pacemaker. *Science* 314 1941-1944.

Lincoln GA, Dayawansa N, Ratnasooriya WD 1994 Characteristics of the antler cycle in male axis deer (Axis axis) living in Sri Lanka close to the Equator. In Recent developments in deer biology pp 213-214 Ed: JA Milne. Moredun Research Institute, Edinburgh.

Lincoln GA, Johnston JD, Andersson H, Wagner G, Hazlerigg DG 2005 Photorefractoriness in mammals: dissociating a seasonal timer from the circadian-based photoperiod response. *Endocrinology* 146 3782-3790.

Lincoln GA Libre EA, Merriam GR 1989 Long-term reproductive cycles in rams after pinealectomy or superior cervical ganglionectomy. J reprod Fertil 85 687-704.

Lincoln GA, Ratnasooriya WD 1996 Testosterone secretion, musth behaviour and social dominance in captive male Asian elephants living near the equator. *J Reprod Fertil* 108 107-113.

Loudon ASI & Curlewis JD 1988 Cycles in antler and testicular growth in a aseasonal tropical deer (Axis axis). *J Reprod Fert* 83 729-738

Loudon ASI & Jabbour HN 1994 Seasonal rhythms in the physiology of deer: endogenous clocks and target tissues. In Recent developments in deer biology pp 197-207 Ed: JA Milne. Moredun Research Institute, Edinburgh.

Macgregor DJ, Lincoln GA 2008 A physiological model of a circannual oscillator. *J Biol Rhythms* 23 252-264.

Martinet L, Mondain-Monval M, Monnerie R 1992 Endogenous circannual rhythms and photorefractoriness of testis activity, moult and prolactin concentrations in mink (*Mustela vison*). *J Reprod Fertil* 95 325-38.

Miyazaki Y, Nisimura T, Numata H 2007 Phase resetting and phase singularity of an insect circannual oscillator. *J Comp Physiol A Neuroethol Sens Neural Behav Physiol* 193 1169-1176.

Miyazaki Y, Nisimura T, Numata H 2009 A circadian system is involved in photoperiodic entrainment of the circannual rhythm of *Anthrenus verbasci*. *J Insect Physiol* 55 494-498.

Miyazaki Y, Nisimura T, Numata H 2005 A phase response curve for circannual rhythm in the varied carpet beetle *Anthrenus verbasci*. *J Comp Physiol* A 191 883-887. 494-498.

Monecke S, Saboureau M, Malan A, Bonn D, Masson-Pevet M, Pevet P 2009 Circannual phase-response curves to short and long photoperiod in the European hamster. *J Biol Rhyth* 24 413-426.

Mrosovsky N 1970 Mechanism of hibernation cycles in ground squirrels: circannian rhythm or sequence of stages. *Pennsylvania Acad Sci* 44 172-175.

Mrosovsky N 1978 Circannual cycles in hibernators pp21-65. In: Strategies in cold: natural torbidity and thermogenesis. Eds: LCH Wang, Hudson JW. Academic Press, New York.

Nakao N, Ono H, Yamamura T, Anraku T, Takagi T, Higashi K, Yasuo S, Katou Y, Kageyama S, Uno Y, Kasukawa T, Iigo M, Sharp PJ, Iwasawa A, Suzuki Y, Sugano S, Niimi T, Mizutani M, Namikawa T, Ebihara S, Ueda HR, Yoshimura T 2008 Thyrotrophin in the pars tuberalis triggers photoperiodic response. *Nature* 452 317-322.

Nisimura J Numata H 2002 Evaluation of the frequency demultiphication hypothesis of circannual pupation rhythm in the varied carpet beetle *Anthrenus verbasci* (Coleoptera: Dermestidae). *Biol Rhythm Res* 33 255-260.

Nottebohm F 1989 From bird song to neurogenesis. *Sci Am* 260 74-79.

O'Brien GM 1993 Seasonal reproduction in flying foxes, reviewed in the context of other tropical mammals. *Reprod Fertil Dev* 5499-521. Review.

Ono H, Nakao N, Yoshimura T 2009 Identification of the photoperiodic signaling pathway regulating seasonal reproduction using the functional genomics approach. *Gen Comp Endocrinol* 163 2-6. Review.

Pengelley ET, Asmundson SJ 1974 Circannual Rhythmicity in hibernating animals. Circannual Clocks pp 96-120 Ed ET Pengelly. San Francisco: Academic Press.

Piersma T, Brugge M, Spaans B, Battley PF 2008 Endogenous circannual rhythmicity in body mass, molt and plumage of great knots (*Calidris tenuirostris*). *The Auk* 125 140-148.

Poole JH 1987 Rutting behavior of African elephants: the phenomina of musth. *Behaviour* 102 283-316.

Poole JH Moss CJ 1981 Musth in the African elephant, *Loxodonta Africana*. *Nature* 292 830-831.

Pravosudov VV, Kitaysky AS, Omanska A 2006 The relationship between migratory behaviour, memory and the hippocampus: an intraspecific comparison. *Proc Biol Sci* 273 2641-2649.

Pyter LM, Reader BF, Nelson RJ 2005 Short photoperiods impair spatial learning and alter hippocampal dendritic morphology in adult male white-footed mice (Peromyscus leucopus). *J Neurosci* 25 4521-4526.

Randall CF, Bromage NR, Duston J, Symes J 1998 Photoperiod-induced phase-shifts of the endogenous clock controlling reproduction in the rainbow trout: a circannual phase-response curve. *J Reprod Fertil* 112 399-405.

Reppert SM, Weaver DR 2002 Coordination of circadian timing in mammals. *Nature* 418 935-941.

Schneider MR, Schmidt-Ullrich R, Paus R 2009 The hair follicle as a dynamic miniorgan. *Curr Biol* 19 R132-142. Review.

Sundararaj BI, Vasal S, Halberg F 1982 Circannual rhythmic ovarian recrudescence in the catfish *Heteropneustes fossilis* (Bloch). *Adv Biosci* 41 319-337.

Wagner GC, Johnston JD, Clarke IJ, Lincoln GA, Hazlerigg DG 2008 Redefining the limits of day length responsiveness in a seasonal mammal. *Endocrinology* 149 32-39.

Wehr TA 2001 Photoperiodism in humans and other primates: evidence and implications. *J Biol Rhythms* 16 348-64. Review.

Wickings EJ, Nieschlag E 1980 Seasonality in endocrine and exocrine testicular function of the adult rhesus monkey (Macaca mulatta) maintained in a controlled laboratory environment. *Int J Androl* 1980 3 87-104.

Wikelski M, Martin LB, Scheuerlein A, Robinson MT, Robinson ND, Helm B, Hau M, Gwinner E 2008 Avian circannual clocks: adaptive significance and possible involvement of energy turnover in their proximate control. *Phil Trans Roy Soc B Biol Sci* 363 411-423.

Wittkowski W, Bockmann J, Kreutz MR, Böckers TM 1999 Cell and molecular biology of the pars tuberalis of the pituitary. *Int Rev Cytol* 185 157-94. Review

Woodfill CJ, Wayne NL, Moenter SM, Karsch FJ 1994 Photoperiodic synchronization of a circannual reproductive rhythm in sheep: identification of season-specific time cues. *Biol Reprod* 50 965-976.

Xu Y, Tamamaki N, Noda T, Kimura K, Itokazu Y, Matsumoto N, Dezawa M, Ide C 2005 Neurogenesis in the ependymal layer of the adult rat 3rd ventricle. *Exp Neurol* 192 251-264.

Zucker I 2001 Circannual Rhythms: mammals. In Handbook of Neurology, vol 12, Circannual Clocks pp 509-528 Eds JS Takashi, FW Turek, RY Moore. New York: Plenum Publishers.

Introduction of the George Eric Lamming Memorial Lecture

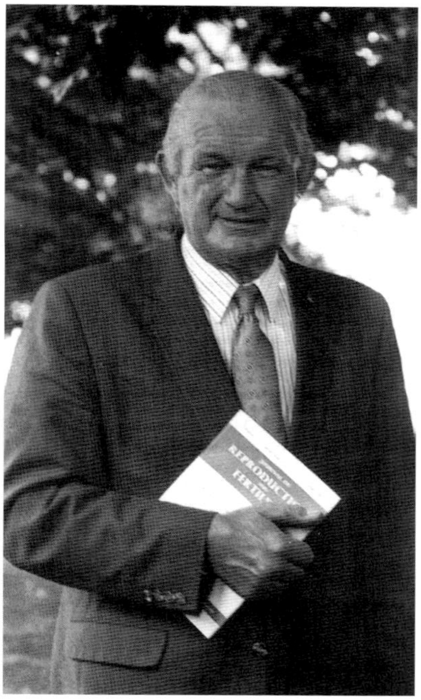

The work presented by Dr. William Murdoch today includes a sequence of carefully designed investigations into the ovulatory process and is a fitting tribute to the career of Eric Lamming. Although best known for his work on anabolic agents in reproduction and his pioneering studies of the use of progesterone in milk to diagnose reproductive status in the dairy cow, Dr. Lamming was a student of broader aspects of ovarian function in ruminants. Much of his work was related to regulation of luteal function, but he contributed papers relating to follicles, including roles of the gonadotropins in induction of ovulation, and feed effects on ovulation rate.

George Eric Lamming was born in Swallow, Lincolnshire on April 14, 1927. He earned his B. Sc. in dairying from Nottingham University , and then an M. Sc. in agricultural economics and a Ph. D. in reproductive physiology at the University of Illinois. His doctoral dissertation was on the effects of vitamin A deficiency in the rabbit.

He returned to Britain in 1951, joining Sir John Hammond's laboratory at Cambridge, and then moved back to Sutton Bonington in 1953. He progressed from Lecturer to Senior Lecturer during 1953 to 1964, and served as Professor of Animal Physiology from 1964 through 1992, then continued his laboratory in reproduction as Professor Emeritus. He played a major part in building an international reputation for Sutton Bonington as a premier School of Agriculture at the University of Nottingham.

As this series of Symposia on Reproduction in Domestic Ruminants developed, Dr. Lamming was one of the forces behind expansion of the breadth of coverage beyond the sheep and cow. His broad interests in the areas of nutrition, growth and reproduction, and the endocrinology of reproduction led him to challenge many students over the years. Quoting from his obituary, "Eric Lamming was a man of powerful intellect and strong personality who made important contributions to research on animal fertility and reproduction, and to the application of that research to veterinary and farming practice."

The work that Dr. Murdoch presents today is important in contexts other than ruminant reproduction. First, it represents the type of studies in animals that can attract support from sources related to human health in an era when support for agricultural animal research has declined severely. Second, it has provided possible insight into a devastating disease that has touched many of our lives. Dr. William Hansel, who was presented with the Upjohn Lifetime Achievement Award at an earlier symposium in this series at Colorado Springs, lost his beloved wife, Millbury, to ovarian cancer. He has devoted his research to this disease in recent years. I personally lost a vibrant young cousin, Cathy Bowyer, not yet 50 years of age, to ovarian cancer in 2009.

Dr. Murdoch earned his B. S. at Delaware Valley College in 1975, and his M. S. in 1977 and Ph. D. in 1980 from West Virginia University. He has carried out his academic career at the University of Wyoming. It gives me great pleasure to introduce Professor William J. Murdoch to present this year's Lamming Memorial Lecture.

Keith Inskeep,
Division of Animal and Nutritional Sciences,
West Virginia University

Mechanisms and pathobiology of ovulation

WJ Murdoch, CJ Murphy, EA Van Kirk and Y Shen

Reproductive Biology Program, University of Wyoming, Laramie, WY USA 82071

The ovulatory process is extraordinary in that it constitutes a hormone-induced injury. Gonadotropin delivered via the follicular vascular wreath stimulates secretion of plasminogen activator by contiguous ovarian surface epithelial cells. A consequent elevation in interstitial plasmin activates collagenases and cleaves tumor necrosis factor α from its anchors on endothelium. Collagen fibril degradation and cellular death at the apex of the preovulatory follicle are hallmarks of impending ovulation. Follicular contractions rupture the weakened fabric at the apex, and the ovum, which has been disconnected from the underlying granulosa, is expelled; these components of the cascade are prostaglandin-mediated. Ovulation is required for fertility; unfortunately, it imparts a cancer risk to the ovarian surface epithelium. DNA-damaging reactive oxygen species are generated by inflammatory cells attracted into the vicinity of the ovulatory stigma. An ischemia-reperfusion flux coincident with ovulation and wound repair also contributes to genotoxicity. Potentially mutagenic lesions in DNA are normally reconciled by TP53 tumor suppressor-dependent cell-cycle arrest and base excision repair mechanisms; it is a unifocal escape that could be problematic. Epithelial ovarian cancer is a deadly insidious disease because it typically remains asymptomatic until it has metastasized to vital abdominal organs.

Introduction

A follicle recruited to ovulate emerges along the ovarian cortex and comes into apposition with the surface epithelium. The initiating signal for ovulation is the surge in secretion of luteinizing hormone (LH) that occurs during the late follicular phase. Proteolytic enzymes and inflammatory mediators liberated at the follicular-ovarian surface interface degrade collagen matrices and provoke cellular death. Follicular contractions facilitate rupture and ovum expulsion (Murdoch, 2000).

More than 90% of cancers of the ovary are thought to arise from the surface epithelium. Circumstances that avert ovulation protect against epithelial ovarian cancer (Bandera, 2005). Damages to DNA caused by oxyradicals are a major cause of cancer (Valko *et al.*, 2004). Indeed, reactive oxygen species produced during the periovulatory period compromise the DNA integrity of bystander ovarian surface cells. These cells proliferate and migrate to mend the void in the ovarian epithelium created by ovulation. It is conceivable that clonal expansion of a cell with unrepaired DNA is an initiating factor in the etiology of ovarian cancer (Murdoch, 2008). Early-stage disease is characterized by formation of an inclusion cyst which contains surface epithelial cells that have invaded the ovary (Feeley and Wells, 2001). Apparently the

Corresponding author E-mail: wmurdoch@uwyo.edu

microenvironment of the inclusion is conducive to metaplastic changes that precede cancer. Malignant cells seed the abdominal cavity when a cyst ruptures. A mutant cell exfoliated during the mechanics of ovulation may account for cases of diffuse intraperitoneal disease in which the ovaries remain relatively uninvolved (Hamilton, 1992).

Objectives of this chapter are to provide overviews of the mechanisms and carcinogenic implications of ovulation with an emphasis on research using an ovine model.

Experimental paradigm

Mature western-range ewes were penned with vasectomized rams and observed for standing estrus (Day 0). Animals were treated on Day 14 with prostaglandin (PG) $F_2\alpha$ to synchronize luteal regression. An agonistic analog of gonadotropin-releasing hormone (GnRH) was administered 36 h after $PGF_2\alpha$ to elicit a preovulatory surge of LH. The dominant follicle within the pair of ovaries will consistently ovulate approximately 24 h after GnRH and form a normal corpus luteum. A translucent stigma develops within 2 h of ovarian rupture (Roberts *et al.*, 1985).

Ovulation: Proteolytic enzymes and tumor necrosis factor

Interstitial (type I) collagen constitutes the primary connective tissue component of the follicular theca and tunica albuginea. Basement membranes that circumscribe thecal capillary beds and support mural granulosa and ovarian surface cells are composed of type IV collagen (Luck, 1994). Fibrillar collagens are comprised of three polypeptide chains coiled into a helix; nascent α-chains consist of repeating triplets of glycine-X-Y, where X and Y are often proline or hydroxyproline (Shoulders and Raines, 2009). Type IV collagen forms a flexible mesh-like scaffold to which matrix constituents (laminin, entactin, perlecan) and epithelial cells attach (LeBleu *et al.*, 2007). Collagen breakdown within the apex of the preovulatory follicle is predictive of ovulation.

Two principal families of enzymes, plasminogen activators/plasmin and matrix metalloproteinases (MMPs), govern tissue dissolution during ovulation. Plasmin (fibrinolysin) is a pleiotropic serine protease that is derived from its zymogen by enzymatic activation. Two forms of plasminogen activator (PA) have been characterized in vertebrates: urokinase (u) and tissue (t) types. Most studies indicate that uPA mediates tissue degradation and carcinogenesis, whereas tPA (that has an affinity for fibrin) modulates thrombolysis (Andreasen *et al.*, 2000). Collectively the zinc/calcium-dependent MMPs ($n \geq 28$) degrade collagens, elastin, proteoglycans, and adhesion molecules. Classical mammalian collagenases truncate each of the polypeptide chains of fibrillar collagens at sites near the carboxyl end (3/4, 1/4 fragments). Matrix metalloproteinases share many structural and functional attributes but differ somewhat in substrate specificities. Types I and IV collagens are the prototype substrates for types I (MMP-1) and IV (MMP-2, gelatinase A; MMP-9, gelatinase B) collagenases. Matrix-degrading effects of metalloproteinases depend upon de novo production, proteolytic activation, and endogenous tissue inhibitor concentrations. Excision of latent collagenases (e.g., by plasmin), permitting a second autolytic cleavage of the Cys-Zn^{2+} bond that stabilizes the propeptide, exposes the catalytic domain of the enzyme. Tissue inhibitors of MMPs (TIMPs 1-4), which noncovalently interact on a 1:1 stoichiometric basis with enzymatic substrate-binding sites, limit the degree of extracellular damage that otherwise would be inflicted by untempered proteolysis (Nagase and Woessner, 1999).

Sheep ovarian surface epithelial cells secrete uPA toward the tunica albuginea and apical follicular wall in response to LH. Receptors for LH on ovarian surface cells are up-regulated at proestrus by estradiol of preovulatory follicular origin (Murdoch *et al.*, 1999a). Ovarian epithelium in close proximity to the preovulatory follicle is exposed to surge concentrations of LH due to an acute histamine-mediated increase (4-12 h after GnRH) in permeability of and blood flow through the thecal vascular wreath (Halterman and Murdoch, 1986; Cavender and Murdoch, 1988).

An increase in plasmin within the apical hemisphere of preovulatory ovine follicles at 12 h after GnRH was attributed to secretion of uPA by ovarian surface epithelial cells (tPA was undetectable). When ovarian surface epithelium was removed surgically at 8 h following GnRH treatment, the follicular rise in uPA and ovarian rupture were negated. Furthermore, ovulation was suppressed by intrafollicular injection of uPA (but not tPA) antibodies at 8 h (Colgin and Murdoch, 1997) or α_2-antiplasmin at 16 h (Murdoch, 1998a) after GnRH. Plasminogen activators also were increased within the apices of preovulatory porcine (Smokovitis *et al.*, 1988) and rat (Peng *et al.*, 1993) follicles. Both uPA and tPA contribute to ovarian plasmin production and ovulatory efficiency in rodents (Hagglund *et al.*, 1996).

Collagenolysis was associated with apical accumulation of plasmin in preovulatory ovine follicles (Murdoch and McCormick, 1992). Explants of follicular wall released hydroxyproline-containing peptides (degraded collagen) after exposure to plasmin and injection of antiplasmin into preovulatory follicles repressed collagenase bioactivity of tissue extracts. The effect of plasmin on collagen breakdown was not transcription-dependent, but rather was related to proenzyme activation (Murdoch, 1998a). Collagenolysis also was elevated preferentially within the apex of preovulatory human follicles (Fukumoto *et al.*, 1981). Morphological observations indicate that preovulatory connective tissue disruption begins at the ovarian surface and advances inward to encompass the apical follicular wall (Bjersing and Cajander, 1975; Talbot *et al.*, 1987). Tunica/thecal fibroblasts and follicular steroidogenic (theca, granulosa) cells are sources of procollagenases (Tadakuma *et al.*, 1993). General chemical inhibitors of collagenases suppressed ovulation in rodents (Reich *et al.*, 1985; Butler *et al.*, 1991). Mice with a mutation in the type I collagen gene, conferring resistance to collagenase, are infertile due to anovulation (Liu *et al.*, 1995).

Tumor necrosis factor (TNF) α, by promoting collagenase gene expression and (at relatively higher concentrations) cellular death, is an intermediary of ovulation. The precursor cytokine is a transmembrane protein that upon cleavage yields a bioactive extracellular subunit. Mature (soluble) TNFα is a noncovalent homotrimer. Target tissue effects of TNFα are receptor subtype- and concentration-dependent. Plasma membrane glycoprotein receptors for TNFα (RI, RII) are present on virtually all nucleated cells. Receptors bind trimeric ligand through a homologous extracellular amino terminal motif. The cytoplasmic segment of TNFRI contains a death domain that upon receptor aggregation can evoke a caspase cascade leading to apoptotic (internucleosomal) DNA fragmentation and pyknosis. Nonlethal transcriptional events (to include collagenase gene up-regulation) also can be activated by TNFRI and TNFRII ligation. It remains unclear what mechanisms dictate pathways of signal transduction outcome - toward genomic stimulation with or without programmed death. At high tissue concentrations, TNFα initiates microvascular coagulation associated with necrotic cellular death and acute inflammation (Larrick and Wright, 1990; Baker and Reddy, 1996).

Tumor necrosis factor α was localized to thecal endothelial cells of preovulatory ovine follicles by fluorescence microscopy. Immunostaining of endothelium within the follicular apex declined abruptly with the approach of ovulation (cells within the counterpart basal wall were unaffected). Plasmin truncated TNFα, releasing it into the site of rupture (Murdoch *et al.*, 1997, 1999). Preovulatory follicles of other species (rat, bovine, human) also secrete TNFα (Terranova, 1997; deMola *et al.*, 1998). Urokinase and basement membrane-degrading MMPs were secreted from human ovarian surface epithelial cells stimulated by TNFα (Yang *et al.*, 2004). Human TNFα is liberated from cells by a metalloproteinase disintegrin (Black *et al.*, 1997).

Types I and IV collagenases were induced in sheep follicular tissues by TNFα; these responses were abrogated by the transcriptional inhibitor actinomycin D (Johnson *et al.*, 1999; Gottsch *et al.*, 2000). Therefore, it appears that TNFα potentiates ovulatory collagenolysis by assuring that sufficient quantities of (pro) MMPs are synthesized. Intrafollicular injection of TNFα antibodies at 10-12 h after GnRH inhibited collagen degradation (Johnson *et al.*, 1999) and blocked ovulation (Murdoch *et al.*, 1997). Moreover, progressive (16-24 h post-GnRH) increases in apoptotic and necrotic cells within the ovarian surface epithelium, tunica albuginea, and apical follicular wall were nullified by immunoneutralization of TNFα (Murdoch 1994, 1995a,b; Murdoch *et al.*, 1997, 1999b). Secretion into the follicular fluid of low (nonlethal) concentrations of TNFα by the oocyte-cumulus complex facilitated collagen breakdown throughout the follicular wall (Johnson *et al.*, 1999). Microinjection of high concentrations of TNFα into the apical wall of explanted sheep follicles (to mimic the local extracellular milieu near ovulation) provoked stigma development (Murdoch *et al.*, 1999b). Addition of TNFα to perfusates of rat ovaries enhanced ovulation rates elicited by LH (Brannstrom *et al.*, 1995). Ovulation occurred in TNFα RI knockout mice during the peripuberal period; however, ovarian cyclicity was disrupted by 6 months of age (the peak in reproductive performance) (Roby *et al.*, 1999). Tumor necrosis factor α-induced hyaluronate-binding protein-6 was expressed in preovulatory rat (Yoshioka *et al.*, 2000), equine (Sayasith *et al.*, 2007), and porcine (Nagyova *et al.*, 2009) follicles.

Net proteolysis during ovulation is controlled by relative balances of enzymes to inhibitors. In theca of periovulatory rat follicles membrane type 1-MMP activates pro-MMP-2 by complexing with TIMP-2 (Jo *et al.*, 2004). Increased production of TIMP-1 and α_2-macroglobulin by granulosa cells serves to confine the extent of ovulatory tissue destruction and assure that a viable corpus luteum can be formed (Curry and Smith, 2006).

Ovulation: Progesterone and prostaglandins

During the preovulatory period, steroidogenic function of the follicle shifts from an estrogen- to progesterone-producing gland. It has been recognized for many years that the rise in progesterone is more than just an index of transition toward the luteal phase. Inhibitors of progesterone biosynthesis/action suppress ovulation (Zalanyi, 2001). That inhibition of follicular prostaglandin (PG) production (by nonsteroidal antiinflammatory agents, most notably indomethacin) inhibits ovulation also is well established. Progesterone and prostaglandins have been implicated as effectors of collagenase production (Murdoch *et al.*, 1986, 1993).

A marked increase in progesterone in preovulatory ovine follicles occurred at 16 h after GnRH. The initial rise in prostaglandin production at 8 h favored PGE_2. Prostaglandin E_2 mediates losses in contacts among mural granulosa and cumulus cells (Murdoch, 1988). Progesterone subsequently induces 9-ketoreductase, which converts PGE_2 to $PGF_2\alpha$ (Murdoch and Farris, 1988). Prostaglandin $F_2\alpha$ stimulates contractile elements within the theca externa (Murdoch *et al.*, 1993). Expressions throughout the bovine follicular wall of prostaglandin receptors predict diverse actions in the ovulatory cascade (Bridges and Fortune, 2007).

Ovulatory mechanisms: Model and additional considerations

An integrative scheme is presented (Figure 1) whereby: 1) gonadotropic stimulation of uPA secretion by ovarian surface epithelial cells conjoined with the preovulatory follicle elicits a localized increase in tissue plasmin, which activates latent collagenases and releases TNFα from its anchors along thecal endothelium; 2) soluble TNFα augments collagenolysis by induction of MMP gene expression and causes epithelial/vascular dissolution; 3) progesterone and prostaglandins facilitate collagenolysis and mediate oocyte delivery to the ovarian surface; 4) weakening of the apical follicular wall leads to stigma formation and ovarian rupture; 5) collagen remodeling, migration of interstitial cells, and neovascularization during differentiation of the sheep corpus luteum were dependent upon TNFα-induced MMP-2 production (Gottsch *et al.*, 2000).

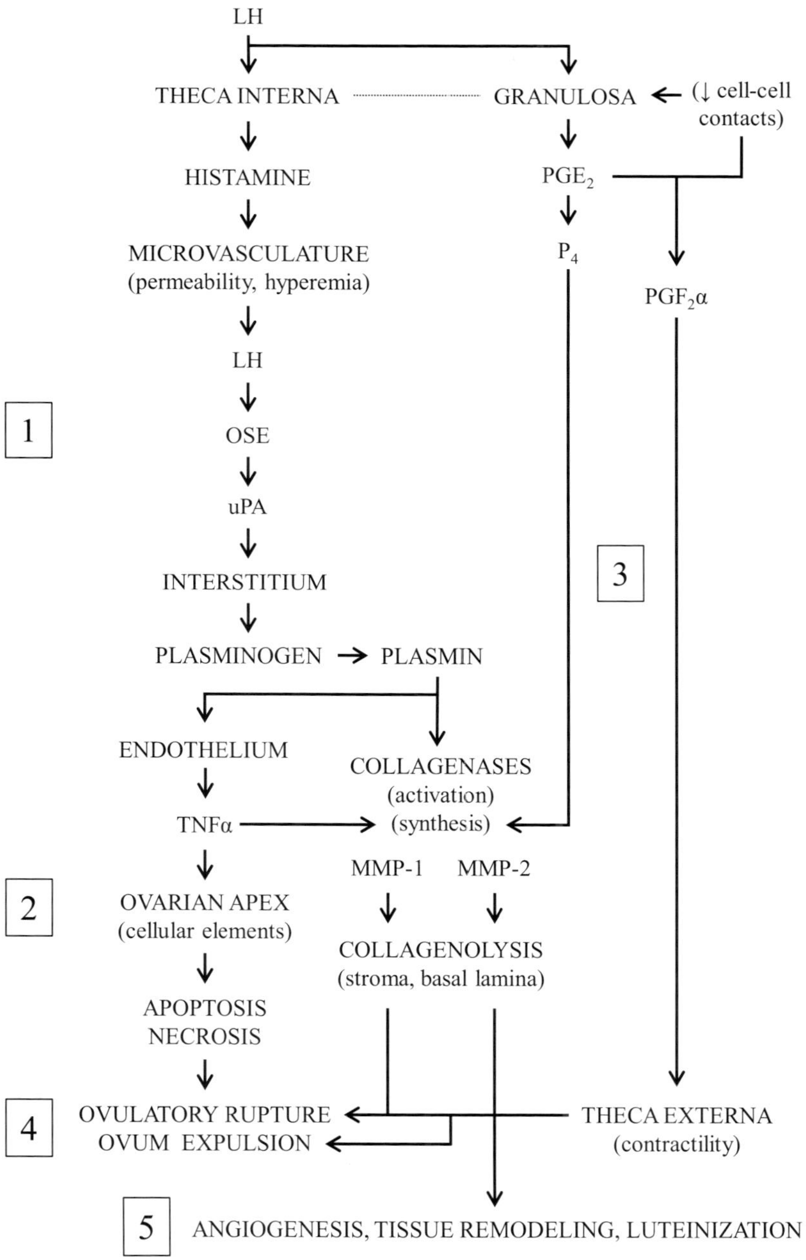

Fig. 1. Sequences of events dictating the ovulatory folliculo-luteal transition in the ewe. OSE, ovarian surface epithelium. P_4, progesterone. See text for explanations (1-5).

Proteases other than PAs/plasmin, MMP-1, and MMP-2 are potential regulators of ovulation. Matrix metalloproteinase-9 was elevated in fluid of preovulatory follicles of pigs (Driancourt *et al.*, 1998) and horses (Riley *et al.*, 2001). Collagenase-3 (MMP-13), which degrades collagens I-III, was increased in preovulatory rat follicles (Balbin *et al.*, 1996; Komar *et al.*, 2001). Cathepsin L, a lysosomal cysteine protease member of the papain family, and ADAMTS-1, a disintegrin and metalloproteinase with thrombospondin-like motifs, were induced in preovulatory follicles of rodents. Mice with a mutant progesterone receptor gene, which failed to ovulate, expressed MMP-2, -9, and -13 upon gonadotropic stimulation, however, mRNAs encoding cathepsin L and ADAMTS-1 were reduced (Robker *et al.*, 2000). Anovulation in a rat polycystic ovarian disease model has been related to increased expression of a lysyl oxidase that initiates cross-link formation of collagen and elastin (Endo *et al.*, 2001).

Thromboxanes and lipoxygenase products of arachidonate catabolism also have been implicated in the mechanisms of ovulation (Carvalho *et al.*, 1989; Wilken *et al.*, 1990). Functional cyclooxygenase and lipoxygenase pathways overlapped in a murine model of ovulation (Kurusu *et al.*, 2009).

Ovulation-cancer connection: Circumstantial evidence

Common (surface epithelial) cancer of the ovary is an ovulation-related disease. Inhibition of ovulation conferred by oral contraceptive use, pregnancy, and lactation safeguard against ovarian cancer (Bandera, 2005).

An ovulation-cancer hypothesis was first proposed by Fathalla in 1971, who suggested that "incessant" ovulations (without intervening dormant periods afforded by pregnancy) caused transformation of the ovarian epithelium. Exposure to estrogen-rich follicular fluid and injury were suspected causes.

Positive correlations among lifetime ovulations, ovarian precursor lesions, and carcinoma have been documented for women. In one analysis (Purdie *et al.*, 2003) there was a 6% increase in cancer risk with each ovulatory year. It appears that the most aggressive/damaging ovulations occur during the peak reproductive years and that ovulations have a more significant impact in premenopausal- than postmenopausal-onset ovarian cancer (Tung *et al.*, 2005).

Assisted reproductive programs that implement ovulation-inducing protocols would presumably increase the carcinogenic risk. Yet data relating use of fertility drugs to ovarian cancer have been inconclusive. Some have concluded that women who do not become pregnant and are subjected to multiple treatments are at an elevated risk, while others suggest weak or no significant correlations (Mahdavi *et al.*, 2006; Chene *et al.*, 2009). Overall rates of ovarian cancer have remained relatively constant despite the widespread application of ovulatory stimulants. Because the latency between initiation (at ovulation) and manifestation of established disease can be quite long (30-40 years or more), it will be important to continue to monitor recipients of superovulation regimens.

Support for the ovulation-cancer concept comes from observations of intensive egg-laying hens. These animals ovulate nearly every day and progress to carcinomatosis at a high frequency (4-40% depending on reproductive history and age) (Fredrickson, 1978; Damjanov, 1989; Rodriguez-Burford *et al.*, 2001). Inhibition of ovulation with a progestin protected hens from ovarian cancer (Barnes *et al.*, 2002).

There are essentially no published data on spontaneous rates of ovarian cancer among nonhuman mammals. One would expect incidences to be low because females of most species are either pregnant, lactating, or seasonally-anestrus for most of their reproductive lives. Inclusion bodies of surface epithelium have been reported in ovaries of ewes (Murdoch, 1994). In rodents, ovarian surface epithelial stratifications, invaginations, and cysts were related to lifetime ovulations (Clow *et al.*, 2002; Tan *et al.*, 2005) and cycles of ovulation induction or estrogen administration (Celik *et al.*, 2004; Burdette *et al.*, 2006, 2007; Gotfredson and Murdoch, 2007). Advancement to cancer occurred in superovulated rats whose ovaries were exposed to a mutagen (Stewart *et al.*, 2004).

Ovulation has been likened to an acute inflammatory reaction (Espey, 1994). Whether inflammation is involved in ovarian carcinogenesis is a subject of recent attention (Shan and Liu, 2009).

Carcinogenic implication of ovulatory genotoxicity

Base damages to DNA caused by reactive oxygen species are an inevitable by-product of physiological metabolism. To combat this predicament, animals have evolved elaborate enzymatic antioxidant defense mechanisms (superoxide dismutase, glutathione perioxidase, catalase); however, these are less than perfect, and toxic oxidants find their way to DNA targets (Collins, 1999).

The N7-C8 bond of guanine is particularly susceptible to attack by the unpaired electron of hydroxyradical. Arguably, 8-oxoguanine is the most important mutagenic lesion in DNA; mispairing with adenine during replications can yield GC-to-TA transversions often detected in tumor cells (Grollman and Moriya, 1993; Cunningham, 1997; Fortini *et al.*, 2003). Ovarian surface epithelial cells isolated from the perimeters of ovulated sheep, human, and hen follicles contained concentrations of 8-oxoguanine that exceeded those of cells obtained from extrinsic areas not affected by ovulation (Murdoch *et al.*, 2001, 2005; Murdoch and Martinchick, 2004). Reactive oxidants are generated by leukocytes which are attracted (by fragments of collagen) into the vicinity of the ovulatory stigma and undergo a respiratory burst (Murdoch and McCormick, 1993). Another contributing determinant of genotoxicity is the ischemia-reperfusion flux that coincides with ovulation and wound reparation (Murdoch et al., 1983; Cavender and Murdoch, 1988). Challenges to the genetic integrity of the ovarian surface epithelium were negated by pharmacological ovulation blockade (Murdoch *et al.*, 2001).

A defective tumor suppressor gene, such as those that overexpress competitive mutant forms of the growth-inhibitory BRCA1/2 or TP53, is a probable basis for developing ovarian neoplasia as a result of ovulation (Aunoble *et al.*, 2000; Cvetkovic, 2003). Oxidative damages to guanine persisted in ovine ovarian surface epithelial cells that were affected by ovulation in vivo and in which synthesis of TP53 was then negated in culture by an antisense oligonucleotide; this was related to discordant cellular growth rates and expression of the cancer antigen CA-125 (Murdoch, 2003). Chromosomal anomalies and metaplasia have been detected in repetitive subcultures (to mimic recurrent ovulation-wound repair) of ovarian surface epithelial cells of rodents (Godwin *et al.*, 1992; Roby *et al.*, 2000).

Fortunately, corruptions to DNA instigated by ovulation are normally conciliated by housekeeping cell-cycle arrest and base-excision repair mechanisms. TP53 allots the time required for repair and proof-reading (Vousden and LU, 2002). Polymerase ß performs the penultimate gap-filling function in the short-patch pathway (Fortini *et al.*, 2003; Sung and Demple, 2006). TP53 and polymerase ß were up-regulated in response to the oxidative stress of ovulation imposed upon the ovarian surface epithelium of sheep (Murdoch *et al.*, 2001). Production of TP53 and polymerase ß were enhanced by progesterone (Murdoch an Van Kirk, 2002). Progesterone also stimulated poly(ADP-ribose) polymerase (PARP) in ovine cells (Murdoch, 1998b). Poly(ADP-ribose) polymerase serves as an adjunct in DNA repair. Binding of PARP and synthesis of branched polymers of ADP-ribose in areas adjacent to a single-strand interruption functions as an antirecombinogenic element (Lindahl and Wood, 1999). Progesterone inhibited proliferation (Wright *et al.*, 2002) and induced apoptosis (Rodriguez, 2003) in cultures of ovarian surface epithelial cells of macaques. The cells of the ovarian epithelium bordering postovulatory follicles of hens (which do not form a corpus luteum) undergo apoptosis and are resorbed during follicular atresia (Murdoch *et al.*, 2005). Ovarian inclusion bodies of surface epithelium can evidently be eliminated via the Fas apoptotic system (Ghahremani *et al.*, 1999).

Antioxidants and ovarian cancer prophylaxis?

There is epidemiological evidence suggesting an inverse relationship between consumption of the antioxidant vitamin E and risk of ovarian carcinoma (Fairfield *et al.*, 2001; McCann *et al.*, 2001). Similar reports have advocated protective effects of vitamin E against cancers of the lung, colorectum, cervix, and prostate gland (Tamini *et al.*, 2002). It appears that in general incidences of oxidative DNA lesions and susceptibility to cancer are potentiated by micronutrient (e.g., antioxidant vitamin) deficiencies (Ames and Wakimoto, 2002). The circulatory antioxidant status of ovarian cancer patients was reduced compared to age-matched controls (Senthil *et al.*, 2004).

DNA of ovarian surface epithelial cells associated with the ovulation stigma of ewes was protected from oxidative base damage by pretreatment with natural-source vitamin E; programmed death within the surface epithelium, ovulation, and pregnancy outcome were not affected (Murdoch and Martinchick, 2004). Oxoguanine-positive surface cells of gonadotropin-primed/superovulated ewes treated with the tumor suppressor disruptor dimethylbenzanthracene and the mitogen estradiol-17ß hypersecreted uPA and formed ovarian inclusion cysts containing proliferative epithelium; these responses were circumvented by pretreatment with vitamin E (Murdoch *et al.*, 2008). Ischemia-reperfusion injury to grafts of ovarian tissues was reduced by vitamin E (Nugent *et al.*, 1998).

Vitamin E is an effective chain-breaking antioxidant in cellular membranes and thereby contributes to membrane phospholipid stability and safeguards intracellular molecules against damage caused by free radicals (Herrera and Barbas, 2001). Vitamin E also can act via mechanisms beyond its oxidant-quenching properties (Kline *et al.*, 2001; Azzi *et al.*, 2002). Nitric oxide production by endothelial cells and superoxide release by leukocytes were suppressed by vitamin E. Nonredox modes of α-tocopherol action include inhibitory and stimulatory effects on rates of mitosis and removal of damaged DNA, respectively. Therefore, vitamin E could act during the postovulatory period to impede untoward proliferative responses of ovarian surface epithelial cells until repairs to DNA can be accomplished.

Ovulation and ovarian cancer: Model and additional considerations

The DNA of ovarian surface epithelial cells contiguous with the site of ovulation is compromised by oxyradicals. It is proposed that this constitutes a first step in the etiology of ovarian tumorigenesis (Figure 2). To fend off accumulations of potentially harmful mutations it is essential that accurate restoration or proficient removal of anomalous cells occurs. The level of danger hence escalates when a cell (as a prelude to mutation) averts (due to a malfunctional tumor suppressor) repair or death. Perhaps the ovarian epithelium is vulnerable to genetic damages that are not reconciled because it has not been under evolutionary pressure to respond to superfluous ovulations (Auersperg *et al.*, 1998). Lifetime ovulations in most animals are kept to a minimum by pregnancy and anestrus.

It remains uncertain why, in particular, the ovarian surface epithelium is so prone to neoplastic transformation; after all, it represents only a small fraction of the diverse cell-types that populate the ovary. Susceptibility may hinge on the fact that (normal) ovarian surface epithelial cells are of an uncommitted phenotype. Unlike the Mullerian epithelia of the female reproductive tract, development of ovarian surface cells is arrested at an immature pluripotent/stem stage (Auersperg *et al.*, 2001).

OVULATION

↓

OXIDATIVE DAMAGE TO DNA OF OSE

malfunctional tumor suppressor genes
steroid hormonal imbalance: $\uparrow E_2 : P_4$

↓

DEFECTIVE DNA REPAIR/APOPTOTIC MECHANISMS

proteases > epithelial inclusion > metaplasia > mutagenesis

↓

MALIGNANT TRANSFORMATION

↓

CLONAL EXPANSION

↓

METASTATIC SPREAD

Fig. 2. Hypothetical role of ovulation in the chronology of epithelial ovarian cancer. E_2, estradiol.

The sequences of events that lead to common ovarian cancer are multifactorial. Several aberrant phases are undoubtedly required to yield a malignant phenotype with distinct growth and metastatic advantages (Figure 2). Ovarian cancer is generally considered to have some level of hormonal involvement; progestins are protective and gonadotropins, androgens, and estrogens are facilitative (Salehi *et al.*, 2008). Paracrine-autocrine modulators (growth factors and cytokines) can also influence ovarian cancer cell behaviors (Auersperg *et al.*, 2001). Metastatic spread is protease-dependent; urokinase and downstream matrix metalloproteinases, that digest basement membranes and interstitial connective tissues, are of particular importance (McDonnel Smedts *et al.*, 2005). Vascular endothelial growth/permeability factor is secreted by ovarian cancer cells and has been related to ascites formation and metastasis (Bamberger and Perrett, 2002).

Because the prognosis for ovarian cancer patients with metastatic disease is so poor, and early detection has proven elusive, it is imperative that methods of chemoprevention be explored. Perhaps supplemental vitamin E could be of value to individuals at risk for the development of ovarian cancer (e.g., those with a genetic predisposition who are not using a contraceptive that inhibits ovulation).

It is important to emphasize in closing that a correlative association between ovulation and the initiation of common ovarian cancer does not prove causal effect and that an "ovulation model" is not absolute and does not explain the genesis of all epithelial ovarian tumors. For example: protection is conferred by tubal ligation or hysterectomy in spite of uninterrupted ovulation; protection provided by one gestation with breast feeding or short-term oral contraceptive use is superior to the predicted benefits of those missed ovulations that would have occurred; reduced numbers of ovulatory cycles due to menstrual irregularities and infertility (e.g., polycystic ovarian syndrome) are independent risk factors for ovarian cancer; and in addition to ovulation, other inflammatory responses (endometriosis and exposure of the ovarian surface to exogenous irritants such as talc, pesticides, or viruses) have been linked to ovarian cancer (Holschneider and Berek, 2000; Ness *et al.*, 2000; Salehi *et al.*, 2008; Shan and Liu, 2009).

References

Ames BN, Wakimoto P 2002 Are vitamins and mineral deficiencies a major cancer risk? *Nature Reviews Cancer* **2** 694-704.

Andreasen PA, Egelund R, Petersen HH 2000 The plasminogen activation system in tumor growth, invasion, and metastasis. *Cellular and Molecular Life Sciences* **57** 25-40.

Aunoble B, Sanches R, Didier E, Bignon YJ 2000 Major oncogenes and tumor suppressor genes involved in epithelial ovarian cancer. *International Journal of Oncology* **16** 567-576.

Auersperg N, Edelson MI, Mok SC, Johnson SW, Hamilton TC 1998 The biology of ovarian cancer. *Seminars in Oncology* **25** 281-304.

Auersperg N, Wong AST, Choi KC, Kang SK, Leung PCK 2001 Ovarian surface epithelium: biology, endocrinology, and pathology. *Endocrine Reviews* **22** 255-288.

Azzi A, Ricciarelli R, Zingg JM 2002 Non-antioxidant molecular functions of alpha-tocopherol (vitamin E). *FEBS Letters* **519** 8-10.

Baker T, Reddy E 1996 Transducers of life and death: TNF receptor superfamily and associated proteins. *Oncogene* **12** 1-9.

Balbin M, Fueyo A, Lopez JM, Diez-Itza I, Velasco G, Lopez-Otin C 1996 Expression of collagenase-3 in the rat ovary during the ovulatory process. *Journal of Endocrinology* **149** 405-415.

Bamberger ES, Perrett CW 2002 Angiogenesis in epithelial ovarian cancer. *Molecular Pathology* **55** 348-359.

Bandera CA 2005 Advances in understanding of risk factors of ovarian cancer. *Journal of Reproductive Medicine* **50** 399-406.

Barnes MN, Berry WD, Straughn JM, Kirby TO, Leath CA, Huh WK, Grizzle WE, Partridge EE 2002 A pilot study of ovarian cancer chemoprevention using medroxyprogesterone acetate in an avian model of spontaneous ovarian carcinogenesis. *Gynecologic Oncology* **87** 57-63.

Bjersing L, Cajander S 1975 Ovulation and the role of the ovarian surface epithelium. *Experentia* **31** 605-608.

Black RA, Rauch CT, Kozlosky CJ, Peschon JJ, Slack JL, Wolfson MF, Castner BJ, Stocking KL, Reddy P, Srinivasan S, Nelson N, Boiani N, Schooley KA, Gerhart M, Davis R, Fitzner JN, Johnson RS, Paxton RJ, March CJ, Cerretti DP 1997 A metalloproteinase disintegrin that releases tumour necrosis factor-α from cells. *Nature* **385** 729-733.

Brannstrom M, Bonello N, Wang LJ, Norman RJ 1995 Effects of tumour necrosis factor α on ovulation in the rat ovary. *Reproduction Fertility and Development* **7** 67-73.

Bridges PJ, Fortune JE 2007 Regulation, action and transport of prostaglandins during the periovulatory period in cattle. *Molecular and Cellular Endocrinology* **263** 1-9.

Burdette JE, Kurley SJ, Kilen SM, Mayo KE, Woodruff TK 2006 Gonadotropin-induced superovulation drives ovarian surface epithelia proliferation in CD1 mice. *Endocrinology* **147** 2338-2345.

Burdette JE, Oliver RM, Ulyanov V, Kilen SM, Mayo KE, Woodruff TK 2007 Ovarian epithelial inclusion cysts in chronically superovulated CD1 and Smad2 dominant-negative mice. *Endocrinology* **148** 3595-3604.

Butler TA, Zhu C, Mueller RA, Fuller GC, LeMaire WJ, Woessner JF 1991 Inhibition of ovulation in the perfused rat ovary by the synthetic collagenase inhibitor SC 44463. *Biology of Reproduction* 44 1183-1188.

Carvalho CB, Yeik BS, Murdoch WJ 1989 Significance of follicular cyclooxygenase and lipoxygenase pathways of metabolism of arachidonate in sheep. *Prostaglandins* **37** 553-558.

Cavender JL, Murdoch WJ 1988 Morphological studies of the microcirculatory system of periovulatory ovine follicles. *Biology of Reproduction* **39** 989-997.

Celik C, Gezginc K, Aktan M, Acar A, Yaman ST, Gungor S, Akyurek C 2004 Effects of ovulation induction on ovarian morphology: an animal study. *International Journal of Gynecological Cancer* **14** 600-606.

Chene G, Penault-Llorca F, Le Bouedec G, Mishellany F, Dauplat MM, Jaffeux P, Aublet-Cuvelier B, Pouly JL, Dechelotte P, Dauplat J 2009 Ovarian epithelial dysplasia after ovulation induction: time and dose effects. *Human Reproduction* **24** 132-138.

Clow OL, Hurst PR, Fleming JS 2002 Changes in the mouse ovarian surface epithelium with age and ovulation number. *Molecular and Cellular Endocrinology* **191** 105-111.

Colgin DC, Murdoch WJ 1997 Evidence for a role of the ovarian surface epithelium in the ovulatory mechanism of the sheep: secretion of urokinase-type plasminogen activator. *Animal Reproduction Science* **47** 197-204.

Collins AR 1999 Oxidative DNA damage, antioxidants, and cancer. *Bioessays* **21** 238-246.

Cunningham RP 1997 DNA repair: caretakers of the genome. *Current Biology* **7** R576-579.

Curry TE, Smith MF 2006 Impact of extracellular matrix remodeling on ovulation and the folliculo-luteal transition. *Seminars in Reproductive Medicine* **24** 228-241.

Cvetkovic D 2003 Early events in ovarian oncogenesis. *Reproductive Biology and Endocrinology* **1** 68.

Damjanov I 1989 Ovarian tumours in laboratory and domestic animals. *Current Topics in Pathology* **78** 1-10.

deMola JRL, Goldfarb JM, Hecht BR, Baumgardner GP, Babbo CJ, Friedlander MA 1998 Gonadotropins induce the release of interleukin-1, interleukin-6 and tumor necrosis factor-α from the human preovulatory follicle. *American Journal of Reproductive Immunology* **39** 387-390.

Driancourt MA, Quesnel H, Meduri G, Prunier A, Hermier D 1998 Luteinization and proteolysis in ovarian follicles of Meishan and Large White gilts during the preovulatory period. *Journal of Reproduction and Fertility* **114** 287-297.

Endo HHT, Nagasawa K, Hayashi T, Chida M, Akutagawa N, Iwasaki M, Kitajima Y, Kiya T, Nishikawa A, Manase K, Kudo R 2001 Lysyl oxidase and MMP-2 expression in dehydroepiandrosterone-induced polycystic ovary in rats. *Biology of Reproduction* **64** 157-162.

Espey LL 1994 Current status of the hypothesis that mammalian ovulation is comparable to an inflammatory reaction. *Biology of Reproduction* **50** 233-238.

Fairfield KM, Hankinson SE, Rosner BA, Hunter DJ, Colditz GA, Willett WC 2001 Risk of ovarian carcinoma and consumption of vitamins A, C, and E and specific carotenoids. *Cancer* **92** 2318-2326.

Fathalla MF 1971 Incessant ovulation - a factor in ovarian neoplasia? *Lancet* **2** 163.

Feeley KM, Wells M. 2001 Precursor lesions of ovarian epithelial malignancy. *Histopathology* **38** 87-95.

Fortini P, Pascucci B, Parlanti E, D'Errico M, Simonelli V, Dogliotti E 2003 8-Oxoguanine DNA damage: at the crossroad of alternative repair pathways. *Mutation Research* **531** 127-139.

Fredrickson TN 1978 Ovarian tumors of the hen. *Environmental Health Perspective* **73** 35-51.

Fukumoto M, Yajima Y, Okamura H, Midorikawa O 1981 Collagenolytic enzyme activity in human ovary: an ovulatory enzyme system. *Fertility and Sterility* **36** 746-750.

Ghahremani M, Foghi A, Dorrington JH 1999 Etiology of ovarian cancer: a proposed mechanism. *Medical Hypotheses* **52** 23-26.

Godwin AK, Testa JR, Handel LM, Liu Z, Vanderveer LA, Tracey PA, Hamilton TC 1992 Spontaneous transformation of rat ovarian surface epithelial cells: association with cytogenetic changes and implications of repeated ovulation in the etiology of ovarian cancer. *Journal of the National Cancer Institute* **84** 592-601.

Gotfredson GS, Murdoch WJ 2007 Morphologic responses of the mouse ovarian surface epithelium to ovulation and steroid hormonal milieu. *Experimental Biology and Medicine* **232** 277-280.

Gottsch ML, Van Kirk EA, Murdoch WJ 2000 Tumour necrosis factor α up-regulates matrix metalloproteinase-2 activity in periovulatory ovine follicles: metamorphic and endocrine implications. *Reproduction, Fertility and Development* **12** 75-80.

Grollman AP, Moriya M 1993 Mutagenesis by 8-oxoguanine: an enemy within. *Trends in Genetics* **9** 246-249.

Hagglund AC, Ny A, Liu K, Ny T 1996 Coordinated and cell-specific induction of both physiological plasminogen activators creates functionally redundant mechanisms for plasmin formation during ovulation. *Endocrinology* **137** 5671-5677.

Halterman SD, Murdoch WJ 1986 Ovarian function in ewes treated with antihistamines. *Endocrinology* **119** 2417-2421.

Hamilton TC 1992 Ovarian cancer, biology. *Current Problems in Cancer* **16** 5-57.

Herrera E, Barbas C 2001 Vitamin E: action, metabolism and perspectives. *Journal of Physiology and Biochemistry* **57** 43-56.

Holschneider CH, Berek JS 2000 Ovarian cancer: epidemiology, biology, and prognostic factors. *Seminars in Surgical Oncology* **19** 3-10.

Jo M, Thomas LE, Wheeler SE, Curry TE 2004 Membrane type 1-matrix metalloproteinase (MMP)-associated MMP-2 activation increases in the rat ovary in response to an ovulatory dose of human chorionic gonadotropin. *Biology of Reproduction* **70** 1024-1032.

Johnson ML, Murdoch J, Van Kirk EA, Kaltenbach JE, Murdoch WJ 1999 Tumor necrosis factor α regulates collagenolytic activity in preovulatory ovine follicles: relationship to cytokine secretion by the oocyte-cumulus cell complex. *Biology of Reproduction* **61** 1581-1585.

Kline K, Yu W, Sanders BG 2001 Vitamin E: mechanisms of action as tumor cell growth inhibitors. *Journal of Nutrition* **131** 161S-163S.

Komar CM, Matousek M, Mitsube K, Mikuni M, Brannstrom M, Curry TE 2001 Effects of genistein on the periovulatory expression of messenger ribonucleic acid for matrix metalloproteinases and tissue inhibitors of metalloproteinases in the rat ovary. *Reproduction* **121** 259-265.

Kurusu S, Jinno M, Ehara H, Yonezawa T, Kawaminami M 2009 Inhibition of ovulation by a lipoxygenase inhibitor involves reduced cyclooxygenase-2 expression and prostaglandin E2 production in gonadotropin-primed immature rats. *Reproduction* **137** 59-66.

Larrick JW, Wright SC 1990 Cytotoxic mechanism of tumor necrosis factor-α. *FASEB Journal* **4** 3215-3223.

LeBleu VS, Macdonald B, Kalluri R 2007 Structure and function of basement membranes. *Experimental Biology and Medicine* **232** 1121-1129.

Lindahl T, Wood RD 1999 Quality control by DNA repair. *Science* **286** 1897-1905.

Liu X, Wu H, Byrne M, Jeffrey J, Krane S, Jaenisch R 1995 A targeted mutation at the known collagenase cleavage site in mouse type I collagen impairs tissue remodelling. *Journal of Cell Biology* **130** 227-237.

Luck MR 1994 The gonadal extracellular matrix. *Oxford Reviews of Reproductive Biology* **16** 34-85.

Mahdavi A, Pejovic T, Nezhat F 2006 Induction of ovulation and ovarian cancer: a critical review of the literature. *Fertility and Sterility* **85** 819-826.

McCann SE, Moysich KB, Mettlin C 2001 Intakes of selected nutrients and food groups and risk of ovarian cancer. *Nutrition and Cancer* **39** 19-28.

McDonnel Smedts A, Curry TE, Murdoch WJ 2005 Proteolytic enzymes and their inhibition in epithelial ovarian cancer. *Current Enzyme Inhibition* **1** 157-170.

Murdoch J, Van Kirk EA, Murdoch WJ 1999 Hormonal control of urokinase plasminogen activator secretion by sheep ovarian surface epithelial cells. *Biology of*

Reproduction **61** 1487-1491.

Murdoch WJ 1988 Disruption of cellular associations within the granulosal compartment of periovulatory ovine follicles: relationship to maturation of the oocyte and regulation by prostaglandins. *Cell and Tissue Research* **252** 459-462.

Murdoch WJ 1994 Ovarian surface epithelium during ovulatory and anovulatory ovine estrous cycles. *Anatomical Record* **240** 322-326.

Murdoch WJ 1995a Programmed cell death in preovulatory ovine follicles. *Biology of Reproduction* **53** 8-12.

Murdoch WJ 1995b Endothelial cell death in preovulatory ovine follicles: possible implication in the biomechanics of rupture. *Journal of Reproduction and Fertility* **105** 161-164.

Murdoch WJ 1998a Regulation of collagenolysis and cell death by plasmin within the formative stigma of preovulatory ovine follicles. *Journal of Reproduction and Fertility* **113** 331-336.

Murdoch WJ 1998b Perturbation of sheep ovarian surface epithelial cells by ovulation: evidence for roles of progesterone and poly(ADP-ribose) polymerase in the restoration of DNA integrity. *Journal of Endocrinology* **156** 503-508.

Murdoch WJ 2000 Proteolytic and cellular death mechanisms in ovulatory ovarian rupture. *Biological Signals and Receptors* **9** 102-114.

Murdoch WJ 2003 Metaplastic potential of p53 downregulation in ovarian surface epithelial cells affected by ovulation. *Cancer Letters* **191** 75-81.

Murdoch WJ 2008 Ovulatory factor in ovarian carcinogenesis. *Advances in Experimental Medicine and Biology* **622** 119-128.

Murdoch WJ, Farris ML 1988 Prostaglandin E_2-9-ketoreductase activity of preovulatory ovine follicles. *Journal of Animal Science* **66** 2924-2929.

Murdoch WJ, Martinchick JF 2004 Oxidative damage to DNA of ovarian surface epithelial cells affected by ovulation: carcinogenic implication and chemoprevention. *Experimental Biology and Medicine* **229** 553-559.

Murdoch WJ, McCormick RJ 1992 Enhanced degradation of collagen within apical vs. basal wall of ovulatory ovine follicle. *American Journal of Physiology* **263** E221-E225.

Murdoch WJ, McCormick RJ 1993 Mechanisms and physiological implications of leucocyte chemoattraction into periovulatory ovine follicles. *Journal of Reproduction and Fertility* **97** 375-380.

Murdoch WJ, Van Kirk EA 2002 Steroid hormonal regulation of proliferative, p53 tumor suppressor, and apoptotic responses of sheep ovarian surface epithelial cells. *Molecular and Cellular Endocrinology* **186** 61-67.

Murdoch WJ, Colgin DC, Ellis JA 1997 Role of tumor necrosis factor-α in the ovulatory mechanism of ewes. *Journal of Animal Science* **75** 1601-1605.

Murdoch WJ, Hansen TR, McPherson LA 1993 Role of eicosanoids in vertebrate ovulation. *Prostaglandins* **46** 85-115.

Murdoch WJ, Nix KJ, Dunn TG 1983 Dynamics of ovarian blood supply to periovulatory follicles of the ewe. *Biology of Reproduction* **28** 1001-1006.

Murdoch WJ, Peterson TA, Van Kirk EA, Vincent DL, Inskeep EK 1986 Interactive roles of progesterone, prostaglandins and collagenase in the ovulatory mechanism of the ewe. *Biology of Reproduction* **35** 1187-1194.

Murdoch WJ, Townsend RS, McDonnel AC 2001 Ovulation-induced DNA damage in ovarian surface epithelial cells of ewes: prospective regulatory mechanisms of repair/survival and apoptosis. *Biology of Reproduction* **65** 1417-1424.

Murdoch WJ, Van Kirk EA, Alexander BM 2005 DNA damages in ovarian surface epithelial cells of ovulatory hens. *Experimental Biology and Medicine* **230** 429-433.

Murdoch WJ, Van Kirk EA, Murdoch J 1999a Plasmin cleaves tumor necrosis factor α exodomain from sheep follicular endothelium: implication in the ovulatory process. *Biology of Reproduction* **60** 1166-1171.

Murdoch WJ, Van Kirk EA, Shen Y 2008 Pathogenic reactions of the ovarian surface epithelium to ovulation, dimethylbenzanthracene, and estrogen are negated by vitamin E. *Reproductive Sciences* **15** 839-845.

Murdoch WJ, Wilken C, Young DA 1999b Sequence of apoptosis and inflammatory necrosis within the formative ovulatory site of sheep follicles. *Journal of Reproduction and Fertility* **117** 325-329.

Nagase H, Woessner JF 1999. Matrix metalloproteinases. *Journal of Biological Chemistry* **274** 21491-21494.

Nagyova E, Nemcova L, Prochazka R 2009 Expression of tumor necrosis factor alpha-induced protein 6 messenger RNA in porcine preovulatory ovarian follicles. *Journal of Reproduction and Development* **55** 231-235.

Ness RB, Grisso JA, Cottreau C, Klapper J, Vergona R, Wheeler JE, Morgan M, Schlesselman JJ 2000 Factors related to inflammation of the ovarian epithelium and risk of ovarian cancer. *Epidemiology* **11** 111-117.

Nugent D, Newton H, Gallivan L, Gosden RG 1998 Protective effect of vitamin E on ischaemia-reperfusion injury in ovarian grafts. *Journal of Reproduction and Fertility* **114** 341-346.

Peng XR, Hsueh AJW, Ny T 1993 Transient and cell-specific expression of tissue-type plasminogen activator and plasminogen activator-inhibitor type 1 results in controlled and directed proteolysis during gonadotropin-induced ovulation. *European Journal of Biochemistry* **214** 147-156.

Purdie DM, Bain CJ, Siskind V, Webb PM, Green AC 2003 Ovulation and risk of epithelial ovarian cancer. *International Journal of Cancer* **104** 228-232.

Reich R, Tsafriri A, Mechanic GL 1985 The involvement of collagenolysis in ovulation in the rat. *Endocrinology* **116** 522-527.

Riley SC, Gibson AH, Leask R, Mauchline DJW, Pedersen HG, Watson ED 2001 Secretion of matrix metalloproteinases 2 and 9 and tissue inhibitor of metalloproteinases into follicular fluid during follicle development in equine ovaries. *Reproduction* **121** 553-560.

Roberts AJ, Dunn TG, Murdoch WJ 1985 Induction of ovulation in proestrous ewes: identification of the ovulatory follicle and functional status of the corpus luteum. *Domestic Animal Endocrinology* **2** 207-210.

Robker RL, Russell DL, Yoshioka S, Sharma SC, Lyndon JP, O'Malley BW, Espey LL, Richards JS 2000 Ovulation: a multi-gene, multi-step process. *Steroids* **65** 559-570.

Roby KF, Son DS, Terranova PF 1999 Alterations of events related to ovarian function in tumor necrosis factor receptor type I knockout mice. *Biology of Reproduction* **61** 1616-1621.

Roby KF, Taylor CC, Sweetwood JS, Cheng Y, Pace JL, Tawfik O, Persons DL, Smith PG, Terranova PF 2000 Development of a syngeneic mouse model for events related to ovarian cancer. *Carcinogenesis* **21** 585-591.

Rodriguez G 2003 New insights regarding pharmacologic approaches for ovarian cancer prevention. *Hematology/Oncology Clinics of North America* **17** 1007-1020.

Rodriguez-Burford C, Barnes MN, Berry W, Partridge EE, Grizzle WE 2001 Immunohistochemical expression of molecular markers in an avian model: a potential model for preclinical evaluation of agents for ovarian cancer chemoprevention. *Gynecologic Oncology* **81** 373-379.

Salehi F, Dunfield L, Phillips KP, Krewski D, Vanderhyden BC 2008 Risk factors for ovarian cancer: an overview with emphasis on hormonal factors. *Journal of Toxicology and Environmental Health, Part B: Critical Reviews* **11** 301-321.

Sayasith K, Dore M, Sirois J 2007 Molecular characterization of tumor necrosis alpha-induced protein 6 and its human chorionic gonadotropin-dependent induction in theca and mural granulosa cells of equine preovulatory follicles. *Reproduction* **133** 135-145.

Senthil K, Aranganathan S, Nalini N 2004 Evidence of oxidative stress in the circulation of ovarian cancer patients. *Clinica Chimica Acta* **339** 27-32.

Shan W, Liu J 2009 Inflammation: a hidden path to breaking the spell of ovarian cancer. *Cell Cycle* **8** 3107-3111.

Shoulders MD, Raines RT 2009 Collagen structure and stability. *Annual Review of Biochemistry* **78** 929-958.

Smokovitis A, Kokolis N, Alexaki-Tzivanidou E 1988 The plasminogen activator activity is markedly increased mainly at the area of the rupture of the follicular wall at the time of ovulation. *Animal Reproduction Science* **16** 285-294.

Stewart SL, Querec TD, Ochman AR, Gruver BN, Bao R, Babb JS, Wong TS, Koutroukides T, Pinnola AD, Klein-Szanto A, Hamilton TC, Patriotis C 2004 Characterization of a carcinogenesis rat model of ovarian preneoplasia and neoplasia. *Cancer Research* **64** 8177-8183.

Sung JS, Demple B 2006 Roles of base excision repair subpathways in correcting oxidized abasic sites in DNA. *FEBS Journal* **273** 1620-1629.

Tadakuma H, Okamura H, Kitaoka M, Iyama K, Usuku G 1993 Association of immunolocalization of matrix metalloproteinase 1 with ovulation in hCG-treated rabbit ovary. *Journal of Reproduction and Fertility* **98** 503-508.

Talbot P, Martin GG, Ashby H 1987 Formation of the rupture site in preovulatory hamster and mouse follicles: loss of surface epithelium. *Gamete Research* **17** 287-302.

Tamini RM, Lagiou P, Adami HO, Trichopoulos D 2002 Prospects for chemoprevention of cancer. *Journal of Internal Medicine* **251** 286-300.

Tan OL, Hurst PR, Fleming JS 2005 Location of inclusion cysts in mouse ovaries in relation to age, pregnancy, and total ovulation number: implications for ovarian cancer? *Journal of Pathology* **205** 483-490.

Terranova PF 1997 Potential roles of tumor necrosis factor-α in follicular development, ovulation, and the life span of the corpus luteum. *Domestic Animal Endocrinology* **14** 1-15.

Tung KH, Wilkens LR, Wu AH, McDuffie K, Nomura AM, Kolonel LN, Terada KY, Goodman MT 2005 Effect of anovulation factors on pre- and postmenopausal ovarian cancer risk: revisiting the incessant ovulation hypothesis. *American Journal of Epidemiology* **161** 321-329.

Valko M, Izakovic M, Mazur M, Rhodes CJ, Tesler J 2004 Role of oxygen radicals in DNA damage and cancer incidence. *Molecular and Cellular Biochemistry* **266** 37-56.

Vousden KH, Lu X 2002 Live or let die: the cell's response to p53. *Nature Reviews Cancer* **2** 595-604.

Wilken C, Van Kirk EA, Slaughter RG, Ji TH, Murdoch WJ 1990 Increased production of ovarian thromboxane in gonadotropin-treated immature rats: relationship to the ovulatory process. *Prostaglandins* **40** 637-646.

Wright JW, Toth-Fejel S, Stouffer RL, Rodland KD 2002 Proliferation of rhesus ovarian surface epithelial cells in culture: lack of mitogenic response to steroid or gonadotropic hormones. *Endocrinology* **143** 2198-2207.

Yang WL, Godwin AK, Xu XX 2004 Tumor necrosis factor-alpha-induced matrix proteolytic enzyme production and basement membrane remodeling by human ovarian surface epithelial cells: molecular basis linking ovulation and cancer risk. *Cancer Research* **64** 1534-1540.

Yoshioka S, Ochsner S, Russell DL, Ujioka T, Fujii S, Richards JS, Espey LL 2000 Expression of tumor necrosis factor-stimulated gene-6 in the rat ovary in response to an ovulatory dose of gonadotropin. *Endocrinology* **141** 4114-4119.

Zalanyi S 2001 Progesterone and ovulation. *European Journal of Obstetrics and Gynecology and Reproductive Biology* **98** 152-159.

The earliest stages of follicular development: Follicle formation and activation

JE Fortune, MY Yang and W Muruvi

Dept. of Biomedical Sciences, Cornell University, Ithaca, NY, USA 14853

The formation of primordial follicles to establish a reservoir of resting follicles and the gradual depletion of that reservoir to provide a succession of growing follicles are key to female fertility, but little is known about the regulation of these early stages of follicular development. This review summarizes the efforts of our laboratory to elucidate these critical processes in cattle. Primordial follicles first appear in fetal ovaries around the end of the first trimester of pregnancy (Day 90), during a decline in fetal ovarian production of estradiol and progesterone. In ovarian cortical pieces from 90 to 120-day-old fetuses, follicles form *in vitro* and estradiol or progesterone inhibits follicle formation, whereas the non-aromatizable androgen 5α-dihydrotestosterone (DHT) does not. Newly formed bovine follicles are not capable of activating within 2 days *in vitro*, but they can acquire the capacity to activate during a longer culture; estradiol and progesterone inhibit the acquisition of their capacity to activate. When primordial follicles first form in cattle, their oocytes are not yet in meiotic arrest and acquisition of competence to activate is correlated with their progression to meiotic arrest at the diplotene stage of first prophase. After they acquire the competence to activate, bovine primordial follicles can be stimulated to activate *in vitro* by insulin or kit ligand, whereas anti-Mullerian hormone (AMH) is inhibitory. Although few follicles progress to the secondary stage *in vitro*, addition of testosterone or vascular endothelial growth factor (VEGF) dramatically increased the incidence of that transition. Regulation of the earliest stages of follicular development is complex and far from understood; better understanding could lead to new interventions to enhance fertility.

Introduction

Mammalian ovaries have a stockpile of primordial follicles. Primordial follicles are non-growing and consist of an oocyte surrounded by a single layer of granulosa cells (Fig. 1A). Once this follicular reservoir has been formed, follicles gradually exit the resting stage to become growing, primary follicles (Fig. 1A). Establishment of the follicular reserve of primordial follicles and the gradual depletion of that resting pool to provide a steady supply of growing follicles are processes critical for female reproduction. Yet little is known about the signals that initiate follicle assembly or those that initiate follicular growth, especially in non-rodent mammalian

---

Corresponding author E-mail: JF11@cornell.edu

species. Our laboratory has developed *in-vitro* models for studying the regulation of follicle formation, the acquisition of follicular capacity to activate (i.e. initiate growth), follicle activation, and the primary to secondary follicle transition. This review will summarize the results obtained with these models.

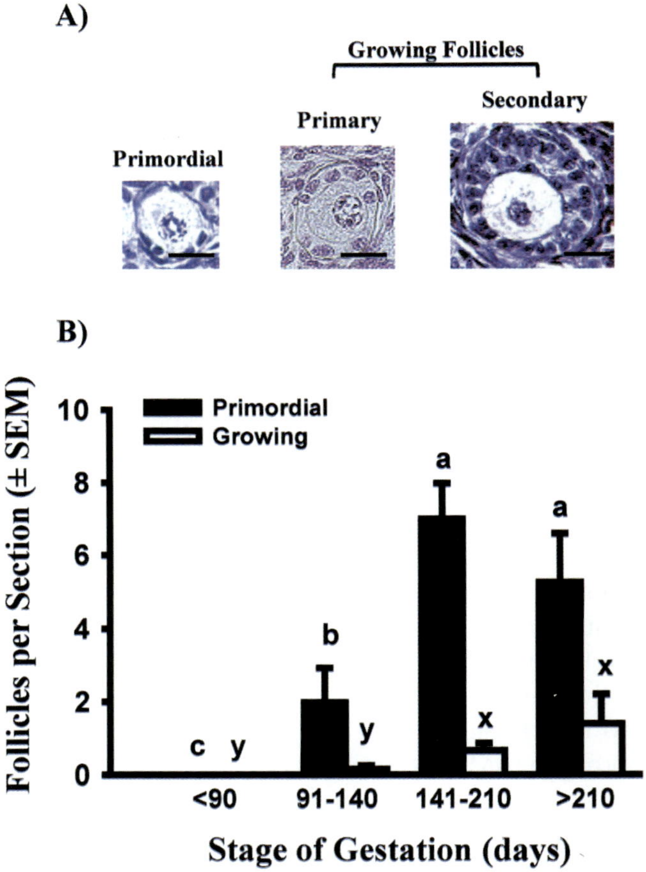

Fig. 1. A) Photomicrographs of early stages of bovine follicular development. Bar = 20 µm. B) Numbers of primordial and growing follicles (only primary follicles before Day 211; primary plus occasional secondary follicles after Day 210) in freshly isolated bovine cortical pieces (means ± SEM). Black bars show data for primordial follicles, and white bars represent growing follicles. Means with different letters within follicle type (primordial: a, b, c; growing: x, y) across gestational stage are significantly different ($P < 0.05$). (Adapted from Yang & Fortune 2008, with permission.)

Summary of experimental methods

Ovaries are dissected from bovine fetuses at a nearby abattoir (Cargill Regional Beef, Wyalusing, PA) and transported to the laboratory at ambient temperature. At the laboratory, the ovarian cortex is microdissected from the underlying medulla and the cortex is cut into small pieces of about 0.5 mm^3. Pieces are cultured for the desired time period on culture inserts (2 pieces/insert) in the wells of 24-well plates in 300 µl of Waymouth›s medium MB 752/1 containing

ITS+ (Insulin, Transferrin, and Selenium + BSA and linoleic acid) in a humidified incubator gassed with 5% CO_2:95% air at 38.5 C. Within each experimental replicate (fetus), treatments *in vitro* are applied to duplicate wells. Some medium (200 µl) is removed and replaced with fresh medium every other day. Cortical pieces are retrieved at the end of culture, fixed in Tousimis fixative (glutaraldehyde and formaldehyde), and processed for embedding in LR White plastic. Serial sections (2 µm) are cut with an ultramicrotome and every 20th section is analyzed for numbers and types of follicles and follicular health. Further methodological details are available in Wandji *et al.* (1996) and Yang & Fortune (2008). Departures from these basic methods will be noted in the sections below.

Follicle formation in cattle

In rats and mice, follicles form fairly synchronously shortly after birth. However, in ruminants and primates, follicles form during fetal life and in an apparently less synchronous fashion than in rodents. Exactly when follicles begin to form in cattle is unclear, since estimates by different laboratories vary from day 74 to day 130 of gestation, even within the same breed (Erickson 1966; Russe 1983; Dominguez *et al.* 1988; Tanaka *et al.* 2001; Garverick *et al.* 2010). The reason for these discrepancies is not clear, but they may be due to how crown-rump length (used to estimate gestational age) was measured and/or the number of fetal time points examined. Because of the lack of consistency in the literature, we re-examined the timing of follicular formation and the first appearance of activated (primary) follicles during bovine gestation, as a prelude to further studies. Primordial follicles have an oocyte and a single flattened layer of granulosa cells; their activation produces primary follicles with a single layer of cuboidal granulosa cells and a growing oocyte (Fig. 1A). Only occasionally were primordial follicles observed in fetal ovaries obtained before day 90 of pregnancy. Between day 91 and day 140, the number of primordial follicles increased, but then numbers appeared to level off between day 141 and day 180 (Fig. 1B). Primary follicles were observed only rarely until after day 140 (Fig. 1B).

When we cultured pieces of ovarian cortex from ovaries obtained at day 91-140 of gestation in medium containing ITS+, the results indicated that follicles formed during the 10-day culture period (Fig. 2, Day 0 *vs.* Control) and this suggested that we could use this *in-vitro* model to study the regulation of follicle formation. Studies by Pepling's laboratory have provided evidence that supports the hypothesis that follicles form shortly after birth in mice in response to withdrawal from the inhibitory effects of circulating maternal steroids (Jefferson *et al.* 2006; Chen *et al.* 2007). Experiments with newborn rat ovaries suggested that progesterone and estradiol also inhibit follicle assembly in that species (Kezele *et al.* 2003; Nilsson *et al.* 2006). There is evidence in the older literature that fetal bovine ovaries produce steroids, especially during the first trimester of pregnancy, before follicle formation commences (Shemesh *et al.* 1978; Dominguez *et al.* 1988) and the ovaries of cattle and sheep have mRNA and protein for SF-1 and steroidogenic enzymes (Quirke *et al.* 2001; Garverick *et al.* 2010). Therefore, we determined the effects of estradiol and progesterone (both at 10^{-6} M) on the number of follicles after 10 days of culture. Both steroids completely inhibited the increase in follicular number that occurred in control cultures (Fig. 2). Nilsson & Skinner (2009) also reported an inhibitory effect of progesterone on the assembly of bovine follicles.

To determine whether our results *in vitro* are consistent with changes in fetal ovarian steroid production *in vivo*, we next measured secretion of estradiol and progesterone during a 24-hour culture by whole minced ovaries from different stages of gestation (see Yang & Fortune 2008 for experimental details). The results showed that estradiol production declined dramatically

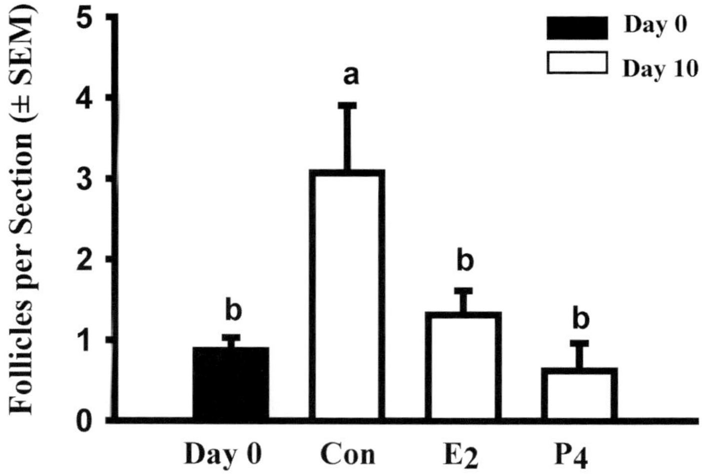

Fig. 2. Effects of steroids on bovine follicle formation *in vitro*. Numbers of follicles (primordial + primary) in ovarian cortical pieces from around day 100 of gestation after 0 (black bar) or 10 (white bar) days in culture with control medium (Con), estradiol (E_2) or progesterone (P_4; both at 10^{-6} M). Data are means ± SEM; means with different letters (a, b) differ significantly ($P < 0.05$; n = 2 fetuses).

between day 80 to 100 of gestation, the period when follicle formation begins, and declined to even lower levels between day 100 to 140, when the first primary follicles appear (Fig. 3). Although progesterone production appeared to decline between day 80 and 140, the pattern was more erratic and the differences were not significant (Fig. 3). The higher levels of both progesterone and estradiol during later gestation are likely due to the increasing number of growing (sometimes antral) follicles at that time. In contrast to the results for estradiol and progesterone, concentrations of testosterone and androstenedione were always very low in the culture medium (Yang & Fortune 2008). It is important to note that the data in Fig. 3 are expressed per ovary and that ovarian size changes greatly over the sampling period. We are currently weighing ovaries before experiments on steroid production and indeed, the changes in ovarian steroid production appear much more pronounced expressed per wt. ovarian tissue, as recently illustrated for progesterone by Nilsson & Skinner (2009). One might wonder whether maternal steroids influence developmental events in the fetal ovary. Circulating maternal estradiol is very low during bovine pregnancy and although progesterone concentrations vary, the highest levels are not very different from levels during the luteal phase of the cycle (Senger 2003). In addition, fetal red blood cells have a powerful 20α-reductase, which converts progesterone to 20α-dihydroprogesterone (P.W. Nathanielsz, personal communication).

In summary, the data support the hypothesis that estradiol and/or progesterone made by the fetal ovary inhibit follicle formation in cattle and that the decline in ovarian production of one or both steroids provides an intra-ovarian signal that initiates follicle formation. Clearly there is much more work to be done to confirm this hypothesis and to determine the steroids involved *in vivo* and the mechanisms of steroid action.

Acquisition by primordial follicles of the capacity to activate

As mentioned above, newly formed primordial follicles do not proceed to primary stage (activate) *in vivo* until around day 141 of gestation (Fig. 1). Thus there is about a 50 day gap between

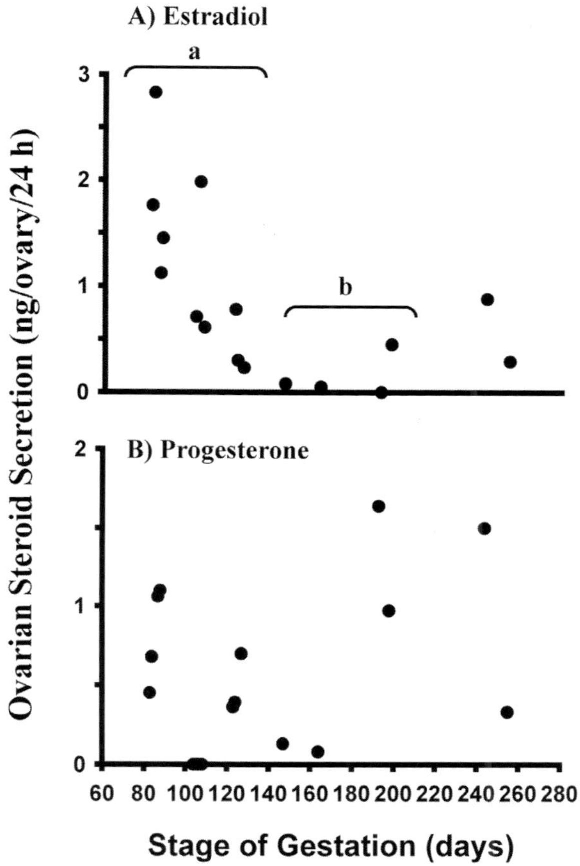

Fig. 3. Estradiol and progesterone secretion (ng/ovary/24 h) *in vitro* by ovaries from bovine fetuses at different gestational ages (means ± SEM). Ovaries were cut into pieces (0.5 - 1 mm^3). The pieces were then cultured for 24 h and steroid concentrations in the culture medium were determined by RIA. a,b: mean estradiol levels differ ($P<0.05$). (From Yang & Fortune 2008, with permission.)

follicle formation and the first observed follicle activation *in vivo*. There are similar gaps between these two developmental events, of 25 and 40 days, in fetal sheep and human ovaries, respectively (van Wagenen & Simpson 1965; McNatty *et al.* 1995). We hypothesized that the gap might occur because 1) the follicles are incapable of activating, 2) they are capable, but an activation signal is missing, or 3) they are capable, but activation is inhibited by a circulating or local factor until a certain stage of gestation. To begin to test these hypotheses, we cultured ovarian cortical pieces from ovaries at day 91-140 of gestation. Although primordial follicles in cortical pieces from fetal ovaries older than day 140, or from adult cattle, can activate within 2 days of culture (Wandji *et al.* 1996; BrawTal & Yossefi 1997), primordial follicles from 91-140 day-old fetuses did not (Fig. 4). However, when the culture period was extended to 10 days, about 65% of the follicles had activated by day 10 of culture (Fig. 4).

The data in Fig. 4 show that newly formed primordial follicles acquire the capacity to activate once they are removed from the milieu of the whole ovary *in vivo* and this suggests that *in vivo* there is an inhibitor(s) that prevents them from developing the capacity to activate. Based on results for newborn mouse ovaries (Jefferson *et al.* 2006; Chen *et al.* 2007) and the temporal patterns of fetal ovarian production of estradiol and progesterone in cattle (Fig. 3), the effects

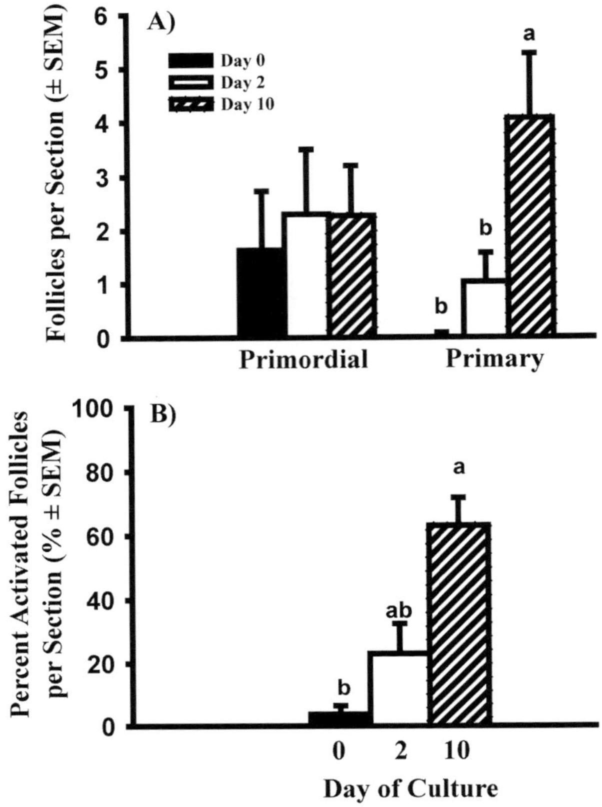

Fig. 4. Effects of length of culture on follicle activation in bovine cortical pieces dissected from fetuses at 91-140 days of gestation. A) Number of primordial and primary follicles in fetal bovine ovarian cortex after 0, 2 and 10 days in culture. B) Percent activated (primary) follicles. Data are means ± SEM; within each panel means with no common letters (a, b) differ significantly across culture period (0, 2, and 10 days) ($P < 0.05$; n = 4 fetuses). (From Yang & Fortune 2008, with permission.)

of adding estradiol, progesterone, or the non-aromatizable androgen DHT (10^{-6}M) to cortical cultures derived from 91-140 day-old fetuses were tested. After 10 days of culture, about 45-60% of follicles had progressed to the primary stage (activated) in control medium (containing ITS+) or medium with DHT (Fig. 5; Yang & Fortune 2008). In contrast, in the presence of estradiol or progesterone, the number of primary follicles and the percentage of follicles that had activated were much lower and not significantly different from the day 0 control (Fig. 5). More recent experiments have shown that the effects of estradiol and progesterone are dose-dependent and that the effect of estradiol on follicle activation can be reversed when estradiol is removed from the culture medium (Fig. 6; Yang & Fortune, unpublished data).

Although there is disagreement among authors about when bovine oocytes finally reach meiotic arrest in the diplotene stage of first prophase of meiosis (Henricson & Rajakoski 1959; Erickson 1966; Baker & Franchi 1967; Russe 1983), Baker & Franchi (1967) reported that bovine primordial follicles form before their oocytes have achieved meiotic arrest. Therefore, we hypothesized that the gap between the first appearance of primordial and primary follicles is necessary to allow the first meiotic prophase to progress to the diplotene stage. Ovaries obtained from fetuses at various stages of gestation were fixed in Bouin's, embedded in paraf-

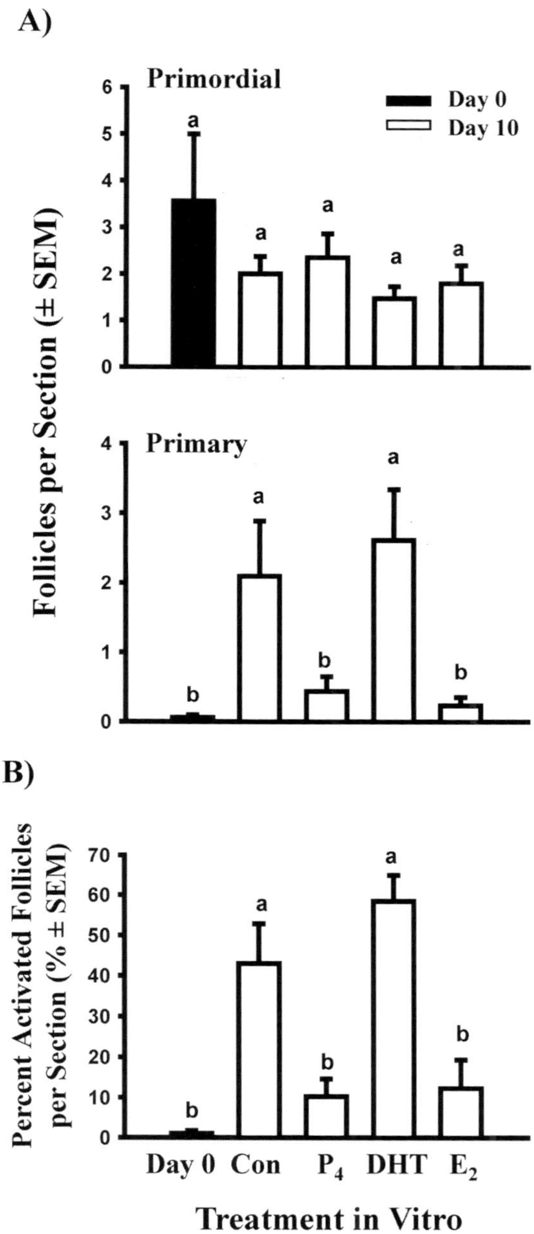

Fig. 5. Effects of control medium (Con), progesterone (P_4), 5α-dihydrotestosterone (DHT), and estradiol (E_2; all at 10^{-6} M) on follicle activation *in vitro* in ovarian cortical pieces from 91 to 140-day-old fetal calves cultured for 10 days. A) Number of primordial and primary follicles in fetal bovine ovarian cortex after 0 or 10 days in culture. B) Percent activated (primary) follicles. Data are means ± SEM; within each panel means with no common letters (a, b) differ significantly ($P < 0.05$; n = 4 fetuses). (From Yang & Fortune 2008, with permission.)

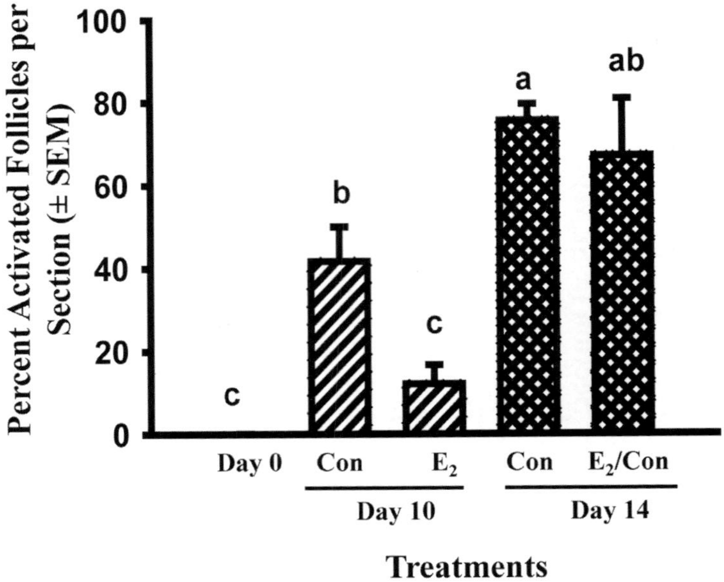

Fig. 6. Percentage of activated follicles in bovine cortical pieces cultured with control medium (Con) or estradiol (E_2; 10^{-6} M) for 10 or 14 days (means ± SEM). E_2/Con: Day 0-10 cultured with E_2 and Day 10-14 with control medium. Cortical pieces were dissected from 100 to 120-day-old fetal calves. Means with no common letters (a, b, c) differ significantly ($P < 0.05$; n = 2 fetuses).

fin, sectioned at 5 μm, and stained with hematoxylin and eosin to allow visualization of the chromatin under light microscopy (Yang & Fortune 2008). The results showed that between 91-140 days of gestation most oocytes are at pre-diplotene stages (mostly pachytene), but after day 140 most oocytes are at the resting, diplotene stage (Fig. 7). In addition, when cortical pieces at similar fetal ages were analyzed for levels of mRNA for YBX2, a biochemical marker for diplotene oocytes, the results reflected closely the change in the proportion of diplotene *vs.* pre-diplotene oocytes that occurred between day 91-140 and after day 140 (Yang & Fortune 2008). The results of more recent experiments showed that when estradiol inhibits follicle activation, there is also an inhibition of the progression of first meiotic prophase and this inhibition is reversed when cortical pieces are switched to control medium (Yang & Fortune, unpublished data).

Regulation of follicle activation after capacity to activate has been acquired

When whole newborn mouse ovaries are cultured, a subset of the newly formed follicles activates and a subset of those primary follicles proceeds to the secondary stage (with two or more layers of granulosa cells) within 8 days *in vitro*, roughly similar to the progression of follicular development during the same time period *in vivo* (Eppig & O'Brien 1996; Gigli *et al.* 2005). About 15 years ago, in collaboration with Dr. Eppig, our laboratory developed methods for studying bovine follicle activation *in vitro*. Small pieces of ovarian cortex (about the same size as newborn mouse ovaries) were isolated from fetal ovaries late in gestation (i.e., a time after primordial follicles acquire the capacity to activate) and cultured in a system similar to

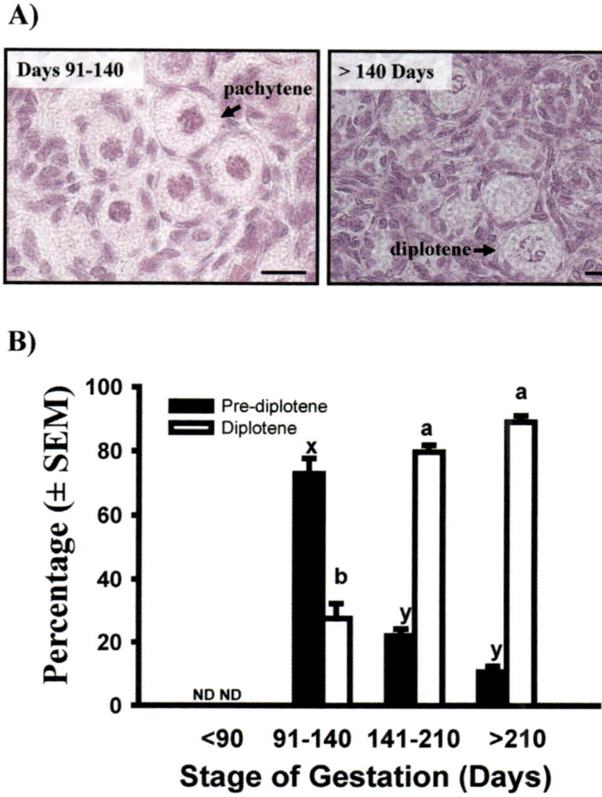

Fig. 7. A) Photomicrographs showing bovine primordial follicles with oocytes at the pachytene or diplotene stage of first meiotic prophase. Bar = 20 µm B) Percentage of oocytes in primordial follicles at pre-diplotene (leptotene, zygotene, or pachytene) and diplotene stages of first meiotic prophase in bovine fetal ovaries collected at different stages of gestation (means ± SEM). Means with no common letters within meiotic stage across gestational stage (pre-diplotene: x, y; diplotene: a, b) are significantly different ($P < 0.05$; n = 3-6 fetuses per gestational stage; with 46-207 oocytes in primordial follicles examined per fetus). ND: not detected. (Adapted from Yang & Fortune 2008, with permission.)

that used for newborn mouse ovaries (the culture system under "Summary of experimental methods" above). At the beginning of culture, most follicles were at the primordial stage, but after 2 days, the number of primordial follicles was much lower than at time 0 and there was a concomitant increase in the number of primary follicles (Wandji *et al.* 1996). The spontaneous wholesale activation *in vitro* was surprising and it did not seem to be due to the fetal nature of the cortical pieces, since Braw-Tal & Yossefi (1997) reported similar results with cortical pieces from adult cattle.

Is there an inhibitor of follicle activation in cattle?

It seemed possible that an inhibitor emanating from the medullary tissue might regulate the rate of follicle activation *in vivo*, so that in the absence of medullary tissue in the cortical cultures most follicles would activate. Co-culture of medullary tissue with cortical pieces had no effect on the number of activated follicles, but this result is not definitive since the inhibitor might not be present in sufficient concentrations in the co-culture situation. In 1999 Themmen's group reported that mice null-mutant for anti-Mullerian hormone (AMH) had more growing follicles early in life, but prematurely depleted their stock of primordial follicles, compared with wild type controls (Durlinger *et al.* 1999). These interesting data suggested that AMH, which is secreted by ovarian follicles, is an intra-ovarian negative modulator of the rate of follicle activation. We tested the hypothesis that adding AMH to ovarian cortical cultures would decrease the rate of activation. Although AMH did not affect activation in that experiment, it significantly inhibited the growth of activated follicles (Yang *et al.*, unpublished data). However, another experiment, in which bovine cortical pieces were transplanted beneath the chorio-allantoic membrane (CAM) of gonadectomized chick embryos, provided indirect evidence that AMH inhibits bovine follicle activation (details provided in Gigli *et al.* 2005).

Since activation occurs within 24 h in cortical pieces cultured with ITS+ (Fortune *et al.* 2000) and AMH is a large protein, it seemed possible that when cortical pieces were cultured with AMH, the hormone did not penetrate the cortical tissue fast enough to prevent the initiation of activation. To test this hypothesis, we cultured cortical pieces from fetuses at day 91-120 of gestation, a time when follicles do not activate within 2 days *in vitro* (Fig. 4), for 10 days with graded doses of recombinant human AMH (100, 500, or 1000 ng/ml). All three doses decreased the percentage of follicles at the primary stage and increased the percentage at the primordial stage (Yang *et al.*, unpublished data). Immunohistochemical analysis of fetal ovaries at various ages showed staining for AMH only in secondary and small antral follicles, which appear during the last trimester (Yang *et al.*, unpublished data). These results strongly suggest that AMH produced by secondary and later stage follicles inhibits activation and slows the growth of primary follicles.

Insulin and kit ligand stimulate follicle activation in cattle

It appears likely that the activation of bovine follicles is controlled by both inhibitory and stimulatory factors. But it has been difficult to study stimulatory factors because of the high rate of what we considered "spontaneous" activation in our control medium containing ITS+. Figueiredo's group in Brazil has tested various hormones and growth factors for effects on follicle activation in caprine ovarian tissue and they reported that several factors increased the number or percentage of growing follicles (e.g., Celestino *et al.* 2010). However, a high percentage of follicles activated in their control medium, which contained ITS, so the additional effects of added hormones/growth factors were very small. We tested the effects of TS+ (i.e. ITS+ without the insulin) plus graded doses of insulin and found that only the two highest doses (3.25 and 6.5 μg/ml) maximally stimulated follicle activation (Yang & Fortune, unpublished data); the highest dose used is the concentration of insulin in ITS+. Interestingly, TS+ maintained the health of the cortical tissue (Fig. 8, panels A *vs.* C and B *vs.* D), but had no effect on activation (Fig. 8; Muruvi *et al.*, unpublished data).

The data shown in Fig. 8 are interesting because they show that what we had considered "spontaneous activation" was actually insulin-stimulated activation and thus, they have provided us with a new model for studying potential stimulators of bovine follicle activation (i.e. culture of cortical pieces in medium with TS+). We used that culture system to test the hypothesis that kit ligand is a stimulator of follicle activation in cattle. The results showed that kit ligand stimulates follicle activation in the absence of insulin and acts via binding to its receptor (Muruvi *et al.*, unpublished data). This culture system will allow us to test other potential stimulators of bovine follicle activation.

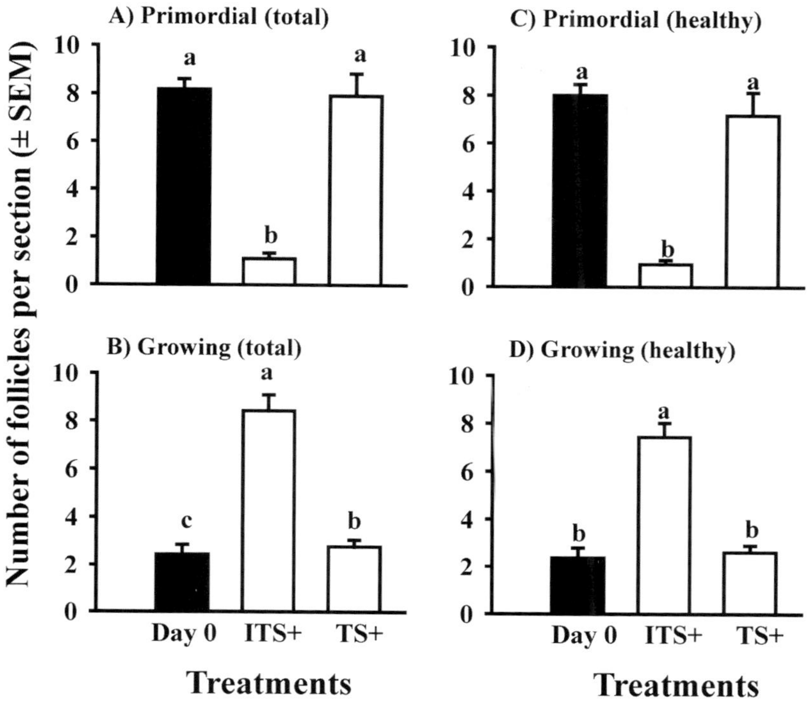

Fig. 8. Effect of insulin on the types and numbers of follicles (mean ± SEM) in ovarian cortical pieces isolated from late-term bovine fetuses. Cortical pieces were cultured for 0 (Day 0; black bar) or 4 (white bars) days in medium supplemented with ITS+ (contains insulin) or with TS+ (identical to ITS+ but without insulin). Within each panel, means (bars) with no common letters (a, b, c) differ significantly ($P < 0.05$; n = 5 fetuses).

The primary to secondary follicle transition

Although the transition from primordial to primary follicle in cattle is readily stimulated in cortical pieces *in vitro* by insulin or kit ligand, as discussed above, this is not the case for the primary to secondary transition. Secondary follicles are preantral follicles with two or more layers of granulosa cells. In whole newborn mouse ovaries placed in organ culture, secondary follicles are evident by day 8 of culture (Eppig & O'Brien 1996) and their numbers are not significantly different from those observed in ovaries of 8-day-old mice *in vivo* (Gigli et *al.* 2005). It is not clear whether the absence of the medulla in the bovine cortical cultures somehow prevents follicles from making the transition or whether the transition involves different signals or conditions in cattle than in mice.

Simply extending the culture period did not increase the percentage of secondary follicles (unpublished data), nor did varying the oxygen concentration *in vitro* (Gigli et *al.* 2006). When cortical pieces were cultured with 0, 2.5, 5, or 10% fetal bovine serum (FBS) in the presence of 0, half-strength, or full-strength ITS+, the combinations most effective at increasing the numbers of secondary follicles were half-strength ITS+ with 5% or 10% FBS (Gigli et *al.* 2006). Because there is evidence that androgens stimulate preantral follicular growth in mice and in rhesus monkeys (Murray et *al.* 1998; Vendola et *al.* 1998; Vendola et *al.* 1999; Wang et *al.*

2001), we cultured bovine cortical pieces with testosterone for 10 days. Testosterone caused a dramatic (about 8-fold), dose-dependent increase in the number of secondary follicles compared to control cultures (Fig. 9 A, B), whereas estradiol had no effect (data not shown), suggesting that testosterone's actions do not require conversion to estradiol (Yang & Fortune 2006). The results of further experiments suggest that androgens play a role *in vivo*. A specific blocker of the androgen receptor (flutamide) completely inhibited testosterone's effects on the development of secondary follicles and immunohistochemistry showed staining for the androgen receptor in both stromal and follicular cells (see Yang & Fortune 2006 for further details). Because vascular endothelial growth factor (VEGF) is an important regulator of angiogenesis and angiogenesis plays an important role in later stages of follicular development (Zeleznik *et al.* 1981; Plendl 2000; Acosta *et al.* 2005), we treated bovine cortical cultures with graded doses of VEGF (1-100 ng/ml in one experiment and 0.1-10 ng/ml in another). The results were similar to those observed in the experiments with testosterone; there was a dose-dependent increase in the number of secondary follicles of about 6-fold compared to control cultures (Fig. 9 C, D) (Yang & Fortune 2007). Thus, we have found that both testosterone and VEGF dramatically increase the primary to secondary transition. However, in both studies most follicles were at the early secondary stage and further experiments are needed to determine how bovine follicles can be "encouraged" to develop beyond that stage.

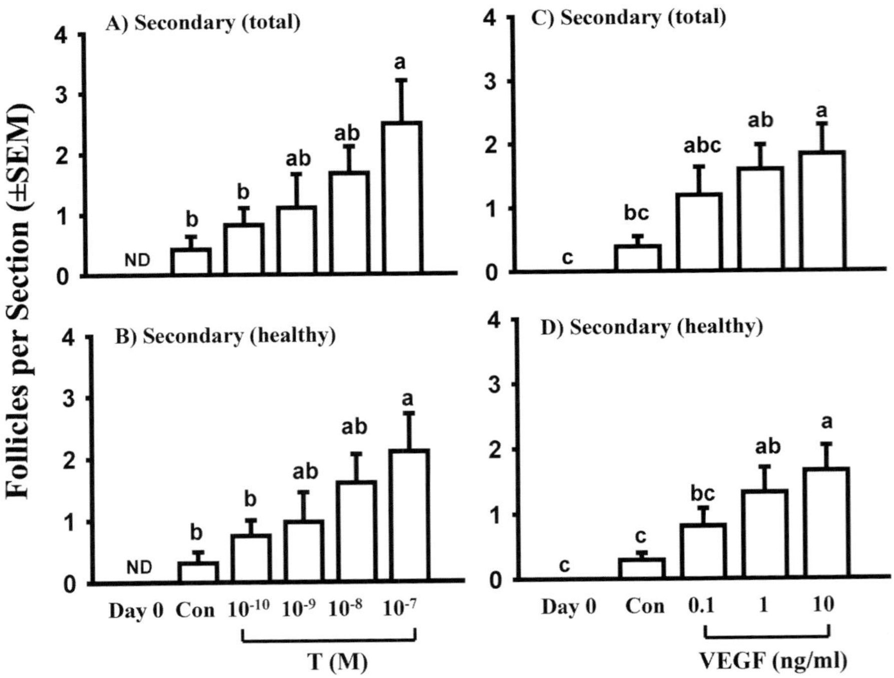

Fig. 9. Effects of graded doses of testosterone (T; 10^{-10} to 10^{-7} M) or vascular endothelial growth factor (VEGF; 0.1 to 10 ng/ml) on numbers of total and healthy follicles in ovarian cortical pieces isolated from late term (5-8 mo. gestation) fetuses and cultured for 10 days (white bars). Secondary follicles were not observed in freshly isolated cortical pieces (Day 0). Con: day 10 controls. Within each panel, means (bars; mean per section ± SEM) with no common letters are significantly different ($P < 0.05$; n = 3 fetuses). ND: not detected. (Data are from Yang & Fortune 2006 and Yang & Fortune 2007.)

Conclusions

The establishment of a pool of resting follicles and their gradual activation to begin growth are essential for female fertility. The results presented in this review suggest that steroid hormones produced by the bovine fetal ovary regulate both follicle formation and the acquisition by newly formed follicles of the capacity to activate. The progression of first prophase of meiosis in the oocytes of primordial follicles can also be regulated by steroids and achievement of meiotic arrest may be an important component of competence of follicles to activate in response to an activation signal. Once follicles have acquired the ability to activate, whether they activate or not probably depends on the balance between inhibitory and stimulatory regulators in their immediate environment. Our studies have provided evidence for AMH as an inhibitor and insulin and kit ligand as stimulators of follicle activation *in vitro*. The primary to secondary follicle transition is also critical for follicular development, but difficult to achieve *in vitro*. In our experiments, supplements to the culture medium (ITS+ and FBS), testosterone, and VEGF increased the number of secondary follicles. At this point, there are many more questions about early follicular development than there are answers. The answers seem worth pursuing, since elucidation of the regulation of early stages of follicular development may lead to new interventions to increase the size of the resting pool of follicles or to methods for enhancing the fertility of valuable domestic animals.

Acknowledgements

The authors thank Cargill Regional Beef for their generous donation of fetal bovine ovaries and Drs. S. S. Suarez and M. E. Pepling for reading the manuscript and for helpful suggestions. This research was supported by National Research Initiative Competitive Grants 2000-35203-9151 and 2003-35203-13532, by the National Institutes of Health (HD060232) and by USDA Multistate project NE-1027.

References

Acosta TJ, Hayashi KG, Matsui M & Miyamoto A 2005 Changes in follicular vascularity during the first follicular wave in lactating cows. *Journal of Reproduction and Development* **51** 273-380.

Baker TG & Franchi LL 1967 The fine structure of chromosomes in bovine primordial oocytes. *Journal of Reproduction and Fertility* **14** 511-513.

BrawTal R & Yossefi S 1997 Studies *in vivo* and *in vitro* on the initiation of follicle growth in the bovine ovary. *Journal of Reproduction and Fertility* **109** 165-171.

Celestino JJ, Bruno JB, Lima-Verde IB, Matos MH, Saraiva MV, Chaves RN, Martins FS, Almeida AP, Cunha RM, Lima LF, Name KP, Campello CC, Silva JR, Bao SN & Figueiredo JR 2010 Steady-state level of kit ligand mRNA in goat ovaries and the role of kit ligand in preantral follicle survival and growth *in vitro*. *Molecular Reproduction and Development* **77** 231-240.

Chen Y, Jefferson WN, Newbold RR, Padilla-Banks E & Pepling ME 2007 Estradiol, progesterone, and genistein inhibit oocyte nest breakdown and primordial follicle assembly in the neonatal mouse ovary *in vitro* and *in vivo*. *Endocrinology* **148** 3580-3590.

Dominguez MM, Liptrap RM & Basrur PK 1988 Steroidogenesis in fetal bovine gonads. *Canadian Journal of Veterinary Research* **52** 401-406.

Durlinger ALL, Kramer P, Karels B, de Jong FH, Uilenbroek JTJ, Grootegoed JA & Themmen APN 1999 Control of primordial follicle recruitment by antiMüllerian hormone in the mouse ovary. *Endocrinology* **140** 5789-5796.

Eppig JJ & O'Brien MJ 1996 Development *in vitro* of mouse oocytes from primordial follicles. *Biology of Reproduction* **54** 197-207.

Erickson BH 1966 Development and radio-response of the prenatal bovine ovary. *Journal of Reproduction and Fertility* **11** 97-105.

Fortune JE, Cushman RA, Wahl CM & Kito S 2000 The primordial to primary follicle transition. *Molecular and Cellular Endocrinology* **163** 53-60.

Garverick HA, Juengel JL, Smith P, Heath DA, Burkhart MN, Perry GA, Smith MF & McNatty KP 2010 Development of the ovary and ontogeny of mRNA and protein for P450 aromatase (arom) and estrogen receptors (ER) alpha and beta during early fetal life in cattle. *Animal Reproduction Science* **117** 24-33.

Gigli I, Byrd DD & Fortune JE 2006 Effects of oxygen tension and supplements to the culture medium on activation and development of bovine follicles *in vitro*.

Theriogenology **66** 344-353.

Gigli I, Cushman RA, Wahl CM & Fortune JE 2005 Evidence for a role for anti-Mullerian hormone in the suppression of follicle activation in mouse ovaries and bovine ovarian cortex grafted beneath the chick chorioallantoic membrane. *Molecular Reproduction and Development* **71** 480-488.

Henricson B & Rajakoski E 1959 Studies of oocytogenesis in cattle. *Cornell Veterinarian* **49** 494-503.

Jefferson W, Newbold R, Padilla-Banks E & Pepling M 2006 Neonatal genistein treatment alters ovarian differentiation in the mouse: inhibition of oocyte nest breakdown and increased oocyte survival. *Biology of Reproduction* **74** 161-168.

Kezele P & Skinner MK 2003 Regulation of ovarian primordial follicle assembly and development by estrogen and progesterone: endocrine model of follicle assembly. *Endocrinology* **144** 3329-3337.

McNatty KP, Smith P, Hudson NL, Heath DA, Tisdall DJ, O WS & BrawTal R 1995 Development of the sheep ovary during fetal and early neonatal life and the effect of fecundity genes. *Journal of Reproduction and Fertility*, Supplement **49** 123-135.

Murray AA, Gosden RG, Allison V & Spears N 1998 Effect of androgens on the development of mouse follicles growing *in vitro*. *Journal of Reproduction and Fertility* **113** 27-33.

Nilsson EE & Skinner MK 2009 Progesterone regulation of primordial follicle assembly in bovine fetal ovaries. *Molecular and Cellular Endocrinology* **313** 9-16.

Nilsson EE, Stanfield J & Skinner MK 2006 Interactions between progesterone and tumor necrosis factoralpha in the regulation of primordial follicle assembly. *Reproduction* **132** 877-886.

Plendl J 2000 Angiogenesis and vascular regression in the ovary. *Anatomia, Histologia, Embryologia* **29** 257-266.

Quirke LD, Juengel JL, Tisdall DJ, Lun S, Heath DA & McNatty KP 2001 Ontogeny of steroidogenesis in the fetal sheep gonad. *Biology of Reproduction* **65** 216-228.

Russe I 1983 Oogenesis in cattle and sheep. *Bibliotheca Anatomica* **24** 77-92.

Senger, P.L. 2003 *Pathways to Pregnancy and Parturition*, second edition. Pullman, WA: Current Conceptions, Inc.

Shemesh M, Allenberg M, Milaguir F, Ayalon N & Hansel W 1978 Hormone secretion by cultured bovine pre and postimplantation gonads. *Biology of Reproduction* **19** 761-767.

Tanaka Y, Nakada K, Moriyoshi M & Sawamukai Y 2001 Appearance and number of follicles and change in the concentration of serum FSH in female bovine fetuses. *Reproduction* **121** 777-782.

van Wagenen G & Simpson ME 1965 *Embryology of the Ovary and Testis. Homo sapiens and Macaca mulatta.* New Haven: Yale University Press.

Vendola K, Zhou J, Wang J, Famuyiwa OA, Bievre M & Bondy CA 1999 Androgens promote oocyte insulin-like growth factor I expression and initiation of follicle development in the primate ovary. *Biology of Reproduction* **61** 353-357.

Vendola KA, Zhou J, Adesanya OO, Weil SJ & Bondy CA 1998 Androgens stimulate early stages of follicular growth in the primate ovary. *Journal of Clinical Investigation* **101** 2622-2629.

Wandji SA, Srsen V, Voss AK, Eppig JJ & Fortune JE 1996 Initiation *in vitro* of growth of bovine primordial follicles. *Biology of Reproduction* **55** 942-948.

Wang H, Andoh K, Hagiwara H, Xiaowei L, Kikuchi N, Abe Y, Yamada K, Fatima R & Mizunuma H 2001 Effect of adrenal and ovarian androgens on type 4 follicles unresponsive to FSH in immature mice. *Endocrinology* **142** 4930-4936.

Yang MY & Fortune JE 2006 Testosterone stimulates the primary to secondary follicle transition in bovine follicles *in vitro*. *Biology of Reproduction* **75** 924-932.

Yang MY & Fortune JE 2007 Vascular endothelial growth factor stimulates the primary to secondary follicle transition in bovine follicles *in vitro*. *Molecular Reproduction and Development* **74** 1095-1104.

Yang MY & Fortune JE 2008 The capacity of primordial follicles in fetal bovine ovaries to initiate growth *in vitro* develops during midgestation and is associated with meiotic arrest of oocytes. *Biology of Reproduction* **78** 1153-1161.

Zeleznik AJ, Schuler HM & Reichert LE Jr. 1981 Gonadotropinbinding sites in the rhesus monkey ovary: role of the vasculature in the selective distribution of human chorionic gonadotropin to the preovulatory follicle. *Endocrinology* **109** 356-362.

The roles of the ovarian extracellular matrix in fertility

RJ Rodgers and HF Irving-Rodgers

Robinson Institute, Research Centre for Reproductive Health, Discipline of Obstetrics and Gynaecology, University of Adelaide, Adelaide, South Australia 5005, Australia

In the mammalian ovary there is considerable and continuous remodelling of tissue during both fetal and adult life, necessitating changes in extracellular matrix. Matrix is a diverse group of molecules varying in its composition and roles, which include regulation of growth factor activity and cell behaviour. Here we discuss four topical aspects of matrices in ovaries. (1) Our current state of knowledge of latent TGFβ binding proteins that can bind the extracellular matrix fibrillins. Fibrillins and latent TGFβ binding proteins may be very important given the genetic linkage data implicating a role for fibrillin 3 in polycystic ovarian syndrome. They will almost certainly be important in the stromal compartments of the ovary by regulating TGFβ bioactivity. (2) Follicles which have an unusual ultrastructural follicular basal lamina and poor quality oocytes. The results suggest that the use of oocytes from these follicles should be avoided in assisted reproductive technologies. (3) Evidence that expression of components of focimatrix correlates with expression of aromatase and cholesterol side-chain cleavage in granulosa cells. Focimatrix is a novel type of basal lamina associated with granulosa cells with expression beginning before deviation and continuing until ovulation. It may be involved in maturation of granulosa cells and selection of the dominant follicle. (4) Evidence is presented in support of a hypothesis that follicular fluid accumulates in follicles due to the osmotic potential of hyaluronan and versican, which are matrices produced by granulosa cells and too large to traverse the follicular antrum. These examples illustrate the diversity of matrix and foreshadow potential important discoveries involving extracellular matrix in ovaries.

Introduction

In the mammalian ovary there is considerable ongoing remodelling of tissue during both fetal and adult life. This includes the formation, activation and growth of follicles which culminates in atresia or ovulation. There is also formation and regression of corpora lutea. These processes are regulated by hormones and growth factors in particular, which have all been well studied. Extracellular matrix also regulates cells and tissues, but its study is relatively limited in the ovary. However it is probably no less important as nearly all cells interact with matrix during development.

Corresponding author E-mail: ray.rodgers@adelaide.edu.au

Extracellular matrix is a very diverse range of molecules that evolved with multicellular organisms and then expanded by gene duplication during the evolution of vertebrates (Huxley-Jones *et al.* 2007). Matrix molecules can be grouped according to which tissue compartment they are located in. The first compartment is that of epithelia, which in the ovary includes surface epithelium and the membrana granulosa, and endothelia as well as some specialized cells such as adipocytes or neurons. Cells in these compartments are surrounded by basal lamina either individually or as groups of cells, providing unique compartments within which these cells reside. In epithelia and endothelia, basal laminas initiate cell polarity, they can control cell proliferation and differentiation and act as barriers to the migration of cells and the passage of molecules across them. They are composed of a lattice-type network of collagen type IV intertwined with a network of laminin, stabilised by the binding of entactin/nidogen-1 or –2 (Schymeinsky *et al.* 2002) to the collagen and laminin. The cells outside these basal laminas are broadly classified as stromal. They contain amongst other cell types fibroblasts and the structural collagens which maintain the integrity of tissues compartments. The non-epithelial or stromal compartments of the ovary include the tunica albuginea, cortical stroma and the specialised theca externa and interna.

Extracellular matrix molecules have many different functions and during evolution matrix also acquired motifs to bind growth factors or their binding proteins. This enabled growth factors to act locally and not as hormones which are broadly dispersed throughout the body upon secretion. We have studied the changing nature of matrix within different compartments of the ovary in several species including bovine, mouse, and human. Here we consider different types of matrix in the bovine ovary and their bearing upon fertility.

Stromal matrix in the ovary

Whilst the theca interna has been well studied the theca externa, tunica albuginea and cortical stroma have received less attention. This is unfortunate as these compartments are altered in human ovaries in the polycystic ovary syndrome (PCOS) which affects up to 5-7% of women in western societies. Women with PCOS often have an increased risk of infertility due to chronic anovulation caused by hyperandrogemia (Balen *et al.* 1995). Up to 20% of women have phenotypically polycystic ovaries, characterized by a multitude of small antral follicles and enlarged theca interna which contributes to the elevated levels of circulating androgens in PCOS women. Interestingly theca cells maintained and passaged in long-term cultures continue to have elevated basal and cAMP-stimulated progesterone, DHEA, 17-hydroxyprogesterone, androstenedione and testosterone production on a per cell basis (Nelson *et al.* 1999), due to elevated expression of steroidogenic enzymes HSD3B and CYP17 (Nelson *et al.* 2001). One conclusion to draw from these studies is that the thecal cells of PCOS ovaries are permanently altered. Another feature of PCOS ovaries is an extremely thickened ovarian capsule or tunica albuginea, and an increased amount of ovarian cortex (Hughesdon 1982). It has been observed that the amount of tunica was increased by 50 per cent in cross sectional area and contained more collagen, while the cortical stromal thickness was increased by one third, and the subcortical stroma, whether deep cortical or medullary, by five fold (Hughesdon 1982). Animal models, including ruminants also exhibit some ovarian features of PCOS (Padmanabhan *et al.* 2006).

It has not been shown if changes to the tunica or or cortical stroma and their collagen content in either women or animal models of PCOS affect their fertility per se, but it is of at least of academic interest to understand their origins and functions. In other normal and fibrotic tissues, Transforming Growth Factor β (TGFβ) stimulates fibroblast function and production and deposition of collagen. During fibrosis of many organs TGFβ activity is also enhanced (Bottinger 2007; Kisseleva & Brenner 2007). TGFβs are part of a superfamily that include activins, bone morphogenic proteins (BMPs), anti-mullerian hormone (AMH or MIS), and growth/differentiation factors (GDF). Members of all of these are expressed in ovaries (Knight & Glister 2006). GDF9 and BMP15 are expressed by oocytes and AMH and activins are expressed by granulosa cells. Studies on expression TGFβ1, 2 and 3 vary somewhat across species. The specialized stromal theca layers of follicles express or contain TGFβ1 (human and sheep), 2 (human, cow and sheep) or 3 (cow) (Chegini & Flanders 1992; Nilsson *et al.* 2003; Juengel *et al.* 2004). The epithelial granulosa cells at different stages of development as well as stroma can express different TGFβ molecules.

Fibrillins are extracellular matrix glycoproteins. Fibrillins form connective tissue microfibrils associated with elastin fibres or extracellular microfilaments (Ramirez & Pereira 1999; Kielty *et al.* 2002). Studies of fibrillin 1 and 2 show that they have a second role, namely they interact with some of the latent TGFß binding proteins (LTBP) (discussed below). The fibrillins and LTBPs can therefore limit local bioavailability and action of TGFβ in a tissue. Direct evidence of this relationship between fibrillins and TGFβs is seen in Marfan's Syndrome and other related syndromes which can be caused by mutations either in fibrillin 1 or in the TGFβ type 2 receptor. Fibrillin 3 is expressed in brain and was only discovered in 2001 and hence much of its activity or roles can only be inferred from our knowledge of fibrillins 1 and 2.

There are four LTBPs. LTBP 1, 3 and 4 can form covalent disulfide complexes with some of the propeptide TGFßs during processing within cells and these are secreted as large latent TGFß complexes (Fig. 1). LTBP 2 does not form such complexes. LTBP 1 and 3 can bind any of the TGFß 1, 2 or 3 propeptides. LTBP 4 can bind only TGFß1 and then less efficiently than LTBP 1 and 3. Secreted LTBPs with or without associated propeptide TGFßs can associate extracellularly with fibrillins at the N terminals. LTBP 2 can dissociate LTBP 1 from fibrillin 1 (Hirani *et al.* 2007) and so can additionally be involved in the regulation of the TGFß bioactivity.

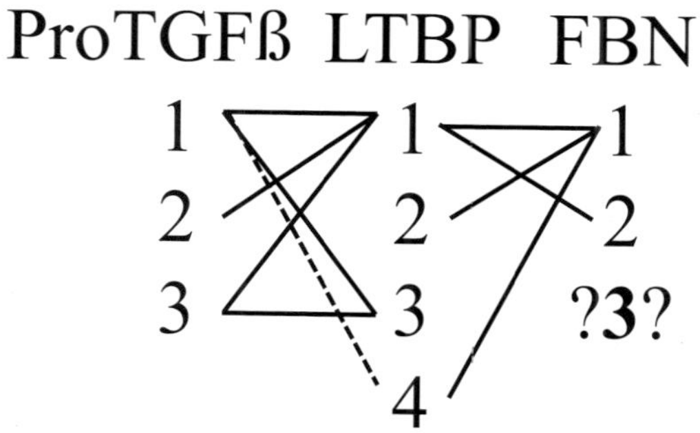

Fig. 1. Interactions between proTGFβ, LTBP and fibrillin (FBN) family members. Lines connect molecules known to interact, and a dashed line indicates weaker association. Associations with fibrillin 3 have not been investigated.

Fibrillin 1, 2 and 3 and LTBP 1 and 2 are expressed in human and bovine (Figs 2 and 3) ovaries (Prodoehl *et al.* 2009a; Prodoehl *et al.* 2009b). However, the expression of fibrillin 3 is very low in both normal and PCOS ovaries and in bovine ovaries. LTBP 3 is also expressed (Penttinen *et al.* 2002) and LTBP 4 has not been examined. The fibillins and LTBPs in bovine ovaries are localized to cells in theca, stroma and tunica albuginea (Prodoehl *et al.* 2009b). The expression patterns appear to be unique with some overlapping co-localization of these proteins while the staining pattern is mostly fibrillar (Figs 2 and 3) (Prodoehl *et al.* 2009b). The expression levels between a number of these genes is highly correlated in ovaries (Prodoehl *et al.* 2009a; Prodoehl *et al.* 2009b), as has been observed in other tissues. Their roles and regulation have not been precisely determined in ovaries but based upon studies in other tissues they are likely to participate in tissue remodelling of stromal compartments during ovarian development and during follicular and luteal development and regression.

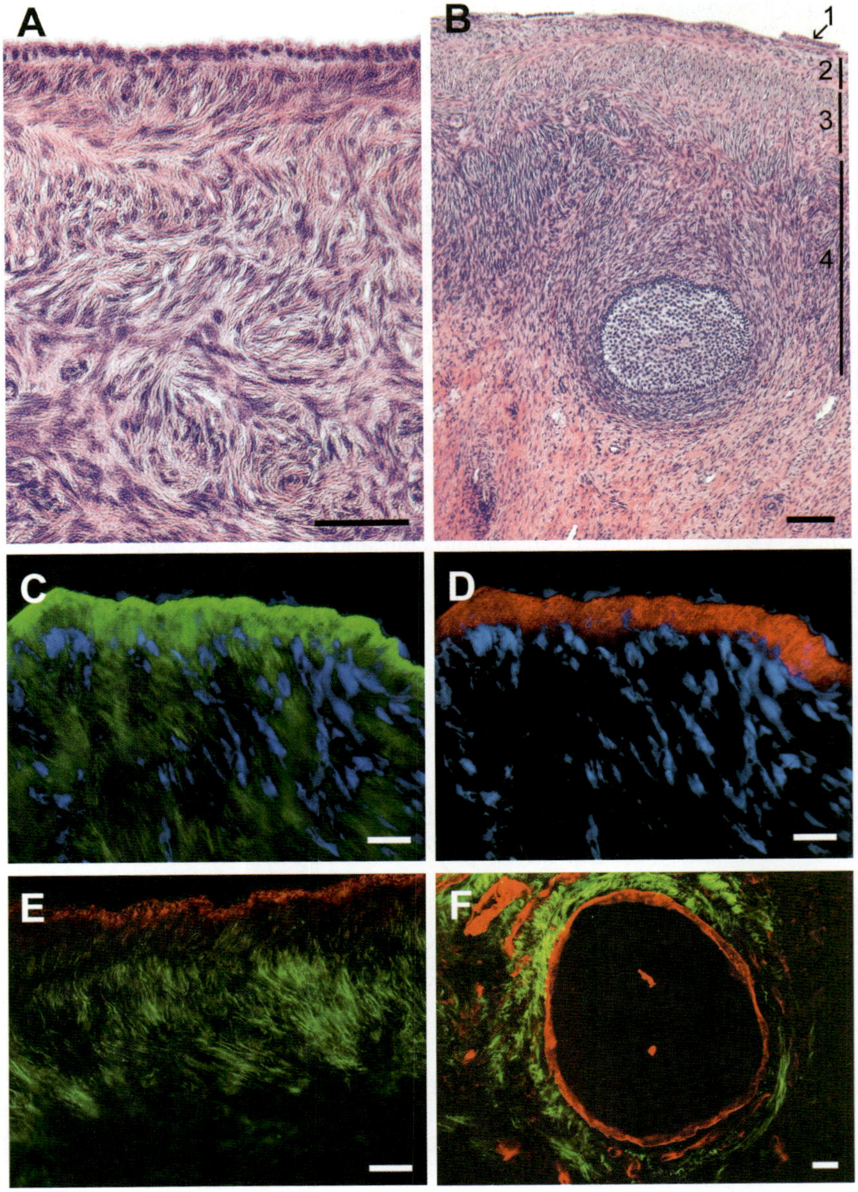

Fig. 2. Localisation of fibrillin 1 and LTBP 1 and 2 in stromal areas of the bovine ovary. Ovarian sections stained with haematoxylin and eosin (A, B) showing surface epithelium (1), the outer (2) and inner (3) regions of the tunica albuginea and the cortical stroma (4). Note the variations in the cellular density and arrangements within the ovary. Fibrillin 1 is most concentrated in the tunica albuginea and less concentrated throughout the cortical stroma (C, green). LTBP2 is present in the tunica albuginea (D and E, red) where it co-localises with fibrillin 1 (C and D are the same section). LTBP 1 is present in the cortical stroma (E, green) and surrounding preantal follicles (F, green; laminin 111 staining in red localizes the follicular basal lamina and sub-endothelial basal laminas). Nuclei are counterstained with DAPI (C, D, blue). Scale bars equal 50 μm (A), 100 μm (B), 20 μm (C, D, F) and 30 μm (E). Parts of this Figure were reprinted with permission from (Prodoehl *et al.* 2009b).

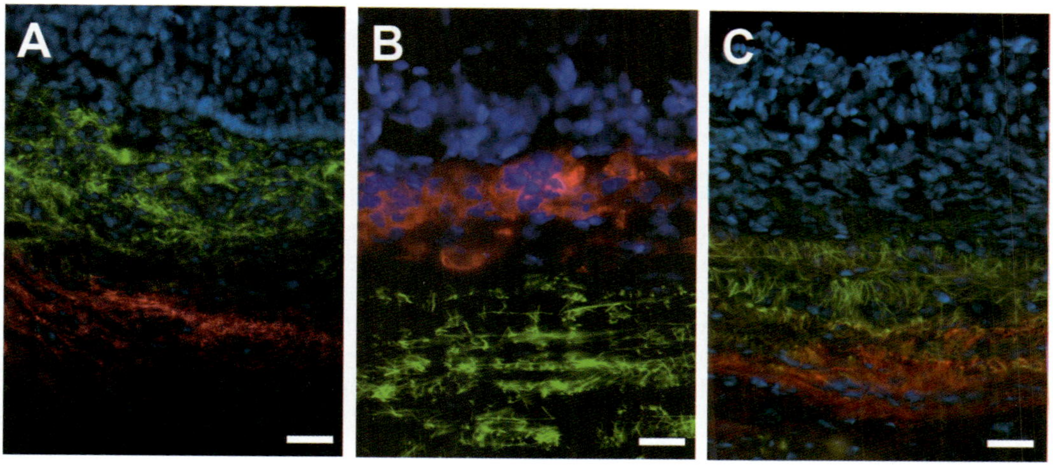

Fig. 3. Localisation of fibrillin 1 and LTBP 1 and 2 in bovine antral follicles. Fibrillin 1 is present in theca interna (A, green). LTBP2 is present in the theca externa (A and C, red). LTBP 1 (B and C, green) present in basal regions of the theca interna and in adjoining theca externa. B, red is CYP17 in theca interna. Nuclei are counterstained with DAPI (blue). Scale bars equal 30 μm (A) and 20 μm (B, C). This Figure was reprinted with permission from (Prodoehl *et al.* 2009b).

Basal laminas and oocyte quality

Generally basal laminas constitute a single layer of lamina densa aligned to the cell surface. However, a number of physiological and pathological conditions lead to different morphological appearances of basal laminas. In patients suffering from diabetes mellitus additional layers of basal lamina are present in kidney, microvasculature, neuronal tissues and the retina (Abrahamson 1986). These expanded multi-layered basal laminas may contribute to the secondary pathology of these organs. In patients with pili annulati, multi layers of basal lamina have been observed in the abnormal hair shafts (Giehl *et al.* 2004). In tadpoles undergoing metamorphosis into frogs, folding of the small intestinal basal lamina has been observed (Murata *et al.* 1994). These changes in morphology of basal laminas presumably reflect or cause changes in basal lamina function.

The follicular basal lamina underlies the membrana granulosa at all stages of development from primordial (van Wezel & Rodgers 1996; Irving-Rodgers *et al.* 2009b), preantral (Irving-Rodgers & Rodgers 2000b; Irving-Rodgers *et al.* 2009b) and antral follicles (Irving-Rodgers & Rodgers 2006) until ovulation when the basal lamina is degraded (Irving-Rodgers *et al.* 2006a). The follicular basal lamina changes in composition during follicular development in bovine (Rodgers *et al.* 2003) and mouse (Irving-Rodgers *et al.* 2010). Extracellular matrix and specifically the follicular basal lamina can influence granulosa cell proliferation and differentiation (Amsterdam *et al.* 1989; Richardson *et al.* 1992; Irving-Rodgers & Rodgers 2006). Additionally, in healthy but not in atretic follicles (Irving-Rodgers *et al.* 2002) the follicular basal lamina excludes capillaries, blood cells and nerve processes from the membrana granulosa.

Different ultrastructural phenotypes of follicular basal lamina have also been observed in follicles in both cattle (Irving-Rodgers & Rodgers 2000a; Irving-Rodgers *et al.* 2002) and humans (Irving-Rodgers *et al.* 2009b). At all follicular stages many follicles have a conventional follicular basal lamina of a single layer which is aligned to the basal surface of the adjacent granulosa cells. At the preantral stage these conventional basal laminas become substantially thicker or even partially laminated in both human and bovine (Irving-Rodgers & Rodgers 2000a; Irving-Rodgers *et al.* 2009b). On atresia the basal lamina is not completely degraded even if macrophages, endothelial cells, and fibroblasts breach the follicular basal lamina as they migrate from the thecal layer into the degrading membrana granulosa. However, on atresia as cells of the membrana granulosa die and the follicle shrinks the follicular basal lamina becomes concertinaed in appearance (McArthur *et al.* 2000; Irving-Rodgers *et al.* 2002).

In addition to changes in the follicular basal lamina during growth and atresia, substantial differences in the ultrastructure of follicular basal laminas have also been observed in follicles of similar developmental stages in both bovine (Irving-Rodgers & Rodgers 2000b) and human (Irving-Rodgers *et al.* 2009b) ovaries. This phenotype occurs in approximately 50% of bovine preantral and antral follicles up to 4 mm diameter (Irving-Rodgers & Rodgers 2000a). The follicular basal lamina of these follicles has additional layers and are referred to as 'loopy' because they have the appearance of having additional 'loops' of basal lamina when observed in cross section by electron microscopy. Unlike in diabetic patients where the pathological changes in basal laminas occur in many organs of the body, these different follicular basal lamina phenotypes exist only in a proportion of ovarian follicles. In diabetics the follicular basal lamina abnormalities are proposed to be due to advanced glycation end-products (Gardiner *et al.* 2003; Goldin *et al.* 2006) or to the action of reactive oxygen species (Meyer zum Gottesberge & Felix 2005), which are likely to affect all organs in the body. If such mechanisms were the cause of the 'loopy' follicular basal laminas then this must be a localised insult, as only a proportion of follicles have a 'loopy' basal lamina.

We have speculated that follicles with a 'loopy' basal lamina have a slowly expanding antrum, and thus produce excess basal lamina that is subsequently shed (Rodgers *et al.* 2001). This implies that when comparing two follicles of the same size the one with the a 'loopy' basal lamina has been growing for longer (Rodgers *et al.* 2001). We subsequently hypothesised that these follicles would contain oocytes of poorer quality, and examined the ability of such oocytes to undergo in vitro maturation, fertilization and development to blastocyst (Irving-Rodgers *et al.* 2009b). Bovine oocytes from follicles (less than 5 mm diameter) with an aligned basal lamina had nearly twice the capacity to develop to blastocyst with a 65% success rate compared to those from a follicle with a 'loopy' basal lamina. How and why such follicles exist is still unknown. It could be that their oocytes are defective in stimulating follicle growth and thus producing the 'loopy' follicular basal lamina. Irrespective of their cause, avoiding these follicles in assisted reproductive technologies should improve success rates.

In these studies we also examined the oocyte quality of atretic follicles. Most of the atretic follicles had a 'loopy' basal lamina which we considered was due to the collapse of the follicle during atresia and therefore was not analogous to the 'loopy' basal laminas of healthy follicles. The small atretic antral follicles had oocytes with a greater developmental capacity than healthy follicles of an equivalent size as has been observed by others previously (Blondin & Sirard 1995; Nicholas *et al.* 2005; Feng *et al.* 2007). Atresia of antral follicles is characterized by death of granulosa cells and it is not until a very advanced stage that the culumus cells (Yang & Rajamahendran 2000) or oocytes (Rajakoski 1960) die, during which time the oocyte could presumably mature, giving them greater capacity to successfully undergo maturation in vitro. Furthermore it has been hypothesised that in cattle atresia mimics preovulatory maturation (Sirard *et al.* 1999). Attempts to utilise this knowledge of the association between atresia and oocyte quality by induction of apoptosis in cumulus cells did not significantly enhance maturation of oocytes (Rubio Pomar *et al.* 2004).

Focimatrix, steroidogenesis and selection of the dominant follicle.

In cows there are two or three waves of development of large antral follicles during an oestrous cycle when a dominant follicle continues to grow as the smaller subordinate follicles in the cohort subsequently regress (Fortune *et al.* 1991; Ginther *et al.* 1996). Dominant follicle development culminates in ovulation, or if the follicular wave is in the luteal phase, atresia ensues. By comparing follicles that are smaller or larger than at which deviation in the growth rate of individual follicles occurs, it has been shown that the expression in granulosa cells of FSH receptor is static or declining, whilst expression of the LH receptor, CYP11A1 (cholesterol side-chain cleavage), 3ß-hydroxysteroid dehydrogenase and CYP19A1 (aromatase) increases [reviewed in (Knight & Glister 2003; Beg & Ginther 2006)]. In follicular fluid there is an increase in oestradiol and progesterone [reviewed in (Knight & Glister 2003; Beg & Ginther 2006)] and free IGF-I and decreased IGFBP-4 and -5 (Mihm *et al.* 2000; Rivera & Fortune 2003; Beg & Ginther 2006) in dominant compared to subordinate follicles.

More recently it has been shown in bovine follicles that a specialised basal lamina-type matrix, focal intra-epithelial matrix (focimatrix) appears before deviation (> 5 mm diameter) and increases in abundance as follicles enlarge to preovulatory sizes (Irving-Rodgers *et al.* 2004; Irving-Rodgers *et al.* 2006b). Focimatrix is deposited as plaques or aggregates of basal lamina material between the epithelial granulosa cells and exists in cattle (Irving-Rodgers *et al.* 2004), sheep (Huet *et al.* 1997), humans (Yamada *et al.* 1999; Alexopoulos *et al.* 2000) and mice (Nakano *et al.* 2007; Irving-Rodgers *et al.* 2010). This matrix is a novel basal lamina because instead of being a sheet enclosing a cell or a group of cells (epithelia or endothelia) and thus creating compartments within tissues, focimatrix exists as aggregates between cells and therefore cannot perform many known functions of basal lamina. Focimatrix in bovine is composed of basal lamina components type IV collagen α1 (COL4A1) and α2, laminin chains α1, β2 (LAMB2) and γ1, perlecan (HSPG2), and nidogen 1 and 2. Like the follicular basal lamina, focimatrix is degraded at ovulation (Irving-Rodgers *et al.* 2006b) hence it is not found in corpora lutea of humans, cattle or mice (Irving-Rodgers *et al.* 2004; Irving-Rodgers *et al.* 2006c; Nakano *et al.* 2007). Thus focimatrix is developmentally regulated and is present before and after follicles deviate in size, suggesting that it may play a role in follicular development including during the period of follicular dominance.

What initiates or controls dominance of one follicle over the others in a cohort has been difficult to determine. Ideally, biopsies would be taken from individual follicles before deviation and then growth monitored until after deviation thus identifying the future dominant and subordinate follicles. Whilst follicular fluids have been sampled in vivo and follicles are apparently unaltered and continue to grow following this procedure (Ginther *et al.* 1997; Mihm *et al.* 2000), taking a biopsy of the wall is likely to ablate the follicle. Therefore most studies have compared dominant and subordinate follicles after deviation, or identified changes that occur during follicle growth at the sizes when follicles deviate.

To investigate if focimatrix is involved in the selection and dominance of ovarian follicles and/or in the maturation of granulosa cells, we quantified focimatrix components in the membrana granulosa and examined the expression of markers of granulosa cells (Irving-Rodgers *et al.* 2009a). Many changes were observed as predicted, due to the size differences between dominant and subordinate follicles. However after statistically removing the effect of follicle size, the volume density of focimatrix components (immunostaining with antibodies to laminin 111) was still significantly elevated in dominant follicles as was the expression of *CYP11A1*. *CYP11A1* mRNA levels were very highly correlated with the genes for focimatrix components and we suggested that focimatrix and *CYP11A1* have a role in follicles gaining dominance (Irving-Rodgers *et al.* 2009a).

To investigate these hypotheses further we examined bovine follicles of equal size before deviation and measured expression of a number of genes as well as the steroid hormone concentrations in follicular fluids (Matti *et al.* 2010). We then sorted the follicles within each animal into two groups for each of three parameters hypothesised to be important in follicular dominance – follicular fluid oestradiol, and TGFß1 (*TGFB1*) and *CYP11A1* expression. One group consisted of follicles with the highest oestradiol concentration or the highest *CYP11A1* expression, which are up regulated during growth, or the lowest *TGFB1*, which is conversely down regulated, and for each parameter the group was compared with a group formed from the remaining follicles. For example, considering the oestradiol groups, for the 14 animals the high group had 14 follicles by taking the follicle with the highest oestradiol level from each animal, and the other group was composed of all the other follicles (n = 21). Similarly for the *CYP11A1* and *TGFB1* comparisons. Before emergence of a dominant follicle, sorting follicles either on *TGFB1* (Fig. 4) or oestradiol levels did not identify a pattern of gene regulation (Matti *et al.* 2010) that would indicate that these parameters were involved in dominance. However, by sorting follicles into two groups on the basis of the levels of *CYP11A1* (Fig. 5) it was clear that one of the follicles in the wave had significantly elevated levels of *CYP11A1*, *CYP19A1*, *COL4A1*, *LAMB2* and *HSPG2* in granulosa cells (Fig. 5) suggesting that the up-regulation of focimatrix and steroidogenic enzymes could be involved in a follicle attaining dominance (Matti *et al.* 2010). Since focimatrix expression precedes deviation and the up-regulation of *CYP11A1* and *CYP19A1*, our current working hypothesis is that focimatrix induces the expression of these steroidogenic enzymes.

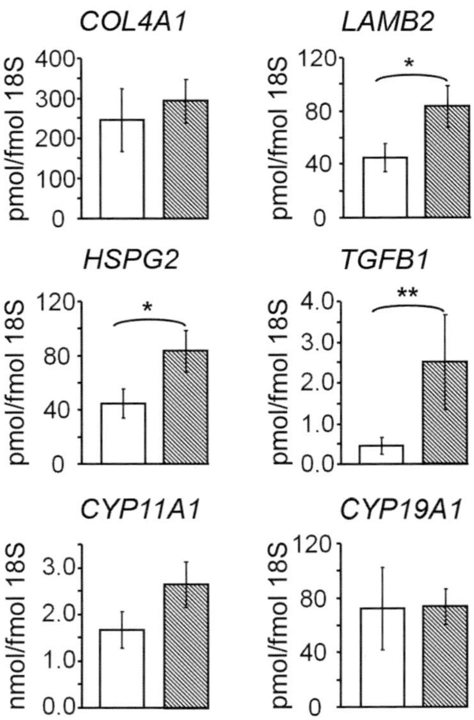

Fig. 4. Expression levels in granulosa cells of predeviated follicles sorted into lowest and higher levels of *TGFB1*. Mean ± SEM levels of all measured parameters when follicles were sorted into groups with the lowest (n = 14) and higher levels (n = 21) of *TFGB1*. $^{*}P<0.05$; $^{**}P<0.01$ significantly different between groups. This Figure was modified and reprinted with permission from (Matti *et al.* 2010).

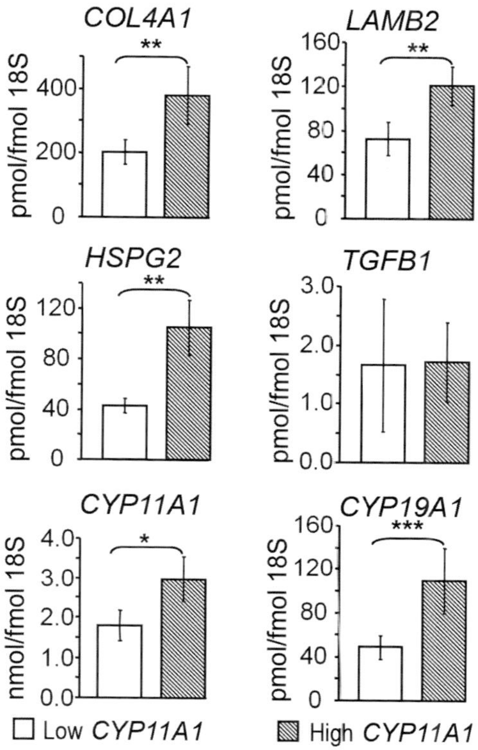

Fig. 5. Expression levels in granulosa cells of predeviated follicles sorted into highest and lower levels of *CYP11A1*. Mean ± SEM levels of all measured parameters when the follicles were sorted into groups with the highest (n = 14) and lower levels (n = 21) of *CYP11A1*. $*P<0.05$; $**P<0.01$; $***P<0.001$ significantly different between groups. This Figure was modified and reprinted with permission from (Matti *et al.* 2010).

Formation of follicular fluid

Formation of follicular fluid and expansion of the follicular antrum are important processes in follicle growth, especially as only large follicles can ovulate. The follicular fluid is probably derived from plasma flowing through thecal capillaries. Capillaries are sparse around primordial follicles (van Wezel & Rodgers 1996; Herrmann & Spanel-Borowski 1998) and generally the stroma surrounding follicles becomes vascularised when the theca and antrum begin to develop. In species with small follicles the thecal capillaries form only a single-layered network, but in species with larger antra the network is multilayered, especially as the follicle increases in size (Yamada *et al.* 1995; Jiang *et al.* 2003). Thus the degree of vascularization of follicles is related to the amount of fluid formed but it is unlikely that vascularisation of theca is a rate limiting step for the formation of follicular fluid since the volume of blood flowing into the thecal capillaries would be considerably greater than the volume needed to fill the antrum. However, there are differences in blood flow or vascularization between dominant and subordinate follicles (Berisha & Schams 2005; Acosta 2007), between follicles with different quality oocytes (Huey *et al.* 1999) and between healthy and atretic follicles (Jiang *et al.* 2003; Clark *et al.* 2004).

Increases in permeability of the thecal capillaries leads to oedema of the thecal tissue, as observed following the LH surge (Espey 1980; Cavender & Murdoch 1988); but transport of fluid from the theca into the follicular antrum requires it to cross the endothelium and sub-endothelial basal lamina before traversing the thecal interstitium, the follicular basal lamina and the membrana granulosa (Fig. 6). In earlier literature both a sodium pump and cleavage of glycoaminoglycans were considered as mechanisms to raise osmotic pressure in the preovulatory follicle and recruit fluid into the centre of the follicle [reviewed by (Gosden *et al.* 1988)]. However, since granulosa cells lack a network of tight junctions an osmotic gradient across the membrana granulosa could not be established with small molecules like sodium. However, it would be possible to establish one with large molecules as there is a nominal 'blood follicle barrier' operating at sizes above 100 kDa (Shalgi *et al.* 1973; Andersen *et al.* 1976). This barrier probably exists largely at the level of the follicular basal lamina.

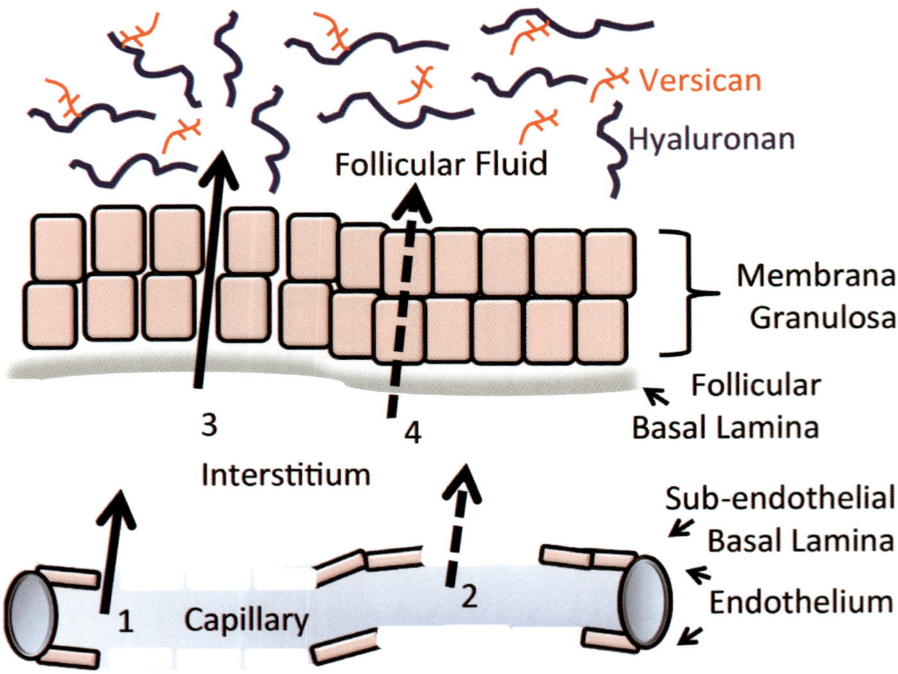

Fig. 6. Drawing illustrating the routes fluid can take from the thecal capillary to the follicular fluid and the potential barriers of the endothelium, sub-endothelial basal lamina, interstitium, follicular basal lamina and membrana granulosa. Routes 1 and 3 show movement of fluid between the cells (solid arrows), and routes 2 and 4 show potential transcellular routes (hatched arrows) which either involve aquaporins or transcytosis. Reprinted with permission from (Rodgers & Irving-Rodgers 2010).

The central hypothesis on how fluid is recruited to the follicular antrum suggests that granulosa cells produce osmotic molecules too large to escape the follicular antrum enabling their osmotic potential to recruit fluid from the thecal vasculature (Fig. 6) (Clarke *et al.* 2006; Rodgers & Irving-Rodgers 2010). In a previous study we found that degradation and removal of the glycosaminoglycans, hyaluronan and chondroitin sulphate/dermatan sulphate, and DNA from follicular fluid resulted in a reduction in osmotic pressure, suggesting that these molecules could contribute to the osmotic potential of the follicular fluid (Clarke *et al.* 2006). The hyaluronan in bovine follicular fluid was found to be up to 2 x 10^6 in molecular weight (Clarke *et al.* 2006), too large to escape from the antral cavity. The chondroitin sulphate proteoglycans identified in our bovine studies were versican (V1 and V0 splice forms) and inter-α-trypsin inhibitor (bikunin with heavy chains 1, 2 and 3), pre-α-trypsin inhibitor (bikunin with heavy chain 3), and inter-α-like trypsin inhibitor (bikunin with heavy chain 2) (Clarke *et al.* 2006). Versican is a large chondriotin sulphate proteoglycan hyalectan expressed in many tissues. It has been shown to be present in extracts of bovine follicles (McArthur *et al.* 2000), follicular fluid of non-ovulating (Clarke *et al.* 2006) and ovulating follicles (Eriksen *et al.* 1999), and in the follicular membrana granulosa (McArthur *et al.* 2000; Irving-Rodgers *et al.* 2004) and is expressed by granulosa cells (Russell *et al.* 2003). Thus versican may directly contribute to the osmotic potential of follicular fluid by virtue of the high sulphation status of chondroitin sulphate side chains. However, versican may also contribute by cross-linking other components like hyaluronan (Zimmermann & Dours-Zimmermann 2008) to form larger molecular weight components, ensuring that both remained trapped in the follicular antrum.

At this stage it is not clear if inter-α-trypsin inhibitor members contribute to the formation of follicular fluid. There are four genes involved in the synthesis of these inter-α-trypsin inhibitor members. The liver expresses these and secretes members of the inter-α-trypsin inhibitor family which are found abundantly in serum. Serum is the source of components of the inter-α-trypsin inhibitor family found in mouse follicular fluid at ovulation (Chen *et al.* 1992). However inter-α-trypsin inhibitor, pre-α-trypsin inhibitor, and inter-α-like trypsin inhibitor exist in bovine (Clarke *et al.* 2006) and porcine (Nagyova *et al.* 2004) follicular fluids well before the LH surge and in follicles that are smaller than pre-ovulatory size. If these molecules are derived from serum they would not contribute to a net gain of fluid by contributing to the osmotic pressure within the antrum, unless actively transported there. However, they may contribute by cross linking to hyaluronan (Rugg *et al.* 2005) ensuring they remain in the follicular antrum. Cross linking of the heavy chains of inter-α-trypsin inhibitor to hyaluronan is catalyzed by tumour necrosis factor-stimulated gene 6 (TNAIFP6) (Milner *et al.* 2007) which is only up regulated after the LH surge at ovulation in pigs (Nagyova *et al.* 2004) and mice (Yoshioka *et al.* 2000). Thus it is unlikely that inter-α-trypsin inhibitor members contribute to the formation of follicular fluid, even if present. Therefore our central hypothesis on follicular fluid formation suggests that production of hyaluronan and versican by granulosa cells generates an osmotic gradient which functions to recruit fluid from the thecal vasculature. Additional studies are required to validate this hypothesis.

Summary

Here we have discussed matrix in ovarian stroma, the follicular basal lamina, focimatrix and follicular fluid and where or how these may impinge upon fertility. That such diverse cellular processes all involve extracellular matrix attests to the complexity and multitude of roles of extracellular matrix. The examples presented also foreshadow many other potential important discoveries to be made involving extracellular matrix in ovaries.

Declaration of interest

The authors declare that there is no conflict of interest that could be perceived as prejudicing the impartiality of the research reported.

Funding

The authors' laboratory is funded by the National Health and Medical Research Council of Australia.

References

Abrahamson DR 1986 Recent studies on the structure and pathology of basement membranes. *J Pathol* **149** 257-78.

Acosta TJ 2007 Studies of follicular vascularity associated with follicle selection and ovulation in cattle. *J Reprod Dev* **53** 39-44.

Alexopoulos E, Shahid J, Ongley HZ & Richardson MC 2000 Luteinized human granulosa cells are associated with endogenous basement membrane-like components in culture. *Mol Hum Reprod* **6** 324-30.

Amsterdam A, Rotmensch S, Furman A, Venter EA & Vlodavsky I 1989 Synergistic effect of human chorionic gonadotropin and extracellular matrix on in vitro differentiation of human granulosa cells: progesterone production and gap junction formation. *Endocrinology* **124** 1956-64.

Andersen MM, Kroll J, Byskov AG & Faber M 1976 Protein composition in the fluid of individual bovine follicles. *J Reprod Fertil* **48** 109-18.

Balen AH, Conway GS, Kaltsas G, Techatrasak K, Manning PJ, West C & Jacobs HS 1995 Polycystic ovary syndrome: the spectrum of the disorder in 1741 patients. *Hum Reprod* **10** 2107-11.

Beg MA & Ginther OJ 2006 Follicle selection in cattle and horses: role of intrafollicular factors. *Reproduction* **132** 365-77.

Berisha B & Schams D 2005 Ovarian function in ruminants. *Domest Anim Endocrinol* **29** 305-17.

Blondin P & Sirard MA 1995 Oocyte and follicular morphology as determining characteristics for developmental competence in bovine oocytes. *Mol Reprod Dev* **41** 54-62.

Bottinger EP 2007 TGF-beta in renal injury and disease. *Semin Nephrol* **27** 309-20.

Cavender JL & Murdoch WJ 1988 Morphological studies of the microcirculatory system of periovulatory ovine follicles. *Biol Reprod* **39** 989-97.

Chegini N & Flanders KC 1992 Presence of transforming growth factor-beta and their selective cellular localization in human ovarian tissue of various reproductive stages. *Endocrinology* **130** 1707-15.

Chen L, Mao SJ & Larsen WJ 1992 Identification of a factor in fetal bovine serum that stabilizes the cumulus extracellular matrix. A role for a member of the inter-alpha-trypsin inhibitor family. *J Biol Chem* **267** 12380-6.

Clark LJ, Irving-Rodgers HF, Dharmarajan AM & Rodgers RJ 2004 Theca interna: the other side of bovine follicular atresia. *Biol Reprod* **71** 1071-8.

Clarke HG, Hope SA, Byers S & Rodgers RJ 2006 Formation of ovarian follicular fluid may be due to the osmotic potential of large glycosaminoglycans and proteoglycans. *Reproduction* **132** 119-31.

Eriksen GV, Carlstedt I, Morgelin M, Uldbjerg N & Malmstrom A 1999 Isolation and characterization of proteoglycans from human follicular fluid. *Biochem J* **340** 613-20.

Espey LL 1980 Ovulation as an inflammatory reaction--a hypothesis. *Biol Reprod* **22** 73-106.

Feng WG, Sui HS, Han ZB, Chang ZL, Zhou P, Liu DJ, Bao S & Tan JH 2007 Effects of follicular atresia and size on the developmental competence of bovine oocytes: a study using the well-in-drop culture system. *Theriogenology* **67** 1339-50.

Fortune JE, Sirois J, Turzillo AM & Lavoir M 1991 Follicle selection in domestic ruminants. *J Reprod Fertil Suppl* **43** 187-98.

Gardiner TA, Anderson HR & Stitt AW 2003 Inhibition of advanced glycation end-products protects against retinal capillary basement membrane expansion during long-term diabetes. *J Pathol* **201** 328-33.

Giehl KA, Ferguson DJ, Dean D, Chuang YH, Allen J, Berker DA, Tosti A, Dawber RP & Wojnarowska F 2004 Alterations in the basement membrane zone in pili annulati hair follicles as demonstrated by electron microscopy and immunohistochemistry. *Br J Dermatol* **150** 722-7.

Ginther OJ, Kot K, Kulick LJ & Wiltbank MC 1997 Sampling follicular fluid without altering follicular status in cattle: oestradiol concentrations early in a follicular wave. *J Reprod Fertil* **109** 181-6.

Ginther OJ, Wiltbank MC, Fricke PM, Gibbons JR & Kot K 1996 Selection of the dominant follicle in cattle. *Biol Reprod* **55** 1187-94.

Goldin A, Beckman JA, Schmidt AM & Creager MA 2006 Advanced glycation end products: sparking the development of diabetic vascular injury. *Circulation* **114** 597-605.

Gosden RG, Hunter RH, Telfer E, Torrance C & Brown N 1988 Physiological factors underlying the formation of ovarian follicular fluid. *J Reprod Fertil* **82** 813-25.

Herrmann G & Spanel-Borowski K 1998 A sparsely vascularised zone in the cortex of the bovine ovary. *Anat Histol Embryol* **27** 143-6.

Hirani R, Hanssen E & Gibson MA 2007 LTBP-2 specifically interacts with the amino-terminal region of fibrillin-1 and competes with LTBP-1 for binding to this microfibrillar protein. *Matrix Biol* **26** 213-23.

Huet C, Monget P, Pisselet C & Monniaux D 1997 Changes in extracellular matrix components and steroidogenic enzymes during growth and atresia of antral ovarian follicles in the sheep. *Biol Reprod* **56** 1025-34.

Huey S, Abuhamad A, Barroso G, Hsu MI, Kolm P, Mayer

J & Oehninger S 1999 Perifollicular blood flow Doppler indices, but not follicular pO2, pCO2, or pH, predict oocyte developmental competence in in vitro fertilization. *Fertil Steril* **72** 707-12.

Hughesdon PE 1982 Morphology and morphogenesis of the Stein-Leventhal ovary and of so-called "hyperthecosis". *Obstet Gynecol Surv* **37** 59-77.

Huxley-Jones J, Robertson DL & Boot-Handford RP 2007 On the origins of the extracellular matrix in vertebrates. *Matrix Biol* **26** 2-11.

Irving-Rodgers HF, Catanzariti KD, Aspden WJ, D'Occhio MJ & Rodgers RJ 2006a Remodeling of extracellular matrix at ovulation of the bovine ovarian follicle. *Mol Reprod Dev* **73** 1292-302.

Irving-Rodgers HF, Catanzariti KD, Aspden WJ, D'Occhio MJ & Rodgers RJ 2006b Remodeling of extracellular matrix at ovulation of the bovine ovarian follicle. *Mol Reprod Dev* **73** 1292-1302.

Irving-Rodgers HF, Friden BE, Morris SE, Mason HD, Brannstrom M, Sekiguchi K, Sanzen N, Sorokin LM, Sado Y, Ninomiya Y & Rodgers RJ 2006c Extracellular matrix of the human cyclic corpus luteum. *Mol Hum Reprod* **12** 525-34.

Irving-Rodgers HF, Harland ML & Rodgers RJ 2004 A novel basal lamina matrix of the stratified epithelium of the ovarian follicle. *Matrix Biol* **23** 207-17.

Irving-Rodgers HF, Harland ML, Sullivan TR & Rodgers RJ 2009a Studies of granulosa cell maturation in dominant and subordinate bovine follicles: novel extracellular matrix focimatrix is co-ordinately regulated with cholesterol side-chain cleavage CYP11A1. *Reproduction* **137** 825-34.

Irving-Rodgers HF, Hummitzsch K, Murdiyarso LS, Bonner WM, Sado Y, Ninomiya Y, Couchman JR, Sorokin LM & Rodgers RJ 2010 Dynamics of extracellular matrix in ovarian follicles and corpora lutea of mice. *Cell Tissue Res* **339** 613-24.

Irving-Rodgers HF, Morris S, Collett RA, Peura TT, Davy M, Thompson JG, Mason HD & Rodgers RJ 2009b Phenotypes of the ovarian follicular basal lamina predict developmental competence of oocytes. *Hum Reprod* **24** 936-44.

Irving-Rodgers HF, Mussard ML, Kinder JE & Rodgers RJ 2002 Composition and morphology of the follicular basal lamina during atresia of bovine antral follicles. *Reproduction* **123** 97-106.

Irving-Rodgers HF & Rodgers RJ 2000a Ultrastructure of the basal lamina of bovine ovarian follicles and its relationship to the membrana granulosa. *J Reprod Fertil* **118** 221-8.

Irving-Rodgers HF & Rodgers RJ 2000b Ultrastructure of the basal lamina of bovine ovarian follicles and its relationship to the membrana granulosa. *J Reprod Fertil* **118** 221-8.

Irving-Rodgers HF & Rodgers RJ 2006 Extracellular matrix of the developing ovarian follicle. *Semin Reprod Med* **24** 195-203.

Jiang JY, Macchiarelli G, Tsang BK & Sato E 2003 Capillary angiogenesis and degeneration in bovine ovarian antral follicles. *Reproduction* **125** 211-23.

Juengel JL, Bibby AH, Reader KL, Lun S, Quirke LD, Haydon LJ & McNatty KP 2004 The role of transforming growth factor-beta (TGF-beta) during ovarian follicular development in sheep. *Reprod Biol Endocrinol* **2** 78.

Kielty CM, Sherratt MJ & Shuttleworth CA 2002 Elastic fibres. *J Cell Sci* **115** 2817-28.

Kisseleva T & Brenner DA 2007 Role of hepatic stellate cells in fibrogenesis and the reversal of fibrosis. *J Gastroenterol Hepatol* **22 Suppl 1** S73-8.

Knight PG & Glister C 2003 Local roles of TGF-beta superfamily members in the control of ovarian follicle development. *Anim Reprod Sci* **78** 165-83.

Knight PG & Glister C 2006 TGF-beta superfamily members and ovarian follicle development. *Reproduction* **132** 191-206.

Matti N, Irving-Rodgers HF, Hatzirodos N, Sullivan TR & Rodgers RJ 2010 Differential expression of focimatrix and steroidogenic enzymes before size deviation during waves of follicular development in bovine ovarian follicles. *Mol Cell Endocrinol* **321** 207-14.

McArthur ME, Irving-Rodgers HF, Byers S & Rodgers RJ 2000 Identification and immunolocalization of decorin, versican, perlecan, nidogen, and chondroitin sulfate proteoglycans in bovine small-antral ovarian follicles. *Biol Reprod* **63** 913-24.

Meyer zum Gottesberge AM & Felix H 2005 Abnormal basement membrane in the inner ear and the kidney of the Mpv17-/- mouse strain: ultrastructural and immunohistochemical investigations. *Histochem Cell Biol* **124** 507-16.

Mihm M, Austin EJ, Good TE, Ireland JL, Knight PG, Roche JF & Ireland JJ 2000 Identification of potential intrafollicular factors involved in selection of dominant follicles in heifers. *Biol Reprod* **63** 811-9.

Milner CM, Tongsoongnoen W, Rugg MS & Day AJ 2007 The molecular basis of inter-alpha-inhibitor heavy chain transfer on to hyaluronan. *Biochem Soc Trans* **35** 672-6.

Murata E, Akita M, Kaneko K & Merker HJ 1994 Changes associated with the basal lamina during metamorphosis of Xenopus laevis. *Acta Anat (Basel)* **150** 178-85.

Nagyova E, Camaioni A, Prochazka R & Salustri A 2004 Covalent transfer of heavy chains of inter-alpha-trypsin inhibitor family proteins to hyaluronan in in vivo and in vitro expanded porcine oocyte-cumulus complexes. *Biol Reprod* **71** 1838-43.

Nakano K, Naito I, Momota R, Sado Y, Hasegawa H, Ninomiya Y & Ohtsuka A 2007 The distribution of type IV collagen alpha chains in the mouse ovary and its correlation with follicular development. *Arch Histol Cytol* **70** 243-53.

Nelson VL, Legro RS, Strauss JF, 3rd & McAllister JM 1999 Augmented androgen production is a stable steroidogenic phenotype of propagated theca cells from polycystic ovaries. *Mol Endocrinol* **13** 946-57.

Nelson VL, Qin KN, Rosenfield RL, Wood JR, Penning TM, Legro RS, Strauss JF, 3rd & McAllister JM 2001 The biochemical basis for increased testosterone production in theca cells propagated from patients with polycystic ovary syndrome. *J Clin Endocrinol Metab* **86** 5925-33.

Nicholas B, Alberio R, Fouladi-Nashta AA & Webb R 2005 Relationship between low-molecular-weight insulin-like growth factor-binding proteins, caspase-3 activity, and oocyte quality. *Biol Reprod* **72** 796-804.

Nilsson EE, Doraiswamy V & Skinner MK 2003 Transforming growth factor-beta isoform expression during bovine ovarian antral follicle development. *Mol Reprod Dev* **66** 237-46.

Padmanabhan V, Manikkam M, Recabarren S & Foster D 2006 Prenatal testosterone excess programs reproductive and metabolic dysfunction in the female. *Mol Cell Endocrinol* **246** 165-74.

Penttinen C, Saharinen J, Weikkolainen K, Hyytiainen M & Keski-Oja J 2002 Secretion of human latent TGF-beta-binding protein-3 (LTBP-3) is dependent on co-expression of TGF-beta. *J Cell Sci* **115** 3457-68.

Prodoehl MJ, Hatzirodos N, Irving-Rodgers HF, Zhao ZZ, Painter JN, Hickey TE, Gibson MA, Rainey WE, Carr BR, Mason HD, Norman RJ, Montgomery GW & Rodgers RJ 2009a Genetic and gene expression analyses of the polycystic ovary syndrome candidate gene fibrillin-3 and other fibrillin family members in human ovaries. *Mol Hum Reprod* **15** 829-41.

Prodoehl MJ, Irving-Rodgers HF, Bonner W, Sullivan TM, Micke GC, Gibson MA, Perry VE & Rodgers RJ 2009b Fibrillins and latent TGF□ binding proteins in bovine ovaries of offspring following high or low protein diets during pregnancy of dams. *Molecular and Cellular Endocrinology* **307** 133-144.

Rajakoski E 1960 The ovarian follicular system in sexually mature heifers with special reference to seasonal, cyclical, end left-right variations. *Acta Endocrinol Suppl (Copenh)* **34(Suppl 52)** 1-68.

Ramirez F & Pereira L 1999 The fibrillins. *Int J Biochem Cell Biol* **31** 255-9.

Richardson MC, Davies DW, Watson RH, Dunsford ML, Inman CB & Masson GM 1992 Cultured human granulosa cells as a model for corpus luteum function: relative roles of gonadotrophin and low density lipoprotein studied under defined culture conditions. *Hum Reprod* **7** 12-8.

Rivera GM & Fortune JE 2003 Selection of the dominant follicle and insulin-like growth factor (IGF)-binding proteins: evidence that pregnancy-associated plasma protein A contributes to proteolysis of IGF-binding protein 5 in bovine follicular fluid. *Endocrinology* **144** 437-46.

Rodgers RJ & Irving-Rodgers HF 2010 Formation of the ovarian follicular antrum and follicular fluid. *Biol Reprod* **82** 1021-9.

Rodgers RJ, Irving-Rodgers HF & Russell DL 2003 Extracellular matrix of the developing ovarian follicle. *Reproduction* **126** 415-24.

Rodgers RJ, Irving-Rodgers HF, van Wezel IL, Krupa M & Lavranos TC 2001 Dynamics of the membrana granulosa during expansion of the ovarian follicular antrum. *Mol Cell Endocrinol* **171** 41-8.

Rubio Pomar FJ, Roelen BA, Slot KA, van Tol HT, Colenbrander B & Teerds KJ 2004 Role of Fas-mediated apoptosis and follicle-stimulating hormone on the developmental capacity of bovine cumulus oocyte complexes in vitro. *Biol Reprod* **71** 790-6.

Rugg MS, Willis AC, Mukhopadhyay D, Hascall VC, Fries E, Fulop C, Milner CM & Day AJ 2005 Characterization of complexes formed between TSG-6 and inter-alpha-inhibitor that act as intermediates in the covalent transfer of heavy chains onto hyaluronan. *J Biol Chem* **280** 25674-86.

Russell DL, Ochsner SA, Hsieh M, Mulders S & Richards JS 2003 Hormone-regulated expression and localization of versican in the rodent ovary. *Endocrinology* **144** 1020-31.

Schymeinsky J, Nedbal S, Miosge N, Poschl E, Rao C, Beier DR, Skarnes WC, Timpl R & Bader BL 2002 Gene structure and functional analysis of the mouse nidogen-2 gene: nidogen-2 is not essential for basement membrane formation in mice. *Mol Cell Biol* **22** 6820-30.

Shalgi R, Kraicer P, Rimon A, Pinto M & Soferman N 1973 Proteins of human follicular fluid: the blood-follicle barrier. *Fertil Steril* **24** 429-34.

Sirard MA, Picard L, Dery M, Coenen K & Blondin P 1999 The time interval between FSH administration and ovarian aspiration influences the development of cattle oocytes. *Theriogenology* **51** 699-708.

van Wezel IL & Rodgers RJ 1996 Morphological characterization of bovine primordial follicles and their environment in vivo. *Biol Reprod* **55** 1003-11.

Yamada O, Abe M, Takehana K, Hiraga T, Iwasa K & Hiratsuka T 1995 Microvascular changes during the development of follicles in bovine ovaries: a study of corrosion casts by scanning electron microscopy. *Arch Histol Cytol* **58** 567-74.

Yamada S, Fujiwara H, Honda T, Higuchi T, Nakayama T, Inoue T, Maeda M & Fujii S 1999 Human granulosa cells express integrin alpha2 and collagen type IV: possible involvement of collagen type IV in granulosa cell luteinization. *Mol Hum Reprod* **5** 607-17.

Yang MY & Rajamahendran R 2000 Morphological and biochemical identification of apoptosis in small, medium, and large bovine follicles and the effects of follicle-stimulating hormone and insulin-like growth factor-I on spontaneous apoptosis in cultured bovine granulosa cells. *Biol Reprod* **62** 1209-17.

Yoshioka S, Ochsner S, Russell DL, Ujioka T, Fujii S, Richards JS & Espey LL 2000 Expression of tumor necrosis factor-stimulated gene-6 in the rat ovary in response to an ovulatory dose of gonadotropin. *Endocrinology* **141** 4114-9.

Zimmermann DR & Dours-Zimmermann MT 2008 Extracellular matrix of the central nervous system: from neglect to challenge. *Histochem Cell Biol* **130** 635-53.

Managing the dominant follicle in high-producing dairy cows

MC Wiltbank[1], R Sartori[2], JLM Vasconcelos[3], AB Nascimento[1], AH Souza[4], AP Cunha[1], A Gumen[5], S Sangsritavong[6], JN Guenther[1], H Lopez[7] and JR Pursley[8]

[1]Department of Dairy Science, University of Wisconsin-Madison, Madison, Wisconsin, USA; [2]Department of Animal Science, USP, Piracicaba, São Paulo, Brazil; [3]Department of Animal Production, UNESP, Botucatu, São Paulo, Brazil; [4]Accelerated Genetics, Baraboo, Wisconsin, USA; [5]Department of Obstetrics and Gynecology, University of Uludag, Bursa, Turkey; [6] Central Research Unit, 113 Thailand Science Park, Prathumthani, Thailand; [7]American Breeders Service, DeForest, Wisconsin, USA; [8]Department of Animal Sciences, Michigan State University, E. Lansing, Michigan, USA

Reduced reproductive efficiency has been reported in high-producing dairy cows. Sources of reproductive inefficiency include decreased expression of estrus, increased diameter of the ovulatory follicle and reduced fertility when cows are inseminated after estrus, increased incidence of double ovulation and twinning, and increased pregnancy loss. To overcome some of these inefficiencies, reproductive management programs have been developed that synchronize ovulation and enable effective timed artificial insemination (AI) of lactating dairy cows. Effective regulation of the corpus luteum (CL), follicles, and hormonal environment are critical for optimizing these programs. Recent programs, such as the 5-day CIDR program, Double-Ovsynch, G-6-G, and estradiol benzoate-CIDR programs were designed to more effectively control one or more physiological events. These events include synchronization of a new follicular wave at the beginning of the program, optimization of the circulating progesterone (P4) concentrations and duration of follicular dominance, optimized reductions in P4 and increases in circulating estradiol (E2) concentrations during the preovulatory period, and tightly synchronized ovulation of a follicle of optimal size and fertility for implementation of timed AI. The success of these programs has been remarkable, although there is substantial variability in effectiveness due to environmental, management, nutritional, genetic, and disease factors as well as potential variability in some aspects of reproductive physiology among commercial dairy farms. Future programs will optimize the reproductive physiology while simplifying the protocol implementation and also match specific reproductive management protocols to specific farms and even specific cows (for example primiparous vs. multiparous).

Corresponding author E-mail: wiltbank@wisc.edu

Distinctive aspects of follicular growth in lactating dairy cows

The high-producing dairy cow has unique physiology related to follicular growth that impacts applied aspects of reproductive management programs. Dynamics and regulation of follicular waves have been reviewed previously (Ginther *et al.* 1996b; Adams *et al.* 2008; Aerts & Bols 2010). This review will focus on observations in lactating dairy cows that are relevant to reproductive management. Specific research citations will be used as examples to illustrate concepts. Due to space limitations, there will be no attempt to provide exhaustive literature citations or comparison of all important research studies during the discussion of each concept.

Follicular waves occur throughout pregnancy with each wave preceded by a surge in FSH. The magnitude of the FSH surge increased as pregnancy progressed. The maximum diameter of the dominant follicle, however, decreased as pregnancy progressed from 11.1 mm in Month 4 to 8.5 mm in Month 9 (Ginther *et al.* 1996b). Emergence of the final follicular wave during pregnancy occurred three weeks before parturition (Ginther *et al.* 1996b) whereas the interval from the last peak of FSH until parturition was approximately 12 days. Following parturition, there was a large increase in FSH with average FSH concentrations being 2-fold greater after parturition than average FSH surge concentrations during pregnancy. The interval from parturition to the day of emergence of the first follicular wave post-partum averaged 4 days (range of 2 to 7 days) (Ginther *et al.* 1996b).

Lactating dairy cows have variable intervals to first ovulation that depend on which post-partum follicular wave is ovulated. The dominant follicle from the first post-partum follicular wave has three potential outcomes: ovulation, atresia, or to become a large anovular follicle such as a follicular cyst. For example, Savio *et al.* (1990) reported that 74% of lactating cows ovulated the dominant follicle of the first follicular wave whereas 21% became cystic. In contrast, Butler *et al.* (2006) reported that 31% of cows ovulated the first dominant follicle post-partum, whereas 44% of cows had atresia of the first wave dominant follicle. The formation of atretic follicles was associated with low circulating E2 concentrations. There were 25.4% of cows that had a large anovular follicle that either became cystic (15%) or produced high E2 but did not ovulate (11%). These two papers illustrate the variability (31% vs. 74%) between studies/herds in the fate of the first-wave dominant follicle. The prevailing LH pulse frequency during the dominance phase of the first follicular wave is likely the major driver for growth and E2 production by the dominant follicle. Insufficient LH causes an atretic first dominant follicle with inadequate E2 production (see Crowe, 2008). It is still not clear what physiological changes result in a large anovular follicle with high E2 production during the first post-partum follicular wave. The lack of an adequate GnRH/LH surge in response to increased E2 may underlie the development of these large anovular follicles (Gumen & Wiltbank 2002). Following the first follicular wave post-partum there continue to be follicular waves every 7 to10 days with multiple potential outcomes such as ovulation, atresia, or cyst development, that depend on the physiological status of the cow.

There are a number of intriguing aspects of follicular wave dynamics that are unique to high production lactating dairy cows (Sartori *et al.* 2004). First, higher producing dairy cattle have lower circulating E2 concentrations than would be expected given their size of dominant follicles. For example, Lopez *et al.* (2005) reported decreasing peak circulating E2 concentrations with increasing milk production. Paradoxically lower circulating E2 was associated with greater follicular diameter when milk production increased. This contradiction could be due to reduced E2 production by the dominant follicle or increased E2 metabolism with increasing milk production in ldairy cows. The hypothesis that follicular E2 production varies with milk production has not yet been adequately tested. Greater E2 metabolism with increasing milk production, however, has been demonstrated (Sangsritavong *et al.* 2002). It seems likely that lesser circulating E2 in cows with greater follicular volume is primarily related to greater E2 metabolism in high milk-producing cows (Lopez *et al.* 2005). Greater E2 metabolism is probably caused by greater blood flow through the gastrointestinal tract and liver associated with the greater feed intake that is required to maintain high milk production (Wiltbank *et al.* 2006).

There also appears to be decreased expression of estrus in dairy cattle (Lopez *et al.* 2004). Lesser expression and detection of estrus in lactating dairy cows may reduce reproductive efficiency in the highest producing cows. Timed AI programs allow high- and low-producing dairy cows to be inseminated at a similar efficiency. This aspect makes these programs particularly appealing for herds with high-producing cows. In addition, the time of AI can be optimized in relation to the time of ovulation. Programs based on the expression of estrus may have more variability in the interval from AI to ovulation. A third intriguing aspect of follicular development in lactating dairy cows is that there is an increasing size of the ovulatory follicle with increasing milk production when cows are inseminated to estrus (Wiltbank *et al.* 2006). These differences may be reduced with timed AI programs because GnRH (or other agent) is used to induce ovulation before expression of estrus (discussed below). When cows are inseminated to estrus there may be a delay in ovulation in the highest-producing cows because greater E2 metabolism delays the attainment of sufficient circulating E2 to induce the GnRH/LH surge. Ovulation of larger follicles in higher producing dairy cows may partially explain the reduction in fertility in cows inseminated to estrus (Santos *et al.* 2010).

A fourth intriguing aspect of lactating dairy cows is the large percentage of cows that are anovular. Surprisingly, there is generally no relationship detected between level of milk production and the percentage of anovular cows. The follicular dynamics and physiology underlying different types of anovulation in cattle have been reviewed (Wiltbank *et al.* 2002; Wiltbank *et al.* 2008a). The most common type of anovular lactating dairy cow (~60% of anovular dairy cows) had follicles larger than ovulatory size but smaller than the classically defined cystic size (Wiltbank *et al.* 2002; Gumen *et al.* 2003). Anovular cows of this type probably have hypothalamic resistance to the positive feedback effects of E2 (Wiltbank *et al.* 2002; Gumen & Wiltbank 2005). The timed AI programs discussed below generally will induce ovulation in this type of anovular cow as well as most other types of anovular dairy cows (Wiltbank *et al.* 2008a). Nevertheless, cows that are anovular or have low P4 (proestrous period) at the start of the Ovsynch program have lower fertility than ovular cows with elevated P4 at start of the Ovsynch program (Bisinotto *et al.* 2010a).

A fifth intriguing aspect of follicular development in lactating dairy cows is an increase in double ovulation associated with greater milk production (Lopez *et al.* 2005). A comparison of the hormonal concentrations during the first follicular wave in cows that select a single follicle compared with cows that select two or three dominant follicles has been performed (Lopez *et al.* 2005). The main hormonal differences between cows with single vs. multiple dominant follicles are increased circulating FSH and LH during the 24 h before follicular deviation (largest follicle $\geq$ 8.5 mm). A reduction in circulating E2 does not appear to be the underlying cause of selection of multiple follicles. Circulating E2 is actually greater in cows with two or three dominant follicles than in cows with one dominant follicle during this critical period before deviation. A reduction in circulating P4 during this period may partially explain the increases in FSH and LH and increased selection of co-dominant follicles (see below). Differences in other aspects of reproductive physiology in lactating dairy cows have also been reported, including number and dynamics of follicular waves, CL volume, circulating P4, and reproductive diseases (Thatcher *et al.* 2010). The reader is referred to the many other reviews on related topics such as follicular management of anovular cows, patterns of follicular waves and fertility, and nutritional effects on follicular development and fertility in dairy cattle (Thatcher *et al.* 2002; Macmillan *et al.* 2003; Bilby *et al.* 2006; Leroy *et al.* 2008a; Leroy *et al.* 2008b; Wiltbank *et al.* 2008a).

Management of the follicle for timed AI in lactating dairy cows

Synchronized ovulation combined with timed AI has been a goal of reproductive physiologists for many years (Wiltbank *et al.* 1965; Zimbelman & Smith 1966; Odde 1990; Pursley *et al.* 1995; Thatcher *et al.* 1996; Lauderdale 2009). Obtaining good fertility with timed AI programs requires optimization of at least 5 distinct aspects of reproductive physiology (Fig. 1). First, synchronization of the follicular wave that will produce the dominant follicle for ovulation near the timed AI. Second, optimization of the hormonal environment and length of time during growth of this synchronized follicular wave. Third, optimization of the preovulatory period including synchronized regression of the CL with optimized timing in the reduction in circulating P4 and increases in circulating E2. Fourth, synchronization of ovulation of a dominant follicle with a high fertility oocyte, optimal periovulatory hormonal environment, and optimal timing and placement of high fertility semen in relation to the synchronized ovulation. Fifth, development of an optimal hormonal environment after AI that allows pregnancy establishment and maintenance. All of these physiological aspects of the program, together with management, nutritional, genetic, and disease aspects of the cow and herd, will contribute to the ultimate outcomes from these programs.

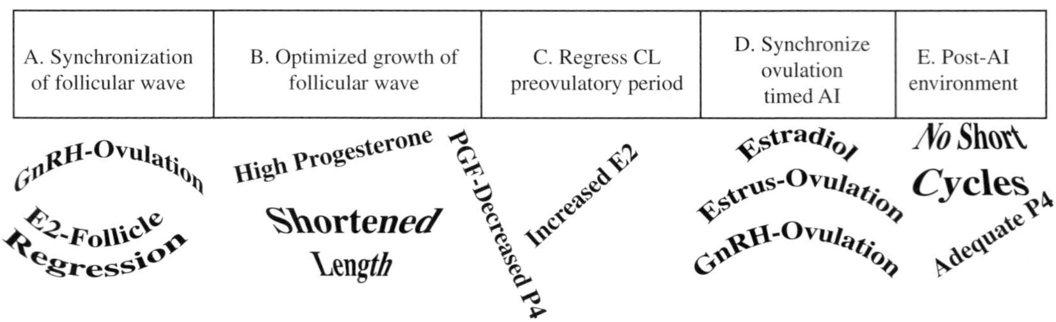

Fig. 1. Schematic of characteristic processes and current methods for timed AI programs.

Initiation of a synchronized follicular wave

One of the major changes with modern reproductive management protocols is the focus on controlling follicular development in addition to control of CL function and circulating P4 concentrations. Detailed studies of the follicular development during synchronization protocols became practical with the development of commercially-available transrectal ultrasound systems. Early ultrasound studies of bovine ovaries clearly showed the dynamics of follicular growth in cows that included follicular waves emerging every 7 to10 days (Savio *et al.* 1988; Sirois & Fortune 1988; Knopf *et al.* 1989). During emergence of a follicular wave, multiple follicles begin growing with the eventual deviation of a single dominant follicle (normally) from this cohort of follicles (Ginther *et al.* 1996a). The size of the follicle at deviation in Holstein dairy cattle averages about 8.5 mm and is associated with a nadir in circulating FSH concentrations. Continued growth of the dominant follicle is dependent on LH secretion. Ovulation depends on the LH surge. The maximal size of the dominant follicle during the estrous cycle or pregnancy and the timing of loss of function of the dominant follicle (i.e., turnover) depend on the hormonal environment and particularly circulating LH concentrations.

Synchronization of a new follicular wave generally entails removal of the functional dominant follicle either by physical destruction, hormonally-induced ovulation, or hormonal inhibition of gonadotropins so that the follicle regresses (Bodensteiner *et al.* 1996). Following aspiration of the dominant follicle there is a rapid increase in circulating FSH caused by the removal of follicle-derived inhibitors of FSH secretion. This FSH "surge" is followed by emergence of a new follicular wave, usually within 1 day. Similarly, induction of ovulation of the dominant follicle either with LH or hCG is followed by an FSH surge and emergence of a new follicular wave. From a practical standpoint, removal of the dominant follicle is usually performed by ovulation of the follicle using GnRH treatment (Thatcher *et al.* 1993; Pursley *et al.* 1995). Treatment with GnRH induces an LH and FSH surge that peaks within 2 h after treatment and returns to nadir concentrations by about 4 h. If this gonadotropin surge causes ovulation then there is a surge in FSH that peaks at about 24 h after the initial GnRH treatment with coincident emergence of a new follicular wave (Bodensteiner *et al.* 1996). Each of these follicular synchronization methods is primarily effective when the dominant follicle is removed, in other words in cows that ovulate in response to GnRH or gonadotropin treatments. Treatment of dairy cows at random stages of the estrous cycle with GnRH results in ovulation in only 50 to 70% of the cows (Pursley *et al.* 1995; Galvao & Santos 2010). Different stages of the estrous cycle have different ovulatory responses with the greatest response on Days 5 to 9 and reduced response earlier and later in the estrous cycle (Vasconcelos *et al.* 1999; Moreira *et al.* 2000; Bello *et al.* 2006). It is unrealistic, therefore, to expect 100% synchronization of follicular waves by using GnRH alone at the beginning of a synchronized ovulation program. Although ovulation to the initial GnRH is not necessarily a requirement for conception with these programs, there is generally a reduction in fertility in cows that do not ovulate to the initial GnRH treatment (Thatcher *et al.* 2002; Galvao & Santos 2010).

One of the methods that is used to increase ovulation to the first GnRH treatment during Ovsynch is to control the day of the cycle at the initiation of Ovsynch. Generally, the best day to give the first GnRH treatment is Day 6 or 7 of the cycle when there is a large dominant follicle (Vasconcelos *et al.* 1999; Moreira *et al.* 2000; Bello *et al.* 2006). There is a high ovulation rate after GnRH on Day 6 or 7 and therefore a synchronized emergence of the new follicular wave. This is one of the key ideas underlying the development of Presynch-Ovsynch (Moreira *et al.* 2001; Ei-Zarkouny *et al.* 2004), G-6-G (Bello *et al.* 2006), and Double-Ovsynch (Souza *et al.* 2008). During Double-Ovsynch, for example, the first Ovsynch protocol synchronizes the cows so that the second Ovsynch procedure is initiated on Day 7 of the cycle.

An alternative method for removing the functional dominant follicle involves inhibiting the gonadotropins that are necessary to sustain dominance. From a practical stand-point this can be accomplished with E2 treatment in the presence of high P4 (Bo *et al.* 1995; Burke *et al.* 2003). It is necessary to have P4 present during E2 treatment to prevent an E2-induced LH surge and ovulation. The combination of E2 and P4 decreases LH and FSH and this reduction in gonadotropin support results in follicular atresia and the regression of dominant follicles within 36 h after treatment (Burke *et al.* 2003; Martinez *et al.* 2005). After treating Holstein cows with 2 mg of E2-benzoate with or without injectable P4 in a CIDR protocol, circulating FSH and LH reached nadir concentrations by ~0.5 days; a time that corresponded with peak circulating E2. The FSH surge occurred at 3 to 4 d after the initial E2 treatments (Cavalieri *et al.* 2003). The length of time from hormonal treatment to emergence of the new follicular wave has been shown to be independent of the stage of follicular development at E2 treatment (Kim *et al.* 2007a). It does depend, however, on the type (Martinez *et al.* 2005) and dose (Burke *et al.* 2003; Colazo *et al.* 2005) of E2 that is used for treatment. The circulating E2 profiles for different esters of E2 are different in cattle (Martinez *et al.* 2005; Souza *et al.* 2005). Although long half-life estrogens (e.g., E2-cypionate) have been successfully used to synchronize the emergence of follicular waves in beef cattle and heifers (Colazo *et al.* 2005), they seem to be less precise for synchronizing wave emergence when used in lactating dairy cows (Thundathil *et al.* 1998) perhaps because of the rapid E2 clearance rates in the liver of high milk-producing cows. The time to emergence of the new follicular wave is reduced with increasing milk production (Souza *et al.* 2009). For example, treatment of cows with 2 mg of E2-benzoate results in follicular wave emergence at 3.8 d in the highest-producing cows but not until 4.5 d in the lowest-producing cows.

Collectively, E2 + P4 protocols will induce synchronous follicular wave emergence in about 70 to 90% of cattle. Most failures in synchronization are related to lack of dominant follicle regression and late wave emergence (Diskin *et al.* 2002; Souza *et al.* 2009). One of the key benefits of synchronizing the follicular wave by inhibiting follicular growth (compared with ovulating the dominant follicle) is that a new CL is not present during the synchronization protocol. This makes incomplete luteal regression less likely in the E2 + P4 protocol compared with the Ovsynch-like protocols (Kim *et al.* 2007b). A downside of not inducing a new ovulation at the beginning of the synchronization procedures is that circulating P4 could be lower in E2 + P4 protocols than needed for optimal oocyte quality in timed AI protocols (Kim *et al.* 2007b; Rutigliano *et al.* 2008).

Optimizing growth of the follicular wave

It is important to optimize the "fertility" of the follicle that will ovulate the oocyte for subsequent fertilization and embryonic development. This optimization involves ovulation of an "optimized" oocyte with production of an "optimized" CL to maintain embryo development and pregnancy. These may be conflicting goals since ovulation of a larger follicle will likely result in a larger CL with greater P4 production. The oocyte from a larger follicle, however, may have reduced fertility (Ahmad *et al.* 1995; Ahmad *et al.* 1996; Revah & Butler 1996). The hormonal environment and duration of growth of this follicle have been found to be key components in optimizing fertility in timed AI programs. Hormonal environment and duration of the follicular wave may impact fertility through its effects on oocyte function, granulosa/thecal cell number or function, oviductal or uterine function, and other potential reproductive functions.

The circulating P4 concentrations have been found to have substantial impact on subsequent fertility. A relationship between pre-AI P4 concentration and subsequent fertility was documented almost 3 decades ago where first service conception rate increased by approximately 10% for every 1 ng/ml increase in average P4 (Fonseca et al. 1983). A study in seasonal dairy herds in New Zealand tested this hypothesis as well (Xu et al. 1997). Cows were synchronized with prostaglandin F2α (PGF) 13 d apart and supplemented or not supplemented with a CIDR for 5 d before the second PGF to increase circulating P4 before AI. There was an increase in percentage of cows that showed estrus after the second PGF (89.6% vs. 82.9%) and percentage pregnant to AI (P/AI) after this estrus (65.1% vs. 59.7%). Analysis of the stage of the estrous cycle at the time of the second PGF demonstrated that the CIDR improved fertility in cows in the earlier (Days 5 to 9; 52.3% vs. 64.8% P/AI) and mid-cycle (Days 10 to13; 59.3% vs. 66.2%) but not later cycle (Days 14 to 19; 71.3% vs. 71.4%). Increasing P4 in cows with lower P4 before PGF synchronization, therefore, improved fertility at the subsequent AI. Indeed, many of the pre-synchronization programs, such as Presynch-Ovsynch, may improve fertility through their effects on P4 during the pre-AI period.

We tested whether P4 concentrations during growth of the preovulatory follicle would alter double ovulation rates (DOV) and fertility in lactating cows (Cunha & Wiltbank, unpublished). Holstein cows (n = 624) were presynchronized before the breeding Ovsynch with an Ovsynch72 protocol (GnRH-7d-PGF-3d-GnRH) but timed AI was not performed (Fig. 2). Cows then began Ovsynch immediately (the 2nd GnRH of the Ovsynch72 was the 1st GnRH of the breeding Ovsynch) (Low-P4; Short Double-Ovsynch) or cows received the first GnRH of the breeding Ovsynch 1 week later (High-P4; Double-Ovsynch; Fig. 2). Ovarian ultrasound and blood sampling were performed in order to assess ovulation, pregnancy status, and circulating P4 concentrations. As expected, cows in the High-P4 group had greater P4 concentrations than cows in the Low-P4 group at the first GnRH of the breeding Ovsynch (1.80 ng/mL vs. 0.38 ng/mL) and at the PGF (4.43 ng/mL vs. 2.51 ng/mL). The DOV was greater in the Low-P4 than in the High-P4 group (20.6% vs. 7.0%; P=0.03). A previous study also reported a reduction in DOV in cows with increased pre-AI P4 concentrations (Rutigliano et al. 2008). Overall P/AI at Day 29 was greater in the High-P4 compared with the Low-P4 group (51.0%, n=292 vs. 37.1%, n=272; P=0.001). Surprisingly, pregnancy loss (between Day 29 to 57) was also less in the High-P4 than the Low-P4 group (6.8% vs. 14.3%; P=0.05). High-P4 during follicular development, therefore, reduced selection of co-dominant follicles and DOV. In spite of ovulating fewer follicles and in spite of a lower P4 concentration after AI, cows treated with the High-P4 protocol had better fertility than those treated with the Low-P4 protocol. These data provide strong evidence for the importance of high P4 during Ovsynch.

A. Double-Ovsynch - High P4 during follicle growth.

Sun	Mon	Tues	Wednesday	Thursday	Friday	Sat
					GnRH	
					PGF	
	GnRH					
	GnRH					
	PGF		GnRH-PM	AI-AM		

B. Short Double-Ovsynch - Low P4 during follicle growth.

Sun	Mon	Tues	Wednesday	Thursday	Friday	Sat
					GnRH	
					PGF	
	GnRH					
	PGF		GnRH-PM	AI-AM		

Fig. 2. Diagrams of a typical weekly calendar for the protocols used in the experiment to test the effect of P4 concentration during the Ovsynch protocol (growth of ovulatory follicle) on fertility and double ovulation rate.

There are many potential physiological mechanisms that may underlie the effect of high P4 during follicular growth to reduce DOV, increase fertility, and reduce pregnancy loss in timed AI protocols. Greater circulating P4 decreases LH pulses (Stumpf *et al.* 1993). In previous studies, low P4 during follicular growth resulted in development of persistent, lower-fertility follicles (Ahmad *et al.* 1994; Ahmad *et al.* 1996; Revah & Butler 1996). For example, lactating dairy cows had lower fertility after development of a persistent follicle compared with control dairy cows (44% vs. 12%; (Ahmad *et al.* 1996). A recent study (Cerri *et al.* 2009) flushed embryos from cows that started Ovsynch on Day 3 or Day 6 of the estrous cycle. Only 7.1% of cows that started Ovsynch on Day 3 ovulated to the first GnRH, whereas 88.6% of cows ovulated to the first GnRH when Ovsynch was started on Day 6. Fertilization rate was similar for the two groups (85 vs. 86%). The percentage of high quality embryos (Grades 1 and 2), however, was greater for cows that started Ovsynch on Day 6 (83.7%) compared with Day 3 (47.0%).

The period of follicular dominance averaged 8.0 d in cows that started Ovsynch on Day 3, and averaged 5.8 d for Day 6 cows. A 2 d increase in follicular dominance, therefore, reduced embryo quality (78% increase in degenerate embryos). In our experiment that used Double-Ovsynch with high or low P4 concentrations, the age of the follicles were identical in the two groups. The preovulatory follicle from the low P4 group, however, would have been exposed to a greater number of LH pulses and this could underlie the low fertility. Thus, reduced fertility can occur in cows that ovulate even minimally persistent follicles or in cows with follicles that may not be older but are overexposed to LH. This may be a critical concept for fertility in normally-ovulating dairy cows or during synchronized breeding protocols.

In an attempt to reduce the duration of follicular dominance, a shortened Ovsynch strategy has been developed. The interval between GnRH and PGF was reduced from 7 to 5 d along with an increase in the proestrous period from 48 to 56 h (time of second GnRH) until 72 h. This strategy has resulted in improved in fertility in beef cattle (Bridges *et al.* 2008). A similar strategy in dairy cattle produced encouraging results. Santos *et al.* (2010) reported an improvement in fertility in the 5-d compared with the 7-d Ovsynch protocol (5-d: 37.9% vs. 7-d: 30.9%). Two treatments with PGF were required, however, for optimizing the synchronization of cows assigned to the 5-d protocol. For the 5-d and the 7-d protocols, timing of the second GnRH and timed AI were both done at 72 h after the PGF (Cosynch-72). This timing of GnRH and AI has been found to reduce fertility in the 7-d protocol (Brusveen *et al.* 2008) but does not alter fertility in the 5-d protocol (Bisinotto *et al.* 2010b) compared with GnRH treatment at 56 h and AI 16 h later. Additional studies are necessary to evaluate the differences between these protocols and to optimize the protocols. It seems likely that protocols with reduced duration of follicular dominance, combined with a longer proestrous period (discussed below), can increase fertility in lactating dairy cows.

Optimizing the hormonal environment during the preovulatory period

The hormonal environment during the proestrous period is critical for reproductive success. First, lack of complete CL regression leads to elevated P4 during the proestrous period and reduced fertility during timed AI protocols (Souza *et al.* 2007). In one study we found that 15% of cows did not have complete CL regression following the Double-Ovsynch protocol. These cows had greatly reduced fertility to the timed AI (Brusveen *et al.* 2009). Treatment with a second injection of PGF, 24 h after the first, resulted in almost all cows having complete CL regression with a slight (~5%) but not significant improvement in fertility.

A second critical factor is to optimize E2 concentrations before AI. In cows treated with GnRH followed seven days later by PGF and then inseminated to estrus, treatment with 1 mg of E2-cypionate at 24 h after PGF, increased E2 concentrations, and increased fertility to the estrus breeding (Cerri *et al.* 2004). To test the effect of E2 during an Ovsynch protocol, we treated cows with Ovsynch (GnRH - 7d - PGF - 56h - GnRH - 16h - timed AI) with or without treatment with 1 mg of E2 (native estradiol-17ß) at 48 h after PGF (8 h before second GnRH treatment and 24 h before timed AI at 72 h) (Souza *et al.* 2007). As expected, there was an increase in expression of estrus in cows treated with E2 (Ovsynch: 44.4% vs. Ovsynch+E2: 80.2%); however, there was no overall improvement in fertility associated with E2 treatment (Ovsynch: 39.4% vs. Ovsynch+E2: 42.4%). Treatment with E2 improved fertility in low body condition score (BCS $\leq$ 2.5) cows (Ovsynch: 28.1% vs. Ovsynch+E2: 40.0%) such that these cows had similar fertility to cows in high BCS (Ovsynch: 43.7% vs. Ovsynch+E2: 43.9%). A sufficient E2 surge, therefore, may be the key rate-limiting step for obtaining high fertility in low BCS cows during timed AI protocols. Treatment with E2 also tended to increase fertility in cows ovulating medium-sized follicles (15 to 19 mm) but not in cows ovulating smaller or larger follicles. This observation is consistent with the concept that increasing circulating E2 may be important for optimizing the preovulatory hormonal environment during timed AI protocols, at least in cows that ovulate an optimized follicle size. Thus, optimizing circulating E2, along with other follicular/luteal optimizations, may improve fertility in cows inseminated to estrus or in cows that are timed AI (Cerri *et al.* 2004; Souza *et al.* 2007).

A third factor to consider for improving fertility is increasing the length of the proestrous period. The importance of increasing the proestrous period has been demonstrated in beef cattle treated with the 5-day protocol (Bridges *et al.* 2010). It seems likely that changes in the proestrous period may alter fertility by affecting the uterine environment and (or) the follicle and oocyte.

Synchronization of ovulation

There are many reasons to synchronize ovulation and perform timed AI rather than wait for estrus. First, higher-producing lactating dairy cows demonstrate less estrous behavior than lower-producing cows (Lopez *et al.* 2004). Timed AI programs, therefore, should result in an increased percentage of higher-producing cows receiving AI compared with programs based on detection of estrus. Second, follicle size could be theoretically optimized during a synchronized ovulation program and this could improve fertility. Third, timing of AI can be optimized in relation to ovulation (one previously designated time in all cows) and this should increase management efficiency and fertility. The first advantage (increased percentage of cows receiving AI) has been reported in direct comparisons of timed AI and estrus programs. Improvements in fertility, however, have not been a consistent result. A meta-analysis done in 2005 (71 trials in 53 research publications with sufficient experimental details for inclusion in the analysis) reported no significant differences in P/AI between Ovsynch compared with various other reproductive management strategies (Rabiee *et al.* 2005).

There are several methods to synchronize the time of ovulation. Any method that will synchronize estrus will also synchronize the time of ovulation; although, synchronization may not be sufficient to allow good success with timed AI. Most timed AI programs use either a GnRH or estradiol treatment to increase the synchrony of ovulation during these programs.

Treatment with GnRH results in an LH surge that reaches a peak by about 2 h and causes ovulation between 24 to 32 h after GnRH (Pursley *et al.* 1995). There are at least 10% of cows that do not ovulate to the second GnRH treatment of Ovsynch (Vasconcelos *et al.* 1999; Bello *et al.* 2006; Souza *et al.* 2007; Brusveen *et al.* 2009; Galvao &v Santos 2010). Two primary reasons explain the lack of synchronized ovulation to the Ovsynch protocol. First, cows may come into estrus before the GnRH treatment and therefore ovulate prematurely because of an endogenous GnRH/LH surge (Vasconcelos *et al.* 1999). Premature ovulation during Ovsynch was only found in cows that started Ovsynch in the later estrous cycle ($\geq$ Day 12) and did not ovulate to the first GnRH treatment of Ovsynch (Vasconcelos *et al.* 1999). Second, cows may not have a dominant follicle at the time of the second GnRH treatment due to initiation of a new follicular wave during the Ovsynch protocol. Immature follicular development at the second GnRH of Ovsynch was found in cows that initiated Ovsynch at various stages of the estrous cycle and in cows that may or may not have ovulated to the first GnRH of Ovsynch (Vasconcelos *et al.* 1999). Obviously, cows that do not ovulate to the second GnRH of Ovsynch have little or no fertility to the timed AI.

Cows that ovulate after Ovsynch may not ovulate an ideal size of follicle. For example, Souza *et al.* (2007) found that only 57.6% cows ovulated a follicle of 14 to 19 mm after Ovsynch.

Twenty percent of cows ovulated a follicle that was too small ($\leq$13 mm) and 22.5% ovulated a follicle that was too large ($\geq$20 mm). Vasconcelos *et al.* (2001) used an aspiration to produce a new follicular wave mid-way through the Ovsynch protocol so that there was ovulation of smaller (~11.5 mm) follicles at the second GnRH of Ovsynch compared with non-aspirated controls (~14.5 mm). The cows ovulating the small follicles had reduced fertility (12% vs. 45% for control). The reduction in fertility in cows ovulating small follicles may be due to reduced E2 before AI, ovulation of a less-mature oocyte, and/or reduced P4 after AI (due to ovulation of a smaller follicle with a subsequently smaller CL). Ovulation of larger follicles may in some cases produce oocytes with reduced fertility (Ahmad *et al.* 1996; Cerri *et al.* 2009). Improvements in fertility to Ovsynch, therefore, are likely to be obtained by increasing the percentage of cows that ovulate an optimally-sized follicle after the final GnRH treatment.

Many studies have used different estrogens to synchronize the time of ovulation in dairy cows treated with E2 + P4 or Ovsynch-like protocols. Estrogens are available for use in synchronization protocols in many countries but are not available in the United States or Europe. Estrogen products are generally sold at a lower price than GnRH products and therefore can be economically attractive for producers. Nevertheless, the increased estrous behavior caused by estrogens is negatively viewed by some producers because of the risk of accidents and the excessive activity observed in the estrogen-treated cows. Estrogens with shorter half-lives (E2 and E2-benzoate) are typically used 24 to 48 h after PGF treatment with AI at about 1 d after E2 treatment. Studies with the Heat-Synch protocol (Pancarci *et al.* 2002; Cerri *et al.* 2004; Stevenson *et al.* 2004) have substituted the longer-acting E2-cypionate 24 h after PGF treatment to synchronize the time of ovulation. Although time of ovulation is shorter after GnRH compared with E2-cypionate treatment, fertility was similar in Heat-Synch vs. Ovsynch protocols. The Heat-Synch protocol has been shown to improve fertility as compared with cows inseminated to estrus (Cerri *et al.* 2004). Interesting, there was improved fertility in cows that showed estrus during the Heat-Synch protocol, although expression of estrus had no effect on fertility in cows that were AI to Ovysnch (Pancarci *et al.* 2002). Some protocols have also used E2-cypionate at the time of PGF/CIDR removal with similar results as observed with synchronized ovulation after a GnRH treatment (Souza *et al.* 2009). Synchronized ovulation occurs around 70 to 75 h after CIDR removal. Data from an earlier trial (Colazo *et al.* 2004) using beef heifers, however, indicated that better fertility is achieved when E2-cypionate was given 24 h after CIDR removal rather than at the time of CIDR removal. Thus, there are a variety of different options for synchronizing ovulation with estrogens. Optimal timing of treatments and of AI can vary based on the half-life of the estrogen, management factors, and the type of protocol used to synchronize follicular/luteal function before the synchronized ovulation.

Post-AI treatments to regulate follicles

Management of follicles after breeding can also be used to regulate reproduction and potentially improve the efficiency of reproductive management programs. Resynchronization of ovulation (Resynch) in cows that did not become pregnant to the first AI can improve reproductive management programs by reducing the time between AI. The physiological aspects of Resynch programs are similar to what has been discussed above; however, some management considerations are critical because of the need to definitively confirm non-pregnancy in cows before treatment with PGF (Galvao *et al.* 2007; Silva *et al.* 2007; Wiltbank *et al.* 2008b).

The use of hCG or GnRH after AI has been tested as a follicular/luteal management strategy to improve fertility in lactating dairy cows (De Rensis *et al.* 2010). Treatment of cattle with these agents at certain times of the cycle can result in ovulation of the dominant follicle. If a follicle is ovulated there should be increased circulating P4 due to the presence of an accessory CL. In addition, hCG could increase circulating P4 due to direct effects of hCG to stimulate luteal function; although, this theoretical hCG effect has not been confirmed experimentally in cattle. The increases in circulating P4 after treatment with hCG on Days 5 to 7 of the estrous cycle have been shown in many studies. For example, Santos *et al.* (2001) treated cows that had been AI to estrus with 3,300 IU of hCG on Day 5 after AI. Treatment with hCG increased circulating P4 and increased fertility (Control: 38.9% vs. hCG: 45.8%). Our recent studies following timed AI protocols found a smaller but significant effect of treatment on Day 5 with hCG on fertility (Control: 37.3% vs. hCG: 40.8%) with significant hCG effects only in first lactation cows (Nascimento, Souza, Bender, Wiltbank, unpublished). Thus, it appears that hCG treatment on Day 5 improves fertility although the physiological reason for this improvement was not defined in these studies. One possibility is that the hCG-induced increase in circulating P4 improves fertility due to P4 effects on the uterus and (or) embryo. A number of studies are consistent with respect to increased P4 increasing embryonic development but the P4 effect appears to be mainly during the early luteal phase (Days 5 to 9) (Mann *et al.* 2006). Treatment with hCG on Day 5 does not increase circulating P4 until Day 8. Perhaps earlier increases in P4 would produce greater improvements in fertility. Another possible effect of hCG treatment is a change in follicular development pattern that could delay luteolysis and thus improve fertility. Ovulation on Day 5 results in a new follicular wave emerging by Day 6 and likely turnover of the dominant follicle of this wave before luteolysis. Thus, the cow is likely to have 3 rather than 2 follicular waves. This change in follicular wave patterns may improve fertility (Townson *et al.* 2002). For example, an absence of circulating E2 from a dominant follicle near the time of normal luteolysis will delay luteolysis until there is sufficient E2 to increase PGF secretion from the uterus (Araujo *et al.* 2009). Changes in follicular wave patterns and timing of luteolysis, therefore, may be part of the mechanism for increased fertility after hCG-induced ovulation of the dominant follicle of the first follicular wave.

Closing remarks

One of the biggest changes in reproductive management research during the last 2 decades has been a focus on precise regulation of follicular development. This was possible because of the availability of high-resolution ultrasound technology allowing evaluation of the dynamic processes of follicular emergence, selection, growth, atresia, and ovulation. Evaluation of the dynamics of follicular development in anovular conditions has provided much greater insight into the physiology of these processes (Wiltbank *et al.* 2002). An understanding of the natural processes regulating follicular development is allowing greater insight into how changes in patterns of follicular development as well as management and nutritional factors may be regulating fertility (Thatcher *et al.* 2002; Townson *et al.* 2002; Macmillan *et al.* 2003; Leroy *et al.* 2008a; Leroy *et al.* 2008b). The most revolutionary of the research changes after introduction of ultrasound may be the many variations of synchronization protocols that are focused on synchronized ovulation of an "optimized follicle". Initial programs resulted in fertility that was similar to breeding to estrus but offered the advantage of a timed AI of all cattle on a preselected day (Pursley *et al.* 1997). Recent, optimized synchronization strategies may result in better fertility in lactating dairy cows than breeding to estrus. Additional research is needed to evaluate these programs in various commercial and experimental conditions. For example, some of these programs may be best for cows in specific physiological circumstances as exemplified by the better conception rates in primiparous than multiparous cows following the Double-Ovsynch protocol (Souza *et al.* 2008). Clearly, a great deal of progress is being made in understanding the physiology of these programs with future progress needed to increase consistency, simplicity, and economic value of these programs for dairy producers.

References

Adams GP, Jaiswal R, Singh J & Malhi P 2008 Progress in understanding ovarian follicular dynamics in cattle. *Theriogenology* **69** 72-80.

Aerts JMJ & Bols PE J 2010 Ovarian follicular dynamics. A review with emphasis on the bovine species. Part II: Antral development, exogenous influence and future prospects. *Reprod Domest Anim* **45** 180-187.

Ahmad N, Beam SW, Butler WR, Deaver DR, Duby RT, Elder DR, Fortune JE, Griel LC, Jones LS, Milvae RA, Pate JL, Revah I, Schreiber DT, Townson DH, Tsang PC W & Inskeep EK 1996 Relationship of fertility to patterns of ovarian follicular development and associated hormonal profiles in dairy cows and heifers. *J Anim Sci* **74** 1943-1952.

Ahmad N, Schrick FN, Butcher RL & Inskeep EK 1994 Fertilization rate and embryo development in relation to rersistent follicles and peripheral estradiol-17-beta in beef cows. *Biol Reprod* **50** 65-65.

Ahmad N, Schrick FN, Butcher RL & Inskeep EK 1995 Effect of persistent follicles on early embryonic losses in beef cows. *Biol Reprod* **52** 1129-1135.

Araujo RR, Ginther OJ, Ferreira JC, Palhao MM, Beg MA & Wiltbank MC 2009 Role of follicular estradiol-17beta in timing of luteolysis in heifers. *Biol Reprod* **81** 426-437.

Bello NM, Steibel JP & Pursley JR 2006 Optimizing ovulation to first GnRH improved outcomes to each hormonal injection of Ovsynch in lactating dairy cows. *J Dairy Sci* **89** 3413-3424.

Bilby TR, Block J, do Amaral BC, Sa O, Silvestre FT, Hansen PJ, Staples CR & Thatcher WW 2006 Effects of dietary unsaturated fatty acids on oocyte quality and follicular development in lactating dairy cows in summer. *J Dairy Sci* **89** 3891-3903.

Bisinotto RS, Chebel RC & Santos JEP 2010a Follicular wave of the ovulatory follicle and not cyclic status influences fertility of dairy cows. *J Dairy Sci* **93** 3578-3587.

Bisinotto RS, Ribeiro ES, Martins LT, Marsola RS, Greco LF, Risco CA, Thatcher WW & Santos JEP 2010b Effect of moment of induced ovulation and progesterone (P4) for resynchronization on fertility of Holstein cows in a 5-d timed AI program. *J Dairy Sci* **93, E-Suppl. 1** 675.

Bo GA, Adams GP, Pierson RA & Mapletoft RJ 1995 Exogenous control of follicular wave emergence in cattle. *Theriogenology* **43** 31-40.

Bodensteiner KJ, Kot K, Wiltbank MC & Ginther OJ 1996 Synchronization of emergence of follicular waves in cattle. *Theriogenology* **45** 1115-1128.

Bridges GA, Helser LA, Grum DE, Mussard ML, Gasser CL & Day ML 2008 Decreasing the interval between GnRH and PGF(2 alpha) from 7 to 5 days and lengthening proestrus increases timed-AI pregnancy rates in beef cows. *Theriogenology* **69** 843-851.

Bridges GA, Mussard ML, Burke CR & Day ML 2010 Influence of the length of proestrus on fertility and endocrine function in female cattle. *Anim Reprod Sci* **117** 208-215.

Brusveen DJ, Cunha AP, Silva CD, Cunha PM, Sterry RA, Silva EPB, Guenther JN & Wiltbank MC 2008 Altering the time of the second gonadotropin-releasing hormone injection and artificial insemination (AI) during ovsynch affects pregnancies per AI in lactating dairy cows. *J Dairy Sci* **91** 1044-1052.

Brusveen DJ, Souza AH & Wiltbank MC 2009 Effects of additional prostaglandin F-2 alpha and estradiol-17 beta during Ovsynch in lactating dairy cows. *J Dairy Sci* **92** 1412-1422.

Burke CR, Mussard ML, Gasser CL, Grum DE & Day ML 2003 Estradiol benzoate delays new follicular wave emergence in a dose-dependent manner after ablation of the dominant ovarian follicle in cattle. *Theriogenology* **60** 647-658.

Butler ST, Pelton SH & Butler WR 2006 Energy balance, metabolic status, and the first postpartum ovarian follicle wave in cows administered propylene glycol. *J Dairy Sci* **89** 2938-2951.

Cavalieri J, Hepworth G, Parker KI, Wright PJ & Macmillan KL 2003 Effect of treatment with progesterone and oestradiol when starting treatment with an intravaginal progesterone releasing insert on ovarian follicular development and hormonal concentrations in Holstein cows. *Anim Reprod Sci* **76** 177-193.

Cerri RLA, Rutigliano HM, Chebel RC & Santos JEP 2009 Period of dominance of the ovulatory follicle influences embryo quality in lactating dairy cows. *Reproduction* **137** 813-823.

Cerri R LA, Santos JEP, Juchem SO, Galvao KN & Chebel RC 2004 Timed artificial insemination with estradiol cypionate or insemination at estrus in high-producing dairy cows. *J Dairy Sci* **87** 3704-3715.

Colazo MG, Kastelic JP, Martinez MF, Whittaker PR, Wilde R, Ambrose JD, Corbett R & Mapletoft RJ 2004 Fertility following fixed-time AI in CIDR-treated beef heifers given GnRH or estradiol cypionate and fed diets supplemented with flax seed or sunflower seed. *Theriogenology* **61** 1115-1124.

Colazo MG, Martinez MF, Small JA, Kastelic JP, Burnley CA, Ward DR & Mapletoft RJ 2005 Effect of estradiol valerate on ovarian follicle dynamics and superovulatory response in progestin-treated cattle. *Theriogenology* **63** 1454-1468.

Crowe MA 2008 Resumption of ovarian cyclicity in post-partum beef and dairy cows. *Reprod Domest Anim* **43** 20-28.

De Rensis F, Lopez-Gatius F, Garcia-Ispierto I & Techakumpu M 2010 Clinical use of human chorionic gonadotropin in dairy cows: An update. *Theriogenology* **73** 1001-1008.

Diskin MG, Austin EJ & Roche JF 2002 Exogenous hormonal manipulation of ovarian activity in cattle. *Domest Anim Endocrin* **23** 211-228.

Ei-Zarkouny SZ, Cartmill JA, Hensley BA & Stevenson JS 2004 Pregnancy in dairy cows after synchronized ovulation regimens with or without presynchronization and progesterone. *J Dairy Sci* **87** 1024-1037.

Fonseca FA, Britt JH, Mcdaniel BT, Wilk JC & Rakes AH 1983 Reproductive traits of Holsteins and Jerseys - effects of age, milk-yield, and clinical abnormalities on involution of cervix and uterus, ovulation, estrous cycles, detection of estrus, conception rate, and days open. *J Dairy Sci* **66** 1128-1147.

Galvao KN & Santos JEP 2010 Factors affecting synchronization and conception rate after the Ovsynch protocol in lactating Holstein cows. *Reprod Domest Anim* **45** 439-446.

Galvao KN, Santos JEP, Cerri RL, Chebel RC, Rutigliano HM, Bruno RG & Bicalho RC 2007 Evaluation of methods of resynchronization for insemination in cows of unknown pregnancy status. *J Dairy Sci* **90** 4240-4252.

Ginther OJ, Kot K, Kulick LJ, Martin S & Wiltbank MC 1996a Relationships between FSH and ovarian follicular waves during the last six months of pregnancy in cattle. *J Reprod Fertil* **108** 271-279.

Ginther OJ, Wiltbank MC, Fricke PM, Gibbons JR & Kot K 1996b Selection of the dominant follicle in cattle. *Biol Reprod* **55** 1187-1194.

Gumen A, Guenther JN & Wiltbank MC 2003 Follicular size and response to Ovsynch versus detection of estrus in anovular and ovular lactating dairy cows. *J Dairy Sci* **86** 3184-3194.

Gumen A & Wiltbank MC 2002 An alteration in the hypothalamic action of estradiol due to lack of progesterone exposure can cause follicular cysts in cattle. *Biol Reprod* **66** 1689-1695.

Gumen A & Wiltbank MC 2005 Follicular cysts occur after a normal estradiol-induced GnRH/LH surge if the corpus hemorrhagicum is removed. *Reproduction* **129** 737-745.

Kim UH, Suh GH, Hur TY, Kang SJ, Kang HG, Park SB, Kim HS & Kim IH 2007a Comparison of two types of CIDR-based timed artificial insemination protocols for repeat breeder dairy cows. *Journal of Reproduction and Development* **53** 639-645.

Kim UH, Suh GH, Hur TY, Kang SJ, Kang HG, Park SB, Kim HS & Kim IH 2007b The effects of administering estradiol benzoate plus progesterone during the growth or static phases of the dominant follicle in CIDR-treated lactating dairy cows. *Journal of Reproduction and Development* **53** 591-596.

Knopf L, Kastelic JP, Schallenberger E & Ginther OJ 1989 Ovarian follicular dynamics in heifers - test of 2-wave hypothesis by ultrasonically monitoring individual follicles. *Domest Anim Endocrin* **6** 111-119.

Lauderdale JW 2009 ASAS Centennial Paper: Contributions in the Journal of Animal Science to the development of protocols for breeding management of cattle through synchronization of estrus and ovulation. *J Anim Sci* **87** 801-812.

Leroy JLMR, Opsomer G, Van Soom A, Goovaerts IGF & Bols P 2008a Reduced fertility in high-yielding dairy cows: Are the oocyte and embryo in danger? Part I - The importance of negative energy balance and altered corpus luteum function to the reduction of oocyte and embryo quality in high-yielding dairy cows. *Reprod Domest Anim* **43** 612-622.

Leroy JLMR, Van Soom A, Opsomer G, Goovaerts IGF & Bols PEJ 2008b Reduced fertility in high-yielding dairy cows: Are the oocyte and embryo in danger? Part II - Mechanisms linking nutrition and reduced oocyte and embryo quality in high-yielding dairy cows. *Reprod Domest Anim* **43** 623-632.

Lopez H, Caraviello DZ, Satter LD, Fricke PM & Wiltbank MC 2005 Relationship between level of milk production and multiple ovulations in lactating dairy cows. *J Dairy Sci* **88** 2783-2793.

Lopez H, Sartori R & Wiltbank MC 2005 Reproductive hormones and follicular growth during development of one or multiple dominant follicles in cattle. *Biol Reprod* **72** 788-795.

Lopez H, Satter LD & Wiltbank MC 2004 Relationship between level of milk production and estrous behavior of lactating dairy cows. *Anim Reprod Sci* **81** 209-223.

Macmillan KL, Segwagwe BVE & Pino CS 2003 Associations between the manipulation of patterns of follicular development and fertility in cattle. *Anim Reprod Sci* **78** 327-344.

Mann GE, Fray MD & Lamming GE 2006 Effects of time of progesterone supplementation on embryo development and interferon-tau production in the cow. *Vet J* **171** 500-503.

Martinez MF, Kastelic JP, Bo GA, Caccia M & Mapletoft RJ 2005 Effects of oestradiol and some of its esters on gonadotrophin release and ovarian follicular dynamics in CIDR-treated beef cattle. *Anim Reprod Sci* **86** 37-52.

Moreira F, de la Sota RL, Diaz T & Thatcher WW 2000 Effect of day of the estrous cycle at the initiation of a timed artificial insemination protocol on reproductive responses in dairy heifers. *J Anim Sci* **78** 1568-1576.

Moreira F, Orlandi C, Risco CA, Mattos R, Lopes F & Thatcher WW 2001 Effects of presynchronization and bovine somatotropin on pregnancy rates to a timed artificial insemination protocol in lactating dairy cows. *J Dairy Sci* **84** 1646-1659.

Odde K G 1990 A review of synchronization of estrus in postpartum cattle. *J Anim Sci* **68** 817-830.

Pancarci SM, Jordan ER, Risco CA, Schouten MJ, Lopes FL, Moreira F & Thatcher WW 2002 Use of estradiol cypionate in a presynchronized timed artificial insemination program for lactating dairy cattle. *J Dairy Sci* **85** 122-131.

Pursley JR, Kosorok MR & Wiltbank MC 1997 Reproductive management of lactating dairy cows using synchronization of ovulation. *J Dairy Sci* **80** 301-306.

Pursley JR, Mee MO & Wiltbank MC 1995 Synchronization

of ovulation in dairy cows using PGF(2-alpha) and GnRH. *Theriogenology* **44** 915-923.

Rabiee AR, Lean IJ & Stevenson MA 2005 Efficacy of Ovsynch program on reproductive performance in dairy cattle: A meta-analysis. *J Dairy Sci* **88** 2754-2770.

Revah I & Butler WR 1996 Prolonged dominance of follicles and reduced viability of bovine oocytes. *J Reprod Fertil* **106** 39-47.

Rutigliano HM, Lima FS, Cerri RLA, Greco LF, Vilela JM, Magalhaes V, Silvestre FT, Thatcher WW & Santos JEP 2008 Effects of method of presynchronization and source of selenium on uterine health and reproduction in dairy cows. *J Dairy Sci* **91** 3323-3336.

Sangsritavong S, Combs DK, Sartori R, Armentano LE & Wiltbank MC 2002 High feed intake increases liver blood flow and metabolism of progesterone and estradiol-17 beta in dairy cattle. *J Dairy Sci* **85** 2831-2842.

Santos JEP, Narciso CD, Rivera F, Thatcher WW & Chebel RC 2010 Effect of reducing the period of follicle dominance in a timed artificial insemination protocol on reproduction of dairy cows. *J Dairy Sci* **93** 2976-2988.

Santos JEP, Thatcher WW, Pool L & Overton MW 2001 Effect of human chorionic gonadotropin, on luteal function and reproductive performance of high-producing lactating Holstein dairy cows. *J Anim Sci* **79** 2881-2894.

Sartori R, Haughian JM, Shaver RD, Rosa GJM & Wiltbank MC 2004 Comparison of ovarian function and circulating steroids in estrous cycles of Holstein heifers and lactating cows. *J Dairy Sci* **87** 905-920.

Savio JD, Boland MP & Roche JF 1990 Development of dominant follicles and length of ovarian cycles in postpartum dairy cows. *J Reprod Fertil* **88** 581-591.

Savio JD, Keenan L, Boland MP & Roche JF 1988 Pattern of growth of dominant follicles during the estrous cycle of heifers. *J Reprod Fertil* **83** 663-671.

Silva E, Sterry RA, Kolb D, Wiltbank MC & Fricke PM 2007 Effect of pretreatment with prostaglandin F-2 alpha before resynchronization of ovulation on fertility of lactating dairy cows. *J Dairy Sci* **90** 5509-5517.

Sirois J & Fortune JE 1988 Ovarian follicular dynamics during the estrous cycle in heifers monitored by real-time ultrasonography. *Biol Reprod* **39** 308-317.

Souza AH, Ayres H, Ferreira RM & Wiltbank MC 2008 A new presynchronization system (Double-Ovsynch) increases fertility at first postpartum timed AI in lactating dairy cows. *Theriogenology* **70** 208-215.

Souza AH, Cunha AP, Caraviello DZ & Wiltbank MC 2005 Profiles of circulating estradiol-17 beta after different estrogen treatments in lactating dairy cows. *Animal Reproduction* **2** 224-232.

Souza AH, Gumen A, Silva EPB, Cunha AP, Guenther JN, Peto CM, Caraviello DZ & Wiltbank MC 2007 Supplementation with estradiol-17 beta before the last gonadotropin-releasing hormone injection of the ovsynch protocol in lactating dairy cows. *J Dairy Sci* **90** 4623-4634.

Souza AH, Viechnieski S, Lima FA, Silva FF, Araujo R, Bo GA, Wiltbank MC & Baruselli PS 2009 Effects of equine chorionic gonadotropin and type of ovulatory stimulus in a timed-AI protocol on reproductive responses in dairy cows. *Theriogenology* **72** 10-21.

Stevenson JS, Tiffany SM & Lucy MC 2004 Use of estradiol cypionate as a substitute for GnRH in protocols for synchronizing ovulation in dairy cattle. *J Dairy Sci* **87** 3298-3305.

Stumpf TT, Roberson MS, Wolfe MW, Hamernik DL, Kittok RJ & Kinder JE 1993 Progesterone, 17-beta-estradiol, and opioid neuropeptides Modulate Pattern of Luteinizing-Hormone in Circulation of the Cow. *Biol Reprod* **49** 1096-1101.

Thatcher WW, delaSota RL, Schmitt EJP, Diaz TC, Badinga L, Simmen FA, Staples CR & Drost M 1996 Control and management of ovarian follicles in cattle to optimize fertility. *Reprod Fert Develop* **8** 203-217.

Thatcher WW, Drost M, Savio JD, Macmillan KL, Entwistle KW, Schmitt EJ, Delasota RL & Morris GR 1993 New Clinical Uses of Gnrh and Its Analogs in Cattle. *Anim Reprod Sci* **33** 27-49.

Thatcher WW, Moreira F, Pancarci SM, Bartolome JA & Santos JEP 2002 Strategies to optimize reproductive efficiency by regulation of ovarian function. *Domest Anim Endocrin* **23** 243-254.

Thatcher WW, Santos JEP, Silvestre FT, Kim IH & Staples CR 2010 Special Issue: 14th Annual Conference of the European Society for Domestic Animal Reproduction (ESDAR) Abstracts. *Reprod Domest Anim* **45** 2-14.

Thundathil J, Kastelic JP & Mapletoft RJ 1998 The effect of estradiol cypionate (ECP) on ovarian follicular development and ovulation in dairy cattle. *Can J Anim Sci* **62** 314-316.

Townson DH, Tsang PCW, Butler WR, Frajblat M, Griel LC, Johnson CJ, Milvae RA, Niksic GM & Pate JL 2002 Relationship of fertility to ovarian follicular waves before breeding in dairy cows. *J Anim Sci* **80** 1053-1058.

Vasconcelos J, Silcox R, Rosa G, Pursley JR & Wiltbank MC 1999 Synchronization rate, size of the ovulatory follicle, and pregnancy rate after synchronization of ovulation beginning on different days of the estrous cycle in lactating dairy cows. *Theriogenology* **52** 1067-1078.

Vasconcelos JLM, Sartori R, Oliveira HN, Guenther JN & Wiltbank MC 2001 Reduction in size of the ovulatory follicle reduces subsequent luteal size and pregnancy rate. *Theriogenology* **56** 307-314.

Wiltbank JN, Zimmerman DR, Ingalls JE & Rowden WW 1965 Use of Progestational Compounds Alone or in Combination with Estrogen for Synchronization of Estrus. *J Anim Sci* **24** 990-998.

Wiltbank M, Lopez H, Sartori R, Sangsritavong S & Gumen A 2006 Changes in reproductive physiology of lactating dairy cows due to elevated steroid metabolism. *Theriogenology* **65** 17-29.

Wiltbank MC, Guenther JN & Fricke PM 2008a Resynchronization strategies in lactating dairy cows. *Proceedings of the Dairy Cattle Reproduction Congress* 9-16.

Wiltbank MC, Gumen A, Lopez H & Sartori R 2008b Management and treatment of dairy cows that are not cycling or have follicular cysts. *Cattle Practice* **16** 14-19.

Wiltbank MC, Gumen A & Sartori R 2002 Physiological classification of anovulatory conditions in cattle. *Theriogenology* **57** 21-52.

Xu ZZ, Burton LJ & Macmillan KL 1997 Reproductive performance of lactating dairy cows following estrus synchronization regimens with PGF2 alpha and progesterone. *Theriogenology* **47** 687-701.

Zimbelman RG & Smith LW 1966 Control of Ovulation in Cattle with Melengestrol Acetate .2. Effects on Follicular Size and Activity. *J Reprod Fertil* **11** 193-201.

Molecular markers of sperm quality

P Sutovsky[1,2] and K Lovercamp[3]

[1]*Division of Animal Sciences, and* [2]*Departments of Obstetrics, Gynecology and Women's Health, University of Missouri-Columbia, Columbia, MO 62511;* [3]*Department of Agriculture, University of Central Missouri, Warrensburg, MO 64093*

Light microscopic semen evaluation provides useful information about a given sperm sample, but due to its subjective nature has limited prognostic value for the reproductive performance of males or the outcome of assisted fertilization. Cryptic sperm abnormalities (occurring at the molecular level) are not easily detectable by light microscopy, but can be revealed by an array of biomarkers. The latter include fluorescent markers of acrosomal status, fluorochromes detecting altered sperm chromatin or DNA integrity, vital dyes revealing sperm mitochondrial activity, probes detecting apoptotic events, and antibodies detecting proteins that are either up- or down-regulated in defective spermatozoa. Many of the above biomarkers are best tested by flow cytometry, permitting rapid, automated, high throughput, objective measurement of the relative abundance of these biomarkers in semen. This review summarizes a strategy for the identification of novel male fertility/sperm quality biomarkers based on proteomic, biochemical and immunocytochemical analyses of defective spermatozoa. This approach identifies proteins or ligands uniquely associated with defective spermatozoa, regardless of whether they carry gross morphological defects or subtle, but critical hidden defects (e.g. DNA strand breaks) not detected with conventional, light microscopic analysis. Such markers, including ubiquitin, sperm thioredoxin SPTRX3/TXNDC8, 15LOX, and Lewis^{y}-terminated N-glycans, are associated with poor semen quality and reduced fertility, warranting a designation of "negative" markers of fertility. The significance of sperm cytoplasmic droplet, a structure that accumulates several of the discussed biomarker proteins, is also discussed with regard to sperm quality and fertility.

Introduction: Novel approaches to semen analysis

Light microscopic evaluation is a cornerstone of semen analysis in both farm animal and human andrology, providing useful information about a sperm sample. However, conventional sperm tests such as motility and morphology assessments rely on subjective evaluation of sperm traits and have limited prognostic value for the reproductive performance of males or for the outcome of assisted fertilization. Consequently, it is difficult to predict the reproductive performance of bulls or boars used for artificial insemination. Similarly, human male infertility could be misdiagnosed as idiopathic, as certain types of sperm abnormalities occur at the molecular level,

Corresponding author E-mail: SutovskyP@missouri.edu

sometimes in the absence of morphological manifestation detectable by light microscopy. To address this problem, structural and molecular anomalies of defective human spermatozoa can be revealed by an array of biomarkers. These latter include fluorescent markers of acrosomal status (e.g. lectins PNA and PSA), fluorochromes detecting altered sperm chromatin or DNA integrity (e.g. acridine orange/SCSA or TUNEL assays), vital dyes revealing sperm mitochondrial activity (JC-1, MitoTracker), probes detecting apoptotic events (FAS ligand, caspase substrates), and antibodies detecting proteins that are either up- or down-regulated in defective spermatozoa. Many of the above biomarkers are best tested by flow cytometry (Fig. 1 A), which in contrast to light microscopic analysis, permits a rapid, automated, and objective measurement of their relative abundance in thousands of cells per sample [reviewed by (Garner, 1997; Gillan et al., 2005)]. Traditional microscopic sperm evaluation allows subcellular localization of specific biomarkers. However, relative intensity of labeling is typically estimated on a small number of cells (e.g. 100-200 per sample) by light microcopy. Collectively, flow cytometry and epifluorescence microscopy, combined with biomarkers of sperm quality/fertility, are quickly becoming useful techniques in andrology. These efforts are now elevated by the introduction of innovative flow cytometric approaches and novel instrumentation. For example, the ImageStream instrument combines the throughput of a flow cytometer with the rapid image acquisition capabilities of a high end CCD camera (Buckman et al., 2009), and the affordable, easy-to-use, but highly accurate capillary-based flow cytometers such as Guava PCA and Guava EasyCyte Plus (Polina et al., 2008) have the potential to be widely used in andrology . However, additional biomarkers of sperm quality are sought, suitable for flow cytometry, and highly correlated with field fertility of male farm animals.

Negative marker approach

We built our strategy for the identification of novel male fertility/sperm quality biomarkers on proteomic, biochemical, and immunocytochemical analyses of defective spermatozoa. We look for proteins or ligands that are uniquely associated with the defective spermatozoa carrying gross morphological defects, or subtle, but critical hidden defects (e.g. DNA strand breaks), not detectable in conventional, light-microscopic analysis. Such markers are associated with poor semen quality and reduced fertility, warranting a designation of "negative" markers of fertility.

To date, we have identified the following potential male fertility markers:

- Ubiquitin (Fig. 1 A, B) is associated with the surface of defective spermatozoa of humans (Sutovsky et al., 2001b), bulls (Sutovsky et al., 2002), boars (Lovercamp et al., 2007a; Sutovsky et al., 2003), stallions (Sutovsky et al., 2003), and rats (Tengowski et al., 2007).
- The 15-lipoxygenase (15LOX) is enriched along with various ubiquitin-interacting components in the cytoplasmic droplets of boar spermatozoa (Fischer et al., 2005) and can be used as a negative marker of boar semen quality (Lovercamp et al., 2007a). Male mice lacking the *15Lox* gene are subfertile, with a significantly increased post-testicular retention of total (i.e. combined proximal and distal) cytoplasmic droplets (Moore et al., 2010).
- We reported that a testis, male germ-line specific thioredoxin SPTRX3/TXNDC8 is associated with superfluous cytoplasm of defective human spermatozoa (Buckman et al., 2009; Jimenez et al., 2004), although this does not seem to be the case for farm animal species.
- In contrast to our negative marker approach, we found that platelet activating factor-receptor (PAFr), present on the normal sperm surface, is under-expressed on the surface of defective bull spermatozoa, although its presence on the surface of leukocytes contaminating some

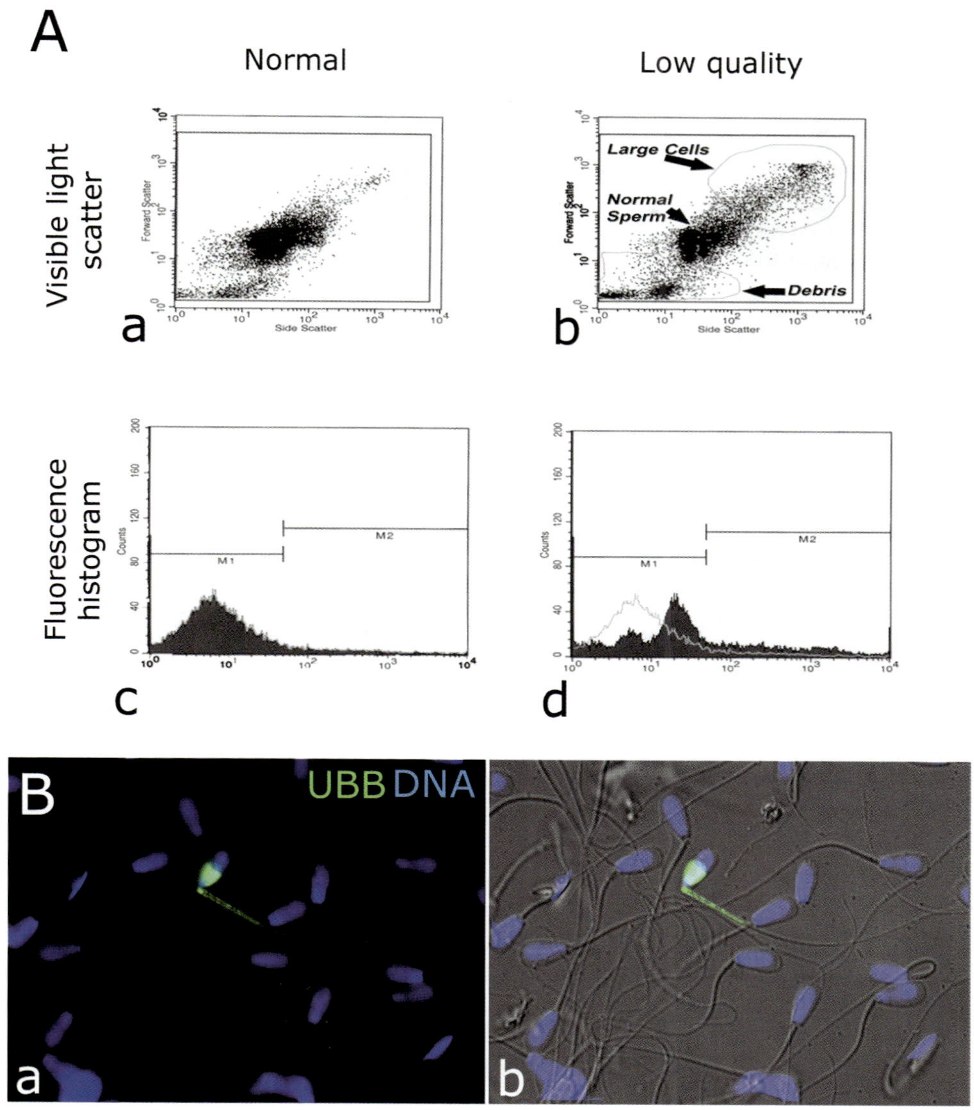

Fig.1. (**A**) Flow cytometric analysis of bull sperm ubiquitin. Normal sperm sample from a fertile bull with median of ubiquitn-induced relative fluorescence (Ubiquitin Median value; no units) of 6.7 is shown on the left (panels *a & c);* right column, panels *b & d,* is a sample from a bull with a high percentage of morphologically abnormal spermatozoa, reflected by Ubiquitin Median value of 20.5. Panels *a* and *b* combine forward and side scatter diagrams of 10,000 cells/events per sample passing through visible light during flow cytometry. Each dot represents one cell/event. The desirable, presumably morphologically normal spermatozoa ("normal sperm" in panel *b)* congregate in the center. Cellular debris is concentrated in the lower left corner. Abnormally large cells are projected in the upper right corner. Panels *c & d,* corresponding to scatter diagrams *a & b,* respectively, are flow cytometric histograms of ubiquitin, reflective of the fluorescence induced by the binding of fluorochrome-conjugated anti-ubiquitin antibodies to the surface of defective spermatozoa. Cells within markers M1 are presumed normal spermatozoa; cells within markers M2 are those tagged with ubiquitin. Note the shift of the histogram peak in panel d, reflective of an increased median value of ubiquitin-induced fluorescence (ubiquitin median) in this sample. (**B**) Immunofluorescence of ubiquitin (green) on the surface of a defective bull spermatozoon surrounded by normal spermatozoa. Sperm nuclear DNA was counterstained with DAPI (blue). In panel *b,* fluorescence is superimposed with differential interference contrast image of the same cells.

of the bull semen samples could cause an artefactual increase the reading of this molecule in samples of poor quality (Sutovsky et al., 2007).

- Arylsufatase A (ASA), another sperm surface protein associated with normal fertility (Wu et al., 2007), is ubiquitinated and thus diminished on the surface of defective bull spermatozoa (unpublished data).
- Various glycan-specific lectins and antibodies are being tested for their ability to recognize altered sperm surface glycosylation in defective spermatozoa. In particular, *Lens cullinaris* agglutinin (LCA) recognizes the surface of ubiquitinated, defective bull spermatozoa (Baska and Sutovsky, 2005); antibodies recognizing the Lewis^y terminated N-glycans bind predominantly to defective human spermatozoa (Pang et al., 2007).
- Acrosome-bining lectins PNA (peanut/ *Arachis hypogaea*-agglutinin) and PSA (*Pisum sativum* agglutinin) recognize glycans present on the outer acrosomal membrane of the sperm acrosome and in the acrosomal matrix, respectively. Consequently, such lectins have been used extensively to determine acrosomal status (intact, capacitated, exocytosed, damaged) in farm animal spermatozoa [e.g. (Cross and Watson, 1994)].

Ubiquitin as a biomarker of male semen quality and fertility

The ubiquitin-proteasome pathway (UPP) regulates many steps of reproductive processes, including, but not limited to, spermatogenesis, epididymal sperm maturation, fertilization, and preimplantation embryo development. Ubiquitin is a small chaperone protein that binds covalently to internal Lys-residues of proteins destined for proteolytic degradation by the 26S proteaome, a multi-subunit proteolytic holoenzyme. Proteins are targeted for ubiquitination due to misfolding, altered glycosylation, oxidation, disulfide-bond reduction, or developmental/cellular programming [reviewed by (Glickman and Ciechanover, 2002)]. Although it is sometimes perceived as a housekeeping pathway, the UPP thus serves a variety of precisely regulated signaling events during the cell cycle, transcriptional control, membrane receptor turnover, and is involved in a variety of cellular pathologies, including Alzheimer's disease, liver cirrhosis, and HIV infection [reviewed by (Hershko and Ciechanover, 1998)]. Ultimately, the tagging of substrate proteins with a multi-ubiquitin chain of four or more ubiquitin molecules predestines such proteins for proteolytic degradation by the 26S proteasome. The latter is a multi-subunit protease complex of ~2 MDa, composed of the 19S regulatory complex (17 subunits; role: ubiquitinated substrate recognition, deubiquitination and priming) and 20S core (14 subunits; role: substrate degradation). Some proteasome-substrate interactions and interactions between 19S subunits are mediated by the 19S ATP-ase subunits which require ATP. Other steps of substrate recognition and priming in the 19S complex (maintenance of non-ATPase 19S subunits), as well as the actual proteolysis in the 20S core, are not ATP-dependent [reviewed by (Voges et al., 1999)].

Consensus is mounting that the proteolysis of ubiquitinated sperm and oocyte proteins by the 26S proteasome is necessary for the success of mammalian fertilization, including acrosomal exocytosis (AE) and sperm-zona pellucida (ZP) penetration (Sakai et al., 2004; Zimmerman and Sutovsky, 2009). The participation of UPP is also required for elimination of paternal mitochondria after fertilization, an observation explaining the basic dogma of developmental and evolutionary biology, namely that of strictly maternal inheritance of human/mammalian mitochondrial DNA (Sutovsky et al., 1999). The validation of ubiquitin as a biomarker of sperm quality was inspired by observations that mammalian spermatozoa with a visible or hidden defect acquire a ubiquitin tag during epididymal sperm maturation (Baska et al., 2008; Sutovsky et al., 2001a). The UPP operates in the mammalian epididymal fluid by virtue of a peculiar apocrine secretion mechanism by which all necessary enzymatic components of UPP are introduced in the epididymal fluid and are in contact with maturing spermatozoa (Baska et al., 2008). Secretion of ubiquitin and other proteins in epididymal fluid occurs through apical blebs (Hermo and Jacks, 2002), large membrane enclosed vesicles of epididymal cell cytoplasm in which both secretory and non-secretory proteins appear to be concentrated. Besides ubiquitin, the ubiquitin activating, ubiquitin-conjugating and deubiquitinating enzymes, as well as various subunits of the ubiquitin dependent protease, the 26S proteasome, have been detected in epididymal fluid (Baska et al., 2008; Jones, 2004). Proteomic analysis also identified ubiquitin in epididymosomes, small epididymal cell-derived vesicles implicated in transferring epididymal proteins to the sperm plasma membrane (Thimon et al., 2008). The concept of ubiquitination and proteasomal degradation occurring on the cell surface or in extracellular space is now being recognized as a non-traditional, extracellular function of UPP, extending beyond the reproductive system (Sakai et al., 2004; Sixt and Dahlmann, 2008).

What makes defective spermatozoa recognizable to UPP? In general, it is protein damage by misfolding/unfolding, oxidation, disulfide bond-reduction, deglycosylation, or sugar trimming (Glickman and Ciechanover, 2002). A classical example is the ubiquitination and degradation of misfolded amyloid proteins in the brain cells, which, when blocked, results in the formation of amyloid plaques and accumulation of undegraded proteins characteristic of Alzheimer's and Huntington's disease. Interestingly, amyloid-like protein aggregates have been recently found in epididymal fluid and proposed to be a part of the epididymal extracellular protein quality control (Cornwall et al., 2007). Regarding altered glycosylation, we observed that defective, ubiquitin tagged bull spermatozoa acquire the ability to bind lectin LCA [(Baska and Sutovsky, 2005) and unpublished data]. Lectin LCA has high affinity for sugar-trimmed mannose-rich glycoproteins known to be ubiquitinated during endoplasmatic-reticulum associated protein quality control [ERAD; reviewed by (Spiro, 2004)]. Perhaps sperm surface glycoproteins could be trimmed in defective epididymal spermatozoa by alpha-mannosidase, one of the abundant glycosidases in epididymal fluid. Alternatively, glycosylases from epididymal fluid could recognize the altered sperm surface and attach immunoprotective glycans to the sperm surface, as observed in defective human spermatozoa (Pang et al., 2007).

Studies of sperm ubiquitination in farm animal species

Flow cytometry has been used as an objective, automated, statistically robust measurement of the relative levels of the above sperm biomarkers in farm animal and human semen. The following observations were made from farm animal field studies:

- Ubiquitin correlates positively with bull sperm DNA fragmentation (Sutovsky et al., 2002).
- Ubiquitin levels change seasonally in stallions, mirroring the seasonality of stallion semen output and quality (Sutovsky et al., 2003).
- Ubiquitin correlates negatively with conventional semen analysis end points (sperm count, motility, percentage of normal morphology), but positively with relative levels of sperm surface associate platelet activating factor-receptor (PAFr) protein in yearling bulls (Sutovsky et al., 2007).
- Semen content of 15LOX measured by flow cytometry correlates negatively with litter size in pigs bred by artificial insemination, whereas ubiquitin has negative correlations with both litter size and farrowing rates. Both 15LOX and ubiquitin correlate positively with the percentage of spermatozoa with a cytoplasmic droplet (CD) in boar semen (Lovercamp et al., 2007a).

Significance of sperm cytoplasmic droplet for farm animal fertility

Ubiquitin and other components of UPP accumulate in bull and boar sperm CD (Fischer et al., 2005; Sutovsky et al., 2001a) and can be used for automated measurement of the semen content of spermatozoa bearing a CD in boars (Lovercamp et al., 2007a). Sperm-borne CD is one of the most widespread and poorly understood sperm abnormalities of boars and bulls. The CD is a membrane-enclosed vesicle of cellular cytoplasm which remains attached to the sperm tail midpiece after completion of spermatogenesis. Mammalian CD are generally spherical and 2-3μm in diameter (Kaplan et al., 1984). During microscopic evaluation, CDs are observed either attached or unattached to the spermatozoa. When attached to the spermatozoon, the CD is associated with the sperm tail midpiece in one of two locations: at the proximal end of the midpiece, i.e. next to the sperm head (proximal CD) located at the distal end of the midpiece (distal CD), or at the junction of the midpiece and principal piece of the sperm tail. The distal CD can also be associated with the sperm tail abnormality known as the distal midpiece reflex, characterized by a 180° bend of the sperm tail around the distal CD at the midpiece/principal piece junction (DMR CD). Finally, the CD can also be detached from the sperm tail and free-floating in the ejaculate (unattached CD). Unattached CDs can be observed individually or as clusters; the latter are present in boar semen.

Formation of CD occurs during spermatogenesis when the haploid round-shaped sperm cell, a round spermatid, matures into an elongated spermatid and eventually into a fully differentiated spermatozoon. Formation of the CD begins when the residual cellular cytoplasm is removed from the elongated spermatid and is retained and destroyed by the Sertoli cell, the nurturing cells of the seminiferous epithelium (Barth and Oko, 1989). When the spermatid stalk, which connects the residual cellular cytoplasm to the presumptive CD is severed, a small amount of cytoplasm remains attached to the sperm midpiece. This small amount of cytoplasm is the CD. All newly formed sperm cells in the testis possess a proximal CD following spermatogenesis (Russell, 1984).

After spermatogenesis, spermatozoa pass from the testis into the epididymis; as spermatozoa pass through epididymis (for 7 to 14 days, depending on the species), they undergo maturation, and become capable of fertilization. During this passage, the CD migrates along the midpiece from the proximal to the distal position. It is not yet understood why, or by what mechanisms, movement of the CD on the sperm tail midpiece occurs during epididymal transit. Following migration to the distal position, the CD can be released in the cauda region of the epididymis in some species. In contrast to the bull and other mammals, the majority of boar spermatozoa in the cauda epididymis still possess a CD in the distal position (Harayama et al., 1996), and some spermatozoa possess a CD in the proximal position. During ejaculation or soon thereafter, CDs can be released from the boar spermatozoa and found free-floating within the seminal plasma (Harayama et al., 1996). Extensive research has analyzed the migration and disposal of the CD in various animal species during epididymal transit, concluding that CDs shed by epididymal spermatozoa are subsequently phagocytosed by epididymal epithelial cells (Axner et al., 2002; Hermo et al., 1988; Temple-Smith, 1984). It is not known whether the CD is formed on the spermatozoa to serve a specific purpose during sperm maturation or fertilization, or if it is simply a rudiment remaining on the sperm cell after spermatogenesis is completed.

Post-epididymal retention of CD has been associated with reduced fertility in both bulls and boars. Both proximal and distal CDs are thought to affect sperm quality/fertility, though individual studies may attribute more weight to one form of CD over the other. Possible factors causing the retention of the CD by ejaculated spermatozoa include suboptimal temperature of semen (Zou and Yang, 2000), environmental temperature of the male (heat stress)(Akbarsha et al., 2000; Huang et al., 2000), reprotoxic chemical exposure (Akbarsha et al., 2000), sexual immaturity (Amann et al., 2000; Arteaga et al., 2001), altered/poor diet (Hassan et al., 2004), disease such as PRRSV in boars (Prieto et al., 1996), photoperiod changes (Sancho et al., 2004) and irregular collection frequency (Pruneda et al., 2005).

There is a negative correlation between sperm cytoplasmic droplet retention by yearling bulls and embryo cleavage following bovine in vitro fertilization (Amann et al., 2000). Spermatozoa from bulls with a high percentage of retained CDs had reduced ability to bind to oocyte zona pellucida, resulting in lower fertilization and cleavage rates in vitro (Thundathil et al., 2001). Sperm-bound CDs in extended boar semen have detrimental relationships with pregnancy rates and litter size (Waberski et al., 1994). Furthermore, these authors noted that CDs represent the most frequent morphological abnormality in boar sperm used for AI. In an *in vitro* study (Petrunkina et al., 2001), using sperm binding to explants of the pig oviductal epithelium of the oviductal sperm reservoir, there was a significant negative correlation of the percentage of sperm with attached CDs and sperm-explant binding. Furthermore, there was a negative correlation between sperm motility and the percentages of spermatozoa with attached CDs. A negative relationship was found between boar sperm CD-frequency, and farrowing rate and total number born in an artificial insemination trial (Lovercamp et al., 2007a; Lovercamp et al., 2007b). Boars with a farrowing rate below the average for the study had a higher number of sperm with attached CDs, and an increased content of sperm ubiquitin compared to the boars above the average farrowing rate.

Conclusions and perspectives

Collectively, the present review illustrates the utility of negative sperm quality markers in male fertility evaluation in large animals. The major advantages of biomarker approach over conventional semen analysis is its ability to accurately, and objectively, measure biomarker levels in a large number of cells per sample, and to uncover hidden sperm defects, not manifested in abnormal morphology. An added advantage of these high precision biomarkers is the ability to discern subtle differences in fertility within the pool of fertile sires, as opposed to extreme differences between fertile and completely infertile animals, revealed by conventional analysis. Of interest is the characterization of biomarker patterns/levels in subfertile animals with compensable vs. non-compensable sperm defects, and the ability to identify sires with superior tolerance to semen cryopreservation, and those that can be distributed in AI doses at higher dilution/lower sperm count per dose. The long-term goal of this work is to determine which markers coincide most closely with pregnancy/non-return rates in cattle, and with pregnancy rates and litter size in pigs. This will facilitate commercialization and dissemination of simple, but highly accurate and objective testing methods for the AI industry and farm animal producers. Further efforts will be focused on understanding how these biomarkers correlate with transient impairments of male infertility caused by heat stress, malnutrition, poisoning or contagious diseases, and permanent fertility disorders caused by testicular or epididymal disfunction, or injury.

Based on the presence of several biomakers on the surface of defective spermatozoa, magnetic nanoparticle-based methods are in development for depletion of defective spermatozoa from semen samples during semen processing for cryopreservation. At the same time, efforts are increasing to promote the use of novel flow cytometric instrumentation in farm animal and human andrology. Besides targeting sperm proteins/surface ligands as biomarkers, genome and transcriptome analyses will increasingly affect the field of andrology. The analysis of sperm-borne RNAs in humans already revealed that, perhaps in parallel to our observations of increased protein ubiquitination in defective spermatozoa, ubiquitin-proteasome pathway gene products are deregulated in the sperm transcriptomes of infertile men (Platts et al., 2007). At the gene level, single nucleotide polymorphisms (SNP) have been found in infertile men within the sequences of the genes encoding for ubiquitin-specific protease USP26 (Stouffs et al., 2005) and ubiquitin activating enzyme UBE2B (Huang et al., 2008). With the help of new SNP chip-technology, the whole genome SNP screening (Van Tassell et al., 2008) is likely to reveal additional genes linked to spermatogenesis and sperm quality traits, in bulls and other species. Some of these newly identified marker genes could translate into biomarker-based assays of sperm quality at the protein level.

Acknowledgements

This work was supported by extramural grants from USDA-NRI, Missouri Life Sciences Trust Fund, and the Food for the 21st Century (F21C) Program of the University of Missouri. Excerpts from this article have been previously published in non-copyrighted meeting proceedings. We acknowledge the following academic and industry collaborators for their essential contributions to the above research: Dr. Tim Safranski (MU), Dr. Klaus van Leyen (Harvard U.), Dr. William Herring (Smithfield, Inc.), Cliff Marshal and Mel De Jarnette (Select Sires Inc.), Eliza Roberts (ABS Global), Dr. John Diehl (Clemson U.), Dr. Bill Plummer (CalPoly), Dr. Mark Tengowski (Pfizer), Dr. Christophe Staub (IMV Technologies), Dr. Eric Schmitt (IV Technologies), and Dr. Henri Clemente (Clemente Associates). Special thanks belong to Dr. Young-Joo Yi, Dr. Gauri Manandhar, Katie Fischer, Kathleen Baska, Kathy Craighead, and Miriam Sutovsky for their essential contributions to our research on sperm quality biomarkers.

Literature cited

Akbarsha, M. A., Latha, P. N. and Murugaian, P. (2000). Retention of cytoplasmic droplet by rat cauda epididymal spermatozoa after treatment with cytotoxic and xenobiotic agents. *J Reprod Fertil* **120**, 385-90.

Amann, R. P., Seidel, G. E., Jr. and Mortimer, R. G. (2000). Fertilizing potential in vitro of semen from young beef bulls containing a high or low percentage of sperm with a proximal droplet. *Theriogenology* **54**, 1499-515.

Arteaga, A., Baracaldo, M. and Barth, A. D. (2001). The proportion of beef bulls in western Canada with mature spermiograms at 11 to 15 months of age. *Canadian Veterinary Journal* **42**, 783-787.

Axner, E., Pukazhenthi, B. S., Wildt, D. E., Linde-Forsberg, C. and Spindler, R. E. (2002). Creatine phosphokinase in domestic cat epididymal spermatozoa. *Mol Reprod Dev* **62**, 265-70.

Barth, A. D. and Oko, R. J. (1989). Abnormal morphology of bovine spermatozoa. Ames, IA: Iowa State University Press.

Baska, K. M., Manandhar, G., Feng, D., Agca, Y., Tengowski, M. W., Sutovsky, M., Yi, Y. J. and Sutovsky, P. (2008). Mechanism of extracellular ubiquitination in the mammalian epididymis. *J Cell Physiol* **215**, 684-96.

Baska, K. M. and Sutovsky, P. (2005). Protein modification by ubiquitination and its consequences for spermatogenesis, sperm maturation, fertilization and pre-implantation embryonic development. In: . In *New impact on protein modifications in the regulation of reproductive system.*, (ed. T. Tokumoto), pp. 83-114. Kerala: Research Signpost. .

Buckman, C., George, T. C., Friend, S., Sutovsky, M., Miranda-Vizuete, A., Ozanon, C., Morrissey, P. and Sutovsky, P. (2009). High throughput, parallel imaging and biomarker quantification of human spermatozoa by ImageStream flow cytometry. *Syst Biol Reprod Med* **55**, 244-51.

Cornwall, G. A., von Horsten, H. H., Swartz, D., Johnson, S., Chau, K. and Whelly, S. (2007). Extracellular quality control in the epididymis. *Asian J Androl* **9**, 500-7.

Cross, N. L. and Watson, S. K. (1994). Assessing acrosomal status of bovine sperm using fluoresceinated lectins. *Theriogenology* **42**, 89-98.

Fischer, K. A., Van Leyen, K., Lovercamp, K. W., Manandhar, G., Sutovsky, M., Feng, D., Safranski, T. and Sutovsky, P. (2005). 15-Lipoxygenase is a component of the mammalian sperm cytoplasmic droplet. *Reproduction* **130**, 213-22.

Garner, D. L. (1997). Ancillary tests of bull semen quality. *Vet Clin North Am Food Anim Pract* **13**, 313-30.

Gillan, L., Evans, G. and Maxwell, W. M. (2005). Flow cytometric evaluation of sperm parameters in relation to fertility potential. *Theriogenology* **63**, 445-57.

Glickman, M. H. and Ciechanover, A. (2002). The ubiquitin-proteasome proteolytic pathway: destruction for the sake of construction. *Physiol Rev* **82**, 373-428.

Harayama, H., Shibukawa, T., Miyake, M., Kannan, Y. and Kato, S. (1996). Fructose stimulates shedding of cytoplasmic droplets from epididymal boar spermatozoa. *Reprod Fertil Dev* **8**, 1039-43.

Hassan, M. E., Smith, G. W., Ott, R. S., Faulkner, D. B., Firkins, L. D., Ehrhart, E. J. and Schaeffer, D. J. (2004). Reversibility of the reproductive toxicity of gossypol in peripubertal bulls. *Theriogenology* **61**, 1171-9.

Hermo, L., Dworkin, J. and Oko, R. (1988). Role of epithelial clear cells of the rat epididymis in the disposal of the contents of cytoplasmic droplets detached from spermatozoa. *Am J Anat* **183**, 107-24.

Hermo, L. and Jacks, D. (2002). Nature's ingenuity: bypassing the classical secretory route via apocrine secretion. *Mol Reprod Dev* **63**, 394-410.

Hershko, A. and Ciechanover, A. (1998). The ubiquitin system. *Annu Rev Biochem* **67**, 425-79.

Huang, I., Emery, B. R., Christensen, G. L., Griffin, J., Peterson, C. M. and Carrell, D. T. (2008). Novel UBE2B-associated polymorphisms in an azoospermic/oligozoospermic population. *Asian J Androl* **10**, 461-6.

Huang, S. Y., Kuo, Y. H., Lee, Y. P., Tsou, H. L., Lin, E. C., Ju, C. C. and Lee, W. C. (2000). Association of heat shock protein 70 with semen quality in boars. *Anim Reprod Sci* **63**, 231-40.

Jimenez, A., Zu, W., Rawe, V. Y., Pelto-Huikko, M., Flickinger, C. J., Sutovsky, P., Gustafsson, J. A., Oko, R. and Miranda-Vizuete, A. (2004). Spermatocyte/spermatid-specific thioredoxin-3, a novel Golgi apparatus-associated thioredoxin, is a specific marker of aberrant spermatogenesis. *J Biol Chem* **279**, 34971-82.

Jones, R. (2004). Sperm survival versus degradation in the mammalian epididymis: a hypothesis. *Biol Reprod* **71**, 1405-11.

Kaplan, M., Russell, L. D., Peterson, R. N. and Martan, J. (1984). Boar sperm cytoplasmic droplets: their ultrastructure, their numbers in the epididymis and at ejaculation and their removal during isolation of sperm plasma membranes. *Tissue Cell* **16**, 455-68.

Lovercamp, K. W., Safranski, T. J., Fischer, K. A., Manandhar, G., Sutovsky, M., Herring, W. and Sutovsky, P. (2007a). Arachidonate 15-lipoxygenase and ubiquitin as fertility markers in boars. *Theriogenology* **67**, 704-18.

Lovercamp, K. W., Safranski, T. J., Fischer, K. A., Manandhar, G., Sutovsky, M., Herring, W. and Sutovsky, P. (2007b). High resolution light microscopic evaluation of boar semen quality sperm cytoplasmic droplet retention in relationship with boar fertility parameters. *Arch Androl* **53**, 219-28.

Moore, K., Lovercamp, K., Feng, D., Antelman, J., Sutovsky, M., Manandhar, G., van Leyen, K., Safranski, T. and Sutovsky, P. (2010). Altered epididymal sperm maturation and cytoplasmic droplet migration in subfertile male Alox15 mice. *Cell Tissue Res.*

Pang, P. C., Tissot, B., Drobnis, E. Z., Sutovsky, P., Morris, H. R., Clark, G. F. and Dell, A. (2007). Expression of bisecting type and Lewisx/Lewisy terminated N-glycans on human sperm. *J Biol Chem* **282**, 36593-602.

Petrunkina, A. M., Gehlhaar, R., Drommer, W., Waberski, D. and Topfer-Petersen, E. (2001). Selective sperm binding to pig oviductal epithelium in vitro. *Reproduction* **121**, 889-96.

Platts, A. E., Dix, D. J., Chemes, H. E., Thompson, K. E., Goodrich, R., Rockett, J. C., Rawe, V. Y., Quintana, S., Diamond, M. P., Strader, L. F. et al. (2007). Success and failure in human spermatogenesis as revealed by teratozoospermic RNAs. *Hum Mol Genet* **16**, 763-73.

Polina, R., Sturgis, C., Patterson, J. and Patterson, B. K. (2008). Rapid, high throughput determination of cervical cytology specimen adequacy using a capillary-based cytometer. *Cytometry B Clin Cytom* **74**, 133-6.

Prieto, C., Suarez, P., Bautista, J. M., Sanchez, R., Rillo, S. M., Simarro, I., Solana, A. and Castro, J. M. (1996). Semen changes in boars after experimental infection with porcine reproductive and respiratory syndrome (PRRS) virus. *Theriogenology* **45**, 383-95.

Pruneda, A., Pinart, E., Dolors Briz, M., Sancho, S., Garcia-Gil, N., Badia, E., Kadar, E., Bassols, J., Bussalleu, E., Yeste, M. et al. (2005). Effects of a high semen-collection frequency on the quality of sperm from ejaculates and from six epididymal regions in boars. *Theriogenology* **63**, 2219-32.

Russell, L. D. (1984). Spermiation - the sperm release process: Ultrastructural observations and unresolved issues. In *Ultrastructure of reproduction*, vol. 2 (eds J. Van Blerkom and P. M. Motta), pp. 46-66. Boston, MA: Martinus Nijhoff Publishers.

Sakai, N., Sawada, M. T. and Sawada, H. (2004). Non-traditional roles of ubiquitin-proteasome system in fertilization and gametogenesis. *Int J Biochem Cell Biol* **36**, 776-84.

Sancho, S., Pinart, E., Briz, M., Garcia-Gil, N., Badia, E., Bassols, J., Kadar, E., Pruneda, A., Bussalleu, E., Yeste, M. et al. (2004). Semen quality of postpubertal boars during increasing and decreasing natural photoperiods. *Theriogenology* **62**, 1271-82.

Sixt, S. U. and Dahlmann, B. (2008). Extracellular, circulating proteasomes and ubiquitin - incidence and relevance. *Biochim Biophys Acta* **1782**, 817-23.

Spiro, R. G. (2004). Role of N-linked polymannose oligosaccharides in targeting glycoproteins for endoplasmic reticulum-associated degradation. *Cell Mol Life Sci* **61**, 1025-41.

Stouffs, K., Lissens, W., Tournaye, H., Van Steirteghem, A. and Liebaers, I. (2005). Possible role of USP26 in patients with severely impaired spermatogenesis. *Eur J Hum Genet* **13**, 336-40.

Sutovsky, P., Moreno, R., Ramalho-Santos, J., Dominko, T., Thompson, W. E. and Schatten, G. (2001a). A putative, ubiquitin-dependent mechanism for the recognition and elimination of defective spermatozoa in the mammalian epididymis. *J Cell Sci* **114**, 1665-75.

Sutovsky, P., Moreno, R. D., Ramalho-Santos, J.,

Dominko, T., Simerly, C. and Schatten, G. (1999). Ubiquitin tag for sperm mitochondria. *Nature* **402**, 371-2.

Sutovsky, P., Neuber, E. and Schatten, G. (2002). Ubiquitin-dependent sperm quality control mechanism recognizes spermatozoa with DNA defects as revealed by dual ubiquitin-TUNEL assay. *Mol Reprod Dev* **61**, 406-13.

Sutovsky, P., Plummer, W., Baska, K., Peterman, K., Diehl, J. R. and Sutovsky, M. (2007). Relative levels of semen platelet activating factor-receptor (PAFr) and ubiquitin in yearling bulls with high content of semen white blood cells: implications for breeding soundness evaluation. *J Androl* **28**, 92-108.

Sutovsky, P., Terada, Y. and Schatten, G. (2001b). Ubiquitin-based sperm assay for the diagnosis of male factor infertility. *Hum Reprod* **16**, 250-8.

Sutovsky, P., Turner, R. M., Hameed, S. and Sutovsky, M. (2003). Differential ubiquitination of stallion sperm proteins: possible implications for infertility and reproductive seasonality. *Biol Reprod* **68**, 688-98.

Temple-Smith, P. D. (1984). Phagocytosis of sperm cytoplasmic droplets by a specialized region in the epididymis of the brushtailed possum, Trichosurus vulpecula. *Biol Reprod* **30**, 707-20.

Tengowski, M. W., Feng, D., Sutovsky, M. and Sutovsky, P. (2007). Differential expression of genes encoding constitutive and inducible 20S proteasomal core subunits in the testis and epididymis of theophylline- or 1,3-dinitrobenzene-exposed rats. *Biol Reprod* **76**, 149-63.

Thimon, V., Frenette, G., Saez, F., Thabet, M. and Sullivan, R. (2008). Protein composition of human epididymosomes collected during surgical vasectomy reversal: a proteomic and genomic approach. *Hum Reprod* **23**, 1698-707.

Thundathil, J., Palasz, A. T., Barth, A. D. and Mapletoft, R. J. (2001). The use of in vitro fertilization techniques to investigate the fertilizing ability of bovine sperm with proximal cytoplasmic droplets. *Anim Reprod Sci* **65**, 181-92.

Van Tassell, C. P., Smith, T. P., Matukumalli, L. K., Taylor, J. F., Schnabel, R. D., Lawley, C. T., Haudenschild, C. D., Moore, S. S., Warren, W. C. and Sonstegard, T. S. (2008). SNP discovery and allele frequency estimation by deep sequencing of reduced representation libraries. *Nat Methods* **5**, 247-52.

Voges, D., Zwickl, P. and Baumeister, W. (1999). The 26S proteasome: a molecular machine designed for controlled proteolysis. *Annu Rev Biochem* **68**, 1015-68.

Waberski, D., Meding, S., Dirksen, G., Weitze, K. F., Leiding, C. and Hahn, R. (1994). Fertility of long-term-stored boar semen: influence of extender (Androhep and Kiev), storage time and plasma droplets in the semen. *Animal Reproduction Science* **36**, 145-151.

Wu, A., Anupriwan, A., Iamsaard, S., Chakrabandhu, K., Santos, D. C., Rupar, T., Tsang, B. K., Carmona, E. and Tanphaichitr, N. (2007). Sperm surface arylsulfatase A can disperse the cumulus matrix of cumulus oocyte complexes. *J Cell Physiol* **213**, 201-11.

Zimmerman, S. and Sutovsky, P. (2009). The sperm proteasome during sperm capacitation and fertilization. *J Reprod Immunol* **83**, 19-25.

Zou, C.-X. and Yang, Z.-M. (2000). Evaluation on sperm quality of freshly ejaculated boar semen during in vitro storage under different temperatures. *Theriogenology* **53**, 1477-88.

Regulation of sperm storage and movement in the ruminant oviduct

PH Hung and SS Suarez

Department of Biomedical Sciences, College of Veterinary Medicine, Cornell University, Ithaca, NY 14853, USA

Three regions of the ruminant oviduct play different roles in the progress of sperm: the uterotubal junction, isthmus, and ampulla. The uterotubal junction acts as a point of selection of sperm, requiring that sperm are progressively motile and express specific proteins in order to enter the oviduct. The isthmus stores sperm, preserving motility and viability until ovulation. Sperm are stored in the isthmus by binding to its mucosal epithelium. In bovine sperm, binding to the oviductal epithelium is promoted by proteins that are secreted by the seminal vesicles and coat the heads of sperm by associating with plasma membrane phospholipids. Putative oviductal receptors for the seminal vesicle proteins are members of the annexin protein family. Release of sperm from the storage site in the isthmus is gradual, which serves to ensure that sperm in the proper physiological state reach the oocytes at the appropriate moment and also to reduce incidence of polyspermic fertilization. The ampulla supports fertilization and may participate in guiding sperm toward the eggs. Further studies are needed to improve our understanding of the interactions between sperm and the female reproductive tract, in order to develop means to improve fertility in ruminants.

Introduction

Mammalian sperm travel a long distance relative to their size in order to reach the site of fertilization in the oviduct. When sperm attempt to enter and pass through the oviduct, they are subjected to selective processes to eliminate those of poor quality. Selective processes also regulate the numbers of sperm that reach the fertilization site, thereby reducing the incidence of polyspermic fertilization (Hunter *et al.* 1982, Hunter & Wilmut 1984). The oviduct acts as well to support fertilization, for instance, by storing sperm and maintaining their viability during storage. Furthermore, the timing of capacitation of sperm may be influenced by the oviduct in order to ensure that capacitated sperm are available at ovulation.

Three regions of the oviduct, uterotubal junction, isthmus, and ampulla (Figure 1) play different roles in selecting and supporting sperm. In this review, the current understanding of the roles of each region will be discussed, particularly with regard to ruminant reproduction.

Corresponding author E-mail: sss7@cornell.edu

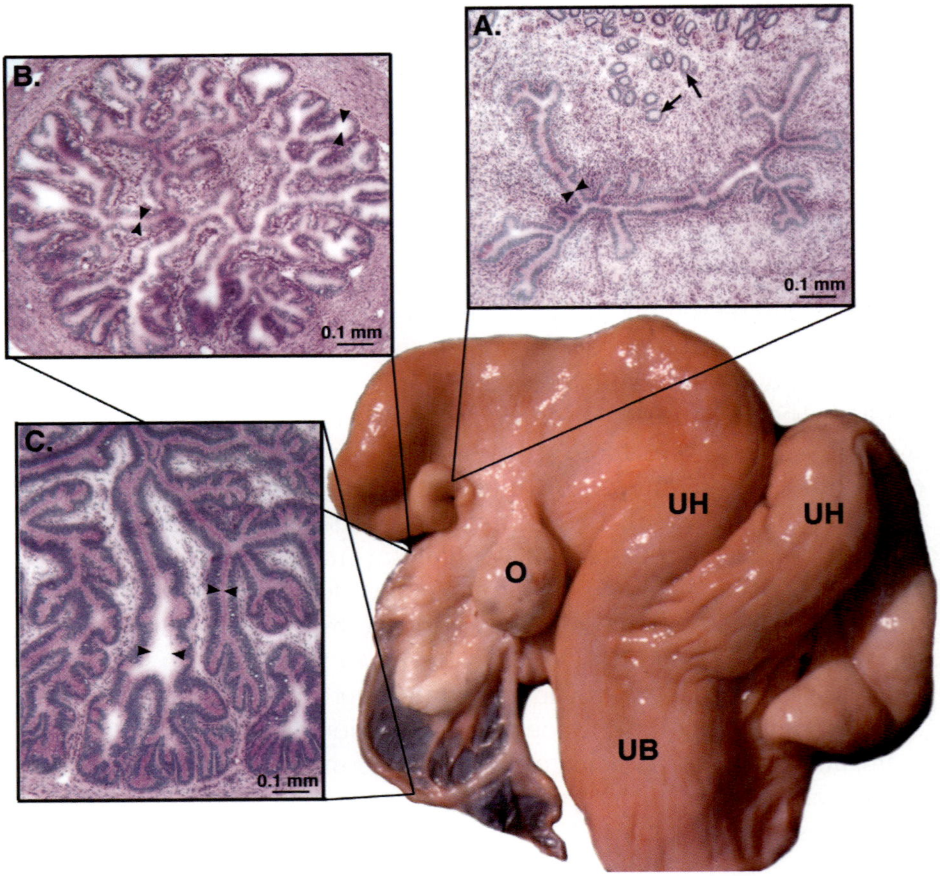

Fig. 1. Regions of the bovine oviduct. On the right, the regions of the bovine female tract are shown (**O**, ovary; **UH** uterine horn; **UB**, lower uterine body). **A.** A frozen section of the bovine uterotubal junction, stained with Periodic Acid Schiff to indicate mucopolysaccharides, and counterstained with hematoxylin. Arrowheads indicate the oviductal lumen, which is narrow and contains mucus. Arrows indicate uterine glands. **B.** A frozen section of the oviductal isthmus, stained as for A. Arrowheads indicate the oviductal lumen. **C.** A frozen section of approximately half of the diameter of the oviductal ampulla, stained as for A. Arrowheads indicate the oviductal lumen. Preparation of these tissues is described in Suarez *et al.* (1997).

The uterotubal junction regulates sperm passage into the oviduct

Regardless of the billions of sperm in the ejaculates of most ruminants, only a minority of several thousand enters the uterotubal junction and passes through it. There may be only a small window of opportunity for sperm to pass through the junction, due to the apparent ability of the junction to close down. In the mouse, patency of the junction can be seen using transillumination of the oviduct and the junction has been observed to close about an hour after mating (Suarez 1987). Three morphological characteristics of the ruminant oviduct indicate that it may do likewise. First, the connective tissue in the bovine junction wall is heavily vascularized and engorgement of the vascular beds may act to compress the lumen (Wrobel *et al.* 1993). Second, the thick smooth muscle layer of the junction could contract to compress the lumen. Third, the tube of the junction is bent into a sigmoidal shape and the muscular ligaments attached to the junction could increase the flexure of the curve to further impede passage of sperm (Hafez & Black 1969, Hook & Hafez 1968).

In the cow, the uterotubal junction is lined with mucosal folds that form channels ending in cul-de-sacs rather than continuing into the isthmus (Figure 2) (Yaniz *et al.* 2000). When muscular and/or vascular action compresses the lumen, these dead ends might form a plug. On the other hand, when the uterotubal junction is not being compressed, the dead ends of the channels could act more like funnels to direct sperm into the isthmus.

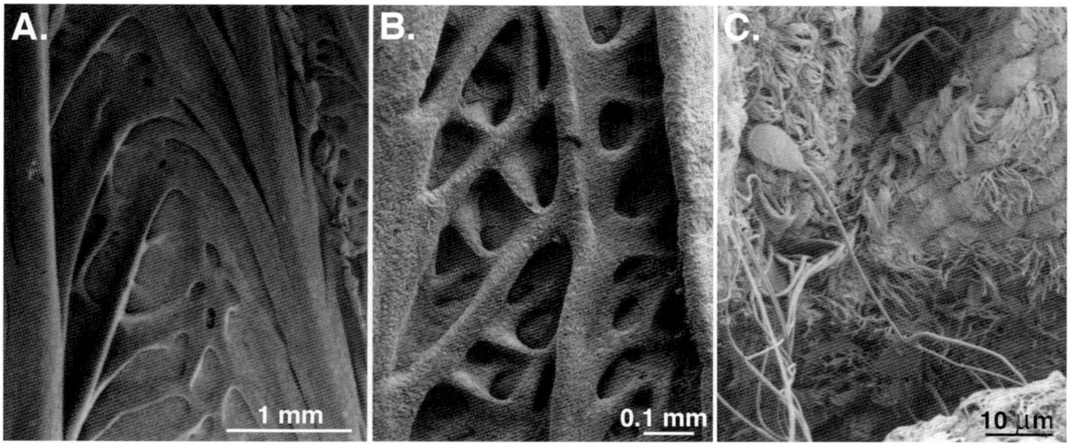

Fig. 2. Scanning electron micrographs of the bovine uterotubal junction and isthmus. **A.** The uterotubal junction is lined with mucosal folds that form channels ending in cul-de-sacs. The bottom of the figure represents the prouterine end of the uterotubal junction. **B.** Mucosal folds in the lower isthmus form pockets in the wall. **C.** Bull sperm binding primarily to cilia on the oviductal epithelium in the lower isthmus to form a reservoir. Figure 2A and 2B are courtesy of Dr. JL Yaniz (Yaniz *et al.* 2000).

When the uterotubal junction is not being closed down by vascular and/or muscular action, the junction is equipped with mechanisms to cause it to act as a point of sperm selection. There are mucous secretions in the lumen of bovine uterotubal junction (Suarez *et al.* 1997) that might filter out sperm with weak motility, as does mucus in the cervical canal (Katz *et al.* 1990). Furthermore, based on null mutant mouse models, there is evidence that mouse sperm must possess certain proteins in order to swim into the uterotubal junction (Nakanishi *et al.* 2004, Yamaguchi *et al.* 2009). For example, calmegin is a spermatogenesis-specific chaperone protein, and the sperm produced by calmegin knockout mice are unable to pass through the uterotubal junction, despite having normal morphology and motility (Ikawa *et al.* 2001). A subsequent study confirmed that each sperm must possess the proteins chaperoned by calmegin, because when females were mated with chimeric males that produced a mixture of developing germ cells in the testis that contained or were missing calmegin, the only sperm that entered into the uterotubal junctions where those in which calmegin had been expressed during development (Nakanishi *et al.* 2004). Calmegin is known to be required for the expression of ADAM3 (a disintegrin and metallopeptidase domain 3) on mature sperm, and sperm from male mice deficient in ADAM3 are also unable to pass through the uterotubal junction (Yamaguchi *et al.* 2009). It is not yet known whether similar proteins are required for ruminant sperm to pass through the uterotubal junction.

In cattle (VanDemark & Moeller 1951), sheep (Mattner & Braden 1963), humans (Kunz *et al.* 1996), and rabbits (Overstreet & Cooper 1978), a small fraction of sperm are transported through the uterus and oviduct to the site of fertilization within a few minutes of mating. This phenomenon, which has been called "rapid sperm transport", may be a consequence of muscular contractions in the female tract that occur during mating, because it occurs too rapidly for it to be the result of sperm swimming and it may not serve to bring competent sperm to the site of fertilization (Hays & VanDemark 1953). For instance, rabbit sperm that underwent rapid transport were found to have sustained damage and thus would be unlikely to fertilize (Overstreet & Cooper 1978, Overstreet & Tom 1982). It is not known whether rapid transport serves any purpose.

Sperm are stored in the isthmus

After sperm pass through the intramural portion of the uterotubal junction, most bind to the epithelium in the extramural portion and/or the lower part of the isthmus of the oviduct to form a storage reservoir. Oviductal reservoirs of sperm have been identified in a broad array of mammals, including sheep (Hunter *et al.* 1982), cattle (Hunter & Wilmut 1984), mice (Suarez 1987), and hamsters (Smith & Yanagimachi 1991). There is evidence that binding to the oviductal epithelium prolongs the motile life span of ruminant sperm. When sperm of cattle (Chian *et al.* 1995, Pollard *et al.* 1991), sheep (Lloyd *et al.* 2008, Lloyd *et al.* 2009), or red deer (Berg *et al.* 2002) were incubated with oviductal epithelium in vitro, higher percentages of the sperm remained motile over time. The mechanism for sustaining motility has been proposed to involve suppression of capacitation, because equine sperm showed delayed capacitation when incubated with oviductal epithelium (Dobrinski *et al.* 1996). Elucidating the mechanism of preservation of motility during storage might suggest new methods for storing sperm in vitro.

There is evidence that sperm at least begin to capacitate while in the oviductal isthmus (Smith & Yanagimachi 1991). It is not fully understood how sperm become capacitated in the oviduct. In vitro, it has been shown that capacitation involves loss of decapacitating factors including cholesterol, a rise in intracellular Ca^{2+}, and an increase in activity of a sperm-specific adenylyl cyclase known as SACY (Sinclair *et al.* 2000). SACY activation results in increased cAMP, which, in turn, activates protein kinase A (PKA) (reviewed by Visconti *et al.* 2002). Through a poorly understood process, activation of PKA, a serine and threonine kinase, leads to increased tyrosine phosphorylation of several sperm proteins (reviewed by Visconti *et al.* 2002), such as testis-specific serine/proline-rich protein, calcium binding protein, and others (Platt *et al.* 2009). Studies in mice (Visconti *et al.* 1995) and cattle (Galantino-Homer *et al.* 1997) have shown that protein tyrosine phosphorylation is correlated with capacitation, confirmed by the ability of sperm to undergo induced acrosome reactions and to fertilize eggs in vitro. Most of the roles of tyrosine phosphorylated proteins in sperm capacitation remain to be determined.

Bull sperm capacitation is facilitated in vitro when heparin is present (Parrish *et al.* 1988). There is evidence that the effect of heparin on sperm is mediated by bovine seminal plasma proteins (binder of sperm, BSP) (Manjunath *et al.* 2009) on the sperm surface, particularly PDC109 (also known as BSPA1/A2) (Manjunath & Therien 2002, Therien *et al.* 1997). BSP proteins are produced by the bovine seminal vesicles and adhere to the sperm surface by associating with phospholipids in the sperm plasma membrane (Desnoyers & Manjunath 1992). BSP proteins are small in mass (14-30 kDa) and each contains a unique N-terminal domain followed by two fibronectin type II domains (Calvete *et al.* 1999). The type II domains contain heparin binding sites (Chandonnet *et al.* 1990) that could be responsible for the stimulation of capacitation by heparin, and phospholipid binding sites that are responsible for binding the BSPs to the sperm surface (Wah *et al.* 2002). BSP homologs have been reported in other ruminant species, including goats (Villemure *et al.* 2003), sheep (Bergeron *et al.* 2005), and bisons (Boisvert *et al.* 2004), and some of the homologs have been demonstrated to bind heparin (Bergeron *et al.* 2005, Boisvert *et al.* 2004, Villemure *et al.* 2003).

The process of capacitation is considered to include hyperactivation of sperm motility. Hyperactivated sperm display asymmetrical, high-amplitude flagellar beating patterns, causing vigorous, and sometimes circular, movement of free-swimming sperm (Suarez *et al.* 1983, Yanagimachi 1970). Hyperactivated motility is required for the penetration of viscoelastic substances in the oviduct (Suarez *et al.* 1991), such as mucus and the matrix of the cumulus oophorus, and for sperm penetration of the zona pellucida (Stauss *et al.* 1995). Hyperactivation is triggered by a rise of intracellular Ca^{2+}, primarily from extracellular sources (reviewed by Suarez 2008). In cattle, sperm can be induced to hyperactivate in vitro by procaine in the presence of extracellular Ca^{2+} and therefore is presumed to operate by stimulating Ca^{2+} influx (Ho & Suarez 2001, Ho & Suarez 2003). In mouse sperm, sperm-specific CatSper proteins are known to form Ca^{2+} channels in the plasma membrane of the principal piece of the flagellum (Carlson *et al.* 2005, Jin *et al.* 2007). Sperm from CatSper-null mice do not hyperactivate (Carlson *et al.* 2005, Jin *et al.* 2007, Qi *et al.* 2007) and cannot fertilize zona pellucida-intact eggs (Quill *et al.* 2003, Ren *et al.* 2001).

BSP proteins play a role in sperm storage

In hamsters (DeMott *et al.* 1995), cattle (Lefebvre *et al.* 1997), and pigs (Wagner *et al.* 2002), studies have shown that sperm-oviductal epithelium interaction is mediated by carbohydrate-recognition mechanisms. Fucose, specifically in the Lewis-A trisaccharide, was identified to be a key component of the receptor for bull sperm binding in the oviduct (Suarez *et al.* 1998). Lewis-A was used in an affinity column to pull proteins from sperm extracts that would play a role in binding sperm to the oviductal epithelium. The main protein identified by this method was PDC109 (Gwathmey *et al.* 2003, Ignotz *et al.* 2001), which is one of the BSP proteins. Gwathmey *et al.* (2006) later reported that two other BSP proteins (BSPA3 and BSP30K), each acting alone, can also induce sperm binding to oviductal epithelium in vitro. This leads to the question: Why do bull sperm need three BSP proteins when they can bind to the oviductal epithelium with any one of the BSP proteins alone? Key functions are often protected by redundancy; however, this apparent redundancy may also provide more intricate control over sperm movement out of the reservoir. Differences in the amino acid sequences of the three BSP proteins result in different patterns of surface charges on the BSP molecules (Gwathmey *et al.* 2006); therefore, it is proposed that each BSP molecule adheres to the surface of sperm and binds sperm to the oviductal epithelium with different affinities and kinetics. Altogether, the BSP proteins may act to provide a gradual release of sperm from the reservoir, in order to ensure that sperm capacitate and reach eggs at the ideal time for fertilization and yet not too many reach the egg at once, which might result in polyspermic fertilization. It is possible that BSP homologs in other ruminant species are also involved in the formation of sperm reservoir; however, this remains to be determined.

Oviductal annexins are possible binding partners of BSP proteins

When BSP proteins were used as bait to pull down oviductal ligands from a mixture of proteins extracted from apical plasma membranes of bovine isthmic epithelium, four annexin proteins (ANXA1, 2, 4, and 5) were captured (Ignotz *et al.* 2007). ANXAs comprise a large, diverse family of Ca^{2+}- and lipid-binding proteins. In other cell types, there is evidence that ANXAs serve as membrane scaffold proteins and are involved in vesicle transport and protein secretion, but much of their functions and secretory pathways are still poorly understood (reviewed by Rescher & Gerke 2004).

In support of the proposal that ANXAs are the oviductal receptors for sperm, all four ANXAs were immunolocalized on the apical surfaces of oviductal epithelium (Ignotz *et al.* 2007). Western blot analysis confirmed that oviductal ANXAs contain fucose, and sperm binding to oviductal epithelium can be inhibited in vitro in the presence of ANXA antibodies (Ignotz *et al.* 2007). There is also evidence that one of the ANXAs (ANXA2) is a sperm binding protein on the porcine oviductal epithelium (Teijeiro *et al.* 2009). Like BSP proteins, ANXAs were also found to bind to heparin (Ishitsuka *et al.* 1998, Shao *et al.* 2006). This interesting finding implicates heparin, or a similar glycosaminoglycan, in the process of binding or release of sperm, particularly since heparin-like molecules have been identified in oviductal fluid (Parrish *et al.* 1989) and have been shown to trigger release of bovine sperm from monolayers of oviductal epithelium in vitro (Gualtieri & Talevi 2000).

Sperm movement beyond the reservoir to the ampulla

In cattle, sperm are stored in the isthmic region of the oviduct for 18-20 hours or more before being released to ascend to the ampulla (Hunter & Wilmut 1984). The release of sperm from the reservoir begins prior to ovulation, which occurs 28-31 hours after the onset of estrus in cattle (Hunter & Wilmut 1984). It is unlikely that the release of sperm is due to the loss of binding sites on the oviductal epithelium, as sperm can bind to oviducts from different stages of estrus cycle (Lefebvre *et al.* 1995). Rather, it is likely that hormonal changes that trigger ovulation also stimulate the release of factors in the oviduct that cause changes in sperm which enable them to release themselves from the oviductal epithelium.

There is evidence that sperm release themselves from the reservoir by two mechanisms: hyperactivation and shedding of sperm surface proteins during capacitation. First, hyperactivation was proposed to play a role in release of mouse and human sperm, (DeMott & Suarez 1992, Pacey *et al.* 1995), because sperm were seen to hyperactivate before pulling away from the epithelial surface. In addition, sperm from CatSper null mice, which are unable to hyperactivate, fail to move beyond the sperm storage reservoir (Ho *et al.* 2009). It is not yet known whether hyperactivation plays such a role in ruminants. Second, sperm may lose binding affinity for the oviductal epithelium by shedding BSP proteins during capacitation. It has been reported that bull sperm shed the BSP protein PDC109 during capacitation in vitro and capacitated sperm are less able to bind to epithelium unless they are treated with purified PDC109 (Gwathmey *et al.* 2003). Less is known of the roles of BSPA3 and BSP30K; however, because capacitated sperm lose binding affinity for the epithelium, one would predict that these two proteins are also shed during capacitation. Because BSPA3 and BSP30K differ from PDC109 in molecular surface charges (Gwathmey *et al.* 2006), we predict that the kinetics of loss during capacitation differs from that of PDC109. Differential loss of BSP proteins could serve to spread out the release of sperm from the reservoir and thus assure that sperm reach eggs shortly after they enter the oviduct, but that not so many reach eggs that polyspermy occurs.

After sperm are released from the reservoir, they are still required to travel a long distance before they reach the fertilization site. Furthermore, as sperm move up the isthmus into the ampulla, the diameter of the tube increases and the shape of the lumen becomes even more complicated by elaboration of the mucosal folds that create narrow, labyrinthine passages (Figure 1). How sperm find their way to the egg is still largely unknown. It has been proposed that chemotaxis serves to guide sperm toward eggs (reviewed by Kaupp *et al.* 2008). The existence of chemotaxis has been well documented in several species of marine invertebrates (reviewed by Hildebrand & Kaupp 2005); therefore, it has been hypothesized that chemotactic factors direct mammalian sperm to eggs. In humans (Cohen-Dayag *et al.* 1995, Spehr *et al.* 2003, Villanueva-Diaz *et al.* 1990) and rabbits (Fabro *et al.* 2002), sperm reportedly turn to swim up a gradient of follicular fluid or putative chemotactic agents, indicating that chemotaxis plays a role in mammalian fertilization; however, unlike the massive response shown by various species of marine invertebrate sperm (Cook *et al.* 1994, Yoshida *et al.* 2003), only small percentages of mammalian sperm (2-12% in humans) have shown this response in vitro (Gakamsky *et al.* 2008). In ruminant species, 8-10% of frozen-thawed bull sperm were reported to orient into a gradient of follicular fluid (Gil *et al.* 2008). Some follicular fluid escapes from the oviduct with the egg mass during fertilization and thus could be present in the ampulla to attract sperm toward the site of fertilization.

Conclusions

Studies from different animal models have helped researchers to better understand the regulation of sperm storage and movement in the oviduct; however, not much research has been done in ruminant species other than *Bos taurus*. There is still much to be learned about how sperm entry through the uterotubal junction is regulated, how sperm fertility is maintained during storage in the oviductal reservoir, how sperm are released from the reservoir, and whether sperm are guided toward eggs in the ampulla by chemotaxis. Such information could prove valuable for developing new methods to improve sperm storage and the success rate of artificial insemination of domestic ruminants and endangered wildlife species.

References

Berg DK, Thompson JG & Asher GW 2002 Development of in vitro embryo production systems for red deer (Cervus elaphus). Part 1. Effect of epithelial oviductal monolayers and heparin on in vitro sperm motility and penetration of in vitro matured oocytes. *Anim Reprod Sci* **70** 65-76.

Bergeron A, Villemure M, Lazure C & Manjunath P 2005 Isolation and characterization of the major proteins of ram seminal plasma. *Molecular Reproduction and Development* **71** 461-470.

Boisvert M, Bergeron A, Lazure C & Manjunath P 2004 Isolation and characterization of gelatin-binding bison seminal vesicle secretory proteins. *Biology of Reproduction* **70** 656-661.

Calvete JJ, Campanero-Rhodes MA, Raida M & Sanz L 1999 Characterisation of the conformational and quaternary structure-dependent heparin-binding region of bovine seminal plasma protein PDC-109. *FEBS Letters* **444** 260-264.

Carlson AE, Quill TA, Westenbroek RE, Schuh SM, Hille B & Babcock DF 2005 Identical phenotypes of CatSper1 and CatSper2 null sperm. *Journal of Biological Chemistry* **280** 32238-32244.

Chandonnet L, Roberts KD, Chapdelaine A & Manjunath P 1990 Identification of heparin-binding proteins in bovine seminal plasma. *Molecular Reproduction and Development* **26** 313-318.

Chian RC, Lapointe S & Sirard MA 1995 Capacitation in vitro of bovine spermatozoa by oviduct epithelial cell monolayer conditioned medium. *Molecular Reproduction and Development* **42** 318-324.

Cohen-Dayag A, Tur-Kaspa I, Dor J, Mashiach S & Eisenbach M 1995 Sperm capacitation in humans is transient and correlates with chemotactic responsiveness to follicular factors. *Proceedings of the National Academy of Sciences of the United States of America* **92** 11039-11043.

Cook SP, Brokaw CJ, Muller CH & Babcock DF 1994 Sperm chemotaxis: Egg peptides control cytosolic calcium to regulate flagellar responses. *Developmental Biology* **165** 10-19.

DeMott RP, Lefebvre R & Suarez SS 1995 Carbohydrates mediate the adherence of hamster sperm to oviductal epithelium. *Biology of Reproduction* **52** 1395-1403.

DeMott RP & Suarez SS 1992 Hyperactivated sperm progress in the mouse oviduct. *Biology of Reproduction* **46** 779-785.

Desnoyers L & Manjunath P 1992 Major proteins of bovine seminal plasma exhibit novel interactions with phospholipid. *Journal of Biological Chemistry* **267** 10149-10155.

Dobrinski I, Suarez SS & Ball BA 1996 Intracellular

calcium concentration in equine spermatozoa attached to oviductal epithelial cells in vitro. *Biology of Reproduction* **54** 783-788.

Fabro G, Rovasio RA, Civalero S, Frenkel A, Caplan SR, Eisenbach M & Giojalas LC 2002 Chemotaxis of capacitated rabbit spermatozoa to follicular fluid revealed by a novel directionality-based assay. *Biology of Reproduction* **67** 1565-1571.

Gakamsky A, Schechtman E, Caplan SR & Eisenbach M 2008 Analysis of chemotaxis when the fraction of responsive cells is small--application to mammalian sperm guidance. *International Joural of Developmental Biology* **52** 481-487.

Galantino-Homer HL, Visconti PE & Kopf GS 1997 Regulation of protein tyrosine phosphorylation during bovine sperm capacitation by a cyclic adenosine 3′5′-monophosphate-dependent pathway. *Biology of Reproduction* **56** 707-719.

Gil PI, Guidobaldi HA, Teves ME, Unates DR, Sanchez R & Giojalas LC 2008 Chemotactic response of frozen-thawed bovine spermatozoa towards follicular fluid. *Animal Reproduction Science* **108** 236-246.

Gualtieri R & Talevi R 2000 In vitro-cultured bovine oviductal cells bind acrosome-intact sperm and retain this ability upon sperm release. *Biology of Reproduction* **62** 1754-1762.

Gwathmey TM, Ignotz GG, Mueller JL, Manjunath P & Suarez SS 2006 Bovine seminal plasma proteins PDC-109, BSP-A3, and BSP-30-kDa share functional roles in storing sperm in the oviduct. *Biology of Reproduction* **75** 501-507.

Gwathmey TM, Ignotz GG & Suarez SS 2003 PDC-109 (BSP-A1/A2) promotes bull sperm binding to oviductal epithelium in vitro and may be involved in forming the oviductal sperm reservoir. *Biology of Reproduction* **69** 809-815.

Hafez ES & Black DL 1969 The mammalian uterotubal junction. In: *The Mammalian Oviduct: Comparative Biology and Methodology*, 85-128. Eds ESE Hafez & RJ Blandau. Chicago: The University of Chicago Press.

Hays RL & VanDemark NL 1953 Spontaneous motility of the bovine uterus. *American Journal of Physiology* **172** 553-556.

Hildebrand E & Kaupp UB 2005 Sperm chemotaxis: a primer. *Annals of the New York Academy of Sciences* **1061** 221-225.

Ho HC & Suarez SS 2001 An inositol 1,4,5-trisphosphate receptor-gated intracellular Ca^{2+} store is involved in regulating sperm hyperactivated motility. *Biology of Reproduction* **65** 1606-1615.

Ho HC & Suarez SS 2003 Characterization of the intracellular calcium store at the base of the sperm flagellum that regulates hyperactivated motility. *Biology of Reproduction* **68** 1590-1596.

Ho K, Wolff CA & Suarez SS 2009 CatSper-null mutant spermatozoa are unable to ascend beyond the oviductal reservoir. *Reproduction, Fertility, and Development* **21** 345-350.

Hook SJ & Hafez ES 1968 A comparative anatomical study of the mammalian uterotubal junction. *Journal of Morphology* **125** 159-184.

Hunter RH, Barwise L & King R 1982 Sperm transport, storage and release in the sheep oviduct in relation to the time of ovulation. *British Veterinary Journal* **138** 225-232.

Hunter RH & Wilmut I 1984 Sperm transport in the cow: peri-ovulatory redistribution of viable cells within the oviduct. *Reproduction Nutrition Development* **24** 597-608.

Ignotz GG, Cho MY & Suarez SS 2007 Annexins are candidate oviductal receptors for bovine sperm surface proteins and thus may serve to hold bovine sperm in the oviductal reservoir. *Biology of Reproduction* **77** 906-913.

Ignotz GG, Lo MC, Perez CL, Gwathmey TM & Suarez SS 2001 Characterization of a fucose-binding protein from bull sperm and seminal plasma that may be responsible for formation of the oviductal sperm reservoir. *Biology of Reproduction* **64** 1806-1811.

Ikawa M, Nakanishi T, Yamada S, Wada I, Kominami K, Tanaka H, Nozaki M, Nishimune Y & Okabe M 2001 Calmegin is required for fertilin α/β heterodimerization and sperm fertility. *Developmental Biology* **240** 254-261.

Ishitsuka R, Kojima K, Utsumi H, Ogawa H & Matsumoto I 1998 Glycosaminoglycan binding properties of annexin IV, V, and VI. *Journal of Biological Chemistry* **273** 9935-9941.

Jin J, Jin N, Zheng H, Ro S, Tafolla D, Sanders KM & Yan W 2007 Catsper3 and Catsper4 are essential for sperm hyperactivated motility and male fertility in the mouse. *Biology of Reproduction* **77** 37-44.

Katz DF, Morales P, Samuels SJ & Overstreet JW 1990 Mechanisms of filtration of morphologically abnormal human sperm by cervical mucus. *Fertility and Sterility* **54** 513-516.

Kaupp UB, Kashikar ND & Weyand I 2008 Mechanisms of sperm chemotaxis. *Annual Review of Physiology* **70** 93-117.

Kunz G, Beil D, Deininger H, Wildt L & Leyendecker G 1996 The dynamics of rapid sperm transport through the female genital tract: evidence from vaginal sonography of uterine peristalsis and hysterosalpingoscintigraphy. *Human Reproduction* **11** 627-632.

Lefebvre R, Chenoweth PJ, Drost M, LeClear CT, MacCubbin M, Dutton JT & Suarez SS 1995 Characterization of the oviductal sperm reservoir in cattle. *Biol Reprod* **53** 1066-1074.

Lefebvre R, Lo MC & Suarez SS 1997 Bovine sperm binding to oviductal epithelium involves fucose recognition. *Biology of Reproduction* **56** 1198-1204.

Lloyd RE, Badia E, Fazeli A, Watson PF & Holt WV 2008 Temporal dynamics of ram sperm binding and survival during 48-h coculture with oviducal epithelial cells. *Reproduction, Fertility, and Development* **20** 835-845.

Lloyd RE, Elliott RM, Fazeli A, Watson PF & Holt WV 2009 Effects of oviductal proteins, including heat shock 70 kDa protein 8, on survival of ram spermatozoa over 48 h in vitro. *Reproduction, Fertility, and Development* **21** 408-418.

Manjunath P & Therien I 2002 Role of seminal plasma phospholipid-binding proteins in sperm membrane lipid modification that occurs during capacitation. *Journal of Reproductive Immunology* **53** 109-119.

Manjunath P, Lefebvre J, Jois PS, Fan J & Wright MW 2009 New nomenclature for mammalian BSP genes. *Biology of Reproduction* **80** 394-397.

Mattner PE & Braden AWH 1963 Spermatozoa in the genital tract of the ewe. I. Rapidity of transport. *Australian Journal of Biological Sciences* **16** 473.

Nakanishi T, Isotani A, Yamaguchi R, Ikawa M, Baba T, Suarez SS & Okabe M 2004 Selective passage through the uterotubal junction of sperm from a mixed population produced by chimeras of calmegin-knockout and wild-type male mice. *Biology of Reproduction* **71** 959-965.

Overstreet JW & Cooper GW 1978 Sperm transport in the reproductive tract of the female rabbit: I. The rapid transit phase of transport. *Biology of Reproduction* **19** 101-114.

Overstreet JW & Tom RA 1982 Experimental studies of rapid sperm transport in rabbits. *Reproduction* **66** 601-606.

Pacey AA, Davies N, Warren MA, Barratt CLR & Cooke LD 1995 Hyperactivation may assist human spermatozoa to detach from intimate association with the endosalpinx. *Human Reproduction* **10** 2603-2609.

Parrish JJ, Susko-Parrish J, Winer MA & First NL 1988 Capacitation of bovine sperm by heparin. *Biology of Reproduction* **38** 1171-1180.

Parrish JJ, Susko-Parrish JL, Handrow RR, Sims MM & First NL 1989 Capacitation of bovine spermatozoa by oviduct fluid. *Biology of Reproduction* **40** 1020-1025.

Platt MD, Salicioni AM, Hunt DF & Visconti PE 2009 Use of differential isotopic labeling and mass spectrometry to analyze capacitation-associated changes in the phosphorylation status of mouse sperm proteins. *J Proteome Res* **8** 1431-1440.

Pollard JW, Plante C, King WA, Hansen PJ, Betteridge KJ & Suarez SS 1991 Fertilizing capacity of bovine sperm may be maintained by binding of oviductal epithelial cells. *Biology of Reproduction* **44** 102-107.

Qi H, Moran MM, Navarro B, Chong JA, Krapivinsky G, Krapivinsky L, Kirichok Y, Ramsey IS, Quill TA & Clapham DE 2007 All four CatSper ion channel proteins are required for male fertility and sperm cell hyperactivated motility. *Proceedings of the National Academy of Sciences of the United States of America* **104** 1219-1223.

Quill TA, Sugden SA, Rossi KL, Doolittle LK, Hammer RE & Garbers DL 2003 Hyperactivated sperm motility driven by CatSper2 is required for fertilization. *Proceedings of the National Academy of Sciences of the United States of America* **100** 14869-14874.

Ren D, Navarro B, Perez G, Jackson AC, Hsu S, Shi Q, Tilly JL & Clapham DE 2001 A sperm ion channel required for sperm motility and male fertility. *Nature* **413** 603-609.

Rescher U & Gerke V 2004 Annexins - unique membrane binding proteins with diverse functions. *Journal of Cell Science* **117** 2631-2639.

Shao C, Zhang F, Kemp MM, Linhardt RJ, Waisman DM, Head JF & Seaton BA 2006 Crystallographic analysis of calcium-dependent heparin binding to annexin A2. *Journal of Biological Chemistry* **281** 31689-31695.

Sinclair ML, Wang XY, Mattia M, Conti M, Buck J, Wolgemuth DJ & Levin LR 2000 Specific expression of soluble adenylyl cyclase in male germ cells. *Mol Reprod Dev* **56** 6-11.

Smith TT & Yanagimachi R 1991 Attachment and release of spermatozoa from the caudal isthmus of the hamster oviduct. *Journal of Reproduction and Fertility* **91** 567-573.

Spehr M, Gisselmann G, Poplawski A, Riffell JA, Wetzel CH, Zimmer RK & Hatt H 2003 Identification of a testicular odorant receptor mediating human sperm chemotaxis. *Science* **299** 2054-2058.

Stauss CR, Votta TJ & Suarez SS 1995 Sperm motility hyperactivation facilitates penetration of the hamster zona pellucida. *Biology of Reproduction* **53** 1280-1285.

Suarez SS 1987 Sperm transport and motility in the mouse oviduct: observations in situ. *Biology of Reproduction* **36** 203-210.

Suarez SS 2008 Control of hyperactivation in sperm. *Human Reproduction Update* **14** 647-657.

Suarez SS, Brockman K & Lefebvre R 1997 Distribution of mucus and sperm in bovine oviducts after artificial insemination: the physical environment of the oviductal sperm reservoir. *Biology of Reproduction* **56** 447-453.

Suarez SS, Katz DF & Overstreet JW 1983 Movement characteristics and acrosomal status of rabbit spermatozoa recovered at the site and time of fertilization. *Biology of Reproduction* **29** 1277-1287.

Suarez SS, Katz DF, Owen DH, Andrew JB & Powell RL 1991 Evidence for the function of hyperactivated motility in sperm. *Biology of Reproduction* **44** 375-381.

Suarez SS, Revah I, Lo M & Kolle S 1998 Bull sperm binding to oviductal epithelium is mediated by a Ca^{2+}-dependent lectin on sperm that recognizes Lewis-a trisaccharide. *Biology of Reproduction* **59** 39-44.

Teijeiro JM, Ignotz GG & Marini PE 2009 Annexin A2 is involved in pig (Sus scrofa) sperm-oviduct interaction. *Molecular Reproduction and Development* **76** 334-341.

Therien I, Soubeyrand S & Manjunath P 1997 Major proteins of bovine seminal plasma modulate sperm capacitation by high-density lipoprotein. *Biology of Reproduction* **57** 1080-1088.

VanDemark NL & Moeller AN 1951 Speed of spermatozoa transport in reproductive tract of estrous cow. *American Journal of Physiology* **165** 674-679.

Villanueva-Diaz C, Vadillo-Ortega F, Kably-Ambe A, Diaz-Perez MA & Krivitzky SK 1990 Evidence that human follicular fluid contains a chemoattractant for spermatozoa. *Fertility and Sterility* **54** 1180-1182.

Villemure M, Lazure C & Manjunath P 2003 Isolation and characterization of gelatin-binding proteins from goat seminal plasma. *Reproductive Biology and Endocrinology* **1** 39.

Visconti PE, Bailey JL, Moore GD, Pan D, Olds-Clarke P & Kopf GS 1995 Capacitation of mouse spermatozoa. I. Correlation between the capacitation state and protein tyrosine phosphorylation. *Development* **121** 1129-1137.

Visconti PE, Westbrook VA, Chertihin O, Demarco I, Sleight S & Diekman AB 2002 Novel signaling pathways involved in sperm acquisition of fertilizing capacity. *Journal of Reproductive Immunology* **53** 133-150.

Wagner A, Ekhlasi-Hundrieser M, Hettel C, Petrunkina A, Waberski D, Nimtz M & Topfer-Petersen E 2002 Carbohydrate-based interactions of oviductal sperm reservoir formation-studies in the pig. *Molecular Reproduction and Development* **61** 249-257.

Wah DA, Fernandez-Tornero C, Sanz L, Romero A & Calvete JJ 2002 Sperm coating mechanism from the 1.8 A crystal structure of PDC-109-phosphorylcholine complex. *Structure* **10** 505-514.

Wrobel KH, Kujat R & Fehle G 1993 The bovine tubouterine junction: general organization and surface morphology. *Cell and Tissue Research* **271** 227-239.

Yamaguchi R, Muro Y, Isotani A, Tokuhiro K, Takumi K, Adham I, Ikawa M & Okabe M 2009 Disruption of ADAM3 impairs the migration of sperm into oviduct in mouse. *Biology of Reproduction* **81** 142-146.

Yanagimachi R 1970 The movement of golden hamster spermatozoa before and after capacitation. *Journal of Reproduction and Fertility* **23** 193-196.

Yaniz JL, Lopez-Gatius F, Santolaria P & Mullins KJ 2000 Study of the functional anatomy of bovine oviductal mucosa. *Anatomical Record* **260** 268-278.

Yoshida M, Ishikawa M, Izumi H, De Santis R & Morisawa M 2003 Store-operated calcium channel regulates the chemotactic behavior of ascidian sperm. *Proceedings of the National Academy of Sciences of the United States of America* **100** 149-154.

Interaction of sperm with the zona pellucida during fertilization

BM Gadella

Department of Farm Animal Health and of Biochemistry & Cell Biology, Faculty of Veterinary Medicine, Utrecht University, Yalelaan 2, 3584 CM Utrecht, The Netherlands

In order to achieve fertilization sperm cells, first need to successfully interact with the zona pellucida. To this end, the sperm surface is extensively remodeled during capacitation and the resulting sperm cells also possess hyperactivated motility. Together, this serves to mediate optimal recognition of the zona pellucida in the oviduct or after in vitro fertilization incubations (primary zona pellucida binding). When the sperm cell attaches to the zona pellucida, it will be triggered to undergo the acrosome reaction which allows the hyperactivated motile sperm cell to drill through the zona pellucida (secondary zona pellucida binding coinciding with sequential local zona pellucida digestion and rebinding). After successful zona penetration, some sperm cells may enter the perivitelline space. This delaying strategy of the oocyte allows only one sperm cell at a given time to bind and fuse with the oocyte (fertilization) and thus minimizes the risk of polyspermy. The fertilization fusion between the oocyte and the first sperm cell is immediately followed by a polyspermic fertilization block, in which the content of the oocyte's cortical granules is released into the perivitelline space. The cortical reaction blocks further sperm-oocyte fusion either by sticking at the oolemma or by the induction of a biochemical reaction of the zona pellucida (zona pellucida hardening). The cortical reaction thus blocks sperm-zona pellucida binding and/or sperm-zona pellucida penetration. This review summarizes the current understanding of sperm-zona pellucida interactions in relation to mammalian fertilization. The lack of knowledge about sperm-zona pellucida binding in ruminants will be critically discussed.

The zona pellucida

The mouse zona pellucida

Most of our current understanding of the zona pellucida is based on data obtained from the mouse species (for a recent review see Wassarman and Litscher 2009). Like in other mammals the extracellular matrix of the oocyte has three peculiar properties: (1) It is quite thick for an extracellular matrix (in rodents around 7 μm); (2) It is not attached directly to the oocyte but to the cumulus cells surrounding the periphery of the oocyte, leaving a cell free space commonly termed perivitelline space between the glycocalyx and the oolemma; and (3) Isolation and solubilization of the zona pellucida revealed that the mouse zona consists of only three zona proteins (ZP1, ZP2, ZP3), all of which are heavily and differentially glycosylated (Wassarman 1988).

Corresponding author E-mail: B.M.Gadella@uu.nl

The mouse zona pellucida is formed by linear filaments of ZP 2 and 3 that are cross linked by ZP1. Zona protein treatments with chymotrypsin, or with reducing agents, altered the functional integrity of ZP1 and as a result filaments of ZP2/ZP3 could be isolated from mouse ZP (Greve and Wassarman 1985). Such filaments are actively being secreted by the oocyte forming linear arrangements attached to the oolemma of developing oocytes (Wassarman and Albertini 1994). At a later phase, the characteristic thick (Wassarman 2008) zona pellucida is formed and between this structure and the oolemma a cavity (the perivitelline space) is created (Wassarman and Albertini 1994). Recent studies on structural features of ZP proteins revealed that, beyond the secretion domain present on the translated preZPs, the secreted ZPs also contain a ZP domain containing a conserved sequence (ZP-N domain at the N terminal end) that is involved in forming polymers that are shared with other extracellular matrix proteins (Jovine et al., 2006). How this ZP-N domain (with PLAC-1 homology Jovine et al., 2007) is involved in ZP polymer formation has recently been elucidated with ultrastructural techniques (Monné et al., 2008).

Solubilization of the zona pellucida (by heat treatment at low pH) and functional studies with the three individual purified zona proteins revealed that ZP3 is the receptor for intact sperm and interacts with sperm surface proteins present in the apical head region (*primary zona pellucida binding*) and that ZP3 is also responsible for induction of the acrosome reaction (Litscher and Wassarman 1996; Buffone et al., 2009a). The c-terminal fragment (ZP-C domain) of ZP3 is also thought to be involved in sperm binding (Wassarman 2008). Specific glycan structures on ZP3 appear to be involved in the zona pellucida-induced acrosome reaction as this response can be mimicked in vitro by adding Lewis X to sperm or by supplementing albumin with covalently linked carbohydrates (neoglycoproteins) (Bendahmane and Tulsiani 2003, Loeser and Tulsiani 1999, Hanna et al., 2004; Kerr et al., 2004, Williams et al., 2007). However, the involvement of *N*- and *O*-glycans on mouse ZP3 for primary sperm binding and fertilization has recently been challenged using transgenic mice that expressed a mutated ZP3 that lacked glycosylation sites. These transgenic mice had normal fertilization rates and normal litter sizes (Gahlay al., 2010).

ZP2 is the receptor that is involved in *secondary zona pellucida binding* as it interacts only with acrosome reacted cells as those cells have exposed acrosomal proteins involved in zona pellucida binding and penetration (Bleil et al., 1988; Howes et al., 2001). While ZP2 is not only involved in the secondary zona pellucida binding event, it also is believed to become cleaved by acrosomal enzymes allowing sperm drilling through the zona pellucida (Moreno et al., 1999) although not much is known about how acrosome proteins mediate zona digestion. For instance it is not known whether the ZP2 processing by acrosomal enzymes is comparable to the formation of ZP2f after fertilization (see section on zona hardening).

Following successful penetration through the zona pellucida, only one sperm will fertilize the oocyte and this one event is immediately followed by the cortical reaction which will initiate *zona pellucida hardening*. Zona pellucida hardening essentially blocks penetrating sperm from proceeding to the perivitelline space. In the mouse, both ZP3 and ZP2 have been shown to be modified into truncated forms: ZP3f and ZP2f, respectively. The ZP3f in its solubilized form did not possess affinity for sperm cells nor the capacity to induce the acrosome reaction (Bleil and Wassarman 1983). The formation of ZP2f is less understood but has been implicated to be functional for zona pellucida hardening (Schroeder et al., 1990; Kalab et al., 1991). Recently, the folding properties of the ZP-N domains of all three ZP proteins has shed new light on the possibility that the cortical reaction mediated modifications to ZP proteins includes re-folding of these domains and thus may be functional in zona hardening (Jovine et al., 2007; Monné et al., 2008). In fact, the folding of ZP2 has been shown to also be essential for primary sperm-zona binding (Gahlay et al., 2010)

Zona pellucida composition in other mammals (especially bovine and porcine)

In pigs, cattle, and other mammalian species the terminology used for ZP proteins varies in the literature despite the fact that the ZP proteins are functionally homologous to the murine system as described by Wassarman (see previous section). Classically, mouse ZP (mZP) proteins have been functionally defined as mZP1 (the cross-linker of linear mZP2-mZP3 polymers), mZP2 (involved in secondary sperm zona binding), and mZP3 (involved in primary sperm-zona binding). In recent literature for human and porcine species, new names for these protein have been proposed based on the length of the cDNA matching each ZP transcript (ZP-A for mZP2; ZP-B for mZP1 and ZPC for mZP3). However, new studies have shown that ZP-B (Conner et al., 2005, Lefièvre et al., 2004; van Gestel et al., 2007) is a fourth ZP protein in primates, porcine, ruminants, and rabbit with sperm binding proteins similar to ZP3 (this protein is absent in murine zonae pellucidae). In recent human literature ZPB is called ZP4 (Gupta et al., 2009, Ganguly et al., 2010) and a pseudogene for this has been found in rodents (Gupta et al., 2009). In cattle, pigs, and humans, ZP3 and ZP4 are involved in sperm binding and induction of the acrosome reaction (Gupta et al., 2009; Chiu et al., 2008a). ZP2 is involved in secondary sperm binding (i.e. after the acrosome reaction; Chiu et al., 2008b) and indirect observations on human material with antibodies raised specifically against ZP1 (this protein is not observed in porcine and bovine zona pellucida) blocked sperm binding but this could be due to steric hindrance of the antibody used towards ZP3/4 binding (Ganguly et al., 2010). In bovine literature, the analogs for human ZP-3 and ZP4 (or ZPB) were called bZP3α and bZP3ß, respectively (Topper et al., 1997) and the 3 forms of the zona protein analogous to human ZP2 were called bZP1, bZP2 and bZP4 (and similar nomenclature was used for porcine zona protein pZPs see Figure 1). As depicted for porcine zona pellucida (Figure 1), the bZP2 has the same polypeptide backbone but lacks a 25 kDa glycoprotein (bZP4) portion of bZP1. The zona pellucida of mouse is composed of ZP1, 2 and 3; however, other rodents such as the hamster also contain ZP4. The human zona pellucida is composed of all four zona proteins (ZP1-4) while bovine and porcine have ZP2, 3 and 4 as proteins, but do not contain ZP1 (Kanai et al., 2008). The older nomenclature should not be used anymore to avoid confusion. For a review of zona pellucida protein composition, nomenclature, and the phylogenetic relationship and diversity of these proteins in vertebrates see Goudet et al., 2008 and Izquierdo-Rico et al., 2009. In all mammalian species mentioned so far, the expressed ZP proteins form a 7 μm thick three dimensional network. In the porcine and bovine species no ultra-structural studies have been conducted to determine whether chymotrypsin or reducing treatments caused dissociation of the three dimensional zona matrix into filaments (as observed for rodents, Greve and Wassarman 1985).

Likely, ZP3 and ZP4 form such filaments by disulfide bridges (Kanai et al. 2008). In vitro, ZP3/ZP4 heteromers have affinity for sperm and are able to induce the acrosome reaction. Glycosylation of these proteins is supposed to be important in both sperm binding as well as in the induction of the acrosome reaction (Chakravarty et al., 2008, Yonezawa et al., 2007). In bovine, α-mannosyl residues on the *N*-linked carbohydrate chains of the zona pellucida glycoproteins have been reported to be essential for sperm binding (Amari et al., 2001). In humans, recombinant ZP4 was sufficient for sperm binding and could induce the acrosome reaction (Chiu et al., 2008a). In fact, the signaling pathways to evoke the acrosome reaction were not identical to that of ZP3. The ZP3 and ZP4 induced acrosome reactions were especially *N*-linked glycosylation dependent and in the sperm they were protein kinase-C, protein tyrosine kinase, T-type Ca^{2+} channels, and extracellular Ca^{2+} dependent. G-proteins also participated in human ZP3- but not in ZP4-induced acrosome reaction (Chiu et al., 2008a). On the other hand, protein kinase-A and L-type Ca^{2+} channels took part only in human ZP4-induced acrosome reaction (Chiu et al., 2008a). Moreover, recombinant bovine or porcine ZP3/ZP4 heterocom

	ZP1	ZP2	ZP3	ZP4
Mouse	+	+	+	-(pseudogen)
Hamster	+	+	+	+
Human	+	+	+	+(ZPB)
Cattle/Pig				
Rabbit/Dog	-	+*	+(ZP3α)	+(ZP3ß or ZPB)
		Secondary zona binding	Primary zona binding	

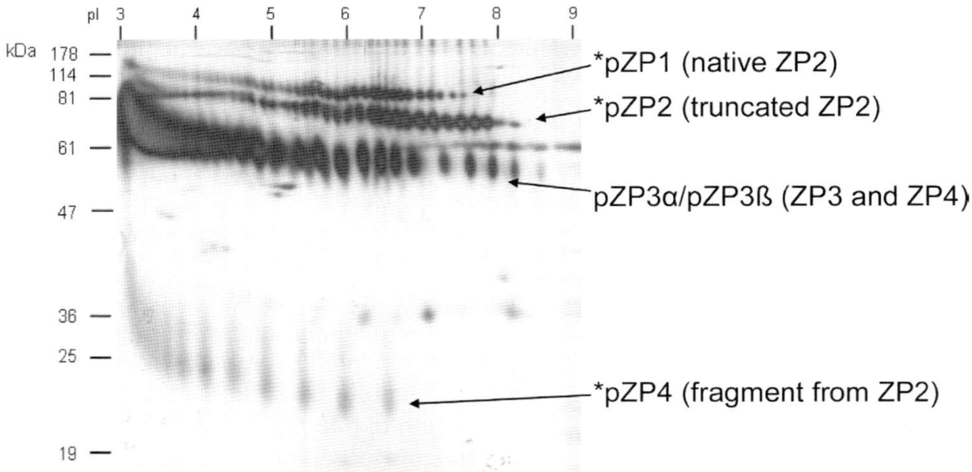

Fig. 1. Upper panel: Comparison of zona pellucida protein composition of the species mentioned in the text. ZP2 is involved in secondary zona binding, whereas, ZP3/ZP4 are involved in primary zona binding and induction of the acrosome reaction. Note the similarity of bovine and porcine zona pellucida protein composition which is different from mouse, hamster, and human in that it does not contain ZP1. **Lower panel: Two dimensional gel electrophoretic separation of solubilized porcine zona proteins**. The multi-glycosylation especially with negative charged carbohydrate chains cause the remarkable acidic shift and the very characteristic so called glycosylation trains of solubilized ZP after 2D IEF/SDS-PAGE of porcine ZP. The porcine nomenclature is indicated with p as a prefix. Between brackets the new nomenclature for ZPB (now named ZP4) is provided. The pZP2 isoform of ZP2 lacks approx. 25 kDa (pZP4) while pZP1 still includes this structure but all three forms are in fact originating from ZP2. The same components as named here were found in bovine ZP with different MW and pI as well as different relative compositions and the same terminology has been used with b as prefix (Topper et al., 1997). Porcine zona proteins are more differentially glycosylated and more charged than bovine or human zona proteins (Hedrick and Wardrip 1986; Koyama et al., 1991). This 2D gel was originally published by van Gestel et al., 2007, and is used with modifications to illustrate the complex carbohydrate nature of the zona pellucida and serves for the reader to appreciate and identify the different zona proteins and isoforms (by permission of Oxford University Press).

plexes expressed in Sf9 cells have an affinity for sperm and induce the acrosome reaction to sperm cells that have bound to these heterocomplexes (Kanai et al., 2007). The pZP4/bZP3 heteromers as well as bZP4/pZP3 heteromers retained sperm binding and acrosome reaction induction properties, which indicates that primary zona binding is conserved between these two species (Kanai et al. 2007) and appears to be similar to the human situation (Chiu et al., 2008b). In addition, a decapeptide of bovine ZP3 can induce a G-protein activation of the acrosome reaction in bovine sperm (Hinsch et al., 2005) showing that specific structures within the zona pellucida are involved in this process. Despite the above mentioned species similarities of synthetic zona proteins in sperm-zona binding and acrosome reaction, it has been shown that differences in *N*-glycosylation of ZP3/ZP4 are responsible for causing bovine and porcine species specific sperm-zona interactions (Yonezawa et al., 2007; Yonezawa et al., 2005). The above study describes the affinity of individual or heteromeric ZP proteins but does not cover all aspects of the zona's affinity for sperm as has been demonstrated by Yurewicz et al., 1998. Based on his observations he concluded that the native ZP texture rather than solubilized and isolated individual zona proteins or ZP3/ZP4 polymers had full affinity for sperm membrane vesicles (Yurewicz et al., 1998). Remarkably, both equine and porcine sperm can bind to the native bovine zona pellucida. Porcine sperm can also induce the acrosome reaction after such binding and the sperm cell is able to penetrate this bovine zona pellucida. In contrast this is not observed for the bound equine sperm to bovine zona pellucida (Sinowatz et al., 2003). A similar phenomenon is described between interspecies sperm zona binding and zona penetration between equine and porcine zona pellucida (Mugnier et al., 2009) and between donkey sperm and bovine zona pellucida (Taberner et al., 2010). These observations challenge the species specificity of both primary and secondary sperm-zona interactions.

In bovine and porcine species, secondary sperm binding needs ZP2 and blocking this interaction prevents fertilization (Hasegawa et al., 2000) and appears to be conserved with human ZP2 (Hinsch et al., 2003). Prior to fertilization a proportion of full sized ZP2 (originally named bZP1 or pZP1) is partially cleaved into a truncated ZP2 (originally named pZP2 or bZP2) and a 25 kDa fragment (originally named pZP4 or bZP4) (Hasegawa et al., 1994; figure 1). The importance of pre-fertilization cleavage of full ZP2 into a truncated and a 25 kDa form for sperm-zona interactions is not yet established. Most likely in porcine and bovine, ZP2 interacts with ZP3 and ZP4 in a species specific manner and is different from mouse, since expressed recombinant porcine ZP2 in transgenic mice does not result in incorporated pZP2 in the resulting zona pellucida (Hasegawa et al., 2006). In contrast to the carbohydrate dependency of bovine primary zona pellucida binding (*N*-acetyllactosamine residues are important), the secondary zona binding to ZP2 was not diminished after ß-galactosidase treatments (Ikeda et al., 2002). Interestingly in humans, acrosome reacted sperm do not bind to the zona pellucida of human oocytes which could imply that primary zona binding involves molecules that are required for establishing secondary zona binding proteins (Liu et al., 2006).

Zona hardening

After primary and secondary sperm zona interactions, sperm will enter the perivitelline space and may interact and fuse with the oolemma and thus fertilize the egg. Immediately after the fertilization fusion, soluble sperm factors (like phospholipase C ξ ; Dale et al., 2010) induce intracellular Ca^{2+} events and oolemma depolarization and this is a permissive step to induce the cortical reaction. The released cortical content will affect the structure of the zona pellucida (zona hardening) preventing sperm from binding to or penetrating the zona pellucida. In mouse, it has been shown that the cortical reaction causes truncations of ZP2 and ZP3 without affecting the molecular weight of ZP1 (Wassarman and Albertini 1994). Recently, evidence has been gathered with transgenic mice expressing mutated ZP2 that lacks the cleavage site so that ZP2 cannot be cleaved into ZP2f during the cortical reaction. The removal of sperm associated to the zona pellucida (normally a result of the cortical reaction) was not detected at the transgenic zona pellucida of two cell stage embryos (Gahlay et al., 2010).

In pigs and cattle, ZP2 is cleaved (Hatanaka et al., 1992, Noguchi et al., 1994) including a change in the disulfide bonds of this zona protein (Iwamoto et al., 1999). In addition, proteases (Hoodbhoy and Talbot 1994) have been found to be responsible for and structural rearrangements in the zona pellucida after fertilization (Funahashi et al., 2000, 2001, Nara et al., 2006). The bovine cortical reaction causes a removal of sialic acid from the carbohydrate moieties of the zona pellucida which causes a reduction in sperm-zona binding and penetration (Velásquez et al., 2007). This effect can be mimicked by adding blocking lectins for sialic acid residues or by adding *N*-acetyl-D-glucosamine (Sakaguchi et al., 2009). Supplementation of *N*-acetyl-D-glucosamine also resulted in increased acrosome reaction induction, increased secondary sperm zona binding and increased polyspermic fertilization. Similar effects were reported for cattle by using fetuin (Landim-Alvarenga et al., 2002). In porcine, the ß-galactosyl residues of the neutral *N*-linked carbohydrate chains of the zona proteins appear to be important for sperm-zona interactions (Yonezawa et al., 2005), indicating that the *N*-glycosylation of the zona pellucida is responsible for species differences between the pig and the cow (Yonezawa et al., 2007). In bovine oocytes, the efficiency of zona hardening and the prevention of polyspermic fertilization are related to the degree of maturation of the oocyte (Santos et al., 2008). In summary, this section of the review describes changes that are supposed to block primary zona binding, the induction of the acrosome reaction, secondary zona binding and sperm penetration. In humans, a fertilized oocyte with a hardened zona pellucida still has the capacity to bind sperm and to induce a voltage-dependent calcium influx along with an acrosome reaction but sperm can not penetrate the hardened zona pellucida (Patrat et al., 2006). Experiments of porcine and bovine fertilized eggs are missing in this regard.

Pre-fertilization zona modifications by oviductal proteins

It is noteworthy that hardened zona ghosts (isolated and purified remnants of ruptured zonae pellucidae) can be used as a binding control when studying sperm-zona interactions with zona ghosts obtained from unfertilized oocytes. The hardened zona ghosts can also be useful to study imperfect polyspermic fertilization blocks such as observed in IVF treatments for pigs. In this light it is interesting that prefertilization hardening of the zona pellucida reduces the risk of polyspermic fertilization in pigs and cows probably by reducing the amount of sperm that bind to the zona pellucida and delaying the speed of zona drilling which in turn will provide the just fertilized oocyte with more time to fulfill its functional cortical reaction (Coy et al., 2008a, Canovas et al., 2009). It is possible that the partial precleavage of ZP2 in porcine and bovine zona pellucida may be relevant for limiting polyspermic fertilization in a similar way (see previous section). Recently it has been acknowledged that the zona pellucida of the ovulated oocyte may be subjected to changes that influence sperm-zona interactions by secretions of the oviduct (Coy and Avilés 2009) but is not clear whether the zona properties are affected or whether the sperm cell functionality is affected (Coy et al., 2010; for review see Killian 2004). Treatments of bovine zona pellucida with antibodies directed against specific oviductal fluid proteins (either osteopontin or lipocalin type prostaglandin D synthetase) inhibited sperm binding and fertilization suggesting that such oviductal proteins at least also interact with the zona pellucida (Gonçalves et al., 2008). Furthermore, the oviduct specific glycoprotein and heparin have been shown to be responsible for post-ovulatory and pre-fertilization modification of the bovine zona pellucida that affect sperm-zona binding and appear to be involved in polyspermy regulation (Coy et al., 2008b). Recently, oviduct-specific glycoprotein has been found as part of the mouse zona pellucida in which it acts as a ZP3 independent sperm adhesion ligand (Lyng and Shur 2009; for a recent review see Avilés et al., 2010); whether or not bovine oviduct specific binding protein works the same remains to be investigated. Similarly, another oviductal protein (also detected in the bovine oviduct) named osteopontin has been reported to reduce polyspermy in porcine (Hao et al., 2006). In addition, another oviduct component is added to the periphery of the ovulated mouse zona pellucida and provides the zona pellucida with additional sperm affinity (independent from sperm ß 1,4-galactosyltransferase I activity; Rodeheffer and Shur 2004; see section on primary sperm binding to zona).

As mentioned above, the zona pellucida proteins (and their differential glycosylation) are a matter of high evolutionary genetic drift (the same is valid for zona binding proteins at the sperm surface or in the sperm acrosome). Therefore, sperm-zona binding can be considered as species specific and variations in this interaction could form the basis of mammalian speciation. Monné et al. 2008 have resolved a specific ZP-N fold structure with implications for overall zona pellucida architecture, the post-fertilization block to polyspermy and speciation. In contrast, the fertilization fusion appears to be much less species specific. For instance, in the hamster oocyte assay in which a zona denuded hamster oocyte is used to assess the fertilization fusion capability of human sperm (Barros et al., 1979). The zona pellucida of mammalian oocytes has to a large extent been studied in only a few species namely domestic animals such as the ewe, cow and sow (from these species ovaries can be obtained relatively easily and from a large amount of animals at a slaughter line) and from laboratory mammals such as the rat, mouse and Guinea-pig. Studies on large quantities of oocytes are required for the type of biochemical studies but provide only a raw view. The ultimate changes of the zona pellucida at the last stages of oocyte maturation (peri-ovulation) and before fertilization in the oviduct are not studied in detail but may well be crucial for obtaining optimal fertilization efficiency both in enhancing the fertilization efficiency (in vitro, this is in the range of 30-60 %; in vivo >85%), but also to prevent polyspermic fertilization (which is relatively frequent in pig IVF) (Hao et al., 2006). Therefore, the use of oviduct secretions in future assisted reproductive technologies is foreseen (Avilés et al., 2010).

The sperm cell

In vitro capacitation:

Before sperm cells enter the isthmus and move up to the ampulla where they may meet the cumulus oocyte complex, they face a series of surface remodeling steps that enables them to interact with the zona pellucida and to induce the acrosome reaction (for review see Tsai and Gadella 2009). Most knowledge on sperm proteins interacting with the zona pellucida has been obtained under in vitro fertilization conditions. Basically, the sperm cell has zona binding properties before ejaculation as has been shown for aspirated sperm from the cauda epididymis (see Tsai and Gadella 2009 for review). In fact, several proteins secreted by the epididymis become adsorbed to the sperm surface (Zanich et al., 2003) and some of them remain hydrophobic interacting (mostly GPI anchored proteins) with sperm after capacitation and have a function in zona binding (Morin et al., 2010; Busso et al., 2007; van Gestel et al., 2007; Shur et al., 2006; Montfort et al., 2002). Aside from these additions, also sperm surface proteins (mostly trans membrane proteins) originate from the testis (Busso et al., 2007, van Gestel et al., 2007).

The above mentioned zona binding proteins reside at the sperm surface but become coated by seminal plasma factors during ejaculation. In the boar this coating serves to modify and stabilize the sperm surface and thus to extend the sperm cell's resistance to stress (see for review Muiño-Blanco et al., 2008), which is probably a physiological requirement for sperm to survive the passage through the female reproductive tract. The seminal coating of glycoproteins also prevents premature activation of sperm cells and therefore can be considered as decapacitation factors (Vadnais and Roberts 2010, Caballero et al., 2005). Recently, decapacitation factors in the mouse were identified by proteomics technology and included plasma membrane fatty acid binding protein, CRISP-1, phosphatidylethonalamine binding protein 1 (Ensslin et al., 1995) and the yet functionally unknown decapacitation factor 10. All four secreted proteins inhibit both zona binding and zona induced acrosome reaction (Nixon et al., 2006).

Remarkably, although bovine seminal plasma proteins also stabilize sperm cells (Manjunath et al., 2007), the knowledge regarding decapacitation factors is very poor for ruminants, probably because inhibiting effects of seminal plasma proteins have not appropriately been tested yet. Instead, a family of gelatin binding proteins are the major secretory proteins recovered from bovine seminal plasma (BSP-A1, BSP-A2, BSP-A3 and BSP-30) and appear to function as pro-capacitation factors under the proper fertilization conditions either in presence of lipoproteins or in presence of heparin (for review see Manjunath et al., 2007). These proteins also form major components of seminal plasma in ram (Bergeron et al., 2005), and in buck (Villemure et al., 2003).

During the processing of sperm for IVF, the sperm are first washed through a discontinuous density gradient (made from isotonic cushions of Percoll, Ficoll or related materials), which for non-ruminant mammals at least serves to remove decapacitation factors rendering such cells responsive to in vitro fertilization incubations. The washed cells are exposed to higher temperature (39 ^{0}C instead of the epididymal 35 ^{0}C) and higher bicarbonate concentrations (>15 mM compared to <5 mM) in the ejaculate and lipid modifying proteins (mostly fatty acid free bovine serum albumin). When incubated for a couple of hours, a subpopulation of sperm cells becomes capacitated (capacitation in vitro) and these types of changes appear to mimic what is happening with sperm cells in the oviduct (for reviews Gadella and Visconti 2006; Tsai and Gadella 2009). This procedure is standard for mammalian IVF and in ruminants the addition of glycosaminoglycans, such as heparin, is required for obtaining full capacitation (Parrish et al., 1986). The IVF procedure is believed to resemble what is happening in the oviduct which is reflected in the name used for the IVF incubation medium called synthetic oviduct fluid (SOF medium). The IVF incubations do not only cause sperm surface stripping of seminal plasma components but include delicate surface alterations (Tsai and Gadella 2009; Gadella et al., 2008) and thus induces a remodeling of lipid membrane protein topology especially in the sperm head. Typically, at the apical ridge area of the sperm surface rearrangements include the aggregation of lipid ordered domains and the build up of a zona binding complex (for reviews see Boerke et al., 2008; Tanphaichitr et al., 2007). Although specific raft forming lipids allow formation and aggregation of rafts, they probably do not play a direct role in zona binding, but more likely form the template for allowing the formation of the zona binding protein complex (for discussion see Nixon et al., 2007). The apical sperm surface specific aggregations of lipid rafts have been observed in capacitating mouse, porcine and bovine sperm (Thaler et al, 2006; van Gestel 2005, 2007, Selvaraj et al., 2007). Our group has shown that capacitation resulted in the exposure and assembly of surface molecules into a high zona affinity complex of proteins in the aggregating lipid ordered apical head surface of porcine sperm (van Gestel et al., 2007). Recently, we also showed that this coincided with the stable docking of the acrosome at the same sperm surface area (Tsai et al., 2007, 2010). Probably this serves as a preparative step of sperm to immediately induce the acrosome reaction after zona recognition.

Primary zona binding

Collectively, the above mentioned in vitro capacitation changes at the sperm head surface are required to establish proper primary zona binding and the immediate induction of the acrosome reaction. Both are induced by ZP3/ZP4 (see zona pellucida section) and are exclusively executed at the apical sperm head surface (Tsai and Gadella 2009). A number of different ways have been described in order to study primary sperm-zona binding (for an overview, see van Gestel et al., 2007). One of the first concerns for a biochemical approach is that once a sperm has attached to the zona pellucida it will undergo the zona-induced acrosome reaction which is immediately followed by the initiation of massive secondary sperm-binding by intra-acrosomal glycoproteins and zona drilling. In order to avoid this, assays have been developed in which primary zona binding is blocked by preincubation of the zona pellucida with (i) the (labeled) sperm protein being studied, peptides derived from the protein of interest, preincubating the sperm with antibodies directed against the protein of study or with preincubating sperm with antibody fragments thereof. Unfortunately, all such approaches can only deliver indirect evidence for the involvement of sperm surface proteins, simply because aspecific capping of the epitopes required for zona recognition may explain inhibited sperm-zona binding. In fact, both the zona pellucida and the apical sperm plasma membrane should be isolated from the sperm and the oocyte, respectively. This allows direct biochemical characterization of primary zona binding proteins from the sperm surface. The two interacting structures can be isolated in large amounts. With this respect, porcine and bovine can be considered as model species since zona material can be obtained directly from the slaughter line in large amounts and both species produce cell rich ejaculates with >85 % normal matured cells (Gadella 2009). These approaches are described Below.

Isolation of the zona pellucida and solubilization of such proteins and immobilization to column material can be followed by affinity chromatography using sperm membrane proteins (Lea et al., 2001; Ensslin et al., 1998). One should be careful to collect ovaries, isolate oocytes from it and purify separated zona pellucida ghosts from that material, without the occurrence of the cortical reaction. The cortical reaction would alter the zona texture and modify the zona proteins (see section about zona hardening). The cortical reaction is prevented routinely by collecting and processing the material in ice cold buffers containing high amounts of EDTA (Dunbar et al., 1980; Topper et al., 1997). Rather than solubilizing the zona pellucida it has been recognized that the complex differential protein glycosylation (see for instance Fig. 1) and the native quarternary structure are essential for accurate primary zona recognition by sperm (Yurewicz et al., 1998; Nakano and Yonezawa 2001) and therefore the native zona isolated from oocytes is preferably used as a template for sperm membrane proteins.

From the sperm cell, only the surface should be used in order to prevent the identification of secondary zona binding proteins from the acrosome (see next section). Two reviews describe pro's and con's for isolating sperm membranes (Gadella 2009; Brewis and Gadella 2010). Basically the method of choice is to perform nitrogen cavitation and differential centrifugation to isolate only the apical sperm plasma membrane; whereas, the acrosome remains intact and distal sperm head membranes as well as plasma membrane of the tail and mid-piece remain associated to the remaining sperm (Flesch et al., 1998). Much less specific results are observed when hypo-osmotic mechanic disruption of sperm is performed as has been done in mammals that produce lower amount of sperm (aspiration from epididymis such as is required for murine species or <30 % normal sperm in case of many primates, for discussion see Gadella 2009).

When zona ghosts and apical sperm membranes are allowed to bind, a number of proteins could be identified as directly involved in primary sperm zona binding proteins using specific membrane proteomics techniques (see van Gestel et al., 2007, Gadella 2009, Brewis and Gadella

2010) and a number of identified proteins were reported in the literature from more indirect methods or with biochemically less specific material. A new approach to identify bovine sperm membrane proteins that interact with receptors on the oocyte and its vestments has not been very successful as membrane proteins are notoriously difficult to solubilize and therefore per definition not so suitable for 2D gel ectrophoretic separation. Consequently, predominantly soluble proteins were identified (Pate et al., 2008). Modern off-gel techniques in combination with the above mentioned isolation of interacting structures will provide functional insights in primary zona binding (Brewis and Gadella unpublished). Currently, a complete compilation of sperm surface proteins involved in primary zona binding is not available for ruminant mammals.

Two transmembrane proteins involved in primary zona binding that originate from testicular germ cells are fertilin ß (previously called ADAM2 or PH30) (Cho et al., 2000; van Gestel et al., 2007) and ß 1,4 galactosyltransferase I (GalTase) (Rodeheffer and Shur 2004, Shur et al., 2006). Interestingly, GalTase is so far the only primary zona binding protein of the sperm surface that is linked to the zona-induced acrosome reaction, which is part of primary zona binding cascade (for a recent review on the zona induced acrosome reaction, see Litscher et al., 2009). GalTase has been reported to act with heterotrimeric G proteins and to cationic channels in order to execute the acrosome reaction (for a model, see Shur et al., 2006). Indeed the acrosome reaction is induced by primary zona binding and signal transduction over the adhered plasma membrane is required for stimulation of this Ca^{2+} driven multiple fusion event. GalTase probably requires additional (and species specific) factors for primary zona binding. One such factor is SED-1 (also called P47), a secretory protein that becomes peripherally associated to the sperm's surface in the epididymis. The interaction with GalTase has been demonstrated (Shur et al., 2006; Copland 2009, Ensslin and Shur 2003) and it is one of the major primary zona binding proteins in our direct binding assay (van Gestel et al., 2007). Other factors associated with the sperm surface include: (i) SPAM 1 (also known as PH20 or 2B1) which also has an epididymal origin but becomes associated to the sperm surface via a glycosylphosphatidylinositol anchored covalent linkage (Morin et al., 2010, Thaler and Cardullo 1995, Seaton et al., 2000, Sleight et al., 2005) although it is also reported to be abundantly expressed in the testis (Hou et al., 1996); (ii) an hyaluronan binding protein called HYBP1, which binds with intrinsic clustered mannose residues to the zona pellucida of ruminants (Ghosh and Datta 2003) and originates at the surface of elongating spermatids in the testis; (iii) Other carbohydrate modifying enzymes associated to the sperm surface are also involved in primary zona binding including *N*-acetylglucosaminidase (Zitta et al., 2006); (iv) fucosyltransferease (Chiu et al., 2007) and (v) arylsulfatase (likely, to originate from seminal vesicles Gadella et al., 1993; for review see Tanphaichitr et al., 2007); (vi) The enzyme carbonyl reductase is secreted and associates to sperm in the epididymis and has been reported to be involved in zona binding in the hamster (Montfort et al., 2002) and was found in our direct porcine zona binding assay (van Gestel et al., 2007); (vii) Similary AQN-3 (one of the porcine spermadhesins) is secreted by the epididymis, coats the sperm surface and remains associated to the isolated apical membrane fraction even under very stringent conditions and has high affinity for the zona pellucida (van Gestel et al., 2007); (viii) Another protein with firm peripheral association to the sperm surface after being secreted in the epididymis is CRISP1 (Busso et al., 2007); (ix) The interaction of sperm surface and acrosome oriented proteasomes with ubiquitinated zona proteins has been implied to be involved in sperm-zona binding (for review see Zimmerman & Sutovsky, 2009). Despite the convincing data set that emerged from this group, their finding requires further investigation since both proteasomes and poly-ubiquitin tags to proteins (recognition signal for the proteasome for protein binding and destruction) are supposed to be restricted to the cytosol (Gallastegui and Groll 2010). Therefore, the reported topologies of proteasomes at the sperm surface and in the lumen of the acrosome and of the polyubiquitin tags at the zona pellucida, which is an extracellular matrix, are both unexpected. (x) Other proteases (Deppe et al., 2008, 2010); and (xi) dipeptidases (Deguchi et al., 2007) have been implied to play a role in zona binding and their activity is partly regulated by the steroids progesterone and estradiol, of which is known (also in ruminants) that their levels are enhanced after ovulation at the period when the acrosome reaction at the zona pellucida takes place in vivo (Lukoseviciute et al., 2007).

Secondary zona binding

After the acrosome reaction a new layer of molecules is exposed for the so called secondary zona binding. The intra-acrosomal zona binding proteins become exposed to the zona pellucida and bind to ZP2. Most of the acrosome content is not released from the acrosome but remains associated with each other in a kind of enzyme matrix (Kim and Gerton 2003).The enzymes are slowly released during sperm zona drilling. The enzyme matrix should have two functionalities namely it should have affinity for ZP2 in the zona pellucida (the drilling sperm with high lateral head displacement properties need to remain attached to the zona pellucida) and the enzyme matrix needs to functionally dissociate the 3D matrix of the zona proteins in order to pave the way for the sperm towards the perivitelline space. Most likely the kinetics of acrosome content release and composition is highly species specific.

Classically the enzyme acrosin has been found to serve the two tasks required for secondary zona binding namely to bind to ZP2 and to cleave proteins as a serine protease (Dunbar et al., 1985) but its function in this process has been questioned as acrosin knock out mice were fertile (Crosby and Barros, 1999) However, considering the complexity of sperm-zona binding in which from the sperm's side multiple proteins are involved, it is possible that redundancy of individual proteins may explain why knock out phenotypes are capable of fertilization. Without redundancy the knock out genotype probably under evolutionary pressure will be less efficient as sperm with a full set of zona binding proteins (see Gadella et al., 2008). A reduced complement may be sufficient for fertilization, but a full complement will provide the sperm with more capability for fertilization. Sperm-zona interactions functionally are selective and create a time delay for sperm to become adjacent to the oolemma. If a sperm is better suited to be the first to bind/fuse with the oolemma it will win the race and after generations that phenotype that maybe referred for generating offspring. In other words, simple knock out mice with a single protein deficiency may still show a fertile phenotype despite the fact the depleted protein has a zona binding function. Another intra-acrosomal protein involved in secondary zona binding and zona penetration is zonadhesin (Lea et al., 2001; Bi et al., 2003) and knock out mice lacking expression of zonadhesin were infertile with impaired sperm zona interactions (Tardif et al., 2010a). Zonadhesin appears to function in a species specific manner (Tardif et al. 2010b), which may be the reason why this protein is under such extreme fast molecular evolution (Herlyn and Zischler 2008) although the latter is also described for acrosin (Raterman and Springer 2008).

Other proteins reported to have secondary zona binding properties include the following: (i) intra acrosomal membrane protein 38 (IAM38 also known as sp38; Mori et al. 1993,1995, Yu et al., 2006), which also has a function in sperm penetration through the zona pellucida; (ii) SAMP14, an acrosomal membrane-associated, glycosylphosphatidylinositol-anchored member of the Ly-6/urokinase-type plasminogen activator receptor superfamily (Shetty et al., 2003); (iii) SAMP32 which is associated with the acrosomal membrane is involved in secondary zona binding and zona penetration (Hao et al., 2002); and (iv) SPAG9 which has a structural homology with c-Jun N terminal kinase interacting protein 3 and is an intra-acrosomal protein with zona affinity and thus can be considered as a secondary zona binding protein (Jagadish et al., 2005).

Remarkably a number of primary zona binding proteins (localized at the sperm surface) are also present in the acrosome often as acrosome specific isoforms. An example of this is SPAM-1, which is 80 kDa in the acrosome (from testicular origin) and at the C-terminus 10 kDa longer than the epidiymal iosoform present at the sperm surface (Morin et al., 2010). Other examples are hyaluronidase and PH20 that are localized in the acrosome and on the sperm surface, respectively (Thaler and Cardullo 1995; Overstreet et al., 1995).

Although secondary zona binding has been postulated to be ZP2 specific, the intra-acrosomal protein sp56 has specific affinity for ZP3 (Buffone et al., 2008a,b). In fact, sp56 was originally believed to be a sperm surface protein, which turned out to be incorrect (for review see Wassarman 2009). It is of interest that sp56 is released from the acrosome as a smaller processed protein with no affinity for the unfertilized zona pellucida (Buffone et al., 2009b). In order for sperm to penetrate the zona pellucida, there must be a mechanism that permits binding of the zona proteins followed by opening of the zona pellucida matrix and renewed binding. If so, the sp56 protein should stop interacting with ZP3 and release of the cleaved form of sp56 might permit renewed binding of intact sp56. The dogma that secondary zona binding is strictly ZP2 specific perhaps needs to be reconsidered. The alternative explanation provides a model in which a sort of preliminary diffusion of sp56 from the acrosome to the sperm surface takes place prior to zona binding (Wassarman 2009; Figure 2). Likewise, the unique role of ZP2 for secondary sperm-zona binding has recently been challenged as the uncleaved form of ZP2 turned out to be required for primary zona binding (Gahlay et al., 2010; Figure 2).

Beyond the protease activity of acrosin and the hyaluronidase activity released from the acrosome during the acrosome reaction, it is not clear what type of modifications are made by the acrosome enzymes to allow sperm penetration through the zona pellucida. Interestingly, relatively high titers of ß *N*-acetylhexosaminidase, ß galactosidase, and ß mannosidase were found in the acrosome of porcine and bovine sperm (Hayashi et al., 2004). Thus, beyond secondary zona binding proteins, specific carbohydrate modifying enzymes might be involved in paving the way for sperm to progress in the voyage towards the oolemma and enable zona penetration (Miller et al., 1993).

Oviduct secretions, follicular fluid and cumulus expansion

Due to the fact that most sperm-zona binding assays are based on preparations derived from epididymal or ejaculated sperm and collected zona pellucida material obtained from washed oocytes derived from follicles, the role of the oviduct, the follicular fluid and the cumulus expansion on the sperm surface have largely been neglected. In vivo the oviduct is the main site of sperm capacitation and has been been an area of intense investigation. Sperm cells entering the oviduct first interact with the oviduct epithelium and after a while are released in the capacitated state (for review on sperm-oviduct binding see Suarez 2008). It is clear that the oviduct can function as an active secretory organ resulting in the release of sperm from the oviduct epithelium (Sostaric et al., 2008). Although these secretions interact with the zona pellucida (see that section), they also interact with the sperm surface and thus could modulate primary sperm-zona binding in two ways. One example is the Glucose-regulated protein 78 (Grp78/BiP), which is secreted by human oviduct epithelial cells and modulates sperm-zona pellucida binding after its association to sperm cells (Marín-Briggiler et al., 2010). The oviduct may also serve to select sperm that have superior properties to fertilize (Gualteri and Talevi 2003) by binding and selectively releasing capacitated sperm (review for porcine and bovine species see Talevi and Gulatieri 2010). In buffalo the mannosylation of the zona pellucida (in part performed by the oviduct) has been found to be important for establishing interactions with the sperm surface

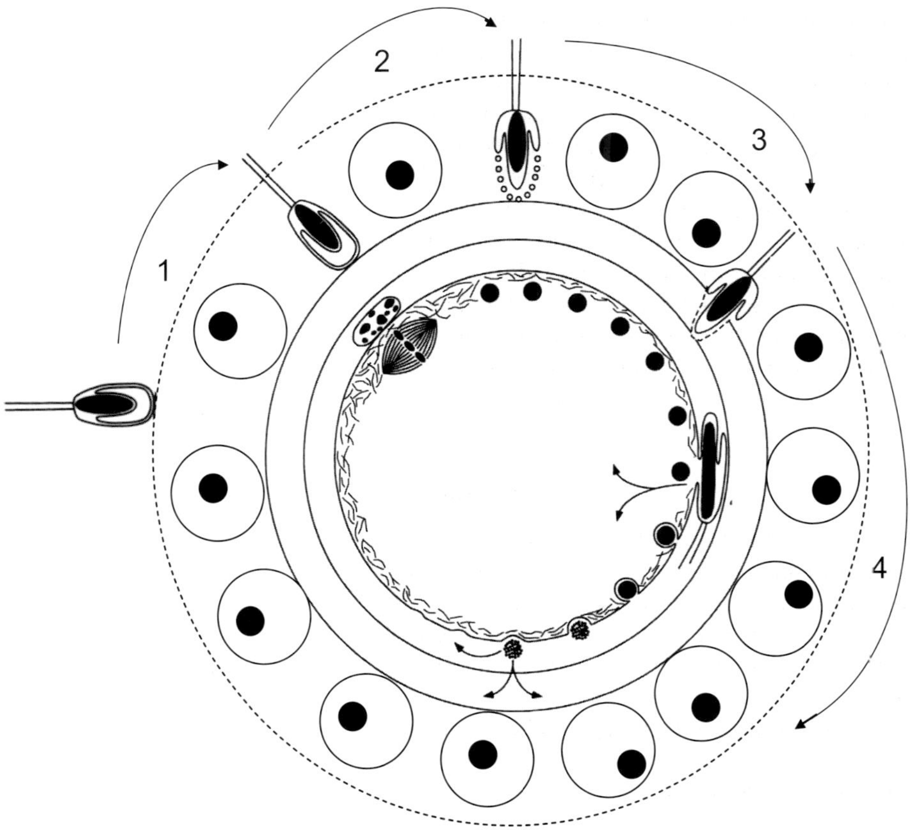

Fig. 2. The proposed sequence of events around fertilization that relate to sperm-zona interactions. Sperm that have entered the oviduct will shed off decapacitation factors that were adhered peripherally to the sperm surface. During this process the acrosome is docked to the sperm plasma membrane and at the docked area the formation of high affinity zona binding complexes are formed (Tsai et al., 2010; van Gestel et al., 2007). **1.** It is not clear whether the resulting sperm which can associate with the extra cellular matrix of the expanded cumulus mass (here represented as one cell layer but in reality composed of more cell layers) surrounding the unfertilized oocyte induces some early steps of acrosomal fusion (proposed by Wassarman 2009) or that acrosome intact sperm are penetrating through the cumulus by the use of hyperactivated motility in combination with surface proteins (Forman and Ducibella 2006). Oviductal secreted proteins are also reported to be important for cumulus and zona pellucida properties (Avilés et al., 2010). **2.** The recognition of the zona pellucida (primary zona binding to ZP3/ZP4) and subsequent inititation of the acrosome reaction (or of the acute secretory phase of it, see point 1) which is induced by the zona pellucida. **3.** The acrosome reaction causes local modifications of zona proteins and the hyperactivated sperm can penetrate this structure due to secondary zona binding (to ZP2). The surface of the penetrating sperm will be further remodeled and this probably serves to enable the fertilization fusion (Tsai and Gadella 2009). **4.** Immediately after the fertilization fusion the cortical reaction causes an overall coating of the oolemma as well as the hardening of the zona pellucida by chemically altering zona proteins. The cleavage of ZP2 appears to be particularly instrumental for the release of sperm from the zona pullicida and to elicit an efficient block to polyspermy (Galthay et al, 2010).

hyaluran binding proteins (HABP-1) and thus for enhancing primary sperm-zona binding (Ghosh and Datta, 2003). It is possible that other non-testicular secretory proteins (for instance those described from the epididymis), known to be involved in primary sperm-zona binding are also secreted by the oviduct and recruited on the sperm surface in order to enhance primary zona binding.

Different glycosylated forms of the glycoproteins glycodelin (previously known as placental protein 14 or progesterone-associated endometrial protein) are present in the oviduct fluid, follicular fluid, and in the cumulus cell layer surrounding the zona pellucida (Yeung et al., 2007). A redistribution and different composition as well as reassociation of three different glycodelin isoforms were noted to occur in the oviduct, by follicular fluid and by the expanded cumulus. This occurs when sperm are progressing towards the zona pellucida and is reported to modulate sperm-zona binding and the zona-induced acrosome reaction (Chiu et al., 2003, 2007, Yeung et al. 2009). For a recent report on the effects of human oviduct fluid on sperm functioning with special attention to zona binding characteristics see Munuce et al., 2009.

Zona contraceptives

Porcine zona pellucida (pZP) can be purified in large quantities (van Gestel et al. 2007). When conjugated to an adjuvant, it can be used to immunize females towards porcine zona proteins (Choudhury et al., 2007). This approach has been used in swine but has also successfully been used across a variety of mammalian species. Currently, pZP vaccination is used to reduce fertility of wildlife populations (Fayrer-Hoskin 2008). However, it is not yet clear how this pZP vaccination works as acontraceptive. One of the possible mechanisms is that anti pZP antibodies block or alter the assembly of the zona pellucida during oocyte maturation. The other possibility is pZP antibodies bind to their epitopes on the normally formed ZP structure. If this epitope is functionally blocking the primary and/or secondary receptor (ZP3/ZP4 and/or ZP2), this will as a consequence prevent sperm recognition, acrosome reaction and/or zona penetration. However, one of the side effects of pZP vaccination is the induction of ovarian failure probably resulting in blocking oocyte development especially at the level of zona pellucida synthesis (Koyama et al., 2005).

Dogmas and new insights

Some dogmas on sperm-zona interactions still prevail in the literature. Several have been mentioned in this overview (see also Figure 2). However, the following dogmas are well accepted: (i) Originally, acrosome intact sperm were supposed to bind to the zona pellucida. On the other hand, the expanded cumulus has the capacity to induce the acrosome reaction (Mattioli et al., 1998) by interacting with a sperm surface glycosylphosphatidylionositol anchored protein (Yin et al., 2009). (ii) Primary sperm zona binding is believed to be ZP3 specific. However, sp56 an intra-acrosomal protein interacts specifically with ZP3 (Buffone et al., 2008a) and although alternative explanations can be given, it probably indicates that also other ZP proteins are involved in secondary sperm-zona binding. (iii) Zona binding is not sufficient to elicit the acrosome reaction and initial zona penetration, which is required to activate a mechano-sensory signal transduction system to evoke the acrosome reaction (Baibakov et al., 2007). How this relates to item (i) remains to be elucidated but it is possible that the premature acrosome reaction is initiated at the cumulus level as proposed by Wassarman (2009), and that subsequent binding to ZP3/ZP4 further induces full acrosome reaction. (iv) Our recently published findings showed that in vitro capacitation not only leads to enhanced zona binding affinity of acrosome intact sperm but also to the stable docking of the outer acrosomal membrane with the apical sperm plasma membrane (Tsai et al., 2010). This could indicate that the zona pellucida binding is required for the induction of the acrosome reaction. (v) Sperm cells that penetrate the cumulus during in vivo fertilization conditions are acrosome intact and probably use sperm surface-associated components for the dispersal of the cumulus mass to ensure sperm penetration (especially PH-20 the GPI anchored form of hyaluronidase which is believed to be responsible, for review see Florman and Ducibella 2006). Effective zona drilling is therefore believed to be achieved only by sperm that were acrosome intact prior to zona binding and premature acrosome reacted sperm will not reach the zona pellucida. (vi) The recent finding on how zona proteins are secreted and folded by the oocyte and which domains and structures are regulatory has shed light on how the zona pellucida is structurally regulated (Monné et al., 2008). These new findings should be placed into the classical concept that ZP1 is the dimeric crosslinker of ZP2/ZP3 hetero-oligomeric filaments. In ruminant and porcine, zona pellucida ZP1, is absent but still a functional 7 um thick zona pelliucida matrix is formed. Probably, the postulated functions of the discrete zona proteins forming the zona pellucida defined earlier need some revisions and the individual properties of each zona protein may turn out to be shared by others. In the review of Florman and Ducibella (2006), alternative cross linking to form the three dimensional zona structure for the human zona pellucida has been depicted. (vii) The uncleaved form of ZP2 is also essential for primary sperm-zona binding in the mouse, and the cortical reaction induces the release of sperm by cleaving ZP2 (Gahlay et al., 2010). It is not clear why in porcine and bovine species a part of ZP2 is already cleaved prior to fertilization and how this relates to in vivo and in vitro control of a block to polyspermy. Moreover, it is also not known how pre- and post-fertilization modifications of zona proteins relate to each other (for instance the cleavage of zona proteins by released proteins from the acrosome when compared with released proteins from cortical granules).

(viii) Lastly, the extremely complicated glycosylation patterns of all zona proteins (see figure 1) and their relevance for the zona structure, sperm binding, acrosome reaction induction, sperm-zona penetration as well as the regulation of polyspermy blockage after the cortical reaction needs to be studied in further detail. To this end, upcoming sperm surface and zona pellucida proteomic approaches will not be sufficient (Brewis and Gadella 2010). Experts from glycobiological disciplines are required and glycomics technologies should be employed to reveal relevant structures and their three dimensional organization during sperm-zona interactions (Vanderschaege et al., 2010).

Author's note after acceptance of manuscript

In humans it has now been shown that ZP1 binds sperm (primary zona binding) and induces the acrosome reaction (Ganguly et al., 2010a) in a similar fashion as is mentioned for ZP4 in the review. Moreover, the glycosylation of ZP1 and a specific ZP domain in that protein are at least in part responsible for this bioactivity (Ganguly et al. 2010b). Therefore, the table in Figure 1 is incomplete as ZP1 has a role in primary zona binding of human sperm.

Acknowledgements

This review is based on the inspiration and experiments and hard labor performed by five successive PhD students that have worked in my group on sperm-zona interactions. Frits Flesch, Renske van Gestel, Edita Sostaric, Jason Tsai and Arjen Boerke, I am warmly grateful for all your support in studying this fascinating topic.

References

Amari S, Yonezawa N, Mitsui S, Katsumata T, Hamano S, Kuwayama M, Hashimoto Y, Suzuki A, Takeda Y & Nakano M 2001.Essential role of the nonreducing terminal alpha-mannosyl residues of the N-linked carbohydrate chain of bovine zona pellucida glycoproteins in sperm-egg binding. *Molecular Reproduction and Development* **59** 221-226.

Avilés M, Gutiérrez-Adán A & Coy P 2010 Oviductal secretions: Will they be key factors for the future ARTs? *Molecular Human Reproduction* [Epub ahead of print].

Baibakov B, Gauthier L, Talbot P, Rankin TL, & Dean J 2007 Sperm binding to the zona pellucida is not sufficient to induce acrosome exocytosis. *Development* **134** 933-943.

Barros C, Gonzalez J, Herrera E & Bustos-Obregon E 1979 Human sperm penetration into zona-free hamster oocytes as a test to evaluate the sperm fertilizing ability. *Andrologia*. **11** 197-210.

Bendahmane M & Tulsiani DR 2003 Capacitated acrosome-intact mouse spermatozoa bind to Sepharose beads coated with functional neoglycoproteins. *Archives of Biochemistry and Biophysics* **415** 203-212.

Bergeron A, Villemure M, Lazure C & Manjunath P 2005 Isolation and characterization of the major proteins of ram seminal plasma *Molecular Reproduction and Development* **71** 461-470.

Bi M, Hickox JR, Winfrey VP, Olson GE & Hardy DM 2003 Processing, localization and binding activity of zonadhesin suggest a function in sperm adhesion to the zona pellucida during exocytosis of the acrosome. *Biochemical Journal* **375** 477-488.

Bleil JD & Wassarman PM 1983 Sperm-egg interactions in the mouse: sequence of events and induction of the acrosome reaction by a zona pellucida glycoprotein. *Developmental Biology* **95** 317-324.

Bleil JD, Greve JM & Wassarman PM 1988 Identification of a secondary sperm receptor in the mouse egg zona pellucida: role in maintenance of binding of acrosome-reacted sperm to eggs. *Developmental Biology* **128** 376-385.

Boerke A, Tsai PS, Garcia-Gil N, Brewis IA & Gadella BM 2008 Capacitation-dependent reorganization of microdomains in the apical sperm head plasma membrane: functional relationship with zona binding and the zona-induced acrosome reaction. *Theriogenology*. **70** 1188-1196.

Brewis IA & Gadella BM 2010 Sperm surface proteomics: from protein lists to biological function. *Molecular Human Reproduction* **16** 68-79.

Buffone MG, Zhuang T, Ord TS, Hui L, Moss SB & Gerton GL 2008a Recombinant mouse sperm ZP3-binding protein (ZP3R/sp56) forms a high order oligomer that binds eggs and inhibits mouse fertilization in vitro. *Journal of Biological Chemistry* **283** 12438-12345.

Buffone MG, Foster JA & Gerton GL 2008b The role of the acrosomal matrix in fertilization. *International Journal of Developmental Biology* **52** 511-522.

Buffone MG, Rodriguez-Miranda E, Storey BT& Gerton GL 2009a Acrosomal exocytosis of mouse sperm progresses in a consistent direction in response to zona pellucida. *Journal of Cellular Physiology* **220** 611-620.

Buffone MG, Kim KS, Doak BJ, Rodriguez-Miranda E & Gerton GL 2009b Functional consequences of cleavage, dissociation and exocytotic release of ZP3R, a C4BP-related protein, from the mouse sperm acrosomal matrix. *Journal of Cell Science* **122** 3153-3160.

Busso D, Cohen DJ, Maldera JA, Dematteis A & Cuasnicu PS 2007 A novel function for CRISP1 in rodent fertilization: involvement in sperm-zona pellucida interaction. *Biology of Reproduction* **77** 848-854.

Caballero I, Vázquez JM, Rodríguez-Martínez H, Gill MA, Calvete JJ, Sanz L, Garcia EM, Roca J & Martínez EA 2005 Influence of seminal plasma PSP-I/PSP-II spermadhesin on pig gamete interaction. *Zygote* **13** 11-16.

Canovas S, Romar R, Grullon LA, Aviles M & Coy P 2009 Pre-fertilization zona pellucida hardening by different cross-linkers affects IVF in pigs and cattle and improves embryo production in pigs. *Reproduction* **137** 803-812.

Chakravarty S, Kadunganattil S, Bansal P, Sharma RK & Gupta SK 2008 Relevance of glycosylation of human zona pellucida glycoproteins for their binding to capacitated human spermatozoa and subsequent induction of acrosomal exocytosis. *Molecular Reproduction and Development* **75** 75-88.

Chiu PC, Koistinen R, Koistinen H, Seppala M, Lee KF & Yeung WS 2003 Zona-binding inhibitory factor-1 from human follicular fluid is an isoform of glycodelin. *Biology of Reproduction* **69** 365-372.

Chiu PC, Chung MK, Koistinen R, Koistinen H, Seppala M, Ho PC, Ng EH, Lee KF & Yeung WS 2007 Glycodelin-A interacts with fucosyltransferase on human sperm plasma membrane to inhibit spermatozoa-zona pellucida binding. *Journal of Cell Science* **120** 33-44.

Chiu PC, Wong BS, Chung MK, Lam KK, Pang RT, Lee KF, Sumitro SB, Gupta SK & Yeung WS 2008a Effects of native human zona pellucida glycoproteins 3 and 4 on acrosome reaction and zona pellucida binding of human spermatozoa. *Biology of Reproduction* **79** 869-877.

Chiu PC, Wong BS, Lee CL, Pang RT, Lee KF, Sumitro SB, Gupta SK & Yeung WS 2008b Native human zona pellucida glycoproteins: purification and binding properties. *Human Reproduction* **23** 1385-1393.

Cho C, Ge H, Branciforte D, Primakoff P & Myles DG 2000 Analysis of mouse fertilin in wild-type and fertilin beta(-/-) sperm: evidence for C-terminal modification, alpha/beta dimerization, and lack of essential role of fertilin alpha in sperm-egg fusion. *Developmental Biology* **222** 289-295.

Choudhury S, Srivastava N, Narwal PS, Rath A, Jaiswal S & Gupta SK 2007 Feasibility and challenges in the development of immunocontraceptive vaccine based on zona pellucida glycoproteins.*Society for Reproduction and Fertility Supplement* **63** 479-493.

Conner SJ, Lefièvre L, Hughes DC & Barratt CL 2005 Cracking the egg:increased complexity in the zona pellucida. *Human Reproduction* **20** 1148-1152.

Copland SD, Murphy AA & Shur BD 2009 The mouse gamete adhesin, SED1, is expressed on the surface of acrosome-intact human sperm. *Fertility and Sterility* **92** 2014-2019.

Coy P & Avilés M 2009 What controls polyspermy in mammals, the oviduct or the oocyte? *Biological Reviews of the Cambridge Philosophical Society* (in press).

Coy P, Grullon L, Canovas S, Romar R, Matas C & Aviles M 2008a Hardening of the zona pellucida of unfertilized eggs can reduce polyspermic fertilization in the pig and cow. *Reproduction* **135** 19-27.

Coy P, Cánovas S, Mondéjar I, Saavedra MD, Romar R, Grullón L, Matás C & Avilés M 2008b Oviduct-specific glycoprotein and heparin modulate sperm-zona pellucida interaction during fertilization and contribute to the control of polyspermy. *Proceedings of the National Academy of Sciences of the USA* **105** 15809-15814.

Coy P, Lloyd R, Romar R, Satake N, Matas C, Gadea J & Holt WV 2010 Effects of porcine pre-ovulatory oviductal fluid on boar sperm function.*Theriogenology* (in press).

Crosby JA & Barros C 1999 Effect of recombinant boar beta-acrosin on sperm binding to intact zona pellucida during in vitro fertilization.*Biology of Reproduction* **61** 1535-1540.

Dale B, Wilding M, Coppola G & Tosti E 2010. How do spermatozoa activate oocytes? *Reproductive Biomedicine Online* [Epub ahead of print]

Deguchi E, Tani T, Watanabe H, Yamada S & Kondoh G 2007 Dipeptidase-inactivated tACE action in vivo: selective inhibition of sperm-zona pellucida binding in the mouse. *Biology of Reproduction* **77** 794-802.

Deppe M, Morales P & Sánchez R 2008 Effect of protease inhibitors on the acrosome reaction and sperm-zona pellucida binding in bovine sperm. *Reproduction of Domestic Animals* **43** 713-719.

Deppe M, Risopatrón J & Sánchez R 2010 Trypsin and chymotrypsin are involved in the progesterone-induced acrosome reaction in canine spermatozoa. *Reproduction of Domestic Animals* 45 453-457.

Dunbar BS, Wardrip NJ & Hedrick JL 1980. Isolation, physicochemical properties, and macromolecular composition of zona pellucida from porcine oocytes. *Biochemistry* **19** 356-365.

Dunbar BS, Dudkiewicz AB & Bundman DS 1985 Proteolysis of specific porcine zona pellucida glycoproteins by boar acrosin. *Biology of Reproduction* 32 619-630.

Ensslin MA & Shur BD 2003 Identification of mouse sperm SED1, a bimotif EGF repeat and discoidin-domain protein involved in sperm-egg binding. *Cell* **114** 405-417.

Ensslin M, Calvete JJ, Thole HH, Sierralta WD, Adermann K, Sanz L & Töpfer-Petersen E 1995 Identification by affinity chromatography of boar sperm membrane-associated proteins bound to immobilized porcine zona pellucida. Mapping of the phosphorylethanolamine-binding region of spermadhesin AWN. *Biological Chemistry Hoppe Seyler* **376** 733-738.

Ensslin M, Vogel T, Calvete JJ, Thole HH, Schmidtke J, Matsuda T & Töpfer-Petersen E 1998 Molecular cloning and characterization of P47, a novel boar sperm-associated zona pellucida-binding protein homologous to a family of mammalian secretory proteins. *Biology of Reproduction* **58** 1057-1064.

Fayrer-Hosken R 2008 Controlling animal populations using anti-fertility vaccines.*Reproduction of Domestic Animals* **43 Suppl 2** 179-185.

Flesch FM, Voorhout WF, Colenbrander B, van Golde LM & Gadella BM 1998 Use of lectins to characterize plasma membrane preparations from boar spermatozoa: a novel technique for monitoring membrane purity and quantity. *Biology of Reproduction* **59** 1530-1539.

Florman HM & Ducibella T 2006 Fertilization in mammals. In: Knobil and Neill's Physiology of Reproduction Third Edition. Neill JD editor, Raven Press, Ltd, New York, pp 55-112.

Funahashi H, Ekwall H & Rodriguez-Martinez H 2000 Zona reaction in porcine oocytes fertilized in vivo and in vitro as seen with scanning electron microscopy. *Biology of Reproduction* 63 1437-1442.

Funahashi H, Ekwall H, Kikuchi K & Rodriguez-Martinez H 2001 Transmission electron microscopy studies of the zona reaction in pig oocytes fertilized in vivo and in vitro *Reproduction* **122** 443-52.

Gadella BM 2009 Sperm surface proteomics. In: Immune Infertility; the impact of immune reactions on human infertility. Edited by Krause WH and Naz RK. Springer-verlag Berlin-Heidelberg (Germany), pp 33-48.

Gadella BM & Visconti P 2006. Regulation of capacitation. In: De Jonge C & Barrett C editors. The Sperm Cell: Production, Maturation, fertilization, Regeneration. Cambridge, UK: Cambridge University Press, pp. 134-169

Gadella BM, Colenbrander B, Van Golde LM & Lopes-Cardozo M 1993 Boar seminal vesicles secrete arylsulfatases into seminal plasma: evidence that desulfation of seminolipid occurs only after ejaculation. *Biology of Reproduction* **48** 483-489.

Gadella BM, Tsai PS, Boerke A & Brewis IA 2008 Sperm head membrane reorganisation during capacitation *International Journal of Developmental Biology* **52** 473-480.

Gahlay G, Gauthier L, Baibakov B, Epifano O & Dean J 2010 Gamete recognition in mice depends on the cleavage status of an egg's zona pellucida protein. *Science* **329** 216-219.

Gallastegui N & Groll M 2010 The 26S proteasome: assembly and function of a destructive machine. *Trends in Biochemical Sciences* [Epub ahead of print]

Ganguly A, Bansal P, Gupta T & Gupta SK 2010a "ZP domain" of human zona pellucida glycoprotein-1 binds to human spermatozoa and induces acrosomal exocytosis. *Reproductive Biology and Endrocrinology* **8**: 110.

Ganguly A, Bukovsky A, Sharma RK, Bansal P, Bhandari B& Gupta SK 2010b In humans, zona pellucida glycoprotein-1 binds to spermatozoa and induces acrosomal exocytosis. *Human Reproduction* **25** 1643-1656.

Ghosh I & Datta K 2003 Sperm surface hyaluronan binding protein (HABP1) interacts with zona pellucida of water buffalo (Bubalus bubalis) through its clustered mannose residues.*Molecular Reproduction and Development* **64** 235-244.

Gonçalves RF, Staros AL & Killian GJ 2008 Oviductal fluid proteins associated with the bovine zona pellucida and the effect on in vitro sperm-egg binding, fertilization and embryo development. *Reproduction in Domestic Animals* **43** 720-729.

Goudet G, Mugnier S, Callebaut I & Monget P 2008 Phylogenetic analysis and identification of pseudogenes reveal a progressive loss of zona pellucida genes during evolution of vertebrates. *Biology of Reproduction* **78** 796-806.

Greve JM & Wassarman PM 1985. Mouse egg extracellular coat is a matrix of interconnected filaments possessing a structural repeat. *Journal of Molecular Biology* **181** 253-264.

Gualtieri R & Talevi R 2003 Selection of highly fertilization-competent bovine spermatozoa through adhesion to the Fallopian tube epithelium in vitro. *Reproduction* **125** 251-258.

Gupta SK, Bansal P, Ganguly A, Bhandari B& Chakrabarti K 2009 Human zona pellucida glycoproteins: functional relevance during fertilization. *Journal of Reproductive Immunology* **83** 50-55.

Hanna WF, Kerr CL, Shaper JH & Wright WW 2004 Lewis X-containing neoglycoproteins mimic the intrinsic ability of zona pellucida glycoprotein ZP3 to induce the acrosome reaction in capacitated mouse sperm. *Biology of Reproduction* **71** 778-789.

Hao Z, Wolkowicz MJ, Shetty J, Klotz K, Bolling L, Sen B, Westbrook VA, Coonrod S, Flickinger CJ & Herr JC 2002 SAMP32, a testis-specific, isoantigenic sperm acrosomal membrane-associated protein. *Biology of Reproduction* **66** 735-744.

Hao Y, Mathialagan N, Walters E, Mao J, Lai L, Becker D, Li W, Critser J & Prather RS 2006 Osteopontin reduces polyspermy during in vitro fertilization of porcine oocytes. *Biology of Reproduction* **75** 726-733.

Hasegawa A, Koyama K, Okazaki Y, Sugimoto M & Isojima S 1994 Amino acid sequence of a porcine zona pellucida glycoprotein ZP4 determined by peptide mapping and cDNA cloning. *Journal of Reproduction and Fertility* **100** 245–255.

Hasegawa A, Tsubamoto H, Hamada Y & Koyama K 2000 Blocking effect of antisera to recombinant zona pellucida proteins (r-ZPA) on *in vitro* fertilization. *American Journal of Reproductive Immunology* **44** 59–64.

Hasegawa A, Kanazawa N, Sawai H, Komori S & Koyama K 2006 Pig zona pellucida 2 (pZP2) protein does not participate in zona pellucida formation in transgenic mice. *Reproduction* **132** 455-464.

Hatanaka Y, Nagai T, Tobita T & Nakano M 1992 Changes in the properties and composition of zona pellucida of pigs during fertilization in vitro. *Journal of Reproduction and Fertility* **95** 431-440.

Hayashi M, Yonezawa N, Katsumata T, Ikeda K, Imai FL, Kikuchi K, Hamano S & Nakano M 2004 Activity of exoglycosidases in ejaculated spermatozoa of boar and bull. *Zygote* **12** 105-109.

Hedrick JL & Wardrip NJ 1986 Isolation of the zona pellucida and purification of its glycoprotein families from pig oocytes. *Analytical Biochemistry* **157** 63–70.

Herlyn H & Zischler H 2008 The molecular evolution of sperm zonadhesin. *International Journal of Developmental Biology* **52** 781-790.

Hinsch E, Groeger S, Oehninger S & Hinsch KD 2003 Localization and functional importance of a conserved zona pellucida 2 protein domain in the human and bovine ovary using monoclonal anti-ZP2 peptide antibodies. *Theriogenology* **60** 1331-1344.

Hinsch E, Aires VA, Hedrich F, Oehninger S & Hinsch KD 2005 A synthetic decapeptide from a conserved ZP3 protein domain induces the G protein-regulated acrosome reaction in bovine spermatozoa. *Theriogenology* **63** 1682-1694.

Hoodbhoy T & Talbot P 1994 Mammalian cortical granules: contents, fate, and function. *Molecular Reproduction and Development* **39** 439-448.

Hou ST, Ma A, Jones R & Hall L 1996 Molecular cloning and characterization of rat sperm surface antigen 2B1, a glycoprotein implicated in sperm-zona binding. *Molecular Reproduction and Development* **45** 193-203.

Howes E, Pascall JC, Engel W & Jones R 2001 Interactions between mouse ZP2 glycoprotein and proacrosin; a mechanism for secondary binding of sperm to the zona pellucida during fertilization. *Journal of Cell Science* **114** 4127-4136.

Ikeda K, Yonezawa N, Naoi K, Katsumata T, Hamano S & Nakano M 2002 Localization of N-linked carbohydrate chains in glycoprotein ZPA of the bovine egg zona pellucida. *European Journal of Biochemistry* **269** 4257-4266.

Iwamoto K, Ikeda K, Yonezawa N, Noguchi S, Kudo K, Hamano S, Kuwayama M & Nakano M 1999 Disulfide formation in bovine zona pellucida glycoproteins during fertilization: evidence for the involvement of cystine cross-linkages in hardening of the zona pellucida. *Journal of Reproduction and Fertility* **117** 395-402.

Izquierdo-Rico MJ, Jimenez-Movilla M, Llop E, Perez-Oliva AB, Ballesta J, Gutierrez-Gallego R, Jimenez-Cervantes C& Aviles M 2009 Hamster zona pellucida is formed by four glycoproteins: ZP1, ZP2, ZP3, and ZP4. *Journal of Proteome Research* 2009 **8** 926-941.

Jagadish N, Rana R, Selvi R, Mishra D, Garg M, Yadav S, Herr JC, Okumura K, Hasegawa A, Koyama K & Suri A 2005 Characterization of a novel human sperm-associated antigen 9 (SPAG9) having structural homology with c-Jun N-terminal kinase-interacting protein. *Biochemical Journal* **389** 73-82.

Jovine L, Janssen WG, Litscher ES & Wassarman PM 2006 The PLAC1-homology region of the ZP domain is sufficient for protein polymerisation. *BMC Biochemistry* **7** 11.

Jovine L, Qi H, Williams Z, Litscher ES & Wassarman PM 2007 Features that affect secretion and assembly of zona pellucida glycoproteins during mammalian oogenesis. *Society of Reproduction and Fertility Supplement* **63** 187-201.

Kalab P, Kopf GS& Schultz RM 1991 Modifications of the mouse zona pellucida during oocyte maturation and egg activation: effects of newborn calf serum and fetuin. *Biology of Reproduction* **45** 783-787.

Kanai S, Yonezawa N, Ishii Y, Tanokura M & Nakano M 2007 Recombinant bovine zona pellucida glycoproteins ZP3 and ZP4 coexpressed in Sf9 cells form a sperm-binding active hetero-complex. *FEBS Journal* **274** 5390-5405.

Kanai S, Kitayama T, Yonezawa N, Sawano Y, Tanokura M & Nakano M 2008 Disulfide linkage patterns of pig zona pellucida glycoproteins ZP3 and ZP4.*Molecular Reproduction and Development* **75** 847-856.

Kerr CL, Hanna WF, Shaper JH & Wright WW 2004 Lewis

X-containing glycans are specific and potent competitive inhibitors of the binding of ZP3 to complementary sites on capacitated, acrosome-intact mouse sperm. *Biology of Reproduction* **71** 770-777.

Killian GJ 2004 Evidence for the role of oviduct secretions in sperm function, fertilization and embryo development. *Animal Reproduction Science* **82-83** 141-153.

Kim KS & Gerton GL 2003 Differential release of soluble and matrix components: evidence for intermediate states of secretion during spontaneous acrosomal exocytosis in mouse sperm. *Developmental Biology* **264** 141-152.

Koyama K, Hasegawa A, Inoue M & Isojima S 1991 Blocking of human sperm-zona interaction by monoclonal antibodies to a glycoprotein family (ZP4) of porcine zona pellucida. *Biology of Reproduction* **45** 727–735.

Koyama K, Hasegawa A, Mochida N & Calongos G 2005 Follicular dysfunction induced by autoimmunity to zona pellucida. *Reproductive Biology* **5** 269-278.

Landim-Alvarenga FC, Boyazoglu SE, Carvalho LR, Choi YH, Squires EL & Seidel GE Jr 2002 Effects of fetuin on zona pellucida hardening, fertilization and embryo development in cattle. *Animal Reproduction Science* **71** 181-191.

Lea IA, Sivashanmugam P & O'Rand MG 2001 Zonadhesin: characterization, localization, and zona pellucida binding. *Biology of Reproduction* **65** 1691-1700.

Lefièvre L, Conner SJ, Salpekar A, Olufowobi O, Ashton P, Pavlovic B, Lenton W, Afnan M, Brewis IA, Monk M, Hughes DC & Barratt CL 2004 Four zona pellucida glycoproteins are expressed in the human. *Human Reproduction* **19**:1580-1586.

Litscher ES & Wassarman PM 1996 Characterization of mouse ZP3-derived glycopeptide, gp55, that exhibits sperm receptor and acrosome reaction-inducing activity in vitro. *Biochemistry* **35** 3980-3985.

Litscher ES, Williams Z & Wassarman PM 2009 Zona pellucida glycoprotein ZP3 and fertilization in mammals. *Molecular Reproduction and Development* **76** 933-941.

Liu DY, Garrett C & Baker HW 2006 Acrosome-reacted human sperm in insemination medium do not bind to the zona pellucida of human oocytes. *International Journal of Andrology* **29** 475-481.

Loeser CR & Tulsiani DR 1999 The role of carbohydrates in the induction of the acrosome reaction in mouse spermatozoa. *Biology of Reproduction* **60** 94-101.

Lukoseviciute K, Bizokas V, Zilinskas H & Januskauskas A 2007 Effect of progesterone and oestradiol on sperm-zona binding and acrosome reaction in bovine spermatozoa after thawing. *Reproduction of Domestic Animals* **42** 320-325.

Lyng R & Shur BD 2009 Mouse oviduct-specific glycoprotein is an egg-associated ZP3-independent sperm-adhesion ligand. *Journal of Cell Science* **122** 3894-3906.

Manjunath P, Bergeron A, Lefebvre J & Fan J 2007 Seminal plasma proteins: functions and interaction with protective agents during semen preservation. *Society of Reproduction and Fertility Supplement* **65** 217-228.

Marín-Briggiler CI, González-Echeverría MF, Munuce MJ, Ghersevich S, Caille AM, Hellman U, Corrigall VM, Vazquez-Levin MH 2010 Glucose-regulated protein 78 (Grp78/BiP) is secreted by human oviduct epithelial cells and the recombinant protein modulates sperm-zona pellucida binding. *Fertility and Sterility* **93** 1574-1584.

Mattioli M, Lucidi P & Barboni B 1998 Expanded cumuli induce acrosome reaction in boar sperm. *Molecular Reproduction and Development* **51** 445-453.

Miller DJ, Gong X & Shur BD 1993 Sperm require beta-N-acetylglucosaminidase to penetrate through the egg zona pellucida *Development* **118** 1279-1289.

Monné M, Han L, Schwend T, Burendahl S & Jovine L 2008 Crystal structure of the ZP-N domain of ZP3 reveals the core fold of animal egg coats. *Nature* **456** 653-657.

Montfort L, Frenette G & Sullivan R 2002 Sperm-zona pellucida interaction involves a carbonyl reductase activity in the hamster. *Molecular Reproduction and Development* **61** 113-119.

Moreno RD, Hoshi M & Barros C 1999 Functional interactions between sulphated polysaccharides and proacrosin: implications in sperm binding and digestion of zona pellucida. *Zygote* **7** 105-111.

Mori E, Baba T, Iwamatsu A & Mori T 1993 Purification and characterization of a 38-kDa protein, sp38, with zona pellucida-binding property from porcine epididymal sperm. *Biochemical and Biophysical Research Communications* **196** 196-202.

Mori E, Kashiwabara S, Baba T, Inagaki Y & Mori T 1995 Amino acid sequences of porcine Sp38 and proacrosin required for binding to the zona pellucida. *Developmental Biology* **168** 575-583.

Morin G, Sullivan R, Laflamme I, Robert C & Leclerc P 2010 SPAM1 isoforms from two tissue origins are differentially localized within ejaculated bull sperm membranes and have different roles during fertilization. *Biology of Reproduction* **82** 271-281.

Mugnier S, Dell'Aquila ME, Pelaez J, Douet C, Ambruosi B, De Santis T, Lacalandra GM, Lebos C, Sizaret PY, Delaleu B, Monget P, Mermillod P, Magistrini M, Meyers SA & Goudet G 2009 New insights into the mechanisms of fertilization: comparison of the fertilization steps, composition, and structure of the zona pellucida between horses and pigs. *Biology of Reproduction* **81** 856-870.

Muiño-Blanco T, Pérez-Pé R & Cebrián-Pérez JA 2008 Seminal plasma proteins and sperm resistance to stress. *Reproduction of Domestic Animals* **43 Supplement 4**:18-31.

Munuce MJ, Serravalle A, Caille AM, Zumoffen C, Botti G, Cabada M & Ghersevich S 2009 Human tubal secretion can modify the affinity of human spermatozoa for the zona pellucida. *Fertility and Sterility* 91 407-413.

Nakano M & Yonezawa N 2001 Localization of sperm ligand carbohydrate chains in pig zona pellucida glycoproteins.*Cells Tissues and Organs* **168** 65-75.

Nara M, Yonezawa N, Shimada T, Takahashi K, Tanokura M, Yumoto F, Nakagawa H, Ohashi K, Hamano S & Nakano M 2006 Fourier transform infrared spectroscopic analysis of the intact zona pellucida of the mammalian egg: changes in the secondary structure of bovine zona pellucida proteins during fertilization. *Experimental Biology and Medicine* **231** 166-171.

Nixon B, MacIntyre DA, Mitchell LA, Gibbs GM, O'Bryan M &Aitken RJ 2006 The identification of mouse sperm-surface-associated proteins and characterization of their ability to act as decapacitation factors.*Biology of Reproduction* **74** 275-287.

Nixon B, Aitken RJ & McLaughlin EA 2007 New insights into the molecular mechanisms of sperm-egg interaction. *Cellular and Molecular Life Sciences* **64** 1805-1823.

Noguchi S, Yonezawa N, Katsumata T, Hashizume K, Kuwayama M, Hamano S, Watanabe S & Nakano M 1994 Characterization of the zona pellucida glycoproteins from bovine ovarian and fertilized eggs. *Biochimica et Biophysica Acta.* **1201** 7-14.

Overstreet JW, Lin Y, Yudin AI, Meyers SA, Primakoff P, Myles DG, Katz DF & Vandevoort CA 1995 Location of the PH-20 protein on acrosome-intact and acrosome-reacted spermatozoa of cynomolgus macaques. *Biology of Reproduction* **52** 105-114.

Parrish JJ, Susko-Parrish JL, Leibfried-Rutledge ML, Critser ES, Eyestone WH & First NL 1986 Bovine in vitro fertilization with frozen-thawed semen. *Theriogenology* **25** 591-600.

Pate BJ, White KL, Chen D, Aston KI, Sessions BR, Bunch TD &Weimer BC 2008 A novel approach to identify bovine sperm membrane proteins that interact with receptors on the vitelline membrane of bovine oocytes. *Molecular Reproduction and Develoment* **75** 641-649.

Patrat C, Auer J, Fauque P, Leandri RL, Jouannet P & Serres C 2006 Zona pellucida from fertilised human oocytes induces a voltage-dependent calcium influx and the acrosome reaction in spermatozoa, but cannot be penetrated by sperm. *BMC Developmental Biology* **6** 59

Raterman D & **Springer MS** 2008 The molecular evolution of acrosin in placental mammals. *Molecular Reproduction and Development* **75** 1196-1207.

Rodeheffer C & Shur BD 2004 Characterization of a novel ZP3-independent sperm-binding ligand that facilitates sperm adhesion to the egg coat. *Development* **131** 503-512.

Sakaguchi Y, Iwata H, Kuwayama T & Monji Y 2009 Effect of N-acetyl-D-glucosamine on bovine sperm-oocyte interactions *Journal of Reproductive Development* **55** 676-684.

Santos P, Chaveiro A, Simões N & Moreira da Silva F 2008 Bovine oocyte quality in relation to ultrastructural characteristics of zona pellucida, polyspermic penetration and developmental competence. *Reproduction of Domestic Animals* **43** 685-689.

Schroeder AC, Schultz RM, Kopf GS, Taylor FR, Becker RB & Eppig JJ 1990 Fetuin inhibits zona pellucida hardening and conversion of ZP2 to ZP2f during spontaneous mouse oocyte maturation in vitro in the absence of serum. *Biology of Reproduction* **43** 891-897.

Seaton GJ, Hall L & Jones R 2000 Rat sperm 2B1 glycoprotein (PH20) contains a C-terminal sequence motif for attachment of a glycosyl phosphatidylinositol anchor. Effects of endoproteolytic cleavage on hyaluronidase activity. *Biology of Reproduction* **62** 1667-1676.

Selvaraj V, Buttke DE, Asano A, McElwee JL, Wolff CA, Nelson JL, Klaus AV, Hunnicutt GR & Travis AJ 2007 GM1 dynamics as a marker for membrane changes associated with the process of capacitation in murine and bovine spermatozoa *Journal of Andrology* **28** 588-599.

Shetty J, Wolkowicz MJ, Digilio LC, Klotz KL, Jayes FL, Diekman AB, Westbrook VA, Farris EM, Hao Z, Coonrod SA, Flickinger CJ & Herr JC 2003 SAMP14, a novel, acrosomal membrane-associated, glycosylphosphatidylinositol-anchored member of the Ly-6/urokinase-type plasminogen activator receptor superfamily with a role in sperm-egg interaction. *Journal of Biological Chemistry* **278** 30506-30515.

Shur BD, Rodeheffer C, Ensslin MA, Lyng R & Raymond A 2006 Identification of novel gamete receptors that mediate sperm adhesion to the egg coat. *Molecular and Cellular Endocrinology* **250** 137-148.

Sinowatz F, Wessa E, Neumüller C & Palma G 2003 On the species specificity of sperm binding and sperm penetration of the zona pellucida. *Reproduction of Domestic Animals* **38** 141-146.

Sleight SB, Miranda PV, Plaskett NW, Maier B, Lysiak J, Scrable H, Herr JC & Visconti PE 2005. Isolation and proteomic analysis of mouse sperm detergent-resistant membrane fractions: evidence for dissociation of lipid rafts during capacitation. *Biology of Reproduction* **73** 721-729.

Sostaric E, Dieleman SJ, van de Lest CH, Colenbrander B, Vos PL, Garcia-Gil N, Gadella BM 2008 Sperm binding properties and secretory activity of the bovine oviduct immediately before and after ovulation. *Molecular Reproduction and Development* **75** 60-74.

Suarez SS 2008 Regulation of sperm storage and movement in the mammalian oviduct. *International Journal of Developmental Biology* **52** 455-462.

Taberner E, Morató R, Mogas T & Miró J 2010 Ability of Catalonian donkey sperm to penetrate zona pellucida-free bovine oocytes matured in vitro. *Animal Reproduction Science* **118** 354-361.

Talevi R & Gualtieri R 2010 Molecules involved in sperm-oviduct adhesion and release.*Theriogenology* **73** 796-801.

Tanphaichitr N, Carmona E, Bou Khalil M, Xu H, Berger T & Gerton GL 2007 New insights into sperm-zona pellucida interaction: involvement of sperm lipid rafts. *Frontiers in Biosciences* **12** 1748-1766.

Tardif S, Akrofi AS, Dass B, Hardy DM & Macdonald CC 2010a Infertility with Impaired Zona Pellucida Adhesion of Spermatozoa from Mice Lacking TauCstF-64. *Biology of Reproduction* [Epub ahead of print]

Tardif S, Wilson MD, Wagner R, Hunt P, Gertsenstein M, Nagy A, Lobe C, Koop BF & Hardy DM 2010b.

Zonadhesin is essential for species specificity of sperm adhesion to the egg's zona pellucida. *Journal of Biological Chemistry* [Epub ahead of print]

Thaler CD & Cardullo RA 1995 Biochemical characterization of a glycosylphosphatidylinositol-linked hyaluronidase on mouse sperm. *Biochemistry* **34** 7788-7795.

Thaler CD, Thomas M & Ramalie JR 2006 Reorganization of mouse sperm lipid rafts by capacitation. *Molecular Reproduction and Development* **73** 1541-1549.

Topper EK, Kruijt L, Calvete J, Mann K, Töpfer-Petersen E, Woelders H 1997 Identification of bovine zona pellucida glycoproteins. *Molecular Reproduction and Development* 46 344-350.

Tsai PS & Gadella BM 2009 Molecular kinetics of proteins at the surface of porcine sperm before and during fertilization. *Society for Reproduction and Fertility* **Supplement 66** 23-36.

Tsai PS, De Vries KJ, De Boer-Brouwer M, Garcia-Gil N, Van Gestel RA, Colenbrander B, Gadella BM & Van Haeften T 2007 Syntaxin and VAMP association with lipid rafts depends on cholesterol depletion in capacitating sperm cells. *Molecular Membrane Biology* **24** 313-324.

Tsai PS, Garcia-Gil N, van Haeften T & Gadella BM 2010 How pig sperm prepares to fertilize: stable acrosome docking to the plasma membrane. *Public Libabry of Sciences One* **5** e11204.

Vadnais ML & Roberts KP 2010 Seminal plasma proteins inhibit in vitro- and cooling-induced capacitation in boar spermatozoa. *Reproduction Fertility and Development.* **22** 893-900.

Vanderschaeghe D, Festjens N, Delanghe J & Callewaert N (2010) Glycome profiling using modern glycomics technology: technical aspects and applications. *Biological Chemistry* **391** 149-161.

van Gestel RA, Brewis IA, Ashton PR, Helms JB, Brouwers JF & Gadella BM 2005 Capacitation-dependent concentration of lipid rafts in the apical ridge head area of porcine sperm cells. *Molecular Human Reproduction* **11** 583-590.

van Gestel RA, Brewis IA, Ashton PR, Brouwers JF & Gadella BM 2007 Multiple proteins present in purified porcine sperm apical plasma membranes interact with the zona pellucida of the oocyte. *Molecular Human Reproduction* 2007 **13** 445-454.

Velásquez JG, Canovas S, Barajas P, Marcos J, Jiménez-Movilla M, Gallego RG, Ballesta J, Avilés M & Coy P 2007 Role of sialic acid in bovine sperm-zona pellucida binding. *Molecular Reproduction and Development* 74 617-628.

Villemure M, Lazure C & Manjunath P 2003. Isolation and characterization of gelatin-binding proteins from goat seminal plasma. *Reproductive Biology and Endocrinology* 2003 **1**:39.

Wassarman PM 1988 Zona pellucida glycoproteins. *Annual Review of Biochemistry* **57** 415-442.

Wassarman PM 2008 Zona pellucida glycoproteins. *Journal of Biological Chemistry* **283** 24285-24289.

Wassarman PM 2009 Mammalian fertilization: the strange case of sperm protein 56. *Bioessays* **31** 153-158.

Wassarman PM & Albertini DF 1994 The mammalian ovum. In: The physiology of Reproduction Second Edition. Edited by Knobil E & Neill JD. Raven Press, Ltd, New York, pp. 79-122.

Wassarman PM & Litscher ES 2009 The multifunctional zona pellucida and mammalian fertilization. *Journal of Reproductive Immunology* **83** 45-49.

Williams SA, Xia L, Cummings RD, McEver RP & Stanley P 2007 Fertilization in mouse does not require terminal galactose or N-acetylglucosamine on the zona pellucida glycans.Journal of Cell Science **120** 1341-1349

Yeung WS, Lee KF, Koistinen R, Koistinen H, Seppala M, Ho PC & Chiu PC 2007 Glycodelin: a molecule with multi-functions on spermatozoa.*Society for Reproduction and Fertililty* **Supplement 63** 143-151.

Yeung WS, Lee KF, Koistinen R, Koistinen H, Seppälä M & Chiu PC 2009 Effects of glycodelins on functional competence of spermatozoa. *Journal of Reproductive Immunology* **83** 26-30.

Yin L, Chung CM, Huo R, Liu H, Zhou C, Xu W, Zhu H, Zhang J, Shi Q, Wong HY, Chen J, Lu Y, Bi Y, Zhao C, Du Y, Ma M, Cai Y, Chen WY, Fok KL, Tsang LL, Li K, Ni Y, Chung YW, Zhou Z, Sha J, Chan HC 2009 A sperm GPI-anchored protein elicits sperm-cumulus cross-talk leading to the acrosome reaction. *Cellular and Molecular Life Sciences* **66** 900-908.

Yonezawa N, Amari S, Takahashi K, Ikeda K, Imai FL, Kanai S, Kikuchi K & Nakano M 2005 Participation of the nonreducing terminal beta-galactosyl residues of the neutral N-linked carbohydrate chains of porcine zona pellucida glycoproteins in sperm-egg binding. *Molecular Reproduction and Development* **70** 222-227.

Yonezawa N, Kanai S & Nakano M 2007 Structural significance of N-glycans of the zona pellucida on species-selective recognition of spermatozoa between pig and cattle. *Society for Reproduction and Fertililty* **Supplement 63** 217-228.

Yu Y, Xu W, Yi YJ, Sutovsky P & Oko R 2006 The extracellular protein coat of the inner acrosomal membrane is involved in zona pellucida binding and penetration during fertilization: characterization of its most prominent polypeptide (IAM38). *Developmental Biology* **290** 32-43.

Yurewicz EC, Sacco AG, Gupta SK, Xu N & Gage DA 1998 Hetero-oligomerization-dependent binding of pig oocyte zona pellucida glycoproteins ZPB and ZPC to boar sperm membrane vesicles. *Journal of Biological Chemistry* **273** 7488-7494.

Zanich A, Pascall JC & Jones R 2003 Secreted epididymal glycoprotein 2D6 that binds to the sperm's plasma membrane is a member of the beta-defensin superfamily of pore-forming glycopeptides. *Biology of Reproduction* **69** 1831-1842.

Zimmerman S & Sutovsky P 2009 The sperm proteasome during sperm capacitation and fertilization. *Journal of Reproductive Immunology* **83** 19-25.

Zitta K, Wertheimer EV & Miranda PV 2006 Sperm N-acetylglucosaminidase is involved in primary binding to the zona pellucida. *Molecular Human Reproduction* **12** 557-563.

Regulation of corpus luteum development and maintenance: specific roles of angiogenesis and action of prostaglandin $F_{2\alpha}$

A Miyamoto[1], K Shirasuna[1], T Shimizu[1], H Bollwein[2] and D Schams[3]

[1] *Graduate School of Animal and Food Hygiene, Obihiro University of Agriculture and Veterinary Medicine, Obihiro 080-8555, Japan;* [2] *Clinic for Cattle, University of Veterinary Medicine Hannover, D-30173 Hannover, Germany;* [3] *Institute of Physiology, Technical University of Munich, Weihenstephaner Berg 3, D-85350 Freising, Germany*

Development of the corpus luteum (CL) in ruminants occurs in a rapid and time-dependent manner within 1 week after ovulation, with morphologic and biochemical changes in the cells of the theca interna and granulosa cells of the preovulatory follicle. These changes involve luteinisation of steroidogenic cells and angiogenesis to establish normal luteal function (progesterone secretion). The CL is composed of a large number of vascular endothelial cells, large and small steroidogenic luteal cells, smooth muscle cells, pericytes, fibrocytes and immune cells, indicating that the CL is a heterogeneous tissue. Moreover, the CL produces and secretes growth factors (fibroblast growth factor, vascular endothelial growth factor and insulin-like growth factor), vasoactive factors (nitric oxide, angiotensin II and endothelin-1), steroids (progesterone is important for its own production), oxytocin and prostaglandins ($PGF_{2\alpha}$ and PGE_2) to regulate luteal formation and development. Clearly, the main function of the CL is to produce progesterone, which is a prerequisite for survival of the embryo, implantation and maintenance of pregnancy. Inadequate luteinisation and angiogenesis during the early luteal phase results in poor progesterone secretion and causes compromised embryo development and reduced fertility. Secretion of adequate amounts of progesterone during luteal development requires "precise luteinisation" of theca and granulosa cells to form luteal cells, neovascularization, and the establishment of a blood supply (angiogenesis). $PGF_{2\alpha}$ in the developing CL acts as a local regulator to enhance progesterone secretion directly and indirectly by stimulating angiogenic factors, VEGF and FGF2. The preceding role of $PGF_{2\alpha}$ may explain why the developing CL does not acquire luteolytic capacity until several days following ovulation. The balance between luteotrophic and luteolytic factors as well as stimulation and inhibition of angiogenic factors during luteal formation, development and maintenance can have a profound effect on the fate of the CL.

Corresponding author E-mail: akiomiya@obihiro.ac.jp

A brief historical overview of corpus luteum research in ruminants

As summarized by McCracken *et al.* (1999), Coiter (1573) described the presence of cavities filled with a yellow solid in the rodent ovary. De Graaf and Mullierum (1943) provided the first definitive description of these structures and noted that the number appeared to be related to the number of fetuses in the uterus. Malpighi (1897) provided an accurate microscopic description of these structures and was the first to name the corpus luteum (CL). Subsequently, Beard (1897) postulated that CL were responsible for the suppression of ovulation and oestrus during pregnancy.

Frenkel (1903) demonstrated that corpora lutea are necessary for implantation and the subsequent maintenance of pregnancy in rabbits. Corner & Allen (1929) prepared a relatively pure alcoholic extract of the CL from sows and demonstrated that the extract could maintain pregnancy in ovariectomized rabbits. In 1934, isolation of the pure crystalline hormone was reported by different groups (Slotta *et al.* 1934; Wintersteiner & Allen 1934). Slotta *et al.* (1934) named the compound progesterone and suggested the structure. In 1960, about 27 papers concerning the CL with only one in ruminants were cited according to PubMed. From 1960 onwards, countless studies have been performed on different aspects of luteal formation, maintenance, function and regression during the oestrous cycle and pregnancy. A critical advance in the field has been development of sophisticated methods for measuring progesterone in tissue, culture supernatants, and peripheral blood. Research activities have been directed towards the topics listed below (Fig. 1).

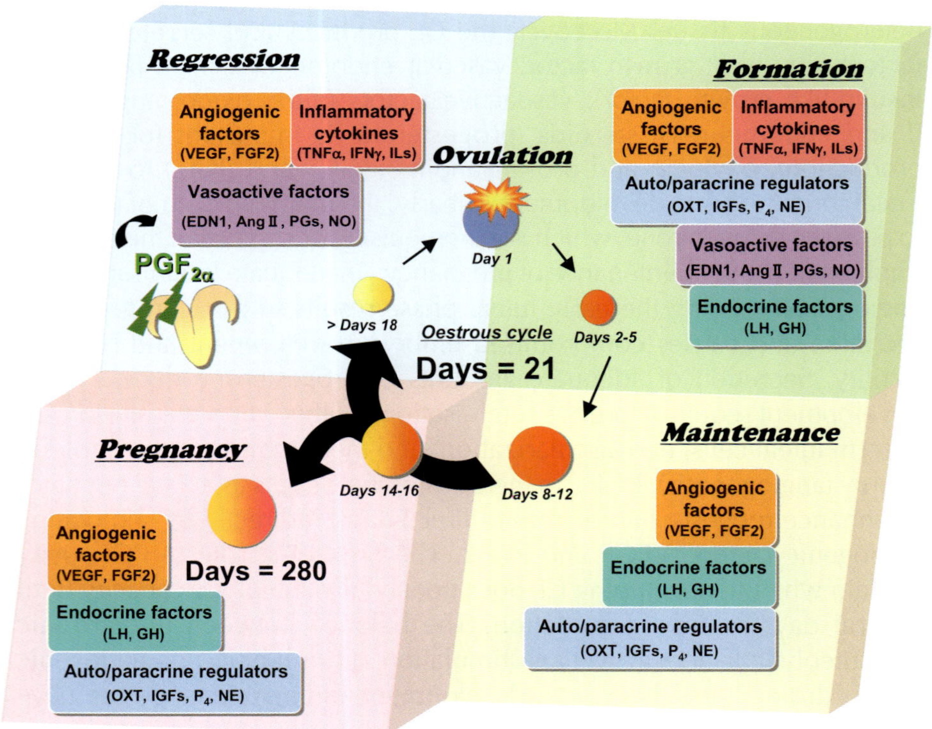

Fig. 1. Schematic presentation of possible involvement of various functional factors during different stages of CL activity. The CL at each stage is regulated by a complex mechanism that consists of endocrine factors, auto/paracrine factors, angiogenic factors, vasoactive factors and inflammatory cytokines. The balance between luteotrophic and luteolytic factors as well as stimulation and inhibition of angiogenic factors is the basic mechanism for CL development, maintenance and regression.

Development of the corpus luteum

An essential step in early CL development is vascularisation of granulosa-lutein cells through angiogenesis. Angiogenesis is defined as the generation of new blood vessels through sprouting from preexisting blood vessels. This process includes breakdown of basement membranes, proliferation and migration of endothelial cells into the extracellular matrix and formation of new capillary lumina along with functional maturation which is regulated by a complex of stimulation and inhibition of angiogenic factors (Schams & Berisha 2004). In cows, sprouting endothelial cells invade the developing CL and continue to grow throughout the first third of the ovarian cycle, and the mature CL is characterized by a dense network of vessels with gradually decreasing vessel density. During luteolysis, all newly formed blood vessels regress, thus luteal angiogenesis is a suitable experimental system to study endothelial cells in sprouting and regressing blood vessels (Augustin *et al.* 1995).

Molecular control of luteal secretion of progesterone

The synthesis and secretion of progesterone are regulated by two morphologically and biochemically distinct steroidogenic cell types in the CL. Small luteal cells respond to luteinising hormone (LH) or cAMP with an increase in secretion of progesterone. Large luteal cells secrete a high basal concentration of progesterone ($\geq$85%), do not respond to LH or cAMP and contain receptors for prostaglandin (PG) $F_{2\alpha}$, growth hormone (GH) and other proteins. Progesterone secretion is regulated by two second messenger pathways. Phosphorylation of steroid acute regulatory (StAR) protein by protein kinase A (PKA) stimulates cholesterol transport, whereas phosphorylation by PKC appears to inhibit this process and induces cell death (Niswender *et al.* 2000).

Trophic regulation of luteal function

Both LH and GH are necessary for normal luteal development and function (Niswender *et al.* 2000; Schams & Berisha 2004). Local regulators such as growth factors (insulin-like growth factors, IGFs; fibroblast growth factors, FGFs), ovarian peptides (oxytocin; angiotensin II, Ang II; endothelin-1, EDN1), and steroids (noradrenalin and prostaglandins ($PGF_{2\alpha}$ and PGE_2): Schams & Berisha 2004) play modulatory roles acting in an autocrine/paracrine fashion.

Luteal regression (luteolysis)

After induction of luteolysis by endometrial $PGF_{2\alpha}$, a cascade of events occurs within the CL, leading to functional and structural luteolysis. The acute changes in vasoactive factors suggest that modulation of vascular stability is a critical component of luteolysis (Miyamoto *et al.* 2009). Other cascades after $PGF_{2\alpha}$-induced luteolysis that occur in parallel or subsequent to changes in vascularity include: (i) luteal nitric oxide (NO) release and blood flow, (ii) up-regulation of inflammatory cytokines and luteal cell apoptosis factors, (iii) up-regulation of vasoactive peptides in luteal cells, (iv) extracellular matrix proteases associated with CL tissue remodelling and (v) invasion by immune cells (monocytes, macrophages, T-lymphocytes) from the blood stream after monocyte chemoattractant protein-1 up-regulation.

There are currently (PubMed) about 14,813 papers concerning the CL in different species. About 4,238 of these papers concern domestic ruminants. However, there are a number of important issues relating to luteal function that require further research. For example, a clearer understanding of how the balance between luteotrophic and luteolytic factors as well as stimulation and inhibition of angiogenic factors affects luteal function is essential. In addition, we need to better understand the role of proteolytic processes (e.g. tissue remodelling), and modulation by the immune system in the regulation of the CL. A schematic of possible involvement of these factors in different stages of the luteal phase is shown in Fig. 1. In this review, we focus on CL development and maintenance in ruminants with specific emphasis on luteal angiogenesis and the action of prostaglandins.

Introduction

Ovulation occurs in response to a cascade of morphological, biochemical, and physiological changes in the Graafian follicle following the LH surge, resulting in expulsion of the matured oocyte and subsequent development of the CL. The bovine CL develops rapidly within 2-3 d after ovulation and is supported by differentiation and hypertrophy of steroidogenic cells, angiogenesis and neovascularisation; it is functional for 17-18 d in the non-pregnant cow. If pregnancy does not occur successfully, the CL must regress within a few days to allow for subsequent ovulation to occur. In non-pregnant cows, luteolysis is caused by pulses of $PGF_{2\alpha}$ that are secreted by the endometrium around d 17-19 of the oestrous cycle (Ginther *et al.* 2009). $PGF_{2\alpha}$ induces a decrease in luteal blood flow which results in a decrease in progesterone released from the CL as well as a decrease in CL volume (Acosta *et al.* 2002; Niswender *et al.* 1976).

The preovulatory follicle is compartmentalised into a highly vascular thecal layer and a non-vascular granulosal layer that are separated by a basal membrane and independently regulated by LH and FSH. The CL is composed of a large number of vascular endothelial cells that can account for up to 50% of all luteal cells. Large and small steroidogenic luteal cells constitute about 30% of all cells of CL (O'Shea *et al.* 1989), and the majority of steroidogenic cells are adjacent to one or more capillaries (Zheng *et al.* 1993). The bovine CL also consists of various cell types such as smooth muscle cells, pericytes, fibrocytes and immune cells, indicating that it is a heterogeneous tissue (Farin *et al.* 1986). The bovine CL produces steroid hormones, PGs (Miyamoto *et al.* 1993; Shemesh & Hansel 1975), a number of angiogenic factors, and other local regulators (Reynolds *et al.* 2000; Schams & Berisha 2004).

Changes in the dominant follicle before and after the LH surge

Preovulatory changes induced by the LH surge

The time between the LH surge and ovulation is a critical period for the rapid start of differentiation of the preovulatory follicle. The CL is formed after ovulation from remaining follicular cells. The preparation of luteal cells for progesterone synthesis begins before ovulation. Luteinisation and secretion of progesterone can occur in the absence of ovulation in cattle (Kesler *et al.* 1981) and sheep (Murdoch & Dunn 1983), indicating that mechanisms associated with luteinisation are not dependent on follicular rupture. Following the preovulatory LH surge but before ovulation, follicular cells begin morphological, endocrinological and biochemical changes associated with luteinisation. The critical roles of PGs in ovulation have been demonstrated by an experiment in which an inhibitor of PG biosynthesis effectively inhibited ovulation in cattle (Algire *et al.* 1992). Injection of an ovulatory dose of hCG induced expression of cyclooxygenase-2 (COX-2) in the granulosa cells of bovine preovulatory follicles (Sirois 1994). The levels of $PGF_{2\alpha}$ and PGE_2 increased by more than 100-fold at 25 h after the endogenous LH surge in bovine preovulatory follicular fluid (Short *et al.* 1995). Additionally, Ang II, a potent vasoconstrictive factor, as well as $PGF_{2\alpha}$ acutely increased around the time of ovulation in the bovine mature follicle in vivo (Acosta *et al.* 2000). FGF2 protein is up-regulated beginning with the LH surge, and the maximum levels were observed at 20 h after GnRH injection in the bovine follicle (Berisha *et al.* 2006). Interestingly, FGF2 localisation changed dramatically from the theca (cytoplasm of endothelial cells) to the nucleus of granulosa cells after the LH surge, suggesting an essential role for survival of granulosa cells or for transition of granulosa cells to luteal cells (Berisha *et al.* 2006). Oxytocin also plays important autocrine/paracrine roles in the follicular/luteal transition of steroidogenesis from estradiol/androgen to progesterone production. Oxytocin not only stimulates progesterone, but also inhibits oestradiol secretion by granulosa cells before the LH surge, but not after the LH surge (Berndtson *et al.* 1996; Voss & Fortune 1991). In addition, oxytocin stimulates progesterone release from early developing CL as examined with the microdialysis system (Miyamoto & Schams 1991).

Vascular changes are associated with the cyclic remodelling of ovarian tissue that occurs during final stages of follicular growth, ovulation and CL development (Acosta *et al.* 2002; Moor *et al.* 1975). The principal angiogenic factors controlling follicular angiogenesis are FGF2 and VEGFA (Berisha *et al.* 2000b). Systemic administration of a VEGF antagonist prevented the development of preovualtory follicles. This inhibition was associated with a decrease in thecal layer vasculature, granulosa cell proliferation, antral formation and steroidogenesis (Wulff *et al.* 2002). Conversely, ovarian injection of VEGFA gene fragments into gonadotropin-stimulated prepubertal pigs increased thecal vascularisation and the number of preovulatory follicles (Shimizu *et al.* 2003). The follicular VEGFA concentration in the fluid and tissue increased in the bovine follicles during final maturation and was associated with increased vascular density in the thacal layer (Berisha *et al.* 2000b). Vessel permeability increased along with neovascularisation of the follicular periphery, thereby supplying a larger effective dose of LH to that particular follicle. LH stimulated VEGFA expression in bovine cultured granulosa cells in a dose dependent manner (Schams *et al.* 2001). As VEGFA mRNA expression is not altered by the LH surge during the periovulatory interval, LH is thought to act at a post-transcriptional level to regulate VEGFA production (Hazzard *et al.* 1999). Capillaries induced by VEGF develop perforations through which blood cells and platelets escape when ovulation occurs. Shortly before ovulation, blood flow stops in a small area of the ovarian surface overlying the bulging follicles. This area, known as the stigma, then ruptures (Findlay 1986).

Follicular luteinisation after ovulation

After follicular rupture, there is a dramatic invagination of the follicular wall that presumably facilitates migration of fibroblasts, endothelial cells and theca interna cells into the central regions of the developing CL. Tissue remodelling and cellular migration are facilitated by breakdown of the basement membrane that separates the avascular granulosa cell layer from the theca interna layer. Small and large luteal cells are derived exclusively from theca and granulosa cells, respectively. However, some small luteal cells may differentiate into large luteal cells (Alila & Hansel 1984). Conversely, some large luteal cells may differentiate into small luteal cells (Fisch *et al.* 1989). In sheep, small luteal cells can stimulate angiogenesis (Grazul-Bilska *et al.* 1991).

The differentiation of granulosa and theca cells into large and small luteal cells is characterized by increased progesterone production. The preovulatory LH surge initiates distinct changes in both expression and regulation of steroidogenic enzymes and is a key event in the luteinisation process. Aromatase cytochrome P-450 enzyme (P450arom) is a key enzyme in oestradiol biosynthesis, catalyzing aromatisation of C19 androgens of theca cell origin to C18 oestrogens within granulosa cells. P450arom mRNA decreases in bovine follicles collected at approximately 20 h after the LH surge (Voss and Fortune 1993). Within the bovine CL, 3ß-hydroxysteroid-dehydrogenase (3ß-HSD) mRNA and enzyme activity increases throughout most of oestrus and then decreases during luteolysis (Couet *et al.* 1990). Moreover, 3ß-HSD enzyme activity is greater in the bovine CL than in preovulatory follicles (Couet *et al.* 1990). Thus, 3ß-HSD activity within the CL facilitates high rates of progesterone biosynthesis.

During luteinisation, the changes in gene expression associated with steroid production in steroidogenic cells are regulated by transcription factors such as Ad4BP/SF-1 and DAX-1. The decrease in DAX-1, a suppressor of Ad4BP/SF-1, is involved in acquisition of the ability to produce progesterone when granulosa cells are luteinising (Shimizu *et al.* 2009). However, during luteinisation of theca cells in culture, suppression of CYP 17 genes was induced by an increase in DAX-1 transcription factor (Murayama *et al.* 2008). Thus, DAX-1 likely contributes to the expression of specific genes to shift steroid production during luteinisation of granulosa and theca cells.

Corpus luteum development and angiogenesis

Vasculature of the developing CL

After ovulation, a rich vascular network is established within the CL to support differentiation of follicular cells and progesterone secretion from luteal cells during the early luteal phase. Functionally, luteal blood vessels can be divided roughly into two types of blood vessels. One type is arteriolovenous vessels, i.e., arteriola (diameter: about 40 μm) and venula vessels (diameter: about 30 μm), which have a smooth muscle layer and exhibit a vasorelaxant effect. In the circulation of blood, the arteriola connects to microcapillary vessels followed by venulae (Kashiwagi *et al.* 2002). It has been reported that in the rabbit CL, arteriolovenous vessels exist in the periphery of the CL (Wiltbank *et al.* 1988), and luteal blood flow is observed mainly in the periphery of the bovine CL in color Doppler images (Acosta *et al.* 2002). The other types are capillary vessels having no smooth muscle layer and thus exhibit little vasorelaxant effect. In the bovine and ovine CL, the number of arteriolovenous and microcapillary vessels drastically increases from the early to mid-luteal phase (Bauer *et al.* 2003; Hojo, *et al.* 2009; Shirasuna *et al.* 2010a), indicating active angiogenesis during this period. A recent study indicated that further angiogenesis does not occur throughout the period of early maternal recognition in the cow (Beindorff *et al.* 2010).

Role of angiogenic factors in the developing CL

Angiogenesis is a critical component of normal luteal function. In 1906, Loeb (1906) indicated that the CL closely resembles "transitory tumors", and the rate of luteal growth is equivalent to the fastest growing tumors. Therefore, the growth of blood vessels and establishment of a blood supply are essential during early luteal development. Indeed, the mature CL has the densest capillary network system in the whole body and each luteal cell is adjacent to one or more capillaries.

One of the major angiogenic factors, FGF2, is generally involved in cell growth, differentiation, transformation and angiogenesis. Gospodarowicz *et al,.* (1985) showed that FGF2 is produced in the bovine CL and stimulates neovascularization and proliferation of a variety of cells such as vascular smooth muscle cells, granulosa cells and endothelial cells. The mRNA expression of FGF2 and its receptor is highest during the early luteal phase (Berisha *et al.*

2000a; Schams *et al.* 1994). FGF2 concentrations in CL tissue are high during the early luteal phase, and decrease significantly in the mid-luteal phase during the oestrous cycle in the cow (Schams *et al.* 1994). FGF2 stimulates progesterone secretion from the early bovine CL as determined using a microdialysis system (Miyamoto *et al.* 1992). In a recent study investigating the impact of FGF2 on bovine CL development and function, an FGF2 antibody was injected directly into the CL (Yamashita *et al.* 2008). This treatment markedly suppressed CL volume and progesterone synthesis (plasma progesterone concentrations and mRNA expression of StAR) as well as decreased mRNA expression of key factors related to angiogenesis ($VEGF_{120}$, FGF2, FGFR-1) and increased the ratio of angiopoietin-2/angiopoietin-1 (an index of instability of vessels), all of which promote angiolysis (Yamashita *et al.* 2008). This suggests that FGF2 promotes the establishment of a new vascular network and luteal function during CL formation in the cow.

The greatest mRNA expression for VEGFA and VEGFR-2 in the CL was detected during the early luteal phase followed by a significant decrease in expression during the mid and late-luteal phase, with further decreases after luteal regression in the cow (Berisha *et al.* 2000b). In contrast, VEGFR-1 mRNA expression did not change during the oestrous cycle (Berisha *et al.* 2000b). The concentration of VEGF protein was increased during the early luteal phase and then decreased, especially in the regressing CL (Berisha *et al.* 2000b). VEGFA can stimulate progesterone secretion from the bovine CL (Kobayashi *et al.* 2001). An injection of VEGF antibody into an intact bovine CL suppressed the increase in CL volume and progesterone synthesis in the early CL (Yamashita *et al.* 2008). These findings are in agreement with the previous report that neutralisation of VEGF using an antibody during the early luteal phase in marmoset monkeys inhibits proliferation of endothelial cells and plasma progesterone concentrations (Fraser *et al.* 2000).

Robinson *et al*,. (2008) investigated the angiogenic and luteotropic roles of FGF2 and VEGF in the bovine CL using an in vitro culture system for luteal angiogenesis. Luteal FGF2 concentration was highest from d 1-2 compared with d 3-4, 5-6 and 8-12 of the oestrous cycle, while luteal VEGF concentration gradually increased from the early to midcycle CL, and then decreased in the regressing CL in the cow (Robinson *et al.* 2009). In a luteal angiogenesis culture system (includes luteal cells, endothelial cells and smooth muscle cells), a physiological dose (1 ng/ml) of FGF2 and VEGF stimulated the extent of the endothelial cell network (Fig. 2; Robinson *et al.* 2008). Using this culture system, a VEGFR2 inhibitor resulted in lower numbers of endothelial networks compared with the control (60% of the control; Woad *et al.* 2009). However, even in the presence of VEGF, a FGFR1 inhibitor drastically reduced the number of vascular networks by more than 90%, suggesting that FGF2 is more crucial than VEGF for forming luteal vascular networks (Fig. 2; Woad *et al.* 2009). The preceding findings indicate that FGF2 plays a key role in the initiation of angiogenesis during very early luteal development in the cow.

In the early CL, FGF2 was localised to endothelial cells but the localization changed to the cytoplasm of luteal cells after 5 to 7 d (Schams *et al.* 1994). VEGFA (mainly localised in the cytoplasm of luteal cells) plays a fundamental role in maintenance of the luteal vasculature following cessation of luteal growth when active angiogenesis is no longer occurring. Indeed, VEGF enhanced endothelial platelet-derived growth factor (PDGF)-BB, a potent stimulator of neovascularisation; whereas, FGF2 enhanced PDGF receptor expression in pericytes and smooth muscle cells surrounding vasculature (Kano *et al.* 2005). Stimulation with VEGF and FGF2 caused a significant pericyte/muscle cell recruitment and formation of vasculature compared with single-agent stimulation, indicating a different contribution of both factors in neovascularisation (Kano *et al.* 2005).

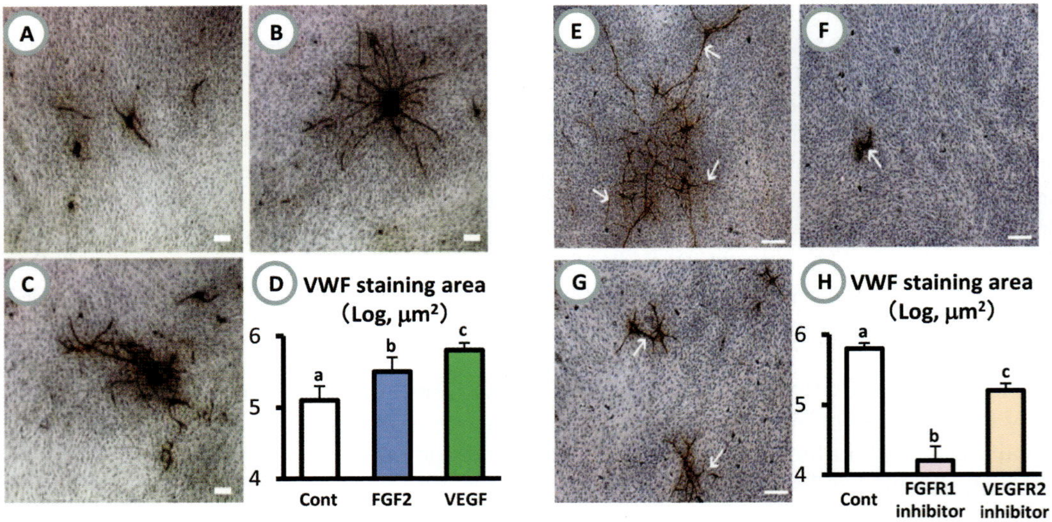

Fig. 2. The effect of FGF2, VEGFA and inhibitors of angiogenesis on the development of the luteal endothelial network in vitro (modified from Robinson *et al.*, 2009; Woad *et al.*, 2009). Luteal cells were dispersed from early CLs. In Figure 2D, luteal cells were treated with control (open bar, Fig. 2A), 1 ng/ml FGF2 (blue bar, Fig. 2B), and 1 ng/ml VEGFA (green bar, Fig. 2C) for 9 days. In Figure 2H, the luteal cells were treated either with control medium containing 1 ng/ml FGF2 and VEGFA (Cont, open bar), plus 1 μM FGFR1 inhibitor (SU5402, pink bar) and 2 μM VEGFR2 inhibitor (SU1498, orange bar) for 9 days. The endothelial cells were immunostained (brown) with von Willbrand Factor (VWF). The scale bar represents 50 μm. Following image analysis and quantification of VWF immunostaining, the effects of angiogenic factors and inhibitors of angiogenesis are shown on total area of VWF in Fig. 2D and 2H. The significant differences ($P < 0.05$) between treatment groups are indicated by different letters and the values are meant + S.E.M.

Potential interaction between cytokines and angiogenesis in the developing CL

The early CL produces angiogenic and luteotropic factors. Tumor necrosis factor-α (TNFα) is recognised as a tumoricidal factor produced by activated macrophages and luteal cells; TNFα and its receptors are detected in the early CL (Sakumoto *et al.* 2000). TNFα is a representative angiogenic factor regulating VEGF and FGF2 in bovine retinal cells (Yoshida *et al.* 2004). Interleukin (IL)-1 and IL-8, mainly produced by activated monocytes and macrophages, are also good candidates as angiogenic factors. Indeed, IL-1α and IL-1β can up-regulate VEGF expression in endometriotic stromal cells (Li *et al.* 1995). Koch *et al.,* (1992) indicated that IL-8 can induce the same levels of chemotaxis, proliferation and angiogenesis in human endothelial cells as FGF2. These findings lead to the hypothesis that various cytokines effectively coordinate to promote angiogenesis and ensure luteal development and function.

Extracellular matrix (ECM) is crucial for angiogenesis and tissue remodeling. Matrix metalloproteinases (MMPs) cleave specific components of the ECM and are inhibited by tissue inhibitors of metalloproteinases (TIMPs). MMPs and TIMPs play a major role in the process of follicular development and atresia, ovulation and CL development, maintenance and regression. A detailed mechanism of MMP-TIMP system in the ruminant CL was nicely reviewed previously (Curry & Smith 2006; Smith *et al.* 1999).

Distinct regulatory mechanisms of $PGF_{2\alpha}$ in the early and midcycle CL

An intriguing question concerning bovine CL function in recent years is "Why is the developing CL (d 1 to 5 of the oestrous cycle) resistant to the luteolytic action of $PGF_{2\alpha}$; whereas, after d 5 exogenous $PGF_{2\alpha}$ can induce rapid luteolysis?" (Henricks *et al.* 1974; Levy *et al.* 2000). To investigate the mechanisms underlying the different actions of $PGF_{2\alpha}$ in the early CL ($PGF_{2\alpha}$-resistant) versus midcycle CL ($PGF_{2\alpha}$-responsive) in domestic animals, several studies have focused on potential differences in steroidogenesis (Tsai & Wiltbank 1998), prostaglandin synthesis (Silva *et al.* 2000; Tsai & Wiltbank 1997b), immune function (Tsai *et al.* 1997a) and vasoactive factors (Choudhary *et al.* 2004; Levy *et al.* 2000; Wright *et al.* 2001). Although $PGF_{2\alpha}$ acutely decreased mRNA expression of 3β-HSD in both the early and midcycle CL, $PGF_{2\alpha}$ decreased StAR mRNA expression in the midcycle CL but not in the early CL (Tsai & Wiltbank 1998), indicating that StAR may be a key factor in reduced steroidogenesis following $PGF_{2\alpha}$ administration in the cow.

Prostaglandin $F_{2\alpha}$ receptor (FPr) mRNA is expressed in the CL at high levels throughout the oestrous cycle (Sakamoto *et al.* 1995; Wiltbank *et al.* 1995). Shirasuna et al., (2008) showed that FPr was localised to luteal cells but also to large blood vessels (mainly endothelial cells) in the periphery of the early and midcycle CL. The presence of FPr in the early CL can induce a specific tissue response (Levy *et al.* 2000; Tsai & Wiltbank 1998). Indeed, these previous reports indicated that FPr mRNA expression was decreased by $PGF_{2\alpha}$ administration at both stages (Levy *et al.* 2000; Tsai & Wiltbank 1998). Thus, the refractoriness of the early CL to the luteolytic effect of $PGF_{2\alpha}$ is not caused by a lack of the FPr.

Angiogenic factors

In a study focusing on the response of angiogenic factors to $PGF_{2\alpha}$ administration, $PGF_{2\alpha}$ injection down-regulated mRNA expression of VEGFA and FGF2 in the midcycle CL (Shirasuna *et al.* 2010b), suggesting that inhibiting angiogenesis may initiate or at least contribute to luteolysis. $PGF_{2\alpha}$ administration drastically decreased VEGF protein expression, in the bovine midcycle CL, after 30 min (Berisha *et al.* 2010). Interestingly, in the early CL (d 4 of the oestrous cycle), $PGF_{2\alpha}$ stimulated mRNA expression of VEGFs and FGF2 (Shirasuna *et al.* 2010b) and $PGF_{2\alpha}$ up-regulated VEGF transcription in human cancer cells (Sales *et al.* 2005). Moreover, both the production of $PGF_{2\alpha}$ and mRNA expression of COX-2 were higher in the early CL compared to other stages of the luteal phase (Kobayashi *et al.* 2001; Milvae & Hansel 1983). Importantly, in the bovine early CL, $PGF_{2\alpha}$ clearly stimulated progesterone secretion (Miyamoto *et al.* 1993; Okuda *et al.* 1998), and VEGF and FGF2 stimulated $PGF_{2\alpha}$ and progesterone secretion (Kobayashi *et al.* 2001). Consequently, it is proposed that $PGF_{2\alpha}$, in the early CL, acts as a local regulator to enhance progesterone secretion directly and also indirectly by stimulating VEGF and FGF2 (Fig. 3). The preceding mechanism may be one of the main reasons why the early CL is resistant to the luteolytic effects of $PGF_{2\alpha}$ (Miyamoto *et al.* 2009).

Insulin-like growth factors

The insulin-like growth factor (IGF) system is essential for support of progesterone secretion from luteal cells. The bovine and ovine CL have been identified as sites of IGF-I and IGF-II mRNA expression as well as peptide production and action throughout the luteal phase (Einspanier *et al.* 1990; Khan-Dawood *et al.* 1994; Sauerwein *et al.* 1992). The mRNA expression of IGF-I

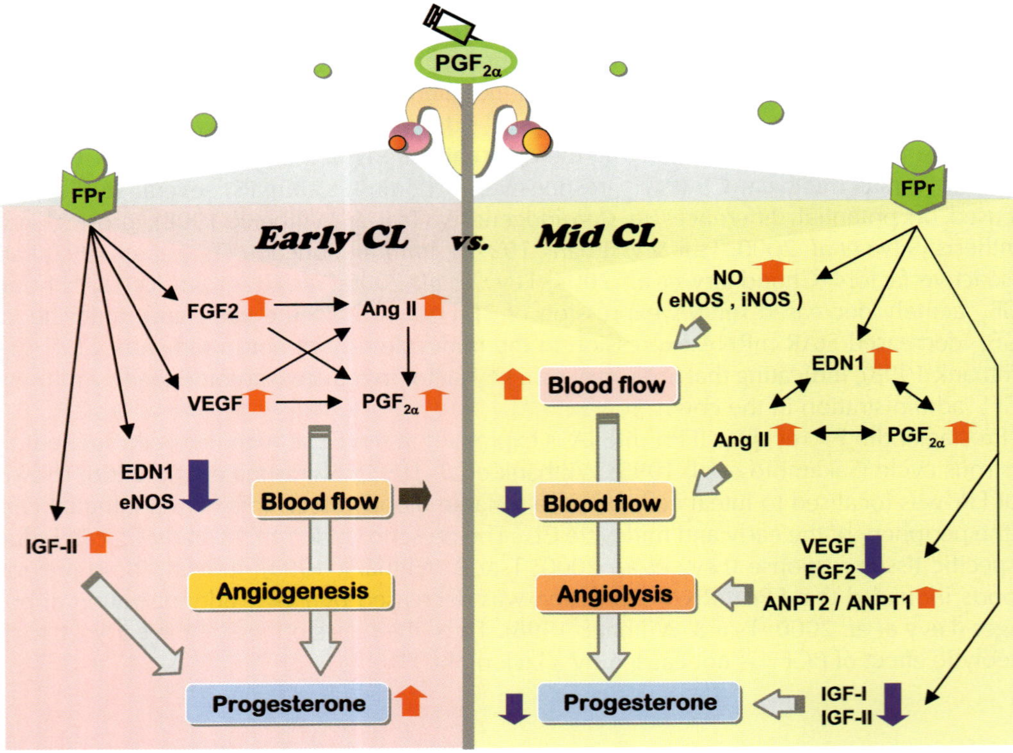

Fig. 3. Proposed model for the differential response of the early and mid-cycle CL to $PGF_{2\alpha}$ administration in the cow. After $PGF_{2\alpha}$ injection, $PGF_{2\alpha}$ enters into the CL via bloodstream. In the early CL, $PGF_{2\alpha}$ acutely stimulates VEGF, FGF2 and IGF-II expression in the bovine CL. VEGF and FGF2 stimulate luteal Ang II and $PGF_{2\alpha}$, and Ang II stimulates luteal $PGF_{2\alpha}$. This local positive feedback system between angiogenic and vasoactive factors supports angiogenesis and progesterone secretion within the CL; consequently, the early CL exhibits resistance to the luteolytic effect of $PGF_{2\alpha}$. Additionally, $PGF_{2\alpha}$ acutely suppresses EDN1 and eNOS expression in the bovine early CL, probably contributing to no response in blood flow.

In the midcycle CL, $PGF_{2\alpha}$ suppresses VEGF and FGF2 expression and creates the increased ratio of ANPT2/ANPT1 (an index of unstability of vessels), initiating angiolysis within the CL. In addition, $PGF_{2\alpha}$ decreases IGF-I and IGF-II expression directly causing a reduction in progesterone. A luteolytic dose of $PGF_{2\alpha}$ stimulates NO production by eNOS and iNOS expression in the CL, thus the luteal blood flow (one of the earliest physiological signs of the luteolytic cascade in the cow) is acutely increased as a result of vasodilation by NO action. Coincidently, vasoactive factors such as EDN1, Ang II and luteal $PGF_{2\alpha}$ start to increase within the CL to induce severe vasoconstriction. These events are coordinated and induce directly or indirectly the drastic decrease in progesterone secretion.

and IGF-II are higher in the early CL than other stages of the bovine luteal phase (Schams *et al.* 2002). Also, IGF-I was localised to both large and small luteal cells, whereas, IGF-II was localised to the perivascular fibroblasts of large blood vessels and pericytes of capillaries in the bovine CL (Amselgruber *et al.* 1994). Although $PGF_{2\alpha}$ significantly inhibited mRNA expression of both IGF-I and IGF-II in the midcycle CL, IGF-II mRNA expression was stimulated by $PGF_{2\alpha}$ in the early CL (Shirasuna *et al.* 2010b). Importantly, the stimulatory effect on progesterone secretion of IGF-II was greater than that of IGF-I in bovine CL tissue culture (Green *et al.* 2007). Additionally, IGF-II stimulated the chemotactic motility of endothelial progenitor cells in a dose-dependent manner and increased neovascularisation in the mouse (Maeng *et al.* 2009). These data suggest that $PGF_{2\alpha}$ may have potential as an angiogenic and luteotrophic agent in the early CL.

Vasoactive factors

Vasoactive factors: EDN1, Ang II and NO are involved in the process of luteal regression in ruminants (Acosta *et al.* 2009; Girsh *et al.* 1996a; Hayashi & Miyamoto 1999; Hinckley & Milvae 2001; Miyamoto *et al.* 1997; Skarzynski *et al.* 2000). In fact, EDN1, Ang II and NO can inhibit progesterone secretion in the bovine (Girsh *et al.* 1996b; Miyamoto *et al.* 1997; Stirling *et al.* 1990) and ovine (Hinckley & Milvae 2001) CL *in vitro*. Moreover, $PGF_{2\alpha}$ stimulated biosynthesis of EDN1 (and EDN1 mRNA expression), Ang II (and ACE mRNA expression) and NO (and eNOS/iNOS mRNA expression) *in vivo* and *in vitro* (Acosta *et al.* 2009; Girsh *et al.* 1996a; Hayashi & Miyamoto 1999; Hinckley & Milvae 2001; Miyamoto *et al.* 1997). A recent study indicated that $PGF_{2\alpha}$ stimulated mRNA expression of EDN1, ACE, eNOS and iNOS in the midcycle CL (Shirasuna *et al.* 2010b). Contrary to the midcycle CL, $PGF_{2\alpha}$ significantly decreased EDN1 and eNOS mRNA expression in the early CL (Shirasuna *et al.* 2010b). Therefore, $PGF_{2\alpha}$ likely has a dual function depending on the stage of the luteal phase, acting as a luteotrophic factor (in the early CL) and a luteolytic factor (in the midcycle CL) in the cow (Fig. 3).

Conclusions

Development of the bovine CL occurs rapidly and in a time dependent manner within 1 week after ovulation, with morphologic and biochemical changes in the cells of the theca interna and granulosa cells of the preovulatory follicle. These changes involve luteinisation of steroidogenic cells and angiogenesis to establish luteal function (progesterone secretion). Angiogenic factors such as FGF2 and VEGF have a crucial role in CL development in ruminants. Additionally, the luteolysin $PGF_{2\alpha}$ has a stage-specific action depending on the stage of luteal development (early vs. mid) during the oestrous cycle in the cow. Taken together, $PGF_{2\alpha}$ appears to possess a dual function, acting as a luteotrophic or an anti-luteolytic factor by stimulating angiogenic factors in the early CL but acting essentially as a luteolytic factor by stimulating vasoactive- and PG-related factors and by inhibiting angiogenic factors, in the midcycle CL in the cow.

Clearly, the main function of the CL is to produce progesterone, which is a prerequisite for survival of the embryo, implantation and maintenance of pregnancy. In the cow, maternal concentrations of progesterone have a marked influence on the development of the embryo and its ability to produce interferon τ (IFNτ). Mann *et al.* (1999) indicated that a late rise in progesterone after post-ovulation or inadequate progesterone secretion during the early luteal phase resulted in the development of compromised embryos with limited ability to produce IFNτ during the maternal recognition period (d 16 after insemination). In contrast, d 16 embryos of cows with an earlier rise in progesterone secretion were more elongated and produced large amounts of IFNτ (Mann *et al.* 1999). Moreover, the progesterone concentration in milk of pregnant cows was significantly higher than cows that were mated but not pregnant cows on d 6 after insemination (Mann *et al.* 1999). These findings strongly suggest that an effective and immediate increase in progesterone is critical in stimulating proper embryo development and IFNτ synthesis.

Secretion of adequate amounts of progesterone during luteal development requires proper differentiation and luteinisation of theca and granulosa cells into luteal cells, growth of blood vessels, and the establishment of a blood supply (angiogenesis). Inadequate luteinisation and angiogenesis during the early luteal phase results in poor progesterone secretion causing compromised embryo development and a reduction in fertility. Further investigation into the precise role of luteinisation and angiogenesis during luteal formation and development may provide new insight for better fertility in the cow.

Acknowledgements

Authors acknowledge Dr. Michael F. Smith, University of Missouri, MO, USA for constructive criticisms to improve the manuscript. This study was supported by a Grant-in-Aid for Scientific Research of the Japan Society for the Promotion of Science (JSPS) and the Global Center of Excellence (GCOE) Program, Ministry of Education, Culture, Sports, Science and Technology, Japan. K. S. was supported by JSPS Research Fellowships for Young Scientists.

References

Acosta TJ, Bah MB, Korzekwa A, Woclawek-Potocka I, Markiewicz W, Jaroszewski JJ, Okuda K & Skarzynski DJ 2009 Acute changes in circulating concentrations of progesterone and nitric oxide and partial pressure of oxygen during prostaglandin F2alpha-induced luteolysis in cattle. *Journal of Reproduction and Development* **55**, 149-155.

Acosta TJ, Ozawa T, Kobayashi S, Hayashi K, Ohtani M, Kraetzl WD, Sato K, Schams D & Miyamoto A 2000 Periovulatory changes in the local release of vasoactive peptides, prostaglandin F2alpha, and steroid hormones from bovine mature follicles in vivo. *Biology of Reproduction* **63**, 1253-1261.

Acosta TJ, Yoshizawa N, Ohtani M & Miyamoto A 2002 Local changes in blood flow within the early and midcycle corpus luteum after prostaglandin F2alpha injection in the cow. *Biology of Reproduction* **66**, 651-658.

Algire JE, Srikandakumar A, Guilbault LA & Downey BR 1992 Preovulatory changes in follicular prostaglandins and their role in ovulation in cattle. *Canadian Journal of Veterinary Research* **56**, 67-69.

Alila HW & Hansel W 1984 Origin of different cell types in the bovine corpus luteum as characterized by specific monoclonal antibodies. *Biology of Reproduction* **31**, 1015-1025.

Amselgruber W, Sinowatz F, Schams D & Skottner A 1994 Immunohistochemical aspects of insulin-like growth factors I and II in the bovine corpus luteum. *Journal of Reproduction and Fertility* **101**, 445-451.

Augustin HG, Braun K, Telemenakis I, Modlich U & Kuhn W 1995 Ovarian angiogenesis. Phenotypic characterization of endothelial cells in a physiological model of blood vessel growth and regression. *American Journal of Pathology* **147**, 339-351.

Bauer M, Schilling N & Spanel-Borowski K 2003 Development and regression of non-capillary vessels in the bovine corpus luteum. *Cell Tissue Research* **311**, 199-205.

Beard J 1897 The span of gestation and the cause of birth: a study of the critical period and its effects in mammalia.

Beindorff N, Nagai K, Shirasuna K, Herzog K, Hoeffmann K, Sasaki M, Bollwein H, Miyamoto A 2010 Vascular changes in the corpus luteum during early pregnancy in the cow. *Journal of Reproduction and Development* **56**, 263-270.

Berisha B, Meyer H & Schams D 2010 Effect of prostaglandin F2alpha on local luteotropic and angiogenic factors during induced functional luteolysis in the bovine corpus luteum. *Biology of Reproduction*, **82**, 940-947.

Berisha B, Schams D, Kosmann M, Amselgruber W & Einspanier R 2000a Expression and localisation of vascular endothelial growth factor and basic fibroblast growth factor during the final growth of bovine ovarian follicles. *Journal of Endocrinology* **167**, 371-382.

Berisha B, Schams D, Kosmann M, Amselgruber W & Einspanier R 2000b Expression and tissue concentration of vascular endothelial growth factor, its receptors, and localization in the bovine corpus luteum during estrous cycle and pregnancy. *Biology of Reproduction* **63**, 1106-1114.

Berisha B, Steffl M, Amselgruber W & Schams D 2006 Changes in fibroblast growth factor 2 and its receptors in bovine follicles before and after GnRH application and after ovulation. *Reproduction* **131**, 319-329.

Berndtson AK, Weaver CJ & Fortune JE 1996 Differential effects of oxytocin on steroid production by bovine granulosa cells. *Molecular and Cellular Endocrinology* **116**, 191-198.

Choudhary E, Costine BA, Wilson ME, Inskeep EK & Flores JA 2004 Prostaglandin F2alpha (PGF2alpha) independent and dependent regulation of the bovine luteal endothelin system. *Domestic Animal Endocrinology* **27**, 63-79.

Coiter V 1573 Externarum et internarum principalium humani corporis partium tabulae microform: atque exercitationes observationesque, novis, diversis, ac artificosissimus figeris illustratae, philosophis, medicis, in primis autem anatomico studio addictis summe utiles. *In Officina Theodorici Gerlatzeni.*

Corner GW & Allen WM 1929 Normal growth and implantation of embryos after very early ablation of the ovaries, under the influence of extracts of the corpus luteum. *American Journal of Physiology* **88**, 340-346.

Couet J, Martel C, Dupont E, Luu-The V, Sirard MA, Zhao HF, Pelletier G & Labrie F 1990 Changes in 3 beta-hydroxysteroid dehydrogenase/delta 5-delta 4 isomerase messenger ribonucleic acid, activity and protein levels during the estrous cycle in the bovine ovary. *Endocrinology* **127**, 2141-2148.

Curry TE, Jr. & Smith MF 2006 Impact of extracellular matrix remodeling on ovulation and the folliculo-luteal transition. *Seminars in Reproductive Medicine* **24**, 228-241.

De Graaf R & Mullierum D 1943 Organis Generationi Inservientibus. Leyden, 1672, translated by G. W. Corner. *Essays in Biology, Univ. of California Press.*

Einspanier R, Miyamoto A, Schams D, Muller M & Brem G 1990 Tissue concentration, mRNA expression and stimulation of IGF-I in luteal tissue during the oestrous cycle and pregnancy of cows. *Journal of Reproduction and Fertility* **90**, 439-445.

Farin CE, Moeller CL, Sawyer HR, Gamboni F & Niswender GD 1986 Morphometric analysis of cell types in the ovine corpus luteum throughout the estrous cycle. *Biology of Reproduction* **35**, 1299-1308.

Findlay JK 1986 Angiogenesis in reproductive tissues. *Journal of Endocrinology* **111**, 357-366.

Fisch B, Margara RA, Winston RM & Hillier SG 1989 Cellular basis of luteal steroidogenesis in the human ovary. *Journal of Endocrinology* **122**, 303-311.

Frenkel L 1903 Die Funktion des Corpus luteum. *Archiv. Gynaekol. (Munich)* **68**, 438-443.

Fraser HM, Dickson SE, Lunn SF, Wulff C, Morris KD, Carroll VA & Bicknell R 2000 Suppression of luteal angiogenesis in the primate after neutralization of vascular endothelial growth factor. *Endocrinology* **141**, 995-1000.

Ginther OJ, Araujo RR, Palhao MP, Rodrigues BL & Beg MA 2009 Necessity of sequential pulses of prostaglandin F2alpha for complete physiologic luteolysis in cattle. *Biol Reprod* **80**, 641-648.

Girsh E, Milvae RA, Wang W & Meidan R 1996a Effect of endothelin-1 on bovine luteal cell function: role in prostaglandin F2alpha-induced antisteroidogenic action. *Endocrinology* **137**, 1306-1312.

Girsh E, Wang W, Mamluk R, Arditi F, Friedman A, Milvae RA & Meidan R 1996b Regulation of endothelin-1 expression in the bovine corpus luteum: elevation by prostaglandin F2alpha. *Endocrinology* **137**, 5191-5196.

Gospodarowicz D, Cheng J, Lui GM, Baird A, Esch F & Bohlen P 1985 Corpus luteum angiogenic factor is related to fibroblast growth factor. *Endocrinology* **117**, 2383-2391.

Grazul-Bilska AT, Redmer DA & Reynolds LP 1991 Secretion of angiogenic activity and progesterone by ovine luteal cell types in vitro. *Journal of Animal Science* **69**, 2099-2107.

Green MP, Mann GE & Hunter MG 2007 Luteal characteristics and progesterone production on day 5 of the bovine oestrous cycle. *Reproduction in Domestic Animal* **42**, 643-647.

Hayashi K & Miyamoto A 1999 Angiotensin II interacts with prostaglandin F2alpha and endothelin-1 as a local luteolytic factor in the bovine corpus luteum in vitro. *Biology of Reproduction* **60**, 1104-1109.

Hazzard TM, Molskness TA, Chaffin CL & Stouffer RL 1999 Vascular endothelial growth factor (VEGF) and angiopoietin regulation by gonadotrophin and steroids in macaque granulosa cells during the peri-ovulatory interval. *Molecular Human Reproduction* **5**, 1115-1121.

Henricks DM, Long JT, Hill JR & Dickey JF 1974 The effect of prostaglandin F2alpha during various stages of the oestrous cycle of beef heifers. *Journal of Reproduction and Fertility* **41**, 113-120.

Hinckley ST & Milvae RA 2001 Endothelin-1 mediates prostaglandin F2alpha-induced luteal regression in the ewe. *Biology of Reproduction* **64**, 1619-1623.

Hojo T, Al-Zi'abi MO, Skarzynski DJ, Acosta TJ & Okuda K 2009 Changes in the vasculature of bovine corpus luteum during the estrous cycle and prostaglandin F2alpha-induced luteolysis. *Journal of Reproduction and Development* **55**, 512-517.

Kano MR, Morishita Y, Iwata C, Iwasaka S, Watabe T, Ouchi Y, Miyazono K, Miyazawa K 2005 VEGF-A and FGF-2 synergistically promote neoangiogenesis through enhancement of endogenous PDGF-B-PDGFRbeta signaling. *Journal of Cell Science* **118**, 3759-3768.

Kashiwagi S, Kajimura M, Yoshimura Y & Suematsu M 2002 Nonendothelial source of nitric oxide in arterioles but not in venules: alternative source revealed in vivo by diaminofluorescein microfluorography. *Circulation Research* **91**, e55-64.

Kesler DJ, Elmore RG, Brown EM & Garverick HA 1981 Gonadotropin releasing hormone treatment of dairy cows with ovarian cysts. I. Gross ovarian morphology and endocrinology. *Theriogenology* **16**, 207-217.

Khan-Dawood FS, Gargiulo AR, Dawood MY 1994 In vitro microdialysis of the ovine corpus luteum of pregnancy: effects of insulin-like growth factor on progesterone secretion. *Biology of Reproduction* **51**, 1299-1306.

Kobayashi S, Berisha B, Amselgruber WM, Schams D & Miyamoto A 2001 Production and localisation of angiotensin II in the bovine early corpus luteum: a possible interaction with luteal angiogenic factors and prostaglandin F2alpha. *Journal of Endocrinology* **170**, 369-380.

Koch AE, Polverini PJ, Kunkel SL, Harlow LA, DiPietro LA, Elner VM, Elner SG, Strieter RM 1992 Interleukin-8 as a macrophage-derived mediator of angiogenesis. *Science* **258**, 1798-1801.

Levy N, Kobayashi S, Roth Z, Wolfenson D, Miyamoto A & Meidan R 2000 Administration of prostaglandin F2alpha during the early bovine luteal phase does not alter the expression of ET-1 and of its type A receptor: a possible cause for corpus luteum refractoriness. *Biology of Reproduction* **63**, 377-382.

Li J, Perrella MA, Tsai JC, Yet SF, Hsieh CM, Yoshizumi M, Patterson C, Endege WO, Zhou F & Lee ME 1995 Induction of vascular endothelial growth factor gene expression by interleukin-1 beta in rat aortic smooth muscle cells. *Journal of Biological Chemistry* **270**, 308-312.

Loeb L 1906 The formation of the corpus luteum in the guinea pig. *Journal of American Medical Association* **46**, 416-423.

Maeng YS, Choi HJ, Kwon JY, Park YW, Choi KS, Min JK, Kim YH, Suh PG, Kang KS, Won MH, Kim YM & Kwon YG 2009 Endothelial progenitor cell homing: prominent role of the IGF2-IGF2R-PLCbeta2 axis. *Blood* **113**, 233-243.

Malpighi M 1897 *De Structura Glandarum Conglobatarum*.

Mann GE, Lamming GE, Robinson RS & Wathes DC 1999 The regulation of interferon-tau production and uterine hormone receptors during early pregnancy. *Journal of Reproduction and Fertility Supplement* **54**, 317-328.

McCracken JA, Custer EE & Lamsa JC 1999 Luteolysis: a neuroendocrine-mediated event. *Physiological Reviews* **79**, 263-323.

Milvae RA & Hansel W 1983 Prostacyclin, prostaglandin F2alpha and progesterone production by bovine luteal cells during the estrous cycle. *Biology of Reproduction* **29**, 1063-1068.

Miyamoto A, Kobayashi S, Arata S, Ohtani M, Fukui Y & Schams D 1997 Prostaglandin F2alpha promotes the inhibitory action of endothelin-1 on the bovine luteal function in vitro. *Journal of Endocrinology* **152**, R7-11.

Miyamoto A, Okuda K, Schweigert FJ & Schams D 1992 Effects of basic fibroblast growth factor, transforming growth factor-beta and nerve growth factor on the secretory function of the bovine corpus luteum in vitro. *Journal of Endocrinology* **135**, 103-114.

Miyamoto A & Schams D 1991 Oxytocin stimulates progesterone release from microdialyzed bovine corpus luteum in vitro. *Biology of Reproduction* **44**, 1163-1170.

Miyamoto A, Shirasuna K & Sasahara K 2009 Local regulation of corpus luteum development and regression in the cow: impact of angiogenic and vasoactive factors. *Domestic Animal Endocrinology* **37**, 159-169.

Miyamoto A, von Lutzow H & Schams D 1993 Acute actions of prostaglandin F2alpha, E2, and I2 in microdialyzed bovine corpus luteum in vitro. *Biology of Reproduction* **49**, 423-430.

Moor RM, Hay MF & Seamark RF 1975 The sheep ovary: regulation of steroidogenic, haemodynamic and structural changes in the largest follicle and adjacent tissue before ovulation. *Journal of Reproduction and Fertility* **45**, 595-604.

Murayama C, Miyazaki H, Miyamoto A & Shimizu T 2008 Involvement of Ad4BP/SF-1, DAX-1, and COUP-TFII transcription factor on steroid production and luteinization in ovarian theca cells. *Molecular and Cellular Biochemistry* **314**, 51-58.

Murdoch WJ & Dunn TG 1983 Luteal function after ovulation blockade by intrafollicular injection of indomethacin in the ewe. *Journal of Reproduction and Fertility* **69**, 671-675.

Niswender GD, Juengel JL, Silva PJ, Rollyson MK & McIntush EW 2000 Mechanisms controlling the function and life span of the corpus luteum. *Physiological Reviews* **80**, 1-29.

Niswender GD, Reimers TJ, Diekman MA & Nett TM 1976 Blood flow: a mediator of ovarian function. *Biology of Reproduction* **14**, 64-81.

O'Shea JD, Rodgers RJ & D'Occhio MJ 1989 Cellular composition of the cyclic corpus luteum of the cow. *Journal of Reproduction and Fertility* **85**, 483-487.

Okuda K, Uenoyama Y, Lee KW, Sakumoto R & Skarzynski D 1998 Progesterone stimulation by prostaglandin F2alpha involves the protein kinase C pathway in cultured bovine luteal cells. *Journal of Reproduction and Development* **44**, 79-84.

Reynolds LP, Grazul-Bilska AT & Redmer DA 2000 Angiogenesis in the corpus luteum. *Endocrine* **12**, 1-9.

Robinson RS, Hammond AJ, Mann GE & Hunter MG 2008 A novel physiological culture system that mimics luteal angiogenesis. *Reproduction* **135**, 405-413.

Robinson RS, Woad KJ, Hammond AJ, Laird M, Hunter MG & Mann GE 2009 Angiogenesis and vascular function in the ovary. *Reproduction* **138**, 869-881.

Sakamoto K, Miwa K, Ezashi T, Okuda-Ashitaka E, Okuda K, Houtani T, Sugimoto T, Ito S & Hayaishi O 1995 Expression of mRNA encoding the prostaglandin F2alpha receptor in bovine corpora lutea throughout the oestrous cycle and pregnancy. *Journal of Reproduction and Fertility* **103**, 99-105.

Sakumoto R, Berisha B, Kawate N, Schams D & Okuda K 2000 Tumor necrosis factor-alpha and its receptor in bovine corpus luteum throughout the estrous cycle. *Biology of Reproduction* **62**, 192-199.

Sales KJ, List T, Boddy SC, Williams AR, Anderson RA, Naor Z & Jabbour HN 2005 A novel angiogenic role for prostaglandin F2alpha-FP receptor interaction in human endometrial adenocarcinomas. *Cancer Research* **65**, 7707-7716.

Sauerwein H, Miyamoto A, Gunther J, Meyer HH & Schams D 1992 Binding and action of insulin-like growth factors and insulin in bovine luteal tissue during the oestrous cycle. *Journal of Reproduction and Fertility* **96**, 103-115.

Schams D, Amselgruber W, Einspanier R, Sinowatz F & Gospodarowicz D 1994 Localization and tissue concentration of basic fibroblast growth factor in the bovine corpus luteum. *Endocrine* **2**, 907-912.

Schams D & Berisha B 2004 Regulation of corpus luteum

function in cattle: an overview. *Reproduction in Domestic Animal* **39**, 241-251.

Schams D, Berisha B, Kosmann M & Amselgruber WM 2002 Expression and localization of IGF family members in bovine antral follicles during final growth and in luteal tissue during different stages of estrous cycle and pregnancy. *Domestic Animal Endocrinology* **22**, 51-72.

Schams D, Kosmann M, Berisha B, Amselgruber WM & Miyamoto A 2001 Stimulatory and synergistic effects of luteinising hormone and insulin like growth factor 1 on the secretion of vascular endothelial growth factor and progesterone of cultured bovine granulosa cells. *Experimental and Clinical Endocrinology & Diabetes* **109**, 155-162.

Shemesh M & Hansel W 1975 Stimulation of prostaglandin synthesis in bovine ovarian tissues by arachidonic acid and luteinizing hormone. *Biology of Reproduction* **13**, 448-452.

Shimizu T, Jiang JY, Iijima K, Miyabayashi K, Ogawa Y, Sasada H & Sato E 2003 Induction of follicular development by direct single injection of vascular endothelial growth factor gene fragments into the ovary of miniature gilts. *Biology of Reproduction* **69**, 1388-1393.

Shimizu T, Sudo N, Yamashita H, Murayama C, Miyazaki H & Miyamoto A 2009 Histone H3 acetylation of StAR and decrease in DAX-1 is involved in the luteinization of bovine granulosa cells during in vitro culture. *Molecular and Cellular Biochemistry* **328**, 41-47.

Shirasuna K, Asahi T, Sasaki M, Shimizu T & Miyamoto A 2010a Distribution of arteriolovenous vessels, capillaries and eNOS expression in the bovine corpus luteum during the estrous cycle: a possible implication of different sensitivity by luteal phase to PGF2alpha in the increase of luteal blood flow. *Journal of Reproduction and Development* **56**, 124-130.

Shirasuna K, Sasahara K, Matsui M, Shimizu T & Miyamoto A 2010b Prostaglandin F2alpha differentially affects mRNA expression relating to angiogenesis, vasoactivation and prostaglandins in the early and mid corpus luteum in the cow. *Journal of Reproduction and Development* **56**, 428-436.

Shirasuna K, Watanabe S, Asahi T, Wijagunawardane MPB, Sasahara K, Jiang C, Matsui M, Sasaki M, Shimizu T, Davis JS & Miyamoto A 2008 Prostaglandin F2alpha increases endothelial nitric oxide synthase in the periphery of the bovine corpus luteum: the possible regulation of blood flow at an early stage of luteolysis. *Reproduction* **135**, 527-539.

Short RE, Staigmiller RB, Bellows RA & Ford SP 1995 Endocrine responses in cows fed Ponderosa pine needles and the effects of stress, corpus luteum regression, progestin, and ketoprofen. *Journal of Animal Science* **73**, 198-205.

Silva PJ, Juengel JL, Rollyson MK & Niswender GD 2000 Prostaglandin metabolism in the ovine corpus luteum: catabolism of prostaglandin F2alpha (PGF2alpha) coincides with resistance of the corpus luteum to PGF2alpha. *Biology of Reproduction* **63**, 1229-1236.

Sirois J 1994 Induction of prostaglandin endoperoxide synthase-2 by human chorionic gonadotropin in bovine preovulatory follicles in vivo. *Endocrinology* **135**, 841-848.

Skarzynski DJ, Kobayashi S & Okuda K 2000 Influence of nitric oxide and noradrenaline on prostaglandin F2alpha-induced oxytocin secretion and intracellular calcium mobilization in cultured bovine luteal cells. *Biology of Reproduction* **63**, 1000-1005.

Slotta K, Ruschig H & Fels E 1934 Reindarstellung der Hormone aus dem corpus luteum. *Berich. Dtsch. Chem. Gesellschaft* **67**, 1270.

Smith MF, McIntush EW, Ricke WA, Kojima FN & Smith GW 1999 Regulation of ovarian extracellular matrix remodelling by metalloproteinases and their tissue inhibitors: effects on follicular development, ovulation and luteal function. *Journal of Reproduction and Fertility Supplement* **54**, 367-381.

Stirling D, Magness RR, Stone R, Waterman MR & Simpson ER 1990 Angiotensin II inhibits luteinizing hormone-stimulated cholesterol side chain cleavage expression and stimulates basic fibroblast growth factor expression in bovine luteal cells in primary culture. *Journal of Biological Chemistry* **265**, 5-8.

Tsai SJ, Juengel JL & Wiltbank MC 1997a Hormonal regulation of monocyte chemoattractant protein-1 messenger ribonucleic acid expression in corpora lutea. *Endocrinology* **138**, 4517-4520.

Tsai SJ & Wiltbank MC 1997b Prostaglandin F2alpha induces expression of prostaglandin G/H synthase-2 in the ovine corpus luteum: a potential positive feedback loop during luteolysis. *Biology of Reproduction* **57**, 1016-1022.

Tsai SJ & Wiltbank MC 1998 Prostaglandin F2alpha regulates distinct physiological changes in early and mid-cycle bovine corpora lutea. *Biology of Reproduction* **58**, 346-352.

Voss AK & Fortune JE 1991 Oxytocin secretion by bovine granulosa cells: effects of stage of follicular development, gonadotropins, and coculture with theca interna. *Endocrinology* **128**, 1991-1999.

Voss AK & Fortune JE 1993 Levels of messenger ribonucleic acid for cytochrome P450 17 alpha-hydroxylase and P450 aromatase in preovulatory bovine follicles decrease after the luteinizing hormone surge. *Endocrinology* **132**, 2239-2245.

Wiltbank MC, Dysko RC, Gallagher KP & Keyes PL 1988 Relationship between blood flow and steroidogenesis in the rabbit corpus luteum. *Journal of Reproduction and Fertility* **84**, 513-520.

Wiltbank MC, Shiao TF, Bergfelt DR & Ginther OJ 1995 Prostaglandin F2alpha receptors in the early bovine corpus luteum. *Biology of Reproduction* **52**, 74-78.

Wintersteiner O & Allen WM 1934 Crystalline progestin. *Journal of Biological Chemistry* **107**, 321-336.

Woad KJ, Hammond AJ, Hunter M, Mann GE, Hunter MG & Robinson RS 2009 FGF2 is crucial for the development of bovine luteal endothelial networks in vitro. *Reproduction* **138**, 581-588.

Wright MF, Sayre B, Keith Inskeep EK & Flores JA 2001 Prostaglandin F2alpha regulation of the bovine corpus luteum endothelin system during the early and midluteal phase. *Biology of Reproduction* **65**, 1710-1717.

Wulff C, Wilson H, Wiegand SJ, Rudge JS & Fraser HM 2002 Prevention of thecal angiogenesis, antral follicular growth, and ovulation in the primate by treatment with vascular endothelial growth factor Trap R1R2. *Endocrinology* **143**, 2797-2807.

Yamashita H, Kamada D, Shirasuna K, Matsui M, Shimizu T, Kida K, Berisha B, Schams D & Miyamoto A 2008 Effect of local neutralization of basic fibroblast growth factor or vascular endothelial growth factor by a specific antibody on the development of the corpus luteum in the cow. *Molecular Reproduction and Development* **75**, 1449-1456.

Yoshida S, Yoshida A & Ishibashi T 2004 Induction of IL-8, MCP-1, and bFGF by TNF-alpha in retinal glial cells: implications for retinal neovascularization during post-ischemic inflammation. *Graefes Arch Clin Exp Ophthalmol* **242**, 409-413.

Zheng J, Redmer DA & Reynolds LP 1993 Vascular development and heparin-binding growth factors in the bovine corpus luteum at several stages of the estrous cycle. *Biology of Reproduction* **49**, 1177-1189.

Inter- and intra-cellular mechanisms of prostaglandin $F_{2\alpha}$ action during corpus luteum regression in cattle

DJ Skarzynski[1] and K Okuda[2]

[1]Department of Reproductive Immunology and Pathology, Institute of Animal Reproduction and Food Research, Polish Academy of Sciences, Olsztyn, Tuwima-St. 10, 10-747 Olsztyn, Poland; [2]Laboratory of Reproductive Endocrinology, Graduate School of Natural Science and Technology, Okayama University, Okayama 700-8530, Japan

The bovine corpus luteum (CL) grows very fast and regresses within a few days at luteolysis. Mechanisms controlling development and secretory function of the bovine CL may involve many factors that are produced both within and outside the CL. In the cow, luteolysis is initiated by uterine prostaglandin (PG)$F_{2\alpha}$ released at the late luteal stage. It can also be induced by injection of exogenous $PGF_{2\alpha}$ given at the mid luteal stage. Luteolysis consists of a phase of rapid decrease in progesterone (P4) production by the CL, followed by a phase of structural regression. Although uterine $PGF_{2\alpha}$ is known to be the main luteolytic factor, its direct action on the CL is mediated by the products of accessory luteal cells: immune cells, endothelial cells, pericytes and fibroblasts. There are studies showing that beside endothelin-1, cytokines (tumor necrosis factor-α, interferons) and nitric oxide play critical roles in functional and structural luteolysis in cattle by stimulating leukotrienes and $PGF_{2\alpha}$, decreasing P4 secretion and apoptosis induction. Because of luteal blood flow and P4 concentrations decrease in parallel during both spontaneous and $PGF_{2\alpha}$-induced luteolysis, a decrease in luteal blood flow resulting in hypoxia has been proposed as one of the main luteolytic mechanisms in the cow. Hypoxia inhibits P4 synthesis in luteal cells by inhibiting the steroidogenic enzymes and promotes apoptosis of luteal cells by increasing pro-apoptotic proteins. Although reduction of luteal blood flow and hypoxia contribute to the late events of luteolysis, little is known about the physiological relevance and the cause of the transient increase in luteal blood flow and reactive oxygen species during the initial step of luteolysis.

Introduction

When animals do not become pregnant, regression of the corpus luteum (CL), named luteolysis, is essential for the normal cyclicity as it allows for the development of a new ovulatory follicle. Luteolysis occurs when there is no pregnancy on Day 16–18 after oestrus in cattle (McCracken *et al.* 1999). In the cow, luteolysis is initiated by prostaglandin (PG)$F_{2\alpha}$ released from the uterus at the late luteal stage (McCracken *et al.* 1999). During luteolysis, $PGF_{2\alpha}$ of uterine origin enters the ovarian artery from the utero-ovarian vein via a countercurrent exchange mechanism (Mc-Cracken *et al.* 1999). This allows uterine $PGF_{2\alpha}$ to pass directly into the ovary, without entering the pulmonary circulation, where it is enzymatically inactivated in the lungs. It has been shown

Corresponding author E-mail: d.skarzynski@pan.olsztyn.pl

that *in vivo* and *in vitro* $PGF_{2\alpha}$ induces a number of mechanisms leading to the regression of the CL, i.e. a decrease in progesterone (P4) secretion, down-regulation of receptors for luteotropic hormones, inhibition of cholesterol cellular uptake, inhibition of cholesterol transport through the cell and/or across the mitochondrial membranes, inhibition of steroidogenic enzymes expression and activity, and finally increase of free calcium ions [Ca^{2+}] in both types of steroidogenic luteal cells (Davis *et al.* 1987; Alila *et al.* 1990; Skarzynski & Okuda 1999). Although *in vivo* $PGF_{2\alpha}$ decreases P4 concentrations in number of species (McCracken *et al.* 1999), it is even luteotropic in the monolayer cultured steroidogenic luteal cells (Alila *et al.* 1988; Okuda *et al.* 1998; Korzekwa *et al.* 2008a). In the cultured bovine luteal cells, supplied with lipoprotein (LP)s as a source of cholesterol-enhancing P4 secretion, $PGF_{2\alpha}$ treatment decreased only LH- and LPs-stimulated P4 secretion (Pate & Condon 1989; Wiltbank *et al.* 1990). Thus, the direct influence of $PGF_{2\alpha}$ on steroidogenesis in luteal cells is still controversial and depends on the methodology of examination. Therefore, the luteolytic action of $PGF_{2\alpha}$ within the bovine CL seems to be mediated by the products of the immune and endothelial luteal cells (reviewed by Pate & Keyes 2001; Meidan *et al.* 2005; Berisha & Schams 2005).

The bovine CL is composed of a heterogeneous mixture of cell types. There are at least two types of steroidogenic cells, large and small luteal cells, which originate from the granulosa and thecal cells of the follicle ruptured at ovulation, respectively. The bovine CL consists of not only steroidogenic luteal cells but also non-steroidogenic cells (accessory cells), *i.e.* vascular endothelial cells, pericytes and fibroblasts, and immune cells such as lymphocytes and macrophages (Lei *et al.* 1991; Hojo *et al.* 2009). Pate and her colleague suggested that immune cells and their products fulfill the part of luteolytic $PGF_{2\alpha}$ action on steroidogenic luteal cells (reviewed by Pate & Keyes 2001; Pate 2003). Additionally, nitric oxide (NO) and leukotriene (LT)C4 are suggested to serve as $PGF_{2\alpha}$ mediators during luteolysis in cattle (Blair *et al.* 1997; Jaroszewski & Hansel 2000; Skarzynski *et al.* 2003a, b; Korzekwa *et al.* 2006). Luteolytic action of $PGF_{2\alpha}$ may also be mediated by endothelin-1 (EDN1), the main product of the luteal endothelial cells (Girsh *et al.* 1996; Davis *et al.* 2003; Meidan *et al.* 2005). The above data strongly indicate that the contact between different types of luteal cells seems to be necessary for its regression. This review focuses on inter-, intracellular, as well receptor mechanisms of uterine $PGF_{2\alpha}$ secretion and action on bovine CL. Furthermore, some of our and others' data on intraluteal mediators of luteolytic actions of $PGF_{2\alpha}$ on bovine CL during luteolysis have also been reviewed. Moreover, the regulation of the blood flow into the CL as an important mechanisms of regression of bovine CL is also discussed.

Uterine prostaglandin $F_{2\alpha}$ is the main luteolytic factor in ruminants

The importance of the uterus in the control of luteal regression was first reported by Loeb (1923), who demonstrated that hysterectomy abolished the oestrous cycle and caused abnormal persistence of the CL in guinea pig. It has also been demonstrated in the cow that the CL is maintained after bilateral hysterectomy (Wiltbank & Casida 1956). In 1970, Lukaszewska & Hansel (1970) showed that a low-molecular-weight substance, extracted from the uterus, has a luteolytic action. Finally, this substance was identified as an arachidonic acid metabolite, *i.e.* $PGF_{2\alpha}$ (Hansel *et al.* 1975). The importance of uterine $PGF_{2\alpha}$ in the functional and structural demise of the bovine CL has been well established (reviewed by McCracken *et al.* 1999; Okuda *et al.* 2002).

Prostaglandins are produced from arachidonic acid (AA) liberated from phospholipid stores through the action of phospholipase (PL)s. Arachidonic acid is then converted into prostaglandin endoperoxide H_2 (PGH_2) by prostaglandin G/H synthases (PTGS, previously known as cyclooxygenase - COX). Two isoforms of the PTGS enzyme, types 1 and 2, are coded by different genes and catalyze the double oxygenation and reduction of AA. Among several enzymes capable of converting PGH_2 into $PGF_{2\alpha}$ (PGF-synthase, PGFS), in the endometrium of cyclic cows around the time of luteolysis only AKR1B5, an aldose reductase also exhibiting 20α-hydroxysteroid dehydrogenase (20α-HSD) activity, was shown to be up-regulated and expressed in significant amounts [Madore *et al.* 2003]. According to Madore *et al.* (2003), AKR1B5 has the ability to combine two converging functions: inactivation of P4 and generation of $PGF_{2\alpha}$. This makes AKR1B5 a multifunctional enzyme with complementary action in the endometrium during luteolysis and delivery, when P4 secretion and luteal function is terminated.

For a long time, the factor(s) that can induce the luteolytic $PGF_{2\alpha}$ output for the bovine uteri have been defined and discussed (reviewed by McCracken et al. 1999; Okuda et al. 2002). It was established in the 80´s in the previous century that $PGF_{2\alpha}$ stimulates oxytocin (OT) released from the ovine CL, and that OT stimulates endometrial PG production (Flint & Sheldrick 1982). Therefore, at the time of luteolysis, CL-derived OT and uterus-derived $PGF_{2\alpha}$ were believed to create a positive feedback loop in ruminants. In fact, the importance of ovarian and / or hypohysial OT in the control of luteolysis in cows was first reported by Armstrong & Hansel (1956). Later, Newcomb *et al.* (1977) reported that injection of OT increased $PGF_{2\alpha}$ secretion in cows. Finally, it has been demonstrated that OT-stimulated $PGF_{2\alpha}$ secretion is associated with the activity of protein kinase (PK)C (Burs *et al.* 1997, Skarzynski *et al.* 2000a) and the gene expression of several enzymes involving in PGs synthesis, e.g., PLA2, PTGS-2, and PGFS (Madore *et al.* 2003). However, there is increasing evidence that OT is not essential for the initiation of $PGF_{2\alpha}$ output during luteolysis in the cow (Parkinson *et al.* 1992; Kotwica *et al.* 1997, 1998; Douglas & Britt 2000). Concentrations of OT in blood (Parkinson et al. 1992; Kotwica et al. 1998), and in intact (Parkinson et al. 1992) and microdialyzed CL (Douglas & Britt 2000) are extremely low at the time of spontaneous luteolysis. Moreover, the blockade of uterine OT receptors with a specific OT antagonist from Day 15 to Day 22 of the cycle affected neither luteolysis nor the duration of the oestrous cycle in heifers (Kotwica *et al.* 1997). Therefore, $PGF_{2\alpha}$ secretion by the endometrium may be regulated not only by OT but also by one or more other factors (i.e. cytokines, steroids and peptide hormones) in cattle (reviewed by Okuda et al. 2002).

Tumor necrosis factor-α (TNF) and its receptors have been demonstrated to be present in the bovine cyclic endometrium (Miyamoto *et al.* 2000; Okuda *et al.* 2010). TNF stimulates $PGF_{2\alpha}$ output by the bovine uterus *in vitro* (Miyamoto *et al.* 2000; Skarzynski et al. 2000a; Murakami *et al.* 2001) as well as in the conscious cows (Skarzynski *et al.* 2003b; 2007; 2009). Moreover, we have shown that the infusion of the lower dose of TNF (1 mg) increased plasma concentrations of PGFM (metabolite of luteolytic $PGF_{2\alpha}$) and inhibited P4 production finally resulting in shortening of the oestrous cycle (Skarzynski *et al.* 2003b). Furthermore, the inhibition of PG production in the bovine uterus and/or CL by a non-selective PTGS inhibitor (indomethacin) preinfusion has completely withdrawn the luteolytic action of TNF showing that action on TNF on the bovine oestrous cycle is mediated by PG production and action (Skarzynski et al. 2007). This cytokine augmented $PGF_{2\alpha}$ production only in the bovine endometrial stromal cells via the activation of PLA_2 and NO synthase *in vitro* (Skarzynski *et al.* 2000a) and *in vivo* (Skarzynski *et al.* 2007), as well as via increasing *PTGS-2* mRNA expression (Okuda et al. 2004a). Because the expression of TNF protein and mRNA have been found only in epithelial cells of the bovine endometrium, TNF seems to play a role as a paracrine factor for regulating endometrial function in the cow (Okuda *et al.* 2010). Therefore, we have proposed a hypothesis that endometrial (Okuda *et al.* 2010) and / or luteal TNF (Shaw & Britt 1995; Sakumoto *et al.* 2000) is a trigger for the output of $PGF_{2\alpha}$ from the uterus in the initiation of luteolysis (Fig. 1).

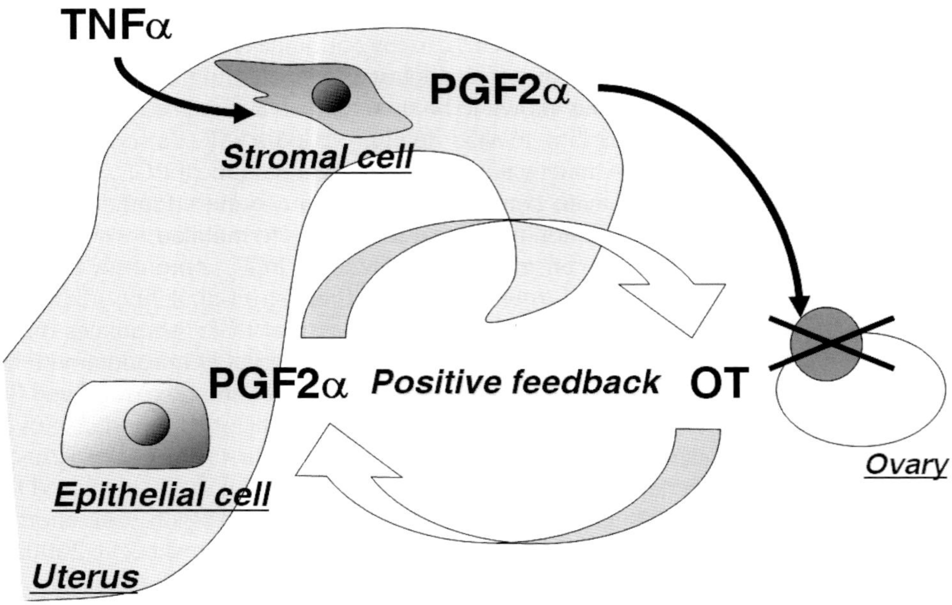

Fig. 1. Hypothetical model of the regulation of prostaglandin (PG)$F_{2\alpha}$ secretion by the bovine endometrium during luteolysis (see text for details).

For the initiation of bovine luteal regression, the pulsatile character of $PGF_{2\alpha}$ is much more important and plays a mandatory role rather than its absolute levels (Schramm et al. 1983; Lamsa *et al* 1989; Ginther *et al.* 2009, 2010). $PGF_{2\alpha}$ released from the endometrium, especially the inter-caruncular region of the surface epithelium of the uterus (Asselin et al. 1998), in a pulsatile manner causes regression of the bovine CL (Ginther *et al.* 2009, 2010). It has recently been shown, that the excessive, bolus $PGF_{2\alpha}$ doses may stimulate nonphysiologic P4 responses and only sequential $PGF_{2\alpha}$ pulses are required and able to stimulate the natural luteolysis in cattle (Ginther *et al.* 2009, 2010). In fact, such a long-lasting and permanent exposition of CL to $PGF_{2\alpha}$ action desensitized the ovine (Lamsa *et al.* 1989) and bovine CL (Skarzynski & Okuda 1999; Bah *et al.* 2006) on the luteolytic effect of supplementary-extraordinary $PGF_{2\alpha}$. A rest period of 6 h is required to restore the normal response to $PGF_{2\alpha}$ (Lamsa *et al.* 1989). However, TNF in concert with other inflammatory mediators including NO may sensitize the bovine CL to luteolytic $PGF_{2\alpha}$ action (Skarzynski *et al.* 2000b; Ohtani *et al.* 2004).

Intra- and intercellular mechanisms of $PGF_{2\alpha}$ action

The receptor for $PGF_{2\alpha}$ (FPr) is coupled to phospholipase C, generating two second messengers, inositol triphosphate (IP3), which is involved in the release of intracellular [Ca^{2+}] and diacylglycerol (DAG), an activator of PKC (Sakamoto *et al.* 1995). FPr was cloned in the bovine species by Sakamoto *et al.* (1994). This receptor was considered as a contractile receptor with two well recognized isoforms (FPr-α and FPr-β), and generated by alternative splicing of C terminal of a single gene identified in ovine and bovine CL (Ezashi *et al.* 1997). Bovine FPr-β and other, new discovered FPr isoforms may act as a negative regulator to attenuate the normal FPr-α-mediated protein kinase C function. However, the data on FPr-β and other FPr isoforms (FPr-δ, -γ, -ε and -ζ) in the bovine CL are at a preliminary stage (Akabane et al. 2008).

As mentioned, the effects of $PGF_{2\alpha}$ in bovine CL appear to be mediated through the PKC second messenger system (Davis *et al.* 1987; Wiltbank *et al.* 1990; Sen *et al.* 2005; Choundhary *et al.* 2005). $PGF_{2\alpha}$ activates PLC, which causes hydrolysis of membrane phosphatidylinositol (PIP2) to IP3 and DAG. IP3 stimulates the release of [Ca^{2+}] from intracellular stores, while DAG enhances the affinity of PKC for calcium, resulting in an increase of free intracellular [Ca^{2+}] concentration and activation of PKC (Davis *et al.* 1987). It has been demonstrated that $PGF_{2\alpha}$ activates the Raf/MEK1/mitogen-activated protein kinase signaling cascade in bovine luteal cells (Chen *et al.* 1998; Arvisais *et al.* 2010). Treatment of midluteal-phase cows *in vivo* with a luteolytic dose of $PGF_{2\alpha}$ resulted in a rapid increase in ERK and mammalian target of rapamycin (mTOR)/p70 ribosomal protein S6 kinase (p70S6K1) signalling and a rapid suppression of Akt phosphorylation in luteal tissue (Arvisais *et al.* 2010). Also *in vitro* treatment of primary cultures of luteal cells with $PGF_{2\alpha}$ as well, resulted in an increase in ERK and mTOR/p70S6K1 signalling and a diminished capacity of IGF-I to stimulate PI3K, Akt, and PKC (Arvisais *et al.* 2010). In fact, the actions of $PGF_{2\alpha}$ were mimicked by a PKC activator (PMA). Therefore, the activation of Raf/MEK1/mitogen-activated protein kinase by $PGF_{2\alpha}$ may provide a mechanism to transduce signals initiated by FPr_B on the cell surface into the nucleus and may be associated with transcriptional activation of luteal genes (Chen *et al.* 1998; Arvisais *et al.* 2010).

The phosphorylation events associated with the activation of PKC and the IP3-mediated sustained elevations of [Ca^{2+}] are believed to regulate OT secretion, to inhibit P4 and cause a cytotoxic effect (Wiltbank *et al.* 1990). Therefore, the luteolytic action of $PGF_{2\alpha}$ is attended by PKC and [Ca^{2+}] as secondary messengers inside the steroidogenic luteal cells (Sen *et al.* 2005; Choundhary *et al.* 2005). Nevertheless, it has been shown that PKC also mediates the luteotropic action of $PGF_{2\alpha}$ in the steroidogenic cell culture from the mid stage of oestrous cycle (Alila *et al.* 1990; Okuda *et al.* 1998). Thus, it should be emphasized that the various actions of $PGF_{2\alpha}$ on the bovine CL upon binding to its G protein-coupled receptor are initiated by the same PLC / DAG-IP3 / Ca^{2+} - PKC pathway.

The possible reason for such different effects are differences in the cell culture system and consequently differences in the cell-to-cell contact, gap junctions and connection-communication between large and small luteal cells and immune or/and endothelial cells (Okuda et al. 1998; Korzekwa *et al.* 2004, 2008a; Miyamoto *et al.* 1993; Sen *et al.* 2006; Shibaya *et al.* 2005; Bah *et al.* 2006). In contrast from the monolayer long-term system of the culture (at least 48-h of culture) used in the study by Okuda *et al.* (1998), Tsai & Wiltbank (1997) and Sen *et al.* (2006) conducted their experiments in luteal cell suspension, incubated and stimulated the cells for a shorten time. Luteal cells cultured in such a system of suspension are in contact with each other and keep their original shape during culture, thus the cytoskeleton works correctly (Shibaya *et al.* 2005). The cytoskeleton keeps a variety of cellular components in place and it has been implicated in a variety of cellular processes, such as cell motility, cell migration, spatial distribution of cell organelles, intracellular communication and cellular responses to membrane events (Shibaya *et al.* 2005). We have shown that the aggregate culture system that ensures three-dimensional, cell-to-cell contact created more physiological conditions for cell function than the *in vitro* monolayer system (Shibaya *et al.* 2005; Korzekwa *et al.* 2008a). Thus, the cell culture suspension system is better than the monolayer one to show the inhibitory effect of $PGF_{2\alpha}$ during luteolysis. The disorders in the cell shape and organization and in the gap junctions may disturb the action of PKC in the cells. Therefore, the model ensuring cell-to-cell contact and shape seems to be necessary for studying the influence of some biologically active substances (i.e. cytokines, $PGF_{2\alpha}$, END1, LT, NO) on bovine luteal function during luteolysis

(Skarzynski & Okuda 1999; Shibaya *et al.* 2005; Sen *et al.* 2006; Korzekwa *et al.* 2008a). Korzekwa *et al.* (2008a) have shown that the cell coculture model, including the main types of CL cells (i.e. steroidogenic, immune and endothelial luteal cells), is the most approximate to study $PGF_{2\alpha}$ role *in vitro* (Fig. 2). The cell-to-cell contact and interactions between endothelial and immune cells with steroidogenic CL cells are needed for luteolytic $PGF_{2\alpha}$ action within the bovine CL *in vitro*. Moreover, concerning *in vivo* studies, Ginther *et al.* (2009) pointed out that such unexpected observed dose-sensitive effects apparently represented a non-physiologic response to unnatural doses and delivery of $PGF_{2\alpha}$. It seems that many of the reported studies during the past few decades on the nature of the luteolytic process in cattle may have resulted in dubious interpretations, owing to potential artifactual or pharmacologic responses to unnatural doses or unnatural delivery of $PGF_{2\alpha}$ to the CL. Therefore, a dose and method of delivery that approximated the endogenous system is needed to study $PGF_{2\alpha}$ action on the bovine CL (Ginther *et al.* 2009). Nevertheless, as suggested by the authors, some reservations are required, owing to the unnatural time of treatment during mid luteal phase.

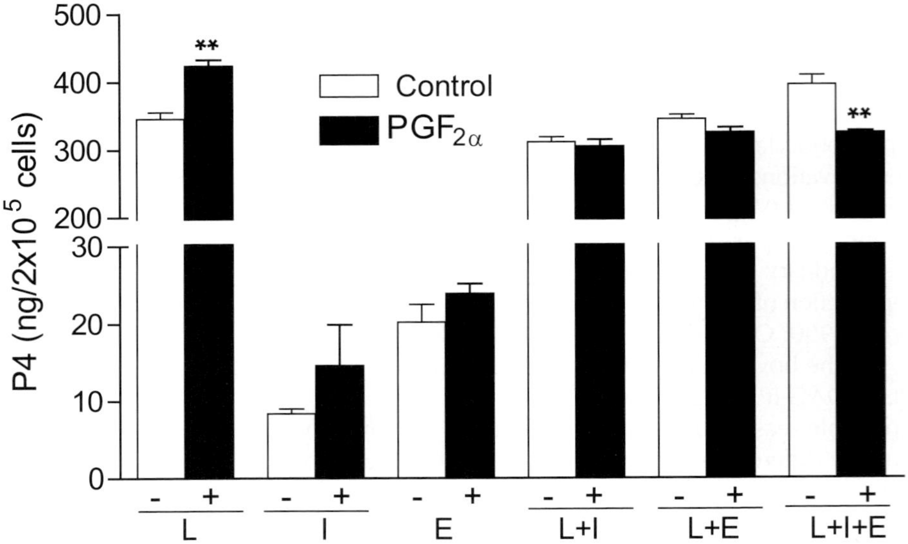

Fig. 2. Effect of prostaglandin (PG)$F_{2\alpha}$ on progesterone (P4) secretion by co-cultured bovine luteal cells (steroidogenic cells-L, endothelial cells-E and/or immune cells-I) obtained on Day 15/16 of the oestrous cycle. The cells were enzymatically isolated, pre-incubated in glass tubes in a shaking water bath for 2 h and then exposed to $PGF_{2\alpha}$ (10-6M) for 22 h. Asterisks indicate significant differences ($P < 0.05$) between the $PGF_{2\alpha}$-treated and Control. Modified from Korzekwa *et al.* 2008a.

Intraluteal mediators of luteolytic $PGF_{2\alpha}$ action

It was previously observed that $PGF_{2\alpha}$ stimulated (Alila *et al.* 1988; Okuda *et al.* 1998; Korzekwa *et al.* 2004), inhibited (Pate & Condon 1989) or had no direct effect on P4 secretion in cultured steroidogenic luteal cells. Therefore, it is suggested that the luteolytic action of $PGF_{2\alpha}$ on bovine CL is mediated by local factors, i.e. EDN1, cytokines and NO. However, the secretory functions of bovine luteal cells are regulated not only by PGs but also by others AA metabolites - LTs (Milvae *et al.* 1986, Korzekwa *et al.* 2010a, b). We have shown that LTs are produced and released in the bovine CL and modulate the production of P4 and PGs in the bovine reproductive tract during the oestrous cycle, influence on the lifespan of CL and may serve as luetolitic mediators (Jaroszewski *et al.* 2003b; Skarzynski et al. 2003b, Korzekwa et al. 2008b, 2010a, c). In addition, prokineticin 1 (PROK1, also termed endocrine gland-derived vascular endothelial growth factor - endocrine gland-derived VEGF) is involved in the recruitment of monocytes to regressing CL and their consequent activation therein (Kisliouk *et al.* 2007). Apelin (APJ, putative receptor protein related to angiotensin type 1 receptor - a G-protein-coupled receptor) and its receptors have been also identified as a novel regulators of blood flow and as an angiogenic factor during luteolysis in cattle (Shirasuna *et al.* 2008a). Moreover, Berisha *et al.* (2010) have recently shown that *in vivo* during $PGF_{2\alpha}$-induced luteolysis, insulin growth factor-1 (IGF1) and vascular endothelial growth factor (VEGFA) protein already decreased after 0.5 h after an analogue of $PGF_{2\alpha}$ treatment. By contrast, angiopoietin-2 (ANGPT2) protein and mRNA, as well as the *IGFBP1 mRNA* significantly increased during the first 2 h of $PGF_{2\alpha}$-induced luteolysis, followed by a steep decrease after 4 h. Moreover, tissue OT peptide and *OTR* mRNA decreased significantly after 2 h, followed by a continuous decrease of *OT* mRNA. Taking together Berisha *et al.* (2010) data, the acute decrease in luteotropic (P4, OT, IGF1) as well pro-angiogenic factors (i.e. VEGF, IGF1) with acute increase in capillary destabilization factors (i.e. ANGPT2) and modulation of vascular stability may be a key components in the cascade of the early events leading to functional luteolysis

Endothelin-1 and vasoactive peptides

Endothelin-converting enzyme 1 (ECE-1) is a key enzyme in the biosynthesis of EDN1, a potent regulator/modulator of $PGF_{2\alpha}$ action during luteolysis in cattle (Levy *et al.* 2000). The rapid increase in EDN1 during luteal regression, the ability of EDN1 to inhibit steroidogenesis *in vitro* and *in vivo*, and the inhibition of the luteolytic effects of $PGF_{2\alpha}$ by pretreatment with type A EDN1 (ETA) receptor antagonists suggest that this peptide functions as an important component of the luteolytic cascade (Girsh *et al.* 1996; Miyamoto *et al* 1997; Ohtani *et al.* 1998; Levy *et al.* 2001). In fact, a pivotal role for the main endothelial cells product - EDN1 in $PGF_{2\alpha}$-induced luteal regression in cows has been well documented by Meidan's group (Girsh *et al.* 1996; Mamluk *et al.* 1999; Meidan *et al.* 2005; Levy *et al.* 2000, 2003; Rosiansky-Sultan *et al.* 2006). mRNA expression of *EDN1* as well as its concentration in bovine CL increased at 2-10 h after $PGF_{2\alpha}$ treatment (Ohtani *et al.* 1998; Wright *et al.* 2001; Shirasuna *et al.* 2004). EDN1 inhibited P4 secretion, in a dose dependent manner via selective EDN1 bindings sites (EBN_A). The expression of members of the EDN system (EDN1, EDN converting enzymes, and EDN_A and EDN_B receptors) increases during luteal regression (Levy et al. 2001; Rosiansky-Sultan *et al.* 2006). Moreover, $PGF_{2\alpha}$ up-regulates EDN1 and EDN_A expression within the CL (Mamluk *et al.* 1999). Besides EDN1, other vasoactive peptides (i.e. angiothensin 2 – ANG2, atrial natriuretic peptide – ANP) are considered important factors in mediating $PGF_{2\alpha}$ luteolytic action (Berisha and Schams 2005; Berisha et al. 2010). These vasoactive peptides decreased blood flow and triggered the luteolytic cascade and consequently inhibited P4 secretion (Shirasuna *et al.* 2004; Miyamoto *et al.* 2005).

However, it has been showed that the EDN1 system (EDN1, EDN_A and EDN converting enzymes) exists in the bovine CL through the oestrous cycle and $PGF_{2\alpha}$ increased *EDN1* mRNA expression *in vivo* only at 10 h after treatment (Wright *et al.* 2001). In fact, up-regulation of EDN1 and ANG2 occurred mainly during structural luteal regression (Berisha & Schams 1995). Therefore, EDN1 seems to be additionally involved in the process of structural egression of the bovine CL by promoting leukocyte migration and stimulating macrophages to release cytokines (i.e. TNF, IFNG; Friedman et al. 2000; Meidan et al. 2005).

Cytokines

The increase in the immune cell numbers in the bovine CL has been observed during luteolysis (Lobel & Levy 1968; Penny *et al.* 1999; Towson *et al.* 2002). Moreover, production of monocyte chemoattractant protein 1 (MCP1), which stimulated proliferation and activation of the immune cells, was observed in the bovine CL from days 12-18 of the oestrous cycle (Townson et al. 2002). The number of leukocytes (i.e. T lymphocytes, macrophages) increased at the time of structural luteolysis and play a central role in structural luteolysis of both steroidogenic and endothelial luteal cells (Benyo & Pate 1992; Friedman et al. 2000; Pate & Keyes 2001; Pate 2003). The most important immune factors involved in the process of regression of bovine CL are pro-inflamatory cytokines: TNF and interferon-γ (IFNG) (Pate & Keyes 2001; Skarzynski *et al.* 2008). Shaw & Britt (1995) using a microdialysis of bovine CL system showed that TNF is released during spontaneous and $PGF_{2\alpha}$-induced luteolysis in cows. mRNAs for *TNF* and its specific receptors (*TNFR type-I*) has clearly been shown to be present in the bovine CL during luteolysis (Sakumoto *et al.* 2000; Neuvians *et al.* 2004; Korzekwa *et al.* 2008b). TNF acting via TNFR type-I in combination IFNG, reduced P4 production, induced apoptosis and $PGF_{2\alpha}$ production by luteal cells *in vitro* (Sakumoto *et al.* 2000; Petroff *et al* 2001; Korzekwa *et al.* 2006). Specific binding sites for TNF are also present in endothelial cells derived from bovine CL (Okuda *et al.* 1999). Furthermore, TNF induces EDN1 production by endothelial cells that may lead to the structural regression of the CL (Okuda *et al.* 1999; Friedman *et al.* 2000). However, mostly all *in vitro* studies indicated that TNF induces luteolysis only in combination with INFG or other intraluteal factors i.e. EDN1 (reviewed by Pate & Keyes 2001; Meidan *et al.* 2005; Skarzynski *et al.* 2008). Therefore, we tested *in vivo* whether TNF acts as a luteolytic factor *in vivo*, and whether it changes the lifespan of bovine CL (Skarzynski *et al.* 2003a). Lower doses of TNF increased $PGF_{2\alpha}$ and nitrite/nitrate (stable metabolites of NO), decreased P4 level and consequently resulted in shortening of the oestrous cycle. Surprisingly, higher doses of TNF stimulated the synthesis of P4 and PGE_2 and consequently resulted in prolongation of the lifespan of bovine CL (Skarzynski *et al.* 2003a; Skarzynski *et al.* 2007; Korzekwa *et al.* 2008b). However, it is difficult to state how these observed concentrations/doses relate to the local concentrations achieved at the CL and the endometrium, because very high TNF concentrations may be achieved locally to exert paracrine and autocrine effects. Thus TNF, depending on its concentrations, influences the secretory function of the CL and uterus in cattle (Skarzynski *et al.* 2009).

TNF belongs to the TNF super family (TNF-SF), which consists of eighteen members and as a classical cytokine is pleiotropic in nature. Regulating reproductive processes, TNF also has a diverse spectrum of biological activities, including stimulation of cell proliferation and differentiation, induction of cell apoptotic death (reviewed by Terranova *et al.* 1995). The pleiotropic TNF properties may depend on the differences in receptors and second messenger actions. Two immunologically distinct TNFRs have now been identified, TNFRI and TNFRII have different intracellular signalling pathways (Beutler & Van Huffel 1994). TNFRI contains an intracellular death domain, which is required for signalling pathways associated with apoptosis. In contrast, TNFRII can induce gene transcription for cell survival, growth, and differentiation (Beutler & Van Huffel 1994). Therefore, TNF may play multiple physiological roles in reproductive tract (Terranova *et al.* 1995; Pate & Keyes 2001; Skarzynski *et al.* 2008).

In our *in vivo* study, we have shown that the inhibition of PG synthesis by indomethacin, a non-specific PTGS inhibitor, injected into the *aorta abdominalis*, blocked the actions of TNF indicating that TNF acts mainly through mediation of AA metabolites (Skarzynski *et al.* 2007). In addition to TNFR, other cytokine membrane receptors, second messengers, including $[Ca^{2+}]$ and regulatory proteins are involved in apoptosis of steroidogenic and endothelial luteal cells (Friedman *et al.* 2000; Petroff *et al.* 2001; Taniguchi *et al.* 2002). Fas ligand (FASL), a member of the TNF super family, primarily engages its receptors (FAS) to induce apoptosis (Taniguchi *et al.* 2002; Okuda *et al.* 2004b). The expression of *FAS* mRNA was increased by IFNG, and TNF augmented the stimulatory action of IFNG on *FAS* expression (Taniguchi *et al.* 2002). Moreover, apoptotic bodies were observed in the luteal cells treated with FASL in the presence of IFNG and/or TNF, showing that leukocyte-derived TNF and IFNG play important roles in FASL-FAS-mediated luteal cell death in the bovine CL.

Leukotrienes

Leukotrienes, especially LTB_4 and LTC_4 could be engaged in the process of luteolysis (Milvae *et al.* 1986). Blair *et al.* (1997) showed using a microdialysis system *in vivo* that at Day 12 of the oestrous cycle after $PGF_{2\alpha}$ infusion increased both LTC_4 and LTB_4 levels in luteal perfusate. Other *in vivo* and *in vitro* studies also indicated that the levels of LTC_4 in the perfusate of bovine CL (Jaroszewski & Hansel 2000; Jaroszewski *et al.* 2003a,b), cultured luteal cells (Jaroszewski *et al.* 2003a; Korzekwa *et al.* 2010a), as well as in the blood of conscious cattle (Jaroszewski & Hansel 2000; Jaroszewski *et al.* 2003a,b; Skarzynski *et al.* 2003b) are elevated after $PGF_{2\alpha}$, NO and TNF treatment at the late luteal phase of oestrous cycle, suggesting that LTs play some role in luteolysis.

Leukotrienes are synthesized by 5-lipoxygenase (5-LO) and commonly known as potential inflammatory factors that cause oedema in respiratory tract diseases, but they also have got the roles in reproduction and may enhance the action of PGs. Receptors for LTs are classified into two separate groups in respect of structure and cell location: LTRI for LTB_4 and LTRII for cysteinyl LTs (LTC_4, LTD_4 and LTE_4). There are two isoforms of receptors for LTB_4 and at least two receptors for cysteinyl LTs (Izumi *et al.* 2002). We have recently shown that mRNA for *5-LO* and *LT receptors* are expressed in the bovine ovarian cell types, i.e. steroidogenic and endothelial luteal, and granulosa cells (Korzekwa *et al.* 2010b). Leukotriene B_4 seems to play a luteotropic role in the bovine CL, stimulating P4 and PGE_2 secretions, whereas LTC_4 stimulates the secretion of luteolytic $PGF_{2\alpha}$ and may enhance the luteolytic cascade (Korzekwa *et al.* 2010a). These *in vitro* results has been recently supported by *in vivo* studies (Korzekwa *et al.* 2010c). Thus, LTs were found to be auto / paracrine factors modulating the secretory functions of ovarian cells depending on the stage of the cycle and type of LTs (Blair *et al.* 1997; Korzekwa *et al.* 2010a, c).

The highest level of mRNA expressions for *LTRs* and *5-LO* in luteal tissue were observed on Day 16-18 of the cycle (Korzekwa *et al.* 2010a). More specifically, a similar pattern of mRNA expression of *LTRs* and *5-LO* and production/secretion of LTs during the cycle was described recently by us in two main cell population of bovine luteal steroidogenic and endothelial cells (Korzekwa *et al.* 2010a, b). The greatest mRNA expression for *LTR-II* and *5-LO* was found at the late luteal phase of the cycle in endothelial luteal cells, whereas *LTR-I* mRNA expression did not differ among cell types. These findings indicate that endothelial cells possess the greatest potential for LTs production among ovarian cells, being these cells the main source of LTs in the bovine ovary (Korzekwa *et al.* 2010a, b). Our most recent data indicate that endogenous LTC_4 inhibits P4 secretion in the oestrous cycle, since Azelastine a specific LTC_4 antagonist, elevated P4 output and prolonged the lifespan of bovine CL i*n vivo* (Korzekwa *et al.* 2010c). Consequently, the data obtained in the recent studies strengthen the concept that LTs are factors regulating reproductive processes as auto- and/or paracrine factors in CL during the oestrous cycle (Korzekwa *et al.* 2010a,b,c). We have shown: (i) LTs production and secretion in luteal tissue and its localization in the ovary; and (ii) the influence of LTs on PGs secretion and action during the estrous cycle. Based on the above findings, LTs action on the bovine reproductive tract has been suggested to be dependent on the LT type, and LTC_4 may serve as a mediator of luteolytic $PGF_{2\alpha}$ action (Milvae *et al.* 1986; Blair *et al.* 1997; Jaroszewski *et al.* 2003 Skarzynski *et al.* 2003b; Korzekwa *et* *al.* 2008b, 2010a,c). Although we have shown that LTC_4 was strongly elevated in the bovine CL between 2- and 4-h after the pharmacological dose of an analogue of $PGF_{2\alpha}$ infusion (dinoprost, 5 mg; Jaroszewski *et al.* 2003b), no stimulatory effect of the luteolytic dose of TNF on LTC_4 output was observed during 4-h (Skarzynski *et al.* 2003b). Moreover, the peaks of luteolytic LTC_4 have been demonstrated in bovine CL on Day 18 after ovulation in heifers undergoing spontaneous luteolysis (Milvae *et al.* 1986), and their frequency increased within the 12-h period during which the onset of P4 decline occurred (Blair *et al.* 1997). Therefore, the release of LTC_4 from the CL may be one of the late results of the activation of the luteolytic cascade induced by uterine $PGF_{2\alpha}$.

Nitric oxide

Nitric oxide which plays roles in a variety of physiological mechanisms, including blood flow regulation appears to be a good candidate to mediate the $PGF_{2\alpha}$ action during the first steps of the luteolytic cascade in cattle (Skarzynski *et al.* 2003a; Shirasuna *et al* 1998; Acosta *et al.* 2009). NADPH-d localization (a marker for nitric oxide synthase - NOS) and immunostaining of both isoforms of NOS (inducible - iNOS and endothelial - eNOS) were detected in steroidogenic cells and in blood vessels of the bovine CL during the entire estrous cycle with increasing activity from the early to the late luteal phases (Skarzynski *et al.* 2003b). However, other studies presented the highest level of eNOS mRNA and protein expression in the early bovine CL (Rosiansky-Sultan *et al.* 2006; Shirasuna *et al.* 2010). Luteolytic or luteotropic actions of NO on the bovine CL during the oestrous cycle is strictly dependent on the stage of CL, and cell interactions (cell-to-cell contact) and composition (Jaroszewski *et al.* 2003a; Weems *et al.* 2004; Klipper *et al.* 2004; Rosiansky-Sultan *et al.* 2006). NO donor (S-NAP) stimulated PGE_2 secretion by steroidogenic luteal cells in the early and mid-luteal phases (Skarzynski & Okuda 2000; Skarzynski *et al.* 2000b). These data show that there is an inverse relationship between NOS and EDN1 throughout the life span of bovine CL, and imply that this pattern may be the result of their interaction between luteal endothelial and immune cells. Thus, NOS are expressed in a physiologically relevant manner: elevated NO at an early luteal stage is likely to play an important role in angiogenesis, whereas reduced levels of eNOS during luteal regression may facilitate the sustained upregulation of EDN1 levels during luteolysis (Rosiansky-Sultan *et al.* 2006; Shirasuna *et al.* 2010). During the development and maintenance of the CL, $PGE_{2,}$ which is both luteotropic and antiluteolytic, may stimulate NO production. Moreover, NO donors and EDN1 increased PGE_2 secretion by bovine luteal slices *in vitro* on Days 13-14 of the cycle without any direct effect on P4 secretion (Weems *et al.* 2004). Therefore, the increased NO production during early stages of the cycle and pregnancy is likely to play a role in the development and angiogenesis of bovine CL (Skarzynski & Okuda 2000; Weems *et al.* 2004; Rosiansky-Sultan *et al.* 2006) and suggests multiple roles of NO in the regulation of the bovine luteal function (Skarzynski *et al.* 2008). However, Shirasuna *et al.* (2010) have observed many of eNOS positive areas in the periphery of the mid, late and regressing bovine CL, where many arteriolovenous vessels are located. As suggested by the authors, the distribution of capillaries, arteriolovenous and eNOS expression differs between early, mid, late and regressing bovine CL. Thus, this structural change from the early (homogeneous, regarding cell types distribution and vasculature composition) to late (heterogeneous) luteal phase is related to the differences in the CL response to $PGF_{2\alpha}$ due to the blood regulating factors, including NO. Moreover, it has been recently shown that not only eNOS is involved in NO production during luteolysis in cattle (Lee et al. 2009). Bovine endothelial luteal cells are a target for $PGF_{2\alpha}$ and that $PGF_{2\alpha}$ stimulates iNOS expression and iNOS activity. Stimulation of the NO generating system and iNOS activity by $PGF_{2\alpha}$ may result in increasing local NO production followed by luteolysis (Lee *et al.* 2009). This *in vitro* observation has been supported by the *in vivo* data (Acosta *et al.* 2009). We have shown *in vivo* that after $PGF_{2\alpha}$ application, concentrations of NO metabolites in the ovarian artery blood plasma preceded the rise in the systemic circulation by about 15 to 30 min (Fig. 3). Thus, it appears that an ovary bearing a CL responds to PGF$_{2\alpha}$ injection within a shorter period of time compared with other organs. This supports the idea that the CL produces a considerable amount of NO in response to PGF$_{2\alpha}$ and that increased NO is responsible for the acute increase in luteal blood flow observed in cattle. Moreover, in the late luteal phase, PGF$_{2\alpha}$ might simulate a shear stress-like reaction of endothelial luteal cells resulting in compensative NO release during the first steps of luteolysis - up to 2-4 h after PGF$_{2\alpha}$ treatment (Skarzynski *et al.* 2003a; Acosta *et al.* 2009). These data suggest that NO produced by two NOS isoforms is involved in structural and functional changes that occur in the bovine CL during lutolysis.

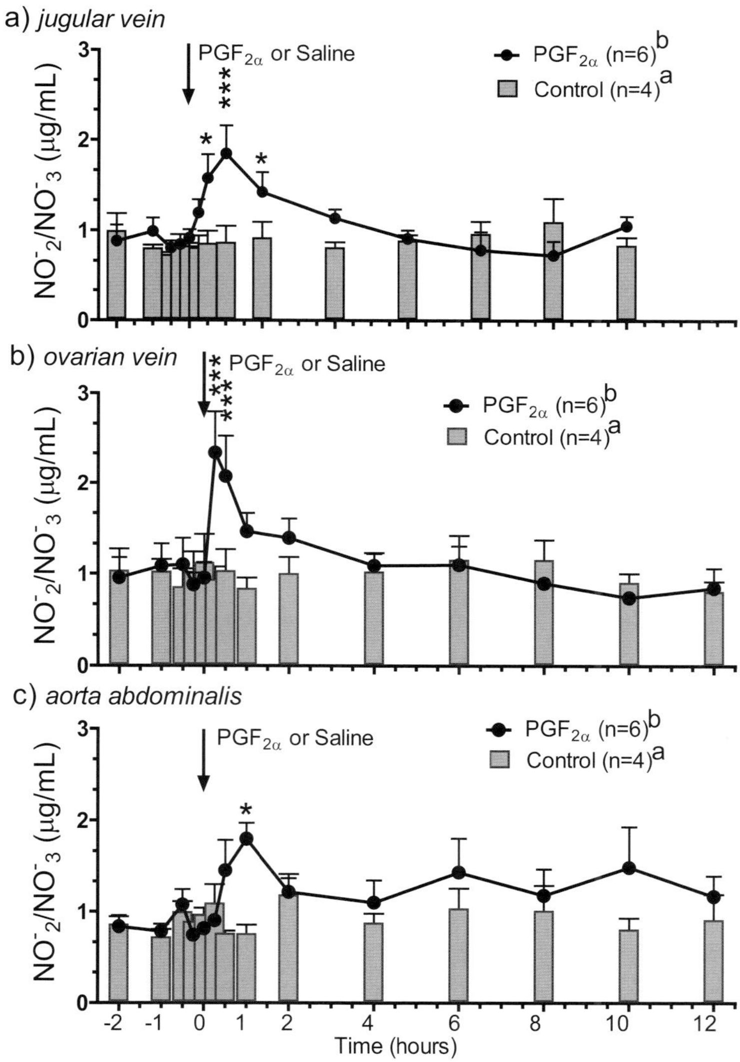

Fig. 3. Effects of prostaglandin (PG)F$_{2\alpha}$ on the concentrations of nitrite/nitrate (NO^-_2/NO^-_3), the stable metabolites of nitric oxide, in blood plasma collected from the (a) jugular vein, (b) ovarian vein and (c) *aorta abdominalis*. Cows were treated with a PGF$_{2\alpha}$ analogue (cloprostenol, 500 µg) or Saline (Controls) intramuscularly on Day 10 of the oestrous cycle. Asterisks indicate significant differences ($P<0.05$) compared with the pretreatment period (baseline). Different superscript letters indicate significant differences ($P<0.05$) between the PGF$_{2\alpha}$-treated and Control. Reprinted from Acosta *et al.* (2009).

Intra-luteal administration of a NOS inhibitor (L-NAME) during the late luteal phase increased P4 secretion and prolonged the functional lifespan of bovine CL (Jaroszewski & Hansel 2000; Shirasuna *et al.* 2008b). When an analogue of $PGF_{2\alpha}$ (cloprostenol) was injected on Day 15 of the cycle in combination with L-NAME, the luteolytic effect of $PGF_{2\alpha}$ was counteracted by the NOS inhibitor (Fig. 4; Skarzynski *et al.* 2003a; Jaroszewski *et al.* 2003b). Nitric oxide has been found as the most potent inhibitor of P4 secretion *in vitro* (Skarzynski *et al.* 2000; Korzekwa *et al.* 2004, 2006) and *in vivo* (Shirasuna *et al.* 2008b). Moreover, a NO donor (Spermine NONOate) strongly stimulated production of $PGF_{2\alpha}$ and LTC_4 by bovine CL both *in vitro* and *in vivo,* showing that NO is involved in the process of luteal regression by bovine CL (Jaroszewski *et al.* 2003a; Korzekwa *et al.* 2004, 2006; Shirasuna *et al.* 2008b) suggesting the role of NO in luteolysis initiation in cows. TNF and $PGF_{2\alpha}$ induce NO synthesis during $PGF_{2\alpha}$-induced luteolysis (Skarzynski *et al.* 2003a,b, 2007, 2009; Acosta *et al.* 2009) Nitric oxide is also involved in structural luteolysis stimulating *BAX* mRNA expression in the steroidogenic luteal cells (Korzekwa *et al.* 2006). Consequently, the ratio of *BCL2* to *BAX* decreased. Moreover, NO stimulates expression and activity of caspase-3. Thus, in concert with END1 and cytokines action, NO seems to play a crucial role in both functional luteolysis (inhibition of the basal and LH-stimulated P4 synthesis; blood flow) and structural luteolysis (induction of apoptosis of the luteal cells). However, Acosta *et al.* (2009) showed that *in vivo* $PGF_{2\alpha}$ induced P4 decline followed with the significant (maintaining only 0.5-2h) NO output by CL-containing ovary. Therefore, luteolytic action of NO might be limited only to the first steps of $PGF_{2\alpha}$-induced luteolytic cascade. Expression of *NOS* mRNA in bovine CL gradually reduced from two until 60-h after $PGF_{2\alpha}$ analogue injection (Neuvians *et al.* 2004; Rosiansky-Sultan *et al.* 2006). Thus, in the late stages of luteal regression, a classical - inverse relationship between $PGF_{2\alpha}$, EDN1 and NO system may exist and reduced levels of NO may facilitate the sustained up-regulation of EDN1 system in the CL (Klipper *et al.* 2004; Rosiansky-Sultan *et al.* 2006).

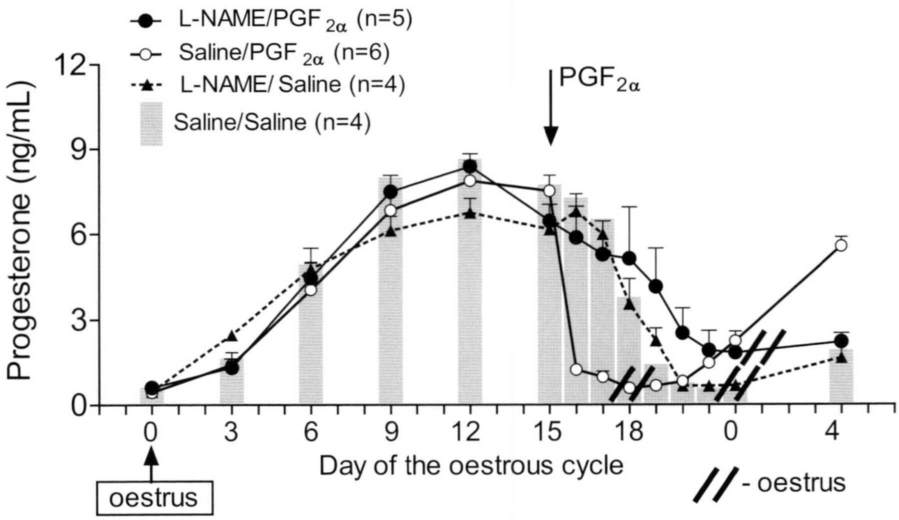

Fig. 4. The effect of 2 h infusion of saline or a nitric oxide synthase inhibitor (L-NAME; 400 mg/1h) and injection of Saline or a prostaglandin $F_{2\alpha}$ analogue ($PGF_{2\alpha}$; cloprostenol, 100 μg) at 30 min of infusion on progesterone concentrations in peripheral blood plasma of heifers on Day 15 of the oestrous cycle. Different subscript letters indicate significant differences ($P<0.05$). Modified from Skarzynski et al. (2003a).

Role of blood flow and hypoxia in the regression of bovine CL

The dynamic changes in the ovarian blood flow have been well demonstrated in ruminants until today. Classical studies found that ovarian blood flow was low just after ovulation, gradually increased toward the luteal stage, then decreased during luteal regression in cattle (Ford & Chenault 1981; Wise *et al.* 1982). These findings have been found by using electromagnetic probes. Recently, intraovarian blood flow was monitored by color-doppler ultrasound sonography (Acosta *et al.* 2002; Ginther *et al.* 2007). These studies found that blood flow increased rapidly and temporally (up to 2h), and then decreased (after 4-8h), when a luteolytic $PGF_{2\alpha}$ was injected to cows. The rapid increase of blood flow has been suggested to be induced by vasodilators, such as PGE_2 (Miyamoto *et al.* 2005) and NO (Skarzynski *et al.* 2003a). In support, it has been shown that intraluteal application of a NO donor drastically increase luteal blood flow (Shirasuna *et al.* 2008b).

As discussed previously, NO, one of the reactive oxygen species (ROS), has been suggested to play critical roles in luteolysis in cows, because it decreases P4 secretion (Korzekwa *et al.* 2006; Shirasuna *et al.* 2008b) and promotes apoptosis in bovine luteal cells (Korzekwa *et al.* 2006). In cattle, we recently observed that an injection of $PGF_{2\alpha}$ induces a transient (1-2 h) increase in the concentrations of NO and partial pressure of O_2 (pO_2) in ovarian venous blood, and that the pO_2 of venous blood is higher in the ovarian vein than in the jugular vein (Acosta *et al.* 2009). Therefore, the luteal micro-environment seems to be high oxygen condition, especially during a short period of time (1-2 h) following $PGF_{2\alpha}$ injection. Interestingly, $PGF_{2\alpha}$ stimulates the NO generating system by increasing inducible iNOS mRNA and protein expression, and NOS activity in cultured luteal endothelial cells (Lee *et al.* 2009) as well as eNOS expression in the periphery of the bovine CL (Shirasuna *et al.* 2008b). In addition to NO, the other ROS, such as hydrogen peroxide (H_2O_2), superoxide anion (O_2^-) and oxygen (O_2) have been implicated in the luteolytic process (Agarwal *et al.* 2005). H_2O_2 has been shown to inhibit P4 secretion and to induce apoptotic changes in cultured bovine luteal cells (Nakamura *et al.* 2001). Therefore, generation of ROS following the changes in the blood flow may be deeply related to the local mechanisms of functional and structural luteolysis in the cow.

Following the rapid increase after $PGF_{2\alpha}$ injection to cows, blood flow decreases in a short time, *i.e.* a significant decrease was observed 8 h after $PGF_{2\alpha}$ injection (Acosta *et al.* 2002; Fig. 5). In both spontaneous and $PGF_{2\alpha}$-induced luteolysis, a decrease in luteal blood flow begins in parallel with systemic P4 concentrations (Ford & Chenault 1981; Wise *et al.* 1982). Furthermore, the pO_2 in the blood collected from the ovarian vein began to decrease at the late luteal stage (Wise *et al.* 1982). Therefore, we hypothesized that O_2 shortage (hypoxia) caused by a decrease of blood supply is one of the factors promoting luteolysis in the cow (Fig. 5). We found that hypoxia inhibits P4 synthesis in cultured bovine luteal cells by inhibiting the steroidogenic enzyme P450scc (Nishimura *et al.* 2006). Hypoxia also promotes apoptosis of luteal cells by increasing a pro-apoptotic protein BNIP3 expression, and by activating caspase-3 (Nishimura *et al.* 2008). These findings suggest that hypoxia promotes both functional luteolysis (P4 decrease) and structural luteolysis (apoptosis), and revealed that O_2 deficiency caused by a decreasing blood supply in bovine CL is one of the factors contributing to luteolysis in the cow (Hojo *et al.* 2009). However, $PGF_{2\alpha}$ is able to inhibit P4 secretion even though pO_2 remains still high and pCO_2 is not up-regulated in the bovine reproductive tract (Acosta *et al.* 2009). Moreover, Watanabe *et al.* (2006) showed that P4 decreased even when blood flow remained high in the bovine CL. Therefore, O_2 deficiency due to decreased blood flow is not mandatory for the induction of both functional and structural luteolysis in cows, but may play such a supporting role in the final steps of bovine luteal regression.

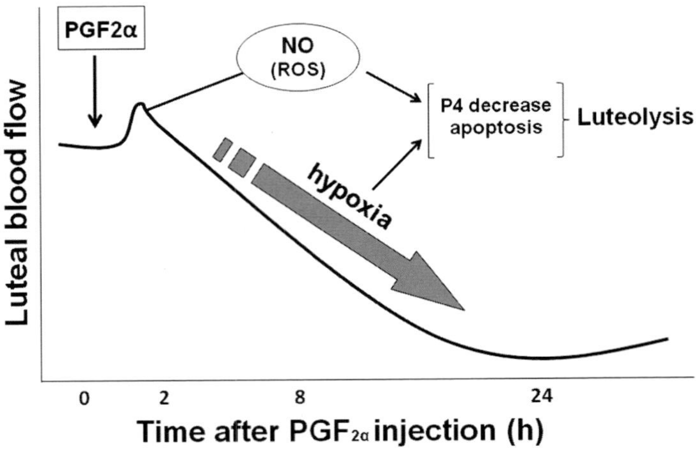

Fig. 5. Scheme of the relationship between luteal blood flow and luteolysis related factors, reactive oxygen species (ROS) and hypoxia. We propose that the temporal increase of blood flow induces ROS including nitric oxide (NO), and that the following decrease of blood flow makes hypoxic conditions in corpus luteum. Since both NO and hypoxia have been shown to decrease P4 synthesis and to induce apoptosis of bovine luteal cells, the changes of blood flow are strongly related to luteolysis by affecting these factors.

Concluding remarks

The pulsatile $PGF_{2\alpha}$ secretion in cattle was previously proposed to be generated by a positive feedback loop between ovarian and/or hypophyseal OT and endometrial $PGF_{2\alpha}$. However, since some data suggest that OT is not essential for the initiation of luteolysis, the importance of a $PGF_{2\alpha}$-OT feedback loop remains less certain in cattle. The bovine endometrium seems to possess endogenous mechanisms for initiation of $PGF_{2\alpha}$ secretion. The mechanism controlling the development, maintenance and secretory function of the CL may involve factors that are produced both within the CL and outside the ovary. Some of these regulators seem to be prostaglandins and other arachidonic acid metabolites (PGE_2, $PGF_{2\alpha}$, LT), neuropeptides, peptide hormones (OT, EDN1), growth factors and hormones (VEGF, FGF, GH, PRL) and steroids (P4 and 17β-oestradiol) that act as autocrine and/or paracrine factors. Although $PGF_{2\alpha}$ is known to be a principal luteolytic factor, its action on the CL is mediated by other intra-ovarian factors cytokines, leukotrienes, EDN1, NO (Fig 6). Nitric oxide, and TNF in combination with IFNG reduced P4 secretion, increased luteal $PGF_{2\alpha}$ production, and induced apoptosis of the luteal cells (Fig. 6). As recently suggested by Berisha et al. (2010) the cascades connected with $PGF_{2\alpha}$-induced luteolysis are: 1) luteal NO release and blood flow up-regulation, 2) up-regulation of inflammatory cytokines and luteal cell apoptosis factors, 3) strong up-regulation of vasoactive peptides in luteal cells, and 4) extracellular matrix proteases associated with luteal tissue remodelling. In addition, the decrease in luteal blood flow and hypoxia has been proposed as an important luteolytic mechanisms in the cow. Hypoxia inhibits P4 synthesis in the bovine luteal cells by inhibiting the steroidogenic enzymes and promotes apoptosis of luteal cells by increasing pro-apoptotic proteins. Although reduction of luteal blood flow and hypoxia contribute to the late events of luteolysis, little is known about the physiological relevance and the cause of the transient increase in luteal blood flow and reactive oxygen species during the initial step of luteolysis.

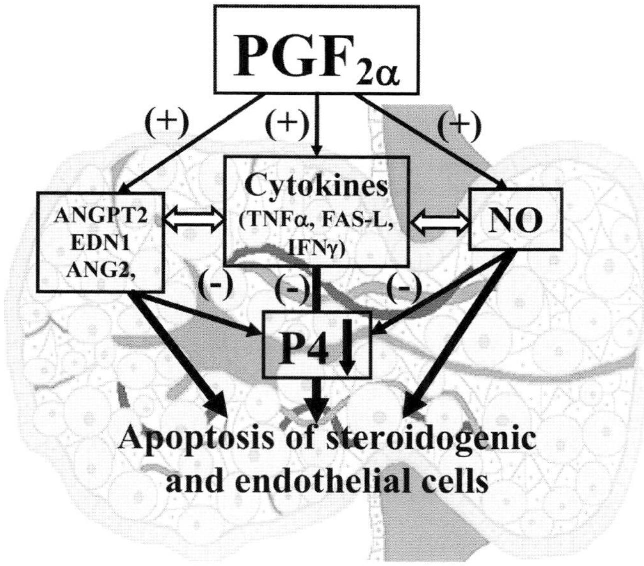

Fig. 6. Hypothetical model of the structural and functional regression of the CL (see text for the details; adapted from Skarzynski *et al.* 2008)

Acknowledgments

The work was supported by the grants-in-aid from the Polish Ministry of Sciences and Higher Education (N308 3279 33) and Japan Society for Promotion of Sciences (JSPS B 22380148). The authors are grateful to Prof. Graça Ferreira-Dias (Technical University of Lisbon, Portugal) for critical reading and editing language of the manuscript. We thank Ilona Kowalczyk-Zieba (Institute of Animal Reproduction & Food Research in Olsztyn, Poland) for technical assistance in preparation the Figures. The authors declare that they have no conflict of interest that would prejudice the impartiality of the scientific word.

References

Acosta TJ, Yoshizawa N, Ohtani M & Miyamoto A 2002 Local changes in blood flow within the early and midcycle corpus luteum after $PGF_{2\alpha}$ injection in the cow. *Biology of Reproduction* **66** 651-658.

Acosta TJ, Bah MM, Korzekwa A, Woclawek-Potocka I, Markiewicz W, Jaroczewski JJ, Okuda K & Skarzynski DJ 2009 Acute changes in circulating concentrations of progesterone and nitric oxide and partial pressure of oxygen during $PGF_{2\alpha}$-induced luteolysis in cattle. *Journal of Reproduction and Development* **55** 149-155.

Agarwal A, Gupta S & Sharma RK 2005 Role of oxidative stress in female reproduction. *Reproductive Biology and Endocrinology* **14** 3-28.

Akabane Y, Shirasuna K, Sasaki M, Matsui M, Berisha B, Schams D, Shimizu T & Miyamoto A 2008 The expression of prostaglandin $F_{2\alpha}$ receptor and its isoforms during the estrous cycle and luteolysis in the bovine corpus luteum. *Biology of Reproduction* **78** *(1 Supplement) 148.*

Alila HW, Dowd JP, Corradino RA, Harris WV & Hansel W 1988 Control of progesterone production in small and large bovine luteal cells separated by flow cytometry. *Journal of Reproduction and Fertility* **82** 645-655.

Alila HW, Davis JS, Dowd JP, Corradino RA & Hansel W 1990 Differential effects of calcium on progesterone production in small and large bovine luteal cells. *Journal of Steroid Biochemistry* **28** 687-693.

Armstrong DT & Hansel W 1959 Alteration of the bovine estrous cycle with oxytocin. *Journal Dairy Sciences* **42** 533-542.

Arvisais E, Hou X, Wyatt TA, Shirasuna K, Bollwein H, Miyamoto A, Hansen TR, Rueda BR & Davis JS 2010 Prostaglandin $F_{2\alpha}$ represses IGF-I-stimulated IRS1/phosphatidylinositol-3-kinase/AKT signaling in the corpus luteum: Role of ERK and P70 ribosomal S6 kinase. *Molecular Endocrinology* **24** 632-643.

Asselin E, Drolet P & Fortier MA 1998 In vitro response to oxytocin and interferon-τ in bovine endometrial cells from caruncular and inter-caruncular areas. *Biology of Reproduction* **59** 241-247.

Bah MM, Acosta TJ, Pilawski W, Deptula K, Okuda K & Skarzynski DJ 2006 Role of intraluteal prostaglandin $F_{2\alpha}$, progesterone and oxytocin in basal and pulsatile progesterone release from developing bovine corpus luteum. *Prostaglandins & other Lipid Mediators* **79** 218-229.

Benyo DF & Pate JL 1992 Tumor necrosis factor-α alters bovine luteal cell synthetic capacity and viability. *Endocrinology* **130** 854-860.

Berisha B & Schams D 2005 Ovarna function in ruminants. *Domestic Animal Endocrinology* **29** 305-217.

Berisha B, Meyer HMM & Schams D 2010 Effect of Prostaglandin $F_{2\alpha}$ on local luteotropic and angiogenic factors during induced functional luteolysis in the bovine corpus luteum. *Biology of Reproduction* **82** 940-947.

Beutler B & Van Huffel C 1994 Unraveling function in the TNF ligand and receptor families. *Sciences* **264** 667-668.

Blair RM, Saatman R, Liou SS, Fortune JE & Hansel W 1997 Roles of leukotrienes in bovine corpus luteum regression: an in vivo microdialysis study. *Proceedings of Society for Experimental Biology and Medicine* **216** 72-80.

Burns PD, Graf GA, Hayes SH & Silvia WJ 1997Cellular mechanisms by which oxytocin stimulates uterine $PGF_{2\alpha}$ synthesis in bovine endometrium: roles of phospholipases C and A_2. *Domestic Animal Endocrinology* **14** 181-191.

Chen D-B, Westfall SD, Fong HW, Roberson MS, & Davis JS 1998 Prostaglandin $F_{2\alpha}$ stimulates the Raf/MEK1/ Mitogen-activated protein kinase signaling cascade in bovine luteal cells. *Endocrinology* **139** 3876-3885.

Choudhary E, Sen A, Inskeep EK & Flores JA 2005 Developmental sensitivity of the bovine corpus luteum to prostaglandin $F_{2\alpha}$ ($PGF_{2\alpha}$) and endothelin-1 (ET-1): Is ET-1 a mediator of the luteolytic actions of $PGF_{2\alpha}$ or a tonic inhibitor of progesterone secretion? *Biology of Reproduction* **72** 633-642.

Davis JS, Weakland LL, Farese RV & West LA 1987 Prostaglandin $F_{2\alpha}$ stimulates phosphatidylinositol 4,5-bisphosphate hydrolysis and mobilizes intracellular Ca^{2+} in bovine luteal cells. *Proceedings of the National Academy of Sciences USA* **84** 3728-3732.

Davis JS, Rueda BR & Spanel-Borowski K 2003 Microvascular endothelial cells of the corpus luteum. *Reproductive Biology & Endocrinology* 10 1-89.

Douglas WS & Britt JH 2000 In vivo oxytocin release from microdialyzed bovine corpora lutea during spontaneous and prostaglandin-induced regression. *Biology of Reproduction* **62** 726-730.

Ezashi T, Sakamoto K, Miwa K, Okudaashitaka E, Ito S & Hayaishi O 1997 Genomic organization and characterization of the gene encoding bovine prostaglandin F receptor *Gene* **190** 271-278.

Flint APF & Sheldrick EL 1982 Ovarian secretion of oxytocin is stimulated by prostaglandin. *Nature* **297** 587-588.

Ford SP & Chenault JR 1981 Blood flow to the corpus luteum-bearing ovary and ipsilateral uterine horn of cows during the oestrous cycle and early pregnancy. *Journal of Reproduction & Fertility* **62** 555-562.

Friedman A, Weiss S, Levy N & Meidan R 2000 Role of tumor necrosis factor-α and its type-1 receptor in luteal regression: induction of programmed cell death in bovine corpus luteum-derived endothelial cells. *Biology of Reproduction* **63** 1905-1915.

Ginther OJ, Silva LA, Araujo RR & Beg MA 2007 Temporal associations among pulses of 13,14-dihydro-15-keto-$PGF_{2\alpha}$, luteal blood flow, and luteolysis in cattle. *Biology of Reproduction* **76** 506-513.

Ginther OJ, Araujo RR, PalhãoMP, Rodrigues BL & Beg MA 2009 Necessity of sequential pulses of prostaglandin $F_{2\alpha}$ for complete physiologic luteolysis in cattle *Biology of Reproduction* **80** 641-648.

Ginther OJ Shrestha HK, Fuenzalida MJ, Shahiduzzaman AKM & Beg MA 2010 Characteristics of pulses of 13,14-Dihydro-15-Keto-prostaglandin $F_{2\alpha}$ before, during, and after spontaneous luteolysis and temporal intrapulse relationships with progesterone concentrations in cattle *Biology of Reproduction* **82** 1049-1056.

Girsh E, Milvae RA, Wang W & Meidan R 1996 Effect of endothelian-1 on bovine luteal cell function: Role in prostaglandin $F_{2\alpha}$-induced antisteroidogenic action. *Endocrinology* **137** 1306-1312.

Hansel W, Shemesh M, Hixon J & Lukaszewska J 1975 Extraction, isolation and identification of a luteolytic substance from bovine endometrium. *Biology of Reproduction* **13** 30-37.

Hojo T, Al-Zi'Abi MO, Skarzynski DJ, Acosta T & Okuda K 2009 Changes in the vasculature of bovine corpus luteum during the estrous cycle and prostaglandin $F_{2\alpha}$-induced luteolysis. *Journal of Reproduction and Development* **55** 512-517.

Izumi T, Yokomizo T, Obinata H, Ogasawara H & Shimizu T 2002 Leukotriene receptors: classification, gene expression, and signal transduction. *Journal of Biochemistry* **132** 1-6.

Jaroszewski JJ & Hansel W 2000 Intraluteal administration of a nitric oxide synthase blocker stimulates progesterone and oxytocin secretion and prolongs the life span of the bovine corpus luteum. *Proceedings of Society for Experimental Biology and Medicine* **224** 50-55.

Jaroszewski JJ, Skarzynski DJ, Blair RM & Hansel W 2003a: Influence of nitric oxide on the secretory function of the bovine corpus luteum: dependence on cell composition and cell-to-cell communication. *Experimental Biology and Medicine* **228** 741-748.

Jaroszewski JJ, Skarzynski DJ & Hansel W 2003b Nitric oxide as a local mediator of prostaglandin $F_{2\alpha}$-induced regression in bovine corpus luteum: an *in vivo* study. *Experimental Biology and Medicine* **228** 1057-1062.

Kisliouk T, Friedman A, Klipper E, Zhou QY, Schams D, Alfaidy N & Meidan R 2007 Expression pattern of prokineticin 1 and its receptors in bovine ovaries during the estrous cycle: involvement in corpus luteum regression and follicular atresia. *Biology of Reproduction* **76** 749-58.

Klipper E, Gilboa T, Levy N, Kisliouk T, Spanel-Borowski K & Meidan R 2004 Characterization of endothelin-1 and nitric oxide generating systems in corpus luteum-derived endothelial cells. *Reproduction* **128** 463-473.

Korzekwa A, Jaroszewski JJ, Bogacki M, Deptula KM, Maslanka TS, Acosta TJ, Okuda K, Skarzynski DJ. 2004 Effects of prostaglandin $F_{2\alpha}$ and nitric oxide on the secretory function of bovine luteal cells. *Journal of Reproduction & Development* **50** 411-417.

Korzekwa A, Shuko M, Jaroszewski J, Izabela Wocławek-Potocka, Okuda K, Skarzynski DJ 2006 Nitric oxide induces programmed cell dead in the bovine corpus luteum: mechanism of action. Journal of Reproduction & Development **52** 353-361.

Korzekwa AJ, Jaroszewski JJ, Woclawek-Potocka I, Bah MM & Skarzynski DJ 2008a Luteolytic effect of prostaglandin $F_{2\alpha}$ on bovine corpus luteum depends on cell composition and contact. *Reprouction in Domestic Animals* **43** 464–472.

Korzekwa A, Murakami S, Wocławek-Potocka I, Bah MM, Okuda K & Skarzynski DJ 2008b The influence of tumor necrosis factor-α (TNF) on the secretory function of bovine corpus luteum: TNF and its receptors expression during the estrous cycle. *Reproductive Biology* **8** 245-262.

Korzekwa A, Lukasik K & Skarzynski DJ 2010a Leukotrienes are auto-/paracrine factors in the bovine corpus luteum: an *in vitro* study. *Reproduction in Domestic Animals* **in press.**

Korzekwa AJ, Acosta TJ, Miklewicz M, Lee SH, Okuda K & Skarzynski DJ 2010b What is the target for leukotrienes action within bovine ovary? *Reproduction in Domestic Animals* **in press.**

Korzekwa AJ, Bah MM, Kurzynowski A, Lukasik K, Groblewska A & Skarzynski DJ. 2010c Leukotrienes modulate secretion of progesterone and prostaglandins during the estrous cycle and early pregnancy in cattle: an in vivo study. *Reproduction* **in press.**

Kotwica J, Skarzynski D, Bogacki M, Melin P & Starostka B 1997 The use of an oxytocin antagonist to study the function of ovarian oxytocin during luteolysis in cattle. *Theriogenology* **48** 1287-1299.

Kotwica J, Skarzynski D, Jaroszewski J, Williams GL & Bogacki M 1998 Uterine secretion of prostaglandin $F_{2\alpha}$ stimulated by different doses of oxytocin and released spontaneously during luteolysis in cattle. *Reproduction Nutrition & Development* **38** 217-226.

Lamsa JC, Kot SJ, Eldering JA, Nay MG & McCracken JA 1989 Prostaglandin $F_{2\alpha}$-stimulated release of ovarian oxytocin in the sheep in vivo: Threshold and dose dependence. *Biology of Reproduction* **40** 1215-1223.

Lee SH, Acosta TJ, Yoshioka S & Okuda K 2009 Prostaglandin $F_{2\alpha}$ regulates nitric oxide generating system in bovine luteal endothelial cells. *Journal of Reproduction & Development* **55** 418-424.

Lei ZM, Chegini N & Rao ChV 1991 Quantitative cell composition of human and bovine corpora lutea from various reproductive states. *Biology of Reproduction* **44** 1148-1156.

Levy N, Kobayashi S, Roth Z, Wolfenson D, Miyamoto A & Meidan R 2000 Administration of prostaglandin $F_{2\alpha}$ during the early bovine luteal phase does not alter the expression of ET-1 and its type A receptors: a possible cause for corpus luteum refractoriness. *Biology of Reproduction* **63** 377-382.

Levy N, Gordin M, Mamluk R, Yanagisawa M, Smith MF, Hampton JH & Meidan R 2001 Distinct cellular localization and regulation of Endothelin-1 and Endothelin-converting enzyme-1 expression in the bovine corpus luteum: implications for luteolysis. *Endocrinology* **142** 5254-5260.

Levy N, Gordin M, Smith MF, Bolden-Tiller O-U & Meidan R 2003 Hormonal regulation and cell-specific expression of endothelin-converting enzyme 1 isoforms in bovine ovarian endothelial and steroidogenic cells *Biology of Reproduction* **68** 1361-1368.

Lobel BL & Levy E 1968 Formation, development and involution of corpora lutea *Acta Endocrinologica* **132** 35-51.

Loeb L 1923 The effect of extirpation of the uterus on the life and function of the corpus luteum in the guinea pig. *Proceedings of Society for Experimental Biology and Medicine* **20** 441-443.

Lukaszewska JH & Hansel W 1970 Extraction and partial purification of luteolytic activity from bovine endometrial tissue. *Endocrinology* **86** 261-270.

Madore E, Harvey N, Parent J, Chapdelaine P, Arosh JA & Fortier MA 2003 An aldose reductase with 20 α-hydroxysteroid dehydrogenase activity is most likely the enzyme responsible for the production of prostaglandin $F_{2\alpha}$ in the bovine endometrium. *Journal of Biology and Chemistry* **278** 11205-11212.

Mamluk R, Levy, Ruead B, Davis JS & Meidan R 1999: Characterization and regulation of type A endothelin receptor gene expression in bovine luteal cells types. *Endocrinology* **40** 2110-2116.

McCracken JA, Custer EE & Lamsa JC. 1999 Luteolysis: a neuroendocrine-mediated event. *Physiological Reviews* **79** 263-323.

Meidan R, Levy N, Kisliouk T, Podlovny L, Rusiansky M & Klipper E 2005 The yin and yang of corpus luteum-derived endothelial cells: Balancing life and death. *Domestic Animal Endocrinology* **29** 318-328.

Milvae RA, Alila HW & Hansel W 1986 Involvement of lipoxygenase products of arachidonic acid metabolism in bovine luteal function. *Biology of Reproduction* **35** 1210-1215.

Miyamoto A, Kobayashi S, Arata S, Ohtani M, Fukui Y & Schams D 1997 *Prostaglandin $F_{2\alpha}$ promotes the inhibitory effects of endothelin-1 on the bovine luteal function in vitro. Journal of Endocrinology* **152** R7-*R11.*

Miyamoto A, Lützow HV & Schams D 1993 Acute actions of prostaglandin $F_{2\alpha}$, E_2, and I_2 in microdialyzed bovine corpus luteum in vitro. *Biology of Reproduction* **49** 423-430.

Miyamoto A, Shirasuna K, Wijayagunawardane MP, Watanabe S, Hayashi M, Yamamoto D, Matsui M & Acosta TJ 2005 Blood flow: A key regulatory component of corpus luteum function in the cow. *Domestic Animal Endocrinology* **29** 329-339.

Miyamoto Y, Skarzynski DJ & Okuda K 2000 Is tumor necrosis factor-α a trigger for the initiation of prostaglandyn $F_{2\alpha}$ releasse at luteolysis in cattle? *Biology of Reproduction* **62** 1109-1115.

Murakami S, Miyamoto Y, Skarzynski DJ & Okuda K 2001 Effects of tumor necrosis factor-α on secretion of prostaglandin E_2 and $F_{2\alpha}$ in bovine endometrium throughout the estrous cycle. *Theriogenology* **55** 1667-1678.

Nakamura T, Ishigami T, Makino N & Sakamoto K 2001 The down-regulation of glutathione peroxidase causes bovine luteal cell apoptosis during structural luteolysis. *Journal of Biochemistry* **129** 937-942.

Neuvians TP, Schams D, Berisha B & Pfaffl MW 2004 Involvement of pro-inflammatory cytokines, mediators of inflammation, and basic fibroblast growth factor in prostaglandin α-induced luteolysis in bovine corpus luteum. *Biology of Reproduction* **70** 473-480.

Newcomb R, Booth WD & Rowson LE 1977 The effect of oxytocin treatment on the levels of prostaglandin F in the blood of heifers. *Journal of Reproduction & Fertility* **49** 17-24.

Nishimura R, Sakumoto R, Tatsukawa Y, Acosta TJ & Okuda K 2006 Oxygen concentration is an important factor for modulating progesterone synthesis in bovine corpus luteum. *Endocrinology* **147** 4273-4280.

Nishimura R, Komiyama J, Tasaki Y, Acosta TJ & Okuda K 2008 Hypoxia promotes luteal cell death in bovine corpus luteum. *Biology of Reproduction* **78** 529-536.

Ohtani M, Kobayashi S, Miyamoto A, Hayashi K & Fukui Y 1998 Real-time relationships between intraluteal and plasma concentrations of endothelin, oxytocin and progesterone during prostaglandin $F_{2\alpha}$-induced luteolysis in the cow. *Biology of Reproduction* **58** 103-108.

Ohtani M, Takase S, Wijayagunawardane MPB., Tetsuka M & Miyamoto A 2004 Local interaction of prostaglandin $F_{2\alpha}$ with endothelin-1 and tumor necrosis factor on the release of progesterone and oxytocin in ovine corpora lutea *in vivo*: A possible implication for a luteolytic cascade. *Reproduction* **127** 117-124.

Okuda K, Uenoyama Y, Lee KW, Sakumoto R & Skarzynski DJ 1998 Progesterone stimulation by prostaglandin $F_{2\alpha}$ involves the protein kinase C pathway in cultured bovine luteal cells. *Journal of Reproduction and Development* **44** 79-84.

Okuda K, Sakumoto R, Uenoyama Y, Berisha B, Miyamoto A & Schams D 1999 Tumor necrosis factor-α receptors in microvascular endothelial cells from bovine corpus luteum. *Biology of Reproduction* **61** 1017-1022.

Okuda K, Miyamoto Y & Skarzynski DJ 2002 Regulation of endometrial prostaglandyn $F_{2\alpha}$ synthesis during luteolysisi and early pregnancy in cattle. *Domestic Animal Endocrinology* **23** 255-264.

Okuda K, Kasahara Y, Murakami S, Takahashi H, Woclawek-Potocka I & Skarzynski DJ 2004a Interferon-τ blocks the stimulatory effect of TNF-α on prostaglandin $F_{2\alpha}$ synthesis by bovine endometrial stromal cells. *Biology of Reproduction* **70** 191-197.

Okuda K, Korzekwa A, Shibaya M, Murakami S, Nishimura R, Tsubouchi M, Woclawek-Potocka I & Skarzynski DJ 2004b Progesterone is a suppressor of apoptosis in bovine luteal cells. *Biology of Reproduction* **71** 2065-2071.

Okuda K, Sakumoto R, Okamoto N, Acosta TJ, Abe H, Okada H, Sinowatz F & Skarzynski DJ 2010 Cellular localization of genes and proteins for tumor necrosis factor-α (TNF), TNF receptor types I and II in bovine endometrium. *Molecular and Cellular Endocrinology* **in press,** doi:10.1016/j.mce.2010.07.025.

Parkinson TJ, Wathes DC, Jenner LJ & Lamming GE 1992 Plasma and luteal concentrations of oxytocin in cyclic and early-pregnant cattle. *Journal of Reproduction & Fertility* **94** 161-167.

Pate JL 2003 Lives in the balance: responsiveness of the corpus luteaum to uterine and embryonic signals. *Reproduction Supp* **61** 207-217.

Pate JL & Condon WA 1989 Regulation of steroidogenesis and cholesterol synthesis by prostaglandin $F_{2\alpha}$ and lipoproteins in bovine luteal cells. *Journal of Reproduction & Fertility* **87** 439-446.

Pate JL & Keyes PL 2001 Immune cells in the corpus luteum: friends or foes? *Reproduction* **122** 665-676.

Penny LA, Armstrong D, Bramley TA, Webb R, Collins RA & Watson ED 1999 Immune cells and cytokine production in the bovine corpus luteum throughout the oestrous cycle and after induced luteolysis. *Journal of Reproduction & Fertility* **115** 87-96.

Petroff MG, Petroff BK & Pate JL 2001 Mechanisms of cytokine-induced death of cultured bovine luteal cells. Reproduction **121** 753-760.

Rosiansky-Sultan M, Klipper E, Spanel-Borowski K & Meidan R 2006 Inverse relationship between nitric oxide synthases and endothelin-1 synthesis in bovine corpus luteum: Interactions at the level of luteal endothelial cell *Endocrinology* **147** 5228-5235.

Sakamoto K, Miwa K, Ezashi T, Okuda-Ashitaka E, Okuda K, Houtani T, Sugimoto T, Ito S & Hayaishi O 1995 Expression of mRNA encoding the prostaglandin $F_{2\alpha}$ receptor in bovine corpora lutea throughout the oestrous cycle and pregnancy. *Journal of Reproduction & Fertility* **103** 99-105.

Sakamoto K, Ezashi T. Miwa K. Okuda-Ashitaka E. Houtani T. Sugimoto T, Ito S & Hayaishi O 1994 Molecular cloning and expression of a cDNA of the bovine prostaglandin $F_{2\alpha}$ receptor. *Journal of Biological Chemistry* **269** 3881-3886.

Sakumoto R, Berisha B, Kawate N, Schams D & Okuda K 2000 Tumor necrosis factor-α and its receptors in bovine corpus luteum throughout the estrous cycle. *Biology of Reproduction* **62** 192-199.

Schramm W, Bovaird L, Glew ME, Schramm G & McCracken JA 1983 Corpus luteum regression induced by ultra-low pulses of prostaglandin $F_{2\alpha}$. *Prostaglandins* **26** 347-364.

Sen A, Choudhary E, Inskeep EK & Flores JA 2005 Effects of selective protein kinase C isozymes in prostaglandin $F_{2\alpha}$-induced Ca signaling and luteinizing hormone-induced progesterone accumulation in the mid-phase bovine corpus luteum. *Biology of Reproduction* **72** 976–84.

Sen A, Wright M, Inskeep EK & Flores JA 2006 Participation of specific PKC isozymes in the inhibitory effect of ET-1 on progesterone accumulation in cells isolated from early- and mid-phase corpora lutea. *Domestic Animal Endocrinology* **31** 284-299.

Shaw DW & Britt JH 1995 Concentrations of tumor necrosis factor-α and progesterone within the bovine corpus luteum sampled by continuous-flow microdialysis during luteolysis in vivo. *Biology of Reproduction* **53** 847-854.

Shibaya M, Deptula KM, Korzekwa A, Okuda K & Skarzynski DJ 2005 Involvement of the cytoskeleton in oxytocin secretion by cultured bovine luteal cells. *Biology of Reproduction* **72** 200-205.

Shirasuna K, Asaoka H, Acosta TJ, Wijayagunawardane MPB, Ohtani M, Hayashi M, Matsui M & Miyamoto A 2004 Real-time relationships in intraluteal release among prostaglandin $F_{2\alpha}$, endothelin-1, and angiotensin II during spontaneous luteolysis in the cow. *Biology of Reproduction* **71** 1706-1711.

Shirasuna K, Shimizu T, Sayama K, Asahi T, Sasaki M, Berisha B, Schams D & Miyamoto A 2008a Expression and localization of apelin and its receptor APJ in the bovine corpus luteum during the estrous cycle and prostaglandin $F_{2\alpha}$-induced luteolysis *Reproduction* **135** 519-525.

Shirasuna K, Watanabe S, Asahi T, Wijayagunawardane MP, Sasahara K, Jiang C, Matsui M, Sasaki M, Shimizu T, Davis JS & Miyamoto A 2008b Prostaglandin $F_{2\alpha}$ increases endothelial nitric oxide synthase in the periphery of the bovine corpus luteum: the possible regulation of blood flow at an early stage of luteolysis. *Reproduction* **135** 527-539.

Shirasuna K, Asahi T, Sasaki M, Shimizu T, & Miyamoto A 2010 Distribution of arteriolovenous vessels, capillaries and eNOS expression in the bovine corpus luteum during the estrous cycle: a possible implication of different sensitivity by luteal phase to $PGF_{2□}$ in the increase of luteal llood llow. *Journal of Reprodcution & Development* **56** 124-130.

Skarzynski DJ & Okuda K 1999 Sensitivity of bovine corpora lutea to prostaglandin $F_{2\alpha}$ is dependent on progesterone, oxytocin and prostaglandins. *Biology of Reproduction* **60** 1292-1298.

Skarzynski DJ & Okuda K 2000 Different actions of noradrenaline and nitric oxide on the output of prostaglandins and progesterone in cultured bovine luteal cells. *Prostaglandins & other Lipid Mediators* **60** 35-47.

Skarzynski DJ, Miyamoto Y & Okuda K 2000a Production of prostaglandin $F_{2\alpha}$ by cultured bovine endometrial cells in response to tumor necrosis factor-α: cell type specificity and intracellular mechanisms. *Biology of Reproduction* **62** 1116-1120.

Skarzynski DJ, Kobayashi S & Okuda K 2000b: Influence of nitric oxide and noradrenaline on prostaglandin $F_{2\alpha}$-induced oxytocin secretion and intracellular calcium mobilization in cultured bovine luteal cells. *Biology of Reproduction* **63** 1000-1005.

Skarzynski DJ, Jaroszewski JJ, Bah MM, Deptuła KM, Barszczewska B, Gawronska B & Hansel W 2003a Administration of a nitric oxide synthase inhibitor counteracts prostaglandin $F_{2\alpha}$-induced luteolysis in cattle. *Biology of Reproduction* **68** 1674-1681.

Skarzynski DJ, Bah MM, Deptula KM, Woclawek-Potocka I, Korzekwa A, Shibaya M, Pilawski W & Okuda K 2003b Roles of tumor necrosis factor of the estrous cycle in cattle: an in vivo study. *Biology of Reproduction* **69** 1907-1913.

Skarzynski DJ, Woclawek-Potocka I, Korzekwa A, Bah MM, Piotrowska K, Barszczewska B & Okuda K 2007 Infusion of exogenous tumor necrosis factor dose dependently alters the length of the luteal phase in cattle: differential responses to treatment with indomethacin and L-NAME, a nitric oxide synthase inhibitor. *Biology of Reproduction* **76** 619-627.

Skarzynski DJ, Ferreira-Dias GM & Okuda K 2008 Regulation of luteal function and corpus luteum regression: hormonal control, immune mechanisms, and intercellular communication. *Reproduction in Domestic Animals* **43** 57-65.

Skarzynski DJ, Piotrowska K, Bah MM, Korzekwa A, Woclawek-Potocka I, Sawai K & Okuda K 2009 Effects of tumor necrosis factor-α (TNFα) on the secretory function of the bovine reproductive tract depend on TNFα achieved concentrations. *Reproduction in Domestic Animals* **44** 371-379.

Taniguchi H, Yokomizo Y & Okuda K 2002 Fas-fas ligand system mediates luteal cell death in bovine corpus luteum. *Biology of Reproduction* **66** 754-759.

Terranova PF, Hunter VJ, Roby KF & Hunt JS 1995 Tumor necrosis factor-α in the female reproductive tract. *Proceedings in Society for Experimental Biology and Medicicne* **209** 325-342.

Towson DH, O'Connor CL & Pru JK 2002 Expression of MCP-1 and distribution of immune cells populations in the bovine corpus luteum through the estrous cycle. *Biology of Reproduction* **66** 361-366.

Tsai S-J & Wiltbank MC 1997 Prostaglandin $F_{2\alpha}$ induces expression of prostaglandin G/H synthase-2 in the ovine corpus luteum: a potential positive feedback loop during luteolysis. *Biology of Reproduction* **57** 1016-1022.

Watanebe S, Shirasuna K, Matsui M, Yamamoto D, Berisha B, Schams D & Miyamoto A 2006 Effect of intraluteal injection of endothelin type A receptor antagonist on $PGF_{2□}$-induced luteolysis in the cow. *Journal of Reproduction & Development* **52** 551-559.

Weems YS, Randel RD, Tatman S, Lewis AW, Neuendorff DA & Weems CW 2004 Effects of estrous synchronization on the response to nitric oxide donors, nitric oxide synthase inhibitors, and endothelin-1 *in vitro*. *Prostaglandins & Other Lipid Mediators* **74** 45-59.

Wiltbank JN & Cassida LE 1956 Alteration of ovarian activity by hysterectomy. *Journal of Animal Sciences* **15** 134-140.

Wiltbank MC, Diskin MG, Flores JA & Niswender GD 1990 Regulation of the corpus luteum by protein kinase C II. Inhibition of lipoprotein-stimulated steroidogenesis by prostaglandin. *Biology of Reproduction* **42** 239-45.

Wise TH, Caton D, Thatcher WW, Barron DH & Fields MJ 1982 Ovarian function during the estrous cycle of the cow: ovarian blood flow and progesterone release rate. *Journal of Animal Sciences* **55** 627-637.

Wright MF, Sayre B, Keith Inskeep EK & Flores JA 2001 Prostaglandin $F_{2\alpha}$ regulation of the bovine corpus luteum endothelin system during the early and midluteal phase. *Biology of Reproduction* **65** 171-1717.

Endocrine actions of interferon-tau in ruminants

TR Hansen[1], LK Henkes[1], RL Ashley[1], RC Bott[1], AQ Antoniazzi[1, 2] and H Han[3]

[1]Animal Reproduction and Biotechnology Laboratory, Department of Biomedical Sciences and [2]BioRep, Departamento de Clínica de Grandes Animais, Centro de Ciências Rurais, Universidade Federal de Santa Maria, 97105-900, Santa Maria, RS, Brazil; [3]Department of Animal Sciences, Colorado State University, Campus Delivery 1683, Fort Collins, CO 80523, USA

The ovine conceptus releases interferon-τ (IFNT), which prevents upregulation of the endometrial estrogen receptor (ESR1) and, consequently, oxytocin receptor (OXTR), thereby disrupting pulsatile release of prostaglandin F2α (PGF) in response to oxytocin. IFNT, through paracrine action on the endometrium, protects the corpus luteum (CL) during maternal recognition of pregnancy. Pregnancy also induces IFN stimulated genes (ISGs) in peripheral blood mononuclear cells (PBMCs), which is interpreted to reflect a "prompted" antiviral and immune cell response peripherally in ruminants. IFNT was recently demonstrated to be released from the uterus in amounts of ~ 200 μg (2 x 10^7 U)/24 h via the uterine vein and to induce ISGs in the CL during maternal recognition of pregnancy. Delivery of recombinant ovine (ro) IFNT into the uterine vein in a location that is upstream of the utero-ovarian plexus from Day 10 to 17 maintained serum progesterone concentrations and extended normal 16-17 d estrous cycles to beyond 32 d. It is concluded from these studies that IFNT is released into the uterine vein and initiates a peripheral antiviral response to protect pregnancy from maternal viral infection. It also may have endocrine action through inducing luteal resistance to PGF and longer-term survival of the CL and maintenance of pregnancy.

Introduction

The timing of release and composition of signals from the conceptus are critical for maintenance of the CL and pregnancy. For example, transferring a Day 5-9 embryo into the uterus of Day 5 estrous cycling ewes extends luteal lifespan (Moor & Rowson 1966b). If a Day 12-13 embryo is transferred into a recipient ewe later than 12 d post-estrus, the chances of the pregnancy surviving to term are drastically reduced (Moor & Rowson 1964, Moor & Rowson 1966a). Therefore, the uterus must receive and respond to a signal from the conceptus by Day 12, after which time it becomes unable to maintain pregnancy. In ewes with one surgically isolated uterine horn, only the CL ipsilateral to the gravid horn survived (Moor & Rowson 1966a), suggesting that the embryo has a local effect on the gravid uterus. Embryos transferred to an isolated horn of ewes with CL on both ovaries only maintained the CL on the side ipsilateral to the embryo (Moor & Rowson 1966a). These experiments were interpreted to indicate that a "local unilateral relationship between the embryo and the corpus luteum" existed and that a systemic response to the conceptus was not necessary to maintain early pregnancy. Hansen et

Corresponding author E-mail: thomas.hansen@colostate.edu

al. reported an interestrous interval of 19 d when conceptuses were flushed on Day 13 and an extension to 35 d when flushed on Day 17 (Hansen *et al.* 1985). These data are interpreted to mean that signals from the conceptus are necessary by Day 12-13 and need to continue until Day 17 to protect the CL from lytic release of uterine-derived PGF.

The major conceptus secretory protein was initially termed protein X and is secreted during Days 10-12 (Godkin *et al.* 1982, Bazer & Roberts 1983). Protein X, was renamed ovine trophoblast protein-1, and later IFNT as reviewed in (Bazer *et al.* 1991, Roberts *et al.* 1992). Peak secretion of IFNT from the ovine conceptus occurs between Days 15-17 of pregnancy (Hansen *et al.* 1985, Ashworth & Bazer 1989, Roberts 1989). IFNT acts through the Type I interferon receptor which shares two subunits, IFNAR1 and IFNAR2. These subunits are expressed in the luminal epithelium, sub-luminal glandular epithelium, and stroma of the ovine uterus in Day 14-15 cyclic and pregnant ewes (Rosenfeld *et al.* 2002). Paracrine action of IFNT on the endometrium has been shown to alter (ewe) (Zarco *et al.* 1988a, Zarco *et al.* 1988b) or attenuate (cow) (Meyer *et al.* 1995) luteolytic pulses of PGF (based on detection of PGFM). Nonpregnant ewes secrete PGF in a pulsatile fashion, while pregnant ewes have a more constant, slowly increasing pattern in the release of PGF (Peterson *et al.* 1976, Zarco *et al.* 1988b). However, more PGF is found exiting the uterus through the uterine vein in Day 13 pregnant vs cyclic ewes (Wilson *et al.* 1972). This antiluteolytic mediation in release of PGF from the endometrium during pregnancy is regulated by conceptus-derived IFNT.

Because the release of PGF from the endometrium is not completely ablated and the CL produces PGF (Silva *et al.* 2000), several groups have described the CL of pregnancy to be more resistant to lytic effects of PGF compared to the CL of the estrous cycle (Inskeep *et al.* 1975, Mapletoft *et al.* 1976, Pratt *et al.* 1977, Silvia & Niswender 1984). Exactly why and how this luteal resistance to PGF occurs during pregnancy is unknown. Also, whether the actions of intraluteal PGF or PGF that continues to be delivered into the uterine vein need to be blocked during early pregnancy is unknown. This review examines endocrine action of pregnancy in ruminants. It is proposed that endocrine release of IFNT into the uterine vein upregulates peripheral antiviral and immune cell responses, which when further challenged with viral infection, immediately respond and protect the pregnancy. A second endocrine action of IFNT during early pregnancy is proposed through induction of interferon-stimulated genes (ISGs) in the CL, which contributes to luteal resistance to PGF.

Luteal cells and luteolysis

Late in the ovine luteolytic process (Day 16), release of progesterone diminishes because of PGF action on large luteal cells. Oxytocin release by large luteal cells and action of oxytocin on small luteal cells further inhibits secretion of progesterone and stimulates intracellular levels of calcium and apoptosis (Niswender *et al.* 2007). PGF also is released from large luteal cells, possibly through a PG transporter (SLCO2A1), and binds PGF receptor (PTGFR) on large luteal cells to further stimulate oxytocin release, increases in intracellular calcium concentrations and, consequently, death of the CL (Davis *et al.* 2010). Luteolysis may also include PGF activation of protein kinase C (PKC) and RAF/MEK1/ERK-mediated increase in early growth response 1 (EGR1) and transforming growth factor B (TGFB1) (Hou *et al.* 2008) as well as repression of insulin like growth factor (IGF-1) and cell-survival responses (phosphoinositide 3-kinase; PI3K and protein kinase B; Akt) (Arvisais *et al.* 2010).

Paracrine action of IFNT

Ruminant conceptuses are free-floating in the uterus during maternal recognition of pregnancy. Thus, paracrine action of IFNT regulates endometrial gene expression and indirectly induces antiluteolytic responses (Godkin *et al.* 1984a, Godkin *et al.* 1984b). In addition to the classical JAK/STAT pathway (Hansen *et al.* 1999, Perry *et al.* 1999, Binelli *et al.* 2001, Pru *et al.* 2001b), Type I IFN also activates PI3K and Akt pathways (Rani *et al.* 2002, Badr *et al.* 2010). IFNT silences up-regulation of ovine *ESR1* (Spencer *et al.* 1995, Spencer & Bazer 1996, Fleming *et al.* 2001) and, consequently, *OXTR* (Spencer & Bazer 1996, Chen *et al.* 2006) in the endometrium. Decreased transcription of the *OXTR* is likely due to the decrease in ESR1 caused by IFNT, as *OXTR* is not directly regulated by IFNT (Fleming *et al.* 2006). Suppressed ESR1 and OXTR in the endometrium causes alteration (ewe) (Zarco *et al.* 1988a, Zarco *et al.* 1988b) or attenuation (cow) (Meyer *et al.* 1995) of luteolytic pulses of PGF (based on detection of PGFM).

Several ISGs have been identified in the ruminant uterus such as 2′, 5′-oligoadenylate synthetase (*OAS*) (Mirando *et al.* 1991, Schmitt *et al.* 1993, Johnson *et al.* 2001), myxovirus (influenza virus) resistance (*Mx*) (Ott *et al.* 1998), and IFN-stimulated gene 15 (*ISG15*) (Naivar *et al.* 1995, Austin *et al.* 1996, Johnson *et al.* 1999b). One conserved primate (Bebington *et al.* 1999a, Bebington *et al.* 1999b, Bebington *et al.* 2000), mouse (Austin *et al.* 2003, Bany & Cross 2006), and bovine (Austin *et al.* 1996, Hansen *et al.* 1997, Johnson *et al.* 1998, Perry *et al.* 1999, Thatcher *et al.* 2001) uterine response to pregnancy is induction of the ubiquitin homolog, ISG15. ISG15 mediates processes such as RNA splicing, chromatin remodeling/polymerase II transcription, cytoskeletal organization and regulation, stress responses, translation and viral replication (Malakhova *et al.* 2003, Giannakopoulos *et al.* 2005, Zhao *et al.* 2005, Takeuchi *et al.* 2006).

Intrauterine delivery of roIFNT delays return to estrus

Because IFNT acts locally on endometrial release of PGF, models were developed in sheep to test effects of intrauterine infusion of IFNT on interestrous interval. Intrauterine infusion of 50 μg native IFNT twice daily extended interestrous interval to 27 d (Vallet *et al.* 1988). Intrauterine infusion of 340 μg roIFNT for 8 d extended return to estrus from 25-64 d in four out of five ewes (Martal *et al.* 1990). Likewise, intrauterine infusion of 1.4 x 10^7 U/d roIFNT from Day 10-18 delayed return to estrus to 33 ± 14 d (Green *et al.* 2005). These studies were interpreted to mean that IFNT acted in paracrine action to extend the luteal phase by attenuating pulses of PGF and, thereby, protect the CL through antiluteolytic action. Importantly, the potential entry of exogenous IFNT from the intrauterine infusion studies was not evaluated in the context of endocrine action through its potential direct impact on the maintenance of CL function.

Endocrine action of IFNT

Systemic delivery of roIFNT induces hyperthermia, but has varied impact on fertility

Delivery of Type I IFN, via intramuscular or subcutaneous injection also was examined by several groups for capacity to extend interestrous interval and increase fertility (Nephew *et al.* 1990, Martinod *et al.* 1991, Schalue-Francis *et al.* 1991, Davis *et al.* 1992). These studies employed mg quantities of rIFN administered through twice daily injections (subcutaneous), which may not reflect physiological levels of IFNT released by the uterus. These quantities (mg) of rIFN induced hyperthermia, and no effect or a decline in fertility. For example, Ott and colleagues (Ott *et al.* 1997) observed an induction of mild hyperthermia following subcutaneous injections of 2, 4 or 6 mg rIFNT on Day 12 post estrus. These investigators also injected 1, 2 or 4 mg roIFNT/d on Days 11-15 and described a modest delay in onset of estrus after adjusting for previous length of estrous cycle. These doses of roIFNT were subsequently reduced to 2 x 10^7 U (200 μg) in intrauterine deliveries to avoid hyperthermia and high death loss of ewes (Spencer *et al.* 1999).

Subcutaneous (Spencer *et al.* 1999) and intramuscular injection (2 mg) (Chen *et al.* 2006) of roIFNT given between Days 11-17 stimulated ISG15 expression within the ovine CL. Chen and colleagues (Chen *et al.* 2006) reported an inter-estrus interval of 32.7 d in ewes that received intrauterine infusions of 200 μg roIFNT, but an average interval of only 17 and 22 d in ewes that were injected i.m. with 200 μg or 2 mg roIFNT, respectively. These investigators also described an increase in endometrial ISG15 expression in response to infusion of roIFNT and injection of 2 mg roIFNT, but not following injection of 200 μg roIFNT. None of these systemic methods of roIFNT treatment prolonged return to estrus for more than a few days.

Induction of ISGs in blood cells during early pregnancy

Until recently (Oliveira *et al.* 2008, Bott *et al.* 2010), IFNT was thought to be sequestered within the uterine lumen and not present in peripheral circulation in high enough concentrations to be detected. Although, IFN-alpha has been shown to suppress tumor necrosis factor α and IFNγ-stimulated prostaglandin production by cultured luteal cells (Pate 1995). Likewise, culture of luteal cells with IFN-alpha and in concentrations of progesterone similar to those observed during early pregnancy also suppressed IFNγ-induction of MHC class II glycoproteins. Pate (1995) concluded from these studies that a signal similar to trophoblast-derived IFNT might reach the ovary and act directly to protect the CL.

ISGs such as MX1 (Ott *et al.* 1998), ISG15 (Johnson *et al.* 1999a, Johnson *et al.* 1999b) and OAS-1 (Johnson *et al.* 2001) have been shown to be upregulated in uterine cross sections as deep as the myometrium. For this reason, IFNT was suspected to induce a secondary mediator in the myometrium. This secondary mediator of IFNT action was called an "interferon-medin" (Spencer *et al.* 1996).

PBMCs from pregnant sheep have increased concentrations of ISGs mRNA (Yankey *et al.* 2001) compared to nonpregnant sheep, which also is the case in cattle (Han *et al.* 2006, Gifford *et al.* 2007). Presence of ISGs in extrauterine tissues such as jugular PBMCs provoked study of ISGs in uterine vein and uterine artery blood as well as the CL (Oliveira *et al.* 2008, Bott *et al.* 2010). Concentrations of ISG15 mRNA in jugular vein on Day 15 of pregnancy were similar to uterine vein and artery ISG15 concentrations suggesting endocrine induction of ISGs through the presence of the conceptus and release of either IFNT or an interferon-medin from the uterus.

Very little is known about the genes that are regulated in blood cells during early pregnancy and no studies have been done to compare blood and endometrial gene expression in response to pregnancy. We hypothesized that several genes would be upregulated by pregnancy on Day 18 of bovine pregnancy in endometrial and blood cells. Several hundred endometrial (674 genes upregulated and 721 downregulated $\geq$ 1.5 fold; $P < 0.05$) and blood cell (375 genes upregulated and 784 downregulated $\geq$ 1.2 fold; $P < 0.05$) genes were differentially expressed based on pregnancy status on Day 18 of pregnancy (United States Patent Application: 20100035270 and Fig. 1). Upregulated ISGs in endometrium (Fig. 1) were similar to other reports using microarray (Klein *et al.* 2005), (Bauersachs *et al.* 2006, Chen *et al.* 2006, Bauersachs *et al.* 2008) and conventional molecular biology approaches (Johnson *et al.* 1999a, Pru *et al.* 2001a, Rempel *et al.* 2005).

A **Endometrial Genes** **Blood Genes**

Fold	P <	Identity	Name	Fold	P <	Identity	Name
9.1	0.0002	BE723335	IRF7	1.5	0.01	BE683272	IRF7
57.6	0.0002	NM_174366	ISG15	3.1	0.01	NM_174366	ISG15
14.1	0.00002	CK966909	UBE1L	1.9	0.002	CK966909	UBE1L
124.7	0.00001	NM_173941	MX2	1.8	0.01	NM_173941.2	MX2
14.7	0.001	CB432365	RIGI	1.7	0.01	CB432365	RIGI
15.4	0.0001	CK960499	OAS	4.5	0.001	CK960499	OAS
1.9	0.03	NM_175827.2	CCL5	2.1	0.02	NM_175827.2	CCL5
48.7	0.001	CB422521	IFI44	1.9	0.03	CB422521	IFI44
10.7	0.0005	NM_174007	CCL8	2.1	0.05	AW659977	TCRb
10.7	0.002	CB419326	GBP5	1.8	0.04	CK945023	CD3D
1.5	0.01	NM_173893.1	B2MG	1.8	0.02	NM_174015	CD8
48.5	0.0001	CB427688	~EIF4E	2.1	0.02	AB008616	MHC-1
-18.4	0.02	NM_174816	OXTR	-2.2	0.04	CK775610	Homer 2

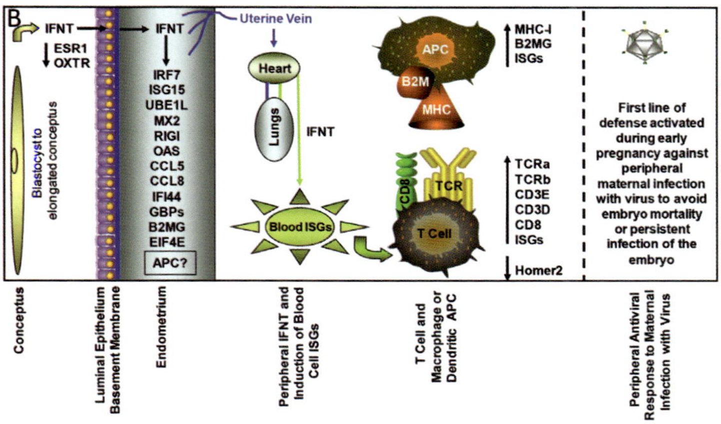

Fig. 1. Hypothetical model of conceptus-induced preemptive maternal resistance to viral infection. Panel A contains fold changes and identities for genes described in Panel B. Cows were artificially inseminated on Day 0. Presence of a conceptus was confirmed on Day 32 post AI by using ultrasound. Blood was collected from lactating Holstein Dairy cows 18 days following AI (4 pregnant and 3 nonpregnant cows) and processed to purify RNA for microarray screening according to the QiaAMP procedure (Qiagen, Inc.). Because of excessive costs in collecting the uterus from lactating dairy cows, Angus-Gelbvieh beef cows were used for endometrial studies. Endometrial RNA was isolated from cows on Day 18 of pregnancy (3 cows; conceptus identified) or the estrous cycle (3 cows; not inseminated) following slaughter and submitted for microarray analysis. The bovine Affymetryx gene chip was screened at the University of Colorado Health Sciences Center (UCHSC) DNA Microarray Core facility. Data were analyzed using GCOS and GeneSifter software. Statistical significance was determined using the t-test calculated from Robust Multichip Average data (Irizarry *et al.* 2003). A 1.5-fold cut off was used to identify all differentially expressed genes in endometrium. A 1.2-fold cut off was used to identify all differentially expressed genes in blood because there were fewer affected genes in the blood and identification of shared gene expression between blood and endometrium was one primary focus of the experiment. Panel B provides hypothesized role of IFNT in activating a peripheral maternal antiviral response. IFNT is released from the conceptus that initiates a local (*i.e.*, paracrine) type I IFN response through up-regulation of ISGs, chemokines, and other genes in the endometrium and myometrium before exiting the uterus by the uterine vein. In endocrine fashion, IFNT then transcriptionally upregulates ISGs and genes involved in activation of T cell and antigen presenting cells (APC) such as macrophages and dendritic cells. The conceptus, therefore, coordinates both local and systemic immunomodulatory events that allow the mother to cope with potential viral infections as more aggressive cytotoxic responses that may be detrimental to the histocompatibly distinct embryo are concomitantly curbed.

Virus induces retinoic acid-induced gene I (RIG-I) and melanoma differentiation-associated protein 5 (MDA-5) which contain RNA helicase domains that bind viral dsRNA and response elements that activate interferon regulatory factors (IRF3 and IRF7), which then induce synthesis of Type I IFN. Several other *ISGs* are induced to regulate viral infection such as OAS-1, which activates endoribonuclease to degrade virus; protein kinase R (PKR) to phosphorylate eukaryotic initiation factor (eIF)-2, which in turn inhibits translation and replication of virus; and ISG15 (Lenschow *et al.* 2007) and MX (MacMicking 2004). This pathway of genes is known to be required for cellular resistance to viral infection. Likewise, several indicators of T cell activation in blood cells were identified.

Homer protein homolog 2 (*HOMER2)* was a major downregulated gene in both endometrium and blood in response to pregnancy. In T cells, *HOMER2* is upregulated after T cell activation (Diehn *et al.* 2002), however it is considered a negative regulator of T cell activation and production of IL-2 (Huang *et al.* 2008). A downregulation of *HOMER2* would allow better access for stimulation of nuclear factor of activated T cells (NFAT) by calcineuron (Huang *et al.* 2008). Other indicators that T cells are activated in response to IFNT include upregulation of many T cell receptor (TCRA, TCRB, TCRG) components such as T cell surface glycoproteins CD3D, CD3E and CD8. IRF7 is a key regulator of Type I IFN-dependent activation of CD8 positive T cells (Honda *et al.* 2005). Both *CD8* and *IRF7* were upregulated in blood in response to pregnancy. CD8 is known to function as a co-receptor with TCR when interacting with major histocompatibility complex (MHCI) on target cells.

Type I IFNs also induce MHCI on many cell types and activate not only T cells, but also natural killer cells. Based on the microarray data, *MHCI* was upregulated in blood cells from Day 18 pregnant when compared to nonpregnant cows and is normally upregulated in professional antigen presenting cells such as dendritic cells and tissue macrophages. The apparent upregulation of blood cell MHCI in response to pregnancy is based on hybridization to probe sets in the microarray and may have been caused by different MHC haplotypes that were expressed by the limited number of cows used in this study (Davies *et al.* 1994). However, beta-2-microglobulin (B2MG) was upregulated in endometrium, but not in blood cells, which might reflect expression of this binding partner for MHCI in tissue followed by homing or translocation of pre-antigen presenting blood cells. Following viral infection of these cells, massive upregulation of RIGI and MDA5 RNA helicases would assist in degrading viral RNA. Processing of viral coat proteins and presentation of antigen would be facilitated through existing upregulation of MHCI and B2MG as well as enhancing the presence of activated CD8 T cells.

Upregulation of CD8 and TCR activated T cells and MHCI/B2MG antigen presenting cells could be detrimental because the conceptus expresses foreign antigens that would clearly be recognized by these cells. However, in ruminants at this very early stage of pregnancy, the conceptus has developed only very peripheral adhesion complexes to the uterine lumen with no penetration of the basement membrane of the endometrium. For this reason, the uterine lumen remains isolated from any circulating T cells. Also *B2MG* and MHC class I genes are silenced in ovine endometrial luminal epithelium and trophectoderm even though they are upregulated in other endometrial layers (Choi *et al.* 2003). Very few immune cells are localized to the endometrium during this stage of pregnancy in ruminants (Vander Wielen & King 1984). This might be caused by lack of specific chemokine receptors on these cells and/or lack of endometrial production of chemokines that would specifically recruit these cells to the endometrium. Alternatively, this could be accounted for by increased expression or presence of immune cell repulsive factors.

However, we described macrophage inflammatory protein (CXCL2) (Hansen *et al.* 1999) and granulocyte chemotactic protein-2 (CXCL6) (Teixeira *et al.* 1997) to be induced by pregnancy and IFNT in bovine endometrium. Also, other groups demonstrated that CXCL9, CXCL10, CXCL11 and CXCR3 are localized to the maternal-fetal interface in sheep during early pregnancy (Imakawa *et al.* 2006). Likewise, monocyte chemotactic protein (Asselin *et al.* 2001) and IFN-gamma inducible protein 10 (Nagaoka *et al.* 2003) have been shown to be expressed in endometrium in response to pregnancy. Based on enclosed microarray analysis, chemokine receptor mRNA concentrations were not upregulated in blood cells from Day 18 pregnant when compared to nonpregnant cows. Chemokine ligand 5 (*CCL5*) was the only major chemokine mRNA that was significantly upregulated in blood. Likewise, only three chemokine ligands, *CCL8, CXCL10 and CCL5* were extensively upregulated in the endometrium. CCL5 induces recruitment of T cells to the lung following viral lung disease (Culley *et al.* 2006). CCL8 is chemotactic for monocytes and CD8+ as well as CD4+ T cells (Taub *et al.* 1995) and might recruit these cells to the endometrium in the event of infection. However, if the associated chemokine receptors are not differentially expressed on these T cells, then very few of these cells would be actively recruited to the endometrium, unless there was a maternal-peripheral infection with virus. Because these maternal antiviral T cells and antigen presenting cells are activated through exposure to Type I IFN from the conceptus, they would immediately be recruited to the endometrium where a first or last line of defense would be established to inhibit virus from passing through the endometrial basement membrane and infecting the conceptus (Fig. 1).

Direct endocrine action of IFNT on the corpus luteum

Endocrine release of conceptus-derived IFNT into the uterine vein. Lymph nodes draining the uterus (iliac) and the head (submandibular) from Day 15 pregnant ewes were examined and found not to differ in ISG gene expression (Antoniazzi et al., unpublished results); suggesting that IFNT was not released into uterine lymphatic drainage and this was not a pathway through which IFNT induced PBMC ISGs. This also was consistent with previous reports describing no antiviral activity in lymph draining the uterus during pregnancy (Lamming *et al.* 1995). However, Godkin and co-workers demonstrated that infusion of radiolabeled IFNT into the uterine lumen resulted in escape of very low levels into the blood (Godkin *et al.* 1984a). Schalue-Francis (Schalue-Francis *et al.* 1991) described antiviral activity in the uterine vein, although levels reported were very low. For these reasons we re-examined the uterine vein as a source for endocrine delivery of IFNT. Antiviral activity was evaluated in uterine vein blood from Day 15 pregnant sheep, which revealed significant amounts of Type I IFN ($\sim 200 \mu g/24h$) on Day 15 of pregnancy (Oliveira *et al.* 2008). Also, pre-adsorption of uterine vein blood from Day 15 pregnant ewes with antibody against roIFNT significantly reduced antiviral activity (Bott *et al.* 2010). It was concluded from these studies that IFNT is released into the uterine vein on Day 15 of pregnancy. Other than Day 15, the timing and concentration of IFNT in uterine vein blood is unknown and is a focus of ongoing study.

Endocrine induction of ISGs in large luteal cells. ISG15 mRNA concentrations were uregulated in CL from Day 15 pregnant compared to nonpregnant ewes (Fig. 2) (Oliveira *et al.* 2008, Bott *et al.* 2010). ISG15 protein and conjugation of ISG15 to targeted proteins also were upregulated in CL in response to pregnancy. ISG15 was predominantly localized to large luteal cells on Day 15 of pregnancy, with less, but significant localization to small luteal cells. Also, large luteal cells isolated on Day 10 of the estrous cycle and cultured with roIFNT for 24 h showed significant induction of ISG15 (Oliveira *et al.* 2008). Finally, IFNAR1 and IFNAR2 mRNA are expressed in the ovine CL (Antoniazzi et al., unpublished results). It was concluded from these studies that in addition to extensively characterized paracrine action on the endometrium, IFNT also likely has direct endocrine action on extrauterine tissues such as blood cells and the CL.

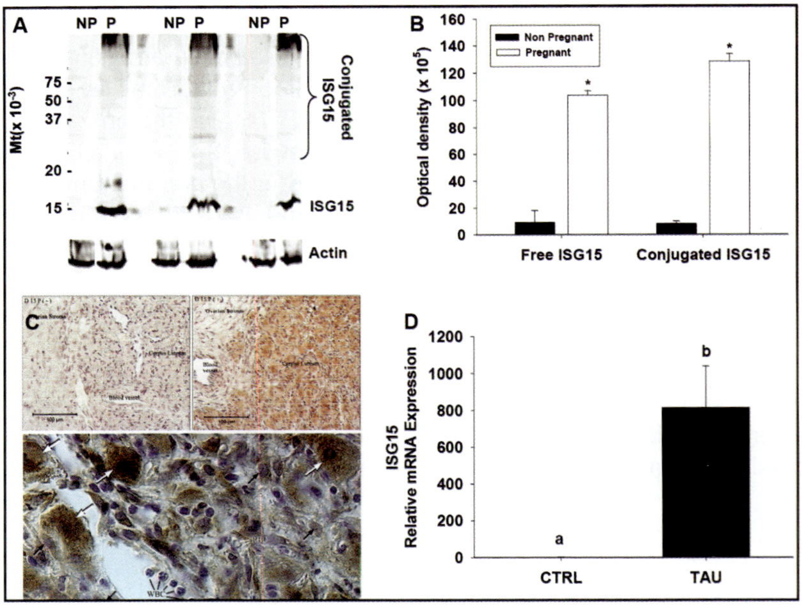

Fig. 2. Western blot of ISG15 (15-kDa) and its conjugates (A, B), immunohistochemical localization of ISG15 in CL (C) and induction of ISG15 following culture of isolated large luteal cells (Day 10 of estrous cycle) with 100 ng/ml roIFNT for 24 h (D). Both free and conjugated ISG15 were induced (*; $P < 0.05$) by pregnancy and in response to culture with roIFNT (a, b; $P < 0.05$). Imunohistochemical staining for ISG15 was upregulated in cross-sections from CL on Day 15 of pregnancy (C: top right panel). Panel C Upper left: no primary antibody control. Localization of ISG15 was most intense in large luteal cells (lower panel in C; white arrows). For more details please see (Oliveira *et al.* 2008). Copyright 2008, The Endocrine Society.

Endocrine delivery of 200 μg roIFNT/d into the uterine vein for 7 d delayed return to estrus. Release of IFNT into the uterine vein on Day 15 of pregnancy was estimated previously to be ~ 200 μg/d (Oliveira *et al.* 2008). For this reason, osmotic pumps loaded to deliver 200 μg/d into the uterine vein for seven consecutive days were surgically installed. Estimated blood volume in sheep was 3.48 L based on average weight of 60 kg and blood volume of 58 ml/kg. Thus, on Day 15 of pregnancy, systemic levels in circulation would stabilize around 2.4 ng/ml/h. This is biologically relevant considering the dissociation constant (Kd) of 3.7×10^{-10} M (Li & Roberts 1994) and estimated 50% occupancy of the receptor at 6.3 ng IFNT/ml.

Osmotic pumps delivering 200 μg roIFNT into the uterine vein/d were surgically installed on Day 10 of the estrous cycle in sheep (Fig. 3). Eighty percent (4/5) of ewes infused with roIFNT for 7 d had extended estrous cycles and luteal phase serum progesterone concentrations through 32 d (Bott *et al.* 2010). In the nonresponder ewe, serum progesterone concentrations were declining at the time of installation of the pump, which was interpreted as onset of luteal regression prior to endocrine delivery of roIFNT. To our knowledge this is the first report of such small endocrine concentrations of IFNT to induce a significant long-term delay in return to estrus.

There was no effect of 24 h endocrine delivery of roIFNT into the uterine vein starting on Day 10 of the estrous cycle on serum progesterone concentrations (Fig. 4) (Bott *et al.* 2010). A sub-luteolytic dose of PGF (4 mg/58 kg), described previously to cause a significant decline in serum progesterone without complete luteolysis (Silvia & Niswender 1984, Silvia & Niswender 1986, Silva *et al.* 2000, Bott *et al.* 2010), was injected 12 h following delivery of roIFNT into the uterine vein. PGF caused a significant decline in serum progesterone concentrations within 6 h, even in ewes with 12 h pre-exposure to delivery of roIFNT into the uterine vein. However, by 8-12 h after injection of PGF serum progesterone returned to concentrations in roIFNT-infused ewes that were intermediate and not different from BSA- or roIFNT-infused ewes in the absence of PGF injection. Endocrine delivery of IFNT also induced upregulation of ISG15 mRNA in the endometrium and the CL. This "recovery" in serum progesterone concentrations was suggested to reflect induction of luteal resistance to PGF through endocrine delivery of IFNT.

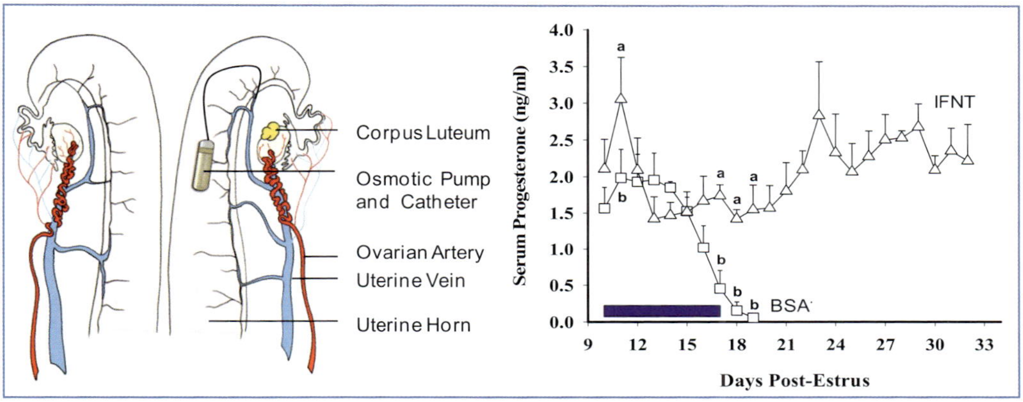

Fig. 3. Osmotic pump delivery (Left Panel) of 200 μg roIFNT (2 x 10^7 IU)/d roIFNT or BSA for 7 d into the uterine vein caused extension of the estrous cycle and maintenance of serum progesterone concentrations (Right Panel) in 80% of ewes. Shaded bar represents time of osmotic pump infusion (Days 10-16). Adapted from Bott *et al.* 2010.

Intraluteal prostaglandins

Concentrations of 15 hydroxyprostaglandin dehydrogenase (PGDH) and prostaglandin-endoperoxide synthase 2 (PTGS2) mRNAs increase in CL on Day 13 of pregnancy compared to the estrous cycle suggesting that the CL of pregnancy is better able to degrade endogenous PGs in the face of increased synthesis via PTGS2 (Silva *et al.* 2000). This upregulation of PTGS2 might contribute to reduced luteal sensitivity to PGF through shifting biosynthesis to PGE2 (Costine *et al.* 2007) through PGE synthase (PTGES).

PGDH, PTGES, PGFS, and PTGS2 mRNA concentrations did not change following 24 h infusion of IFNT into the uterine vein (Bott *et al.* 2010). This was interpreted to suggest that IFNT does not induce luteal resistance through inhibiting mRNAs encoding intraluteal biosynthesis of PGs, at least on Day 10 of the estrous cycle. SLCO2A1 facilitates transport of PGs across membranes (Chan *et al.* 1998, Schuster 1998, Endo *et al.* 2002, Schuster 2002). PGF is transported through SLCO2A1 in the ovine endometrim (Banu *et al.* 2008) and through countercurrent exchange in the utero-ovarian plexus (Lee *et al.* 2010). One action of IFNT might be to downregulate SLCO2A1 in the utero-ovarian plexus and thus disrupt delivery of PGF to the CL. SLCO2A1 may also regulate release of PGF from large luteal cells during autocrine activation of PTGFR to induce luteolysis (Niswender *et al.* 2007). Downregulation of SLCO2A1 in large luteal cells might impair release of PGF and, consequently, autocrine action of PGF on large luteal cell apoptosis. Another target in the CL for development of resistance to luteolysis is downregulation of the PGTFR. However, it has been reported that PTGFR mRNA (Juengel

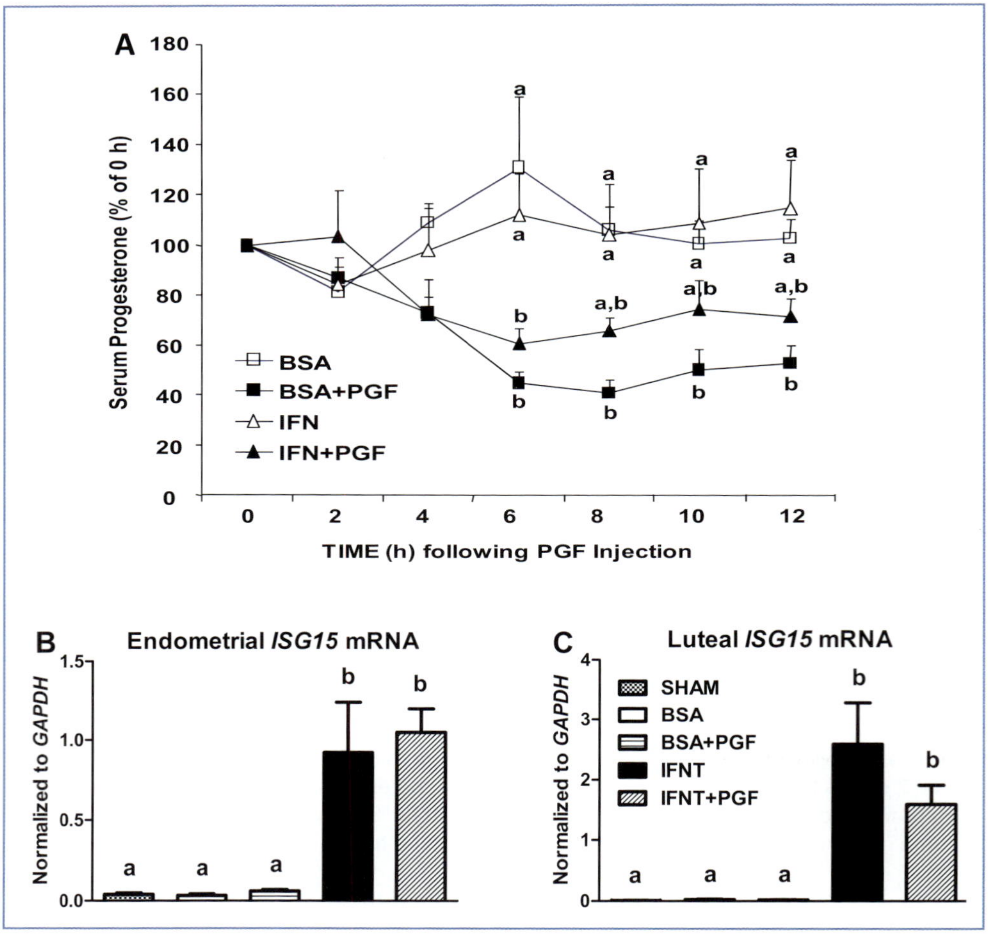

Fig. 4. Endocrine delivery of IFNT into the uterine vein protects the CL from PGF through attenuating the decline in serum progesterone (A) and possibly through induction of ISGs in the endometrium (B) and CL (C). BSA or roIFNT (200 μg/24h) were infused into the uterine vein in 24 ewes (12 ewes per treatment). Half of these ewes were injected with PGF (4mg/58 kg bw) 12 h later. Panel A describes a decrease in serum progesterone concentrations 6 h following PGF regardless of infusion treatment. However, in roIFNT infused ewes, serum progesterone concentration increased after 6 h to levels not different from controls. Data are the mean (n = 6 ewes per treatment) $\pm$ SE. Significant differences ($P < 0.05$) in treatments and time are denoted with different letters. Endometrium and CL (Panel C) were collected and examined for ISG15 mRNA concentrations, which increased following endocrine delivery of roIFNT. Means differ ($P < 0.05$) when designated by different superscripts. Adapted from Bott *et al.* 2010.

et al. 1998), protein (Wiepz *et al.* 1992) and affinity constant (Wiepz *et al.* 1992) are not attenuated during maternal recognition of pregnancy in sheep. These nicely designed studies concluded that the mechanism through which the ovine CL achieves resistance to PGF during early pregnancy does not involve PTGFR. Prostaglandin E2 receptor (PTGER2) is coupled to the cAMP signal transduction pathway, which stimulates steroidogenesis and production of progesterone in cultured human luteinized granulosa (Chandras *et al.* 2007). PTGER4 also is a G-protein receptor coupled to cAMP as reviewed in (Sugimoto & Narumiya 2007), but to our knowledge, functional coupling of this receptor subtype to synthesis of progesterone has not been studied in the CL. Upregulation of PGE2 receptors coupled to cAMP signaling in the CL during pregnancy might also contribute to luteal resistance to PGF. Regardless of the specific PTGERs involved, the general steroidogenic action of PGE2 has been extensively studied since the first report that it induces adenylate cyclase in bovine CL (Marsh 1971).

Conclusions

IFNs were discovered as antiviral cytokines (Isaacs & Lindenmann 1957). Viral infection of a pregnant cow can result in vertical transmission to the fetus (Casaro *et al.* 1971). A significant upregulation of Type I IFN and ISGs has been described in PBMC following infection of pregnant heifers with bovine viral diarrhea virus prior to and following development of the fetal immune system (Smirnova *et al.* 2008, Shoemaker *et al.* 2009, Smirnova *et al.* 2009). This defense to viral infection also is initiated through release of IFNT from the conceptus during early pregnancy. Through prompting, but not completely activating maternal antiviral responses, peripheral maternal resistance may protect the pregnancy in the event that viral infection occurs.

Why the ruminant conceptus produces IFNT, a Type I IFN, in amounts large enough to induce systemic responses has been proposed to be related to maternal mediation of inflammatory and immune responses that might be detrimental to the "foreign" conceptus (Roberts *et al.* 1992). A variation in this theme is suggested herein, where the local endometrial and peripheral maternal immune responses become primed during early pregnancy through conceptus-derived IFNT to express *ISGs* that could more effectively recognize virus, mount an antiviral response and consequently prohibit transfer of any maternal viral infection to the conceptus or fetus. This antiviral mechanism is important in ruminants in context of the epitheliochorial placenta and the lack of transport of maternal antibodies to the embryo or fetus and would facilitate more rapid maternal defense to spread of viral infection to the unprotected pregnancy. Pregnancy-induced antiviral mechanisms may also exist in other mammalian species despite different modes of maternal recognition of pregnancy and implantation.

The CL required during pregnancy for 50 days in sheep and 6-8 months in cattle (Senger 2003). One critical early mechanism to protect this CL during maternal recognition of pregnancy is the release of IFNT from the conceptus and paracrine action on the endometrium to disrupt upregulation of ESR1, OXTR and luteolytic pulsatile release of PGF. IFNT also is released into the uterine vein and has endocrine action on the CL as well as PBMC. It functions to induce ISGs in the CL which are hypothesized to provide resistance to continued exposure to PGF from the uterus as well as from the CL. The CL becomes resistant to PGF in response to pregnancy (Inskeep *et al.* 1975, Mapletoft *et al.* 1976, Pratt *et al.* 1977, Silvia & Niswender 1984). Mechanisms associated with resistance to PGF might include modification of PGF receptor coupling to G-proteins, activation of PKC and associated apoptotic responses; endometrial (Banu *et al.* 2008), uterine vein (Lee *et al.* 2010) and intraluteal transport of PGF through SLCO2A1 and upregulation of receptors and luteotrophic responses to PGE2 (PTGERs) (Antoniazzi et al., unpublished results). Type I IFN, which are closely related to IFNT, protect immune cells from apoptosis through activating the PI3Kδ, Akt, Rho-A and NFκB (Badr *et al.* 2010). Cell death and apoptotic genes are induced by PGF during luteolysis (reviewed in (Niswender *et al.* 2007)). PGF-mediated induction of the PKC-Raf-MEK1-Erk pathway entails blocking the cell survival Akt pathway (Arvisais *et al.* 2010). We suspect that endocrine action of IFNT might stabilize the cell survival Akt pathway. Endocrine delivery of IFNT into the uterine vein induced a significant extension of estrous cycles (>32 d) using the lowest amounts of IFNT to date that are relevant in context of the Kd of the IFN type I receptor. Systemic delivery of similar biochemically relevant doses of IFNT might be tested in future experiments to improve embryo survival.

Acknowledgements

We thank the following collaborators: Dr. Russell Anthony, Dr. Jason Bruemmer, Dr. Gordon Niswender, Dr. Natalia Smirnova, Dr. Brett Webb, Dr. Cristina Weiner, and Dr. Ann Hess (Colorado State University); Dr. James Pru (Washington State University), Ms. Kathleen Austin (University of Wyoming); Dr. Fuller Bazer and Dr. Tom Spencer (Texas A&M University), and Dr. João Francisco Oliveira (Universidade Federal de Santa Maria, Brazil). All experiments using animals were reviewed and approved by the Colorado State University and the University of Wyoming IACUC. Research was funded by USDA-NIFA-NRI grant 2006-35203-17258.

References

Arvisais E, Hou X, Wyatt TA, Shirasuna K, Bollwein H, Miyamoto A, Hansen TR, Rueda BR & Davis JS 2010 Prostaglandin F2alpha represses IGF-I-stimulated IRS1/phosphatidylinositol-3-kinase/Akt signaling in the corpus luteum: role of ERK and P70 ribosomal S6 kinase. *Mol Endocrinol* **24** 632-643.

Ashworth CJ & Bazer FW 1989 Changes in ovine conceptus and endometrial function following asynchronous embryo transfer or administration of progesterone. *Biol Reprod* **40** 425-433.

Asselin E, Johnson GA, Spencer TE & Bazer FW 2001 Monocyte chemotactic protein-1 and -2 messenger ribonucleic acids in the ovine uterus: regulation by pregnancy, progesterone, and interferon-tau. *Biol Reprod* **64** 992-1000.

Austin KJ, Bany BM, Belden EL, Rempel LA, Cross JC & Hansen TR 2003 Interferon-stimulated gene-15 (Isg15) expression is up-regulated in the mouse uterus in response to the implanting conceptus. *Endocrinology* **144** 3107-3113.

Austin KJ, Ward SK, Teixeira MG, Dean VC, Moore DW & Hansen TR 1996 Ubiquitin cross-reactive protein is released by the bovine uterus in response to interferon during early pregnancy. *Biol Reprod* **54** 600-606.

Badr G, Saad H, Waly H, Hassan K, Abdel-Tawab H, Alhazza IM & Ahmed EA 2010 Type I interferon (IFN-alpha/beta) rescues B-lymphocytes from apoptosis via PI3Kdelta/Akt, Rho-A, NFkappaB and Bcl-2/Bcl(XL). *Cell Immunol* **263:**31-40.

Banu SK, Lee J, Satterfield MC, Spencer TE, Bazer FW & Arosh JA 2008 Molecular cloning and characterization of prostaglandin (PG) transporter in ovine endometrium: role for multiple cell signaling pathways in transport of PGF2alpha. *Endocrinology* **149** 219-231.

Bany BM & Cross JC 2006 Post-implantation mouse conceptuses produce paracrine signals that regulate the uterine endometrium undergoing decidualization. *Dev Biol* **294** 445-456.

Bauersachs S, Mitko K, Ulbrich SE, Blum H & Wolf E 2008 Transcriptome studies of bovine endometrium reveal molecular profiles characteristic for specific stages of estrous cycle and early pregnancy. *Exp Clin Endocrinol Diabetes* **116** 371-384.

Bauersachs S, Ulbrich SE, Gross K, Schmidt SE, Meyer HH, Wenigerkind H, Vermehren M, Sinowatz F, Blum H & Wolf E 2006 Embryo-induced transcriptome changes in bovine endometrium reveal species-specific and common molecular markers of uterine receptivity. *Reproduction* **132** 319-331.

Bazer FW & Roberts RM 1983 Biochemical aspects of conceptus--endometrial interactions. *J Exp Zool* **228** 373-383.

Bazer FW, Thatcher WW, Hansen PJ, Mirando MA, Ott TL & Plante C 1991 Physiological mechanisms of pregnancy recognition in ruminants. *J Reprod Fertil Suppl* **43** 39-47.

Bebington C, Bell SC, Doherty FJ, Fazleabas AT & Fleming SD 1999a Localization of ubiquitin and ubiquitin cross-reactive protein in human and baboon endometrium and decidua during the menstrual cycle and early pregnancy. *Biol Reprod* **60** 920-928.

Bebington C, Doherty FJ & Fleming SD 1999b Ubiquitin cross-reactive protein gene expression is increased in decidualized endometrial stromal cells at the initiation of pregnancy. *Mol Hum Reprod* **5** 966-972.

Bebington C, Doherty FJ & Fleming SD 2000 Ubiquitin and ubiquitin-protein conjugates are present in human cytotrophoblast throughout gestation. *Early Pregnancy* **4** 240-252.

Binelli M, Subramaniam P, Diaz T, Johnson GA, Hansen TR, Badinga L & Thatcher WW 2001 Bovine interferon-tau stimulates the Janus kinase-signal transducer and activator of transcription pathway in bovine endometrial epithelial cells. *Biol Reprod* **64** 654-665.

Bott RC, Ashley RL, Henkes LE, Antoniazzi AQ, Bruemmer JE, Niswender GD, Bazer FW, Spencer TE, Smirnova NP, Anthony RV & Hansen TR 2010 Uterine vein infusion of interferon tau (IFNT) extends luteal life span in ewes. *Biol Reprod* **82** 725-735.

Casaro AP, Kendrick JW & Kennedy PC 1971 Response of the bovine fetus to bovine viral diarrhea-mucosal disease virus. *Am J Vet Res* **32** 1543-1562.

Chan BS, Satriano JA, Pucci M & Schuster VL 1998 Mechanism of prostaglandin E2 transport across the plasma membrane of HeLa cells and Xenopus oocytes expressing the prostaglandin transporter "PGT". *J Biol Chem* **273** 6689-6697.

Chandras C, Harris TE, Bernal AL, Abayasekara DR & Michael AE 2007 PTGER1 and PTGER2 receptors mediate regulation of progesterone synthesis and type 1 11beta-hydroxysteroid dehydrogenase activity by prostaglandin E2 in human granulosa lutein cells. *J Endocrinol* **194** 595-602.

Chen Y, Green JA, Antoniou E, Ealy AD, Mathialagan N, Walker AM, Avalle MP, Rosenfeld CS, Hearne LB & Roberts RM 2006 Effect of interferon-tau administration on endometrium of nonpregnant ewes: a comparison with pregnant ewes. *Endocrinology* **147** 2127-2137.

Choi Y, Johnson GA, Spencer TE & Bazer FW 2003 Pregnancy and interferon tau regulate major histocompatibility complex class I and beta2-microglobulin expression in the ovine uterus. *Biol Reprod* **68** 1703-1710.

Costine BA, Inskeep EK, Blemings KP, Flores JA & Wilson ME 2007 Mechanisms of reduced luteal sensitivity to prostaglandin F2alpha during maternal recognition of pregnancy in ewes. *Domest Anim Endocrinol* **32** 106-121.

Culley FJ, Pennycook AM, Tregoning JS, Dodd JS, Walzl G, Wells TN, Hussell T & Openshaw PJ 2006 Role of CCL5 (RANTES) in viral lung disease. *J Virol* **80** 8151-8157.

Davies CJ, Joosten I, Andersson L, Arriens MA, Bernoco D, Bissumbhar B, Byrns G, van Eijk MJ, Kristensen B, Lewin HA & et al. 1994 Polymorphism of bovine MHC class II genes. Joint report of the Fifth International Bovine Lymphocyte Antigen (BoLA) Workshop, Interlaken, Switzerland, 1 August 1992. *Eur J Immunogenet* **21** 259-289.

Davis MA, Ott TL, Mirando MA, Moser MT & Bazer FW 1992 Effect of recombinant alpha interferons on fertility and interestrous interval in sheep. *Theriogenology* **38** 867-875.

Davis TL, Bott RC, Slough TL, Bruemmer JE & Niswender GD 2010 Progesterone inhibits oxytocin- and prostaglandin F2alpha-stimulated increases in intracellular calcium concentrations in small and large ovine luteal cells. *Biol Reprod* **82** 282-288.

Diehn M, Alizadeh AA, Rando OJ, Liu CL, Stankunas K, Botstein D, Crabtree GR & Brown PO 2002 Genomic expression programs and the integration of the CD28 costimulatory signal in T cell activation. *Proc Natl Acad Sci U S A* **99** 11796-11801.

Endo S, Nomura T, Chan BS, Lu R, Pucci ML, Bao Y & Schuster VL 2002 Expression of PGT in MDCK cell monolayers: polarized apical localization and induction of active PG transport. *Am J Physiol Renal Physiol* **282** F618-622.

Fleming JA, Choi Y, Johnson GA, Spencer TE & Bazer FW 2001 Cloning of the ovine estrogen receptor-alpha promoter and functional regulation by ovine interferon-tau. *Endocrinology* **142** 2879-2887.

Fleming JG, Spencer TE, Safe SH & Bazer FW 2006 Estrogen regulates transcription of the ovine oxytocin receptor gene through GC-rich SP1 promoter elements. *Endocrinology* **147** 899-911.

Giannakopoulos NV, Luo JK, Papov V, Zou W, Lenschow DJ, Jacobs BS, Borden EC, Li J, Virgin HW & Zhang DE 2005 Proteomic identification of proteins conjugated to ISG15 in mouse and human cells. *Biochem Biophys Res Commun* **336** 496-506.

Gifford CA, Racicot K, Clark DS, Austin KJ, Hansen TR, Lucy MC, Davies CJ & Ott TL 2007 Regulation of interferon-stimulated genes in peripheral blood leukocytes in pregnant and bred, nonpregnant dairy cows. *J Dairy Sci* **90** 274-280.

Godkin JD, Bazer FW, Moffatt J, Sessions F & Roberts RM 1982 Purification and properties of a major, low molecular weight protein released by the trophoblast of sheep blastocysts at day 13-21. *J Reprod Fertil* **65** 141-150.

Godkin JD, Bazer FW & Roberts RM 1984a Ovine trophoblast protein 1, an early secreted blastocyst protein, binds specifically to uterine endometrium and affects protein synthesis. *Endocrinology* **114** 120-130.

Godkin JD, Bazer FW, Thatcher WW & Roberts RM 1984b Proteins released by cultured Day 15-16 conceptuses prolong luteal maintenance when introduced into the uterine lumen of cyclic ewes. *J Reprod Fertil* **71** 57-64.

Green MP, Spate LD, Bixby JA, Ealy AD & Roberts RM 2005 A comparison of the anti-luteolytic activities of recombinant ovine interferon-alpha and -tau in sheep. *Biol Reprod* **73** 1087-1093.

Han H, Austin KJ, Rempel LA & Hansen TR 2006 Low blood ISG15 mRNA and progesterone levels are predictive of non-pregnant dairy cows. *J Endocrinol* **191** 505-512.

Hansen PJ, Anthony RV, Bazer FW, Baumbach GA & Roberts RM 1985 In vitro synthesis and secretion of ovine trophoblast protein-1 during the period of maternal recognition of pregnancy. *Endocrinology* **117** 1424-1430.

Hansen TR, Austin KJ & Johnson GA 1997 Transient ubiquitin cross-reactive protein gene expression in the bovine endometrium. *Endocrinology* **138** 5079-5082.

Hansen TR, Austin KJ, Perry DJ, Pru JK, Teixeira MG & Johnson GA 1999 Mechanism of action of interferon-tau in the uterus during early pregnancy. *J Reprod Fertil Suppl* **54** 329-339.

Honda K, Yanai H, Negishi H, Asagiri M, Sato M, Mizutani T, Shimada N, Ohba Y, Takaoka A, Yoshida N & Taniguchi T 2005 IRF-7 is the master regulator of type-I interferon-dependent immune responses. *Nature* **434** 772-777.

Hou X, Arvisais EW, Jiang C, Chen DB, Roy SK, Pate JL, Hansen TR, Rueda BR & Davis JS 2008 Prostaglandin F2alpha stimulates the expression and secretion of transforming growth factor B1 via induction of the early growth response 1 gene (EGR1) in the bovine corpus luteum. *Mol Endocrinol* **22** 403-414.

Huang GN, Huso DL, Bouyain S, Tu J, McCorkell KA, May MJ, Zhu Y, Lutz M, Collins S, Dehoff M, Kang S, Whartenby K, Powell J, Leahy D & Worley PF 2008 NFAT binding and regulation of T cell activation by the cytoplasmic scaffolding Homer proteins. *Science* **319** 476-481.

Imakawa K, Imai M, Sakai A, Suzuki M, Nagaoka K, Sakai S, Lee SR, Chang KT, Echternkamp SE & Christenson RK 2006 Regulation of conceptus adhesion by endometrial CXC chemokines during the implantation period in sheep. *Mol Reprod Dev* **73** 850-858.

Inskeep EK, Smutny WJ, Butcher RL & Pexton JE 1975 Effects of intrafollicular injections of prostaglandins in non-pregnant and pregnant ewes. *J Anim Sci* **41** 1098-1104.

Irizarry RA, Hobbs B, Collin F, Beazer-Barclay YD, Antonellis KJ, Scherf U & Speed TP 2003 Exploration, normalization, and summaries of high density oligonucleotide array probe level data. *Biostatistics* **4** 249-264.

Isaacs A & Lindenmann J 1957 Virus interference. I. The interferon. *Proc R Soc Lond B Biol Sci* **147** 258-267.

Johnson GA, Austin KJ, Collins AM, Murdoch WJ & Hansen TR 1999a Endometrial ISG17 mRNA and a related mRNA are induced by interferon-tau and localized to glandular epithelial and stromal cells from pregnant cows. *Endocrine* **10** 243-252.

Johnson GA, Austin KJ, Van Kirk EA & Hansen TR 1998 Pregnancy and interferon-tau induce conjugation of bovine ubiquitin cross-reactive protein to cytosolic uterine proteins. *Biol Reprod* **58** 898-904.

Johnson GA, Spencer TE, Hansen TR, Austin KJ, Burghardt RC & Bazer FW 1999b Expression of the interferon tau inducible ubiquitin cross-reactive protein in the ovine uterus. *Biol Reprod* **61** 312-318.

Johnson GA, Stewart MD, Gray CA, Choi Y, Burghardt RC, Yu-Lee LY, Bazer FW & Spencer TE 2001 Effects of the estrous cycle, pregnancy, and interferon tau on 2′,5′-oligoadenylate synthetase expression in the ovine uterus. *Biol Reprod* **64** 1392-1399.

Juengel JL, Melner MH, Clapper JA, Turzillo AM, Moss GE, Nett TM & Niswender GD 1998 Steady-state concentrations of mRNA encoding two inhibitors of protein kinase C in ovine luteal tissue. *J Reprod Fertil* **113** 299-305.

Klein C, Bauersachs S, Ulbrich SE, Einspanier R, Meyer HH, Schmidt SE, Reichenbach HD, Vermehren M, Sinowatz F, Blum H & Wolf E 2005 Monozygotic Twin Model Reveals Novel Embryo-Induced Transcriptome Changes of Bovine Endometrium in the Pre-Attachment Period. *Biol Reprod.*

Lamming GE, Wathes DC, Flint AP, Payne JH, Stevenson KR & Vallet JL 1995 Local action of trophoblast interferons in suppression of the development of oxytocin and oestradiol receptors in ovine endometrium. *J Reprod Fertil* **105** 165-175.

Lee J, McCracken JA, Banu SK, Rodriguez R, Nithy TK & Arosh JA 2010 Transport of prostaglandin F(2alpha) pulses from the uterus to the ovary at the time of luteolysis in ruminants is regulated by prostaglandin transporter-mediated mechanisms. *Endocrinology* **151** 3326-3335.

Lenschow DJ, Lai C, Frias-Staheli N, Giannakopoulos NV, Lutz A, Wolff T, Osiak A, Levine B, Schmidt RE, Garcia-Sastre A, Leib DA, Pekosz A, Knobeloch KP, Horak I & Virgin HWt 2007 IFN-stimulated gene 15 functions as a critical antiviral molecule against influenza, herpes, and Sindbis viruses. *Proc Natl Acad Sci U S A* **104** 1371-1376.

Li J & Roberts RM 1994 Interferon-tau and interferon-alpha interact with the same receptors in bovine endometrium. Use of a readily iodinatable form of recombinant interferon-tau for binding studies. *J Biol Chem* **269** 13544-13550.

MacMicking JD 2004 IFN-inducible GTPases and immunity to intracellular pathogens. *Trends Immunol* **25** 601-609.

Malakhova OA, Yan M, Malakhov MP, Yuan Y, Ritchie KJ, Kim KI, Peterson LF, Shuai K & Zhang DE 2003 Protein ISGylation modulates the JAK-STAT signaling pathway. *Genes Dev* **17** 455-460.

Mapletoft RJ, Del Campo MR & Ginther OJ 1976 Local venoarterial pathway for uterine-induced luteolysis in cows. *Proc Soc Exp Biol Med* **153** 289-294.

Marsh J 1971 The effect of prostaglandins on the adenyl cyclase of the bovine corpus luteum. *Ann N Y Acad Sci* **180** 416-425.

Martal J, Degryse E, Charpigny G, Assal N, Reinaud P, Charlier M, Gaye P & Lecocq JP 1990 Evidence for extended maintenance of the corpus luteum by uterine infusion of a recombinant trophoblast alpha-interferon (trophoblastin) in sheep. *J Endocrinol* **127** R5-8.

Martinod S, Maurer RR, Siegenthaler B, Gerber C & Hansen PJ 1991 The effects of recombinant bovine interferon-alpha on fertility in ewes. *Theriogenology* **36** 231-239.

Meyer MD, Hansen PJ, Thatcher WW, Drost M, Badinga L, Roberts RM, Li J, Ott TL & Bazer FW 1995 Extension of corpus luteum lifespan and reduction of uterine secretion of prostaglandin F2 alpha of cows in response to recombinant interferon-tau. *J Dairy Sci* **78** 1921-1931.

Mirando MA, Short EC, Jr., Geisert RD, Vallet JL & Bazer FW 1991 Stimulation of 2′,5′-oligoadenylate synthetase activity in sheep endometrium during pregnancy, by intrauterine infusion of ovine trophoblast protein-1, and by intramuscular administration of recombinant bovine interferon-alpha I1. *J Reprod Fertil* **93** 599-607.

Moor RM & Rowson LE 1964 Influence of the Embryo and Uterus on Luteal Function in the Sheep. *Nature* **201** 522-523.

Moor RM & Rowson LE 1966a The corpus luteum of the sheep: functional relationship between the embryo and the corpus luteum. *J Endocrinol* **34** 233-239.

Moor RM & Rowson LE 1966b Local maintenance of the corpus luteum in sheep with embryos transferred to various isolated portions of the uterus. *J Reprod Fertil* **12** 539-550.

Nagaoka K, Sakai A, Nojima H, Suda Y, Yokomizo Y, Imakawa K, Sakai S & Christenson RK 2003 A chemokine, interferon (IFN)-gamma-inducible protein 10 kDa, is stimulated by IFN-tau and recruits immune cells in the ovine endometrium. *Biol Reprod* **68** 1413-1421.

Naivar KA, Ward SK, Austin KJ, Moore DW & Hansen TR

1995 Secretion of bovine uterine proteins in response to type I interferons. *Biol Reprod* **52** 848-854.

Nephew KP, McClure KE, Day ML, Xie S, Roberts RM & Pope WF 1990 Effects of intramuscular administration of recombinant bovine interferon-alpha I1 during the period of maternal recognition of pregnancy. *J Anim Sci* **68** 2766-2770.

Niswender GD, Davis TL, Griffith RJ, Bogan RL, Monser K, Bott RC, Bruemmer JE & Nett TM 2007 Judge, jury and executioner: the auto-regulation of luteal function. *Soc Reprod Fertil Suppl* **64** 191-206.

Oliveira JF, Henkes LE, Ashley RL, Purcell SH, Smirnova NP, Veeramachaneni DN, Anthony RV & Hansen TR 2008 Expression of interferon (IFN)-stimulated genes in extrauterine tissues during early pregnancy in sheep is the consequence of endocrine IFN-tau release from the uterine vein. *Endocrinology* **149** 1252-1259.

Ott TL, Fleming JG, Spencer TE, Joyce MM, Chen P, Green CN, Zhu D, Welsh TH, Jr., Harms PG & Bazer FW 1997 Effects of exogenous recombinant ovine interferon tau on circulating concentrations of progesterone, cortisol, luteinizing hormone, and antiviral activity; interestrous interval; rectal temperature; and uterine response to oxytocin in cyclic ewes. *Biol Reprod* **57** 621-629.

Ott TL, Yin J, Wiley AA, Kim HT, Gerami-Naini B, Spencer TE, Bartol FF, Burghardt RC & Bazer FW 1998 Effects of the estrous cycle and early pregnancy on uterine expression of Mx protein in sheep (Ovis aries). *Biol Reprod* **59** 784-794.

Pate JL 1995 Involvement of immune cells in regulation of ovarian function. *J Reprod Fertil Suppl* **49** 365-377.

Perry DJ, Austin KJ & Hansen TR 1999 Cloning of interferon-stimulated gene 17: the promoter and nuclear proteins that regulate transcription. *Mol Endocrinol* **13** 1197-1206.

Peterson AJ, Tervit HR, Fairclough RJ, Havik PG & Smith JF 1976 Jugular levels of 13, 14-dihydro-15-keto-prostaglandin F and progesterone around luteolysis and early pregnancy in the ewe. *Prostaglandins* **12** 551-558.

Pratt BR, Butcher RL & Inskeep EK 1977 Antiluteolytic effect of the conceptus and of PGE2 in ewes. *J Anim Sci* **45** 784-791.

Pru JK, Austin KJ, Haas AL & Hansen TR 2001a Pregnancy and interferon-tau upregulate gene expression of members of the 1-8 family in the bovine uterus. *Biol Reprod* **65** 1471-1480.

Pru JK, Rueda BR, Austin KJ, Thatcher WW, Guzeloglu A & Hansen TR 2001b Interferon-tau suppresses prostaglandin F2alpha secretion independently of the mitogen-activated protein kinase and nuclear factor kappa B pathways. *Biol Reprod* **64** 965-973.

Rani MR, Hibbert L, Sizemore N, Stark GR & Ransohoff RM 2002 Requirement of phosphoinositide 3-kinase and Akt for interferon-beta-mediated induction of the beta-R1 (SCYB11) gene. *J Biol Chem* **277** 38456-38461.

Rempel LA, Francis BR, Austin KJ & Hansen TR 2005 Isolation and sequence of an interferon-tau-inducible, pregnancy- and bovine interferon-stimulated gene product 15 (ISG15)-specific, bovine ubiquitin-activating E1-like (UBE1L) enzyme. *Biol Reprod* **72** 365-372.

Roberts RM 1989 Conceptus interferons and maternal recognition of pregnancy. *Biol Reprod* **40** 449-452.

Roberts RM, Cross JC & Leaman DW 1992 Interferons as hormones of pregnancy. *Endocr Rev* **13** 432-452.

Rosenfeld CS, Han CS, Alexenko AP, Spencer TE & Roberts RM 2002 Expression of interferon receptor subunits, IFNAR1 and IFNAR2, in the ovine uterus. *Biol Reprod* **67** 847-853.

Schalue-Francis TK, Farin PW, Cross JC, Keisler D & Roberts RM 1991 Effect of injected bovine interferon-alpha I1 on estrous cycle length and pregnancy success in sheep. *J Reprod Fertil* **91** 347-356.

Schmitt RA, Geisert RD, Zavy MT, Short EC & Blair RM 1993 Uterine cellular changes in 2′,5′-oligoadenylate synthetase during the bovine estrous cycle and early pregnancy. *Biol Reprod* **48** 460-466.

Schuster VL 1998 Molecular mechanisms of prostaglandin transport. *Annu Rev Physiol* **60** 221-242.

Schuster VL 2002 Prostaglandin transport. *Prostaglandins Other Lipid Mediat* **68-69** 633-647.

Senger PL 2003 *Pathways to pregnancy and parturition.* Pullman, WA: Current Conceptions.

Shoemaker ML, Smirnova NP, Bielefeldt-Ohmann H, Austin KJ, van Olphen A, Clapper JA & Hansen TR 2009 Differential expression of the type I interferon pathway during persistent and transient bovine viral diarrhea virus infection. *J Interferon Cytokine Res* **29** 23-35.

Silva PJ, Juengel JL, Rollyson MK & Niswender GD 2000 Prostaglandin metabolism in the ovine corpus luteum: catabolism of prostaglandin F(2alpha) (PGF(2alpha)) coincides with resistance of the corpus luteum to PGF(2alpha). *Biol Reprod* **63** 1229-1236.

Silvia WJ & Niswender GD 1984 Maintenance of the corpus luteum of early pregnancy in the ewe. III. Differences between pregnant and nonpregnant ewes in luteal responsiveness to prostaglandin F2 alpha. *J Anim Sci* **59** 746-753.

Silvia WJ & Niswender GD 1986 Maintenance of the corpus luteum of early pregnancy in the ewe. IV. Changes in luteal sensitivity to prostaglandin F2 alpha throughout early pregnancy. *J Anim Sci* **63** 1201-1207.

Smirnova NP, Bielefeldt-Ohmann H, Van Campen H, Austin KJ, Han H, Montgomery DL, Shoemaker ML, van Olphen AL & Hansen TR 2008 Acute non-cytopathic bovine viral diarrhea virus infection induces pronounced type I interferon response in pregnant cows and fetuses. *Virus Res* **132** 49-58.

Smirnova NP, Ptitsyn AA, Austin KJ, Bielefeldt-Ohmann H, Van Campen H, Han H, van Olphen AL & Hansen TR 2009 Persistent fetal infection with bovine viral diarrhea virus differentially affects maternal blood cell signal transduction pathways. *Physiol Genomics* **36** 129-139.

Spencer TE & Bazer FW 1996 Ovine interferon tau suppresses transcription of the estrogen receptor and oxytocin receptor genes in the ovine endometrium. *Endocrinology* **137** 1144-1147.

Spencer TE, Becker WC, George P, Mirando MA, Ogle TF & Bazer FW 1995 Ovine interferon-tau inhibits estrogen receptor up-regulation and estrogen-induced luteolysis in cyclic ewes. *Endocrinology* **136** 4932-4944.

Spencer TE, Ott TL & Bazer FW 1996 tau-Interferon: pregnancy recognition signal in ruminants. *Proc Soc Exp Biol Med* **213** 215-229.

Spencer TE, Stagg AG, Ott TL, Johnson GA, Ramsey WS & Bazer FW 1999 Differential effects of intrauterine and subcutaneous administration of recombinant ovine interferon tau on the endometrium of cyclic ewes. *Biol Reprod* **61** 464-470.

Sugimoto Y & Narumiya S 2007 Prostaglandin E receptors. *J Biol Chem* **282** 11613-11617.

Takeuchi T, Inoue S & Yokosawa H 2006 Identification and Herc5-mediated ISGylation of novel target proteins. *Biochem Biophys Res Commun* **348** 473-477.

Taub DD, Proost P, Murphy WJ, Anver M, Longo DL, van Damme J & Oppenheim JJ 1995 Monocyte chemotactic protein-1 (MCP-1), -2, and -3 are chemotactic for human T lymphocytes. *J Clin Invest* **95** 1370-1376.

Teixeira MG, Austin KJ, Perry DJ, Dooley VD, Johnson GA, Francis BR & Hansen TR 1997 Bovine granulocyte chemotactic protein-2 is secreted by the endometrium in response to interferon-tau (IFN-tau). *Endocrine* **6** 31-37.

Thatcher WW, Guzeloglu A, Mattos R, Binelli M, Hansen TR & Pru JK 2001 Uterine-conceptus interactions and reproductive failure in cattle. *Theriogenology* **56** 1435-1450.

Vallet JL, Bazer FW, Fliss MF & Thatcher WW 1988 Effect of ovine conceptus secretory proteins and purified ovine trophoblast protein-1 on interoestrous interval and plasma concentrations of prostaglandins F-2 alpha and E and of 13,14-dihydro-15-keto prostaglandin F-2 alpha in cyclic ewes. *J Reprod Fertil* **84** 493-504.

Vander Wielen AL & King GJ 1984 Intraepithelial lymphocytes in the bovine uterus during the oestrous cycle and early gestation. *J Reprod Fertil* **70** 457-462.

Wiepz GJ, Wiltbank MC, Nett TM, Niswender GD & Sawyer HR 1992 Receptors for prostaglandins F2 alpha and E2 in ovine corpora lutea during maternal recognition of pregnancy. *Biol Reprod* **47** 984-991.

Wilson L, Jr., Butcher RL & Inskeep EK 1972 Prostaglandin F2alpha in the uterus of ewes during early pregnancy. *Prostaglandins* **1** 479-482.

Yankey SJ, Hicks BA, Carnahan KG, Assiri AM, Sinor SJ, Kodali K, Stellflug JN & Ott TL 2001 Expression of the antiviral protein Mx in peripheral blood mononuclear cells of pregnant and bred, non-pregnant ewes. *J Endocrinol* **170** R7-11.

Zarco L, Stabenfeldt GH, Basu S, Bradford GE & Kindahl H 1988a Modification of prostaglandin F-2 alpha synthesis and release in the ewe during the initial establishment of pregnancy. *J Reprod Fertil* **83** 527-536.

Zarco L, Stabenfeldt GH, Quirke JF, Kindahl H & Bradford GE 1988b Release of prostaglandin F-2 alpha and the timing of events associated with luteolysis in ewes with oestrous cycles of different lengths. *J Reprod Fertil* **83** 517-526.

Zhao C, Denison C, Huibregtse JM, Gygi S & Krug RM 2005 Human ISG15 conjugation targets both IFN-induced and constitutively expressed proteins functioning in diverse cellular pathways. *Proc Natl Acad Sci U S A* **102** 10200-10205.

The development of reproductive management practices in New Zealand: what will the future hold in a consumer-focused, environmentally-conscious, export-driven marketplace?

CR Burke and GA Verkerk

DairyNZ Limited, Private Bag 3221, Hamilton 3240, New Zealand

The New Zealand (NZ) economy and its dairy industry are sensitive to global consumer perception of farming practices used to generate milk products because milk exports account for >25% of national export earnings and >90% of milk produced is exported as products. Astute management of product image and market risk is, therefore, important for the viability of the industry and country. More than 95% of milk produced in NZ comes from strictly seasonal, pasture-based systems, with associated constraints on reproductive performance. Increasing herd sizes, operational changes and genetic selection priorities have further challenged dairy farmers to achieve optimal levels of herd fertility. Reproductive management practices have developed to address the need to maintain a 365-day inter-calving interval, essentially through maximizing the number of cyclic cows during the breeding period and minimizing the duration of the seasonal calving period. Aspects of the hormonal interventions developed and routinely used to achieve these objectives have been the subject of product quality and market risk concerns forcing the industry to explore alternative ways of achieving reproductive performance goals. One approach has been to exploit the inherently high level of fertility in NZ dairy herds. This approach has seen the inclusion of fertility-related traits in the national genetic evaluation system to prevent further decline in genetic fertility. More recently, a nationally coordinated extension program has been adopted to support farmers and their advisors to identify, prioritize and improve on key management areas for incremental gains in herd reproductive performance. Advances in automation and bio-sensing are yet to make a significant impact, but remain potentially valuable additions in supporting the dairy farmer to manage the areas having the largest effects on reproductive performance.

Corresponding author E-mail: chris.burke@dairynz.co.nz

Introduction

More than 90% of milk produced in NZ is exported in about 200 different product forms. In 2009, the dairy industry earned NZ$11.3 billion: 42% of primary and 27% of total exports. The majority of the 11,000 dairy farms are operated seasonally with a high reliance on grazed pasture. Producers have a strong profit focus achieved by low production costs.

Low-cost milk production is supported by utilization of pasture *in situ*. Herd nutritional demand is managed to match supply. The feed supply and demand balance requires a condensed calving in spring to minimize herd feed demand during low pasture growth in winter and match peak feed intake with peak growth in spring (Figure 1). The development of reproductive management practices has been influenced by the unique challenges of maintaining a 365-day inter-calving interval in this seasonal system (Holmes 2001). Science innovation and farmer perception of the value of new technologies have also directed technology development that ranged through genetic selection, information technologies, feed management systems, and hormonal control of pregnancy reestablishment and calving. Reproductive practices have also been influenced by international regulatory constraints on food safety and local community pressures on environmental stewardship and animal welfare protection.

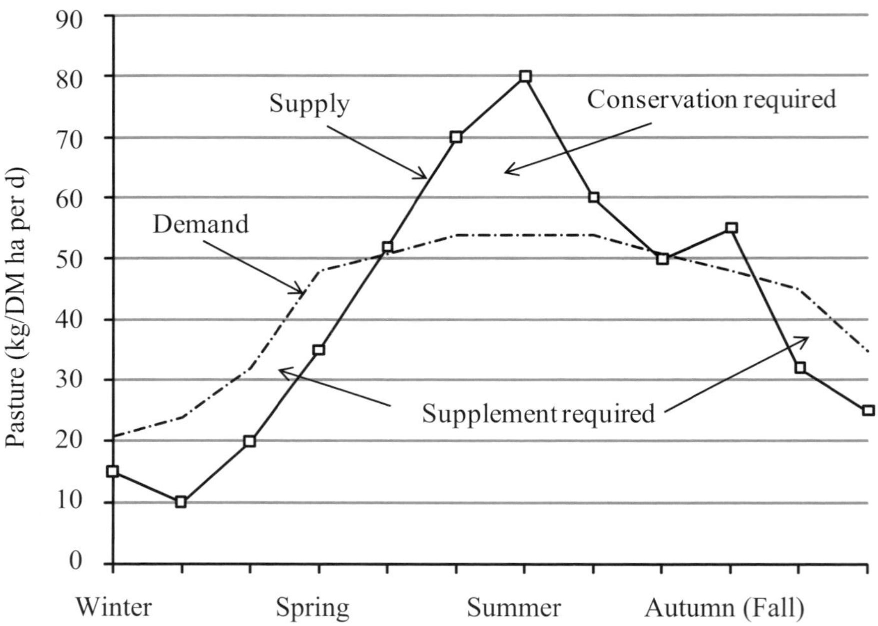

Fig. 1. Representation of the annual pasture supply/demand curve for the pasture-based, seasonal dairy production system in New Zealand (adapted from Macdonald et al. 2008).

This paper describes how reproductive management technologies in NZ have developed and how local and export requirements have influenced these practices. Future efforts to achieve a level of fertility that supports dairy farming goals is discussed in this context.

Reproductive constraints in the seasonal, pasture-based dairy system

The seasonal, pasture-based dairying system

The low-cost pastoral system is central to economic success in an environment not distorted by agricultural subsidies. The pasture that provides 90% of dry matter on most farms is dominated by ryegrass, which has rapid spring growth but moderate summer and low winter growth. Pasture quality varies with season and growing conditions (Roche et al. 2009), and the amount a cow can readily eat constrains milk production (Kolver & Muller 1998).

To achieve a 365-day inter-calving interval, cows must resume cyclicity, display estrual behavior, and be successfully mated during a defined breeding period beginning 12 weeks after a designated "planned start of calving" date for the herd. Cows that cannot maintain this calving interval are generally culled. Artificial insemination (AI) is typically used during the first 4 to 6 weeks of the mating season to generate replacement stock, followed by natural bull mating for a total breeding period of 10 to 14 weeks.

Changes in farm size and operating structure

The average NZ dairy herd in 2008 had 351 cows. Although 200 to 249-cow herds were most common, 19% had more than 500 cows, and 10% of cows were in herds greater than 1,000 (New Zealand Dairy Statistics 2008-09). Business structures have changed with increased herd size, with corporate farm ownership more common where shareholders have no day-to-day involvement, and staff roles are specialized (e.g., feeding and milk harvesting, employed managers provided with consultancy advice). Large herds present additional challenges, particularly for estrous detection and calving management.

Changes in breed and genotype prevalence

Shifts in breed prevalence and crossbreeding feature strongly in the history of NZ dairying (Holmes 2001). By the early 1970s, the dominant breed had changed from Jersey to a Friesian that had been selected under local conditions from animals imported from the United States of America before 1925 (Harris & Kolver 2001). From the 1960s, North American Holstein-Friesian (NAHF) genetics were introduced with an expectation that traits for very high production would be expressed in NZ conditions. The mean proportion of these NAHF genetics in the replacement female population increased from 1.7% in 1970 to 40.6% in 2000 (Harris & Kolver 2001).

The NAHF genotype is capable of producing a large quantity of milk, but on a pasture system alone, this strain of dairy cow mobilizes large amounts of body reserves, which results in a reduced lactation length and reproductive performance (Harris & Kolver 2001; Harris & Winkelman 2000). Crossbreeding was adopted to mitigate the deleterious effect of NAHF on reducing fertility (Harris & Kolver 2001). Farmers focused on breeding cows more suited to pasture-based systems (Montgomerie 2004) and also took advantage of heterosis effects, including those that improve fertility (Harris 2005). More recently, semen from elite crossbred sires ('KiwiCross') has been available. These sires were used for 17.4% of AI breeding in 2008 (New Zealand Dairy Statistics 2008-09). Inclusion of a fertility breeding value into genetic worth estimations (Harris *et al.* 2006) could be expected to halt any further decline in genetic fertility (Montgomerie 2004).

Reproductive management practices

Calving induction

Following the discovery that calving could be pharmaceutically induced prematurely (Adams 1969), the practice of induced calving in cows that conceived late in the breeding period was widely adopted to maintain condensed calving patterns and increase final pregnancy rates by extending the mating period (Welch 1973). Compared with cows calving spontaneously, these cows produced 8% less milk over the lactation, had a 5% lower conception rate to first service, and a 2% greater non-pregnancy rate (Hayes *et al.* 1998). Some of this penalty is probably a consequence of the greater risk of periparturient disorders following induced calving (Malmo 1993). Despite these losses, inductions proved to be beneficial both biologically and economically, compared with much delayed spontaneous calving (Chesterton & Marchant 1985; Malmo 1993; Stevens *et al.* 2000). Use peaked in the 1990s with 7 to 12 % of the national herd being induced annually (Verkerk *et al.* 1997; Hayes 1998; Stevens *et al.* 2000; Xu & Burton 2003).

In an early survey of farmer attitudes, 66% of farmer respondents that did not induce (24% of total) identified welfare concerns as their reason (Williamson 1993). Most farmers that used calving induction disagreed with the statement that "Inductions cause unnecessary suffering to the cow", but did agree to concerns about calf welfare. Of the farmers that induced, 95% said that their primary motivator was to bring late calving cows into earlier production and 71% thought induced cows had more problems. Another survey conducted in 1999 (Stevens *et al.* 2000) reported that above average physical and financial performance can be achieved without the calving induction practice, although there was a positive economic benefit for the practice of inducing. This survey preceded voluntary reduction targets aiming for an industry-wide prevalence of no more than 2% induced cows by 2010.

After voluntary reduction targets had been introduced, views of farmers were again surveyed (Blackett *et al.* 2006). Regardless of whether inductions were practiced, lower non-pregnancy rates and shortening calving spread were consistent goals. Farmers expressed strong views that calving induction and hormone treatments for anestrous cows were "unpleasant" and "unnatural". Inductions were considered to mask systemic problems, affect cow health adversely, and euthanasia of premature calves was acknowledged as a distressing task. Farmers supporting the use of calving induction believed that high non-pregnancy rates and loss of high genetic merit cows were their primary barriers to reducing induction, whereas farmers with 'nil' and 'reducing' induction practices believed that their policy had not affected productivity to any great extent. Whereas some farmers were irritated that local community and overseas customers were able to influence farm practices, they recognized that their future depended on satisfying their markets.

Botha and Verkerk (2002) also explored factors influencing induction decisions and found that the most important consideration was a desire to make spring management easier and to maximize economic returns. The complexities of managing a system subject to the vagaries of weather and its influence on seasonal feed supply (Figure 1) were acknowledged as a barrier to induction reduction.

Factors external to the farm are now driving change, as this reproductive management practice could affect access to international markets (Bodecker 1998). An industry-led initiative to encourage voluntary reduction of calving induction set targets on a national basis at "5% by 2005 and 2% by 2010". After a regulatory review in 2002 concluded that the procedure carries significant risk to animal welfare, a 'Code of Practice' was introduced in 2005 that specified selection criteria for candidates and procedures for animal management. This code has improved welfare outcomes and calving induction rates have fallen to approximately 5%, but in areas of rapid dairy expansion, individual herd induction rates continue to be high. The Code is currently under review, with continuing community pressure to eliminate this practice on the basis of ethical unacceptability. More stringent procedures have recently been established with industry self-regulation supporting further reductions, such that from mid-2012, no more than 4% of cows within a herd should be induced.

Anestrous cow therapy

Initial treatments for anestrous cows were estradiol cypionate and intra-uterine iodine infusion, but were found to be detrimental to fertility (Fielden *et al.* 1973). It was not until progesterone was used that anestrous-cow treatments became efficacious. The first treatment protocols involved insertion of a controlled internal drug-releasing (CIDR) device impregnated with progesterone for 4 to 7 days, with or without an injection of equine chorionic gonadotropin at CIDR removal; a 61% conception rate among the 85% of cows inseminated on detection of estrus was achievable (Macmillan & Peterson, 1993; Macmillan & Burke, 1986). A number of systematic changes in drug type and timing for the progesterone-based treatment were subsequently reported, all with the aim of regulating ovarian development and maximizing the proportion of treated animals being detected in estrus (McDougall *et al.* 1992; Xu *et al.* 1997; Xu *et al.* 2000). Submission rates to AI of 90% within a few days after treatment were achievable (Rhodes *et al.* 2003), and the recommended protocol became progesterone treatment for 8 days with 2 mg estradiol benzoate injected at the start of the protocol, and 1 mg estradiol benzoate injected 24 hours after progesterone withdrawal. Using this protocol, a 28-day submission rate of 93% and first-service conception rate of 47% were demonstrated in field trials; as compared with 70% and 45%, respectively, in anestrous cows left untreated (McDougall & Compton 2005). Lower conception rates compared with those routinely achieved in cycling cows are considered a consequence of insemination at the first postpartum estrus (Rhodes *et al.* 1999), rather than a treatment effect *per se*.

Although a 'GnRH-prostaglandin $F_{2\alpha}$-GnRH' treatment (GPG, e.g. 'OvSynch') was promoted as a less expensive alternative, the omission of progesterone resulted in a poorer conception rate when used in anestrous cows (McDougall 2010a). 'Progesterone priming' appears to be required to reactivate behavioral centers in the brain (McDougall *et al.* 1992) and also supports premature luteolysis (Burke *et al.* 1994). Failure of the first GnRH injection to induce formation of a functional corpus luteum, and failure of $PGF_{2\alpha}$ (7 days after GnRH) to induce complete luteolysis were seen as substantial risks when treating anestrous cows with a standard GPG protocol.

In 2007, food safety regulations changed in European Union countries and estrogen treatments for dairy cows were banned in NZ. Treatments were revised, with the most obvious change being to substitute estradiol with GnRH, while retaining progesterone as the basis of treatment (McDougall 2010a).

Although submission and pregnancy rates to AI during the first few weeks of mating were improved for anestrous cows treated with a progesterone-based protocol, it became apparent that these treatments were not improving the 6-week in-calf rate nor the non-pregnancy rate of anestrous cows (McDougall & Compton 2005; McDougall 2010a), which are the key measures of overall herd-level reproductive performance promoted by the New Zealand National Herd Fertility Project (InCalf; Blackwell 2008).

A range of alternative approaches to mitigating an anestrous problem has also been explored. Providing additional feed to high-genetic merit cows appears of limited value, because much of the additional energy is partitioned into milk production, especially in early lactation (Roche *et al.* 2006; Lucy *et al.* 2009), without benefit to cow fertility (Burke & Roche 2007; Lucy 2007). Improved feeding of cows with a higher risk of being anestrus is substantially more successful during the dry period (Burke *et al.* 1995; Chagas *et al.* 2006), when extra intake can be partitioned toward improving body condition at calving, thus reducing the postpartum anovulatory interval (Burke & Roche 2007). Burke *et al.* (2010) reported that feeding a postpartum diet with a high proportion of non-structural carbohydrate reduced the interval to first ovulation by 8 days, although other studies have not detected a benefit of concentrate feeding on fertility (Kennedy *et al.* 2003; DE Dalley *personal communication*).

Once-daily milking is a lactational management strategy that is becoming increasingly popular to reduce energy demand (Figure 1) on the cow through a 20% reduction in milk production. Reducing milking frequency, even for only several weeks postpartum, reduces tissue mobilization and loss of body condition (McNamara et al. 2003), and 3-week submission rates to AI were observed to be 10% greater with this strategy (Rhodes et al. 1998). Cows milked once-daily for the entire lactation also had an 11% lower anestrous rate, an 8% greater 3-week submission rate to AI, and a 5-day shorter interval between calving and conception (Clark et al. 2006). Farmers view once-daily milking in early lactation as a key strategy for cows that calve in poor body condition, with the additional benefit of reducing labor requirements to offset the loss in milk revenue.

Cautionary addendums to these approaches is the positive economic argument for the individual cow by use of an effective anestrous treatment (McDougall 2010b), and likelihood that the observed responses to alternate approaches might not be achievable in all circumstances.

The possibility of a 'bull effect' as a non-hormonal strategy for anestrous cows has been explored by farmers, despite a lack of scientific evidence that bull presence can stimulate ovulation in high-genetic merit, lactating anestrous dairy cows. Norton (2008) reported a study of the reproductive performance of lactating dairy cows not seen in estrus before the start of mating when either comingled with vasectomized bulls for the first 3 weeks of mating, or with tail paint and observation only to aid heat detection. Cows exposed to bulls had a greater 3-week submission rate to AI (78% vs. 71%) and 4-week pregnancy rate (42% vs. 36%), but this strategy did not improve the 6-week pregnancy rate or the final non-pregnancy rate (Norton 2008). The costs and inconvenience of managing vasectomized bulls were noted, but not quantified, and farmer-participants believed that increased performance was due to improved heat detection.

Advances in semen processing and artificial breeding services

The importance of AI for genetic gain was recognized in the 1950s, but the intense seasonal demand was challenging (James 1957), and led to extended-life fresh semen technology with low sperm doses that facilitated use of teams of elite sires (Shannon 1968). Much later, poly-L-lysine encapsulated semen was tested, but proved inferior to the routine use of Caprogen as a semen life extender (Vishwanath *et al.* 1996). By the early 1970s, 60% of herds used AI with conception rates routinely exceeding 60% (Macmillan 1974). Use of AI peaked at 85% of the national herd in the 1990s, but has recently declined to 75% (New Zealand Dairy Statistics 2008-09).

Most AI is performed by a network of professional technicians using mobile electronic recording systems, synchronized daily to the National Database records. This incorporates a tool to match sires to individual cows to reduce deleterious major gene effects and inbreeding (Lopez-Villalobos *et al.* 2004), a recognized threat where semen technologies disseminate elite genetics widely (Stichbury 1968; Lucy 2007).

Sex-sorted semen is available from within NZ (using local sires) and overseas. The economic case for sex-sorted semen is sensitive to additional costs of semen production and poorer conception rates (Underwood *et al.* 2010), so currently routine use is limited (WH McMillan *personal communication*). Increasing community concerns about surplus dairy calves slaughtered for veal and leather, or an acute shortage of replacement females, may see this re-evaluated.

Estrous detection

Widespread use of AI has made heat detection a critical skill. Although the concentrated mating period is conducive to high estrous detection efficiency, as sexually active groups form easily and cows have optimal under-foot conditions to express mounting behavior, this remains the most labor intensive and skilled task in reproduction programs. Poor detection of estrus results from errors in sensitivity and specificity (Xu and Burton 1996). Errors in sensitivity (missing cows in estrus) manifest as later calving in the subsequent season with lower production, and fewer AI-bred replacement heifers, are estimated to cost NZ$160 each during the AI period. Errors in specificity (inseminating cows not in estrus) is an immediate waste of semen and time spent inseminating, provides misleading information that may influence future estrous detection and potentially terminates pregnancy if the cow has already conceived (Macmillan *et al.* 1977; Sturman *et al.* 2000; Burke *et al.* 2005).

Estrous detection efficiency in high-yielding cows managed intensively is less than 50% (Senger 1994). Although some of this inefficiency may be management-related, faster clearance rates of circulating estradiol may also lead to a weaker signal for estrus (Sangsritavong et al. 2002; Lopez et al. 2004; Wiltbank et al. 2006). Although per cow production of milksolids (fat plus protein yield) in NZ has increased by about 25% over the last 2 decades (New Zealand Dairy Statistics 2008-09), peak milk yields from well-managed high-genetic merit cows are only 25 to 35 kg/d, less even than what overseas studies define as 'low producers'! Higher producing NZ cows are unlikely to have attained the level of production that would reduce expression of estrous behavior. At a phenotypic level, there is no evidence of a negative association between milksolids (fat and protein yields) production and fertility in NZ dairy cattle (Xu & Burton 2003, Pryce & Harris, 2006).

Estrous detection efficiencies in different strains of HF dairy cattle were compared using milk progesterone measurements (Macdonald *et al.* 2008; Lucy *et al.* 2009). Overall detection efficiency averaged 84% with 16% of anticipated estruses missed, and 16% of recorded estrous observations being false positives. An increased difficulty in detecting estrus in the NAHF genetic strain was not supported by these data.

Increasing herd size reduces estrous detection performance and satisfactory levels cannot be achieved without technological aids (Senger 1994; Diskin & Shreenan 2000; Rae 2002). Tail paint is the most widely used estrous detection method in NZ, but estrous mount detector products attached to the tail-head are also popular. These aids assist with heat detection, but none advance the farmer beyond visual identification.

External influences on reproduction management practices

Influences beyond the farm gate increasingly affect management practices on the dairy farm. The comprehensive NZ industry strategy for dairy farming's future (DairyNZ 2009) identifies external influences originating from; (1) the NZ Public; (2) Consumers and Trade; (3) Government and Regulations; and (4) Stewardship and Social Responsibility (Figure 2). On-farm factors are partitioned into those that influence production, including resource use, and those arising as a consequence of human capability in farm management activities, both of which are influenced externally.

The New Zealand public

Local citizens draw their views of animal production systems from their collective knowledge, and given that the degrees of separation in the urban-rural divide in NZ are fewer than in more urbanized countries, their local knowledge tends to increase their level of trust of farmers, such that they may be more 'forgiving' of the way that production systems interact with the animals; they are, however, much less tolerant of farm practices that affect the quality of the environment, especially water quality. Regional authorities are more strictly regulating land and water use, and proposed caps on the level of nitrate leaching in some areas is forcing farmers to consider changes to their farming systems. These proposals may ultimately constrain stocking rates and milk productivity, but technological solutions to these issues without constraining milk production are more likely to result in changes to management systems in which cows spend a proportion of their time off pasture. Changes that lead to longer periods of confinement on hard surfaces, especially during the spring breeding period, may reduce estrous detection efficiency such that traditional methods used now (Macmillan *et al.* 1988) may no longer be adequate. Investment in constructed areas to stand cows off pasture for periods of time gives farmers greater flexibility for feed inputs other than pasture, and as the proposed changes to reduce levels of calving induction also take effect, there is a likelihood that some NZ farmers will consider a shift away from a strictly spring calving towards longer lactations involving both autumn and spring calving herds.

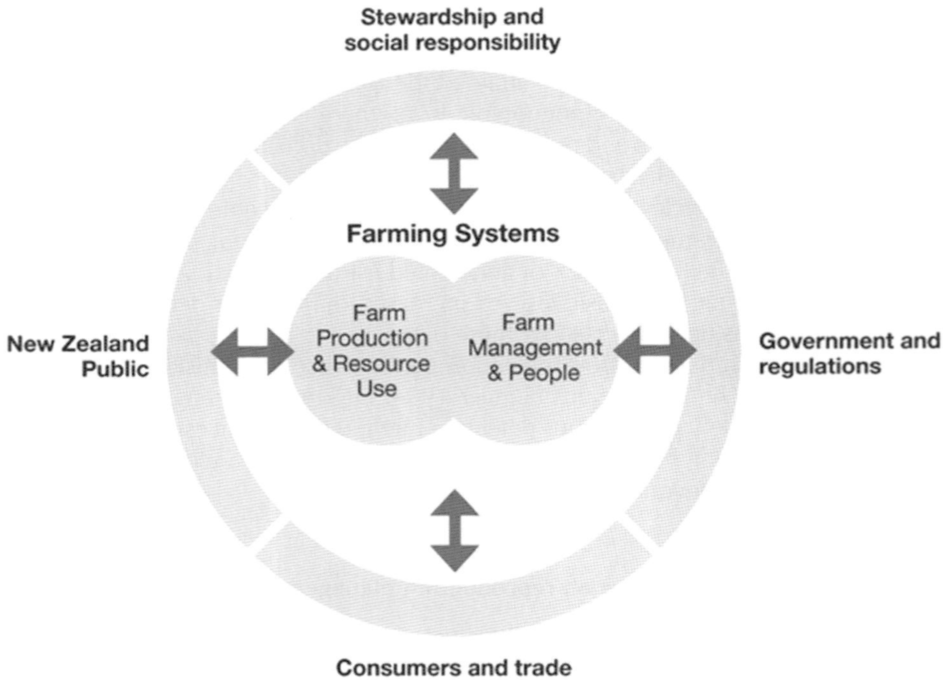

Fig. 2. The comprehensive New Zealand industry strategy for dairy farming's future (*www.dairynz.co.nz/file/fileid/14354*): sources of external influence over dairy farm systems in New Zealand (DairyNZ 2009).

Consumers and trade

Martin *et al.* (2009) referred to the increasing consumer demand for animal products that are "Clean, green and ethical" (CGE), suggesting social-sexual signaling, nutrition and genetic selection strategies as possibilities for remaining productive and profitable while delivering a 'CGE product'. Matthews (2007) noted that key international drivers for change in livestock welfare, and associated welfare regulations, included: demands and activities of non-governmental organizations, corporate and retailer actions, and international trade/animal welfare policies. Farm management practices noted as welfare sensitive issues included AI and early calf separation (Matthews 2007). Seasonally-related changes in body condition reserves associated with seasonal variation in quality and quantity of feed, inadequate protection from adverse climates, and the number of animals per stockperson are also identified among community concerns about animal welfare.

External pressure to improve performance in certain areas (e.g. to improve body condition) would tend to be congruent with industry recommendations to improve reproduction performance, but other practices noted as potential welfare topics (AI and early calf separation) are likely to be defended vigorously by mainstream industry, as these practices are considered indispensible to future success of the dairy farm business.

Government and regulations

The establishment of the New Zealand Food Safety Authority (NZFSA) followed similar United Kingdom initiatives to create a transparent separation between the regulatory and compliance processes that protect food safety and those that manage food production. The consequence is that greater weight is given to consumer arguments in debates on the acceptability of products and practices that can influence food safety. For example, it was a European Community decision that led to the NZFSA ban on the use of estradiol in NZ. To some extent, processing companies can manage specific residue-related issues by segmenting their processing systems. In the case of estradiol, however, widespread use made it logistically impossible to segment the proportion of supply going to the European Union market.

Stewardship and social responsibilities

Farmers in NZ have long understood that they must meet the needs of their marketplace and are generally also prepared to meet the challenges posed by the local community around resource management and animal welfare. Recently (Feb. 2010), the NZ Ministry of Agriculture and Forestry released a 'Code of Welfare for Dairy Cattle' as a tertiary regulation under the 1999 Animal Welfare Act (*www.dairynz.co.nz/file/fileid/20167*). This new code describes minimum standards of care and recommended best-practice for the management of dairy cattle. It was developed collaboratively with the dairy industry, but represents an agreed position across the wider community as to expectations for the care of dairy cattle. The code serves at a regulatory level in the prosecution of farmers that fail to meet standards, and is an important definition of expectations for 'stewardship and social responsibility'.

Managing reproductive performance in the future

Reproductive management practices will inevitably continue to be influenced by external factors associated with food safety, animal welfare and environmental resource management, key factors that influence the perceptions of consumers. In managing these risks, there will be an increased emphasis on strategies that prevent, rather than treat, reproductive failure.

Exploiting the inherent fertility from the pasture-grazed, seasonal system

Large-scale studies in Australia (Morton 2010) and NZ (Xu & Burton 2003) reported substantial variation in reproductive performance among herds within similar climates and with similar genetic compositions (Figure 3). Managerial factors were largely responsible for the variance and these studies provided crucial data to establish a hierarchy of measures from the overall measures of 6-week in-calf rate and final non-pregnancy rate to the underlying drivers (i.e. submission and conception rates) and other quantifiable areas of management that contribute to reproductive performance (Figure 4). The Australian study lead to an extension program, called 'InCalf' (Morton *et al.* 2003), to support farmers and their advisers achieve incremental gains in herd reproductive performance. This program has been adapted for use in NZ (Burke *et al.* 2008a & 2008b; Blackwell 2008). Success requires that farmers monitor and actively manage the areas that influence reproductive performance at herd level (Figure 4). They are encouraged to make full use of their advisory network, which collectively has the expertise to support the multifactorial complexity of improving reproductive performance.

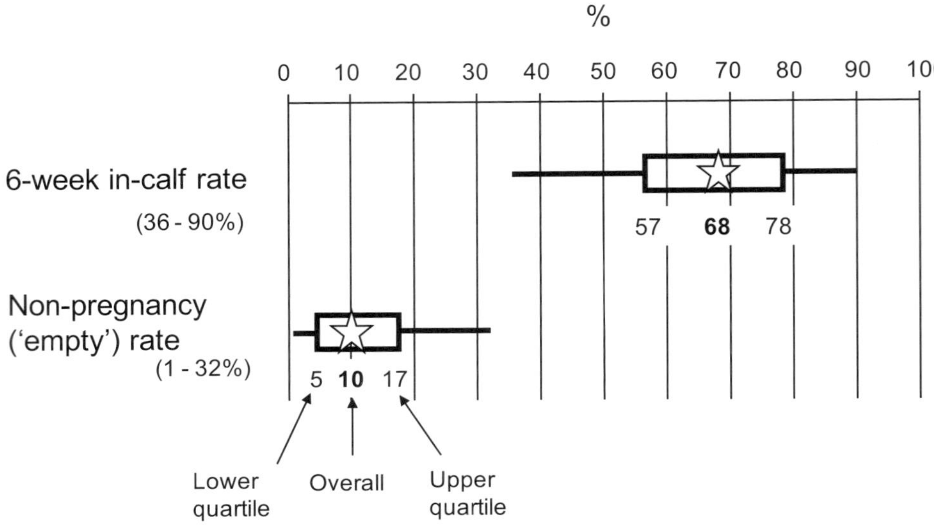

Fig. 3. Distribution and quartile levels of performance for the 6-week in-calf rate and non-pregnancy ('empty') rate from an industry survey involving 101,185 cow records during the 1998 to 2000 seasons in New Zealand (Xu & Burton 2003).

Inherent fertility associated with both genetics and AI practices is one of the eight managerial ingredients that influence herd reproductive performance (Figure 4). Farmers have choice over breed, and can also prioritize their preferred traits. Herd improvement companies and the national evaluation system must ensure that genetic fertility does not unwittingly decline further (Grosshans *et al.*1997; Montgomerie 2004), while acknowledging that the inclusion of multiple measures of fertility in genetic evaluation is hampered by cost and impracticality. Genomic selection methods and particular gene markers may mitigate some of these issues and advance the rate of gain in particular traits of interest (Gatley 2008). Genomic predictions increase the reliability of the breeding value for fertility by 3-4% in proven bulls, and by 20% (32 to 52%) in unproven bulls (Harris & Johnson 2010), allowing bulls as young as 2 years old to be promoted with associated increases in the rate of genetic gain.

The other seven managerial areas influencing reproductive performance at herd level are depicted in Figure 4. It can be argued that commonly used 'reproductive technologies' do not improve herd fertility. For example, hormonal treatment of noncycling cows does not improve 'overall reproductive performance' (McDougall & Compton 2005 & 2006; McDougall 2010a), and if the underlying problem is ignored, the herd becomes a 'symptomatic reactor' on an annual cycle. In contrast, reducing the proportion of late calving cows and ensuring that calving body condition score targets are achieved reduces the incidence of noncycling (McDougall *et al.* 1995; Roche *et al.* 2007), and hence improves overall reproductive performance (Xu & Burton 2003). Although most farmers and veterinarians intuitively agree, the InCalf extension program has a mandate to 'remind' and facilitate a wider adoption of this strategic approach to improving herd-level reproductive performance.

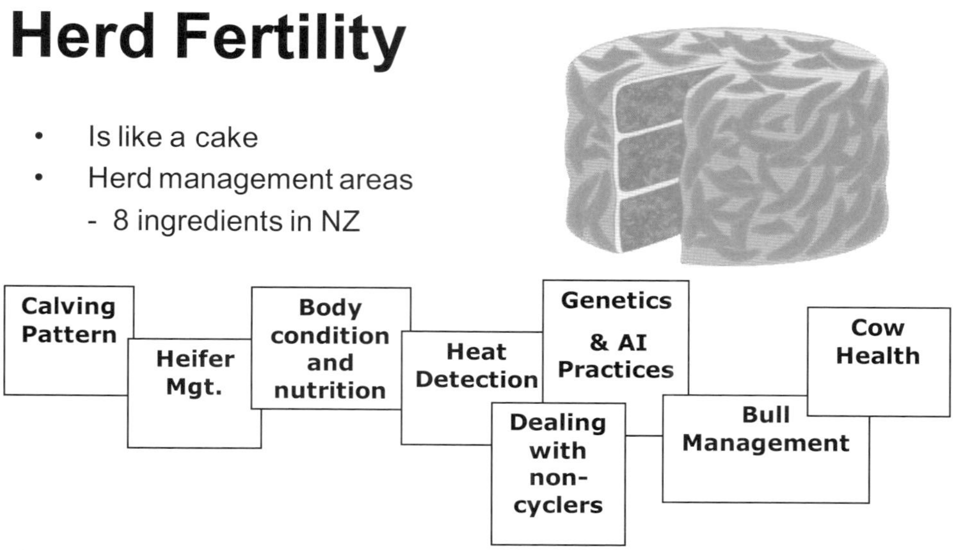

Fig. 4. Schematic used for the 'InCalf'extension program depicting the 8 management areas ('ingredients of the herd fertility cake') identified as being the most influential on dairy herd reproductive performance in New Zealand (Morton *et al.* 2003; Burke *et al.* 2008a).

Advances in automation, information technology, and biosensing

There are some time-consuming tasks in fertility management that must be performed to a high standard, and automation technologies present an opportunity to improve performance in these areas.

Substantial opportunities exist to automate estrous detection. Current technologies do not fully meet performance expectations, as they still require substantial labor input, are expensive, fragile, and can be unreliable. The major problem with current methods (viz. visually with aid of tail paint) is the laborious and somewhat skilled nature of the task (CR Burke & MB Blackwell *unpublished*). Farms may be more affected where multiple or novice staff have responsibility for estrous detection as compared with the more traditional farm managed by a single experienced operator. Farmer expectations are that an automated estrous detection system would remove the 'human' element by identifying and drafting estrous cows accurately, quickly and reliably, without disturbing the flow of the milking operation. Significant progress with automated estrous detection in NZ is reported, including use of a camera (Hempstalk *et al.* 2010) and activity-based monitoring systems (Harris *et al.* 2010).

As robotic milking systems develop for pasture-based farming, more dairy cows in NZ will be milked through robots. Robotic milking has been associated with a longer interval to first service (Kruip *et al.* 2002). It was speculated that less farmer-cow contact contributed to this difference and that cow fertility *per se* was not compromised. High levels of reproductive performance were consistently achieved in a NZ pasture-based, seasonal robotically milked herd (J. Jago *personnel communication*). The difficulty for estrous detection in this system is a lack of forced group movement, cows located at multiple sites and an overriding objective to minimize labor inputs (Burke *et al.* 2005).

Advances in information technology are expected to assist farmers, as monitoring systems and high quality records are required for managing for good reproductive performance. Information technology continues to develop with radio-frequency identification (RFID) systems to identify individual cows as part of a national animal identification and traceability initiative (NAIT), integrated with walkover weighing, and systems to draft pre-determined animals directly after milking (e.g. Protrack; LIC, Hamilton, NZ). These systems are increasingly viewed in larger herds as essential equipment, but issues remain with the integrity of tags and tag readers, which do not achieve 100% perfection in their operation.

Biosensing technologies offer opportunities for direct assessment of reproductive activity and performance indicators in areas that influence reproductive performance, such as nutrition and energy status (Miglior *et al.* 2009). When combined with automation, these technologies should aid farmer decision-making, especially in the context of minimal individual cow attention and scarcity of skilled labor. The cost-benefit argument will remain a major hurdle to widespread adoption on NZ farms.

Conclusions

As the seasonal, pasture-based dairying system in NZ has developed, one fortunate aspect has been that a relatively high level of cow fertility has been retained. Product image and market risk factors have influenced and will continue to influence on-farm reproductive management practices. Current trends suggest that future approaches to managing reproduction will favor preventative strategies that circumvent the need to intervene with hormones, and avoid practices that have an adverse effect on perceptions of animal welfare, food safety, and the environment. Advances in strategic information capture and automation will assist farmers with the monitoring and decision-making tasks required to effectively manage fertility in the herd.

References

Adams WM 1969 The elective induction of labor and parturition in cattle. *Journal of the American Veterinary Medical Association* **154** 261-265.

Blackett P, Compton C & Glassey C 2006 To induce or not to induce? Insights into important influences on dairy farmer decision making over induced calving. *Proceedings of the New Zealand Society of Animal Production* **66** 350-354.

Blackwell MB 2008 The InCalf Programme in New Zealand. *Proceedings of the Society of Dairy Cattle Veterinarians* p. 9-13.

Bodecker PCW 1998 Combined industry approach to reduction of the use of induction in the national herd. *Proceedings of the Society of Dairy Cattle Veterinarians* p. 79-93.

Botha CAJ & Verkerk GA 2002 Factors influencing decision-making in dairy cows: a case study of scientists' and producers' views. *Proceedings of the New Zealand Society of Animal Production* **62** 257-260.

Burke CR, Blackwell MB & Little S 2008a The InCalf Book for New Zealand dairy farmers. DairyNZ, Hamilton, New Zealand.

Burke CR, Davis KL & Jago J 2005 Predicting next oestrous date and capturing automatically milked cows for artificial insemination. *Proceedings of the New Zealand Society of Animal Production* **65** 231-235.

Burke CR, Fowler C & Tiddy RM 2008b Building towards the InCalf Programme for New Zealand. *Proceedings of the Society of Dairy Cattle Veterinarians* p. 1-8.

Burke CR, Kay JK, Phyn CVC, Meier S, Lee JM & Roche JR 2010 Short communication: Effects of dietary nonstructural carbohydrates pre- and postpartum on reproduction of grazing dairy cows. *Journal of Dairy Science* **93** *(In press)*.

Burke CR, McDougall S & Macmillan KL 1995 Effects of breed and calving liveweight on postpartum ovarian activity in pasture-fed heifers. *Proceedings of the New Zealand Society of Animal Production* **55** 76-78.

Burke CR, Mihm M, Macmillan KL & Roche JF 1994 Some effects of prematurely elevated concentrations of progesterone on luteal and follicular characteristics during the oestrus cycle in heifers. *Animal Reproduction Science* **35** 27-39.

Burke CR & Roche JR 2007 Effects of pasture feeding during the periparturient period on post-partum anovulation in grazed dairy cows. *Journal of Dairy Science* **90** 4304-4312.

Chagas LM, Rhodes FM, Blache D, Gore PJS, Macdonald KA & Verkerk GA 2006 Precalving effects on metabolic responses and postpartum anestrus in grazing primiparous dairy cows. *Journal of Dairy Science* **89** 1981-1989.

Chesterton RN & Marchant RM 1985 Early induction of dairy cows. *Proceedings of the Society of Dairy Cattle Veterinarians* p. 52-58.

Clark DA, Phyn CVC, Tong MJ, Collis SJ & Dalley DE 2006 A systems comparison of once- versus twice-daily milking of pastured dairy cows. *Journal of Dairy Science* **89** 1854-1862.

DairyNZ 2009 Strategy for New Zealand dairy farming. *www.dairynz.co.nz/file/fileid/14354.*

Diskin MG & Shreenan JM 2000 Expression and detection of oestrus in cattle. *Reproduction, Nutrition & Development* **40** 481-491.

Fielden ED, Macmillan KL & Watson JD 1973 The anoestrous syndrome in New Zealand dairy cattle. 1. A preliminary investigation. *New Zealand Veterinary Journal* **21** 77-81.

Gatley P 2008 DNA proven genetics. *Proceedings of the Society of Dairy Cattle Veterinarians* p. 157-160.

Grosshans T, Xu ZZ, Burton LJ, Johnson DL & Macmillan KL 1997 Performance and genetic parameters for fertility of seasonal dairy cows in New Zealand. *Livestock Production Science* **51** 41-51.

Hempstalk K, Harris BL & Lopdell TJ 2010 Automatic reading of Kamars for heat detection in dairy herds. *Proceedings of the New Zealand Society of Animal Production* **70** 8-12.

Harris BL 2005 Breeding dairy cows for the future in New Zealand. *New Zealand Veterinary Journal* **53** 384-389.

Harris BL, Hempstalk K, Dela Rue, BT, Jago JG & McGowan JE 2010 Improving the power of activity-based heat detection using additional automatically captured data. *Proceedings of the New Zealand Society of Animal Production* **70** 299-302.

Harris BL & Johnson DL 2010 Genomic predictions for New Zealand dairy bulls and integration with national genetic evaluation. *Journal of Dairy Science* **93** 1243-1252.

Harris BL & Kolver ES 2001 Review of Holsteinization on intensive pastoral dairy farming in New Zealand. *Journal of Dairy Science* **84** E56-E61.

Harris BL, Pryce JE, Xu ZZ & Montgomerie WA 2006 Development of a new fertility breeding value in the dairy industry. *Proceedings of the New Zealand Society of Animal Production* **66** 107-112.

Harris BL & Winkelman AM 2000 Influence of North American Holstein genetics on dairy cattle performance in New Zealand. *Proceedings of the Large Herds Australia Conference* p.122-136.

Hayes DP 1998 Reproductive performance of New Zealand herds. *Proceedings of the Society of Dairy Cattle Veterinarians* p. 189-205.

Hayes DP, Pfeiffer DU & Morris RS 1998 Effects of calving induction on subsequent milk yield and reproductive performance of cows from seasonally mated New Zealand dairy herds. *New Zealand Veterinary Journal* **46** 97-101.

Holmes CW 2001 Managing fertility in the New Zealand dairy herd. *Proceedings of the New Zealand Society of Animal Production* **61** 135-140.

James JP 1957 The progress and prospects of artificial breeding in New Zealand. *Proceedings of the New Zealand Society of Animal Production* **17** 5-19.

Kennedy J, Dillon P, O'Sullivan K, Buckley F & Rath M 2003 The effect of genetic merit for milk production and concentrate feeding level on the reproductive performance of Holstein-Friesian cows in a grass-based system. *Animal Science* **76** 297-308.

Kolver ES & Muller LD 1998 Performance and nutrient intake of high producing Holstein cows consuming pasture or total mixed ration. *Journal of Dairy Science* **81** 1403-1411.

Kruip TAM, Morice H, Robert M & Ouweltjes W 2002 Robotic milking and its effect on fertility and cell counts. *Journal of Dairy Science* **85** 2576-2581.

Lopez H, Satter LD & Wiltbank MC 2004 Relationship between level of milk production and estrous behavior of lactating dairy cows. *Animal Reproduction Science* **81** 209-223.

Lopez-Villalobos N, Harris BL & Pryce JE 2004 Mate selection to control inbreeding and maximize farm profit of commercial dairy cattle. *Proceedings of the New Zealand Society of Animal Production* **64** 122-126.

Lucy MC 2007 Fertility in high-producing dairy cows: Reasons for decline and corrective strategies for sustainable improvement. Pp. 237-254. In: Reproduction in Domestic ruminants. Eds: Juengel JL, Murray JF & Smith MF. Nottingham University Press, Nottingham, UK.

Lucy MC, Verkerk GA, Whyte BE, Macdonald KA, Burton L, Cursons RT, Roche JR & Holmes CW 2009 Somatotropic axis components and nutrient partitioning in genetically diverse dairy cows managed under different feed allowances in a pasture system. *Journal of Dairy Science* **92** 526-539.

Macdonald KA, Penno JW, Lancaster JAS & Roche JR 2008 Effect of stocking rate on pasture production, milk production, and reproduction of dairy cows in pasture-based systems. *Journal of Dairy Science* **91** 2151-2163.

Macdonald KA, Verkerk GA, Thorrold BS, Pryce JE, Penno JW, McNaughton LR, Burton LJ, Lancaster JAS, Williamson JH & Holmes CW 2008 A comparison of three strains of Holstein-Friesian grazed on pasture and managed under different feed allowances. *Journal of Dairy Science* **91** 1693-1707.

Macmillan KL 1974 The application of artificial breeding as a reproductive technique in cattle *Proceedings of the New Zealand Society of Animal Production* **34** 158-166.

Macmillan KL & Burke CR 1986 Effects of oestrous cycle control on reproductive efficiency. *Animal Reproduction Science* **42** 307-320.

Macmillan KL, Fielden ED & Curnow RJ 1977 Factors influencing A.B. conception rates. VIII. Effects of non-oestrous inseminations and return patterns after second inseminations. *New Zealand Journal of Experimental Agriculture* **5** 123-127.

Macmillan KL & Peterson AJ 1993 A new intravaginal progesterone releasing device for cattle (CIDR-B) for oestrus synchronization, increasing pregnancy rates and the treatment of post-partum anoestrus. *Animal Reproduction Science* **33** 1-25.

Macmillan KL, Taufa VK, Barnes DR, Day AM & Henry R 1988 Detecting estrus in synchronized heifers using tailpaint and an aerosol raddle. *Theriogenology* **30** 1099-1114.

Malmo J 1993 Calving induction. *Proceedings of Society of Dairy Cattle Veterinarians* p. 225-238.

Martin GB, Durmic Z, Kenyon PR & Vercoe PE 2009 'Clean, green and ethical' animal reproduction: extension to sheep and dairy systems in New Zealand. *Proceedings of the New Zealand Society of Animal Production* **69** 140-147.

Mathews LR 2007 International drivers for animal welfare change and implications for New Zealand. *Proceedings of the New Zealand Society of Animal Production* **67** 226-231.

McDougall S 2010a Effects of treatment of anestrous dairy cows with gonadotropin-releasing hormone, prostaglandin, and progesterone. *Journal of Dairy Science* **93** 1944-1959.

McDougall S 2010b Comparison of diagnostic approaches, and a cost-benefit analysis of different diagnostic approaches and treatments of anoestrous dairy cows. *New Zealand Veterinary Journal* **58** 81-89.

McDougall S, Burke CR, Macmillan KL & Williamson NB 1992 The effect of pre-treatment with progesterone on the oestrous response to oestradiol-17β benzoate in the post-partum dairy cow. *Proceedings of the New Zealand Society of Animal Production* **52** 157-160.

McDougall S, Burke CR, Williamson NB & Macmillan KL 1995 The effect of stocking rate and breed on the period of postpartum anoestrum in grazing dairy cattle. *Proceedings of the New Zealand Society of Animal Production* **55** 236-238.

McDougall S & Compton CWR 2005 Reproductive performance of anestrous dairy cows teated with progesterone and estradiol benzoate. *Journal of Dairy Science* **88** 2388-2400.

McDougall S & Compton CWR 2006 Reproductive performance in the subsequent lactation of dairy cows previously treated for failure to be detected in oestrus. *New Zealand Veterinary Journal* **54** 132-140.

McNamara S, Mee J, O'Mara F, Boland M, & Murphy J 2003 Effects of altering energy balance by varying milking frequency on production and reproduction in Holstein-Friesian cows. *Reproduction in Domestic Animals* **38** 331-332.

Miglior F, Wiggans GR, Faust MA & Van Doormaal BJ 2009 Impact of new on-farm technologies in dairy cattle breeding. *ICAR Technical Series* **13** 213-214.

Montgomerie WA 2004 Future genetic progress of dairy cattle in New Zealand. *Proceedings of the New Zealand Society of Animal Production* **64** 96-100.

Morton JM 2010 Interrelationships between herd-level reproductive performance measures based on intervals from initiation of the breeding program in year-round and seasonal calving dairy herds. *Journal of Dairy Science* **93** 901-910.

Morton J, Larcombe M & Little S 2003 The InCalf Book for dairy farmers. Dairy Australia, Australia.

New Zealand Dairy Statistics 2008-09. www.dairynz.co.nz/dairystatistics.

Norton C 2008 Canterbury teaser bull study. *Proceedings of the Society of Dairy Cattle Veterinarians* p. 143-149.

Pryce JE & Harris BL 2006 Genetics of body condition score in New Zealand dairy cows. *Journal of Dairy Science* **89** 4424-4432.

Rae DO 2002 Bovine estrus: Tools for detection and understanding. p. 7-21, In: Factors Affecting Calf Crop: Biotechnology of Reproduction. Eds: Fields M, Sand R & Yelich J, CRC Press LLC, Boca Raton, Florida.

Rhodes FM, Clark BA, Macmillan KL & McDougall S 1998 Use of once daily milking or treatment with progesterone and oestradiol benzoate in anoestrous cows. *Proceedings of the New Zealand Society of Animal Production* **58** 44-45.

Rhodes FM, Clark BA, McDougall S & Macmillan KL 1999 Insemination at the second of two induced oestrous periods in anoestrous dairy cows increases conception rates to first service. *New Zealand Veterinary Journal* **47** 39-43.

Rhodes FM, McDougall S, Burke CR, Verkerk GA & Macmillan KL 2003 Invited review: Treatment of cows with an extended postpartum anestrous interval. *Journal of Dairy Science* **86** 1876-1894.

Roche JR, Berry DP & Kolver ES 2006 Holstein-Friesian strain and feed effects on milk production, body weight, and body condition score profiles in grazing dairy cows. *Journal of Dairy Science* **89** 3532-3543.

Roche JR, MacDonald KA, Burke CR, Lee JM & Berry DP 2007 Associations among body condition score, body weight, and reproductive performance is seasonal-calving dairy cattle. *Journal of Dairy Science* **90** 376-391.

Roche JR, Turner LR, Lee JM, Edmeades DC, Donaghy DJ, Macdonald KA, Penno JW & Berry DP 2009 Weather, herbage quality and milk production in pastoral systems. 2. Temporal patterns and intra-relationships in herbage quality and mineral concentration parameters. *Animal Production Systems* **49** 200-210.

Sangsritavong S, Combs DK, Sartori R, Armentano LE & Wiltbank MC 2002 High feed intake increases liver blood flow and metabolism of progesterone and estradiol-17β in dairy cattle. Journal of Dairy Science ***85*** 2831-2842.

Senger PL 1994 The estrus detection problem: New concepts, technologies, and possibilities. *Journal of Dairy Science* **77** 2745-2753.

Shannon P 1968 Advances in semen dilution. *Proceedings of the New Zealand Society of Animal Production* **28** 23-31.

Stevens J, Burton L & Rendel J 2000 Induced calving. *Proceedings of the Society of Dairy Cattle Veterinarians* **17** 79-93.

Stichbury JW 1968 Genetic implications of advances in semen dilution. *Proceedings of the New Zealand Society of Animal Production* **28** 32-39.

Sturman H, Oltenacu EAB & Foote RH 2000 Importance of inseminating only cows in estrus. *Theriogenology* **53** 1657-1667.

Underwood SL, Bathgate R, Ebsworth M, Maxwell WM & Evans G 2010 Pregnancy loss in heifers after artificial insemination with frozen-thawed, sex-sorted, re-frozen-thawed dairy bull sperm. *Animal Reproduction Science* **118** 7-12.

Verkerk GA, Goble G, McDougall S, Woods M & Clark B 1997 Induction of parturition in dairy cows: a survey from spring 1996 in the Waikato region. *Proceedings of the New Zealand Society of Animal Production* **57** 231-233.

Vishwanath R, Xu ZZ & Macmillan KL 1996 Prospects for overcoming the physiological limits of dairy cow fertility. *Proceedings of the New Zealand Society of Animal Production* **56** 355-357.

Welch RAS 1973 Induction of parturition in cattle with corticosteroids: an analysis of field trials. *New Zealand Veterinary Journal* **21** 103-108.

Williamson NB 1993 Calving induction programmes for cattle and farmer attitudes to them. *Proceedings of the Society of Dairy Cattle Veterinarians* p. 195-201.

Wiltbank N, Lopez H, Satori R, Sangsritavong S & Gümen A 2006 Changes in reproductive physiology of lactating dairy cows due to elevated steroid metabolism. *Theriogenology* **65** 17-29.

Xu ZZ & Burton LJ 1996 Reproductive efficiency in lactating dairy cows. *Proceedings of the New Zealand Society of Animal Production* **56** 34-37.

Xu ZZ & Burton LJ 2003 Reproductive performance of dairy cows in New Zealand: Monitoring Fertility Report. *www.aeu.org.nz/page.cfm?id=58&nid=26*

Xu ZZ, Burton LJ & Macmillan KL 1997 Treatment of post-partum anoestrous dairy cows with progesterone, oestradiol and equine chorionic gonadotrophin. *New Zealand Veterinary Journal* **45** 205-207.

Xu ZZ, Verkerk GA, Mee J, Morgan S, Clark BA, Burke CR & Burton LJ 2000 Progesterone and follicular changes in postpartum noncyclic dairy cows after treatment with progesterone and oestradiol or with progesterone, GnRH, PGF2α, and oestradiol. *Theriogenology* **54** 272-282.

Physiological differences and implications to reproductive management of *Bos taurus* and *Bos indicus* cattle in a tropical environment

R Sartori[1], MR Bastos[2], PS Baruselli[3], LU Gimenes[3], RL Ereno[4] and CM Barros[4]

[1]Department of Animal Science, ESALQ, University of São Paulo (USP), Piracicaba, SP, Brazil, 13418-900. [2]Department of Animal Reproduction and Radiology, FMVZ, São Paulo State University (UNESP), Botucatu, SP, Brazil, 18618-000. [3]Department of Animal Reproduction, FMVZ, University of São Paulo (USP), São Paulo, SP, Brazil, 05508-000.[4]Department of Pharmacology, IBB, São Paulo State University (UNESP), Botucatu, SP, Brazil, 18618-000

In the current review the main fundamental biological differences in reproductive function between *Bos taurus* and *Bos indicus* cattle are discussed. Breed differences regarding puberty, estrous cycle patterns, estrous behavior, acquisition of ovulatory capacity, ovarian structures and reproductive hormones are presented. The main physiological differences that *Bos indicus* cattle present relative to *Bos taurus* cattle include: delayed age at puberty; higher circulating concentrations of hormones such as estradiol, progesterone, insulin and IGF-I, despite having smaller ovulatory follicle size and corpora lutea; greater population of small follicles and smaller size of the dominant follicle at deviation; and greater sensitivity of follicles to gonadotropins. Knowledge of the differences between *Bos indicus* and *Bos taurus* breeds help explain different management procedures and responses to hormonal treatments associated with artificial insemination, ovarian superstimulation, and in vivo and in vitro embryo production.

Introduction

Over the years, cattle have been raised and selected especially for meat and dairy production and the majority of breeds are either *Bos taurus* or *Bos indicus* (Zebu). Some of the *Bos taurus* breeds, such as Holstein and Jersey, have been selected for high milk production, and others for beef production. Due to intensive selection, *Bos taurus* breeds are very efficient for food production as compared to other breeds; however, they are not well adapted to tropical environments and cannot maximize their potential for production in the tropics. The main problem with *Bos taurus* cattle in the tropics is the very low tolerance to heat stress. As compared to *Bos taurus*, *Bos indicus* (Zebu) breeds experience a less severe reduction in feed intake, growth rate, milk yield and reproductive function in response to heat stress (Adeyemo *et al.* 1979; Bennett *et al.* 1985; Pegorer *et al.* 2007).

Corresponding author E-mail: sartori@esalq.usp.br

Although *Bos taurus* breeds are more precocious, Zebu cattle are extensively used in the tropics, especially in Brazil, due to their thermo tolerance and resistance to parasites. In fact, Brazil alone has nearly 200 million cattle of which 80% are Zebu or crossbred Zebu animals. The extensive systems of management which predominate in South America have continually exposed these cattle to a tropical climate and nutritional environment resulting in increased tolerance to that environment through selection pressure. This environmental tolerance means that Zebu cattle can thrive where *Bos taurus* cattle may not.

To overcome or minimize problems related to decreased production of purebred *Bos taurus* cattle in tropical regions, one strategy has been to produce *Bos taurus* X *Bos indicus* crossbreds. Zebu cattle are known to be less fertile and have lower levels of milk production than *Bos taurus* breeds, but are better adapted to the environmental conditions which makes them more likely to reproduce successfully in the tropics. Crossbreds incorporate the environmental adaptation of Zebu cattle and the higher production of *Bos taurus* cattle (Negussie *et al.* 1999) as well as the benefit of hybrid vigor.

Because most of the reproductive physiology studies in cattle have been performed with *Bos taurus* breeds in countries with a temperate climate, strategies for reproductive management that have been used in Zebu cattle were adapted from those studies and may not be ideal for *Bos indicus*. Therefore, the increase in knowledge of the physiological differences between *Bos taurus* and *Bos indicus* breeds has been useful to develop specific protocols or strategies for reproductive management to maximize production in different breeds of cattle raised in a tropical environment.

Similarities and differences in reproductive physiology of *Bos taurus* and *Bos indicus* cows and heifers

Puberty

Puberty is defined by the animal's ability to reproduce as a result of the development of hypothalamic neurons that secrete GnRH at the appropriate frequency and in sufficient quantities to release gonadotropins and promote gametogenesis. Although the first ovulatory estrus is the main marker of puberty (Rawlings *et al.* 2003), heifers usually only reach maximum fertility on their third estrus (Byerley *et al.* 1987). Increased LH pulse frequency in the circulation, which is the determining factor for sexual maturity of heifers, is due to decreased hypothalamic sensitivity to the negative feedback of estradiol (Day *et al.* 1987) which is influenced by genetic and environmental factors (Martin *et al.* 1992; Nogueira 2004).

Most heifers reared in the tropics are subjected to low quality forages and suffer from protein, energy and/or mineral deficiencies. Therefore, most of these animals cannot reach puberty until 2 years of age, while those in a temperate climate reach puberty around 9 to 12 months of age (Fajersson *et al.* 1991). According to Nogueira (2004), independent of nutrition, there also seems to be a genetic factor associated with puberty in Zebu cattle, since 30% of Nelore heifers (12 of 37) became pregnant at 16 months of age but there was no difference in age or weight from the group mean at first ovulation.

There are also clear differences in age at puberty between *Bos taurus* and *Bos indicus* cattle. Generally, Zebu heifers reach sexual maturity and puberty later than *Bos taurus* heifers. This was demonstrated in the study by Rodrigues *et al.* (2002), where the cessation of inhibition of LH pulses by estradiol occurred simultaneously with the onset of puberty in heifers of both genotypes, but it happened earlier in *Bos taurus* heifers, especially during the initial period of weight gain (16 to 18 months of age). The estimated age at puberty for Zebu in the tropics and subtropics is between 16 and 40 months, with a mean of 25 months, i.e., 6 to 12 months later than *Bos taurus* (Abeygunawardena & Dematawewa 2004; Nogueira 2004). Moreover, smaller breeds, such as the Zebu breeds, normally reach puberty at an older age and heavier body weight than *Bos taurus* heifers (Martin *et al.* 1992; Bagley 1993). Finally, regardless of size and nutrition level, Zebu cattle are less precocious in regards to puberty because the selection pressure for puberty has been much less intensive than in *Bos taurus* cattle (Eler *et al.* 2002), even though there is a high correlation between scrotal circumference in *Bos indicus* bulls and younger age of puberty in their daughters (Forni & Albuquerque 2005; Eler *et al.* 2006). Moreover, age at first conception was highly heritable (h^2 = 0.44 to 0.67; Pereira *et al.* 2007) as was heifer pregnancy (h^2 = 0.58 to 0.66; Eler *et al.* 2006; Pereira *et al.* 2007). There was also a high genetic correlation between age at first calving and interval from the onset of breeding season to calving in the subsequent year (Forni & Albuquerque 2005). Therefore, the potential to improve age of puberty and shorten postpartum anestrus interval through selection in *Bos indicus* cattle does exists.

Estrous cycle and follicular dynamics

During the estrous cycles of heifers and cows, there is growth and regression of follicles in a wave-like pattern (Pierson & Ginther 1984; Savio *et al.* 1988). Studies in *Bos taurus* cattle have described the occurrence of two to four follicular waves during the estrous cycle, with a predominance of two waves, and very rarely four waves (Sirois & Fortune 1988; Townson *et al.* 2002; Sartori *et al.* 2004). In a study with *Bos indicus* cattle in Brazil, Figueiredo *et al.* (1997) observed two- and three-wave cycles in Nelore cattle, with the majority of cows having two (83.3%) and heifers having three (64.7%) follicular waves. Other studies in Nelore heifers (Mollo *et al.* 2007), Gir cows (Gambini *et al.* 1998, Viana *et al.* 2000), and Brahman cows (Zeitoun *et al.* 1996) have detected a predominance of three waves, but also observed animals with two, four, and even a few with five waves during a cycle.

Although, several studies evaluated estrous cycle patterns in *Bos taurus* and *Bos indicus* cattle, very few have directly and simultaneously compared these genetic groups under the same environmental and management conditions. An experiment performed in Florida compared multiparous lactating Angus (temperate *Bos taurus*; n = 12), Brahman (tropical *Bos indicus*; n = 12), and Senepol (tropical *Bos taurus*; n = 12) cows throughout an estrous cycle during the summer (Alvarez *et al.* 2000). In this study, the majority of Angus and Brahman cows had two follicular waves during the estrous cycle (72.7% and 55.6%, respectively) and 70% of the cycles of Senepol cows had three waves.

A study in our laboratory compared estrous cycle patterns between *Bos indicus* and *Bos taurus* cows (Bastos *et al.* 2010). From January to April 2010, 5 to 10 year old multiparous nonlactating cows (n = 12 Nelore and 12 Holstein cows) were managed in individual stalls and fed a total mixed maintenance ration (TMR) according to the NRC (2000). The TMR consisted of 42.8% sugar cane bagasse, 45.7% corn, 5.7% molasses, 3.2% soybean hulls, 1.2% urea, and 1.4% mineral salt. Nelore and Holstein cows had a BCS (scale from 1 to 5) of 3.1 ± 0.1 and 2.8 ± 0.2, and a body weight of 508 ± 17 and 575 ± 20 kg, respectively. After a 14 to 21-d period of adaptation, estrus was synchronized and cows were monitored daily by ovarian ultrasonography throughout an entire estrous cycle. Moreover, during the first follicular wave, ultrasound scanning was performed twice a day. Daily blood samples from the jugular vein were also collected for hormone assays during the entire period of study, except in two occasions in which blood was collected immediately before and 4 hours after feeding during the follicular and luteal phases. In this study, 80% of Nelore cows and 60% of Holstein cows presented three waves of follicular development during the estrous cycle. All the remaining cows had two waves. Moreover, average estrous cycle length was 23 d (range of 21 to 26 d) and was similar between Nelore and Holstein cows (P > 0.05).

From other data, the average interestrous interval was 21 d, for both *Bos taurus* and *Bos indicus* cattle (discussed by Bó *et al.* 2003 and Sartori *et al.* 2004), and two-wave cycles were shorter than three-wave cycles (Savio *et al.* 1988, 1990; Sirois & Fortune 1988; Alvarez *et al.* 2000; Townson *et al.* 2002; Sartori *et al.* 2004). There were, however, exceptions, in which high-producing lactating Holstein cows tended to have a longer estrous cycle (23 d), due to a prolonged time between luteolysis and ovulation (discussed by Sartori *et al.* 2004).

Although there are similarities in estrous cycle length and follicular wave patterns between *Bos taurus* and *Bos indicus* cattle, differences in antral follicle population between genetic groups are well documented and are illustrated in Figure 1. At the onset of each follicular wave, approximately 24 small (2 to 5 mm) viable antral follicles were detected in *Bos taurus* cattle (Ginther *et al.* 1996), however, in *Bos indicus* cattle, there were greater numbers of small follicles during wave emergence. Buratini Jr. *et al.* (2000) described the occurrence of approximately 50 small follicles in the ovaries of Nelore heifers. High numbers of small follicles were also observed in the ovaries of Sindhi (*Bos indicus*) heifers (49.0 ± 6.4, n = 14) and lactating cows (64.0 ± 5.1, n = 34; MCC Mattos, unpublished observations). By directly comparing number of small follicles (3 to 5 mm) in the ovaries between *Bos taurus* and *Bos indicus* cattle, Alvarez *et al.* (2000) observed a greater number of follicles at wave emergence in Brahman (39 ± 4) compared to Senepol (33 ± 4), or Angus (21 ± 4) multiparous lactating cows. Recent studies performed with both genetic groups in contemporary environmental and nutritional conditions showed that *Bos indicus* had a greater number of follicles at wave emergence compared to *Bos taurus* cattle (Carvalho *et al.* 2008; Gimenes *et al.* 2009). Carvalho *et al.* (2008) synchronized ovulation in Nelore and Angus heifers and Gir and Holstein heifers, using a progesterone intravaginal device and 2 mg of estradiol benzoate with or without PGF2α at the beginning of the treatment. There was no interaction of breed, therefore, genetic group was combined. In this trial, *Bos indicus* cattle recruited 33.4 ± 3.2 follicles, while *Bos taurus* heifers recruited 25.4 ± 2.5 follicles (P = 0.09). Gimenes *et al.* (2009), synchronized Nelore and Holstein heifers using a norgestomet auricular implant and 2 mg of estradiol benzoate with or without a 50 mg injection of progesterone. Nelore heifers had 29.7 ± 3.1 follicles at wave emergence; whereas, Holstein heifers had 15.0 ± 2.8 follicles (P < 0.01). Similarly, Bastos *et al.* (2010) detected significant differences in number of antral follicles between Nelore and Holstein cows. At wave emergence, the number of 2 to 5 mm follicles present on the ovaries was 42.7 ± 5.9 for Nelore (range of 25 to 100) and 19.7 ± 3.2 for Holstein (range of 5 to 40) cows (P < 0.05).There was little variation in number of small follicles throughout the entire estrous cycle in both breeds as reported by Alvarez *et al.* (2000) and Buratini Jr. *et al.* (2000). Significant differences in ovarian follicle population between *Bos indicus* and *Bos taurus* breeds may be associated with higher circulating concentrations of insulin and IGF-I in *Bos indicus* cattle, as described by Alvarez *et al.* (2000) and Bastos *et al.* (2010).

Follicular deviation and selection of the dominant follicle

After follicular wave emergence in cattle, there is a mechanism of selection in which only one follicle becomes dominant, inhibiting the growth of other follicles on the ovary (subordinate follicles; Ginther *et al.* 1996). Follicular deviation has been used to refer to the time at which differences in the growth rate between the future dominant and the future subordinate follicles become apparent (Ginther *et al.* 1996). In *Bos taurus* breeds, such as Holstein, follicular deviation occurs when the largest developing follicle reaches 8.5 to 9.0 mm in diameter (Ginther *et al.* 1996; Sartori *et al.* 2001), whereas, in Zebu cattle, such as Nelore, deviation occurs when the largest growing follicle reaches 5 to 7 mm (Castilho *et al.* 2007; Figueiredo *et al.* 1997; Sartorelli *et al.* 2005; Ereno 2008; Gimenes *et al.* 2008). There are exceptions, however, in both genetic groups of animals. When comparing high-producing lactating Holstein cows to nulliparous Holstein heifers, Sartori *et al.* (2004) observed that deviation occurred when the largest growing follicle reached 9.8 mm and 8.3 mm in lactating cows and heifers, respectively ($P < 0.05$). Likewise, Bastos *et al.* (2010) detected that follicular deviation occurred when the largest developing follicle reached 7.0 ± 0.2 and 8.9 ± 0.4 mm in nonlactating Nelore and Holstein cows, respectively ($P < 0.05$).

Although follicle size at deviation differs substantially between breeds, the time of deviation during the first follicular wave in *Bos indicus* relative to the preceding ovulation (2.3 to 2.8 d; Sartorelli *et al.* 2005; Ereno 2008; Gimenes *et al.* 2008) was similar to that reported in *Bos taurus* cattle (Ginther *et al.* 1996; Sartori *et al.* 2001). In fact, when comparing Nelore to Holstein cows, Bastos *et al.* (2010) observed that deviation occurred, on average, 2.3 d after ovulation, independent of breed.

The mechanisms that control selection of the dominant follicle are complex and not fully understood. Ovarian theca cells express LH receptors (LHR) from preantral to preovulatory sizes (Xu *et al.* 1995). Although it is clear that LHR expression occurs in granulosa cells of dominant follicles (Xu *et al.* 1995; Bao *et al.* 1997), there is some controversy about the time when these cells start to express functional LHR and whether it is required to support dominant follicle growth at the time of deviation when FSH levels are declining or low. LHR mRNA abundance measured by real-time PCR was higher in granulosa cells from the largest follicle of the wave compared with the second largest follicle before morphological deviation, suggesting that acquisition of LH responsiveness by granulosa cells is part of the deviation process (Beg *et al.* 2001). Other studies utilizing *in situ* hybridization, failed to detect LHR mRNA in granulosa cells around deviation (Evans & Fortune 1997; Fortune *et al.* 2001; Garverick *et al.* 2002), which is in agreement with previous reports showing binding of LH to granulosa cells of only selected dominant follicles (Ireland & Roche 1982; Webb & England 1982).

The LHR gene in sheep and cattle follicles is subject to alternative splicing, and variants with deletion of exon 10 and/or partial deletion of exon 11 were reported (Bacich *et al.* 1994; Abdennebi *et al.* 2002; Robert *et al.* 2003). Although functional properties of LHR splice variants have not been fully elucidated, the variant with a partial deletion of exon 11 has been shown to be translated into a protein that is not translocated to the cell membrane (Bacich *et al.* 1999; Kawate 2004), and deletion of exon 10 resulted in impaired activation by LH in comparison with hCG in humans (Gromoll *et al.* 2000; Muller *et al.* 2003). Therefore, PCR strategies amplifying exon fragments present in all transcripts should permit quantification of LH receptor expression without identifying each of the variant forms. In a recent study assessing expression of LHR alternative transcripts by PCR in granulosa cells from crossbred Nelore cows, all isoforms were only detected in follicles at 7 mm in diameter or larger, and mRNA abundance increased with follicle size (Nogueira *et al.* 2007a). In Nelore cattle, follicle deviation occurs when the dominant follicle reaches 5 to 7 mm in diameter; therefore, these results suggest that expression of functional LHR only occurs in granulosa cells after deviation. In a follow up study using the same PCR strategy, Barros *et al.* (2009) assessed LHR expression in granulosa cells from the two largest follicles in the ovary of Nelore heifers taken before (Day 2 of the wave), during (Day 2.5), and after (Day 3) the expected time of follicular deviation. LHR mRNA expression was detected only in two out of seven largest follicles obtained on Day 2.5 (both in 7 mm follicles), but not on Day 2. Moreover, the majority of the largest follicles obtained on Day 3 expressed LHR (64% positive follicles from 8 to 14 mm). Therefore, data obtained in Nelore cattle suggest that expression of functional LHR occurs after follicular deviation and is a consequence, rather a means of selection (Part of the review above was presented at the Annual Meeting of the IETS/2010 by Barros *et al.* 2010).

Acquisition of ovulatory capacity

Although follicle deviation occurs in *Bos indicus* when the dominant follicle reaches 5 to 7 mm in diameter (Figueiredo *et al.* 1997; Sartorelli *et al.* 2005; Castilho *et al.* 2007; Gimenes *et al.* 2008; Bastos *et al.* 2010) compared to 8 to 9 mm in *Bos taurus* (Ginther *et al.* 1996; Sartori *et al.* 2001; Bastos *et al.* 2010), it is possible that additional growth is necessary for the dominant follicle to acquire ovulatory capacity in both breeds.

Sartori *et al.* (2001) observed that Holstein cows with follicles 7 or 8.5 mm in diameter did not ovulate, even after administration of high doses of pLH (40 mg). However, 80% of the cows with follicles ≥ 10 mm ovulated after pLH administration. Conversely, Gimenes *et al.* (2008) reported that administration of 25 mg pLH in *Bos indicus* heifers induced ovulation in 33.3, 80.0 and 90.0% of animals with follicles that were 7.0 to 8.4, 8.5 to 10 and > 10 mm in diameter, respectively. These results were not unexpected, and corroborate the data showing differences in size of the growing follicle at follicular deviation between *Bos indicus* and *Bos taurus* cattle.

This relationship between follicular diameter, acquisition of ovulatory capacity and gene expression of LHR isoforms, was recently investigated (Simões, 2009). In the first experiment, the minimum pLH dose (Lutropin-V, Bioniche Animal Health Inc, Belleville, ON, Canada) necessary to induce ovulation in Nelore cows that had a first wave dominant follicle of 10 to 11 mm in diameter was found to be 3.125 mg. In the second experiment, 6.25 mg of pLH was utilized to induce ovulation of first wave dominant follicles of 7 to 8.0, 8.1 to 9.0 and 9.1 to 10 mm in diameter. In a third experiment, theca and granulosa cells, obtained from abattoir-derived ovarian follicles, were separated for total RNA extraction, and gene expression of LHR isoforms was measured by semiquantitative RT-PCR using GAPDH as the internal control. Simões (2009) observed that with the increase in follicle diameter (7.0 to 8.0, 8.1 to 9.0 and 9.1 to 10.0 mm) in Nelore or crossbred Nelore females, there was a corresponding increase in ovulation rates (9.0, 36.0 and 90.0%, respectively) and expression of LHR isoforms in granulosa cells (16.5, 21.0 and 37.6; mRNA LHR/mRNA GAPDH), but not in theca cells. It was concluded that in Zebu cattle ovulatory capacity is related to an increase in follicle diameter and expression of LH receptors in granulosa cells.

Maximum size of dominant/ovulatory follicle and CL and circulating hormones

Ginther *et al.* (1989), working with Holstein females, observed that heifers with two follicular waves had dominant follicles with maximum diameters of 17.1 and 16.5 mm for the first and second wave, respectively. In contrast, in *Bos indicus* females, the diameters reported were 11.3 and 12.3 mm, respectively (Figueiredo *et al.* 1997; Sartorelli *et al.* 2005; Figure 1). Similarly, in Zebu cattle, the size of the CL ranged from 17 to 21 mm in diameter (Segerson *et al.* 1984, Rhodes *et al.* 1995, Figueiredo *et al.* 1997); whereas, in *Bos taurus* cattle diameters of 20 to 30 mm were detected (Ginther *et al.* 1989). Although there seem to be clear differences in size of ovarian structures between *Bos taurus* and *Bos indicus*, follicle size, and consequently CL size may be determined by factors other than breed.

Studies have reported that dairy cows develop larger ovulatory follicles, but have lower serum estradiol concentrations than heifers (Sartori *et al.* 2004; Wolfenson *et al.* 2004) or dry cows (De La Sota *et al.* 1993), suggesting an increased steroid metabolism in dairy cows, as reported by Sangsritavong *et al.* 2002). In relation to serum concentration of estradiol, there are few data comparing *Bos indicus* to *Bos taurus*. In the study by Alvarez *et al.* (2000), there were no differences in maximum circulating estradiol among Brahman, Angus, and Senepol cows (8.9 ± 1.6, 9.1 ± 1.4, and 8.7 ± 1.4 pg/mL, respectively). This seems to be the only study in which the maximum diameter of the ovulatory follicle was greater in *Bos indicus* (15.6 ± 0.5 mm) than in *Bos taurus* cattle (12.8 ± 0.4 and13.6 ± 0.4 mm for Angus and Senepol, respectively). Conversely, Segerson *et al.* (1984) compared Angus to Brahman cattle and observed higher serum concentrations of estradiol-17ß and progesterone in *Bos taurus* cows.

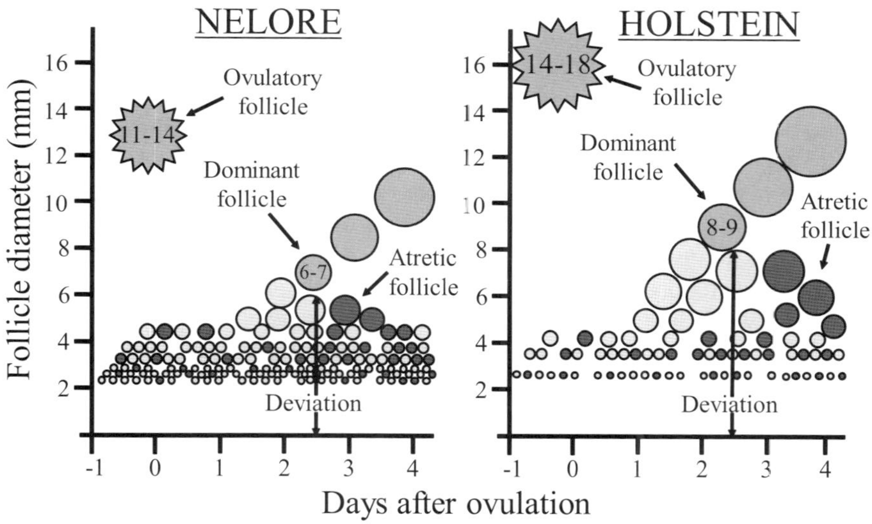

Fig. 1. Schematic representation of follicle development in Nelore (*Bos indicus*) and Holstein (*Bos taurus*) cows based on data from the literature and personal data. *Bos indicus* (Nelore) have a greater population of small (2 to 5 mm) follicles in the ovaries throughout the entire estrous cycle than *Bos taurus* (Holstein) cattle. Moreover, although both breeds present follicle deviation between Day 2 and 3 after ovulation, the diameter of the future dominant follicle at deviation is greater in Holstein cattle. The diameter of the ovulatory follicle is also greater in Holsteins than in Nelore cows.

According to Randel (1976) *Bos indicus* and *Bos indicus* crossbred females had lower progesterone concentration per gram of luteal tissue than in *Bos taurus* females. However, Segerson et *al.* (1984) did not detect differences in progesterone concentration in the CL between Brahman and Angus cows (75.8 ± 11.3 and 65.9 ± 5.3 μg/g of CL, respectively; $P > 0.10$). Conversely, studies performed in Brazil detected higher circulating progesterone in *Bos indicus* (Nelore or Gir) compared to *Bos taurus* (Angus or Holstein) cattle. Carvalho *et al.* (2008) compared *Bos indicus* (Nelore and Gir), *Bos taurus* (Angus and Holstein) and crossbreds (Angus x Nelore and Gir x Holstein) throughout the period of an estrus synchronization protocol. Two PGF2α treatments, 12 days apart were performed 24 and 12 days before treatment with an intravaginal source of progesterone was initiated. On Day 0, each heifer received a progesterone intravaginal device plus estradiol benzoate. During that period (with a progesterone device), serum progesterone concentrations were higher in *Bos indicus* heifers. Similarly, Bastos *et al.*

(2010) reported that although the maximum diameter of the ovulatory follicle (15.7 $\pm$ 0.3 mm *vs* 13.4 $\pm$ 0.3 mm; Figure 1) and the maximum CL volume (7610.5 $\pm$ 512.0 mm^3 *vs* 4916.6 $\pm$ 548.1 mm^3) were greater in Holsteins, plasma peak estradiol (7.70 $\pm$ 0.67 *vs* 12.71 $\pm$ 0.98 pg/mL) and progesterone (4.06 $\pm$ 0.18 *vs* 4.64 $\pm$ 0.40 ng/mL) concentrations were higher in Nelore cows. This suggests that *Bos indicus* females may be slower to metabolize estradiol and progesterone.

Estrous behavior

Behavioral signs of estrus can be observed in cattle and used for estrus detection for the purposes of artificial insemination (AI). However, these characteristics are influenced by age, milk yield, environment and hierarchy (revised in Landaeta-Hernández *et al.* 2004). Additionally, differences can be noted among breeds (Rae *et al.* 1999), and even among genetic groups (*Bos indicus vs Bos taurus*).

Mizuta (2003) compared the reproductive behavior of Nelore cows with Angus cows using radiotelemetry (Heat-Watch). Nelore cows exhibited a shorter estrus compared to Angus cows (12.9 $\pm$ 2.9 *vs* 16.3 $\pm$ 4.8 hours, respectively). Additionally, more than 50% of Nelore cows showed estrus during the evening and night (between 6:00 PM and 6:00 AM; Pinheiro *et al.* 1998; Membrive 2000), and about 30% exhibited estrus only during darkness (Pinheiro *et al.* 1998). These factors decrease the efficacy of estrous detection for traditional AI. However, short estrus duration has been observed in high-producing Holstein cows. In a recent study evaluating the association between levels of milk production and estrous behavior, Lopez *et al.* (2004) observed a shorter duration (6.2 versus 10.9 hours) and intensity (6.3 versus 8.8 mounts) of estrus in cows with higher (> 39.5 kg/d) compared to lower (< 39.5 kg/d) milk production. These differences within the same breed may be related to lower circulating concentrations of estradiol in higher *vs* lower milk producing cows (Lopez *et al.* 2004) as well as in lactating cows compared to heifers (Sartori *et al.* 2002, 2004). Based on such results, Wiltbank *et al.* (2006) hypothesized that high producing cows (above 40 kg of milk/d) have low circulating estradiol due to a high metabolism of this steroid. The effect of higher metabolism on estrus behavior was also observed in beef cattle. Nelore heifers submitted to high dietary intake exhibited less intense and shorter duration of estrus as compared with Nelore heifers receiving low dietary intake (Mollo *et al.* 2007).

Although there are differences between *Bos taurus* and *Bos indicus* in duration and intensity of estrus, other factors such as feed intake, body size, and steroid metabolism may exert profound effects over this behavior.

Tolerance to heat stress

Heat stress is a particularly severe problem in cattle reproduction because of reduction in estrus expression, lower fertilization rates, increased embryonic loss and, consequently, lower fertility. Over 50% of the bovine population is located in the tropics and it is estimated that heat stress causes severe economic loss in approximately 60% of dairy farms around the world (Wolfenson *et al.* 2000). The magnitude of this effect on reproduction in dairy cattle is increasing, as augmented milk yield enhances susceptibility of cows to the deleterious effects of heat stress (Al-Katanani *et al.* 1999; Sartori *et al.* 2002; Lopez-Gatius 2003).

Bos indicus breeds experience a less severe reduction in reproductive function in response to heat stress than *Bos taurus* breeds (Adeyemo *et al.* 1979; Bennett *et al.* 1985; Rocha *et al.* 1998; Barros *et al.* 2006). Most of this adaptation to elevated temperature is due to superior ability of thermo-tolerant breeds to regulate body temperature (Adeyemo *et al.* 1979; Gaughan *et al.* 1999) as well as intrinsic cellular resistance to elevated temperature (Malayer & Hansen 1990; Sartorelli *et al.* 2006). High environmental temperature and humidity resulted in a marked decline in oocyte quality from Holstein and crossbred Angus cows (Rocha *et al.* 1998). In contrast, a high percentage of oocytes retrieved from Brahman cows exhibited normal morphology and yielded a high proportion of blastocysts, regardless of season (Rocha *et al.* 1998). Although *Bos indicus* cattle are more resistant to heat stress than *Bos taurus* cattle, exposure of Gir cows to a 28-d period of heat stress exerted a delayed effect on reproductive function, manifested by an increased incidence of large follicles, more follicular codominance, and reductions in estrous cycle length, progesterone concentrations, and oocyte developmental capacity (Torres-Junior *et al.* 2008).

Infertility in the male caused by heat stress can be eliminated through the use of AI with semen collected and frozen from males in cool environments. In females, transfer of in vivo or in vitro produced (IVP) embryos have been utilized as an attempt to bypass effects of heat stress (Hammond *et al.* 1996; Al-Katanani *et al.* 2002; Sartori *et al.* 2006). For example, a retrospective study was performed in high-producing Holstein cows (average milk production 28.4 ± 2.3 kg/d) submitted to ET (n = 2112) or AI (n = 7501) during the period of 2000 to 2003 (Rodrigues *et al.* 2004). Estrus was detected in cows, which were subjected to AI 12 hours later or ET 7 d later. Pregnancy rates were higher in those receiving embryos than those undergoing AI during the summer months, but no differences were observed during the cooler months.

Using *Bos indicus* genotype embryos during summer months can also improve fertility. In vitro studies have shown that *Bos indicus* embryos submitted to heat shock at early stages of development are better able to survive as compared to *Bos taurus* embryos (Malayer *et al.* 1990; Kamwanja *et al.* 1994; Barros *et al.* 2006; Sartorelli *et al.* 2006). More recently, effects of heat stress on embryonic development in culture were evaluated in Nelore and crossbred (*Bos indicus* X *Bos taurus*) oocytes fertilized with Nelore or Angus (*Bos taurus*) spermatozoa. The decrease in blastocyst development rates caused by exposure to 41°C during 12 hours was more evident when the heat shock was applied at earlier stages of development, particularly for embryos that had a predominant *Bos taurus* genotype (Erberhardt *et al.* 2009). In the study reported by Sartorelli *et al.* (2006), embryos from Angus or Nelore cows produced using oocytes obtained by ovum pickup (OPU) procedures were exposed to a culture temperature of 41°C for 12 hours beginning 96 hours after fertilization. Thereafter, embryos were transferred at the blastocyst stage to crossbred recipient heifers. Pregnancy rates after transfer were: 29.4% (15/51) for non-stressed Nelore embryos, 29.0% (11/38) for stressed Nelore embryos, 21.4% (6/28) for non-stressed Angus embryos and 7.1% (1/14) for stressed Angus embryos. These results and previous reports (Malayer *et al.* 1990; Erberhardt *et al.* 2009) clearly indicate that Nelore embryos are better able to survive during heat stress at early stages of development and more capable of establishing pregnancies following heat stress than Angus embryos.

Although heat stress induces a deleterious effect on *Bos taurus* oocytes and embryos, this sensitivity differs between categories, i.e. heifers (H), high-producing cows in peak lactation (PL) and repeat-breeders (RB; Ferreira *et al.* 2010). In this study, previously cited categories of Holstein cattle were evaluated during summer heat stress. At OPU, heifers had greater number of follicles than PL cows (H = 18.5 ± 1.9[a], PL = 12.4 ± 1.1[b], RB = 17.2 ± 2.0[ab]; P = 0.04). Heifers also had greater number of total oocytes (H = 9.6 ± 1.6[a], PL = 5.0 ± 0.9[b], RB = 8.8 ± 13[ab]; P = 0.03) and viable oocytes (H = 7.6 ± 1.5[a], PL = 3.6 ± 0.8[b], RB = 6.8 ± 1.2[ab]; P = 0.05) recovered at OPU than PL cows. During IVP, embryos from heifers performed better than PL and RB embryos (cleavage at Day 3: H = 47.8%[a], PL = 31.1%[b], RB = 35.4%[b], P = 0.008; blastocyst at Day 7: H = 21.0%[a], PL = 4.1%[b], RB = 3.8%[b], P < 0.0001; and grade I embryos: H = 1.3 ± 0.4[a], PL = 0.3 ± 0.2[b], RB = 0.5 ± 0.2[b], P = 0.04). The differences observed among heifers and cows are probably related to their metabolism under heat stress, comprising oocyte number and quality. Also, although RB had similar results at OPU (number of oocytes) as heifers, they probably had compromised oocytes, because their in vitro production or performance was poorer.

Reproductive management

Use of Bos indicus genotype

The utilization of thermo tolerant breeds has been employed by the beef industry in countries with a hot climate. However, the short duration of estrus in Zebu cattle is one of the major factors that limit the widespread use of AI in these breeds. This problem can be overcome with the use of fixed-time artificial insemination (FTAI) protocols, developed or adapted specifically for these cattle. Additionally, in vivo and in vitro embryo production has been increasing in tropical countries like Brazil, particularly in the Nelore breed (Viana & Camargo 2007).

Fixed-time artificial insemination (FTAI)

Although AI is a good alternative to introduce *Bos taurus* genetics into a *Bos indicus* herd, its traditional use limits the widespread application and success of this breeding technology. Factors already mentioned, such as short duration of estrus and estrus expression during the night reduce the estrus detection rate and consequently decrease pregnancy success. Postpartum cyclicity is influenced primarily by suckling and poor nutrition which are difficult to overcome in *Bos indicus* cattle. Suckling results in inhibition of GnRH/LH pulse frequency and reduces follicular development (reviewed by Willians *et al.* 1996). Poor nutrition delays the development of large ovarian follicles in postpartum cows reducing the maximum diameter and persistence of dominant follicles (reviewed by Bó *et al.* 2003).

For these reasons, FTAI has become a tool for increasing the efficiency of AI, since it eliminates the need for estrus detection. Estradiol and progestogen/progesterone treatments have been used increasingly over the past years in estrus synchronization programs in cattle (Macmillan & Peterson 1993; Macmillan & Burke 1996). This association promotes regression of antral follicles and the emergence of a new follicular wave, on average, 4 d after the beginning of the protocol, depending on the estradiol source utilized (reviewed in Bó *et al.* 2003). However, the successful application of AI in *Bos indicus* cattle, not only has to overcome the problem of estrus detection but also the problem of nutritionally and suckling-induced anestrus. One alternative to increase pregnancy rates in FTAI programs in anestrus *Bos indicus* cattle may be the addition of 300 to 500 IU of equine chorionic gonadotropin (eCG) at the time of removal of the progesterone releasing devices (Macmillan & Peterson 1993; Macmillan & Burke 1996; Baruselli *et al.*, 2004).

Other differences between *Bos indicus* and *Bos taurus* cattle emphasize the need for different strategies to manipulate the estrous cycle. Carvalho *et al.* (2008) observed that *Bos indicus* heifers can maintain higher circulating progesterone concentrations than *Bos taurus* or crossbred heifers. Therefore, these authors hypothesized that *Bos indicus* heifers are more sensitive to high concentrations of circulating progesterone, which may have a suppressive effect on LH pulsatility and, consequently, reduce follicular growth during a synchronization protocol. In this study, the administration of PGF2α at the beginning of a synchronization protocol in the *Bos indicus* protocol decreased circulating progesterone concentrations during treatment and increased follicular growth rate, dominant follicle diameter and ovulation rate. Another alternative is the use of norgestomet implants in *Bos indicus* heifers instead of progesterone devices, because of a reduced suppressive effect of norgestomet on LH pulsatility (Kojima *et al.* 1992). In a previous study of follicular dynamics using cyclic Nelore heifers treated with a norgestomet ear implant or progesterone-releasing intravaginal device (CIDR), follicular growth, maximum diameter of the dominant follicle, and ovulation rate were greater in norgestomet-treated heifers (Sá Filho *et al.* 2005).

Treatments to induce multiple ovulations

Barros & Nogueira (2001) examined the efficacy of different superstimulatory protocols in which the expected time of ovulation was postponed by 6 to 12 hours and ovulation was induced by administration of LH or GnRH (Barros & Nogueira 2001; Nogueira *et al.* 2002). Although these protocols did not significantly increase the quantity of viable embryos compared to estrus detection protocols, it was possible to control the time of ovulation with hormonal treatments, allowing the use of FTAI. From these experiments, a new protocol was developed called the P-36 protocol (Barros & Nogueira 2005). The protocol included insertion of a CIDR for 36 hours after PGF2α administration and induction of ovulation with exogenous LH, administered 12 hours after CIDR removal (48 hours after PGF2α administration). FTAI was performed 12 and 24 hours later since ovulation occurs between 24 and 36 hours after LH administration (Nogueira & Barros, 2003). The effectiveness of the P-36 protocol has been confirmed (Barros & Nogueira 2001, 2005; Baruselli *et al.* 2006), and more recently, an average of 13.3 $\pm$ 0.75 total structures and 9.4 $\pm$ 0.63 viable embryos, with a viability rate of 71.0% (1279/1807) following 136 embryo collections in Nelore cows has been reported (Nogueira *et al.* 2007b). These results were comparable to those reported in studies in which Nelore cows were inseminated 12 and 24 hours after onset of behavioral estrus (Nogueira *et al.* 2002; Nogueira & Barros 2003).

A variation of the P-36 protocol in which the progesterone device is removed 24 hours after PGF2α (protocol P-24) and LH is administered 24 hours later (48 hours after PGF2α), has been utilized in Nelore females, apparently with comparable results to those obtained with P-36 protocol (Zanenga *et al.* 2003; Baruselli *et al.* 2006).

The use of the P-36 protocol in *Bos taurus* breeds has resulted in a decrease in the number of viable embryos in comparison with conventional protocols with estrus detection. In Holstein (Martins *et al.* 2005; Rodrigues *et al.* 2005; Baruselli *et al.* 2006) and Angus donors (Bó *et al.* 2006; Chesta *et al.* 2007), viable embryo production was increased with the P-36 protocol when the ovulation induction treatment (LH or GnRH) was administered at 60 hours (P-36/LH60), rather than 48 hours (P-36/LH48) after PGF2α administration. Similarly, the results obtained by Barcelos *et al.* (2006), in Bonsmara donors (5/8 Afrikaner and 3/8 Hereford/Shorthorn) indicated that the P-36/LH60 protocol was more efficacious.

On the other hand, even though delaying ovulation for 12 hours in the P-36 protocol in *Bos taurus* breeds (P-36/LH60 protocol) had positive effects on embryo production, the opposite occurred when used in *Bos indicus* breeds.The P-36/LH60 protocol caused a decrease in embryo production when compared to P-36/LH48 protocol (Baruselli *et al.* 2006). Therefore, it can be inferred that ovulation in superstimulation protocols must be induced earlier in *Bos indicus* donors; whereas, in *Bos taurus* donors, it seems necessary to delay treatment with an ovulation inducer, thereby allowing an increase in follicle size, and acquisition of LH receptors.

Bos indicus breeds have a reduced capacity for LH secretion and a greater sensitivity to exogenous gonadotropins than *Bos taurus* cattle (Randel 1984). Superovulatory response was evaluated in Nelore cows submitted to three different doses of Folltropin-V (100, 133 or 200 mg) in a crossover design. There were no significant differences in any of the variables evaluated, indicating that it is possible to reduce the dose of FSH to 100 mg in Nelore cows submitted to a FTAI superstimulatory protocol, without compromising superovulatory response and embryo production (Baruselli *et al.* 2006). Others studies in Nelore heifers successfully induced superovulation and embryo production using a smaller dose of FSH (70 mg; Sartori *et al.* 2009), which is very unlikely to be effective in *Bos taurus* cattle.

In vitro embryo production

Especially due to the greater antral follicle population in *Bos indicus* cattle in relation to *Bos taurus* cattle, in vitro embryo production is much more successful in *Bos indicus* cattle (Viana & Camargo, 2007). In a recent study, (Pontes *et al.* 2010) Gir, Holstein and crossbreds (1/4 Holstein x 3/4 Gir or 1/2 Holstein-Gir) were compared for total and viable (good and regular quality grades according to Seneda *et al.* 2001) oocyte yield, and *in vitro* embryo production. The number of total and viable oocytes, and embryos produced were greater in Gir than in Holstein cattle (17.1 *vs* 11.4; 12.1 *vs* 8.0; 3.2 *vs* 2.2, respectively). Moreover, embryo production (5.5 blastocysts) was even greater in Holstein-Gir crossbreds compared to the other breeds.

A recent study was conducted comparing *Bos indicus* and *Bos taurus* cattle in which Nelore and Holstein heifers were submitted to a synchronization protocol to induce the emergence of a new follicular wave. Follicles were aspirated 1, 3 or 5 d after expected wave emergence (Gimenes *et al.* 2010). There was no effect of time of OPU on the variables evaluated. However, more oocytes were recovered and more embryos were produced from Nelore than Holstein heifers, as demonstrated in Table 1.

Table 1. Effect of genetic group on oocyte recovery and quality, and developmental competence of *Bos indicus* (Nelore) and *Bos taurus* (Holstein) heifers.

	GENETIC GROUP	
	Nelore (n = 9)	Holstein (n = 9)
Number of Replicates	6	6
OOCYTE RECOVERY AND QUALITY		
Visualized follicles	41.0 ± 2.1^a	22.1 ± 1.3^b
Total oocytes	37.1 ± 2.6^a	15.4 ± 1.2^b
Recovery rate (%)	82.3 ± 2.5^a	66.8 ± 2.8^b
Oocytes submitted to IVC	25.6 ± 1.8^a	9.1 ± 0.9^b
DEVELOPMENTAL COMPETENCE		
Cleaved structures	21.1 ± 1.6^a	5.2 ± 0.5^b
Cleavage rate (%)	82.6 ± 1.6^a	59.9 ± 3.6^b
Blastocysts 7 d after IVF	7.3 ± 0.9^a	1.1 ± 0.2^b
Blastocyst rate (%)	28.3 ± 2.8^a	14.1 ± 2.9^b

$^{a,b}P < 0.05$.

Similar results were found in another recent study (Sales *et al.*, 2010). Oocyte quality and quantity of nonlactating cattle was evaluated. In this study, 14 Gir and 14 Holstein cows were submitted to eight successive OPU sessions performed every 14 d. Gir cows had a greater number and better quality of oocytes recovered by OPU than Holstein donors (Table 2).

Ovarian superstimulation with gonadotropins has been reported to increase the number of oocytes retrieved by OPU as compared to nonstimulated *Bos taurus* cattle (Blondin *et al.*, 1997, 2002). However, this beneficial effect of superestimulation has not been confirmed in *Bos indicus* females (Seneda *et al.* 2004; Monteiro *et al.* 2009).

Evidence suggests that when *Bos taurus* cattle experience a "coasting" period (i.e. deprivation of FSH to induce follicle atresia) between hormonal stimulation and slaughterhouse ovary collection (Goodhand *et al.* 1999) and from ovary collection to oocyte aspiration (Blondin *et al.* 1997) in vitro developmental potential of cumulus-oocyte complex (COC) is effected. In both situations, follicles driven into phases of pseudodominance or early atresia provided COC with an ideal environment in which to acquire developmental competence (Blondin *et al.* 2002). A very high blastocyst rate (80%) was reported by Blondin *et al.* (2002) after superestimulating Holstein heifers with FSH and delaying COC retrieval by OPU using a coasting period of 48 hours. Additionally, LH was administered 6 hours before OPU in an attempt to render the COC more competent. Recently, the same protocol proposed by Blondin *et al.* (2002) was simultaneously compared to other protocols used for OPU and in vitro embryo production (IVP) in Nelore cattle (Monteiro *et al.* 2009). Their results indicate that ovarian superstimulation associated with deprivation of FSH and OPU did not increase in vitro embryo production in Nelore cattle. On the contrary, the highest rate of hatched blastocysts was observed in oocytes from nonstimulated cows.

Table 2. Effect of genetic group on oocyte recovery and quality of nonlactating *Bos indicus* (Gir) and *Bos taurus* (Holstein) cows.

	GENETIC GROUP	
	Gir (n = 14)	Holstein (n = 14)
Number of Replicates	8	8
Visualized follicles	25.5 ± 1.2	23.8 ± 1.1
Total oocytes	23.4 ± 1.6^a	14.9 ± 0.9^b
Recovery rate (%)	91.2^a (2604/2856)	61.1^b (1633/2673)
Oocyte quality		
Grade 1	5.3 ± 0.5^a	1.6 ± 0.2^b
Grade 2	9.8 ± 0.7^a	5.2 ± 0.4^b
Grade 3	4.8 ± 0.5	4.3 ± 0.4
Grade 4	0.9 ± 0.2	1.0 ± 0.2
Apoptosis by TUNEL (%)	16.6^b (21/117)	40.6^a (34/82)

$^{a,b}P < 0.05$.

Further experiments are necessary to understand why Nelore cattle did not respond as well as *Bos taurus* breeds to the protocol proposed by Blondin *et al.* (2002). It may be necessary to adjust FSH dosage and the "coasting" period to obtain better results in *Bos indicus* cattle. On the other hand, perhaps the fact that Nelore females usually have a larger number of follicles available for OPU precludes the use of superestimulatory protocols that might be useful for animals with lower number of follicles (*Bos taurus*).

Final considerations

Bos indicus and *Bos taurus* cattle have been mainly used for milk and beef production all over the world. Although, in general, *Bos taurus* cattle have been more intensely selected for production, a better adaptation to the tropical and sub-tropical environments makes *Bos indicus* cattle and crossbreds feasible options for production.

There are, however, significant differences in the reproductive physiology of those genetic groups, as seen in Table 3, that affect the application of adequate tools for reproductive management. For example, *Bos taurus* in general reach puberty sooner and have a shorter gestation length as compared to *Bos indicus* cattle (Paschal et al, 1991). Therefore, in order to have a 12 month calving interval, *Bos indicus* cows must conceive 10 d earlier than *Bos taurus* cattle.

Table 3. Main differences on reproductive physiology of *Bos taurus* and *Bos indicus* females.

Physiology	Bos indicus	References	Bos taurus	References
Age at puberty (months)	16 to 40	Abeygunawardena & Dematawewa (2004) Nogueira (2004)	9 to 12	Fajersson et *al*. (1991)
Duration of estrus (hours)	10.9 to 12.9	Pinheiro et *al*. (1998) Mizuta (2003)	16.3	Mizuta (2003)
Number of small follicles	30 to 60	Alvarez et *al*. (2000) Buratini Jr. et *al*. (2000) Carvalho et *al*. (2008) Gimenes et *al*. (2009) Bastos et *al*. (2010)	15 to 33	Ginther et *al*. (1996) Alvarez et *al*. (2000) Carvalho et *al*. (2008) Gimenes et *al*. (2009) Bastos et *al*. (2010)
Diameter of dominant follicle at deviation (mm)	5.4 to 7.0	Sartorelli et *al*. (2005) Castilho et *al*. (2007) Ereno et *al*. (2008) Gimenes et *al*. (2008) Bastos et *al*. (2010)	8.3 to 9.8	Ginther et *al*. (1996) Sartori et *al*. (2001) Sartori et *al*. (2004) Bastos et *al*. (2010)
Diameter of largest subordinate follicle at deviation (mm)	5.3 to 5.9	Sartorelli et *al*. (2005) Castilho et *al*. (2007) Gimenes et *al*. (2008)	7.2	Ginther et *al*. (1996)
Diameter related to acquisition of ovulatory capacity (mm)	7.0 to 8.5	Gimenes et *al*. (2008)	10.0	Sartori et *al*. (2001)
Diameter of ovulatory follicle (mm)	11.3 to 14.0	Figueiredo et *al*. (1997) Sartorelli et *al*. (2005) Mollo et *al*. (2007)	13.9 to 17.1	Ginther et *al*. (1989) Sartori et *al*. (2004)
Diameter of corpus luteum (mm)	17 to 21	Segerson et *al*. (1984) Rhodes et *al*. (1995) Figueiredo et *al*. (1997) Bastos et *al*. (2010)	20 to 30	Ginther et *al*. (1989) Kastelic et *al*. (1990) Bastos et *al*. (2010)

Differences in estrus behavior and ovarian function also make some adjustments of reproductive management necessary, such as the use of FTAI in postpartum cows. These strategies are also very useful for high milk-producing cows, due to their lower circulating estradiol. Moreover, the greater antral follicle population and sensitivity to gonadotropins in *Bos indicus* cattle, make the use of superovulation much more affordable than in *Bos taurus* cattle especially in vitro situations. Finally, greater sensitivity to the negative feedback of steroid hormones on the hypothalamus/pituitary makes a dose reduction necessary during hormone treatments in *Bos indicus cattle*.

Acknowledgements

We thank all the students, institutions and companies that have collaborated with our research groups, as well as EMBRAPA and the funding agencies FAPESP, CNPq and CAPES of Brazil.

References

Abdennebi L, Lesport AS, Remy JJ, Grebert D, Pisselet C, Monniaux D & Salesse R 2002 Differences in splicing of mRNA encoding LH receptor in theca cells according to breeding season in ewes. *Reproduction* **123** 819-826.

Abeygunawardena H & Dematawewa CMB 2004 Pré-pubertal and postpartum anestrus in tropical Zebu cattle. *Animal Reproduction Science* **82-83** 373-387.

Adeyemo O, Heath E, Adadevoh BK, Steinbach J & Olaloku EA 1979 Some physiological and behavioral responses in Bos indicus and Bos taurus heifers acclimatized to the hot humid seasonal equatorial climate. *International Journal of Biometeorology* **23** 231-241.

Al-Katanani YM, Drost M, Monson RL, Rutledge JJ, Krininger CE 3rd, Block J, Thatcher WW & Hansen PJ 2002 Pregnancy rates following timed embryo transfer with fresh or vitrified in vitro produced embryos in lactating dairy cows under heat stress conditions. *Theriogenology* **58** 171-182.

Al-Katanani YM, Webb DW & Hansen PL 1999 Factors affecting seasonal variation in 90 day non-return rate to first service in lactating Holstein cows in a hot climate. *Journal of Dairy Science* **82** 2611-2615.

Alvarez P, Spicer LJ, Chase Jr CC, Payton ME, Hamilton TD, Stewart RE, Hammond AC, OlsonTA &Wetteman RP 2000 Ovarian and endocrine characteristics during the estrous cycle in Angus, Brahman and Senepol cows in a subtropical environment. *Jounal of Animal Science* **78** 1291-1302.

Bacich DJ, Earl CR, O'Keefe DS, Norman RJ & Rodgers RJ 1999 Characterization of the translated products of the alternatively spliced luteinizing hormone receptor in the ovine ovary throughout the oestrous cycle. *Molecular and Cellular Endocrinology* **147** 113-124.

Bacich DJ, Rohan RM, Norman RJ & Rodgers RJ 1994 Characterization and relative abundance of alternatively spliced luteinizing hormone receptor messenger ribonucleic acid in the ovine ovary. *Endocrinology* **135** 735-744.

Bagley CP 1993 Nutritional management of replacement beef heifers: A Review. *Journal of Animal Science* **71** 3155-3163.

Bao B, Garverick HA, Smith GW, Smith MF, Salfen BE & Youngquist RS 1997 Changes in messenger ribonucleic acid encoding luteinizing hormone receptor, cytochrome P450-side chain cleavage, and aromatase are associated with recruitment and selection of bovine ovarian follicles. *Biology of Reproduction* **56** 1158-1168.

Barcelos ACZ, Satrapa RA, Nogueira MFG & Barros CM 2006 Superstimulatory protocol P-36 in Bosmara breed: use of eCG and delay on induction of ovulation with LH. *Acta Scientiae Veterinariae* **34** 513 (abstract).

Barros CM, Ereno R, Machado MF, Buratini Jr J, Pegorer MF, Simões RAL & Satrapa R 2009 Gene expression of luteinizing hormone receptor (LHR) isoforms in granulosa cells of follicles from Nelore heifers before, during and after follicular deviation. *Reproduction Fertility and Development* **21** 245 (abstract).

Barros CM, Ereno RL, Simões RA, Fernandes P, Buratini J & Nogueira MF 2010 Use of knowledge regarding LH receptors to improve superstimulatory treatments in cattle. *Reproduction Fertility and Development* **22** 132-137.

Barros CM & Nogueira MFG 2001 Embryo transfer in Bos indicus cattle. *Theriogenology* **56** 1483-1496.

Barros CM & Nogueira MFG 2005 Superovulation in zebu cattle: protocol P-36. *Embryo Transfer Newsletter* **23** 5-9.

Barros CM, Pegorer MF, Vasconcelos JL, Eberhardt BG & Monteiro FM 2006 Importance of sperm genotype (indicus versus taurus) for fertility and embryonic development at elevated temperatures. *Theriogenology* **65** 210-218.

Baruselli PS, Reis EL, Marques MO, Nasser LF & Bó GA 2004 The use of hormonal treatments to improve reproductive performance of anestrous beef cattle in tropical climates. *Animal Reproduction Science* **82-83** 479-486.

Baruselli PS, de Sá Filho MF, Martins CM, Nasser LF, Nogueira MFG, Barros CM & Bo GA 2006 Superovulation and embryo transfer in Bos indicus cattle. *Theriogenology* **65** 77-88.

Bastos MR, Mattos MCC, Meschiatti MAP, Surjus RS, Guardieiro MM, Mourão GB, Pires AV, Pedroso AM, Santos FAP & Sartori R 2010 Ovarian function and circulating hormones in nonlactating Nelore versus Holstein cows. *Acta Scientiae Veterinariae (Abstract in press).*

Beg MA, Bergfelt DR, Kot K, Wiltbank MC & Ginther OJ 2001 Follicular-fluid factors and granulosa-cell gene expression associated with follicle deviation in cattle. *Biology of Reproduction* **64** 432-441.

Bennett IL, Finch VA & Holmes CR 1985 Time spent in shade and its relationship with physiological factors of thermoregulation in three breeds of cattle. *Applied Animal Behavior Science* **13** 227-236.

Blondin P, Bousquet D, Twagiramungu H, Barnes F &

Sirard MA 2002 Manipulation of follicular development to produce developmentally competent bovine oocytes. *Biology of Reproduction* **66** 38-43.

Blondin P, Guilbault LA & Sirard MA 1997 The time interval between FSH-P administration and slaughter can influence the developmental competence of beef heifer oocytes. *Theriogenology* **48** 803-813.

Bó GA, Baruselli PS, Chesta PM & Martins CM 2006 The timing of ovulation and insemination schedules in superstimulated cattle. *Theriogenology* **65** 89-101.

Bó GA, Baruselli PS & Martinez MF 2003 Pattern and manipulation of follicular development in *Bos indicus* cattle. *Animal Reproduction Sciencie* **78** 307-326.

Buratini Jr J, Price CA, Visintin JA & Bó GA 2000 Effects of dominant follicle aspiration and treatment with recombinant bovine somatotropin (BST) on ovarian follicular development in nelore (Bos indicus) heifers. *Theriogenology* **54** 421-431.

Byerley DJ, Staigmiller RB, Berardinelli JG & Short RE 1987 Pregnancy rates of beef heifers bred either on puberal or third estrus. *Journal of Animal science* **65** 645-650.

Carvalho JB, Carvalho NA, Reis EL, Nichi M, Souza AH & Baruselli PS 2008 Effect of early luteolysis in progesterone-based timed AI protocols in Bos indicus, Bos indicus x Bos taurus, and Bos taurus heifers. *Theriogenology* **69** 167-175.

Castilho C, Garcia JM, Renesto A, Nogueira GP & Brito LF 2007 Follicular dynamics and plasma FSH and progesterone concentrations during follicular deviation in the first post-ovulatory wave in Nelore (*Bos indicus*) heifers. *Animal Reproduction Sciencie* **98** 189-196.

Chesta P, Tribulo L, Tribulo H, Balla E, Baruselli P & Bó G 2007 Effect of time of ovulation induction by gonadotropin-releasing hormone or pituitary luteinizing hormone on ova/embryo production in superstimulated beef cows inseminated at a fixed time. *Reproduction Fertility and Development* **19** 307 (abstract).

Day ML, Imakawa K, Wolfe PL, Kittok RJ & Kinder JE 1987 Endocrine mechanism of puberty in heifers. Role of hypothalamo-pituitary estradiol receptors in the negative feedback of estradiol on luteinizing hormone secretion. *Biology of Reproduction* **37** 1054-1065.

De La Sota RL, Lucy MC, Staples CR & Thatcher WW 1993 Effects of recombinant bovine somatotropin (Sometribove) on ovarian function in lactating and nonlactating dairy cows. *Journal of Dairy Science* **76** 1002-1013.

Eler JP, Ferraz JB, Balieiro JC, Mattos EC & Mourão GB 2006 Genetic correlation between heifer pregnancy and scrotal circumference measured at 15 and 18 months of age in Nellore cattle. *Genetics and Molecular Research* **5** 569-580.

Eler JP, Silva Jr JA, Feraz JBS, Dias F, Oliveira HN, Evans JL & Golden BL 2002 Genetic evaluation of the probability of pregnancy at 14 months for Nelore heifers. *Journal of Animal Science* **80** 951-954.

Erberhardt BC, Satrapa RA, Capinzaiki CRL, Trinca LA & Barros CM 2009 Influence of the breed of bull (Bos taurus indicus vs. Bos taurus taurus) and the breed of cow (Bos taurus indicus, Bos taurus taurus and crossbred) on the resistence of bovine embryos to heat. *Animal Reproduction Science* **114** 54-61.

Ereno RL 2008 Gene expression of luteinizing hormone receptor (LHR) isoforms in granulosa cells of follicles from Nellore heifers before, during and after follicular deviation. PhD thesis, University of Sao Paulo State (Brazil).

Evans AC & Fortune JE 1997Selection of the dominant follicle in cattle occurs in the absence of differences in the expression of messenger ribonucleic acid for gonadotropin receptors. *Endocrinology* **138** 2963-2971.

Fajersson P, Barradas HV, Romanponce H & Cook RM 1991 The effects of dietary protein on age and weight at the onset of puberty in Brown Swiss and Zebu heifers in the tropics. *Theriogenology* **35** 845-855.

Ferreira RM, Ayres H, Ferraz ML, Araújo AB, Chiaratti MR, Sá Filho MF, Calomeni G, Rodrigues CA, Watanabe YF, Vireque AA & Baruselli PS 2010 Ovum pick up and in vitro embryo production during the summer: differences between holstein heifers, high producing hostein cows in peak lactation and repeat breeder Holstein cows. *Reproduction, Fertility and Development* **22** 290 (abstract).

Figueiredo RA, Barros CM, Pinheiro OL & Sole JMP 1997 Ovarian follicular dynamics in Nelore breed (*Bos indicus*) cattle. *Theriogenology* **47** 1489-1505.

Forni S & Albuquerque LG 2005 Estimates of genetic correlations between days to calving and reproductive and weight traits in Nelore cattle. *Journal of Animal Science* **83** 1511-1515.

Fortune JE, Rivera GM, Evans AC & Turzillo AM 2001 Differentiation of dominant versus subordinate follicles in cattle. *Biology of Reproduction* **65** 648-654.

Gambini ALG, Moreira MBP, Castilho C & Barros CM 1998 Follicular development and sychronization of ovulation in Gir cows. *Revista Brasileira de Reprodução Animal* **22** 201-210.

Garverick HA, Baxter G, Gong J, Armstrong DG, Campbell BK, Gutierrez CG & Webb R 2002 Regulation of expression of ovarian mRNA encoding steroidogenic enzymes and gonadotrophin receptors by FSH and GH in hypogonadotrophic cattle. *Reproduction* **123** 651-661.

Gaughan JB, Mader TL, Holt S, Josey MJ & Rowan KJ 1999 Heat tolerance of Boran and Tuli crossbred steers. *Journal of Animal Science* **77** 2398-2405.

Gimenes LU, Fantinato Neto P, Arango JSP, Ayres H & Baruselli PS 2009 Follicular dynamics of *Bos indicus, Bos taurus and Bubalus bubalis* heifers treated with norgestomet ear implant associated or not to injectable progesterone. *Animal Reproduction* **6** 256.

Gimenes LU, Ferraz ML, Araújo, AB, Fantinato Neto P, Chiaratti MR, Mesquita LG, Arango JSP, Raposo M, Souza DC, Calomeni GD, Gardinal R, Rodriguez CLV, Trinca LA, Meirelles FV & Baruselli PS 2010 OPU at different times of a synchronized follicular wave did not affect IVP in Bos indicus, Bos taurus and Bubalus bubalis. *Reproduction, Fertility and Development* **22** 293.

Gimenes LU, Sá Filho MF, Carvalho NAT, Torres-Junior JRS, Souza AH, Madureira EH, Trinca LA, Sartorelli ES, Barros CM, Carvalho JBP, Mapletoft RJ & Baruselli PS 2008 Follicle deviation and ovulatory capacity in *Bos indicus* heifers. *Theriogenology* **69** 852-858.

Ginther OJ, Knopf L & Kastelic JP 1989 Temporal associations among ovarian events in cattle during oestrous cycles with two or three follicular waves. *Journal of Reproduction and Fertility* **87** 223-230.

Ginther OJ, Wiltbank MC, Fricke PM, Gibbons JR & Kot K 1996 Selection of the dominant follicle in cattle. *Biology of Reproduction* **55** 1187-1194.

Goodhand KL,Watt RG, Staines ME, Hutchinson JSM& Broadbent PJ 1999 In vivo oocyte recovery and in vitro embryo production from bovine oocyte donors aspirated at different frequencies or following FSH treatment. *Theriogenology* **51** 951-961.

Gromoll J, Eiholzer U, Nieschlag E & Simoni M 2000 Male hypogonadism caused by homozygous deletion of exon 10 of the luteinizing hormone (LH) receptor: differential action of human chorionic gonadotropin and LH. *Journal of Clinical Endocrinology & Metabolism* **85** 2281-2286.

Hammond AC, Olson TA, Chase Jr CC, Bowers EJ, Randel RD & Murphy CN 1996 Heat tolerance in two tropically adapted Bos taurus breeds, Senepol and Romosinuano, compared with Brahman, Angus, and Hereford cattle in Florida. *Journal of Animal Science* **74** 295-303.

Ireland JJ & Roche JF 1982 Development of antral follicles in cattle after prostaglandin-induced luteolysis: changes in serum hormones, steroids in follicular fluid, and gonadotropin receptors. *Endocrinology* **111** 2077-2086.

Kamwanja LA, Chase Jr CC, Gutierrez JA, Guerriero VJ, Olson TA & Hammond AC 1994 Responses of bovine lymphocytes to heat shock as modified by breed and antioxidant status. *Journal of Animal Science* **72** 438-744.

Kawate N 2004 Studies on the regulation of expression of luteinizing hormone receptor in the ovary and the mechanism of follicular cyst formation in ruminants. *Journal of Reproduction and Development* **50** 1-8.

Kojima N, Stumpf TT, Cupp AS, Werth LA, Roberson MS, Wolfe MW, Kittok RJ, & Kinder JE 1992. Progestins and exogenous progesterone do not mimic the corpus luteum in regulation in LH and 17b-estradiol in circulation of cows. *Biology of. Reprodution* **47** 1009.

Landaeta-Hernández AJ, Palomares-Naveda R, Soto-Castillo G, Atencio A, Chase Jr CC & Chenoweth PJ 2004 Social and breed effects on the expression of a PGF2α induced oestrus in beef cows. *Reproduction in Domestic Animals* **39** 315-320.

Lopez-Gatius F 2003 Is fertility declining in dairy cattle? A retrospective study in northeastern Spain. *Theriogenology* **60** 89-99.

Lopez H, Satter LD & Wiltbank MC 2004 Relationship between level of milk production and estrous behavior of lactating dairy cows. *Animal Reproduction Science* **81** 209-223.

Macmillan KL & Burke CR 1996 Effects of oestrus cycle control on reproductive efficiency. *Animal Reproduction Science* **42** 307-320.

Macmillan KL & Peterson AJ 1993 A new intravaginal progesterone releasing device for cattle (CIDR-B) for oestrus synchronisation, increasing pregnancy rates and the treatment of postpartum anoestrus. *Animal Reproduction Science* **33** 1-25.

Malayer JR & Hansen PJ 1990 Differences between Brahman and Holstein cows in heat-shock induced alterations of protein synthesis and secretion by oviducts and uterine endometrium. *Journal of Animal Science* **68** 266-280.

Martin LC, Brinks JS, Bourdon RM & Cundiff LV 1992 Genetic effects on beef heifer puberty and subsequent reproduction. *Journal of Animal Science* **70** 4006-4017.

Martins CM, Castricini ESC, Reis EL, Torres-Júnior JRS, Gimenes LU, Sa Filho MF & Baruselli PS 2005 Produção embrionária de vacas holandesas a diferentes protocolos de superovulação com inseminação em tempo fixo. *Acta Scientiae Veterinariae* **33** 286 (abstract).

Membrive CMB 2000 *Estudo da sincronização das ondas foliculares e das características de estros, por radiotelemetria, em novilhas cruzadas (Bos indicus x Bos taurus) tratadas com acetato de melengestrol e prostaglandina associados a hCG, GnRH ou 17b estradiol + progesterona.* São Paulo, 2000. 156p. Dissertação (Mestrado) – Faculdade de Medicina Veterinária e Zootecnia, Universidade de São Paulo, São Paulo.

Mizuta K 2003 *Estudo comparativo dos aspectos comportamentais do estro e dos teores plasmáticos de LH, FSH, progesterona e estradiol que precedem a ovulação em fêmeas bovinas Nelore (Bos taurus indicus), Angus (Bos taurus taurus) e Nelore x Angus (Bos taurus indicus x Bos taurus taurus).* São Paulo, 2003. 98 p. Tese (Doutorado) – Faculdade de Medicina Veterinária e Zootecnia, Universidade de São Paulo, São Paulo.

Mollo MR, Rumpf R, Martins AC, Mattos MCC, Lopes Jr, G, Carrijo LHD & Sartori R 2007 Ovarian function in Nelore heifers under low or high feed intake. *Acta Scientiae Veterinariae* **35** 958 (abstract).

Monteiro F, Ferreira M, Potiens J, Eberhardt B, Trinca L & Barros C 2009 Influence of superovulatory protocols on in vitro production of Nellore (Bos indicus) embryos. *Reproduction of Domestic Animals* Apr 1 [Epub ahead of print].

Muller T, Gromoll J & Simoni M 2003 Absence of exon 10 of the human luteinizing hormone (LH) receptor impairs LH, but not human chorionic gonadotropin action. *Journal of Clinical Endocrinology & Metabolism.* **88** 2242-2249.

National Research Council 2000 Nutrient requeriments of beef cattle. 7 rev. ed., update 2000. Washington: National Academy Press 232p.

Negussie B, Brannang E & Rottmann OJ 1999 Reproductive performance and herd life of dairy cattle at Asella livestock farm, Arsi, Ethiopia. II. Crossbreds with 50, 75 and 87.5% European inheritance. *Journal of Animal Breeding and Genetics* **116** 225-234.

Nogueira GP 2004 Puberty in south american *Bos indicus* (Zebu) cattle. *Animal Reproduction Science* **82** 361-372.

Nogueira MFG, Barros BJP, Teixeira AB, Trinca LA, D'Occhio MJ & Barros CM 2002 Embryo recovery and pregnancy rates after the delay of ovulation and fixed time insemination in superstimulated beef cows. *Theriogenology* **57** 1625-1634.

Nogueira MFG & Barros CM 2003 Timing of ovulation in Nelore cows superestimulated with P36 protocol. *Acta Scientiae Veterinariae* **31** 509 (abstract).

Nogueira MFG, Buratini J, Jr., Price CA, Castilho AC, Pinto MG & Barros CM 2007a Expression of LH receptor mRNA splice variants in bovine granulosa cells: changes with follicle size and regulation by FSH in vitro. *Molecular Reproduction & Development* **74** 680-686.

Nogueira MFG, Fragnito PS, Trinca LA & Barros CM 2007b The effect of type of vaginal insert and dose of pLH on embryo production, following fixed-time AI in a progestin-based superstimulatory protocol in Nelore cattle. *Theriogenology* **67** 655-660.

Paschal JC, Sanders JO & Kerr JL 1991 Calving and weaning characteristics of Angus-, Gray Brahman-, Gir-, Indu-Brazil-, Nellore-, and Red Brahman-sired F1 calves. *Journal of Animal Science* **69** 2395-2402.

Pegorer MF, Vasconcelos JLM, Trinca LA, Hansen PJ & Barros CM 2007 Influence of sire and sire breed (Gyr versus Holstein) on establishment of pregnancy and embryonic loss in lactating Holstein cows during summer heat stress. *Theriogenology* **67** 692-697.

Pereira E, Oliveira HN, Eler JP, Silva JA II de V & Van Melis MH 2007 Comparison among three approaches for evaluation of sexual precocity in Nellore cattle. *Animal* **1** 411-418.

Pierson RA & Ginther OJ 1984 Ultrasonography of the bovine ovary. *Theriogenology* **21** 495-504.

Pinheiro OL, Barros CM, Figueredo RA, Valle ER, Encarnação RO & Padovani CR 1998 Estrous behaviour and the estrus-to-ovulation interval in Nelore cattle (*Bos indicus*) with natural estrus or estrus induced with prostaglandin F2α or norgestomet and estradiol valerate. *Theriogenology* **49** 667-681.

Pontes JHF, Silva KCF, Basso AC, Ferreira CR, Santos GMG, Sanches BV, Porcionato JPF, Vieira PHS, Sterza FAM & Seneda MM 2010 Comparison of oocyte and embryo production among *Bos taurus, Bos indicus* and *indicus-taurus* donor cows. *Reproduction, Fertility and Development* **22** 248.

Rae DO, Chenoweth PJ, Giangreco MA, Dixon PW & Bennet FL 1999 Assessment of estrus detection by visual observation and electronic detection methods and characterization of factors associated with estrus and pregnancy in beef heifers. *Theriogenology* **51** 1121-1132.

Randel RD 1976 LH and ovulation in Brahman, Brahman x Hereford and Hereford heifers. *Journal of Animal Science* **43** 300.

Randel RD 1984 Seasonal effects on female reproductive functions in the bovine (Indian breeds). *Theriogenology* **21** 70-85.

Rawlings NC, Evans ACO, Honaramooz A & Bartlewski PM 2003 Antral follicle growth and endocrine changes in prepubertal cattle, sheep and goats. *Animal Reproduction Science* **78** 259-270.

Rhodes FM, De'ath G & Entwistle KW 1995 Animal and temporal effects on ovarian follicular dynamics in Brahman heifers. *Animal Reproduction Science* **38** 265-277.

Robert C, Gagne D, Lussier JG, Bousquet D, Barnes FL & Sirard MA 2003 Presence of LH receptor mRNA in granulosa cells as a potential marker of oocyte developmental competence and characterization of the bovine splicing isoforms. *Reproduction* **125** 437-446.

Rocha A, Randel RD, Broussard JR, Lim JM, Blai RM, Roussel JD, Godke RA & Hansel W 1998 High environmental temperature and humidity decrease oocyte quality in Bos taurus but not in Bos indicus cows. *Theriogenology* **49** 657-665.

Rodrigues CA, Ayres H, Nichi M, Bo GA & Baruselli PS 2004 Artificial insemination and embryo transfer pregnancy rates in high production Holstein breeding under tropical conditions. In 'Proceedings of the 15th International Congress of Animal Reproduction' (Eds P. K. Basrur, P. J. Broadbent, M. Henry and L. E. Pinheiro.) 396 (Elsevier: Porto Seguro, Brazil.) (abstract).

Rodrigues CA, Mancilha RF, Reis EL, Ayres H, Gimenes LU & Sá Filho MF 2005 Efeito do número de implantes de norgestomet e do momento da administração do indutor de ovulação em vacas holandesas superovuladas (abstract). *Acta Scientiae Veterinariae* **33** 229.

Rodrigues HD, Kinder JE & Fitzpatrick LA 2002 Estradiol regulation of luteinizing hormone secretion in heifers of two breed types that reach puberty at different ages. *Biology of Reproduction* **66** 603-609.

Sá Filho MF, Gimenes LU, Ayres H, Carvalho NAT, Carvalho JB & Baruselli PS 2005 Dinâmica folicular de novilhas Bos indicus tratadas com implante auricular de norgestomet ou com dispositivo intravaginal de progesterona. *Acta Scientiae Veterinariae* **33** 266 (abstract).

Sales JNS, Iguma LT, Batista RITP, Gama MAS, Camargo LSA, Gimenes LU, Marques MG, Simões R, Fernandes CB, Viana JHM & Baruselli PS 2010 Effect of different energy levels diet on oocyte quantity and quality of non lactating cows (Bos indicus and Bos taurus) submitted to ovum pick-up. *Acta Scientiae Veterinariae* (Abstract in press).

Sangsritavong S, Combs DK, Sartori R, Armentano LE & Wiltbank MC 2002 High feed intake increases liver blood flow and metabolism of progesterone and estradiol 17 beta in dairy cattle. *Journal of Dairy Science* **85** 2831-2842.

Sartorelli ES, Carvalho LM, Bergfelt DR, Ginther OJ & Barros CM 2005 Morphological characterization of follicle deviation in Nelore (*Bos indicus*) heifers and cows. *Theriogenology* **63** 2382-2394.

Sartorelli ES, Satrapa RA, Barcelos ACZ, Potiens JR & Barros CM 2006 Influence of heat stress on apoptosis rate of in vitro produced bovine embryos (indicus vs taurus) and in their capacity to originate pregnancies. *Acta Scientiae Veterinariae* **34** 474 (abstract).

Sartori R, Fricke PM, Ferreira JC, Ginther OJ & Wiltbank MC 2001 Follicular deviation and acquisition of ovulatory capacity in bovine follicles. *Biology of Reproduction* **65** 1403-1409.

Sartori R, Guardieiro MM, Barros CM, Bastos MR, Machado GM, Leme LO & Rumpf R 2009 Lack of improvement on embryo production by the replacement of the last two doses of pFSH by eCG in superestimulated Nelore heifers. *Reproduction Fertility and Development* **21** 245 (abstract).

Sartori R, Gumen A, Guenther JN, Souza AH, Caraviello D & Wiltbank MC 2006 Comparison of artificial insemination versus embryo transfer in lactating dairy cows. *Theriogenology* **65** 1311-1321.

Sartori R, Haughian JM, Shaver RD, Rosa GJM & Wiltbank MC 2004 Comparison of ovarian function and circulating steroids in estrous cycles of Holstein heifers and lactating cows. *Journal of Dairy Science* **87** 905-920.

Sartori R, Rosa GJM & Wiltbank MC 2002 Ovarian structures and circulating steroids in heifers and lactating cows in summer and lactating and dry cows in winter. *Journal of Dairy Science* **85** 2813-2822.

Savio JD, Boland MP & Roche JF 1990 Development of dominant follicles and length of ovarian cycles in post-partum dairy cows. *Journal of Reproduction and Fertility* **88** 581-591.

Savio JD, Keenan L, Boland MP & Roche JF 1988 Pattern of growth of dominant follicles during the oestrous cycle of heifers. *Journal of Reproduction and Fertility* **83** 663-671.

Segerson EC, Hansen TR, Libby DW, Randel RD & Getz WR 1984 Ovarian and uterine morphology and function in Angus and Brahman cows. *Journal of Animal Science* **59** 1026-1046.

Seneda MM, Blaschi W, Andrade ER, Nonato I, Pontes JHF, Ereno JC & Uvo S 2004 Use of Pluset before follicular aspiration (OPU). Impact on in vitro embryo production in Bos indicus cows. *Acta Scientiae Veterinariae* **2** 186 (abstract).

Seneda MM, Esper CR, Garcia JM, Oliveira JA & Vantini R 2001 Relationship between follicle size and ultrasound-guided transvaginal oocyte recovery. *Animal Reproduction Science* **67** 37-43.

Simões RAL 2009 Determinação da taxa de ovulação e sua correlação com diâmetro folicular e isoformas de RNAm para receptor de LH, em vacas da raça Nelore. Botucatu, 2009. 86 p. Dissertação (Mestrado) - Universidade Estadual Paulista Júlio de Mesquita Filho, Botucatu.

Sirois J & Fortune JE 1988 Ovarian follicular dynamics during the estrous cycle in heifers monitored by real-time ultrasonography. *Biology of Reproduction* **39** 308-317.

Torres-Júnior JRS, Pires MFA, de Sá WF, Ferreira AM, Viana JHM, Camargo LSA, Ramos AA, Folhadella IM, Polisseni J, Freitas C, Clemente CAA, Sá Filho MF, Paula-Lopes FF & Baruselli PS 2008 Effect of maternal heat-stress on follicular growth and oocyte competence in Bos indicus cattle. *Theriogenology* **69** 155-166.

Townson DH, Tsang PCW, Butler WR, Frajblat M, Griel Jr LC, Johnson CJ, Milvae RA, Niksic GM & Pate JL 2002 Relationship of fertility to ovarian follicular waves before breeding in dairy cows. *Journal of Animal Science* **80** 1053-1058.

Viana JHM & Camargo LSA 2007 Bovine embryo production in Brazil: A new scenario. *Acta Scientiae Veterinariae* **35** 920-924.

Viana JHM, Ferreira AM, Sá WF & Camargo LSA 2000 Follicular dynamics in zebu cattle. *Pesquisa Agropecuária Brasileira* **35** 2501-2509.

Webb R & England BG 1982 Identification of the ovulatory follicle in the ewe: associated changes in follicular size, thecal and granulosa cell luteinizing hormone receptors, antral fluid steroids, and circulating hormones during the preovulatory period. *Endocrinology* **110** 873-881.

Willians GL, Gazal OS, Guzmán Vega GA & Stanko RL 1996 Mechanisms regulating suckling-mediated anovulation in the cow. *Animal Reproduction Science* **42** 289-297.

Wiltbank MC, Lopez H, Sartori R, Sangsritavong S & Gümen A 2006 Changes in reproductive physiology of lactating dairy cows due to elevated steroid metabolism. *Theriogenology* **65** 17-29.

Wolfenson D, Inbara G, Rotha Z, Kaimb M, Blocha A & Braw-Tal R 2004 Follicular dynamics and concentrations of steroids and gonadotropins in lactating cows and nulliparous heifers. *Theriogenology* **62** 1042-1055.

Wolfenson D, Roth Z & Meidan R 2000 Impaired reproduction in heat stressed cattle: basic and applied aspects. *Animal Reproduction Science* **60-61** 535-547.

Xu Z, Garverick HA, Smith GW, Smith MF, Hamilton SA & Youngquist RS 1995 Expression of follicle-stimulating hormone and luteinizing hormone receptor messenger ribonucleic acids in bovine follicles during the first follicular wave. *Biology of Reproduction* **53** 951-957.

Zanenga CA, Pedrosa MF, Lima GF, Marques MO, Santos ICC, Valentim R & Baruselli PS 2003 Comparison between two superovulation protocols associated with FTAI, in Nelore cows (*Bos taurus indicus) Acta Scientiae Veterinariae* **31** 626-627 (abstract).

Zeitoun MM, Rodriguez HF, Randel RD 1996 Effect of season on ovarian follicular dynamics in Brahman cows. *Theriogenology* **45** 1577-1581.

Using basic approaches to address applied problems in dairy reproduction

P Lonergan

School of Agriculture, Food Science and Veterinary Medicine, College of Life Sciences, University College Dublin, Belfield, Dublin 4, Ireland

Poor reproductive efficiency is a worldwide problem affecting the dairy industry. There is substantial evidence for an association between high milk production and lower conception rates observed in cows compared to heifers. However, whether the decline in fertility is due directly to the level of milk production or other factors associated with lactation is unclear. There are various checkpoints along the developmental axis which could, in part, contribute to reduced fertility including suboptimal follicle development associated with poor oestrus exhibition, suboptimal oocyte quality, altered sperm transport and fertilization and/or a suboptimal reproductive tract environment incapable of supporting normal embryo development. The challenge is deciphering where the major problems lie. Evidence for the relative contributions of oocyte quality, embryo quality and the reproductive tract environment is discussed in this paper.

Introduction and context

Poor reproductive efficiency is a worldwide problem affecting the dairy industry and has been the subject of numerous excellent reviews (e.g., Lucy 2001, Inskeep & Dailey 2005, Leroy *et al.* 2008a,b, Inskeep & Dailey 2010). While in some locations this situation is exacerbated by problems of heat stress during summer (Hansen 2007), even in more moderate climates a steady decline in fertility has been noted. There is substantial evidence for an association between high milk production and the lower conception rate observed in cows (25-40%) compared to heifers (60-75%) (Sreenan & Diskin 1986, Pursley *et al.* 1997, Lucy 2001, Diskin & Morris 2008). However, whether the decline in fertility is due directly to the level of milk production or other factors associated with lactation is unclear (Chebel *et al.* 2008).

Infertility in dairy cattle is a multifactorial problem which may be linked to various checkpoints along the developmental axis including suboptimal follicle development associated with poor oestrus exhibition, suboptimal oocyte quality, altered sperm transport and fertilization and/or a suboptimal reproductive tract environment incapable of supporting normal embryo development. One of the obstacles to achieving a better understanding of the causes of poor fertility is the difficulty in separating these various issues from each other. For example, while the proportion of pregnancies after AI declined in past 50 years, there has been little change in the average number of oocytes/embryos and transferable embryos produced in embryo transfer (ET) programmes in USA/Canada; furthermore, there has been little change in the proportion of animals that become pregnant following ET over a period of approximately 30 years (Hasler 2006).

Corresponding author E-mail: pat.lonergan@ucd.ie

Approaches to understanding embryo mortality – when does the problem occur?

One approach to identifying at which stage along the developmental axis problems arise has been to inseminate animals and either recover embryos at given stages after insemination to determine fertilization failure and timing of embryonic mortality, or to continually monitor pregnancy to pinpoint the period of embryonic loss. Published data indicate fertilisation rates of 90% and average calving rates of about 55% are normal for heifers and moderate yielding dairy cows, indicating an embryonic and foetal mortality rate of about 35% (Sreenan & Diskin 1986, Diskin *et al.* 2006, Diskin & Morris 2008). Relatively few embryos are thought to be lost between fertilization and Day 8 of gestation (corresponding to the blastocyst stage); 70-80% of the total embryonic loss is estimated to occur between Days 8 and 16 after insemination (corresponding to the day of maternal recognition of pregnancy in cattle); a further 10% between days 16 and 42, by which time implantation is complete, and further 5-8% between day 42 and term.

Dunne *et al.* (2000) reported that embryo survival rates in beef heifers on Days 14, 30 and at full-term were similar (68%, 76%, 72%, respectively), indicating that most embryo loss, at least in beef heifers, occurs before Day 14. Silke *et al.* (2002) reported embryonic loss of 6-7% between Day 28 and 84 of gestation in dairy cows and heifers. Starbuck *et al.* (2004) reported embryonic loss of about 11% between Day 30-60 and related this loss to concentration of progesterone at week 5 of gestation, twin ovulation, body condition, age and sire. Both of these studies provide evidence for a relatively low incidence of late embryonic loss.

The sparse data from flushed early embryos from normally ovulating (i.e., non-superovulated), high-yielding lactating dairy cows indicate that fertilization rate is also high (83%, 610/732 in review by Sartori *et al.* 2010), but few studies have directly compared lactating and nonlactating dairy cows. In the study of Sartori *et al.* (2002), comparing lactating and nonlactating (either nulliparous heifers or dry cows) Holstein cattle, fertilization was only reduced during summer in lactating dairy cows; however, lactating dairy cows had poorer embryo development than nonlactating females, irrespective of season. This last observation is interesting as it suggests that the ability of the reproductive tract to support normal embryo development may be impaired in lactating cows. However, oocyte quality cannot be ruled out as a contributing factor, as it is clear from IVF studies, where typically 80% of inseminated oocytes cleave and 30-40% develop to blastocysts, that fertilization success is no guarantee of future development (Lonergan 2007).

Sartori *et al.* (2010) reviewed data on fertilisation and embryo quality up to Day 7 post AI in single-ovulating and superovulated dairy cows. The authors concluded that fertilisation was not the primary factor reducing viable embryo yield in embryos recovered from non-heat stressed single-ovulating, lactating dairy cows. In contrast, fertilisation failure appeared to be a major cause of reduced embryo yield in superovulated lactating (57%, n=8938) and non-lactating (50%, n=16039) dairy cows (Sartori *et al.* 2010). Summarising recent data (Wiebold 1988, Ryan *et al.* 1993, Sartori *et al.* 2002, Cerri *et al.* 2009a,b,c) the authors concluded that <50% of ova and/or embryos recovered from high-yielding dairy cows are viable 7 days after AI (Sartori *et al.* 2010).

Chebel *et al.* (2008) evaluated factors affecting success of on-farm ET programmes in large dairy herds. Non-lactating dairy cows had a greater response to superovulation, yielded a greater proportion of ova/embryos, an increased number of fertilized oocytes and an increased number of viable embryos compared to lactating dairy cows.

Isolating follicle/oocyte issues – the argument for a guilty oocyte

Following parturition, in association with peak milk yield, high yielding dairy cows enter a variable period of negative energy balance where the energy expenditure for peak milk production is not matched by the energy derived from dry matter intake. During this period of energy deficit, fats are mobilized from endogenous stores resulting in, among other things, increased non esterified fatty acids in circulation and in follicular fluid which has been associated with poor oocyte quality (Leroy *et al.* 2005).

One way of experimentally separating potential issues surrounding the follicle and/or oocyte from issues relating to the reproductive tract environment is to use transvaginal ovum-pick up coupled with IVF. Differences in development seen in this scenario would by definition not be related to post-ovulation issues, i.e., the reproductive tract, but rather reflect the intrinsic quality of the oocyte. While several authors have reported development of ovum-pick up/IVF embryos in dairy cows, e.g., Fouladi-Nashta *et al.* (2007), few have compared development from lactating dairy cows and non-lactating cows or heifers. In one study from our group (Rizos *et al.* 2005) there was no difference in the proportion of good quality oocytes undergoing fertilization and development to the blastocyst stage between lactating cows and heifers. Snjiders *et al.* (2000) found that a lower proportion of oocytes recovered from dairy cows with a higher genetic merit for milk production underwent cleavage or developed to the blastocyst stage in vitro than those from cows of average genetic merit.

Using ovum-pick up and assessment of oocyte morphology, several studies from Virginia (Kendrick *et al.* 1999, Gwazdauskas *et al.* 2000, Walters *et al.* 2002) have demonstrated that conditions related to early lactation have a negative effect on oocyte quality and endocrine measures in dairy cattle. For example, Kenderick *et al* (1999) conducted OPU twice weekly between Day 30 and 100 of lactation and reported that a low energy diet reduced milk yield, BCS and serum P4 and had a negative impact on oocyte quality.

Isolating embryo/reproductive tract issues – the argument for a guilty embryo/reproductive tract

A series of studies from our laboratory and others involving culture of zygotes in vitro or in vivo from the zygote to blastocyst stage have shown that postfertilization culture conditions do not significantly alter the proportion of in vitro derived bovine zygotes developing to the blastocyst stage but can significantly affect the quality of these embryos (Enright *et al.* 2000, Rizos *et al.* 2002, Lonergan *et al.* 2003). Thus, to a large extent, the quality of the oocyte (which will of course itself be affected by the follicular environment in which it develops) dictates its own developmental fate. This is not to say that an excellent quality oocyte can overcome a deleterious uterine environment.

The use of ET technology allows the endogenous oocyte of the cow to be removed as a confounding factor in understanding the cause of infertility and thus bypasses the events of follicle development and oocyte quality, as well as the potential negative effects of lactation associated metabolic stress on these processes. Several studies from Florida have compared ET with AI in order to overcome poor conception rate of lactating dairy cows due to heat stress (Putney *et al.* 1989, Ambrose *et al.* 1999, Drost *et al.* 1999, Al-Katanani *et al.* 2002; reviewed by Rutledge 2001), the notion being that transferring embryos to recipients at a stage when they are less susceptible to heat stress (i.e., on Day 7) may enhance pregnancy rates during periods of heat stress when the cow's endogenous oocyte would be susceptible. In all of these studies, conception rate was higher for ET than AI when fresh or frozen in vivo produced embryos were used; transfer of frozen (Ambrose *et al.* 1999, Drost *et al.* 1999) or vitrified (Al-Katanani *et al.* 2002) IVF embryos had no advantage over AI. Consistent with this, Vasconcelos *et al.* (2006) examined the factors affecting pregnancy rate after ET of in vivo derived fresh embryos to lactating dairy cow recipients. Pregnancy rate, corrected for cows with a CL, were 36.5% (84/230) vs 58.7% (91/155) on Day 25 and 33% (76/230) vs 45.8% (71/155) on Day 46 for AI and ET, respectively. Furthermore, Demetrio *et al.* (2007) reported higher conception rates in lactating Brazilian dairy cows following the transfer of a fresh embryo derived from nonlactating cows compared to after AI. In contrast, Sartori *et al.* (2006) compared ET with AI in dairy cows in Wisconsin at cooler times of the year and found no difference in conception rate. Taken together, these data would suggest that the oocyte is more susceptible to adverse conditions imposed by heat stress and perhaps negative energy balance than the embryo.

Routine ET, such as described above, involves the placement of an embryo, typically on Day 7, into the uterine horn, thus bypassing the oviduct. Up until relatively recently, the oviduct was inaccessible without resorting to major surgery. The recent refinement of endoscopy techniques to allow access to the oviducts of cattle have greatly facilitated the study of early embryo development (Havlicek *et al.* 2005, Wetscher *et al.* 2005, Besenfelder *et al.* 2008). Now it is possible to transfer large numbers of in vitro produced embryos to the oviducts to study development in vivo as well as recovering embryos at specific early stages of development. In studies on beef heifers where 50 – 100 embryos have been transferred to the oviduct ipsilateral to the CL (Tesfaye *et al.* 2007), recovery rates have been in the order of 80%; blastocyst yields have been in the order of 40-50%, in line with what is expected from in vitro derived zygotes.

Until recently, this model of multiple ET had not been attempted in the postpartum dairy cow. We hypothesized that part of the difference in fertility between heifers and post partum lactating dairy cows could be explained by differences in the ability of the reproductive tract (oviduct and uterus) to support early embryo development and that this would be related to circulating progesterone concentration. Testing this hypothesis in single-ovulating animals would be extremely challenging due to the numbers of animals required. Therefore, using endoscopy, we transferred 1800 in vitro produced embryos to the oviducts of nulliparous Holstein-Friesian heifers and post partum lactating Holstein-Friesian cows and assessed their development to the blastocyst stage following recovery on Day 7 (Rizos *et al.* 2010). Recovery rate was lower from cows (57%) compared to heifers (79%) and of the structures recovered only 18% had developed to the blastocyst stage in cows compared to 34% in heifers, providing evidence for an impairment in the ability of the reproductive tract of the post partum cow to support embryo development.

Hasler (2006) reviewed data on embryo production following superovulation in Holstein cattle and subsequent pregnancy rates following fresh ET into Holstein cows and heifers over a 20-25 year period to determine whether the documented decline in fertility of dairy cows has been accompanied by a corresponding decline in the efficacy of superovulation and ET. Little change was reported in either the mean number of transferable embryos resulting from superovulation (which could be interpreted as a proxy for oocyte quality) or in the proportion of recipient animals that became pregnant following ET, although heifers had a higher pregnancy rate than lactating cows. This would suggest that as milk yield has increased over the past several decades, the uterine capacity to support a pregnancy has not changed dramatically and would point to oocyte quality as a significant factor in the decline in dairy cow fertility. Consistent with this, Sartori *et al.* (2002) compared embryo quality on Day 5 from normally ovulating lactating vs nonlactating dairy cows; although fertilization rate was similar (88-90%) the proportion of viable embryos was much lower in lactating cows (53%) than in non-lactating cows (82%).

The ability to separate the contribution of the embryo and the recipient to embryonic survival up to Day 60 of pregnancy has been developed in a model by McMillan (1998) which suggests that variation in recipient quality rather than embryo quality is a major source of variation in pregnancy rates after ET. Based on pregnancy rates after repeated ET, two herds were established ('high' and 'low' pregnancy); significantly more embryos were elongated at Day 14 in the high herd (67%) than the low herd (14%) and this delay was still apparent by Day 17, encompassing the critical window of maternal recognition of pregnancy. Based on subsequent experiments they concluded that the difference in fertility was due to significantly more interferon-tau being secreted by the conceptus acting on a uterus with a reduced capacity to secret prostaglandin, perhaps enabling a wider window for maternal pregnancy recognition.

Isolating embryo/reproductive tract issues – the argument for a guilty reproductive tract and the role of progesterone

The steroid hormone progesterone plays a key role in the reproductive events associated with pregnancy establishment and maintenance. High concentrations of circulating progesterone in the immediate post-conception period have been associated with an advancement of conceptus elongation, an associated increase in interferon-tau production and higher pregnancy rates in cattle (Mann & Lamming 1999, Mann & Lamming 2001, Stronge *et al.* 2005, McNeill *et al.* 2006, Carter *et al.* 2008, Forde *et al.* 2009) and sheep (Ashworth *et al.* 1989, Satterfield *et al.* 2006).

The effects of elevated progesterone shortly after conception on the advancement of conceptus elongation have been convincingly demonstrated in cattle and sheep. Garrett *et al.* (1988) administered 100 mg progesterone on Days 1, 2, 3 and 4 of pregnancy which resulted in an increased peripheral plasma progesterone concentration on Days 2 to 5 and significantly larger conceptuses on Day 14. Using a progesterone implant on Day 3 of pregnancy, Carter *et al.* (2008) significantly elevated progesterone concentrations until Day 8 and this was associated with a larger conceptus recovered at slaughter on Day 16. Similarly, when ewes received daily injections of 25 mg progesterone from 36 h postmating, blastocyst diameter increased by 220% on Day 9 and the time of elongation of blastocysts to a filamentous conceptus on Day 12 was advanced (Satterfield *et al.* 2006); these effects of progesterone treatment on blastocyst development were blocked by administration of RU486, a progesterone receptor antagonist.

From the above, it is clear that the concentration of circulating progesterone has an effect on the developing embryo. This effect is likely as a result of downstream effects of progesterone-induced changes in gene expression in the tissues of the uterus (Bauersachs *et al.* 2006, Satterfield *et al.* 2006, Forde *et al.* 2009) resulting in changes in the composition of histroph to which the developing embryo is exposed. The importance of histotroph for conceptus development was demonstrated in the uterine gland knockout (UGKO) model in sheep in which embryos fail to develop beyond the blastocyst stage in adult UGKO ewes (Spencer *et al.* 2007).

In a series of recent experiments using in vitro and in vivo models we addressed the issue of whether the effects of progesterone on conceptus elongation could be due, at least in part, to a direct effect of progesterone on the embryo (Clemente *et al.* 2009). Progesterone receptor mRNA was present at all stages of embryo development raising the possibility of a direct effect of progesterone on the embryo. Exposure to progesterone in vitro in the absence or presence of oviduct epithelial cells did not affect the proportion of embryos developing to the blastocyst stage, blastocyst cell number or the relative abundance of selected transcripts in the blastocyst. Furthermore, exposure to progesterone in vitro did not affect post-hatching elongation of the embryo following transfer to synchronised recipients and recovery on Day 14. In contrast, transfer of in vitro derived blastocysts to a uterine environment previously primed by elevated progesterone resulted in a 4-fold increase in conceptus length on Day 14. These data provide clear evidence to support the hypothesis that progesterone-induced changes in the uterine environment are responsible for the advancement in conceptus elongation reported previously in cattle and that, interestingly, the embryo does not need to be present during the period of high progesterone in order to exhibit advanced elongation. This is consistent with the fact that administration of progesterone early in the oestrous cycle can advance uterine receptivity for the transfer of older asynchronous embryos (Geisert *et al.* 1991).

Most of these bovine data on the role of progesterone have been generated in nonlactating beef heifers; for example, there are few if any published reports of endometrial gene expression in the lactating dairy cows despite evidence for suboptimal progesterone concentrations in such animals and evidence for increased progesterone metabolism in the liver (Sangsritavong *et al.* 2002). The critical involvement of oestradiol and progesterone in almost every aspect of reproductive physiology makes changes in steroid metabolism an attractive explanation for the numerous changes in reproduction in lactating dairy cows. Similar data on endometrial function in the dairy cow would aid our understanding of factors associated with embryonic mortality.

A number of treatments can be used to increase peripheral concentrations of progesterone after AI including those that increase endogenous function of the existing CL, induce accessory CL, or supplement progesterone directly (see reviews by Lamb *et al.* 2010, Binelli *et al.* 2001, Inskeep 2004). However, data on outcome in terms of pregnancy rate are often conflicting and may reflect timing of treatment as well as the fact that only a proportion of animals with inherently low progesterone may benefit from such treatment. Stevenson *et al.* (2007) assessed effects of a variety of interventions after AI on fertility including administration of GnRH, hCG or an intravaginal progesterone-releasing device (CIDR). GnRH and hCG effectively induced ovulation and increased CL number but only increased circulating progesterone concentrations in hCG-treated cows. Treatment with a CIDR or hCG increased conception rate but only in some herds.

So, is it all down to the endometrium?: maternal-embryonic cross-talk

The ability to transfer an in vitro derived embryo (i.e., one developed in the absence of any contact with the female reproductive tract) to a synchronized recipient and obtain acceptable pregnancy rates would suggest that the embryo is somewhat autonomous for at least the first week of life and that direct contact with the maternal reproductive tract is, to a certain extent, unnecessary.

In support of this, when we compared the transcriptome of the endometrium in pregnant and cyclic heifers on various days from oestrus (Day 5, 7, 13 and 16) we could only detect differentially expressed genes in the endometrium on Day 16, coincident with a filamentous embryo secreting large amount of interferon-tau (Forde *et al.* 2010). This would suggest that the cow, or more specifically her uterus, is always an optimist regarding likelihood of pregnancy i.e., that the temporal changes occurring in the endometrium are similar in pregnant and cyclic cows up the point when luteolysis normally occurs.

The origin of embryo (e.g., in vivo derived following superovulation *vs* in vitro produced following IVF *vs* nuclear transfer) can have a significant impact on the dynamics of embryo mortality. Heyman *et al.* (2002) monitored the evolution of pregnancy following the transfer of embryos derived from somatic cell cloning, embryonic cloning and IVF in order to detect the occurrence of late gestation losses and their frequency. On the basis of progesterone concentrations on Day 21, there were no significant differences in the percentages of initiated pregnancies between the groups (55.6-62.7%). Confirmed pregnancy rate by Day 35 using ultrasound scanning was significantly lower in the two somatic cloned groups (27.5-33.8%) compared with the embryonic clones (49.2%) and IVF embryos (52.9%). This pattern was maintained at Days 50, 70 and 90. The incidence of loss between Day 90 of gestation and calving was 43.7% for adult somatic clones and 33.3% for foetal somatic clones compared with 4.3% after embryonic cloning and 0% after IVF.

Two recent key papers provide strong evidence that the endometrium of the cow reacts differently to different embryo types (Bauersachs *et al.* 2009, Mansouri-Attia *et al.* 2009); in other words, embryos of different quality (i.e., with divergent developmental fates) signal differently to the endometrium and in turn elicit a different response in terms of the transcriptome of the endometrium. In this way, the endometrium can be considered as a biological sensor able to fine-tune its physiology in response to the presence of embryos whose development will become altered much later after the implantation process (Mansouri-Attia *et al.* 2009).

Conclusion

Many factors are likely to impact on the success or otherwise of pregnancy. It is clear that maternal factors (e.g., oocyte quality, reproductive tract environment) can have a strong influence on the likelihood of embryo survival. However, the inherent quality of the embryo can also affect the likelihood of it undergoing early embryonic mortality, for example, by failing to elicit the correct response from the endometrium to ensure an optimal environment.

Acknowledgements

The author's work is supported by Science Foundation Ireland (07/SRC/B1156).

References

Al-Katanani YM, Drost M, Monson RL, Rutledge JJ, Krininger CE, 3rd, Block J, Thatcher WW & Hansen PJ 2002 Pregnancy rates following timed embryo transfer with fresh or vitrified in vitro produced embryos in lactating dairy cows under heat stress conditions. *Theriogenology* **58** 171-182.

Ambrose JD, Drost M, Monson RL, Rutledge JJ, Leibfried-Rutledge ML, Thatcher MJ, Kassa T, Binelli M, Hansen PJ, Chenoweth PJ & Thatcher WW 1999 Efficacy of timed embryo transfer with fresh and frozen in vitro produced embryos to increase pregnancy rates in heat-stressed dairy cattle. *J Dairy Sci* **82** 2369-2376.

Ashworth CJ, Sales DI & Wilmut I 1989 Evidence of an association between the survival of embryos and the periovulatory plasma progesterone concentration in the ewe. *J Reprod Fertil* **87** 23-32.

Bauersachs S, Ulbrich SE, Gross K, Schmidt SE, Meyer HH, Wenigerkind H, Vermehren M, Sinowatz F, Blum H & Wolf E 2006 Embryo-induced transcriptome changes in bovine endometrium reveal species-specific and common molecular markers of uterine receptivity. *Reproduction* **132** 319-331.

Bauersachs S, Ulbrich SE, Zakhartchenko V, Minten M, Reichenbach M, Reichenbach HD, Blum H, Spencer TE & Wolf E 2009 The endometrium responds differently to cloned versus fertilized embryos. *Proc Natl Acad Sci U S A* **106** 5681-5686.

Besenfelder U, Havlicek V, Moesslacher G, Gilles M, Tesfaye D, Griese J, Hoelker M, Hyttel PM, Laurincik J, Brem G & Schellander K 2008 Endoscopic recovery of early preimplantation bovine embryos: effect of hormonal stimulation, embryo kinetics and repeated collection. *Reprod Domest Anim* **43** 566-572.

Binelli M, Thatcher WW, Mattos R & Baruselli PS 2001 Antiluteolytic strategies to improve fertility in cattle. *Theriogenology* **56** 1451-1463.

Carter F, Forde N, Duffy P, Wade M, Fair T, Crowe MA, Evans AC, Kenny DA, Roche JF & Lonergan P 2008 Effect of increasing progesterone concentration from Day 3 of pregnancy on subsequent embryo survival and development in beef heifers. *Reprod Fertil Dev* **20** 368-375.

Cerri RL, Juchem SO, Chebel RC, Rutigliano HM, Bruno RG, Galvao KN, Thatcher WW & Santos JE 2009a Effect of fat source differing in fatty acid profile on metabolic parameters, fertilization, and embryo quality in high-producing dairy cows. *J Dairy Sci* **92** 1520-1531.

Cerri RL, Rutigliano HM, Chebel RC & Santos JE 2009b Period of dominance of the ovulatory follicle influences embryo quality in lactating dairy cows. *Reproduction* **137** 813-823.

Cerri RL, Rutigliano HM, Lima FS, Araujo DB & Santos JE 2009c Effect of source of supplemental selenium on uterine health and embryo quality in high-producing dairy cows. *Theriogenology* **71** 1127-1137.

Chebel RC, Demetrio DG & Metzger J 2008 Factors affecting success of embryo collection and transfer in large dairy herds. *Theriogenology* **69** 98-106.

Clemente M, de La Fuente J, Fair T, Al Naib A, Gutierrez-Adan A, Roche JF, Rizos D & Lonergan P 2009 Progesterone and conceptus elongation in cattle: a direct effect on the embryo or an indirect effect via the endometrium? *Reproduction* **138** 507-517.

Demetrio DG, Santos RM, Demetrio CG & Vasconcelos JL 2007 Factors affecting conception rates following artificial insemination or embryo transfer in lactating Holstein cows. *J Dairy Sci* **90** 5073-5082.

Diskin MG & Morris DG 2008 Embryonic and early foetal losses in cattle and other ruminants. *Reprod Domest Anim* **43 Suppl 2** 260-267.

Diskin MG, Murphy JJ & Sreenan JM 2006 Embryo survival in dairy cows managed under pastoral conditions. *Animal Reproduction Science* **96** 297-311.

Drost M, Ambrose JD, Thatcher MJ, Cantrell CK, Wolfsdorf KE, Hasler JF & Thatcher WW 1999 Conception rates after artificial insemination or embryo transfer in lactating dairy cows during summer in Florida. *Theriogenology* **52** 1161-1167.

Dunne LD, Diskin MG & Sreenan JM 2000 Embryo and foetal loss in beef heifers between day 14 of gestation and full term. *Anim Reprod Sci* **58** 39-44.

Enright BP, Lonergan P, Dinnyes A, Fair T, Ward FA, Yang X & Boland MP 2000 Culture of in vitro produced bovine zygotes in vitro vs in vivo: implications for early embryo development and quality. *Theriogenology* **54** 659-673.

Forde N, Carter F, Fair T, Crowe MA, Evans ACO, Spencer TE, Bazer FW, McBride R, Boland MP, O'Gaora P, Lonergan P & Roche JF 2009 Progesterone-regulated changes in endometrial gene expression contribute to advanced conceptus development in cattle. *Biol Reprod* **81** 784-794.

Forde N, Carter F, Spencer TE, Bazer FW, McBride R, O'Gaora P, Roche JF & Lonergan P 2010 Temporal changes in endometrial gene expression in cattle in response to the presence of a conceptus: how soon does the cow know she is pregnant? *Biol Reprod* in press.

Fouladi-Nashta AA, Gutierrez CG, Gong JG, Garnsworthy PC & Webb R 2007 Impact of dietary fatty acids on oocyte quality and development in lactating dairy cows. *Biol Reprod* **77** 9-17.

Garrett JE, Geisert RD, Zavy MT & Morgan GL 1988 Evidence for maternal regulation of early conceptus growth and development in beef cattle. *J Reprod Fertil* **84** 437-446.

Geisert RD, Morgan GL, Zavy MT, Blair RM, Gries LK, Cox A & Yellin T 1991 Effect of asynchronous transfer and oestrogen administration on survival and development of porcine embryos. *J Reprod Fertil* **93** 475-481.

Gwazdauskas FC, Kendrick KW, Pryor AW & Bailey TL 2000 Impact of follicular aspiration on folliculogenesis as influenced by dietary energy and stage of lactation. *J Dairy Sci* **83** 1625-1634.

Hansen PJ 2007 Exploitation of genetic and physiological determinants of embryonic resistance to elevated temperature to improve embryonic survival in dairy cattle during heat stress. *Theriogenology* **68 Suppl 1** S242-249.

Hasler JF 2006 The Holstein cow in embryo transfer today as compared to 20 years ago. *Theriogenology* **65** 4-16.

Havlicek V, Wetscher F, Huber T, Brem G, Mueller M & Besenfelder U 2005 In vivo culture of IVM/IVF embryos in bovine oviducts by transvaginal endoscopy. *J Vet Med A Physiol Pathol Clin Med* **52** 94-98.

Heyman Y, Chavatte-Palmer P, LeBourhis D, Camous S, Vignon X & Renard JP 2002 Frequency and occurrence of late-gestation losses from cattle cloned embryos. *Biol Reprod* **66** 6-13.

Inskeep EK 2004 Preovulatory, postovulatory, and postmaternal recognition effects of concentrations of progesterone on embryonic survival in the cow. *J Anim Sci* **82 E-Suppl** E24-39.

Inskeep EK & Dailey RA 2005 Embryonic death in cattle. *Vet Clin North Am Food Anim Pract* **21** 437-461.

Inskeep EK & Dailey RA 2010 Maximizing embryonic and early foetal survival in dairy cattle. *WCDS Advances in Dairy Technology* **22** in press.

Kendrick KW, Bailey TL, Garst AS, Pryor AW, Ahmadzadeh A, Akers RM, Eyestone WE, Pearson RE & Gwazdauskas FC 1999 Effects of energy balance of hormones, ovarian activity, and recovered oocytes in lactating Holstein cows using transvaginal follicular aspiration. *J Dairy Sci* **82** 1731-1741.

Lamb GC, Dahlen CR, Larson JE, Marquezini G & Stevenson JS 2010 Control of the estrous cycle to improve fertility for fixed-time artificial insemination in beef cattle: a review. *J Anim Sci* **88** E181-192.

Leroy JL, Opsomer G, De Vliegher S, Vanholder T, Goossens L, Geldhof A, Bols PE, de Kruif A & Van Soom A 2005 Comparison of embryo quality in high-yielding dairy cows, in dairy heifers and in beef cows. *Theriogenology* **64** 2022-2036.

Leroy JL, Opsomer G, Van Soom A, Goovaerts IG & Bols PE 2008a Reduced fertility in high-yielding dairy cows: are the oocyte and embryo in danger? Part I. The importance of negative energy balance and altered corpus luteum function to the reduction of oocyte and embryo quality in high-yielding dairy cows. *Reprod Domest Anim* **43** 612-622.

Leroy JL, Van Soom A, Opsomer G, Goovaerts IG & Bols PE 2008b Reduced fertility in high-yielding dairy cows: are the oocyte and embryo in danger? Part II. Mechanisms linking nutrition and reduced oocyte and embryo quality in high-yielding dairy cows. *Reprod Domest Anim* **43** 623-632.

Lonergan P 2007 State-of-the-art embryo technologies in cattle. *Soc Reprod Fertil Suppl* **64** 315-325.

Lonergan P, Rizos D, Kanka J, Nemcova L, Mbaye AM, Kingston M, Wade M, Duffy P & Boland MP 2003 Temporal sensitivity of bovine embryos to culture environment after fertilization and the implications for blastocyst quality. *Reproduction* **126** 337-346.

Lucy MC 2001 Reproductive loss in high-producing dairy cattle: where will it end? *J Dairy Sci* **84** 1277-1293.

Mann GE & Lamming GE 1999 The influence of progesterone during early pregnancy in cattle. *Reproduction in Domestic Animals* **34** 269-274.

Mann GE & Lamming GE 2001 Relationship between maternal endocrine environment, early embryo development and inhibition of the luteolytic mechanism in cows. *Reproduction* **121** 175-180.

Mansouri-Attia N, Sandra O, Aubert J, Degrelle S, Everts RE, Giraud-Delville C, Heyman Y, Galio L, Hue I, Yang X, Tian XC, Lewin HA & Renard JP 2009 Endometrium as an early sensor of in vitro embryo manipulation technologies. *Proc Natl Acad Sci U S A* **106** 5687-5692.

McMillan WH 1998 Statistical models predicting embryo survival to term in cattle after embryo transfer. *Theriogenology* **50** 1053-1070.

McNeill RE, Diskin MG, Sreenan JM & Morris DG 2006 Associations between milk progesterone concentration on different days and with embryo survival during the early luteal phase in dairy cows. *Theriogenology* **65** 1435-1441.

Pursley JR, Wiltbank MC, Stevenson JS, Ottobre JS, Garverick HA & Anderson LL 1997 Pregnancy rates per artificial insemination for cows and heifers inseminated at a synchronized ovulation or synchronized estrus. *J Dairy Sci* **80** 295-300.

Putney DJ, Drost M & Thatcher WW 1989 Influence of summer heat stress on pregnancy rates of lactating dairy cattle following embryo transfer or artificial insemination. *Theriogenology* **31** 765-778.

Rizos D, Burke L, Duffy P, Wade M, Mee JF, O'Farrell KJ, MacSiurtain M, Boland MP & Lonergan P 2005 Comparisons between nulliparous heifers and cows as oocyte donors for embryo production in vitro. *Theriogenology* **63** 939-949.

Rizos D, Carter F, Besenfelder U, Havlicek V & Lonergan P 2010 Contribution of the female reproductive tract to low fertility in postpartum lactating dairy cows. *J Dairy Sci* **93** 1022-1029.

Rizos D, Ward F, Duffy P, Boland MP & Lonergan P 2002 Consequences of bovine oocyte maturation, fertilization or early embryo development in vitro versus in vivo: implications for blastocyst yield and blastocyst quality. *Mol Reprod Dev* **61** 234-248.

Rutledge JJ 2001 Use of embryo transfer and IVF to bypass effects of heat stress. *Theriogenology* **55** 105-111.

Ryan DP, Prichard JK, Kopel E, Godke RA 1993 Comparing earl;y embryo mortality in dairy cows during hot and cool seasons of the year. *Theriogenology* **39** 719-737.

Sangsritavong S, Combs DK, Sartori R, Armentano LE & Wiltbank MC 2002 High feed intake increases liver blood flow and metabolism of progesterone and estradiol-17beta in dairy cattle. *J Dairy Sci* **85** 2831-2842.

Sartori R, Bastos MR & Wiltbank MC 2010 Factors affecting fertilisation and early embryo quality in single- and superovulated dairy cattle. *Reprod Fertil Dev* **22** 151-158.

Sartori R, Gumen A, Guenther JN, Souza AH, Caraviello DZ & Wiltbank MC 2006 Comparison of artificial insemination versus embryo transfer in lactating dairy cows. *Theriogenology* **65** 1311-1321.

Sartori R, Sartor-Bergfelt R, Mertens SA, Guenther JN, Parrish JJ & Wiltbank MC 2002 Fertilization and early embryonic development in heifers and lactating cows in summer and lactating and dry cows in winter. *J Dairy Sci* **85** 2803-2812.

Satterfield MC, Bazer FW & Spencer TE 2006 Progesterone regulation of preimplantation conceptus growth and galectin 15 (LGALS15) in the ovine uterus. *Biol Reprod* **75** 289-296.

Silke V, Diskin MG, Kenny DA, Boland MP, Dillon P, Mee JF & Sreenan JM 2002 Extent, pattern and factors associated with late embryonic loss in dairy cows. *Anim Reprod Sci* **71** 1-12.

Snijders SE, Dillon P, O'Callaghan D & Boland MP 2000 Effect of genetic merit, milk yield, body condition and lactation number on in vitro oocyte development in dairy cows. *Theriogenology* **53** 981-989.

Spencer TE, Johnson GA, Bazer FW, Burghardt RC & Palmarini M 2007 Pregnancy recognition and conceptus implantation in domestic ruminants: roles of progesterone, interferons and endogenous retroviruses. *Reprod Fertil Dev* **19** 65-78.

Sreenan JM & Diskin MG 1986. The extent and timing of embryonic mortality in cattle. In *Embryonic mortality in farm animals*, pp. 142-158.

Starbuck MJ, Dailey RA & Inskeep EK 2004 Factors affecting retention of early pregnancy in dairy cattle. *Anim Reprod Sci* **84** 27-39.

Stevenson JS, Portaluppi MA, Tenhouse DE, Lloyd A, Eborn DR, Kacuba S & DeJarnette JM 2007 Interventions after artificial insemination: conception rates, pregnancy survival, and ovarian responses to gonadotropin-releasing hormone, human chorionic gonadotropin, and progesterone. *J Dairy Sci* **90** 331-340.

Stronge AJ, Sreenan JM, Diskin MG, Mee JF, Kenny DA & Morris DG 2005 Post-insemination milk progesterone concentration and embryo survival in dairy cows. *Theriogenology* **64** 1212-1224.

Tesfaye D, Lonergan P, Hoelker M, Rings F, Nganvongpanit K, Havlicek V, Besenfelder U, Jennen D, Tholen E & Schellander K 2007 Suppression of connexin 43 and E-cadherin transcripts in in vitro derived bovine embryos following culture in vitro or in vivo in the homologous bovine oviduct. *Mol Reprod Dev* **74** 978-988.

Vasconcelos JL, Demetrio DG, Santos RM, Chiari JR, Rodrigues CA & Sa Filho OG 2006 Factors potentially affecting fertility of lactating dairy cow recipients. *Theriogenology* **65** 192-200.

Walters AH, Pryor AW, Bailey TL, Pearson RE & Gwazdauskas FC 2002 Milk yield, energy balance, hormone, follicular and oocyte measures in early and mid-lactation Holstein cows. *Theriogenology* **57** 949-961.

Wetscher F, Havlicek V, Huber T, Muller M, Brem G & Besenfelder U 2005 Effect of morphological properties of transferred embryonic stages on tubal migration Implications for in vivo culture in the bovine oviduct. *Theriogenology* **64** 41-48.

Wiebold JL 1988 Embryonic mortality and the uterine environment in first-service lactating dairy cows. J Reprod Fertil **84** 393-399

Applying nutrition and physiology to improve reproduction in dairy cattle

JEP Santos, RS Bisinotto, ES Ribeiro, FS Lima, LF Greco, CR Staples and WW Thatcher

Department of Animal Sciences, University of Florida, Gainesville, FL 32611

The establishment and maintenance of pregnancy in lactating dairy cows is a complex biological event that is influenced by a multitude of factors, from the reproductive biology of the cow to managerial aspects of the dairy farm. It is often mentioned in the scientific literature that fertility in dairy cows has declined concurrent with major advances in milk production. Some of this decline is attributed to the negative genetic correlation between milk production and reproduction. In the United States, yearly production per cow has increased steadily at a rate of 1.3% in the last decade and it is likely that this trend will continue in the years to come. At this rate, the average cow in the United States will be producing over 14 tons of milk per year in 2050 and technologies will have to be developed to allow these cows to reproduce to maintain the sustainability of dairy production. Despite high production, it is not uncommon for dairy herds with rolling herd averages for milk yield above 11,000 kg to overcome the challenges of reproduction and obtain satisfactory reproductive performance. Among other things, those herds have been able to mitigate some of the mechanisms that suppress reproduction in dairy cows such as extended postpartum anovulatory period, poor estrous detection, low pregnancy per insemination and, to a lesser extent, the high pregnancy loss. The success of those farms comes from an integrated approach to fertility that includes adequate cow comfort, elaborated transition cow management and nutrition, aggressive postpartum health monitoring program with preventative and curative measures to mitigate the negative effects of diseases on reproduction, and a sound reproductive program that includes manipulation of the ovarian cycle to allow for increased insemination rate. More recently, introduction of fertility traits in selection programs have created new opportunities for improved reproduction without neglecting economically important production traits.

Introduction

Reproductive efficiency is a major component of economic success in dairy herds. The establishment of a pregnancy as well as the loss of pregnancy are extremely valuable particularly

Corresponding author E-mail: jepsantos@ufl.edu

because they determine milk production per day of calving interval and the risk of a cow to be removed from the herd (De Vries, 2006). Unfortunately, fertility in dairy cows involves extremely complex biological events that are influenced by a multitude of environmental and biological factors, as well as the genetic makeup of the dairy cow.

The physiological and environmental stresses faced by high-producing dairy cows under the current production systems compromise estrous detection and their ability to conceive and deliver a viable offspring. Some of the limitations to high fertility are related to the reproductive biology of the high-producing cow which, through homeorrhetic controls, has resulted in adaptations to the increased nutrient needs for milk synthesis and metabolic rate. Although reproduction is critical for perpetuation of the species, from the individual point of view, reproduction is considered an expendable process that has low priority under nutrient restrictions (Wade and Jones, 2004). Considering the nutrient requirements of a high-producing dairy cow which often consumes 4 to 6 times its maintenance needs, it is plausible to suggest that nutrient extraction by the ovaries and the early pregnant uterus is negligible. Nonetheless, signals from splanchnic and adipose tissues coordinate the release of gonadotropins and the support to resumption of ovulation and pregnancy, such that under periods of nutrient restriction, ovulation is impaired and establishment and maintenance of pregnancy compromised. Some of the many limitations to high fertility in dairy cows include: incidence of periparturient diseases, anovulation, reduced estrous behavior, and compromised embryo quality and development; managerial and environmental factors such as nutrition, comfort offered by facilities, and thermal stress; and genetics of the cow. Because of these factors and the complexity of reproduction, the solutions for improving fertility will include both short- and long-term components that address the biology of the cow as well as the environmental events and managerial procedures critical for successful reproduction. In spite of the link suggested between high-production and compromised fertility, it is unlikely that the rate of increase in milk yield per cow will diminish in the following years or decades. In fact, the ongoing trend for increasing milk production and the need for improvements in efficiency of use of resources with higher producing cows (Capper et al., 2009) will make the production of today's cow to be overshadowed by that of future generations. The intent of this manuscript is to present some of the current strategies to overcome poor reproduction in dairy herds.

The paradox of milk yield and fertility

Almost every article on dairy cattle fertility in the scientific literature mentions that the increment in milk production observed in the last 50 years, as consequence of genetic selection and improvements in nutrition and management, has coincided with a corresponding decline in fertility. Geneticists have demonstrated a negative genetic correlation between milk yield and fertility in dairy cattle (Roxström et al., 2001; Hansen et al., 1983), although some have also suggested that the low heritability of fertility traits precludes major antagonisms between selection for milk yield and reduction in reproduction (Hansen, 2000). Because environmental factors and lactation have major impacts on the reproductive efficiency of dairy herds, it is likely that the negative associations between the genetics for production traits and fertility are only observed after the onset of lactation and the consequent shifts in nutrient partition to favor the mammary gland (Bauman and Currie, 1980).

The genetic potential for milk production today for the dairy cow was established in 1998 when LA-Foster Blackstar Lucy 607 completed a 365-day lactation producing 34,144 kg of milk, more than 750 kg of fat, and almost 980 kg of protein (Holstein World, 1999). This was Lucy's fifth lactation at the age of 6 years and 3 months, thereby indicating that this phenomenal cow was able to reproduce on a yearly basis in spite of the massive production of milk. Lucy's production at peak was 116 kg/d, which is the equivalent to 2.5 to 3 times the peak production of the average high-producing Holstein cow today. It is obvious that, today, Lucy is an aberration of the population, but it is also clear that the right genetic selection and environment can result in tremendous production. In fact, studies conducted at the University of Minnesota with a control and a selected line of Holstein cows for milk yield starting in 1964 clearly demonstrated the marked increase in milk yield in 1998 for an entire lactation (10,959 vs. 6,454 kg/year; Hansen, 2000). The selected line of cows has not experienced a depression in fertility, although health traits have been compromised (Hansen et al., 2000).

The rationale for increased production

The major reason for emphasis on production traits is because most of the cash receipts of a dairy farm come from sales of milk, and only a minor portion results from sales of animals, even those destined for dairy production. Using data 2000 to 2007 from two dairy farms with 1,500 cows, each with an annualized mortality of lactating cows of 5.3%/year and an average milk yield of 12,400 kg/cow/year, approximately 88% of the cash receipts were obtained through the sales of milk, 9.1% from sales of prepartum or early lactation cows for dairy purposes, 2.4% from sales of cows destined to slaughter, and only 0.4% from sales of newborn male calves. Historical facts and conventional wisdom maintain that growth and consolidation resulting in large family-owned farms seem to be the present and future of the dairy industry in the United States (LaDue et al., 2003) and other leading dairy countries. In fact, the number of dairy farms with fewer than 100 cows will decline by 92% between 2000 and 2020 (LaDue et al., 2003). This consolidation poses new challenges for reproduction; one of them is the ratio of cows/personnel, thereby resulting in less individual attention and a more group-basis approach for health and reproduction activities. This consolidation is concurrent with the steady increase in the yearly milk production per cow in the United States (Fig. 1). Assuming the same increase in yearly milk yield per cow of 1.3% and the projections for population growth in the United States from the United States Census Bureau (http://www.census.gov/population/www/), it will be possible to reduce the dairy cow population by 11.1% in the next 40 years and still maintain the same milk availability per capita of approximately 270 kg/year.

In addition to the economic component, adoption of technology and modernization of dairy practices to enhance production have substantially reduced the resources needed to produce milk. Capper et al. (2009) estimated that a farm in the US today produces the same amount of milk with 21% of the animals, 23% of the feedstuffs, and 10% of the land required in 1944. Greater milk production per cow dilutes the needs for maintenance and the trend for increased milk per cow will likely continue given the need to sustain a growing population with no additional use of land and other natural resources.

Genotype and fertility

It is no question that genotype and environment need to be matched to optimize production and fertility (Macdonald et al., 2008). Cows with greater potential for production but with restricted nutrient intake suffer greater body weight losses (Macdonald et al., 2008), which depresses fertility (Santos et al., 2009). In fact, cows of greater genetic potential subjected to grazing conditions had reduced pregnancy at the end of the breeding period (Macdonald et al., 2008). It was later demonstrated that cows selected for higher milk production suffered uncoupling of the somatotropic axis characterized by reduced expression of growth hormone (GH)

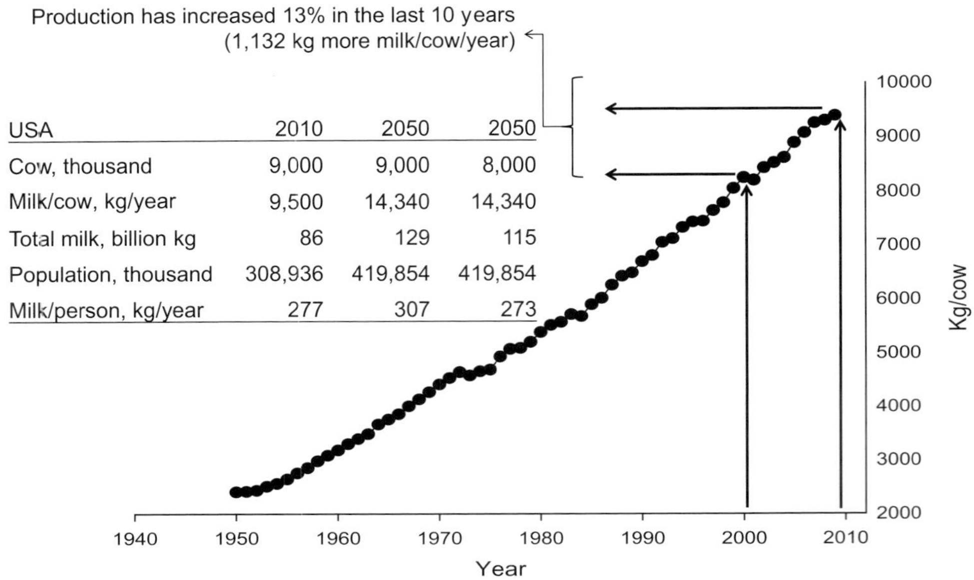

Fig. 1. Continuous increase in the yearly milk production per cow in the United States from 1950 to 2009 and projected production and milk availability per person based on the steady increase of 1.3%/year and the current (2010) and expected population in 2050. It is projected that the average cow in the United States will produce 14,340 kg/year in 2050, which will allow for a reduction in the dairy cow population from 9 to 8 million and still maintain the same per capita milk availability. Information compiled from the population division of the United States Census Bureau and from the United States Department of Agriculture.

receptor in the liver (Lucy et al., 2009). Re-coupling of the GH and insulin-like growth factor-1 (IGF-1) system has a pivotal role to reestablish follicular steroidogenesis and the ovulatory process in dairy cows, which might be related to fertility. As feed intake increases and energy balance improves, the concentrations of insulin in plasma increase because of the greater flux of propionate and synthesis of glucose by the liver, and the increments in plasma insulin and energy balance seem to be some of the signals to reestablish the GH receptor population in the liver of dairy cows (Butler et al., 2003). This re-couples the somatotropic axis and results in substantial increases in plasma concentrations of IGF-1 and in the steroidogenic capacity of ovarian follicles (Butler et al., 2004).

Because selective partition of nutrients favoring the mammary gland can have major implications to the energy reserves of dairy cows and impact future fertility, one could conclude that an obvious solution is to suppress milk yield; however, little of the variation in energy balance of cows is determined by the amount of energy secreted in milk and a much greater proportion is determined by energy intake (**Fig. 2**). Therefore, selecting for less milk yield with no changes in nutrient intake is unlikely to be the most productive method to improve energy status of early lactation dairy cows. Completely abolishing the dry period resulted in a dramatic decline in milk yield in the subsequent lactation with minor effects on nutrient intake (Rastani et al., 2005). Cows devoid of a dry period produced substantially less milk (5.7 to 9 kg/day) than their counterparts with a 28 or 56-day dry period (Rastani et al., 2005). Interestingly, continuous milking resulted in cows undergoing negligible negative energy balance in early lactation and they experienced early postpartum ovulation (Gümen et al., 2005). It is unlikely that such measures will be adopted by dairy producers in an attempt to improve reproduction considering the substantial losses of production. A more reasonable alternative is to develop markers that identify cows that consume more feed in the first weeks of lactation and determine whether this might have a genetic link. It has been suggested that energy balance in early lactation has a genetic component (Friggens et al. 2007); therefore, it might be a possible to select sires of daughters that undergo less exacerbated negative nutrient balance but, at the same time, maintain high production.

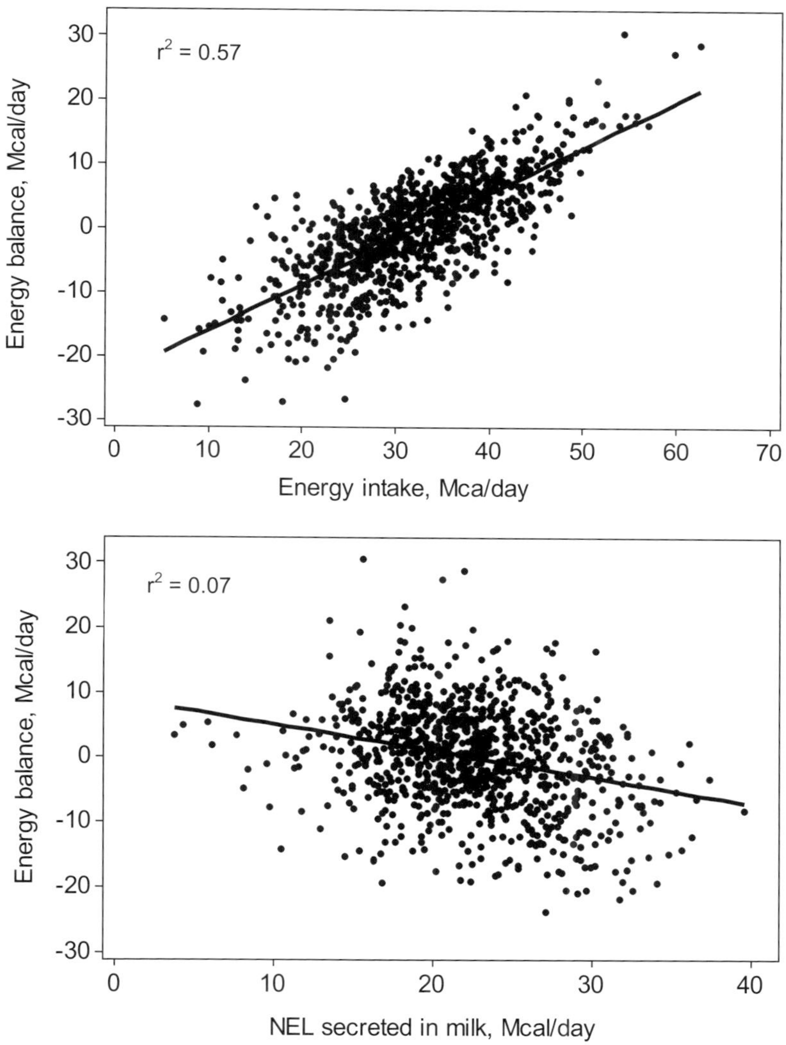

Fig. 2. Regression of energy balance (Mcal/day of net energy for lactation, NEL) and net energy intake (Mcal/day) or NEL secreted in milk in a group of 136 Holstein cows in the first 6 weeks postpartum. Adjusted coefficients of determination (r^2) with energy balance were 0.57 and 0.07 for energy intake and energy secretion in milk, respectively.

Selecting for improved fertility without compromising production

One of the topics often discussed is the possibility of selecting cows for improved fertility at the same time that lactation performance is not compromised. Although heritability values for fertility and some health traits are generally low, there is surprisingly large genetic variation in these traits that allow for selection of cattle (Weigel and Rekaya, 2000). In fact, since the adoption of productive life in the selection program in the United States in the 90's, breeding value of daughters compiled by the Animal Improvement Programs Laboratory of the United States Department of Agriculture has no longer declined and has shown some signs of improvement in the last decade.

Because of the interest for selection of cattle for fertility traits, a fertility index designated as daughter pregnancy rate (DPR) was developed (VanRaden et al., 2004) and incorporated in the selection program in February of 2003 in the United States. This index is derived from days open, which to no surprise has low heritability, approximately 0.04. The calculation is based on the formula: pregnancy rate = 21/(days open - voluntary waiting period + 11), of which 21 represents the length of the estrous cycle in which a cow has the opportunity to become pregnant, days open is the interval between calving and pregnancy, the voluntary waiting period is a determined value of 60 days, and 11 is the midpoint of 21 days for the length of the estrous cycle. The standard 60-day voluntary waiting period has been prone to criticism because this parameter varies widely between and within farms (Chang et al., 2007), and a delay in the eligibility to first insemination would compromise predictions of DPR. Recently, Chang et al. (2007) evaluated 44,901 lactation records to study the number of 21-day opportunity periods required to achieve pregnancy. The duration of the voluntary waiting period ranged from 28 to 74 days and, despite this variability, the predicted transmitting ability (PTA) of the sires using a voluntary waiting period either fixed at 60 days or according to the farm value resulted in very high correlation (0.98), although some sires were ranked differently according to the model used. The same study observed that the daughters of sires with greater PTA for DPR, as computed by the Animal Improvement Programs Laboratory, required fewer 21-day periods to become pregnant (Chang et al., 2007). The relationship between PTA values of DPR and days open is not linear (VanRaden et al., 2004), but most cow populations become pregnant on average after two to five 21-day breeding opportunities. Within that range, the relationship becomes linear, and each point in DPR represents a change in 4 days open (VanRaden et al., 2004).

Data from 626 Holstein bulls that are proven sires included in the active AI list were collected from the August 2010 summaries from the database of the Animal Improvement Programs Laboratory (http://www.aipl.arsusda.gov). Predicted transmitting ability values for production traits, net merit, and DPR were merged with data for bull fertility based on sire conception rate. Simple regression analysis of data from these 626 bulls indicate a weak negative relationship (r^2 = 0.09) between milk yield and DPR. On the other hand, if selection is based on net merit, which takes into account productive, health and reproductive traits, then the relationship became positive with better prediction (**Fig. 3**, panel A). Part of that is because 11% of the value of net merit is attributed to DPR.

Of the 626 Holstein bulls, 382 had data on sire conception rate. No relationship was observed between sire conception rate and DPR; in other words, the fertility of the sire had no relationship with the fertility of its daughters (**Fig. 3**, panel B). Nevertheless, when sires were categorized as low ($\leq$ 1) or high ($>$ 1) sire conception rate, a total of 213 of the 382 bulls were classified as high fertility. There was still a wide variety of bulls to select from with high sire conception rate that resulted in considerable positive PTAs for both net merit and DPR (**Fig. 3**, panel C). The changes in DPR are substantial considering that the range for most of the Holstein sire population goes from -3 to +3, a 6 percentage point value that represents a spread of 24 days open. These data indicate that selection for productive traits such as yield of fat and protein does not need to be accomplished at the expense of current and future fertility of the dairy herd.

Health, body condition, and fertility in dairy cows

Although major emphasis has been given to high milk yield as a potential suppressor of fertility in dairy cows, little or no association has been observed between milk production in early lactation and the risk of anovulation, pregnancy, and pregnancy loss in high-producing dairy cows (Santos et al., 2009). However, a major issue facing dairy cows under intensive systems is the high incidence of health problems, particularly those that affect the reproductive tract and those of metabolic origin.

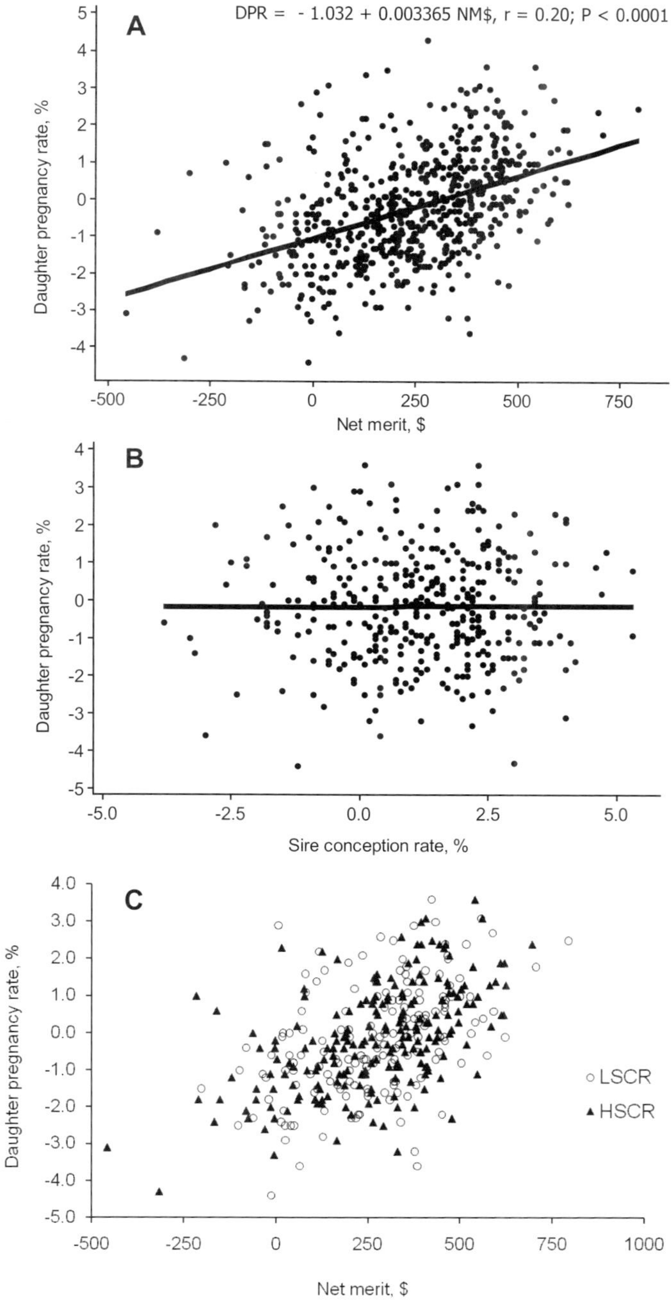

Fig. 3. Relationship between daughter pregnancy rate (DPR) and other selection traits in a population of Holstein bulls that are proven sires included in the active AI list from the august 2010 summaries from the database of the Animal Improvement Programs Laboratory (http://www.aipl.arsusda.gov/). Panel A indicates that selection for net merit results in daughters with better pregnancy rate. Panel B depicts no relationship between sire and daughter fertility. Panel C segregates bulls according to sire conception rate (SCR) as low (< 1; range, -3.8 to 1) or high (> 1; range, 1.1 to 5.3).

Data from 5,719 postpartum dairy cows evaluated daily for health disorders from eight experiments conducted by our group on seven dairy farms were compiled. All cows were evaluated for cyclicity at 65 days postpartum by sequential progesterone analyses in plasma 12 to 14 days apart. These cows were subjected to presynchronized timed AI programs using variations of the Ovsynch protocol. Of the 5,719 dairy cows evaluated, only 55.8% of them were considered healthy and did not develop clinical disease in the first 60 days postpartum. Incidence of diseases (calving related problems, 14.6%; metritis, 16.1%; clinical endometritis, 20.8%; fever, 21.0%; mastitis, 12.2%; ketosis, 10.4%; lameness, 6.8%; digestive problems, 2.8%; pneumonia, 2.0%) was high and 27.0% of the cows were diagnosed with a single disease event, whereas 17.2% had at least 2 disease events in the first 2 months of lactation. At this point, either the genetics of high production has lead to increased risk of health problems or producers have not been able to offer cows the proper preventative health program through nutrition, cow comfort, and general management to minimize the risk of diseases. It is likely that a mismatch between genotype and management conditions at the farm occur in many instances. Interestingly, the diagnosis of diseases in the first 60 days postpartum did not influence milk yield in that lactation, and the 305-day milk yields were 10,919, 11,041, and 10,858 kg for cows considered healthy, those with a single disease, and those with multiple diseases, respectively. In spite of the similar milk yield, cows diagnosed with health problems were less likely to be cyclic at 65 days postpartum (**Table 1**). Calving related disorders and those that affect the reproductive tract were the major contributors for depressed cyclicity.

Table 1. Impact of health problems in the first 60 d postpartum on resumption of estrous cyclicity by 65 d postpartum in dairy cows[1]

Health status	Cyclic, %	Adjusted OR (95% CI)[2]	P
Health problem			
Healthy	84.1	1.00	—
1 case of disease	80.0	0.97 (0.72 – 1.30)	0.83
> 1 case of disease	70.7	0.60 (0.44 – 0.82)	0.001
Type of health problem[3]			
Calving problem	70.5	0.52 (0.40 – 0.68)	< 0.001
Metritis	63.8	0.37 (0.28 – 0.50)	< 0.001
Clinical endometritis	68.9	0.51 (0.37 – 0.71)	< 0.001
Fever postpartum	80.0	0.55 (0.40 – 0.74)	< 0.001
Mastitis	81.5	0.87 (0.55 – 1.36)	0.53
Clinical ketosis	77.7	0.71 (0.47 – 1.07	0.10
Lameness	85.0	0.82 (0.52 – 1.30)	0.40
Pneumonia	88.9	1.78 (0.22 – 14.34)	0.59
Digestive problem	60.7	0.54 (0.25 – 1.17)	0.12

[1] 5,719 postpartum dairy cows evaluated daily for health disorders on seven dairy farms in the United States.
[2] OR = odds ratio; CI = confidence interval.
[3] Calving problem = includes dystocia, twin birth, stillbirth, and retained placenta, which was characterized by presence of fetal membranes 24 h after calving; Metritis = watery fetid uterine discharge in the first 14 days postpartum; Clinical endometritis = vaginal mucus score > 2 (> 10% pus in the mucus); Fever = rectal temperature > 39.5 °C in the first 14 days postpartum; Mastitis = presence of abnormal milk in one of the quarters; Clinical ketosis = lack of appetite and presence of ketonuria using test strips; Pneumonia = increased lung sounds and respiratory frequency concurrent with fever; Digestive problem = indigestion caused by displacement of abomasum, bloat or diarrhea.

Similar to the depression in cyclicity, diagnosis of health disorders in early lactation markedly reduced pregnancy at the first postpartum AI (**Table 2**), and increased the risk of pregnancy loss in the first 60 days of gestation (**Table 3**). On the contrary, healthy cows achieved very high fertility with 51.4% pregnancy per AI at first postpartum insemination (**Table 2**). These data indicate that reduction in morbidity by preventing periparturient diseases has the potential to enhance fertility of dairy cows by improving resumption of postpartum ovulation, increasing pregnancy per AI, and minimizing pregnancy loss.

Table 2. Impact of health problems in the first 60 d postpartum on pregnancy at first postpartum AI of dairy cows[1]

Health status	Pregnant, %	Adjusted OR (95% CI)[2]	*P*
Health problem			
Healthy	51.4	1.00	
1 case of disease	43.3	0.79 (0.69 – 0.91)	0.001
> 1 case of disease	34.7	0.57 (0.48 – 0.69)	< 0.001
Type of health problem[3]			
Calving problem	40.3	0.75 (0.63 – 0.88)	< 0.001
Metritis	37.8	0.66 (0.56 – 0.78)	< 0.001
Clinical endometritis	38.7	0.62 (0.52 – 0.74)	< 0.001
Fever postpartum	39.8	0.60 (0.48 – 0.65)	< 0.001
Mastitis	39.4	0.84 (0.64 – 1.10)	0.20
Clinical ketosis	28.8	0.50 (0.36 – 0.68)	< 0.001
Lameness	33.3	0.57 (0.41 – 0.78)	< 0.001
Pneumonia	32.4	0.63 (0.32 – 1.27)	0.20
Digestive problem	36.7	0.78 (0.46 – 1.34)	0.38

[1] 5,719 postpartum dairy cows evaluated daily for health disorders on seven dairy farms in the United States.
[2] OR = odds ratio; CI = confidence interval.
[3] Calving problem = includes dystocia, twin birth, stillbirth, and retained placenta, which was characterized by presence of fetal membranes 24 h after calving; Metritis = watery fetid uterine discharge in the first 14 days postpartum; Clinical endometritis = vaginal mucus score > 2 (> 10% pus in the mucus); Fever = rectal temperature > 39.5 °C in the first 14 days postpartum; Mastitis = presence of abnormal milk in one of the quarters; Clinical ketosis = lack of appetite and presence of ketonuria using test strips; Pneumonia = increased lung sounds and respiratory frequency concurrent with fever; Digestive problem = indigestion caused by displacement of abomasum, bloat or diarrhea.

One of the consequences of diseases is that cows have reduced appetite and oftentimes lose more body weight. Nutrient intake is the major driver of energy balance (**Fig. 2**), and energy balance is associated with fertility in dairy cows (Butler, 2003). In fact, cows that lost more body condition in the first 65 days postpartum were more likely to be anovular, had decreased pregnancy per AI, and increased risk of pregnancy loss (Santos et al., 2009). In addition, health disorders might have direct impacts on the reproductive tract, particularly uterine diseases and those that result in inflammatory responses such as mastitis and pneumonia. Therefore, it is critical that management of early lactation dairy cows include methods to minimize negative nutrient balance and excessive losses of body condition. Dairy form has a genetic correlation of -0.73 with body condition score (Dechow et al., 2004). Because of this negative genetic correlation, selection indexes now include a penalty for dairy form in an attempt to preserve body condition and improve fertility.

Table 3. Impact of health problems in the first 60 d postpartum on risk of pregnancy loss in the first 60 d of gestation in dairy cows[1]

Health status	Pregnancy loss, %	Adjusted OR (95% CI)[2]	P
Health problem			
Healthy	8.9	1.00	---
1 case of disease	13.9	1.73 (1.25 – 2.39)	< 0.001
> 1 case of disease	15.8	2.08 (1.36 – 3.17)	< 0.001
Type of health problem[3]			
Calving problem	15.9	1.67 (1.16 – 2.40)	< 0.01
Metritis	11.3	1.01 (0.71 – 1.60)	0.76
Clinical endometritis	15.1	1.55 (1.04 – 2.32)	0.03
Fever postpartum	18.0	2.00 (1.24 – 3.14)	< 0.01
Mastitis	19.8	2.62 (1.48 – 4.64)	< 0.001
Clinical ketosis	14.6	1.64 (0.75 – 3.59)	0.22
Lameness	26.4	2.67 (1.38 – 5.12)	< 0.01
Pneumonia	16.7	1.87 (0.40 – 8.69)	0.42
Digestive problem	15.8	1.81 (0.52 – 6.32)	0.35

[1] 5,719 postpartum dairy cows evaluated daily for health disorders on seven dairy farms in the United States.
[2] OR = odds ratio; CI = confidence interval.
[3] Calving problem = includes dystocia, twin birth, stillbirth, and retained placenta, which was characterized by presence of fetal membranes 24 h after calving; Metritis = watery fetid uterine discharge in the first 14 days postpartum; Clinical endometritis = vaginal mucus score > 2 (> 10% pus in the mucus); Fever = rectal temperature > 39.5 °C in the first 14 days postpartum; Mastitis = presence of abnormal milk in one of the quarters; Clinical ketosis = lack of appetite and presence of ketonuria using test strips; Pneumonia = increased lung sounds and respiratory frequency concurrent with fever; Digestive problem = indigestion caused by displacement of abomasum, bloat or diarrhea.

Optimization of reproductive programs as a platform to evaluate nutrition and health effects on fertility

Major advancements in manipulation of the estrous cycle have been achieved to optimize fertility of dairy cows subjected to synchronization of ovulation programs since the advent of the Ovsynch protocol in 1995. These programs were originally designed to improve insemination rate because of the challenges with estrous detection on dairy farms (Lopez et al., 2004); however, new knowledge of the reproductive biology of the dairy cow and the ability to manipulate follicle growth and luteal lifespan has created opportunities to optimize fertility at the same time that insemination is assured.

It is no surprise that adoption of timed AI programs for routine management of reproduction in dairy herds has been widespread, and benefits to reproductive efficiency also have translated into economic advantages to the producer. The average value of a pregnancy has been estimated at $278.00 for farms in the United States (de Vries, 2006). Under intensive systems, implementation of timed AI has been considered economically advantageous to treat anovular cows compared with methods based on detection of estrus (De Vries et al., 2006). When compared with a well-managed natural service breeding program, timed AI resulted in similar reproductive performance (Lima et al., 2009), but greater economic return (Lima et al., 2010). More recently, work from New Zealand in a grazing system clearly demonstrated the economic benefit of timed AI programs at the beginning of the breeding season in cyclic and anovular dairy cows (McDougall, 2010).

Optimizing timed AI programs

Optimizing these programs is important to the reproduction of dairy herds, but also to serve as a platform to test other concepts such as the impact of nutrition on embryo quality and pregnancy (Cerri et al., 2009a). Response to the Ovsynch protocol improves when cows ovulate to the first GnRH of the program and when a responsive CL is present at the $PGF_{2\alpha}$ treatment (Chebel et al., 2006; Moreira et al., 2001; Vasconcelos et al., 1999). These responses benefit pregnancy per AI (Chebel et al., 2006; El-Zarkouny et al., 2004; Moreira et al., 2001) in part because ovulation to the initial GnRH reduces the length of dominance and improves embryo quality (Cerri et al., 2009b). Furthermore, initiating the Ovsynch protocol in early diestrus minimizes the risk of spontaneous regression of the CL and ovulation before completion of the program (El-Zarkouny et al., 2004; Moreira et al., 2001; Vasconcelos et al., 1999). A common method to presynchronize the estrous cycle is the use of $PGF_{2\alpha}$ injections administered 14 days apart with the Ovsynch initiated 12 days later (Moreira et al., 2001; El-Zarkouny et al., 2004). Respecting the interval between presynchronization and initiation of Ovsynch is critical to optimizing ovulation to the initial GnRH treatment and pregnancy (Galvão et al., 2007).

The benefits of this program to fertility go beyond synchronization of the estrous cycle. A large proportion of dairy cows suffer from uterine diseases (Galvão et al., 2009), and intra-uterine antimicrobial therapy has been shown to improve reproduction of cows with endometritis (Leblanc et al., 2002). The issue of milk and tissue residue with antimicrobials is of concern particularly when 15 to 30% of the cows would need to be treated upon diagnosis of endometritis. When cows received routine $PGF_{2\alpha}$ treatments starting after 30 days postpartum, the use of intrauterine cephalosporin after 40 days postpartum had no benefit to uterine health, pregnancy at first AI, pregnancy loss, and the rate of pregnancy in the first 300 days postpartum (Galvão et al., 2009). Therefore, routine use $PGF_{2\alpha}$ helps eliminate uterine infections and inflammation, particularly in cows with a responsive CL, synchronizes estrus for insemination, and presynchronizes the estrous cycle to improve response to timed AI programs.

In many herds, the prevalence of anovular cows is high (Santos et al., 2009), and these cows unlikely benefit from presynchronization with $PGF_{2\alpha}$ (Moreira et al., 2001). A potentially more promising system to improve fertility of anovular cows is the use of GnRH for presynchronization such as in the double Ovsynch program, which has been shown to increase pregnancy per AI of primiparous cows (Souza et al., 2008), which are known to be more prone to anovulation (Santos et al., 2009).

Another aspect is the timing of induction of ovulation after luteolysis and subsequent interval to insemination in these programs. Brusveen et al. (2008) demonstrated that maintaining an interval of 16 hours between induction of ovulation and AI, when GnRH is given at 56 hours after luteolysis, optimized pregnancy per insemination in dairy cows. Finally, optimizing the length of ovulatory follicle dominance by reducing the interval between follicle recruitment and ovulation has been shown to benefit fertility (Santos et al., 2010).

The encouraging aspect of these optimized programs is that pregnancy per AI in high-producing cows is now above 40% and, in some cases, as high as 50%. Furthermore, these programs allow producers to optimize insemination rate with high fertility, which improves the overall pregnancy rate of the herd. Even when no estrous detection is used and cows are inseminated only after timed AI, overall pregnancy rate is high (Lima et al., 2010). These programs do not necessarily solve the underlying problems causing reduced fertility in lactating dairy cows, but they have offered producers an alternative to circumvent the changes in the reproductive biology of the high-producing dairy cow that seem to compromise reproductive performance. They also offer a platform with tightly controlled ovarian cycles to test nutritional interventions that might benefit fertility.

Incorporating nutritional programs to enhance fertility

The transition period from late gestation to early lactation is the most turbulent time in the life of a cow (Drackley, 1999). The endocrine and metabolic adaptations to lactation associated with the decline in feed intake in late gestation contribute to exacerbation in negative nutrient balance in early lactation. Concurrently, this same period is characterized by a high risk of diseases that oftentimes compromise fertility (**Tables 1-3**). From a biological and evolutionary point of view, it is logical that cows prioritize milk production to sustain their offspring rather than resumption of reproductive cycles to reestablish fertility. From a production point of view, both components milk yield and reproduction must be optimized to enhance sustainability of dairy farming. During periods of energy restriction, oxidizable fuels consumed in the diet are prioritized toward essential processes that sustain life (Wade and Jones, 2004). Homeorrhetic controls in early lactation assure that body tissue, primarily adipose stores, is mobilized in support of milk production (Bauman and Currie, 1980). Therefore, the early lactation cow, that is unable to consume enough energy-yielding nutrients to meet the needs of production and maintenance, will sustain high yields of milk components at the expense of body tissues. This poses a problem to reproduction, as energy status is linked with delayed ovulation (Butler, 2003). Energy deprivation reduces the frequency of LH pulses, thereby impairing follicle maturation and ovulation. Furthermore, undernutrition inhibits estrous behavior partly because of reduced estrogen receptor-alpha abundance in the brain (Hileman et al., 1999).

The most important component of energy balance is dry matter intake and not the changes in milk energy secretion (**Fig. 3**). In addition to the obvious influence of the environment, recent studies have proposed that energy balance of early lactation cows has a genetic component (Friggens et al. 2007). The challenge of manipulating energy balance is to understand the mechanisms that control appetite of cows in early lactation (Allen et al., 2009; Drackley, 1999). This becomes particularly important given the notion that glucogenic diets and those with greater energy density might favor resumption of postpartum ovulation in dairy cows (Garnsworthy et al., 2009). This is critical as these diets might suppress dry matter intake because of their effects on satiety (Allen et al., 2009).

Glucogenic diets

Diet composition can be manipulated in an attempt to influence ovarian recrudescence and restoration of fertility in dairy cows. The first postpartum ovulation in dairy cattle occurs approximately 2 weeks after the nadir of negative energy balance (Butler, 2003). Severe weight and body condition losses are associated with anovulation in dairy cattle (Santos et al., 2009), which compromises reproductive performance at first postpartum insemination. Perhaps the major underlying factor for delayed ovulation is the low LH pulsatility that compromises the development of the dominant follicle, its steroidogenesis, and acquisition of ovulatory capacity. Intense catabolism of adipose tissue and lack of adequate concentrations of metabolic cues might further compromise fertility because of potential implications to oocyte competence (Leroy et al., 2008).

Although some cows develop follicles to diameters compatible with those of ovulatory follicles during periods of extensive tissue catabolism, many lose their dominance and regress (Gümen et al., 2003). It is suggested that the re-coupling of the somatotropic axis has a pivotal role to reestablish follicular steroidogenesis and ovulation in dairy cows. Insulin seems to be one of the signals to reestablish the GH receptor population in the liver of cows (Butler et al., 2003), which re-couples the GH/IGF-1 axis causing substantial elevation in plasma IGF-1 and enhancement of the steroidogenic capacity of ovarian follicles (Butler et al., 2004).

Gong et al. (2002) demonstrated that diets rich in starch, also called glucogenic, increased the concentrations of insulin in early lactation and expedited first postpartum ovulation. Van Knegsel et al. (2007) substantiated the positive effects of a glucogenic diet to hasten recrudescence of first postpartum ovulation in dairy cows. Similarly, findings by Garnsworthy et al. (2009) suggested that a combination of a glucogenic diet before the first postpartum ovulation, followed by a diet enriched with lipids resulted in the best reproductive performance. These findings warrant further investigations with large number of cows to confirm that the benefits to first ovulation are also observed for pregnancy. Nevertheless, Garnsworthy et al. (2009) suggested that the benefits of glucogenic diets early in lactation might be detrimental during the breeding period because hyperinsulinemia might compromise oocyte quality and embryo development typically observed in heifers and nonlactating cows (Santos et al., 2008b). Whether this is also true for lactating cows with high nutrient needs remains to be demonstrated.

Caution is needed when excess of fermentable carbohydrates are fed because propionate is a known powerful hypophagic agent in ruminants (Allen et al., 2009). The net flux of propionate from the portal-drained viscera increases immediately after feed consumption (Benson et al., 2002), and propionate is thought to increase oxidative pathways in the hepatocytes that alter firing of the vagus nerve and influence appetite. Intake is determined by meal size (satiety) and inter-meal interval (hunger), and diets high in rapidly fermentable starch stimulate satiety and result in smaller meals (Allen et al., 2009). It is possible that the benefits of an altered diet formulation in the first few weeks postpartum in an attempt to stimulate early recrudescence of ovarian activity might be negated if at the expense of dry matter intake. Therefore, it is important that early lactation diets promote high energy intake, primarily from diets containing substrates that stimulate gluconeogenesis to enhance plasma glucose and insulin. Probably, the critical point is to ensure that every cow has access to feed and is capable of consuming the largest quantity of diet possible, at the same time that a disease prevention and treatment program is implemented to control and treat diseases that suppress appetite.

Supplementation with lipids

Feeding fat to dairy cattle has been shown to improve pregnancy per AI in some, but not all cases (Santos et al., 2008a), and this improvement is likely attributed to the non-caloric effects of certain fatty acids (de Veth et al., 2009; Santos et al., 2008a; Staples et al., 1998). One of the limitations to fatty acid feeding is the extensive rumen biohydrogenation of unsaturated fatty acids; however, even when fatty acids are biohydrogenated, the resulting *trans* fatty acids produced in the rumen might also benefit fertility (de Veth et al., 2009).

Feeding flaxseed, a source rich in linolenic acid (C18:3 n-3), reduced pregnancy loss in dairy cows (Ambrose et al., 2006). Juchem et al. (2010) demonstrated that cows fed a supplement rich in unsaturated fatty acids had 1.5 times greater odds to be pregnant compared with cows fed more saturated fatty acids. Feeding more unsaturated fatty acids increased fertilization and improved embryo quality (Cerri et al., 2009a). In fact, changes in the fatty acid composition of the follicular fluid during early lactation have been associated with alterations in oocyte competence in dairy cows (Leroy et al., 2008). Furthermore, when embryos were produced *in vivo* from super-stimulated dairy cows, those fed fat sources rich in polyunsaturated fatty acids produced more developed embryos (Thangavelu et al., 2007).

Some fatty acids have the ability to modulate the uterine secretion of $PGF_{2\alpha}$ (Staples et al., 1998), which has been proposed as an alternative to improve embryonic survival in cattle (Santos et al., 2008a; Staples et al., 1998). In 3 of 5 experiments described by Santos et al. (2008a), feeding n-3 fatty acids to lactating dairy cows reduced pregnancy losses. More recently, Silvestre et al. (2010a) demonstrated that sequential feeding of a fat supplement containing n-6 fatty acids during the transition period followed by feeding n-3 fatty acids during the breeding period maximized the cumulative proportion of pregnant cows after the first two postpartum inseminations (**Fig. 4**). It was suggested that during remodeling of tissues in early lactation, supplying more n-6 fatty acids might enhance immune response and favor tissue repair (Silvestre et al., 2010b), which can then favor reproduction (Juchem et al., 2010). On the other hand, during the breeding period, attenuating the immune system with n-3 fatty acids might benefit embryonic survival (Silvestre et al., 2010a; Santos et al., 2008a; Santos et al., 2008b). Collectively, these data suggest that feeding moderate amounts of supplemental fat to dairy cows generally improves fertility and responses are mediated by the supply of specific fatty acids for absorption.

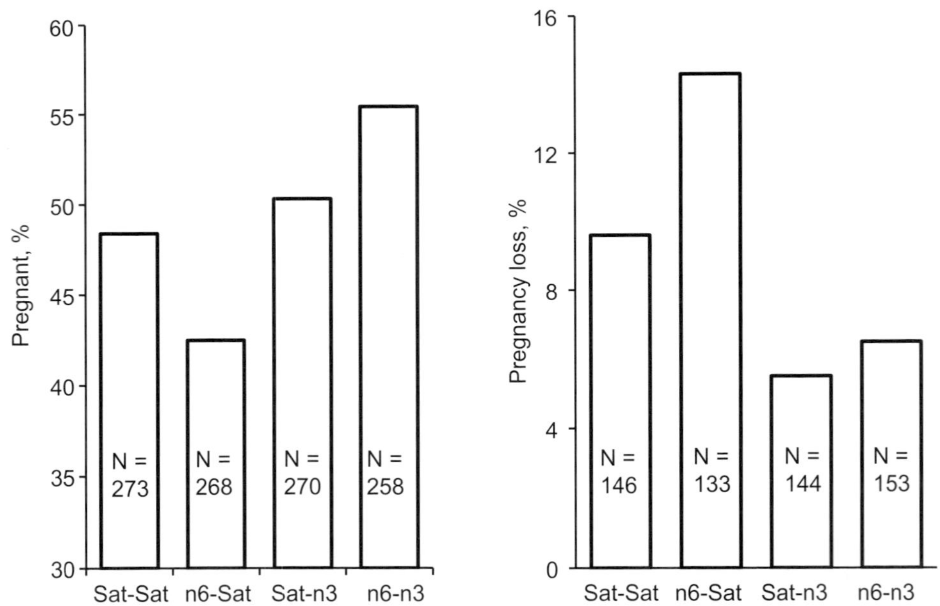

Fig. 4. Effect of feeding Ca salts of either mostly saturated (Sat), mostly omega 6 (n6) or mostly omega 3 (n3) fatty acids during the transition (-30 to 30 days postpartum) or the breeding periods (31 to 160 days postpartum) on pregnancy on day 60 after the first and second AI or pregnancy loss between 32 and 60 days of gestation. Treatments are depicted according to the sequence of fat fed during the transition and breeding periods. Cows fed n3 had greater 52.9 vs. 45.5%, $P < 0.01$ pregnancy per AI than those fed Sat primarily as a result of reduced 6.1 vs. 11.8%, $P < 0.01$ pregnancy loss (Silvestre et al., 2010a).

Conclusions

It is clear that good reproduction in dairy herds require a team approach to the issues facing the high-producing dairy cow. Increased production partitions more nutrients to the mammary gland, which results in less priority to expendable biological processes for the individual cow, one of them being reproduction. Tissue catabolism in early lactation has been implicated in the depression of fertility and it is no surprise that major losses in body weight, particularly body fat, compromise resumption of postpartum ovulation and pregnancy in dairy cows. These effects become even more pronounced following the occurrence of periparturient diseases. A holistic approach to fertility is needed and it is unlikely that a single strategy will solve reproductive problems in dairy herds. Immediate solutions have been developed and optimized to circumvent the challenges with low estrous expression and reduced insemination rates and these programs now allow for high pregnancy per insemination because of improved periovulatory reproductive events of follicle dominance, CL regression and ovulation. Because postpartum health has a dramatic impact on fertility of dairy cows, it is pivotal that nutrition and health programs be designed to minimize the risk and reduce the prevalence of periparturient diseases. Furthermore, specific nutrients targeted at defined periods of the lactation cycle influence signals that favor recrudescence of postpartum ovulation, and establishment and maintenance of pregnancy. The high-yielding cow of today will soon be surpassed by more productive cows, and the gain in production should be concurrent with gains in fertility and health. Matching the genotype with proper management, nutrition and health programs, combined with selection for fertility and the use of breeding technologies will allow producers to cope with the reproductive challenges faced by dairy cows producing well over 11 tons of milk a year.

Acknowledgments

The authors would like to thank their funding agencies and industry partners (National Research Initiative of the United States Department of Agriculture, Southeast Milk Checkoff Program, USDA Formula Funds, National Association of Animal Breeders, Pfizer Animal Health, Intervet/Schering Plough Animal Health, Virtus Nutrition, Arm & Hammer Animal Nutrition, and Select Sires Inc.) that supported much of their work cited in this manuscript.

References

Allen MS, Bradford BJ & Oba M 2009 Board invited review: the hepatic oxidation theory of the control of feed intake and its application to ruminants. *Journal of Animal Science* **87** 3317-3334.

Ambrose DK, Kastelic JP, Corbett R, Pitney PA, Petit HV, Small JA & Zalkovic P 2006 Lower pregnancy losses in lactating dairy cows fed a diet enriched in α-linolenic acid. *Journal of Dairy Science* **89** 3066-3074.

Bauman DE & Currie WB 1980 Partitioning of nutrients during pregnancy and lactation: a review of mechanisms involving homeostasis and homeorhesis. *Journal of Dairy Science* **63** 1514-1529.

Benson JA, Reynolds CK, Aikman PC, Lupoli B & Beever DE 2002 Effects of abomasal vegetable oil infusion on splanchnic nutrient metabolism in lactating dairy cows. *Journal of Dairy Science* **85** 1804-1114.

Brusveen DJ, Cunha AP, Silva CD, Cunha PM, Sterry RA, Silva EPB, Guenther JN & Wiltbank MC 2008 Altering the time of the second gonadotropin-releasing hormone injection and artificial insemination (AI) during Ovsynch affects pregnancies per AI in lactating dairy cows. *Journal of Dairy Science* **91** 1044–1052.

Butler ST, Pelton SH & Butler WR 2004 Insulin increases 17 beta-estradiol production by the dominant follicle of the first postpartum follicle wave in dairy cows. *Reproduction* **127** 537-545.

Butler ST, Marr AL, Pelton SH, Radcliff RP, Butler MC & Butler WR 2003 Insulin restores GH responsiveness during lactation-induced negative energy balance in dairy cattle: effects on expression of IGF-I and GH receptor 1A. *Journal of Endocrinology* **176** 205-217.

Butler WR 2003 Energy balance relationships with follicular development, ovulation and fertility in postpartum dairy cows. *Livestock Production Science* **83** 211-218.

Capper JL, Cady RA & Bauman DE 2009 The environmental impact of dairy production: 1944 compared with 2007. *Journal of Animal Science* **87** 2160-2167.

Cerri RLA, Juchem SO, Chebel RC, Rutigliano HM, Bruno RGS, Galvão KN, Thatcher WW & Santos JEP 2009a Effect of fat source differing in fatty acid profile on metabolic parameters, fertilization and embryo quality in high-producing dairy cows. *Journal of Dairy Science* **92** 1520–1531.

Cerri RLA, Rutigliano HM, Chebel RC & Santos JEP 2009b Period of dominance of the ovulatory follicle influences embryo quality in lactating dairy cows. *Reproduction* **137** 813-823.

Chang YM, González-Recio O, Weigel KA & Fricke PM 2007 Genetic analysis of the twenty-one-day pregnancy rate in US Holsteins using an ordinal censored threshold model with unknown voluntary waiting period. *Journal of Dairy Science* **90** 1987-1997.

Chebel RC, Santos JEP, Cerri RLA, Rutigliano HM & Bruno RGS 2006 Reproduction in dairy cows following progesterone insert presynchronization and resynchronization protocols. *Journal of Dairy Science* **89** 4205-4219.

Dechow CD, Rogers GW, Klei L, Lawlor TJ & VanRaden PM 2004 Body condition scores and dairy form evaluations as indicators of days open in US Holsteins. *Journal of Dairy Science* **87** 3534-3541.

de Veth MJ, Bauman DE, Koch W, Mann GE, Pfeiffer AM & Butler WR 2009 Efficacy of conjugated linoleic acid for improving reproduction: a multi-study analysis in early-lactation dairy cows. *Journal of Dairy Science* **92** 2662-2669.

De Vries A 2006 Economic value of pregnancy in dairy cattle. *Journal of Dairy Science* **89** 3876–3885.

De Vries A, Crane MB, Bartolome JA, Melendez P, Risco CA & Archbald LF 2006 Economic comparison of timed artificial insemination and exogenous progesterone as treatments for ovarian cysts. *Journal of Dairy Science* **89** 3028-3037.

Drackley JK 1999 ADSA foundation scholar award. Biology of dairy cows during the transition period: the final frontier? *Journal of Dairy Science* **82** 2259-2273.

El-Zarkouny SZ, Cartmill JA, Hensley BA & Stevenson JS 2004 Pregnancy in dairy cows after synchronized ovulation regimens with or without presynchronization and progesterone. *Journal of Dairy Science* **87** 1024-1037.

Friggens NC, Berg P, Theilgaard P, Korsgaard IR, Ingvartsen KL, Løvendahl P & Jensen J 2007 Breed and parity effects on energy balance profiles through lactation: evidence of genetically driven body energy change. *Journal of Dairy Science* **90** 5291-5305.

Galvão KN, Greco LF, Vilela JM, Sá Filho MF & Santos JEP 2009 Effect of intrauterine infusion of ceftiofur on uterine health and fertility in dairy cows. *Journal of Dairy Science* **92** 1532-1542.

Galvão KN, Sá Filho MF & Santos JEP 2007 Reducing the interval from presynchronization to initiation of timed AI improves fertility in dairy cows. *Journal of Dairy Science* **90** 4212-4218.

Garnsworthy PC, Fouladi-Nashta AA, Mann GE, Sinclair KD & Webb R 2009 Effect of dietary-induced changes in plasma insulin concentrations during the early post partum period on pregnancy rate in dairy cows. *Reproduction* **137** 759-768.

Gong JG, Lee WJ, Garnsworthy PC & Webb R 2002 Effect of dietary-induced increases in circulating insulin concentrations during the early postpartum period on reproductive function in dairy cows. *Reproduction* **123** 419-427.

Gümen A, Rastani RR, Grummer RR & Wiltbank MC 2005 Reduced dry periods and varying prepartum diets alter postpartum ovulation and reproductive measures. *Journal of Dairy Science* **88** 2401-2411.

Gümen A, Guenther JN & Wiltbank MC 2003. Follicular size and response to Ovsynch versus detection of estrus in anovular and ovular lactating dairy cows. *Journal of Dairy Science* **86** 3184-3194.

Hansen LB 2000 Consequences of selection for milk yield from a geneticist's viewpoint. *Journal of Dairy Science* **83** 1145-1150

Hansen LB, Freeman AE & Berger PJ 1983 Association of heifer fertility with cow fertility and yield in dairy cattle. *Journal of Dairy Science* **66** 306-314.

Hileman SM, Lubbers LS, Jansen HT & Lehman MN 1999 Changes in hypothalamic estrogen receptor-containing cell numbers in response to feed restriction in the female lamb. *Neuroendocrinology* **69** 430-437.

Holstein World 1999 North Carolina cow makes 75,275 lbs of milk. *Holstein World*, February, pp. 12.

Juchem SO, Cerri RLA, Villaseñor M, Galvão KN, Bruno RGS, Rutigliano HM, DePeters EJ, Silvestre FT, Thatcher WW & Santos JEP 2010. Supplementation with calcium salts of linoleic and trans-octadecenoic acids improves fertility of lactating dairy cows. *Reproduction in Domestic Animals* **45** 55–62.

LaDue E, Gloy B & Cuykendall C 2003 Future structure of the dairy industry: historical trends, projections and issues. Research Bulletin 2003-01. Cornell Program on Agricultural and Small Business Finance, Department of Applied Economics and Management, Cornell University, Ithaca, USA, pp. 1-62.

LeBlanc SJ, Duffield TF, Leslie KE, Bateman KG, Keefe GP, Walton JS & Johnson WH 2002 The effect of treatment of clinical endometritis on reproductive performance in dairy cows. *Journal of Dairy Science* **85** 2237-2249.

Leroy JL, Van Soom A, Opsomer G, Goovaerts IG & Bols PE 2008 Reduced fertility in high-yielding dairy cows: are the oocyte and embryo in danger? Part II. Mechanisms linking nutrition and reduced oocyte and embryo quality in high-yielding dairy cows. *Reproduction in Domestic Animals* **43** 623-632.

Lima FS, De Vries A, Risco CA, Santos JEP & Thatcher WW 2010 Economic comparison of natural service and timed artificial insemination breeding programs in dairy cattle. *Journal of Dairy Science* **93** 4404–4413.

Lima FS, Risco CA, Thatcher MJ, Benzaquen ME, Archbald LF, Santos JEP & Thatcher WW 2009 Comparison of reproductive performance in lactating dairy cows bred by natural service or timed artificial insemination. *Journal of Dairy Science* **92** 5456–5466.

Lopez H, Satter LD & Wiltbank MC 2004 Relationship between level of milk production and estrous behavior of lactating dairy cows. *Animal Reproduction Science* **81** 209-223.

Lucy MC, Verkerk GA, Whyte BE, Macdonald KA, Burton L, Cursons RT, Roche JR & Holmes CW 2009 Somatotropic axis components and nutrient partitioning in genetically diverse dairy cows managed under different feed allowances in a pasture system *Journal of Dairy Science* **92** 526-539.

Macdonald KA, Penno JW, Lancaster JA & Roche JR 2008 Effect of stocking rate on pasture production, milk production, and reproduction of dairy cows in pasture-based systems. *Journal of Dairy Science* **91** 2151-563.

McDougall S 2010 Comparison of diagnostic approaches, and a cost-benefit analysis of different diagnostic approaches and treatments of anoestrous dairy cows. *New Zealand Veterinary Journal* **58** 81-89.

Moreira F, Orlandi C, Risco CA, Mattos R, Lopes F & Thatcher WW 2001 Effects of presynchronization and bovine somatotropin on pregnancy rates to a timed artificial insemination protocol in lactating dairy cows. *Journal of Dairy Science* **84** 1646-1659.

Rastani RR, Grummer RR, Bertics SJ, Gümen A, Wiltbank MC, Mashek DG & Schwab MC 2005 Reducing dry period length to simplify feeding transition cows: milk production, energy balance, and metabolic profiles. *Journal of Dairy Science* **88** 1004-1014.

Roxström A, Strandberg E, Berglund B, Emanuelson U & Philipsson J 2001 Genetic and environmental correlations among female fertility traits and milk production in different parities of Swedish Red and White dairy cattle. *Acta Agriculturae Scandinavica Section A - Animal Science* **51** 7-14.

Santos JEP, Narciso CD, Rivera F, Thatcher WW & Chebel RC 2010 Effect of reducing the period of follicle dominance in a timed AI protocol on reproduction of dairy cows. *Journal of Dairy Science* **93** 2976-2988.

Santos JEP, Rutigliano HM & Sá Filho MF 2009 Risk factors for resumption of postpartum cyclicity and embryonic survival in lactating dairy cows. *Animal Reproduction Science* **110** 207-221.

Santos JEP, Bilby TR, Thatcher WW, Staples CR & Silvestre FT 2008a Long chain fatty acids of diet as factors influencing reproduction in cattle. *Reproduction in Domestic Animals* **43 (Supp. 2)** 23-30.

Santos JEP, Cerri RLA & Sartori R 2008b Nutritional management of the donor cow. *Theriogenology* **69** 88-97.

Silvestre FT, Carvalho TSM, Crawford C, Santos JEP, Staples CR, Jenkins T & Thatcher WW 2010a Effects of differential supplementation of fatty acids during the peripartum and breeding periods of Holstein cows: I. uterine and metabolic statuses, reproduction and lactation. *Journal of Dairy Science* **93** *in press*

Silvestre FT, Carvalho TSM, Crawford C, Santos JEP, Staples CR, Jenkins T & Thatcher WW 2010b Effects of differential supplementation of fatty acids during the peripartum and breeding periods of Holstein cows: II. acute phase proteins and neutrophil function. *Journal of Dairy Science* **93** *in press*

Souza AH, Ayres H, Ferreira RM & Wiltbank MC 2008 A new presynchronization system (Double-Ovsynch) increases fertility at first postpartum timed AI in lactating dairy cows. *Theriogenology* **70** 208–215.

Staples CR, Burke JM & Thatcher WW 1998 Influence of supplemental fats on reproductive tissues and performance of lactating cows. *Journal of Dairy Science* **81** 856-871.

Thangavelu G, Colazo MG, Ambrose DJ, Oba M, Okine EK & Dyck MK 2007 Diets enriched in unsaturated fatty acids enhance early embryonic development in lactating Holstein cows. *Theriogenology* **68** 949-957.

Vasconcelos JLM, Silcox RW, Rosa GJ, Pursley JR & Wiltbank MC 1999 Synchronization rate, size of the ovulatory follicle, and pregnancy rate after synchronization of ovulation beginning on different days of the estrous cycle in lactating dairy cows. *Theriogenology* **52** 1067-1078.

van Knegsel ATM, H. van den Brand, Dijkstra J, van Straalen WM, Jorritsma R, Tamming S & Kemp B 2007 Effect of glucogenic vs. lipogenic diets on energy balance, blood metabolites, and reproduction in primiparous and multiparous dairy cows in early lactation. *Journal of Dairy Science* **90** 3397-3490.

VanRaden PM, Sanders AH, Tooker ME, Miller RH, Norman HD, Kuhn MT & Wiggans GR 2004 Development of a national genetic evaluation for cow fertility. *Journal of Dairy Science* **87** 2285-2292.

Wade GN & Jones JE 2004 Neuroendocrinology of nutritional infertility. *American Journal of Physiology - Regulatory Integrative Comparative Physiology* **287** R1277-R1296.

Weigel KA & R Rekaya 2000 Genetic parameters for reproductive traits of Holstein cattle in California and Minnesota *Journal of Dairy Science* **83** 1072–1080.

Controlling the dominant follicle in beef cattle to improve estrous synchronization and early embryonic development

ML Day[1], ML Mussard[1], GA Bridges[2] and CR Burke[3]

[1]*Department of Animal Sciences, The Ohio State University, Columbus OH USA 43210;* [2]*North Central Research and Outreach Center, University of Minnesota, Grand Rapids, MN, USA;* [3]*DairyNZ Limited, Hamilton 3240, New Zealand*

Estrous synchronization and timed ovulation programs that permit AI at a predetermined time (timed AI) rather than as determined by detection of spontaneous estrus are requisite for increased adoption of AI in the beef cattle industry. In the past two decades, significant progress has been achieved in developing programs that synchronize ovulation to address this need. While this progress has been driven by a multitude of fundamental discoveries in reproductive biology, the greatest impact in the past two decades has been the result of enhanced understanding of the pattern of ovarian follicle growth in cattle and development of technologies to coordinate growth and ovulation of the dominant follicle. At present, estrous synchronization programs that result in acceptable timed AI pregnancy rates are available for beef cattle. The capacity to control growth of the dominant follicle and evaluate the impact of various approaches on fertility has resulted in greater understanding of the factors that influence maturity of ovulatory follicles. Modifications to the standard industry breeding programs, with the aim of lengthening and/or increasing the gonadotropic stimulus and estradiol production by preovulatory follicles, have been shown to substantially increase timed AI pregnancy rate in beef cattle. Associations between characteristics of follicular development and fertility have surfaced from application of estrous and ovulation synchronization technologies and led to investigation of the fundamental mechanisms that underlie these relationships.

Introduction

Effective estrous synchronization technologies to facilitate the use of timed AI in beef cattle have been developed (Larson et al, 2006; Sa Filho et al., 2009) and modifications that enhance their efficacy (Bridges et al., 2009; Meneghetti et al., 2009) continue to be discovered (Figure 1). The current technologies reflect the culmination of relevant fundamental discoveries in reproductive physiology that date to the early 1900s, and research in estrous synchronization that has been ongoing for over 60 years. The rapid progress in the field of estrous synchronization and timed AI over the last two decades can be directly linked to the discovery of a wave-like pattern of follicular development in cattle (Savio et al., 1988; Sirois and Fortune,

---

Corresponding author E-mail: day.5@osu.edu

1988; Ginther et al., 1989). Since that time, research has progressed through investigation of the implications of not controlling follicular development, approaches to coordinate follicle development and application of methodology to control growth and ovulation of the dominant follicle in conjunction with other components of estrous synchronization and timed AI programs. The synchronization programs currently used in cattle reflect only a portion of the valuable knowledge gained through this area of research. Through attempts to coordinate follicular development and standardize the timing of ovulation, greater understanding of the impact of variation in follicular development on fertility in cattle has evolved. Various relationships between fertility in cattle and aspects of follicular development, such as follicle size, length of proestrus, follicular estradiol production, and progesterone concentrations during follicular development to fertility in cattle have emerged, and led to fundamental investigations of the mechanisms that underlie these associations.

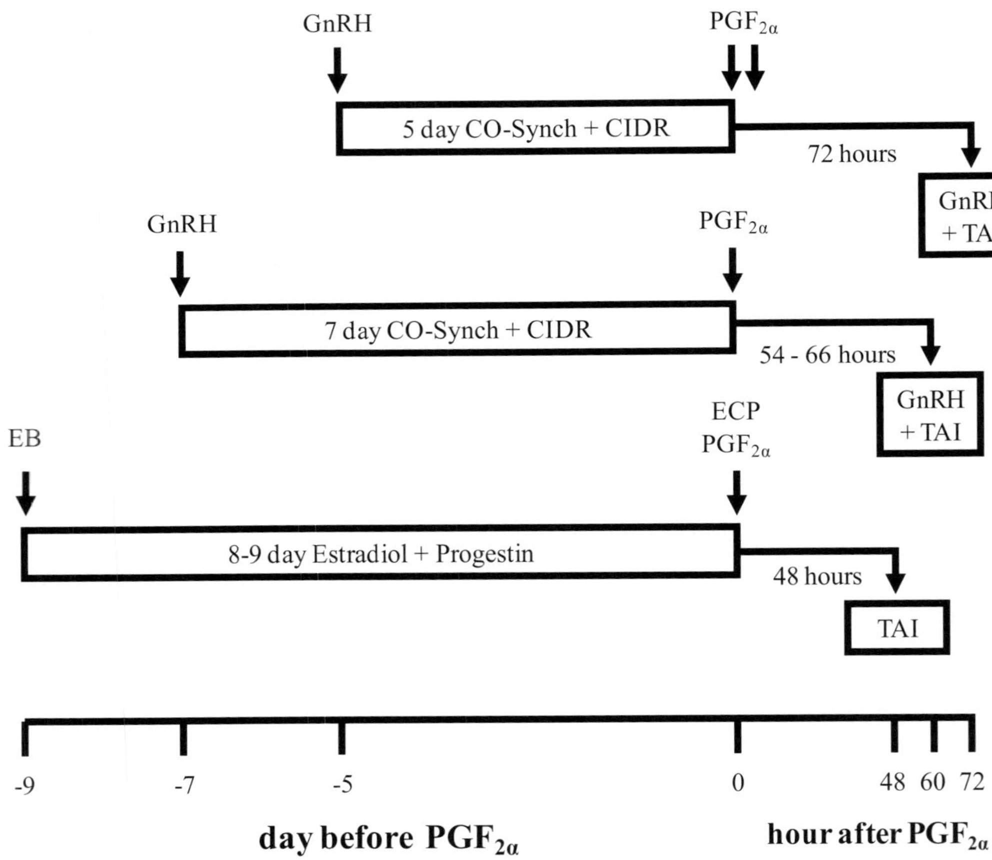

Fig. 1. Common estrous synchronization programs used with timed AI in postpartum beef cows. GnRH = gonadotropin releasing hormone; $PGF_{2\alpha}$ = prostaglandin $F_{2\alpha}$, CIDR = Controlled Internal Drug Release Insert; EB = estradiol benzoate; ECP = estradiol cypionate; TAI = timed AI. With the GnRH-based programs in the USA, the CIDR® is the only available progestin source. With Estradiol + Progestin systems, varying forms of estradiol are used at the start of the progestin treatment. Also timing of $PGF_{2\alpha}$, form and timing of estradiol used to synchronize ovulation, interval to timed AI and source of progestin vary among programs.

Traditional approaches to estrous cycle control in cattle

Early attempts to synchronize estrus in cattle were based on the knowledge that progesterone prevents the occurrence of estrus and ovulation (Christian and Casida, 1948). A variety of progestins were administered in an assortment of methods to attempt to coordinate the timing of estrus in cattle (Trimberger and Hansel, 1955; Zimbelman and Smith, 1966). Progestin treatments of relatively long duration resulted in the most precise timing of estrus since this allowed for spontaneous occurrence of luteolysis during progestin treatment, but fertility was substantially less than would be expected following a spontaneous estrus (Zimbelman et al., 1970; Wishart, 1977). The inverse relationship between duration of progestin treatment and fertility led to development of short-term progestin treatments.

One approach to shortening the duration of progestin treatment was administration of a pharmacological dose of estrogen at the initiation of treatment to induce luteal regression; rather than relying on long-term treatments to allow spontaneous luteolysis (Wiltbank and Kasson, 1968; Mauleon, 1974). Synchrony of estrus and fertility varied with these approaches since the response to estrogen varied by stage of the estrous cycle (Lemon, 1975; Miksch et al., 1978). Development of short-term programs was also aided by identification of $PGF_{2\alpha}$ as a luteolysin (McCracken et al., 1972) and characterization of its efficacy to induce luteolysis (Lauderdale, 1975). However, the timing of estrus after utilizing this approach continued to vary (Wishart, 1974; Thimonier et al., 1975) due to stage of the estrous cycle at which luteal regression was induced (King et al., 1982), and fertility varied due to the stage of the estrous cycle when progestin treatment was initiated (Beal et al., 1988). Although usable estrous synchronization programs existed at this time, the efficacy of most programs was not predictable (Odde, 1990, review).

Coordinating follicular growth for estrous synchronization

Persistent ovarian follicles

Characterization of the wave-like pattern of follicular growth in cattle through the use of ovarian ultrasonography (Savio et al., 1988; Sirois and Fortune, 1988; Ginther et al., 1989) provided insight into challenges associated with earlier approaches to synchronize estrus. Although it had been known for some time that ovarian follicular development was not a random event in cattle (Rajakoski, 1960), controlling this aspect of ovarian function was not an intentional component of most programs. With new insight on the normal pattern of follicular growth and ultrasonographic capabilities, it was demonstrated that administration of a progestin in the absence of a corpus luteum extended the lifespan of the dominant ovarian follicle until the progestin was withdrawn (Sirois and Fortune, 1990). Dominant ovarian follicles with an extended lifespan ('persistent follicles') were shown to develop when practically any type of progestin was administered in the absence of a corpus luteum (Stock and Fortune, 1993; Anderson and Day, 1994), resulting in increased frequency of LH pulses and concentrations of estradiol (Kinder et al., 1996, review). Fertility was reduced if the lifespan of a dominant follicle was prolonged for four days (Mihm et al., 1994) and while fertilization of oocytes was unaffected, the embryo died shortly thereafter (Ahmad et al., 1995). Since the need of a progestin for synchronization of estrus in beef cattle has been well documented (Day, 2004, review), subsequent research focused on preventing ovulation of persistent follicles at the synchronized estrus.

Coordinating follicular development through management of persistent follicles

The discovery that atresia of persistent follicles could be induced by acutely increasing peripheral progesterone concentrations (Stock and Fortune, 1993; Savio et al., 1993), resulting in synchronous emergence of a new follicular wave 3.5 later (Anderson and Day, 1994) provided a potential tool that could be used to manipulate follicular development for estrous synchronization and avoid the infertility inherent to ovulation of persistent follicles. McDowell et al. (1998a) demonstrated that 24 hours of exposure to mid-luteal progesterone concentrations was sufficient to induce atresia of persistent follicles.

The concept of using progesterone delivered via an injection to synchronize atresia of persistent ovarian follicles and coordinate follicular development in herds of cattle was evaluated in a series of experiments (Anderson and Day, 1994, 1998; McDowell et al., 1998b). Experiments varied by progestin source and duration and the use of $PGF_{2\alpha}$ to induce luteal regression. Conclusions from this series of experiments were that induced atresia of persistent follicles with progesterone resulted in a synchronous and fertile estrus and provided a means to coordinate follicular development in cows at random stages of the estrous cycle and in anestrous cows. A limitation of this approach for estrous synchronization was duration of treatment (≥ 14 days) necessary to ensure that most females initially developed persistent follicles. Synchronization programs that exceed 10 days are not acceptable to most producers. Furthermore, injectable progesterone is not commercially available in the USA.

Infertility associated with long term progestin use and development of persistent follicles can be avoided if cattle are not inseminated at the first estrus after progestin withdrawal but are inseminated at a subsequent synchronized estrus. Initial investigation of this approach involved feeding of an oral progestin for 14 days and induction of luteolysis with $PGF_{2\alpha}$ 17 days later (Brown et al., 1988). This presynchronization with a progestin takes advantage of the beneficial effects of progestins and passively coordinates follicular development since a majority of females are in a similar stage of the estrous cycle at the time of $PGF_{2\alpha}$-induced luteal regression. This approach has been further refined (Lamb et al., 2000; Mallory et al., 2010) and effectively synchronizes estrus in cattle. The interval from initiation of progestin treatment to AI with this approach ranges from 33 to 36 days.

Coordination of follicular development with estradiol

An alternative to managing persistent follicles to coordinate growth of the dominant follicle would be to 'reset' follicular development at the outset of an estrous synchronization program and avoid development of persistent follicles altogether. Early evidence that estrogens may function in this manner was that injection of estradiol valerate induced atresia of large ovarian follicles (Engelhardt et al., 1989). It was subsequently demonstrated that injection of estradiol 17ß induced atresia of the dominant follicle of the first follicular wave resulting in emergence of a new follicular wave approximately four days later in all females (Bo et al., 1995) thus providing a valuable tool to control growth of the dominant follicle for estrous synchronization. Several studies have focused on understanding the variation and mechanisms associated with the use of estradiol to reset follicular development using estradiol benzoate (EB; see Day and Burke, 2002 for review). Intramuscular injection of EB consistently induced atresia of dominant follicles and resulted in emergence of a new follicular wave (Burke et al., 2000, 2001), interval from EB to emergence of the new follicular wave increased with dose and EB was effective across stages of the estrous cycle (Day and Burke, 2002). The conception rate of cows administered EB at the initiation of progestin treatment was similar to that of cows exhibiting a spontaneous estrus (Day et al., 2000). Further, it was demonstrated that sustained concentrations of progesterone, for a minimum of 48 h, were necessary for EB to consistently reset follicular development (Burke et al., 1998).

In intact cows, administration of EB during the luteal phase suppressed LH and/or FSH in the periphery and induced an immediate decline in estradiol production by dominant follicles through suppression of aromatase (Burke et al., 2005; 2007). Timing of emergence of the new wave of follicular development was dependent upon the duration of FSH suppression by the exogenously administered estradiol and was dose dependent (Burke et al., 2003). These findings, and others (not cited) clearly established that the administration of exogenous estradiol represents a predictable and highly effective method to coordinate growth of the dominant follicle for estrous synchronization and timed AI in cattle.

Coordination of follicular development with GnRH

A second method to reset follicular development at the outset of an estrous synchronization program is the use of GnRH or its agonists. Injection of GnRH induces an LH surge within 2 hours (Kaltenbach et al., 1974) and, within 1 to 2 days, there is a reduction in the number of large follicles (Thatcher et al., 1989) due to ovulation and subsequent formation of a new corpus luteum (Twagiramungu et al., 1994). Synchronized emergence of a new follicular wave after GnRH (Macmillan and Thatcher, 1991) occurred within 1 to 2 days after GnRH injection (Twagiramungu et al., 1994, 1995).

A challenge of using GnRH for estrous synchronization is that ovulation in response to the first GnRH is induced in only 66% of beef cows (Geary et al., 2000). In heifers, response rates approaching 50% have been reported (Pursley et al., 1995). Variation in response to GnRH has been attributed to day of the estrous cycle (Moreira et al., 2000) and the influence of day of the estrous cycle on ovulatory response and growth of newly emerged dominant follicles in cows and heifers has recently been investigated (Atkins et al., 2008, 2010). Estrous synchronization programs that use GnRH should be structured to minimize the negative impact of uncoordinated follicular development that occurs in 20 to 50% of females treated.

Estrous synchronization programs for timed AI in beef cows

The capacity to coordinate growth of the dominant follicle stimulated a period of intense investigation that led to development of programs currently used for estrous synchronization in beef cattle. The importance of these contributions is recognized, but the focus here is on the current programs used for timed AI in beef cows, their benefits and shortcomings, and ongoing research to improve the current methodology.

Strategy of current timed AI programs

In beef cows, timed AI programs include a progestin source to suppress estrus and for induction of estrous cycles in anestrous females, and $PGF_{2\alpha}$ to induce luteal regression (Figure 1). In the USA, GnRH or its agonist is used to reset follicular development at the initiation of the synchronization program and at the end of the program to synchronize ovulation for timed AI. In many other countries estradiol (either 17ß-estradiol or estradiol benzoate) is used in timed-AI to reset follicular development and estradiol (including estradiol cypionate) is again used at the end of the program to synchronize ovulation.

Regardless of whether programs are GnRH- or estradiol-based, the rationale for the design of current programs is similar. Treatments begin with insertion of an intravaginal progestin device that is accompanied by GnRH or estradiol to reset follicular development. Emergence of a new follicular wave occurs 1 to 2 (GnRH) or 3 to 4 (estradiol) days later. When GnRH is used, emergence of the new follicular wave is accompanied by formation of the GnRH-induced accessory corpus luteum. Due to the difference in time of emergence between GnRH and estradiol, the progestin is withdrawn and $PGF_{2\alpha}$ is given either 7 (GnRH) or 8 to 9 (estradiol) days later. Hence, progesterone is withdrawn 5 to 6 days after emergence of a dominant follicle. The final step is to synchronize ovulation with either GnRH, given 60-66 hours after $PGF_{2\alpha}$, estradiol cypionate which is given at progestin withdrawal, or 17ß-estradiol/EB given 24 to 48 hours after $PGF_{2\alpha}$.

Estrous synchronization and timed AI with GnRH

The standard GnRH-based timed AI program used in the USA is referred to as the "CO-Synch + CIDR" program (Figure 1). Some of the key research that led to development of this program (Macmillan and Thatcher, 1991; Twagiramunga et al., 1995; Pursely et al., 1995; Geary et al., 2001; Lamb et al., 2001) culminated in a large multistate project (Larson et al., 2006) which reported that timed-AI pregnancy rate with the CO-Synch + CIDR program was 54%. This program is a widely used estrous synchronization system for timed AI in beef cows in the USA.

While the CO-Synch + CIDR program has been successful and yielded acceptable timed-AI pregnancy rates, limitations to fertility have been linked to the lack of coordination of follicular development in some females. Failure of the first GnRH to reset follicular development leads to aberrant follicular dynamics during the synchronization program (Geary et al., 2000) and the induced ovulation of small follicles in some animals by the second GnRH (Perry et al., 2005). Cattle induced to ovulate follicles smaller than observed at a spontaneous estrus with the second GnRH have decreased fertility (Lamb et al., 2001; Perry et al., 2005). The capacity of the first GnRH to reset follicular development as well as stage of the estrous cycle at treatment has been linked to size of the dominant follicle at the time of the second GnRH (Atkins et al., 2008, 2010). Hence, pregnancy rate to timed AI with the standard CO-Synch + CIDR program is limited by induced ovulation of compromised follicles.

Follicular maturity and fertility in cattle

The influence of ovulatory follicle maturity on fertility in beef cattle has been investigated (Mussard et al., 2003; 2007; Bridges et al., 2010; Perry et al., 2005). One hypothesis was that diameter of ovulatory follicles was the most appropriate indicator of follicle "maturity" and that cows induced to ovulate small follicles would have decreased fertility compared to cows which are induced to ovulate large dominant follicles. Within each of three experiments (Table 1; Mussard et al., 2003; 2007) this hypothesis was supported, but as data accumulated,from multiple experiments, the relationship of follicle diameter to pregnancy rate appeared inconsistent. In fact, across experiments, the more consistent predictor of pregnancy rate appeared to be the interval from initiation of luteal regression with $PGF_{2\alpha}$ to either a spontaneous or GnRH-induced LH surge (Table 1). Since the stage of a spontaneous estrous cycle between luteal regression and initiation of estrus and the LH surge is typically referred to as proestrus, we, in turn, refer to the interval from $PGF_{2\alpha}$ (and progestin withdrawal when applicable) to GnRH treatment as 'proestrus' in our research. The observed relationship between length of proestrus and conception rate led to an additional experiment (Table 1; Bridges et al., 2010) designed to hold follicle diameter constant and only vary length of proestrus. It was demonstrated that at a constant ovulatory follicle diameter, length of proestrus had a substantial influence on conception rate. Taken together, data from this series of studies suggested a strong positive relationship of duration of proestrus with follicle maturity and fertility, and furthermore, suggested that diameter of the ovulatory follicle, in itself, was not a consistent predictor of follicle maturity. The effect of ovulatory follicle size at GnRH-induced ovulation or at spontaneous ovulation on conception rate has also been evaluated by Perry et al. (2005, 2007). It was reported that diameter of the ovulatory follicle influenced conception rate after detection of estrus in heifers, but not in postpartum cows. In postpartum cows that did not exhibit estrus, diameter of the ovulatory follicle was positively associated with conception rate when ovulation was induced with GnRH. Thus, if a 'complete' spontaneous proestrus occurred in cows (confirmed by exhibition of estrus), diameter of the ovulatory follicle did not impact fertility. The impact of follicle diameter on conception rate was evident when ovulation was induced with GnRH; at a constant duration of proestrus. Since findings suggested that maturity of the ovulatory follicle and probability of conception is perhaps best defined by length of proestrus, we applied this knowledge towards optimizing the existing CO-Synch + CIDR program to take advantage of this relationship.

Table 1. Conception rate, diameter and age of the ovulatory follicle, duration of proestrus, and number of cows included from a series of experiments investigating the effect of follicle maturity on fertility.

Conception rate (%)[a]	Follicle diameter at ovulation (mm)[b]	Duration of proestrus (days)[c]	n	Experiment
4	11.1 ± 0.2	1.0 ± 0.1	45	Mussard et al., 2003a[e]
8	11.1 ± 0.2	1.0 ± 0.1	12	Mussard et al., 2003b[f]
10	12.6 ± 0.2	1.25	10	Bridges et al., 2010[g]
57	13.6 ± 0.2	2.2 ± 0.1	54	Mussard et al., 2003a[e]
67	13.7 ± 0.2	2.0 ± 0.1	12	Mussard et al., 2003b[f]
71	12.9 ± 0.2	2.25	28	Bridges et al., 2010[g]
76	10.7 ± 0.1	3.3 ± 0.1	29	Mussard et al., 2007[d]
100	12.0 ± 0.3	4.7 ± 0.2	24	Mussard et al., 2007[d]

[a] Percentage of animals determined to be pregnant following insemination. Pregnancy determination was conducted via ultrasonography at approximately 30 days post-insemination.
[b] Diameter of the largest ovulatory follicle as determined by ultrasonography conducted either at GnRH administration or estrus.
[c] Interval from PGF_{2a} until GnRH administration.
[d] Cows were either induced with GnRH to ovulate a small (~ 11 mm) follicle or allowed to spontaneously exhibit estrus. Cows were inseminated 12 hours following estrus or GnRH.
[e] Cows were induced to ovulate either a small (~ 11 mm) or large (~ 13 mm) ovarian follicle with GnRH. Animals were inseminated 12 h following GnRH administration.
[f] Cows were induced to ovulate either a small (~ 11 mm) or large (~ 13 mm) ovarian follicle with GnRH. Embryo from non-treated cows were then transferred 7 days after GnRH.
[g] Cows were induced to ovulate an ovarian follicle of similar diameter with GnRH either 1.25 or 2.25 days following PGF_{2a} administration. Animals were inseminated 12 h following GnRH administration. Includes only cows with a luteal phase of normal length.

Lengthening proestrus in the CO-Synch + CIDR program

The length of proestrus (interval from $PGF_{2\alpha}$ to second GnRH and timed AI) with the traditional 7-day CO-Synch + CIDR program was varied from 56 to 72 hours in mature cows without influencing timed AI pregnancy rate, but in younger cows ($\leq$ 3 years of age), greatest pregnancy rates were achieved with timed AI at 56 hours (Dobbins et al., 2009). Others (Busch et al., 2008) have reported that timed AI pregnancy rates were greater when proestrus was 66 than 54 hours. In practice, the second GnRH is given and timed AI is performed in most herds between 54 and 66 hours after $PGF_{2\alpha}$, and there is no evidence that extending this interval beyond 66 hours will increase timed AI pregnancy rate. It was theorized that if the interval from the first GnRH and insertion of the CIDR to $PGF_{2\alpha}$ was shortened to 5 days, proestrus could be lengthened and timed-AI pregnancy rate would increase. In the 5-day CO-Synch + CIDR program (Figure 1), two rather than one injection of $PGF_{2\alpha}$ are administered at CIDR withdrawal, which is 5 days after CIDR insertion and the first GnRH injection. With this approach, the new follicular wave emerges 3 to 4 days before $PGF_{2\alpha}$ is given, which is earlier relative to emergence of the ovulatory follicle (5 to 6 days) in the 7-day CO-Synch + CIDR program. Thus, the dominant follicle enters proestrus at a follicular age when follicular fluid concentrations and capacity of granulosa cells to produce estradiol are greater than with the 7 day program (Valdez et al., 2005). Bridges et al. (2008) determined that the appropriate interval from $PGF_{2\alpha}$ to the second GnRH and timed-AI with the 5 day program was 72 hours. In comparison with the traditional 7 day CO-Synch + CIDR program, the 5-day CO-Synch + CIDR program increased timed-AI pregnancy rate from 59.9 to 70.4% (Bridges et al., 2008). Similarly, a 14% increase in timed-AI pregnancy rate was detected in yearling heifers with the 5-day as compared to 7-day program (Wilson et al., 2007). This substantial increase in timed-AI pregnancy rate with the 5-day program has been achieved using two doses of $PGF_{2\alpha}$ (or cloprostenol sodium, CLP) spaced at 12 hours apart. Pregnancy rate is decreased with a single dose of $PGF_{2\alpha}$ or CLP (Kasimanickam., et al. 2009; Souto et al., 2009) due to failure of a single dose to induce luteal regression in approximately 1/3 of cows (Souto et al., 2009). Cruppe et al. (2010) recently reported that giving two simultaneous doses of $PGF_{2\alpha}$ together at the time of CIDR withdrawal in the 5-day program resulted in pregnancy rates similar to those achieved with two injections, spaced 8 hours apart. Collectively, experiments that have included over 1700 cows across 23 herds and four years, have achieved a mean pregnancy rate of 68.4% with the 5-day CO-Synch + CIDR program using two doses of $PGF_{2\alpha}$ given simultaneously or spaced 2, 7, 8 or 12 hours apart, depending upon individual experimental objectives.

Hormonal impact of lengthened proestrus

Proestrus starts with the diappearance of progesterone and terminates with either a spontaneous or GnRH- induced LH surge. An immediate response to declining progesterone is an increase in the frequency of LH pulses (Kinder et al., 1996), providing the primary stimulus for final development of preovulatory follicles (Ireland and Roche, 1983) and the preovulatory increase in estradiol (Kaneko et al., 1991). Concentrations of estradiol, magnitude of the LH surge, and progesterone concentrations during the ensuing luteal phase were compared in cattle experiencing either a short (SPE) or long (LPE) proestrus (Figure 2; Bridges et al., 2010). Ovulatory follicle size was similar and the magnitude of the GnRH-induced LH surge did not differ between treatments. There tended to be lower concentrations of progesterone in the SPE treatment, however, the most striking difference was the greater concentrations of estradiol in the LPE treatment during the 32 hours preceding GnRH administration (Figure 3). In another model, when proestrus was lengthened in the 5- vs. the 7-day CO-Synch + CIDR program, diameter of the ovulatory follicle did not differ but peak estradiol concentration tended to be greater with the 5-day program (Bridges et al., 2009). It has been concluded that increasing the length of proestrus escalates preovulatory concentrations of estradiol, presumably through prolonged gonadotropic stimulation of the dominant follicle, resulting in increased timed-AI pregnancy rates in the 5-day CO-Sync + CIDR program.

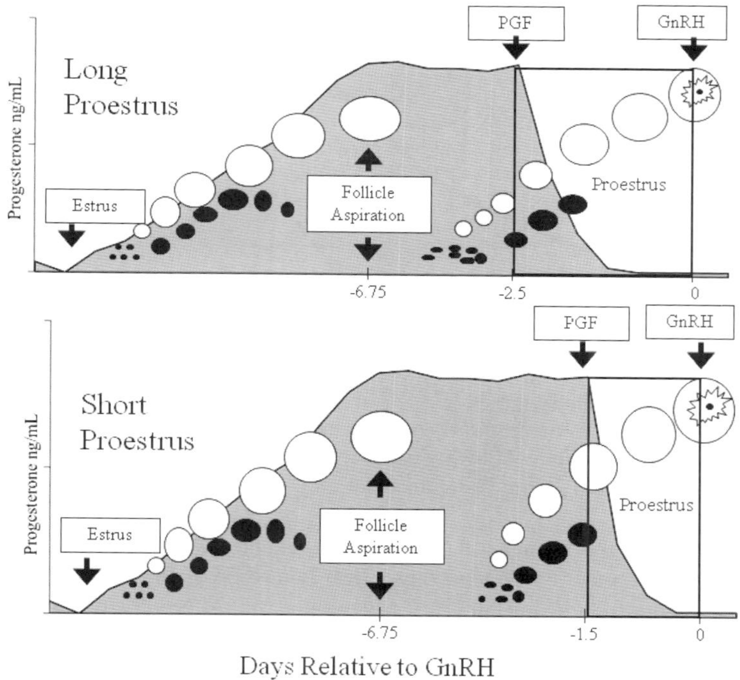

Fig. 2. Animal model used in a series of experiments cited to result in treatments that varied in length of proestrus and prevovulatory estradiol concentrations. Animals were synchronized to a common day of estrus prior to ovarian follicular aspiration. Ovarian follicular aspiration resulted in emergence of a new wave of follicles either 1 or 2 days after aspiration. In the Long Proestrus treatment, $PGF_{2\alpha}$ (PGF) was administered approximately 4 days after aspiration and GnRH given 2.5 days later. In the Short Proestrus treatment, PGF was given 5 days after emergence and GnRH administered 1.5 days later.

Increased gonadotropic stimulus in estradiol-based synchronization programs

Scientists that work with estradiol-based programs (Figure 1) in *Bos indicus* influenced cattle have investigated alternative approaches to enhance gonadotropic stimulation of the dominant follicle during synchronization. The capacity of progesterone to regulate frequency of LH pulses occurs along a continuum of concentrations. If concentrations of progesterone are reduced but not to basal levels, a measurable increase in LH pulse frequency that is capable of stimulating growth of the dominant follicle occurs (Kinder et al., 1996). Therefore, it is conceivable that if progesterone concentrations are less during the period of progestin treatment during estrous synchronization, maturity of the dominant follicle at initiation of proestrus would be advanced and thereby result in increased estradiol concentrations and fertility.

One approach is to induce luteal regression before the end of progestin treatment using $PGF_{2\alpha}$ in order to remove contributions to peripheral progesterone concentrations from the corpus luteum, leaving the exogenous treatment as the only progestin source. When $PGF_{2\alpha}$ was given on the fourth day of an 8-day estradiol based program, pregnancy rate to embryo transfer was enhanced (Moreno et al., 2002). In cyclic cows that received $PGF_{2\alpha}$ on either day 7 or day 9

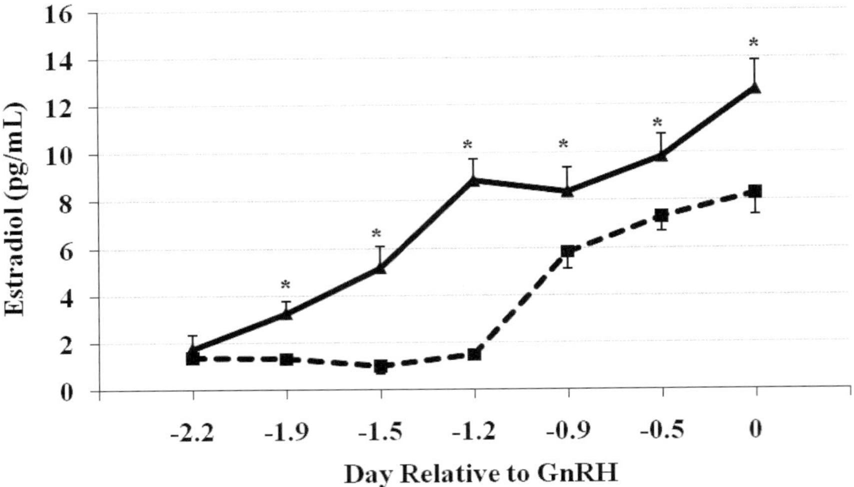

Fig. 3. Preovulatory plasma estradiol concentrations of beef cows that were induced to ovulate a similar sized follicle following either a long (2.2 days; LPE; ▲) or short (1.2 days; SPE; ■) proestrus. Asterisks indicate times that differed ($P < 0.05$) between treatments.

of a 9-day estradiol-based synchronization program (Peres et al., 2009), treatment with $PGF_{2\alpha}$ on day 7 reduced progesterone concentrations on day 9 (just before progestin withdrawal) and increased diameter of the ovulatory follicle and timed-AI pregnancy rate. Alternatively, a device that releases less progesterone, such as a CIDR that has been used previously to synchronize estrus (Martinez et al., 2003), could be inserted to lessen progesterone concentrations during treatment. Diameter of the ovulatory follicle and timed AI pregnancy rate were greater in Nelore heifers that received a twice-used CIDR compared to a new CIDR (Dias et al., 2009). While neither of these approaches technically increases the length of proestrus, the reduction in progesterone concentrations before the onset of proestrus increased follicular diameter, suggesting that the endpoint of increasing maturity of the dominant follicle and timed AI pregnancy rate may have been achieved.

Rather than using the approaches designed to increase endogenous LH listed above, administration of exogenous gonadotropins has also been used enhance follicular maturity. Treatment of beef cows with eCG on the fifth day of an 8-day estradiol based program (Tribulo et al., 2002) increased pregnancy rate of embryo transfer recipients. Likewise, treatment with exogenous eCG at the start of proestrus increased diameter of the ovulatory follicle and timed-AI pregnancy rate in estradiol-based programs (Baruselli et al., 2004; Peres et al., 2009; Dias et al., 2009). With this approach the gonadotropic stimulus is provided exogenously, but a similar net outcome of enhanced follicular growth and fertility is achieved.

Impact of length of proestrus on embryonic mortality

The animal model described in Figure 2 has been used to investigate the impact of length of proestrus and associated changes in preovulatory estradiol concentrations on uterine function and embryo development in cattle (Bridges et al., 2005; 2006a; 2006b; 2010). Due to the impact on estradiol concentrations, hereafter LoE refers to the SPE treatment and HiE refers the LPE treatment. In the first experiment gene expression for oxytocin receptor and cyclooxygenase-2 in the uterus on day 5 of the estrous cycle were greater in LoE than HiE treatment (Bridges et a., 2005) indicating that treatments influence expression of genes known to regulate luteal function. The objective of the second experiment was to determine the effect of decreased preovulatory estradiol concentrations on embryonic development to day 6 of pregnancy (Bridges et al., 2006a). Embryos were collected on day 6 of gestation from cows that were AI following the HiE and LoE treatments. Fertilization rate, embryo grade, total cells per embryo, and accessory sperm cell number were similar between treatments. Although the number of recovered embryos was somewhat limiting, findings indicated that catastrophic defects in early embryo development were not associated with the LoE treatment. In a third experiment, aspects of conceptus and uterine function were compared on day 15.5 of gestation between cows that received the HiE and LoE treatments and were implanted with embryos from untreated cattle on d 15.5 of gestation (Bridges et al., 2006b, Bridges and Day, unpublished). Content of IFN-τ in the uterine lumen and uterine concentrations of mRNA for ISG-15 and MX-1 from pregnant animals did not differ between treatments. Nuclear progesterone receptors, predominantly localized in the deep glandular epithelium were more abundant ($P < 0.05$; Figure 4) in the HiE than LoE treatment. Results of this experiment suggest that up to day 15.5 of pregnancy, decreased preovulatory estradiol concentrations do not impair conceptus development or its ability to induce mRNA for interferon stimulated genes in the uterus. However, alterations in uterine progesterone receptors existed at this stage of pregnancy. Previous research (Table 1) has demonstrated a substantial negative impact of shortened proestrus on pregnancy rate by day 30 after ovulation (either with AI or embryo transfer) and in Experiment 2 (Mussard et al., unpublished) return to estrus following AI for non-pregnant cows with a shortened proestrus was approximately 25 days, suggesting that embryos survived through maternal recognition of pregnancy in some females but were lost shortly thereafter. It is therefore proposed that pregnancy loss in animals that have suboptimal preovulatory estradiol concentrations occurs after maternal recognition of pregnancy during the pre-implantation period but before day 30 of gestation. The hypothesis of ongoing experiments is that decreased preovulatory estradiol concentrations lead to inappropriate gene expression and protein synthesis by the uterus, which results in the inability of the uterus to sustain the conceptus through the pre-implantation period.

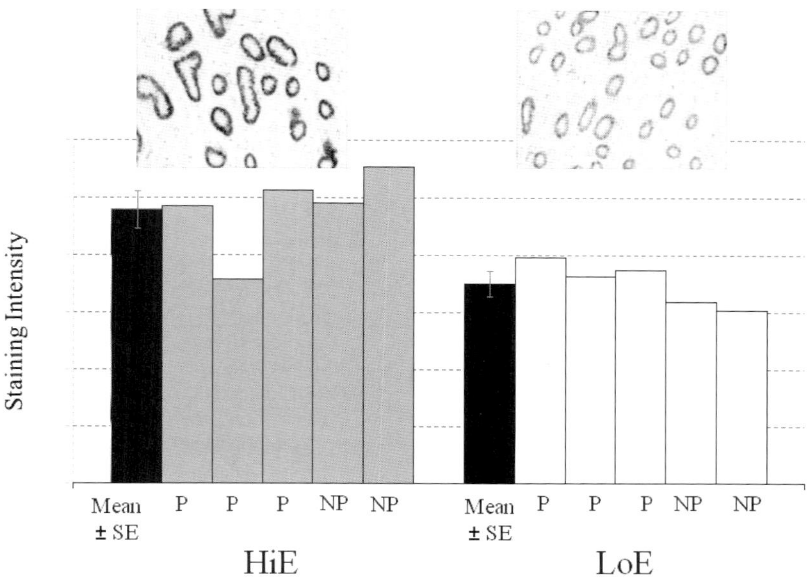

Fig. 4. Nuclear progesterone receptor in the deep uterine glandular epithelium in cattle on day 15.5 of the estrous cycle in pregnant (P) and nonpregnant (NP) heifers that were induced to ovulate a similar sized follicle following either a long proestrus (2.5 days) that increased preovulatory estradiol concentrations (HiE) or a shortened proestrus (1.5 days) that resulted in reduced preovulatory concentrations (LoE). Representative sections from females in each treatment are shown above the respective treatment. Staining intensity differed between treatment, $P < 0.05$.

Conclusions

Significant discoveries in the past two decades in reproductive biology regarding the manner in which ovarian follicles grow, the impact of exogenous intervention on this growth and description of methods to coordinate this process have led to development of estrous synchronization programs that consistently result in timed-AI pregnancy rates of 50% or greater in beef cattle. Recent advancements have pushed this proportion to almost 70% with some programs and emphasize that adequate gonadotropic stimulation of follicular function before ovulation is requisite to optimize fertility. The mechanisms responsible for variation in fertility related to follicular maturity may include influences on oocyte quality, embryonic growth, oviductal function, luteal function or uterine environment, and a combination of some or all of these critical aspects of pregnancy establishment is likely. The findings suggest that the elevated estradiol concentrations that result from increased stimulation of the dominant follicle may be responsible for increased fertility through actions to create a uterine environment capable of sustaining the embryo through to attachment.

Acknowledgements

This project was supported by National Research Initiative Competitive Grants no. 2007-35203-18118 from the USDA National Institute of Food and Agriculture and no. 00-35203-9133 and 94-37203-0923 from the USDA Cooperative State Research, Education, and Extension Service; Select Sires, Plain City, OH; COBA/Select Sires, Columbus, OH; Pfizer Animal Health (New York, NY); and Teva Animal Heath (St Joseph, MO). Salaries and research support provided by State and Federal funds appropriated to the Ohio Agricultural Resource Development Center (OARDC; Manuscript No. 15/10/AS). Appreciation is expressed to graduate students and research personnel that contributed to the project; Les Anderson, Chad McDowell, Valerie Bogacz, Chad Gasser, Lucas Helser, Martin Maquivar, Lucas Souto, Leandro Cruppe, Fernanda Abreu and David Grum.

References

Ahmad N, Schrick FN, Butcher RL & Inskeep EK 1995 Effect of persistent follicles on early embryonic losses in beef cows. *Biology of Reproduction* **52** 1129-1135.

Anderson LH & Day ML 1994 Acute progesterone administration regresses persistent dominant follicles and improves fertility of cattle in which estrus was synchronized with melengestrol acetate. *Journal of Animal Science* **72** 2955-2961.

Anderson LH & Day ML 1998 Development of a progestin-based estrus synchronization program: I. Reproductive response of cows fed melengestrol acetate for 20 days with an injection of progesterone. *Journal of Animal Science* **76** 1267-1272.

Atkins JA, Busch DC, Bader JF, Keisler DH, Patterson DJ, Lucy MC & Smith MF 2008 Gonadotropin-releasing hormone-induced ovulation and luteinizing hormone release in beef heifers: effect of day of the cycle. *Journal of Animal Science* **86** 83-93.

Atkins JA, Smith MF, Wells KJ & Geary TW 2010 Factors affecting pre-ovulatory follicle diameter and ovulation rate to GnRH in postpartum beef cows Part I: Cycling cows. *Journal of Animal Science* **doi:10.2527/j as 2009-2531**.

Baruselli PS, Reis EL, Marques MO, Nasser LF & Bó GA 2004 The use of hormonal treatments to improve reproductive performance of anestrous beef cattle in tropical climates. *Animal Reproduction Science* **82-83** 479-486.

Beal WE, Chenault JR, Day ML & Corah LR 1988 Variation in conception rates following synchronization of estrus with melengestrol acetate and prostaglandin F2α. *Journal of Animal Science* **66** 599-602.

Bo GA, Adams GP, Pierson RA & Mapletoft RJ 1995 Exogenous control of follicular wave emergence in cattle. *Theriogenology* **43** 31-40.

Bridges GA, Mussard ML, Winkler JL, Gasser CL, Grum DE, Pate JL & Day ML 2005 Influence of duration of proestrus on preovulatory estradiol concentrations and uterine gene expression following induced ovulation in cattle. *Proceedings of the 38th Society for the Study of Reproduction Annual Meetings* M451(abstract).

Bridges GA, Mussard ML, Grum DE, Helser LA, Gasser

CL, Dauch DM, Pate JL & Day ML 2006a The influence of pre-ovulatory estradiol concentrations on uterine function in beef cattle. *Journal of Animal Science* **84** (Supplement 2) 101 (abstract).

Bridges GA, Mussard ML, Helser LA, Grum DE, Lantz DM, Ott TL, Pate JL & Day ML 2006b Effect of pre-ovulatory estradiol concentrations on conceptus and uterine development. *Proceedings of the 7th International Ruminant Reproduction Symposium,* 90 (abstract).

Bridges GA, Helser LA, Grum DE, Mussard ML, Gasser CL & Day ML 2008 Decreasing the interval between GnRH and PGF2α from 7 to 5 days and lengthening proestrus increases timed-AI pregnancy rates in beef cows. *Theriogenology* **69** 843–851.

Bridges GA, Mussard ML, Helser LA & Day ML 2009 Comparison of follicular dynamics and hormone concentrations between the 7 d and 5 d CO-Synch + CIDR program in two-year old beef cows. *Journal of Animal Science* **87** (Supplement 2) 372 (abstract).

Bridges GA, Mussard ML, Burke CR & Day ML 2010 Influence of the length of proestrus on fertility and endocrine function in female cattle. *Animal Reproduction Science* **117** 208-215.

Brown LN, Odde KG, LeFever DG, King ME & Neubauer CJ 1988 Comparison of MGA-PGF2α to Syncro-Mate B for estrous synchronization in beef heifers. *Theriogenology* **30** 1–12.

Busch DC, Schafer DJ, Wilson DJ, Mallory DA, Leitman NR, Haden JK, Ellersieck MR, Smith MF & Patterson DJ 2008 Timing of artificial insemination in postpartum beef cows following administration of the CO-Synch + controlled internal drug-release protocol. *Journal of Animal Science* **86** 1519–25.

Burke CR, Morgan S, Clark BA & Rhodes FM 1998 Effect of luteolysis on control of ovarian follicles using oestradiol benzoate and progesterone in cattle. *Proceedings of the New Zealand Society of Animal Production* **58** 89-91.

Burke CR, Day ML, Bunt CR & Macmillan KL 2000 Use of a small dose of estradiol benzoate during diestrus to synchronize development of the ovulatory follicle in cattle. *Journal of Animal Science* **78** 145-151.

Burke CR, Mussard ML, Grum DE & Day ML 2001 Effects of maturity of the potential ovulatory follicle on the provocation of oestrus and ovulation in cattle with oestradiol benzoate. *Animal Reproduction Science* **66** 161-174.

Burke CR, Mussard ML, Gasser CL, Grum DE & Day ML 2003. Estradiol benzoate delays new follicular wave emergence in a dose dependent manner after ablation of the dominant ovarian follicle in cattle. *Theriogenology* **60** 647-658.

Burke CR, Cardenas H, Mussard ML & Day ML 2005 Histological and steroidogenic changes in dominant ovarian follicles during oestradiol-induced atresia in heifers. *Reproduction* **129** 611-620.

Burke CR, Cardenas H, Mussard ML, Gasser CL & Day ML 2007. Steroidogenic changes and expression of messenger RNA encoding steroidogenic enzymes, gonadotrophin receptors and cell-death signaling in the dominant ovarian follicle during oestradiol-induced atresia in cattle. *Animal Reproduction Science* **99** 244-257.

Christian RE & Casida LE 1948 The effect of progesterone in altering the estrual cycle of the cow. *Journal of Animal Science* **7** 540 (abstract).

Cruppe LH, Souto LA, Maquivar M, Gunn P, Mussard ML, Wolfenson D, Pires AV, Bridges GA & Day ML 2010 Use of two coincident doses of PGF2α with the 5-d CO-Synch + CIDR estrous synchronization program. In *ADSA-PSA-AMPA-CSAS-WSASAS-ASAS Joint Annual Meeting,* July 11-15, Denver, Colorado, USA

Day ML 2004 Hormonal induction of estrous cycles in anestrous, Bos taurus beef cows. *Animal Reproduction Science* **82-83** 487-494.

Day ML & Burke CR 2002 Management of follicular growth with progesterone and estradiol within progestin – based estrous synchrony systems. In *Factors Affecting Calf Crop, Biotechnology of Reproduction,* p. 101 Eds Fields MJ, Sand RS & Yelich JV. New York, NY:CRC Press.

Day ML, Burke CR, Taufa VK, Day AM & Macmillan KL 2000. The strategic use of estradiol to enhance fertility and submission rates of progestin based estrus synchronization programs in seasonal dairy herds. *Journal of Animal Science* **78** 523-529.

Dias CC,Wechsler FS, Day ML & Vasconcelos JLM 2009 Progesterone concentrations, exogenous eCG and timing of prostaglandin F2α treatment affect fertility in postpubertal Nelore heifers. *Theriogenology* **72** 378–385.

Dobbins CA, Eborn DR, Tenhouse DE, Breiner RM, Johnson SK, Marston TT &. Stevenson JS 2009 Insemination timing affects pregnancy rates in beef cows treated with CO-Synch protocol including an intravaginal progesterone insert. *Theriogenology* **72** 1009–1016.

Engelhardt H, Walton JS, Miller RB & King GJ 1989 Estradiol-induced blockade of ovulation in the cow: Effects of luteinizing hormone release and follicular fluid steroids. *Biology of Reproduction* **40** 1287-1297.

Geary TW, Downing ER, Bruemmer JE & Whittier JC 2000 Ovarian and estrous response of suckled beef cows to the select synch estrous synchronization protocol. *The Professional Animal Scientist* **16** 1-5.

Geary TW, Salverson RR & Whittier JC 2001 Synchronization of ovulation using GnRH or hCG with the CO-Synch protocol in suckled beef cows. *Journal of Animal Science* **79** 2536-2541.

Ginther O J, Knopf L & Kastelic JP 1989 Temporal associations among ovarian events in cattle during oestrous cycles with two and three follicular waves. *Journal of Reproduction and Fertility* **87** 223-230.

Ireland JJ & Roche JF 1983 Growth and differentiation of large antral follicles after spontaneous luteolysis in heifers: Changes in concentration of hormones in follicular fluid and specific binding of gonadotropins to follicles. *Journal of Animal Science* **57** 157-167.

Kaltenbach CC, Dunn TG, Kiser TE, Corah LR, Akbar AM

& Niswender GD 1974 Release of FSH and LH in beef heifers by synthetic gonadotropin releasing hormone. *Journal of Animal Science* **38** 357-362.

Kaneko H, Terada T, Taya K, Watanabe G, Sasamoto S, Hasegawa Y & Igarashi M 1991 Ovarian follicular dynamics and concentrations of oestradiol-17ß, progesterone, luteinizing hormone and follicle stimulating hormone during the periovulatory phase of the oestrous cycle in the cow. *Reproduction Fertility & Development* **3** 529-535.

Kasimanickam R, Day ML, Rudolph JS, Hall JB & Whittier WD 2009 Two doses of prostaglandin improve pregnancy rates to timed-AI in a 5-day progesterone-based synchronization protocol in beef cows. *Theriogenology* **71** 762-767.

Kinder JE, Kojima FN, Bergfeld EGM, Wehrman ME & Fike KE 1996 Progestin and estrogen regulation of pulsatile LH release and development of persistent ovarian follicles in cattle. *Journal of Animal Science* **74** 1424-1440.

King ME, Kiracofe GH, Stevenson JS & Schalles RR 1982 Effect of stage of the estrous cycle on interval to estrus after PGF2α in beef cattle. *Theriogenology* **18** 191-200.

Lamb GC, Nix DW, Stevenson JS & Corah LR 2000. Prolonging the MGA-Prostaglandin F2α interval from 17 to 19 days in an estrus synchronization system for heifers. *Theriogenology* **53** 691–698.

Lamb GC, Stevenson JS, Kesler DJ, Garverick HA, Broan DR & Salfen BE 2001 Inclusion of an intravaginal progesterone insert plus GnRH and prostaglandin F2a for ovulation control in postpartum suckled beef cows. *Journal of Animal Science* **79** 2253-2259.

Larson JE, Lamb GC, Stevenson JS, Johnson SK, Day ML, Geary TW, Kesler DJ, DeJarnette JM, Schrick FN, DiCostanzo A & Arseneau JD 2006 Synchronization of estrus in suckled beef cows before detected estrus and (or) timed artificial insemination using gonadotropin-releasing hormone (GnRH), prostaglandin F2α (PG), and progesterone (CIDR). *Journal of Animal Science* **84** 332-342.

Lauderdale JW 1975 The use of prostaglandin in cattle. *Annales de Biologie Animale Biochimie Biophysique* **15** 419-425.

Lemon M, Pelletier J, Saumande J & Signoret JP 1975 Peripheral plasma concentrations of progesterone, oestradio-17ß and luteinizing hormone around oestrus in the cow. *Journal of Reproduction and Fertility* **42** 137-140.

Macmillan KL & Thatcher WW 1991 Effects of an agonist of gonadotropin-releasing hormone on ovarian follicles in cattle. *Biology of Reproduction* **45** 883-889.

Mallory DA, Wilson DJ,Busch DC, Ellersieck MR, Smith MF & Patterson DJ 2010 Comparison of long-term progestin-based estrus synchronization protocols in beef heifers *Journal of Animal Science* **doi**:10.2527jas.2010-3084.

Martínez MF, Colazo MG, Kastelic JP & Mapletoft RJ 2003a Effects of estradiol and progesterone on plasma steroid and gonadotropin concentrations in CIDR-treated ovariectomized cows. *Theriogenology* **59** 224 (abstract).

Mauleon P 1974 New trends in the control of reproduction in the bovine. *Livestock Production Science* **1** 117-131.

McCracken JA, Carlson JC, Glew ME, Goding JR, Baird DT, Green K & Samuelsson B 1972 Prostaglandin F2α identified as a luteolytic hormone in sheep. *Nature New Biology* **238** 129-134.

McDowell CM, Anderson LH, Kinder JE & Day ML 1998a Duration of treatment with progesterone and regression of persistent ovarian follicles in cattle. *Journal of Animal Science* **76** 850-855.

McDowell CM, Anderson LH, Lemenager RP, Mangione DA & Day ML 1998b Development of a progestin-based estrus synchronization program: II. Reproductive response of cows fed melengestrol acetate for 14 days with injections of progesterone and prostaglandin F2a. *Journal of Animal Science* **76** 1273-1279.

Meneghetti M, Sa´ Filho OG, Peres RFG, Lamb GC & Vasconcelos JLM 2009 Fixed-time artificial insemination with estradiol and progesterone for Bos indicus cattle: I. Basis for development of protocols. *Theriogenology* **72** 179–189.

Mihm M, Baguisi A, Boland MP & Roche JF 1994 Association between the duration of dominance of the ovulatory follicle and pregnancy rate in beef heifers. *Journal of Reproduction and Fertility* **102** 123-130.

Miksch ED, LeFever DG, Mukembo G, Spitzer JC & Wiltbank JN 1978 Synchronization of estrus in beef cattle. II. Effect of an injection of norgestomet and an estrogen in conjunction with a norgestomet implant in heifers and cows. *Theriogenology* **10** 201-221.

Moreira F, de la Sota RL, Diaz T & Thatcher WW 2000 Effect of day of the estrous cycle at the initiation of a timed artificial insemination protocol on reproductive responses in dairy heifers. *Journal of Animal Science* **78** 1568-1576.

Moreno D, Cutaia L, Tribulo H, Tribulo R, Villata ML, Caccia M & Bo G 2002 Effect of time of prostaglandin administration on pregnancy rates in embryo recipients treated with progesterone vaginal devices and transferred without estrus detection. *Theriogenology* **57** 552 (abstract).

Mussard ML, Burke CR & Day ML 2003 Ovarian follicle maturity at induced ovulation influences fertility in cattle. *Proceedings of the Annual Conference of the Society for Theriogenology* 79-185.

Mussard ML, Burke CR, Behlke EJ, Gasser CL & Day ML 2007 Influence of premature induction of an LH surge with GnRH on ovulation, luteal function and fertility in cattle. *Journal of Animal Science* **85** 937-943.

Odde KG 1990 A review of synchronization of estrus in postpartum cattle. *Journal of Animal Science* **68** 817-830.

Peres RFG, Claro Junior I, Sa´ Filho OG, Nogueira GP &Vasconcelos JLM 2009 Strategies to improve fertility in Bos indicus postpubertal heifers and nonlactating cows submitted to fixed-time artificial insemination. *Theriogenology* **72** 681–689.

Perry GA, Smith MF, Lucy MC, Green JA, Parks TE, MacNeil MD, Roberts AJ, & Geary TW 2005. Relationship between follicle size at insemination and pregnancy success. *Proceedings of the National Academy of Science USA* **5268-5273.**

Perry GA, Smith MF, Roberts AJ, MacNeil MD & Geary TW 2007. Relationship between size of the ovulatory follicle and pregnancy success in beef heifers. *Proceedings of the National Academy of Science USA* **5268-5273.**

Pursley JR, Mee MO & Wiltbank MC 1995 Synchronization of ovulation in dairy cows using PGF2α and GnRH. *Theriogenology* **44** 915-923.

Rajakoski E 1960 The ovarian follicular system in sexually mature heifers with special reference to seasonal, cyclical, and left-right variations. *Acta Endocrinologica* **34** (Supplement 52) 1-68.

Sa´ Filho OG, Meneghetti M, Peres RFG, Lamb GC & Vasconcelos JLM 2009 Fixed-time artificial insemination with estradiol and progesterone for Bos indicus cattle: II. Strategies and factors affecting fertility. *Theriogenology* **72** 210–218.

Savio JD, Keenan L & Boland MP 1988 Pattern of growth of dominant follicles during the oestrous cycle of heifers. *Journal of Reproduction and Fertility* **83** 663-671.

Savio JD, Thatcher WW, Morris GR, Entwistle K, Drost M & Mattiacci MR 1993 Effects of induction of low plasma progesterone concentrations with a progesterone-releasing device on follicular turnover and fertility in cattle. *Journal of Reproduction and Fertility* **98** 77-84.

Sirois J & Fortune JE 1988 Ovarian follicular dynamics during the estrous cycle in heifers monitored by real-time ultrasonography. *Biology of Reproduction* **39** 308-317.

Sirois J & Fortune JE 1990 Lengthening the bovine estrous cycle with low levels of exogenous progesterone: a model for studying ovarian follicular dominance. *Endocrinology* **127** 916-925.

Souto LA, Maquivar M, Mussard ML, Bridges GA, Grum DE & Day ML 2009 Fertility and luteal regression with 5-d CIDR synchronization programs in postpartum beef cows using differing luteolytic treatments. *Journal of Animal Science* **87** (Supplement 2) 372 (abstract).

Stock AE, Fortune JE 1993 Ovarian follicular dominance in cattle: relationship between prolonged growth of the ovulatory follicle and endocrine parameters. *Endocrinology* **132** 1108-1114.

Thatcher WW, Macmillan KL, Hansen PJ & Drost M 1989 Concepts for regulation of corpus luteum function by the conceptus and ovarian follicles to improve fertility. *Theriogenology* **31** 149-164.

Thimonier J, Chupin D & Pelot J 1975 Synchronization of oestrus in heifers and cyclic cows with progestagens and prostaglandin analogues alone or in combination. *Annales de Biologie Animale Biochimie Biophysique* **15** 437-449.

Tribulo H, Moreno D, Cutaia L, Gatti G, Tribulo R, Caccia M & Bo GA 2002 Pregnancy rates in embryo recipients treated with progesterone vaginal devices, and eCG and transferred without estrus detection. *Theriogenology* **57** 563 (abstract).

Trimberger GW & Hansel W 1955 Conception rate and ovarian function following estrus control by progesterone injections in dairy cattle. *Journal of Animal Science* **14** 224-232.

Twagiramungu H, Guilbault LA, Proulx JG & Dufour JJ 1994 Influence of corpus luteum and induced ovulation on ovarian follicular dynamics in postpartum cyclic cows treated with buserelin and cloprostenol. *Journal of Animal Science* **72** 1796-1805.

Twagiramungu H, Guilbault LA & Dufour JJ 1995 Synchronization of Ovarian Follicular Waves with a Gonadotropin-Releasing Hormone Agonist to Increase the Precision of Estrus in Cattle: A Review. *Journal of Animal Science* **73** 3141–3151.

Valdez KE, Cuneo SP, Gorden PJ & Turzillo AM 2005 The role of thecal androgen production in the regulation of estradiol biosynthesis by dominant bovine follicles during the first follicular wave. *Journal of Animal Science* **83** 597-603.

Wiltbank JN & Kasson CW 1968 Synchronization of estrus in cattle with an oral progestational agent and an injection of an oestrogen. *Journal of Animal Science* **27** 113-116.

Wilson KN, Day ML, Whittier WD, Kasimanickam R & Hall JB 2007 Comparison of 5-day or 7-day CIDR-based estrous synchronization systems for fixed-time AI in beef heifers. *Journal of Animal Science* **85** (Supplement 2) 43 (abstract).

Wishart DF 1974 Synchronization of oestrus in cattle using a progestogen (SC21009) and PGF2α. *Theriogenology* **1** 87-90.

Wishart DF 1977 Synchronization of oestrus in heifers using steriod (SC 5914, SC 9880 and SC 21009) treatment for 21 days: The effect of treatment on the ovum collection and fertilization rate and the development of the early embryo. *Theriogenology* **8** 249-269.

Zimbelman RG, Smith LW 1966 Control of ovulation in cattle with melengestrol acetate. II. Effects on follicular size and activity. *Journal of Reproduction and Fertility* **11** 193-201.

Zimbelman RG, Lauderdale JW, Sokolowski JH, Schalk TG 1970 Safety and pharmacologic evaluations of melengestrol acetate in cattle and other animals: A review. *Journal of the American Veterinary Medical Association* **157** 1528-36.

Causes and consequences of the variation in the number of ovarian follicles in cattle

ACO Evans[1], F Mossa[1], T Fair[1], P Lonergan[1], ST Butler[2], AE Zielak-Steciwko[3], GW Smith[4], F Jimenez-Krassel[5], JK Folger[5], JLH Ireland[5] and JJ Ireland[5]

[1]School of Agriculture Food Science and Veterinary Medicine, and the Conway Institute, College of Life Sciences, University College Dublin, Belfield, Dublin 4, Ireland; [2]Moorepark Dairy Production Research Centre, Teagasc, Fermoy, Co. Cork, Ireland; [3]Institute of Animal Breeding, Faculty of Biology and Animal Science, Wroclaw University of Environmental and Life Sciences, 50-375 Wroclaw, Poland; [4]Laboratory of Mammalian Reproductive Biology and Genomics, [5]Molecular Reproductive Endocrinology Laboratory Department of Animal Science, Michigan State University, East Lansing, Michigan 48824, USA

Summary

In cattle we have noted that the antral follicle count (AFC, follicles ≥3 mm in diameter) varies greatly among animals (from 5 to 50), is repeatable within animals, and is highly correlated with the total number of healthy follicles in ovaries. Also, animals with low AFC have higher serum concentrations of FSH and LH, but lower concentrations of Anti-Mullerian Hormone, progesterone and androgens than animals with high AFC. We have investigated the effect of maternal environment during gestation on their offspring AFC by restricting maternal nutrition to 60% of maintenance requirements (compared with 100% in controls) during the first third of gestation. Calves born to nutritionally restricted mothers had 60% lower AFC compared with calves born to mothers fed control diets. In other studies we have evidence to indicate that fertility may be compromised in animals with low AFC due to effects on oocytes, progesterone and the endometrium compared with animals with high AFC. To examine this directly we assessed AFC in post-partum dairy cows and found that cows with a high AFC had higher pregnancy rates, shorter calving to conception intervals and received fewer services during the breeding season compared with cows with a low AFC. In addition, the high variation in follicle numbers in adults may not only be reflective of reproductive disorders and suboptimal fertility, but there is evidence to indicate that it may be associated with alterations in the function of other non-reproductive systems (e.g. cardiovascular) that may have profound effects on the animal's health and welfare.

Corresponding author E-mail: alex.evans@ucd.ie

Introduction

In cattle, growth of ovarian antral follicles from about 300 μm to 5 mm in diameter takes more than 30 days (Lussier *et al.* 1987). Subsequent follicle growth to 15 to 20 mm in diameter is rapid and occurs in a wave-like pattern over the next 4 to 6 days with two or three waves occurring during the normal course of oestrous cycles in cattle (Evans 2003). The wave-like pattern of follicle growth was first proposed by Rajakoski in 1960 after a large study examining the number of follicles >1 mm in diameter in the ovaries of slaughtered cattle on different days of the cycle (Ireland *et al.* 2000). Rajakoski's observation, that the numbers of follicles increased and decreased in a wave-like pattern, gave rise to the two follicle wave hypothesis (Rajakoski 1960). Ireland and Roche used intrafollicular concentrations of oestradiol to progesterone to classify antral follicles ≥ 6 mm in diameter and proposed the three-wave hypothesis for dominant follicle development in cattle (Ireland & Roche 1982, Ireland & Roche 1983b, Ireland & Roche 1983a, Ireland & Roche 1987). The development of ultrasonography as a tool to noninvasively monitor the growth and regression of individual ovarian follicles repeatedly in the same animal (Pierson & Ginther 1984) firmly established that antral follicles grow in cohorts, in two or three wave-like patterns during oestrous cycles in cattle (Pierson & Ginther 1988, Savio *et al.* 1988, Sirois & Fortune 1988). This finding was later extended to other reproductive periods in cattle and to other species (Ireland *et al.* 2000, Evans 2003). Numerous subsequent studies examined the associations among reproductive hormones and follicle growth (Mihm *et al.* 2002). However, the observations that the number of primordial follicles is highly variable in cattle at birth (Erickson 1966b), that the number of different follicle types vary greatly among adult cattle, and that they reliably ovulate one, or occasionally two, follicles during each oestrous cycle prompted further investigations into the variation in ovarian follicle numbers in cattle.

Variation in the numbers of ovarian follicles and associated reproductive hormones

Follicle numbers

Our research groups have now conducted a number of studies that have systematically counted and catalogued the numbers of antral follicles on different days of the oestrous cycle in both beef and dairy heifers and in post-partum dairy cows. We have established that the numbers of follicles in ovarian follicular waves of the oestrous cycle are highly variable among animals but very highly repeatable within individuals (Burns *et al.* 2005, Ireland *et al.* 2007, Ireland *et al.* 2008, Jimenez-Krassel *et al.* 2009) (Mossa *et al.* 2010b). This observation holds true when considering the peak or nadir numbers associated with waves or the mean numbers across all days of the cycle. However, the count must include all the follicles ≥ 3 mm in diameter in both ovaries (the antral follicle count or AFC) and explains why many studies in the last 20 years that have focused on follicles ≥ 5 or 6 mm in diameter have not noted the high variability of follicle numbers growing during follicular waves among animals nor the remarkably high repeatability of follicle numbers during waves in individuals. For example, we have noted that the AFC in both ovaries during different follicular waves of an oestrous cycle may be consistently lower than 5 during follicular waves in some animals and greater than 50 in others (Burns *et al.* 2005, Ireland *et al.* 2007, Mossa *et al.* 2010b) (Figure 1). Moreover, this high repeatability of follicle numbers during waves persists for at least one year (Burns *et al.* 2005).

The observation of the variation in AFC raises questions about the possibility for variation in the total numbers of follicles in the ovaries. To address this, age matched heifers (adult cycling animal 12 to 18 months of age) that had high (≥25) or low (≤15) AFC were identified, and the numbers of all follicles in the ovaries were counted in histological sections (Ireland *et al.* 2008).

This study showed that the AFC reliably predicted the numbers of morphologically healthy follicles in all classes of the stages of folliculogenesis (Ireland *et al.* 2008) (Figure 2). For example, cattle with a low AFC also had a very low total number of healthy primordial, preantral and antral follicles in ovaries compared with cattle with a high AFC (Ireland *et al.* 2008).

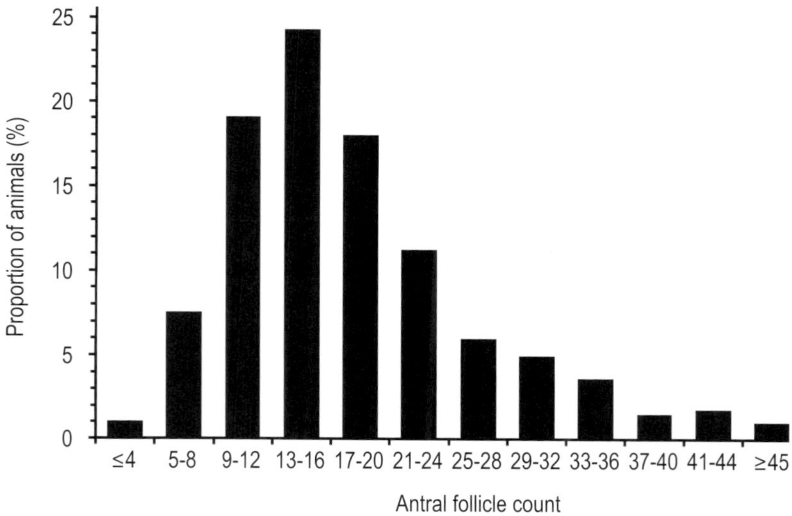

Fig. 1. Frequency distribution of the number of follicles ≥3mm in diameter (Antral Follicle Count) in post-partum Holstein–Friesian dairy cows (n = 383) measured using ultrasonography (Mossa et al unpublished)

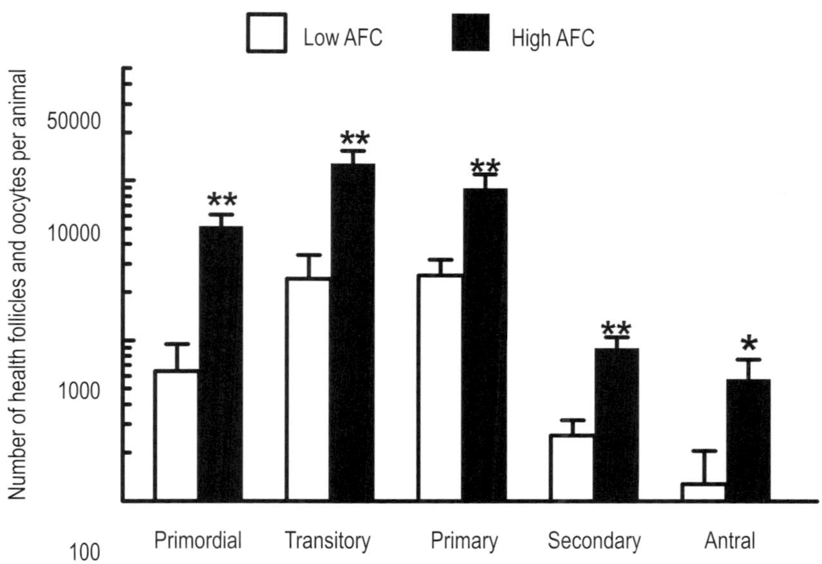

Fig. 2. Number of morphologically healthy primordial, transitory, primary, secondary, and antral follicles in ovaries of cattle with a low (≤15 follicles, n = 5) versus a high (≥25 follicles, n = 5) numbers of follicles ≥3 mm in diameter (Antral Follicle Count, AFC) during ovarian follicular waves. The ovary contralateral to the recent ovulation was removed surgically 1–2 days after ovulation and histologically examined. Asterisks (*$P < 0.05$, **$P < 0.01$) indicate difference between means for the low versus high group. From (Ireland *et al.* 2008).

Hormones

Transient rises in FSH concentrations precede and stimulate the emergence of follicle waves (Adams *et al.* 1992). A number of studies have now shown that FSH concentrations are lower in animals with high AFC compared with animals with low AFC (Burns *et al.* 2005, Ireland *et al.* 2007, Mossa *et al.* 2010b). In addition, circulating LH concentrations during the estrous cycle are chronically higher in young adult cattle with low versus high AFC (Jimenez-Krassel *et al.* 2009). This observation leads to the question as to whether pituitary function differs between the two groups of animals. We tested this notion by examining the response to ovariectomy of cows with high or low AFC and then challenging them with GnRH and follicular fluid (rich source of inhibin) on separate occasions 30 days after ovariectomy (Mossa *et al.* 2010b). The study showed that there was no difference between the two groups in basal FSH or LH secretion or response to the treatments leading to the conclusion that differences in gonadotrophin secretion between cows with high versus low AFC is due to differences in negative feedback hormones and not differences in pituitary function (Mossa *et al.* 2010b).

Evidence that the total number of healthy follicles in ovaries contributes to the endocrine environment is provided by examining Anti-Müllerian Hormone (AMH) concentrations. AMH is produced primarily by granulosa cells of healthy growing follicles (La Marca & Volpe 2006) and is positively associated with follicle numbers in mice (Kevenaar *et al.* 2006) and women (Jayaprakasan *et al.* 2009, van Disseldorp *et al.* 2009). It has recently been shown that AMH concentrations can reliably predict the AFC and the number of healthy follicles and oocytes in age matched young adult cattle (Ireland *et al.* 2008). Furthermore, AMH serum concentrations before superovulation are highly positively correlated with the numbers of ovulations after treatment (Rico *et al.* 2009) and are repeatable within animals (Ireland *et al.* 2008, Rico *et al.* 2009). In comparison to AMH, serum concentrations of both oestradiol and inhibin-A, the main feedback regulators of FSH secretion, are not different between groups of animals with high and low AFC (Burns *et al.* 2005, Ireland *et al.* 2007). This may be explained by the fact that individual follicles from cattle with low AFC have higher follicular fluid concentrations and produce more oestradiol than follicles from animals with high AFC (Ireland *et al.* 2009) and we have speculated that this difference may be a consequence of higher circulating FSH concentrations in the low versus the high AFC groups (Ireland *et al.* 2009). Nonetheless it appears that the total oestradiol negative feedback is similar between the high and low groups as fewer follicles produce more oestradiol in the low AFC animals compared with more follicles producing lower oestradiol in the high AFC group (at least within the limits of sensitivity of our oestradiol assay). Despite not being able to measure a difference in circulating oestradiol concentrations between high and low AFC groups, we have recently shown that circulating androgen concentrations are indeed higher in cattle with high compared with low AFC (Jimenez-Krassel *et al.* 2009). In the absence of an alternative explanation, we suggest that the difference in circulating gonadotrophin concentrations associated with variable AFC is due to differences in ovarian feedback hormones produced by the follicles.

Due to the considerable interest in the contribution of early/mid luteal phase progesterone concentrations for the successful establishment of pregnancy, we compared progesterone concentrations between groups of animals and found that animals with low AFC have much lower progesterone concentrations during oestrous cycles than animals with high AFC (Jimenez-Krassel *et al.* 2009) (Figure 3). Also the ability of both granulosa and luteal cells from animals with low AFC to produce progesterone in vitro was diminished compared with animals with high AFC (Jimenez-Krassel *et al.* 2009). The possible consequences of this difference in progesterone concentrations are discussed below.

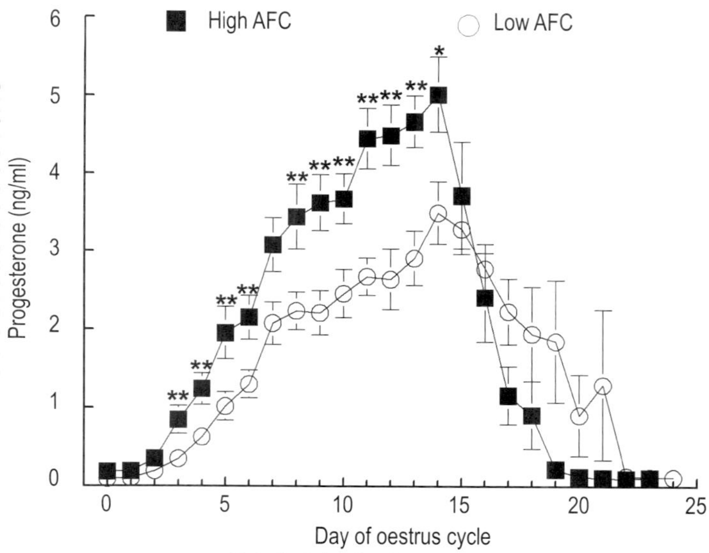

Fig. 3. Alterations in serum concentrations of progesterone during the bovine oestrous cycle (Day 0 = oestrus). Each symbol represents the daily mean (±SEM) progesterone value for animals with a consistently low (≤ 15 follicles per wave, n = 32 oestrous cycles for 25 animals) versus high (≥ 25 follicles per wave, n = 30 cycles for 22 animals) AFC during follicular waves. Asterisks indicate significant differences (** $P < 0.01$) between groups. ANOVA indicated an overall significant effect of group (Low versus High, $P<0.02$), day of cycle ($P<0.001$) and group x day interaction ($P<0.001$). From (Jimenez-Krassel *et al.* 2009).

Causes of the variation in the numbers of ovarian follicles

The cause of the inherently high variation in number of follicles is unknown but a number of explanations are plausible. Firstly, proliferation of oogonia during early embryonic development (that give rise to a fixed pool of non proliferating oocytes within primordial follicles for the lifetime of the animal) may be highly variable resulting in a highly variable pool of follicles. Secondly, proliferation of oogonia may be relatively constant (similar among females) but depletion of this pool may proceed at different rates among individuals giving rise to females with differing AFC at the same age. Thirdly, the variation in follicle numbers among age matched females occurs as a result of a combination of the first two possibilities.

David Barker (the Barker Hypothesis) suggests that environmental influences early in human foetal life are reflected in impaired growth, development and metabolism leading to increased risk for diseases in adulthood (Barker 1992). The hypothesis proposes that some diseases originate through foetal adaptations to malnutrition that permanently alter body function. This hypothesis is supported by animal models (McMillen & Robinson 2005). Most studies have examined the link between malnutrition with cardiovascular disease, obesity and diabetes, but few studies have examined potential links with reproduction. However, poor foetal growth due to the manipulation of maternal diet alters gonadotrophin gene expression in the pituitary and number of follicles in the ovaries of late-gestation lambs (Da Silva *et al.* 2002). In addition, maternal under-nutrition during the first trimester retards foetal ovarian development in sheep (Borwick *et al.* 1997). Hence, it is reasonable to speculate that maternal nutrition during gestation, at the time of ovarian development in their foetuses, may impact oogonia proliferation and thus follicle numbers postnatally. We have recently started to test this hypothesis by restricting nutrition of beef heifers to 0.6 of their maintenance energy requirements, from shortly before conception to the end of the first trimester of pregnancy (period encompassing the peak in oocyte numbers in foetuses (Erickson 1966a)). Results show that calves born to nutritionally restricted mothers have a 60% lower peak, minimum and mean AFC during follicular waves compared with calves born to mothers fed control diets (Mossa *et al.* 2009) (Table 1). In addition, calves born to dams nutritionally restricted also show higher resting arterial blood pressure compared with those born to control mothers (Mossa *et al.* 2009). In addition, similar studies in *Bos indicus* cross heifers support the notion that prenatal maternal nutrition affects ovarian measures in their offspring (Sullivan *et al.* 2009).

Table 1. Mean (± SEM) number of follicles ≥3 mm in diameter (Antral Follicle Count) during follicle waves in heifer calves born to mothers fed a control diet (Control) or who were nutritionally restricted (Restricted, 60% energy requirement) for the first 110 days of gestation. From (Mossa *et al.* 2009).

Heifer age (weeks)	Antral Follicle Count		
	Control (n = 13)	Restricted (n = 10)	P<
7	23.9±2.1	14.1±0.9	0.01
18	26.1±2.9	16.2±1.1	0.01
35	23.9±2.2	16.6±1.2	0.01

The Barker Hypothesis, and supporting data in a variety of animal models, indicates that a negative uterine environment can influence the development of different organs and systems in the foetus including the reproductive system. This observation may have relevance for the dairy industry, since it is well established that selecting dairy cows for increased milk production potential has been associated with a concomitant decrease in fertility and an increase in the susceptibility to some diseases (Beckers *et al.* 2002). In order to have a 365-day calving interval, cows must conceive during the period of their peak lactation. This period of peak metabolic stress is coincident with follicle growth, ovulation, fertilization, early embryonic development and early foetal development. According to the Barker Hypothesis, animals conceived and developing in this nutritionally stressed maternal environment may have compromised development that could affect them for the rest of their lives. We have investigated the relationship between maternal milk production (a proxy for maternal stress) on performance indicators in the first, second, and third lactations of their female offspring using a large Irish database and results have shown that greater milk yield preconception and during gestation is associated with reduced survival and milk yield and greater somatic cell count in their progeny (Berry *et al.* 2008). This shows that maternal environment during gestation in dairy cows does have long-term effects on their female offspring but we have not yet investigated the effects of AFC.

Consequences of the variation in the numbers of ovarian follicles

In women undergoing IVF treatment, the number of antral follicles present before ovarian stimulation is considered a predictor of the ovarian responsiveness to gonadotrophin stimulation, since low numbers of follicles are associated with lower numbers of oocytes recovered and pregnancy rates (Tomas *et al.* 1997, Chang *et al.* 1998, Hsieh *et al.* 2001, Huang *et al.* 2001, Beckers *et al.* 2002). Similarly in cattle the number of follicles prior to superovulatory treatment is correlated with the numbers of follicles and corpora lutea after superovulation, and total ova and transferable embryos recovered (Kawamata 1994, Cushman *et al.* 1999, Taneja *et al.* 2000, Singh *et al.* 2004). Moreover, intrafollicular oestradiol concentrations are about 2-fold higher in animals with a low versus a high AFC (Ireland *et al.* 2009) and this may have detrimental effects on oocyte maturation and developmental competence in cattle with low follicle numbers because high physiological concentrations of oestradiol block maturation of bovine oocytes in vitro (Beker-van Woudenberg *et al.* 2004). In addition, lower circulating concentrations of progesterone in cattle with low AFC are associated with a much lower endometrial thickness from Day 0 to 6 of the oestrous cycle (Jimenez-Krassel *et al.* 2009) and endometrial thickness is positively associated with implantation and pregnancy rates in humans subjected to in vitro fertilization programs (Raga *et al.* 1999). Taken together these findings indicate that AFC is positively associated with fertility in cattle. To test this hypothesis we performed ovarian ultrasonography on 306 dairy cows (aged 3.48 ± 1.66 years) during the first wave of follicular development 1 to 4 months post-partum and recorded their reproductive performances during the breeding season. Cows with a high AFC had higher pregnancy rates, shorter calving to conception intervals and received fewer services during the breeding season compared with cows with a low AFC (Mossa *et al.* 2010a). This is supported by a study in beef heifers showing higher pregnancy rates in heifers with high AFC versus low AFC (Cushman *et al.* 2009).

Conclusion

Improved understanding of the pattern of follicle development in the last 20 years has led to the development of more effective treatments to synchronize (and induce) oestrus behaviour in cattle. The recent studies reviewed here indicate that the variation in number of follicles growing during follicle waves, and in toto in ovaries, may be an important consideration when new methods are developed to manipulate and improve superovulation and fertility in cattle. Moreover, the variation in number of oocytes and follicles in offspring may be determined by the maternal environment during foetal development coincident with development of all the organ systems. Thus, the high variation in follicle numbers in adults may not only be reflective of reproductive disorders and suboptimal fertility, but also alterations in other non-reproductive systems that may have profound effects on the animal's health and welfare.

Grant support

AE, FM, TF and PL are supported by grants from Science Foundation Ireland (07/SRC/B1156) and from the Irish Department of Agriculture, Fisheries and Food, Research Stimulus Fund programme 2006 (RSF 06-328).

SB is supported by funds from the National Development Plan, the Irish Dairy Levy Trust, and Irish Department of Agriculture, Fisheries and Food, Research Stimulus Fund programme 2006 (RSF 06-328).

AEZ-S is supported by a grant from the Polish Ministry of Science and Higher Education (N N311 324136).

GWS is supported by grants from the National Research Initiative Competitive Grant no. 2005-35203-16011 from the USDA National Institute of Food and Agriculture, Agriculture and Food Research Initiative Competitive Grant no. 2009-65203-05700 from the USDA National Institute of Food and Agriculture, and by the Michigan Agricultural Experiment Station

JJI is supported by National Research Initiative Competitive Grants 2001-002255, 2004-01697 and 2007-01289 from the USDA Cooperative State Research, Education and Extension Service and by funds from the Michigan Agriculture Experiment Station.

Acknowledgements

We thank D Berry for his comments on this manuscript.

References

Adams GP, Matteri RL, Kastelic JP, Ko JCH & Ginther OJ 1992 Association between surges of follicle-stimulating hormone and the emergence of follicular waves in heifers. *Journal of Reproduction and Fertility* **94** 177-188.

Barker DJ 1992 The effect of nutrition of the fetus and neonate on cardiovascular disease in adult life. *Proceedings of the Nutrition Society* **51** 135-144.

Beckers NGM, Macklon NS, Eijkemans MJC & Fauser BCJM 2002 Women with regular menstrual cycles and a poor response to ovarian hyperstimulation for in vitro fertilization exhibit follicular phase characteristics suggestive of ovarian aging. *Fertility and Sterility* **78** 291-297.

Beker-van Woudenberg AR, van Tol HTA, Roelen BAJ, Colenbrander B & Bevers MM 2004 Estradiol and its membrane-impermeable conjugate (estradiol-bovine serum albumin) during in vitro maturation of bovine oocytes: effects on nuclear and cytoplasmic maturation, cytoskeleton, and embryo quality. *Biol Reprod* **70** 1465-1474.

Berry DP, Lonergan P, Butler ST, Cromie AR, Fair T, Mossa F & Evans ACO 2008 Negative influence of high maternal milk production before and after conception on offspring survival and milk production in dairy cattle. *Journal of Dairy Science* **91** 329-337.

Borwick SC, Rhind SM, McMillen SR & Racey PA 1997 Effect of undernutrition of ewes from the time of mating on fetal ovarian development in mid gestation. *Reproduction Fertility and Development* **9** 711-715.

Burns DS, Jimenez-Krassel F, Ireland JL, Knight PG & Ireland JJ 2005 Numbers of antral follicles during follicular waves in cattle: evidence for high variation among animals, very high repeatability in individuals, and an inverse association with serum follicle-stimulating hormone concentrations. *Biology of Reproduction* **73** 54-62.

Chang MY, Chiang CH, Hsieh TT, Soong YK & Hsu KH 1998 Use of the antral follicle count to predict the outcome of assisted reproductive technologies. *Fertility and Sterility* **69** 505-510.

Cushman RA, Allan MF, Kuehn LA, Snelling WM, Cupp AS & Freetly HC 2009 Evaluation of antral follicle count and ovarian morphology in crossbred beef cows: investigation of influence of stage of the estrous cycle, age, and birth weight. *Journal of Animal Science* **87** 1971-1980.

Cushman RA, DeSouza JC, Hedgpeth VS & Britt JH 1999 Superovulatory response of one ovary is related to the micro- and macroscopic population of follicles in the contralateral ovary of the cow. *Biology of Reproduction* **60** 349-354.

Da Silva P, Aitken RP, Rhind SM, Racey PA & Wallace JM 2002 Impact of maternal nutrition during pregnancy on pituitary gonadotrophin gene expression and ovarian development in growth-restricted and normally grown late gestation sheep fetuses. *Reproduction* **123** 769-777.

Erickson BH 1966a Development and radio-response of the prenatal bovine ovary. *Journal of Reproduction and Fertility* **11** 97-105.

Erickson BH 1966b Development and senescence of the postnatal bovine ovary. *Journal of Animal Science* **25** 800-805.

Evans ACO 2003 Characteristics of ovarian follicle development in domestic animals. *Reproduction in Domestic Animals* **38** 1-7.

Hsieh Y-Y, Chang C-C & Tsai H-D 2001 Antral follicle counting in predicting the retrieved oocyte number after ovarian hyperstimulation. *Journal of Assisted Reproduction and Genetics* **18** 320-324.

Huang F-J, Chang S-Y, Tsai M-Y, Kung F-T, Wu J-F & Chang H-W 2001 Determination of the efficiency of controlled ovarian hyperstimulation in the gonadotropin-releasing hormone agonist-suppression cycle using the initial follicle count during gonadotropin stimulation. *Journal of Assisted Reproduction and Genetics* **18** 91-96.

Ireland JJ, Mihm M, Austin E, Diskin MG & Roche JF 2000 Historical perspective of turnover of dominant follicles during the bovine estrous cycle: key concepts, studies, advancements, and terms. *Journal of Dairy Science* **83** 1648-1658.

Ireland JJ & Roche JF 1982 Development of antral follicles in cattle after prostaglandin-induced luteolysis: changes in serum hormones, steroids in follicular fluid, and gonadotropin receptors. *Endocrinology* **111** 2077-2086.

Ireland JJ & Roche JF 1983a Development of nonovulatory antral follicles in heifers: changes in steroids in follicular fluid and receptors for gonadotropins. *Endocrinology* **112** 150-156.

Ireland JJ & Roche JF 1983b Growth and differentiation of large antral follicles after spontaneous luteolysis in heifers: changes in concentrations of hormones in follicular fluid and specific binding of gonadotropins to follicles. *Journal of Animal Science* **57** 157-167.

Ireland JJ & Roche JF 1987. Hypotheses regarding development of dominant follicles during a bovine estrous cycle. In *Follicular Growth and Ovulation Rate in Farm Animals*, pp. 1-18.

Ireland JJ, Ward F, Jimenez-Krassel F, Ireland JL, Smith GW, Lonergan P & Evans ACO 2007 Follicle numbers are highly repeatable within individual animals but are inversely correlated with FSH concentrations and the proportion of good-quality embryos after ovarian stimulation in cattle. *Human Reproduction* **22** 1687-1695.

Ireland JJ, Zielak-Steciwko AE, Jimenez-Krassel F, Folger J, Bettegowda A, Scheetz D, Walsh S, Mossa F, Knight PG, Smith GW, Lonergan P & Evans ACO 2009 Variation in the ovarian reserve is linked to alterations in intrafollicular estradiol production and ovarian biomarkers of follicular differentiation and oocyte quality in cattle. *Biology of Reproduction* **80** 954-964.

Ireland JLH, Scheetz D, Jimenez-Krassel F, Themmen

AP, Ward F, Lonergan P, Smith GW, Perez GI, Evans AC & Ireland JJ 2008 Antral follicle count reliably predicts number of morphologically healthy oocytes and follicles in ovaries of young adult cattle. *Biology of Reproduction* **79** 1219-1225.

Jayaprakasan K, Deb S, Batcha M, Hopkisson J, Johnson I, Campbell B & Raine-Fenning N 2009 The cohort of antral follicles measuring 2-6 mm reflects the quantitative status of ovarian reserve as assessed by serum levels of anti-Mullerian hormone and response to controlled ovarian stimulation. *Fertility and Sterility* **In Press** 2009 Nov 2018. [Epub ahead of print].

Jimenez-Krassel F, Folger JK, Ireland JL, Smith GW, Hou X, Davis JS, Lonergan P, Evans ACO & Ireland JJ 2009 Evidence that High Variation in Ovarian Reserves of Healthy Young Adults Has a Negative Impact on the Corpus Luteum and Endometrium During Estrous Cycles in Cattle. *Biology of Reproduction* **80** 1272-1281.

Kawamata M 1994 Relationship between the number of small follicles prior to superovulatory treatment and superovulatory response in Holstein cows. *Journal of Veterinary Medical Science* **56** 965-970.

Kevenaar ME, Meerasahib MF, Kramer P, van de Lang-Born BM, de Jong FH, Groome NP, Themmen AP & Visser JA 2006 Serum anti-mullerian hormone levels reflect the size of the primordial follicle pool in mice. *Endocrinology* **147** 3228-3234.

La Marca A & Volpe A 2006 Anti-Mullerian hormone (AMH) in female reproduction: is measurement of circulating AMH a useful tool? *Clinical Endocrinology* **64** 603-610.

Lussier JG, Matton P & Dufour JJ 1987 Growth rates of follicles in the ovary of the cow. *Journal of Reproduction and Fertility* **81** 301-307.

McMillen IC & Robinson JS 2005 Developmental origins of the metabolic syndrome: prediction, plasticity, and programming. *Physiological Reviews* **85** 571-633.

Mihm M, Crowe MA, Knight PG & Austin EJ 2002 Follicle wave growth in cattle. *Reproduction in Domestic Animals* **37** 191-200.

Mossa F, Butler ST, Berry DP, Jimenez-Krassel F, Lonergan P, Smith GW, Ireland JJ & Evans ACO 2010a. Number of follicles during follicular waves is positively associated with fertility in dairy cows. In *Reproduction in Domestic Ruminants VII*, in this volume.

Mossa F, Jimenez-Krassel F, Walsh S, Berry DP, Butler ST, Folger J, Smith GW, Ireland JL, Lonergan P, Ireland JJ & Evans AC 2010b Inherent capacity of the pituitary gland to produce gonadotropins is not influenced by the number of ovarian follicles > or = 3 mm in diameter in cattle. *Reproduction, Fertility and Development* **22** 550-557.

Mossa F, Kenny D, Jimenez-Krassel F, Smith GW, Berry D, Butler S, Fair T, Lonergan P, Ireland JJ & Evans ACO 2009 Undernutrition of heifers during the first trimester of pregnancy diminishes size of the ovarian reserve in female offspring. *Biology of Reproduction,* **81** (Supplement 1), 135.

Pierson RA & Ginther OJ 1984 Ultrasonography of the bovine ovary. *Theriogenology* **21** 495-504.

Pierson RA & Ginther OJ 1988 Ultrasonic imaging of the ovaries and uterus in cattle. *Theriogenology* **29** 21-37.

Raga F, Bonilla-Musoles F, Casan EM, Klein O & Bonilla F 1999 Assessment of endometrial volume by three-dimensional ultrasound prior to embryo transfer: clues to endometrial receptivity. *Human Reproduction* **14** 2851-2854.

Rajakoski E 1960 The ovarian follicular system in sexually mature heifers with special reference to seasonally, cyclical, and left-right variations. *Acta Endocrinologica* **Supplement 52** 1-68.

Rico C, Fabre S, Medigue C, di Clemente N, Clement F, Bontoux M, Touze JL, Dupont M, Briant E, Remy B, Beckers JF & Monniaux D 2009 Anti-mullerian hormone is an endocrine marker of ovarian gonadotropin-responsive follicles and can help to predict superovulatory responses in the cow. *Biology of Reproduction* **80** 50-59.

Savio JD, Keenan L, Boland MP & Roche JF 1988 Pattern of growth of dominant follicles during the oestrous cycle of heifers. *Journal of Reproduction and Fertility* **83** 663-671.

Singh J, Dominguez M, Jaiswal R & Adams GP 2004 A simple ultrasound test to predict the superstimulatory response in cattle. *Theriogenology* **62** 227-243.

Sirois J & Fortune JE 1988 Ovarian follicular dynamics during the estrous cycle in heifers monitored by real-time ultrasonography. *Biology of Reproduction* **39** 308-317.

Sullivan TM, Micke GC, Greer RM, Irving-Rodgers HF, Rodgers RJ & Perry VE 2009 Dietary manipulation of Bos indicus x heifers during gestation affects the reproductive development of their heifer calves. *Reproduction, Fertility and Development* **21** 773-784.

Taneja M, Bols PE, Van de Velde A, Ju JC, Schreiber D, Tripp MW, Levine H, Echelard Y, Riesen J & Yang X 2000 Developmental competence of juvenile calf oocytes in vitro and in vivo: influence of donor animal variation and repeated gonadotropin stimulation. *Biology of Reproduction* **62** 206-213.

Tomas C, Nuojua-Huttunen S & Martikainen H 1997 Pretreatment transvaginal ultrasound examination predicts ovarian responsiveness to gonadotropins in in-vitro fertilization. *Human Reproduction* **12** 220-223.

van Disseldorp J, Lambalk CB, Kwee J, Looman CW, Eijkemans MJ, Fauser BC & Broekmans FJ 2009 Comparison of inter- and intra-cycle variability of anti-Mullerian hormone and antral follicle counts. *Human Reproduction* **25** 221-227.

Assisted reproduction in Mediterranean wild ruminants: lessons from the Spanish ibex (*Capra pyrenaica*)

J Santiago-Moreno, MA Coloma, A Toledano-Díaz, C Castaño, A Gómez-Brunet and A López-Sebastián

Department of Animal Reproduction, INIA, Avda. Puerta de Hierro km 5.9, 28040 Madrid, Spain

Summary

Despite apparent progress in reproductive technology as applied to wild ruminants, the success achieved in terms of the number of offspring that become healthy adults has remained low. Difficulties often arise through a lack of knowledge regarding appropriate cryopreservation techniques, and indeed through a lack of detailed information on the reproductive physiology of the species in question. The Spanish ibex (*Capra pyrenaica*) is a wild caprid found exclusively in the mountains of Iberia; only two of the original four subspecies still exist. Great efforts need to be made to preserve this species. The endocrine and environmental mechanisms that control its seasonal reproduction need to be properly understood, reproductive technologies (particularly the cryopreservation of gametes) optimised, and genetic resource banks developed. The experience obtained with the Spanish ibex may be useful in *ex situ* conservation strategies designed to preserve other threatened Mediterranean wild ruminants.

Introduction

Many wild ruminant species of the Mediterranean Basin are under threat from the lack of food available where there are high animal population densities, the loss of heterozygosity derived from habitat fragmentation, and other pressures. For example, the Turkish mouflon (*Ovis gmelini anatolica*), which is endemic to central Turkey, is vulnerable to livestock raising and illegal hunting and is currently represented by a single population of 700 animals in the centre-south of the country (Arihan & Bilgin 2001). The Atlas aoudad or Barbary sheep (*Ammotragus lervia lervia*) lives in the mountains of Morocco, northern Algeria and northern Tunisia - although a small population has been introduced into southeastern Spain - and is listed as vulnerable by the IUCN (IUCN 2009). A decline in its numbers in excess of 10% is expected over the next 15 years, mainly as a result of hunting and habitat loss. The original ecotypes of European mouflon (*Ovis orientalis musimon*) inhabiting the islands of Sardinia and Corsica are classified as vulnerable, and reproductive strategies have been established to help preserve the species (Ptak *et al.* 2002). In the early 1900s the Cypriot mouflon (*Ovis orientalis ophion*) came close

---

Corresponding author E-mail: moreno@inia.es

to extinction. Although its numbers have recently become viable it remains threatened by illegal hunting, the introduction of competitive species, climatic factors (excessively warm and dry conditions), and forest fires (Hadjisterkotis 2001).

The Spanish ibex (*Capra pyrenaica*) is an Iberian mountain ungulate, the populations of which have declined significantly over the last few centuries as a result of hunting pressure, habitat fragmentation and agricultural development. The species had disappeared from the French Pyrenees by the mid-nineteenth century, and by around 1890 the subspecies *C. p. lusitanica* became extinct in Portugal (Pérez *et al.* 2002). The Pyrenean subspecies *C. p. pyrenaica* became extinct in January 2000, when the last female died. Thus, only two of the four original subspecies still exit: *C. p. hispanica* and *C. p. victoriae*. Several ibex populations, mainly from southern Spain, have suffered at the hands of sarcoptic mange; in certain cases the mortality rate has been over 95% (Fandos 1991). This disease continues to affect most populations of ibexes in southern Spain, although now with less virulence. The species is protected under the Bern Convention and the EU Habitats and Species Directive. It is listed as Critically Endangered in Portugal, owing to its very small population in that country (Cabral *et al.* 2005). However, recent measures designed to protect the species have played a crucial role in its ongoing recovery in the Iberian Peninsula. A genetic resource bank (GRB) for the different ecotypes of Spanish ibex has also been established, the first of its kind for a Mediterranean mountain ungulate. This will help guarantee the preservation of the species in the face of possible disasters or outbreaks of further disease. The successful use of assisted reproduction technologies with the Spanish ibex may provide a useful model for the *ex situ* conservation of other threatened wild ruminants of the Mediterranean.

Genetic Resource Banks

The long-term cryopreservation of the germplasm of threatened species offers flexibility in their genetic management (Holt 1994) along with a degree of security with respect to disasters or outbreaks of disease that might seriously affect subpopulations (Kirkwood & Colenbrander 2001). A fundamental requirement of any GRB programme is the ability to successfully cryopreserve cells and tissues. Since spermatozoa are more accessible than oocytes or embryos, so they are currently of greater potential in breeding programmes, and at present are the primary cell types preserved in most emerging GRBs. The optimisation of sperm collection methods and the development of more effective cryopreservation protocols of ibex spermatozoa have been a priority.

Sperm collection

Semen collection using artificial vaginas has been used from time to time in wild ruminants maintained in captivity (Gizejewski 2004), but this requires rearing males in close human contact and training these animals in their use. Internal artificial vaginas and vaginal condoms have also been tried (Bainbridge & Jabbour 1998) but in practice their use is very limited. The difficulties associated with sperm recovery in the wild can be partly solved by post-mortem epididymal spermatozoa retrieval or electroejaculation. Viable epididymal spermatozoa can be retrieved from the dead males of a number of wild species (Soler et al. 2003; Perez-Garnelo *et al.* 2004). The time that elapses between death and sperm recovery affects the final sperm quality, and this should be taken into account when sperm doses are prepared for use in assisted reproduction. Frozen-thawed epididymal spermatozoa retrieved from ibexes within eight hours of death offer the maximum guarantee of success in artificial insemination (Santiago-Moreno *et al.* 2006a). The method of sperm collection used may also influence the quality of the spermatozoa. For example, collections can be made by making several small cuts with a scalpel at the tail of the epididymis (Santiago-Moreno *et al.* 2007a). However, spermatozoa thus collected are commonly contaminated with blood and epididymal cells (Martinez-Pastor *et al.* 2006), which may interfere with the optimal cryopreservation of the gametes. Spanish ibex epididymal spermatozoa may also be successfully collected, and with less contamination, by applying air pressure inside the vas deferens. However, high pressure seems to inflict considerable mechanical stress on sperm cells and to have a detrimental effect on their viability (Santiago-Moreno *et al.* 2007b). Alternatively, a larger number of sperm cells more resistant to freezing-thawing can be obtained by retrograde flushing from the vas deferens to the cauda epididymidis employing a Tris, citric acid, glucose, egg yolk-based medium (Santiago-Moreno *et al.* 2009a).

Electroejaculation in living ibexes allows repetitive sperm collection from captive or semi-captive animals. However, the sperm quality is very often poor (Durrant 2009) due to urine contamination, low semen volumes and low sperm concentrations (Giulini *et al.* 2004). A suitable anaesthetic protocol for electroejaculation must be followed to ensure good immobilization and to prevent pain associated with the procedure. The need to select an appropriate anaesthetic is underscored by the fact that several interfere with the neuromuscular mechanisms that control the erectile and ejaculatory functions, while others favour retrograde ejaculation during electrical stimulation (Tecirlioglu *et al.* 2002). In ibexes, an anaesthetic combination based on detomidine 270 µg/kg plus ketamine 1.4 mg/kg has been successfully used; this allows penis protrusion in the majority of animals and minimum urine contamination (Table 1).

Table 1. Effect of anaesthetic protocols on the average number of electrical pulses required for ejaculation, on the percentage of ibexes showing penis protrusion, and on the percentage of ibexes showing urine contamination of the semen.

	Det-Ket-1	Det-Ket-2	Telazol	Det-Ket-Telazol
Electrical pulses	30	40	26	40
Penis protrusion	50%	89%	78%	60%
Urine contamination	11%	14%	10%	9%

Det-Ket-1: detomidine 190 mg/kg and ketamine 2 mg/kg; Det-Ket-2: detomidine 270 mg/kg and ketamine 1.4 mg/kg; Telazol: tiletamine 3.4 mg/kg and zolazepan 3.4 mg/kg; Det-Ket-Telazol: detomidine 100 mg/kg plus ketamine 1 mg/kg plus tiletamine 0.5 mg/kg and zolazepan 0.5 mg/kg. Except when Telazol is used, anaesthesia reversals occur 1-12 min after administration of atipemazole 0.25 mg/kg. All drugs are administered by intramuscular injection.

Breeding seasonality is a limiting factor for successful sperm retrieval in most wild species. Maximum testicular and accessory sex gland activity occur over just a short period of the year, ensuring that sufficient numbers of normal spermatozoa are produced at the right time (rutting season). The identification of this period is important to ensure maximum semen volume retrieval, higher sperm quality, and the greatest resistance to the freezing-thawing process. In Spanish ibex, maximum testicular size and plasma testosterone concentrations occur in October-December (Fig. 1; Toledano-Díaz *et al.* 2007). Surprisingly, the low plasma testosterone concentrations seen during spring and summer do not prevent spermatogenesis in this species, unlike in most other wild ruminants so far studied (Lincoln 1985; Gosch & Fischer 1989). Sperm abnormalities reach their height, however, at this time (Coloma *et al.* 2010).

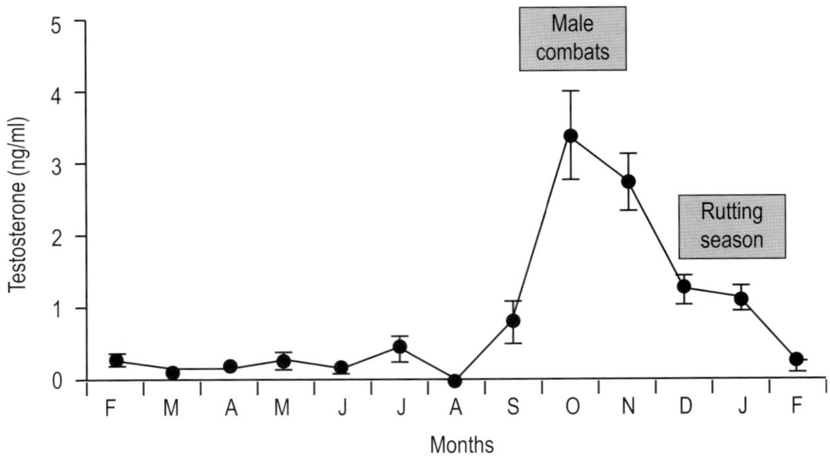

Fig. 1. Changes in plasma concentration of testosterone over the year in the Spanish ibex.

Selective criteria for inclusion of sperm samples in genetic resource banks

The sanitary control of sperm donors avoids the use of contaminated sperm in assisted reproduction (Philpott 1993), reduces the risk of cross-contamination during semen processing (Clarke 1999) and liquid nitrogen storage (Tedder *et al.* 1995; Clarke, 1999), and better maintains values of sperm variables over the freezing-thawing process (Santiago-Moreno *et al.* 2009a). The morphometry of the horns may be a useful criterion for selecting semen samples for GRBs. These secondary sexual characteristics appear to be a sensitive indicator of genetic stress (Parsons 1992) and serve as signals of male vigour that females may use to select mates (Geist 1966, 1991). Certainly, it has been shown that ibexes producing the largest and most symmetrical horns have better sperm quality (Fig. 2; Santiago-Moreno *et al.* 2007b). Reproductive success is therefore related to pre-copulatory strategies such as combat ability associated with horn development, although post-copulatory strategies related to sperm-competition also are involved (Preston *et al.* 2003).

Additives in sperm cryopreservation

The cryoprotection offered by extenders containing different additives has been tested in Ibex sperm samples obtained by electroejaculation and post-mortem collection from the cauda epididymis (Table 2). Egg yolk is beneficial to sperm cryopreservation because it protects against cold shock (Watson 1981); it may also provide certain protection during freezing and thawing (Aboagla & Terada, 2004). Although the replacement of egg yolk with other additives, such as lactose, leads to very low post-thaw motility (Santiago-Moreno *et al.* 2007a), the use of high egg yolk concentrations (12%-20%) can negatively affect the fertilization rate (Santiago-Moreno *et al.* 2006b; 2009b). Thus, the use of extenders containing egg yolk at low concentrations (TCG-6% e.y.) is recommended for the cryopreservation of both epididymal and ejaculated ibex spermatozoa.

The chemical composition of the egg yolks of different avian species varies, particularly in terms of the cholesterol, fatty acid and phospholipid contents (Bair & Marion 1978, Surai *et al.* 1999). This has led to investigations into which type of egg yolk might be more appropriate for use in extenders. Egg yolk from quail has been used successfully in the cryopreservation of

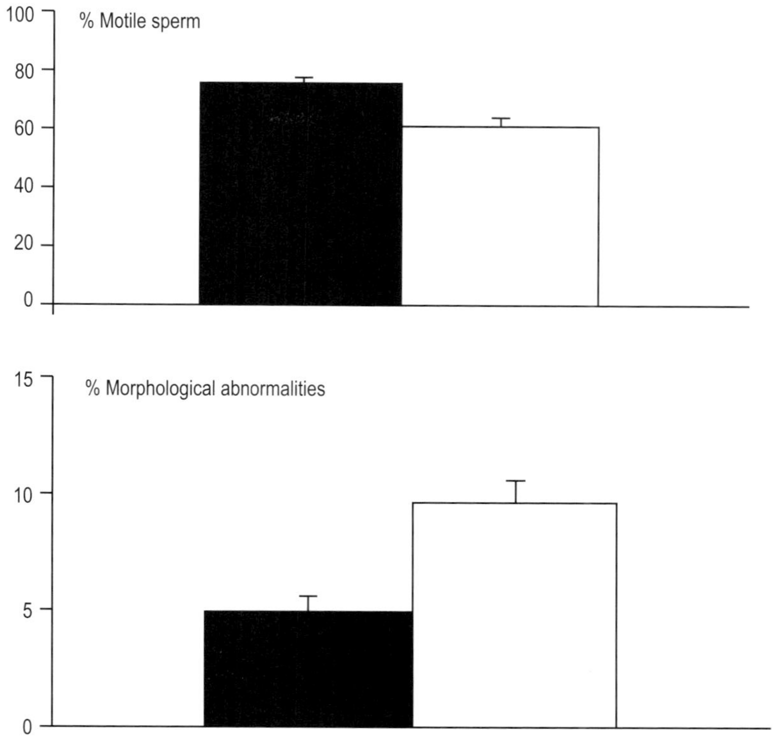

Fig. 2. Percentage of motile spermatozoa and morphological sperm abnormalities from ibexes with good (solid bars) and poor horn condition (open bars). Horn condition is calculated as the sum of the values assigned to the horn length, the horn base perimeter and relative asymmetry between the respective lengths and bases of the left and the right horns, using the method by Luzon *et al.* (2008).

Table 2. Composition of different extenders used to freeze ibex spermatozoa. The best results are usually obtained using TCG-6% egg yolk extender, both with epididymal spermatozoa recovered post mortem and those obtained by electroejaculation.

	Triladyl®	TCG-6% e.y.	TCG-12 % e.y.	TCG-20 % e.y.	TCG-Equex	TTG-6% e.y.	TTG-12% e.y.	TCG-lactose
Glycerol % (v v-1)	6	5	5	5	5	5	5	5
Tris % (w v-1)	?	3.8	3.8	3.8	3.8	1.2	1.2	3.8
Tes % (w v-1)	-	-	-	-	-	4.8	4.8	-
Citric Acid % (w v-1)	?	2.2	2.2	2.2	2.2	-	-	1.7
Glucose % (w v-1)	-	0.6	0.6	0.6	0.6	0.2	0.2	1.3
Fructose % (w v-1)	?	-	-	-	-	-	-	-
Egg yolk % (v v-1)	20	6	12	20	6-20	6	12	-
Lactose % (w v-1)	-	-	-	-	-	-	-	6
Equex Pasta % (v v-1)	-	-	-	-	0.6	-	-	-

sperm in some species, especially equids (Trimeche *et al.* 1997). However, it offers no advantage over chicken egg yolk in the cryopreservation of Spanish ibex epididymal spermatozoa (Santiago-Moreno *et al.* 2008a).

In ibexes, the seminal plasma has a negative effect on sperm survival when egg yolk-based diluents are employed (Coloma *et al.* 2010), an inconvenience also noted with domestic caprine sperm (Iritani & Nishikawa 1963). The problem is caused by a phospholipase secreted from the bulbourethral glands that hydrolyzes the membrane phospholipids of spermatozoa and produces toxic derivates from egg yolk phospholipids (Aamdal *et al.* 1965; Pellicer-Rubio & Combarnous 1998). The removal of the seminal plasma is found to be more beneficial during the time of declining photoperiod than at other times during the year, reflecting the increased activity of the accessory sex glands during the rutting season (Chapman & Chapman 1979).

Artificial insemination in Spanish ibex captive breeding programmes

Factors affecting captive breeding programs

The pregnancy rate in wild ruminant captive breeding programs is usually lower than the natural rate observed in the wild (Asher *et al.* 2000). This is often attributed to the lack of detailed information regarding the reproductive physiology of the species in question. Oestrus and ovulation synchronization protocols should take account the mating period and the characteristics of the sexual cycle defined for each species (Fig. 3). The Spanish ibex is a seasonal, polyoestrous species with alternating periods of oestrous activity and anoestrus. Anoestrus is characterised by low plasma concentrations of progesterone (< 0.5 ng/ml), reflecting complete ovulatory arrest. Ibexes show ovulatory activity with 1 to 3 progesterone cycles (progesterone peaks of 1.4 ± 0.1 ng/ml). The mean duration of the oestrus cycle is 19 days (range: 17–23 days). There is usually one short cycle (10–14 days with average maximum values of 0.8 ± 0.2 ng/ml) prior to or following a cycle of normal duration. The first progesterone cycle takes place between December 3 and 27. The end of seasonal ovulatory activity stretches from January 15 to February 9. Thus, the mean duration of the breeding season is only about 43 days (Santiago-Moreno *et al.* 2003). Furthermore, social interactions may interfere with the use of assisted reproduction techniques in wild species. Indeed, it has been shown that the anovulatory condition in subordinate ibex females (Fig.3) may be related to social status (Santiago-Moreno *et al.* 2007c), with high-ranking females showing a larger number of progesterone cycles. Hence, focusing the use of hormonal treatments on dominant animals might be cost-effective. Stress induced by synchronization treatments can also negatively affect reproduction and, in some cases lead to complete fertilization failure (Morrow *et al.* 2009). Thus, long acclimatization periods are needed under captive conditions, and synchronization protocols requiring minimum handling should be used.

Synchronization of ovulation and artificial insemination

The artificial insemination of ibex females synchronized by administering intravaginal progestagens for 11 days in conjunction with injections of equine chorionic gonadotropin (eCG) and cloprostenol two days before progestagen withdrawal (the standard method used in domestic goats), leads to fertilization rates of just 19-35% (Santiago-Moreno *et al.* 2006a,b). However, protocols based on the injection of luteolytic hormones appear to solve the problems associated with the use of eCG (anti-eCG antibodies are generated in animals repeatedly treated [Baril *et al.* 1996] and premature luteal regression [Saharrea *et al.* 1998]) and intravaginal progestagens (vaginal inflammation). In fact, the synchronization of ovulation in ibex females has been achieved following the IMA-PRO2® method described for dairy goats (Lopez-Sebastian *et al.*

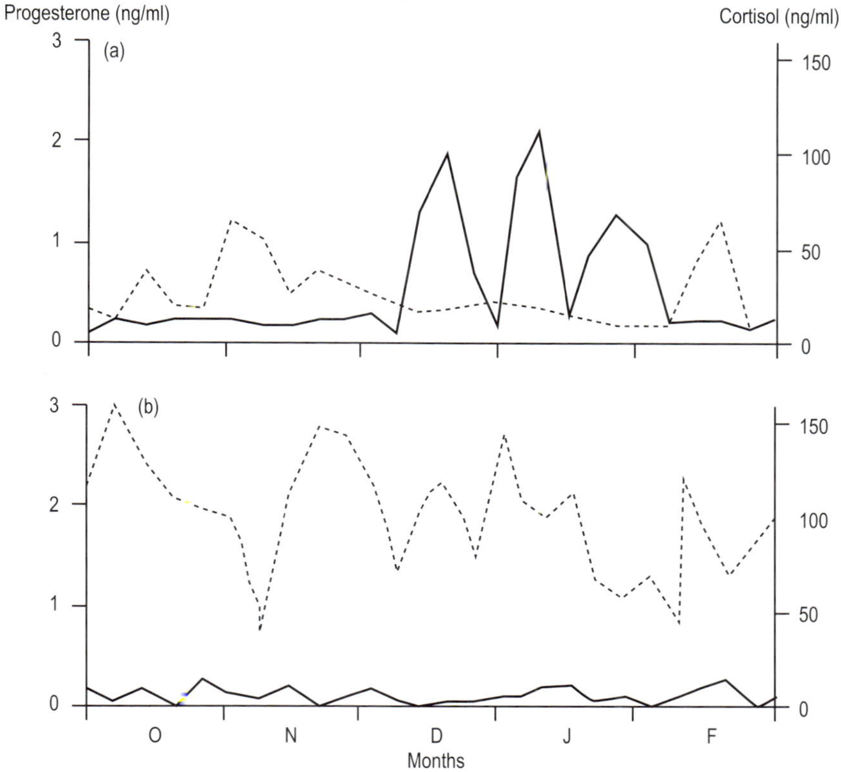

Fig. 3. Progesterone profiles (—) and plasma cortisol concentrations (- - -) in one representative dominant ibex female with cyclic ovulatory activity (a) and in one representative subordinate ibex female with no ovulatory activity (b).

2007). This minimises the number of times an animal is handled and avoids potential vaginal infections. In the breeding season, oestrus and ovulation are synchronised by the intramuscular (i.m.) injection of 25 mg of progesterone (4-pregneno-3,20-dione) in olive oil, plus a 100 μg i.m. injection of cloprostenol on day 0 followed by a single i.m. dose of 100 μg cloprostenol 10 days later. Ibexes are inseminated by laparoscopy with 200 x 10^6 spermatozoa 52 h after the second injection of cloprostenol, allowing fertility rates of 25-63% (Santiago-Moreno *et al.* 2008a,b).

The fertility of the sperm used in artificial insemination must be verified before use. Recent studies have reported the birth of live hybrids (*Capra pyrenaica x Capra hircus*) produced by the insemination of female domestic goats with electroejaculated or epididymal ibex spermatozoa. Along with routine semen analysis, this might be a good way of evaluating fertilising capacity in ibexes (Santiago-Moreno *et al.* 2006a,b). Heterospecific *in vivo* fertilization avoids the use of valuable homologous individuals, and spermatozoa are placed in the domestic female's reproductive tract when conditions are optimal for sperm capacitation, fertilization and embryonic development. The fertilising capacity of frozen-thawed sperm samples of other rare and wild species such as the mouflon (*Ovis gmelini musimon*), the gaur (*Bos gaurus*), Przewlaski's horse (*Equus przewalskii*) or Grant's zebra (*Equus burchelli*) could be tested in domestic sheep (*Ovis aries*), cattle (*Bos taurus*) and horses (*Equus caballus*), respectively.

Future strategies

Although spermatozoa are the primary cell types preserved in most emerging GRBs (because they are far more accessible than oocytes or embryos), embryo cryopreservation and embryo transfer provide ways of maximizing the number of offspring that a valuable female is capable of producing during or even after her lifetime. However, the cryopreservation of the embryos of wild ungulates has not been extensively studied, which may be due to the low rates of embryo recovery following superovulation (Leibo & Songsasen, 2002). Usually, embryo cryopreservation in a wild species involves a standard equilibrium freezing method developed for the embryos of a related domestic species (Leibo 1984; Andrabi & Maxwell, 2007). Interspecific embryo transfer may be a useful strategy in animal conservation programs when there is a lack of suitable female recipients. Interspecific embryo transfer has been successfully performed between the European mouflon (*Ovis orientalis musimon*) and domestic sheep (*Ovis aries*) (Santiago-Moreno *et al.* 2001), urial sheep (*Ovis orientalis*) and domestic sheep, the gaur (*Bos gaurus*) and domestic cattle (Stover *et al.* 1981), and the Spanish ibex and domestic goat (*Capra hircus*) (Fernández-Arias *et al.* 1999).

The Pyrenean ibex (*Capra pyrenaica pyrenaica*) was one of the four subspecies of the Spanish ibex. It has been recently been declared extinct by the Spanish Government, and is listed as such by the IUCN. Prior to the death of the last animal, cells from a skin biopsy were obtained, multiplied and kept frozen in liquid nitrogen. Although recent experiments have been focused on trying to clone this animal, only one recipient female (a hybrid between a Spanish ibex male and a female domestic goat) has maintained pregnancy to term. Unfortunately, the newborn – the first animal of an extinct subspecies to be born - died minutes after birth due to lung defects (Folch *et al.* 2009).

Conclusions

Assisted reproduction technologies may be the only way to guarantee the continued survival of certain species, subspecies or ecotypes at serious risk of extinction. The establishment of conservation plans involving the use of such technologies first requires rigorous studies on the reproductive biology of the taxon in question. Recent advances in our knowledge of seasonal breeding, ovulatory cycles and testicular activity in the Spanish ibex have allowed assisted reproduction technologies to be successfully used. The cryopreservation of sperm is a complex process that involves balancing many factors in order to obtain satisfactory results. Although there are many similarities between ibex and domestic goat sperm, that of the former requires special attention in order to maximise its post-thawing viability. An intricate knowledge of the appropriate methods of sperm collection and the diluents to use is essential to ensure even minimal success. Recent advances in these areas have allowed the establishment of GRBs for the most representative ecotypes of the Spanish ibex. The experience obtained with this species may be useful in *ex situ* conservation strategies designed to preserve other threatened wild ruminants.

Acknowledgements

This research was supported by MCINN grant AGL2008-01747.

References

Aamdal J, Lyngset O & Fossum K 1965 Toxic effect of lysolecithin on sperm. *Nordisk veterinaermedicin (Nor Vet Med)* **17** 633-639.

Aboagla EM & Terada T 2004 Effects of egg yolk during the freezing step of cryopreservation on the viability of goat spermatozoa. *Theriogenology* **62** 1160-1172.

Andrabi SMH & Maxwell WMC 2007 A review on reproductive biotechnologies for conservation of endangered mammalian species. *Animal reproduction Science* **99** 223-243.

Arihan O & Bilgin CC 2001 Population biology and conservation of the Turkish mouflon (*Ovis gmelini anatolica*, Valenciennes, 1856). In *Proceedings of the third International Symposium on mouflon*, pp. 31-36. Eds A Náhlik & W Uloth. Sopron, Hungary: Lövér Print.

Asher GW, Berg DK & Evans G 2000 Storage of semen and artificial insemination in deer. *Animal Reproduction Science* **62** 195-211.

Bainbridge DR & Jabbour HN 1998 Potential of assisted breeding techniques for the conservation of mammalian species in captivity: a review. *Veterinary Record* **143** 159-168.

Bair CW & Marion WW 1978 Yolk cholesterol in eggs from various avian species, Poultry Science **57** 1260-1265.

Baril G, Remy B, Leboeuf B, Beckers JF & Saumande J 1996 Synchronization of estrus in goats: The relationship between eCG binding in plasma, time of occurrence of estrus and fertility following artificial insemination. *Theriogenology* **45** 1553-1559.

Cabral MJ, Almeida J, Almeida PR, Dellinger T, Ferrand de Almeida N., Oliveira ME, Palmeirim JM, Queiroz AI, Rogado L & Santos-Reis M (eds) 2005 *Livro Vermelho dos Vertebrados de Portugal*. Instituto da Conservação da Natureza, Lisboa, Portugal.

Chapman NG & Chapman DI 1979 Seasonal changes in the male accessory glands of reproduction in adult fallow deer (*Dama dama*) *Journal of Zoology (London)* **189** 259-274.

Clarke GN 1999 Sperm cryopreservation: is there a significant risk of cross-contamination? Human Reproduction **14** 2941-2943.

Coloma MA, Toledano-Díaz A, López-Sebastián A & Santiago-Moreno J 2010 The influence of washing Spanish ibex (*Capra pyrenaica*) sperm on the effects of cryopreservation in dependency of the photoperiod. *Theriogenology* **73** 900-908.

Durrant BS 2009 The importance and potential of artificial insemination in CANDES (companion animals, non-domestic, endangered species). *Theriogenology* **71** 113-122.

Fandos P 1991 *La cabra montés en el Parque Natural de las Sierras de Cazorla, Segura y las Villas*. Eds ICONA/CSIC. Madrid, Spain.

Fernández-Arias A, Alabart JL, Folch J & Beckers F 1999 Interspecies pregnancy of Spanish ibex (*Capra pyrenaica*) fetus in domestic goat (*Capra hircus*) recipients induces abnormally high plasmatic levels of pregnancy-associated glycoprotein *Theriogenology* **51** 1419-1430.

Folch J, Cocero MJ, Chesné P, Alabart JL, Domínguez V, Cognié Y, Roche A, Fernandez-Arias A, Martí JI, Sánchez P, Echegoyen E, Beckers JF, Sánchez-Bonastre A & Vignon X 2009 First birth of an animal from an extinct subspecies *(Capra pyrenaica pyrenaica)* by cloning. Theriogenology **71** 1026-1034.

Geist V 1966 The evolutionary significance of mountain sheep horns. *Evolution* **20** 558-566.

Geist V 1991 Bones of contention revisited: did antler enlarge with sexual selection as a consequence of neonatal security strategies? *Applied Animal Behaviour Science* **29** 453-469.

Giulini S, Pesce F, Madgar I, Marsella T, Volpe A, Aloysio D & Battaglia C 2004 Influence of multiple transrectal electroejaculation on semen parameters and intracytoplasmic sperm injection outcome. *Fertility and Sterility* **82** 200-204.

Gizejewski Z 2004 Effect of season on characteristics of red deer (*Cervus elaphus L.*) semen collected using modified artificial vagina. *Reproductive Biology* **4** 51-66.

Gosch B & Fischer K 1989 Seasonal changes of testis volume and sperm quality in adult fallow deer (*Dama dama)* and their relationship to antler cycle. Journal of Reproduction and Fertility **85** 7-17.

Hadjisterkotis E 2001 The Cyprus mouflon, a threatened species in a biodiversity "hotspot" area. In *Proceedings of the third International Symposium on mouflon*. pp. 71-81. Eds A. Náhlik & W Uloth. Sopron, Hungary: Lövér Print.

Holt WV 1994 Reproductive technologies. In *Creative Conservation: Interactive Management of Wild and Captive Animals*, pp. 144-166. Eds. PJS Olney, GM Mace & ATC Feistner. London: Chapman and Hall.

Iritani A & Nishikawa V 1963 Studies on the egg yolk coagulating factor in goat semen. III. Release of some acids accompanied by the coagulating phenomena. *Japanese Journal of Animal Reproduction* **8** 109-112.

IUCN 2009 *IUCN Red List of Threatened Species*. Version 2009.2. Available from: www.iucnredlist.org

Kirkwood JK & Colenbrander B 2001 Disease control measures fro genetic resource banking. In *Cryobanking the Genetic Resource; wildlife conservation for the future?*, pp. 69-84. Eds PF Watson & WV Holt. London: Taylor and Francis.

Leibo SP 1984. One-step method for direct non-surgical transfer of frozen-thawed bovine embryos. *Theriogenology* **21** 767-790.

Leibo SP & Songsasen N 2002 Cryopreservation of gametes and embryos of non-domestic species. *Theriogenology* **57** 303-306.

Lincoln GA 1985 Seasonal breeding in deer. In *Biology of Deer Production*, pp 165-179. Eds K Drew & P Fennessy. Royal Society of New Zealand, Bull 22, Wellington.

Lopez-Sebastian A, Gonzalez-Bulnes A, Carrizosa JA, Urrutia B, Diaz-Delfa C, Santiago-Moreno J & Gomez-Brunet A 2007 New estrus synchronization and artificial insemination protocol for goats based on male exposure, progesterone and cloprostenol. *Theriogenology* **68** 1081-1087.

Luzón M, Santiago-Moreno J, Meana A, Toledano-Díaz A, Pulido-Pastor A, Gómez-Brunet A & López-Sebastián A 2008. Parasitism and horn quality in male Spanish ibex (*Capra pyrenaica hispanica*) from Andalucía based on coprological analysis and muscle biopsy. *Spanish Journal of Agricultural Research* **6** 353-361.

Martinez-Pastor F, Garcia-Macias V, Alvarez M, Chamorro C, Herraez P, de Paz P & Anel L 2006 Comparison of two methods for obtaining spermatozoa from the cauda epididymides of Iberian red deer. *Theriogenology* **65** 471-485.

Morrow CJ, Penfold LM & Wolfe BA 2009 Artificial insemination in deer and non-domestic bovids. *Theriogenology* **71** 149-165.

Parsons P 1992 Fluctuating asymmetry: a biological monitor of environmental and genomic stress. *Heredity* **68** 361-364.

Pellicer-Rubio MT & Combarnous Y 1998 Deterioration of goat spermatozoa in skimmed milk-based extenders as a result of oleic acid released by the bulbourethral lipase BUSgp60. *Journal of Reproduction and Fertility* **112 95-105.**

Pérez JM, Granados JE, Soriguer RC, Fandos P, Márquez FJ & Crampe JP 2002 Distribution, status and conservation problem of the Spanish Ibex, *Capra pyrenaica* (*Mammalia: Artiodactyla*). *Mammal Review* **32** 26-39.

Perez-Garnelo SS, Garde J, Pintado B, Borque C, Talavera C, Delclaux M, Lopez M & de la Fuente Martinez J 2004 Characteristics and in vitro fertilizing ability of Giant Panda (*Ailuropoda melanoleuca*) frozen-thawed epididymal spermatozoa obtained 4 hours postmortem: a case report. *Zoo Biology* **23** 279-85.

Philpott M 1993 The dangers of disease transmission by artificial insemination and embryo transfer. *British Veterinary Journal* **149** 339-369.

Preston BT, Stevenson IR, Pemberton JM, Coltman DW & Wilson K 2003 Overt and covert competition in a promiscuous mammal: the importance of weaponry and testes size to male reproductive success. *Proceedings of the Royal Society of London* **B 270** 633-640.

Ptak G, Clinton M, Barboni B, Muzzeddu M, Cappai P, Tischner M & Loi P 2002 Preservation of the wild European mouflon: the first example of genetic management using a complete program of reproductive biotechnologies. Biology of Reproduction **66** 796-801.

Santiago-Moreno J, González-Bulnes A, Gómez Brunet A, Cocero MJ, del Campo A, García-García R & López Sebastián A 2001 Procedure for successful interspecific embryo transfer between mouflon (*Ovis gmelini musimon*) and Spanish Merino sheep (*Ovis aries*). *Journal of Zoo and Wildlife Medicine* 32 336-341.

Santiago-Moreno J, Gómez-Brunet A, González-Bulnes A, Malpaux B, Chemineau P, Pulido A & López-Sebastián A 2003 Seasonal ovulatory activity and plasma prolactin concentrations in Spanish ibex (*Capra pyrenaica hispanica*) maintained in captivity. *Reproduction Nutrition and Development* **43** 217-224.

Santiago-Moreno J, Toledano-Díaz A, Pulido-Pastor A, Gómez-Brunet A & López-Sebastián A 2006a Birth of live Spanish ibex (*Capra pyrenaica hispanica*) derived from artificial insemination with epididymal spermatozoa retrieved after death. *Theriogenology* **66** 283-291.

Santiago-Moreno J, Toledano-Díaz A, Pulido-Pastor A, Dorado J, Gómez-Brunet A & López-Sebastián A 2006b Effect of egg yolk concentration on cryopreserving Spanish ibex (*Capra pyrenaica*) epididymal spermatozoa. *Theriogenology* **66** 1219-1226.

Santiago-Moreno J, Toledano-Díaz A, Dorado J, Pulido-Pastor A, Coloma MA & López-Sebastián A 2007a Recovery and cryopreservation of Spanish Ibex epididymal spermatozoa. *Archives of Andrology* **53** 309-316.

Santiago-Moreno J, Toledano-Díaz A, Pulido-Pastor A, Gómez-Brunet A, & López-Sebastián A 2007b Horn quality and postmortem sperm parameters in Spanish ibex (*Capra pyrenaica hispanica*). *Animal Reproduction Science* **99** 354-362.

Santiago-Moreno J, Toledano-Díaz A, Gómez-Brunet A, Pulido-Pastor A & López-Sebastián A 2007c Social dominance and breeding activity in Spanish ibex (*Capra pyrenaica*) maintained in captivity. *Reproduction Fertility and Development* **19** 436-442.

Santiago-Moreno J, Coloma MA, Toledano-Díaz A, Dorado J, Pulido-Pastor A & López-Sebastián A 2008a A comparison of the protective action of chicken and quail egg yolk in the cryopreservation of Spanish ibex epididymal spermatozoa. *Cryobiology* **57** 25-29.

Santiago-Moreno J, Toledano-Díaz A, Gómez-Brunet A, Pulido-Pastor A & López-Sebastián A 2008b Synchronization of ovulation and artificial insemination protocol for Spanish Ibex (*Capra pyrenaica*) based in progesterone and cloprostenol. *Spanish Journal of Agricultural Research* **6** 39-41.

Santiago-Moreno J, Astorga RJ, Luque I, Coloma MA, Toledano-Díaz A, Pulido-Pastor A, Gómez-Guillamon F, Salas-Vega R & López-Sebastián A 2009a Influence of recovery method and microbial contamination on the response to freezing-thawing in ibex (*Capra pyrenaica*) epididymal spermatozoa. *Cryobiology* **59** 357-362.

Santiago-Moreno J, Coloma MA, Dorado J, Pulido-Pastor A, Gómez-Guillamon F, Salas-Vega R, Gómez-Brunet A, & López-Sebastián A 2009b Cryopreservation of Spanish ibex (*Capra pyrenaica*) sperm obtained by electroejaculation outside the rutting season. *Theriogenology* **71** 1253-1260.

Saharrea A, Valencia J, Balcázar A, Mejía O, Cerbón JL, Caballero V, Zarco L 1998 Premature luteal regression in goats superovulated with PMSG: effect of hCG or GnRH administration during early luteal phase. *Theriogenology* **50** 1039-1052.

Soler AJ, Pérez-Guzmán MD & Garde JJ 2003 Storage of red deer epididymides for four days at 5°C: Effects on sperm motility, viability, and morphological integrity. *Journal of Experimental Zoology* **295A** 188-99.

Stover J, Evans J & Dolensek EP 1981 Interspecies embryo transfer from gaur to domestic Holstein. In *Annual Proceedings of the American Association of Zoo Veterinarians, pp.* 122-124.

Surai PF, Speake BK, Noble RC & Mezes M 1999 Species-specific differences in the fatty acid profiles of the lipids of the yolk and of the liver of the chick. *Journal of the Science of Food* and *Agriculture* **79** 733-736.

Tecirlioglu RT, Hayes ES & Trounson AO 2002 Semen collection from mice: electroejaculation. *Reproduction Fertility and Development* **14** 363-371.

Tedder RS, Zuckerman MA, Goldstone AH, Hawkins AE, Fielding A, Briggs EM, Irwin D, Blair S, Gorman AM, Patterson KG, Linch DC, Heptonstall J & Brink NS 1995 Hepatitis B transmission from contaminated cryopreservation tank. *Lancet* **346** 137-140.

Toledano-Díaz A, Santiago-Moreno J, Gómez-Brunet A, Pulido-Pastor A & López-Sebastián A 2007 Horn growth related to testosterone secretion in two wild Mediterranean ruminant species Spanish ibex (*Capra pyrenaica hispanica*) and mouflon (*Ovis orientalis musimon*). *Animal Reproduction Science* **102** 300-307.

Trimeche A, Antón M, Renard P, Gandemer G & Tainturier D 1997 Quail egg yolk: a novel cryoprotectant for the freeze preservation of Poitou Jackass sperm. *Cryobiology* **34** 385-393.

Watson PF 1981 The roles of lipid and protein in the protection of ram spermatozoa at 5°C by egg yolk lipoprotein. *Journal Reproduction and Fertility* **62** 483-492.

Enhancing reproductive performance in domestic dairy water buffalo (*Bubalus bubalis*)

L Zicarelli

Dipartimento di Scienze Zootecniche e Ispezione degli Alimenti - Università "Federico II" – Napoli Via Delpino, 1 80137 Napoli, Italy

The purpose of the review is to describe the factors that affect fertility in domestic water buffalo (*Bubalus bubalis*) and the techniques that enable an improvement in reproductive performance. On Italian and Latin American farms where natural mating is practiced and bulls are always present in the herd, the inter-calving interval is approximately 400 days and the culling rate is lower than 15%. The buffalo has a tendency for seasonal reproductive activity. Reproduction is favoured when there is a decrease in day length. Ovarian activity stops if conception does not occur within 3 to 5 ovarian cycles. It is important, therefore, that appropriate management of the transition period is practiced, particularly with respect to the hygienic conditions of the uterus. In tropical countries located north of the equator, feed deficiencies and heat stress are considered the main factors that lead to poor fertility in the summer. In Pakistan, for example, the increase in body condition score during the autumn was associated with the commencement of the breeding season in buffaloes. Anoestrus is observed also in Italy, however, where the average daily temperature during the same period is 13.5 to 23.5°C and feeding is constant throughout the year. The only common element between the two areas is the progressive increase in daylight hours between April and June and the day length greater than 12 hours up to September. In Italian herds that apply an out-of-season breeding strategy, an improvement in fertility (measured as the percentage of corpora lutea corresponding to subsequent pregnancy) is observed when water pools are present on the farm. This demonstrates that an improvement in environmental conditions reduces the incidence of embryonic mortality and/or abnormal cycles. To summarize, in the absence of serious nutritional problems, an improvement in environmental conditions increases fertility in buffalo.

Introduction

Domestic water buffalo (*Bubalus bubalis*) represent a fundamental and irreplaceable resource for tropical countries. Buffalo populations are increasing at a greater rate than those of bovine species. Between 1961 and 2008, the bovine and buffalo populations increased by 43% and 105% and between 1995 and 2007 increased by 2% and 13%, respectively (Faostat.fao.org/faostat). The population data refer to the population present in 43 of 143 countries that currently breed buffalo (Misra & Tyagi 2007).

Corresponding author E-mail: zicarell@unina.it

The majority of the authors believe that the main reproductive characteristics of buffalo are delayed puberty, prolonged postpartum ovarian inactivity, long inter-calving intervals and a tendency for seasonality (Madan 1988; Misra & Tyagi 2007). The reproductive problems depend on the region of the world. In tropical countries north of the equator (TCNE), for example, the majority of the authors assert that the summer anoestrus is caused by heat stress and forage scarcity. In Italy, however, anoestrus is observed in the same period of the year as TCNE (as demonstrated by the calving distribution; Fig. 1) although the diet in Italy is constant throughout the year and the ambient temperatures are milder. The aim of this review is to examine the main factors affecting fertility in buffalo and the strategies that may be adopted to enhance the reproductive performance of buffalo.

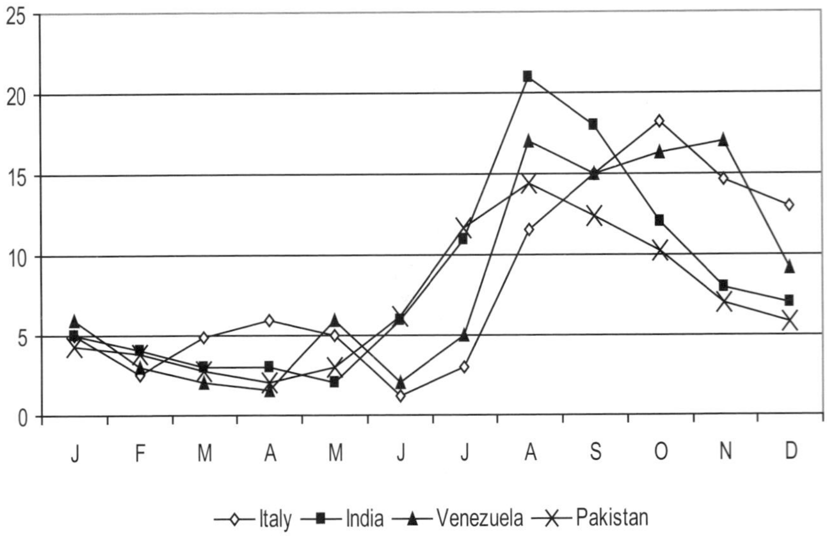

Fig. 1. Monthly calving percentage for Italy (Zicarelli *et al.* 1977), India (Singh, 1988), Venezuela (Zicarelli, 1994), and Pakistan (Hassan *et al.* 2007). Calendar months (single letter abbreviations) are indicated on the x-axis.

Reproductive seasonality

The place of origin and the duration of gestation have undoubtedly influenced the way in which reproductive seasonality occurs. The natural necessity to coincide calving and weaning with the most-suitable time of year represents one of the causes of this 'adaptation' process (Zicarelli 1994). This time of year should satisfy the nutritional requirements of the offspring through a period in which etiologic agents (infectious and parasites) are less aggressive and/ or present. Those born under the most-favourable conditions have brought about the natural selection of individuals endowed with a more ideal reproductive seasonality that promotes the survival of the species (Zicarelli 1997). Spring calving (March to May), which guarantees good availability of forage to offspring in temperate zones north of the equator, occurs when reproduction takes place in autumn in the case of five month gestations (sheep and goats) or in the previous spring in the case of 11 and 12 month gestations (horses and donkeys). The same calving period, therefore, is conditioned by the neuroendocrine system. The reactivation of the reproductive cycle with regard to the length of gestation (short day breeder [negative photoperiod] or long breeder [positive photoperiod]) is therefore controlled.

In tropical zones where the domestic buffalo developed (between 31°N and 2°S) forage availability is usually adequate after the rainy season (July through September). In species like the domestic buffalo, therefore, whose pregnancy lasts 310 to 316 days, the sensitivity to decreasing light stimulus and the reproductive season seems to take place between September and January. Around the equatorial belt, where the light/dark ratio varies little throughout the year, the reproductive season is highly conditioned by forage availability (Vale *et al.* 1990; 1996). There is a tendency towards seasonality in buffalo because buffalo evolved far away from the equator. Moving buffalo to other regions of the world has not modified the sensitivity of the hypothalamic hypophyseal axis to a decreasing light/dark ratio.

In Italy, the seasonality makes it necessary to change the calving calendar in order to meet the milk market demand. This is accomplished by using an out-of-breeding mating strategy (OBMS) that entails the interruption of natural mating or the use of artificial insemination (AI) between October and late January in adult females and between September and late March in heifers. These months are the most-favourable periods for reproductive activity (Zicarelli 1994; Zicarelli 1997; Campanile *et al.* 2009).

In research carried out in Italy (Parmeggiani & Di Palo 1994), it was demonstrated that buffaloes with a tendency towards seasonality showed high plasma melatonin concentrations two hours after sunset even when they were moved to another farm where other females showed low plasma melatonin concentrations and less sensitivity towards light stimulation (Di Palo *et al.* 1997). The plasma melatonin concentrations had a repeatability of 0.733 (Di Palo *et al.* 1993). If the heredity of plasma melatonin turns out to be high, as we expect based on the high repeatability, the plasma melatonin could be incorporated into genetic selection programmes for buffalo (Zicarelli 1994). In an effort to validate this theory, we reported that Romanov 58°N, Karakul 41°N and White-faced 51°N sheep (Lincoln 1992) showed continuous cyclic activity throughout the year even if living at latitudes where other genotypes were sensitive to the light/dark ratio.

In heifers and adult female buffaloes, the differences between night and day concentrations of plasma melatonin in March were less in heifers (5.0 times) compared with adult buffaloes (28.3 times) (Borghese *et al.* 1995). Both buffaloes that calve in spring (Di Palo *et al.* 1993; more adaptable to out-of-breeding-mating-strategy) and the heifers (Borghese *et al.* 1995; less sensitive to the photoperiod; Zicarelli 1994) show the same behavioural pattern.

Heifer fertility is not compromised by the season (Campanile *et al.* 1991; Avallone *et al.* 1994; Zicarelli 1994). During the summer and when daylight hours are more than dark hours, there is an increase in prolactin in the blood but, contrary to assertions by Madan (1988), buffalo regularly conceive. We believe that hyperprolactinemia is a consequence of the hypothyroidism (Campanile *et al.* 1994) during the warm months. The hypothyroidism exerts a positive feedback on thyroid stimulating hormone and hence on thyrotropin releasing hormone. Thyrotropin releasing hormone promotes an increase in prolactin (Zicarelli 1994; 1997).

The majority of authors attribute reproductive seasonality to nutritional factors. The breeding period in areas where 97% of the buffalo population are bred takes place in the months of greater forage availability (Roy *et al.* 1968; Singh *et al.* 1988; Shah 1990; Singh & Lal 1992; Qureshi *et al.* 1999a). Greater forage availability is found during the months of July through November characterized by decreasing daylight length in TCNE.

Recently Hassan *et al.* (2007) reported the different seasonality of Nili-Ravi buffaloes, purebred Sahiwal and cross-bred cattle in Pakistan. The difference between Nili-Ravi buffaloes and purebred Sahiwal was characterized by negative and positive photoperiod sensitivity, respectively. Data similar to those recorded in buffaloes have been observed in cross-bred cattle (Holstein or Jersey x Sahiwal). It cannot be ruled out, however, that the high temperatures (35 to 41°C) and milder temperatures (22 to 28°C) may influence negatively and positively (respectively) the ovarian activity. This finding suggests, moreover, that crossbreeding with *Bos taurus* may modify the seasonality of native bovines, which have the higher incidence of deliveries during the first 5 months of the year and, hence, conceive in the hottest months (April to August).

If heat stress is the main cause of the anoestrus then it should adversely affect the reproductive activity of buffalo compared with *Bos indicus* cattle. In Italy exactly the opposite pattern is observed. For out-of-season mated buffaloes, the conception rate increases between July and September, a period during which Holstein cows shows a low conception rate.

In Italian herds where the OBMS technique is not used (Zicarelli *et al.* 1977) as well as 30 to 40 years ago on the majority of farms (Ferrara 1957), the resumption of the reproductive cycle (RRC) took place from September (decreasing light period) until January (light increasing period but predominantly dark hours) (Fig. 1). Sensitivity to the negative photoperiod is also found on farms where a constant balanced diet is provided year-round (Zicarelli 1994). This type of seasonality, where reproductive events are not synchronised with forage availability, indicates that the buffalo bred in Italy are not autochthonous in the sense that they will sometimes calve during periods of forage scarceness and low temperature which in turn hinders the survival of the calf. Italian findings should be sufficient to define the buffalo as a short day breeder. Indeed, a similar seasonality to that found in Italy and Asian tropical areas is also found in Venezuela (Montiel 2000) and Egypt (Zoheir *et al.* 2007) (Fig. 1).

In southern Brazil (Da Silva & Grodzki 1991; Baruselli *et al.* 2001) and Argentina (L Zicarelli, unpublished observations), the wet season (and consequently, increased pasture availability) starts in October to November and continues until March to April. Pasture scarcity goes from May to June until October to November. The buffalo calving period under these conditions is mainly concentrated from February to May (Fig. 2). The breeding period is from April to July and the calf weaning calf period under free range and suckling calf conditions is from September to December. These events permit the coincidence of forage availability within the first 2 to 4 months of lactation and most of the dry period (October to April). The breeding period, however, is mainly concentrated during the pasture scarcity period (May to July).

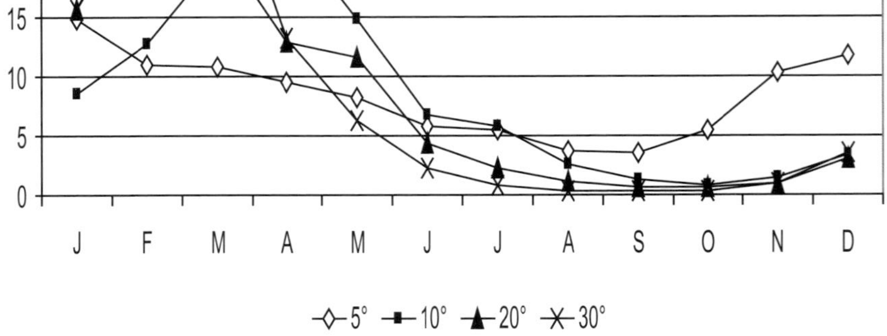

Fig. 2. Monthly calving percentage in Brazil as a function of latitude (°S). Calendar months (single letter abbreviations) are indicated on the x-axis.

Baruselli *et al.* (2001), who evaluated data from the Brazilian Breeders Association, observed that the seasonality is more accentuated from the north (0 to 8 degrees latitude) to the south (24 to 32 degrees latitude) of Brazil (Fig. 2) and hence the calving season is influenced by latitude. From the findings shown here, it can be unequivocally stated that, although the domestic water buffalo shows reproductive activity throughout the year, there is a greater tendency to concentrate reproductive activity in months of decreasing daylight or if increasing, when dark hours prevail.

Reproductive efficiency

Many scientists affirm that the buffalo shows delayed puberty and a long inter-calving interval. These characteristics are affected by several factors, such as year of calving, season of delivery, genotype and heat stress (Zicarelli *et al.* 2007). The delayed puberty and the consequent older age at first calving have been addressed by many authors. In a study performed on 86 farms (30,735 primiparous buffaloes, which calved between 1975 and 2005), it was observed that the mean age at first calving decreased by 1 month every 5 years (Zicarelli 2007). The hormonal pattern in cyclic buffalo is similar to that described in a cyclic *Bos taurus* cow (Seren *et al.* 1994). The main difference between the two species is the percentage of cyclic individuals in the different seasons.

The different reproductive efficiency of buffalo compared with *Bos taurus* is due to several features. These features must be considered because there is a need to modify the calving calendar in the buffalo so that the milk market demand is met. There are fewer primordial and antral follicles (Le Van *et al.* 1989) as well as a lesser ovarian weight and lesser ovarian volume in the buffalo compared with the bovine (Vittoria 1997). The number of oocytes in a buffalo calf is one-fifth that recorded in a bovine calf (Le Van *et al.* 1989; Gasparrini 2002). After calving, there are a low number of ovarian follicles and follicular waves and few cycles occur. If conception does not take place, therefore, an anoestrus of variable length begins (Zicarelli *et al.* 1994). With regard to this topic, the transition period and the postpartum period have a major importance for fertility in buffalo. It should be pointed out that in the farms adopting semi-free housing, the presence of mycotoxins in the roughages, *Clostridia*, *Coxiella burnetii*, and the incorrect input of Ca, P and crude protein in the last two months of pregnancy often lead to the occurrence of vaginal or uterine prolapse which impairs the RRC (Zicarelli 2000). It is not clear whether the seasonality of the species depends on the reduced follicular population or if this latter effect is the cause of buffalo seasonality.

If the calving calendar is not modified, the delayed RRC after calving can be due to the lack of the "bull effect" (Zicarelli *et al.* 1997) and/or to poor nutritional conditions. In small farms in TCNE where the bull is not present, the dry period of the animals (March to June) coincides with the scarcity of forage. South of the equator over the 20th parallel, the dry period (November to March) coincides with the abundance of forage and the bull is always present in the herd. In the first case, prolonged inter-calving intervals are observed (Shah 1990) whereas in the second case inter-calving intervals less than 400 days are recorded (Zicarelli 1994).

These observations suggest that in those areas, the meeeting of nutritional requirements and the absence/presence of the bull are the most important factors (Zicarelli *et al.* 1997), especially taking into account that the protein content of the pastures is very low (6 to 10% of DM) and leguminosae are found in irrigated areas or during the rainy season. In Pakistan, Qureshi *et al.* (1999a, 1999b) reported that the seasonality is influenced by nutritional and non-nutritional factors. Unless the feed deficiencies are serious, however, nutritional factors in general do not play a significant role (Zicarelli 1999; Paul & Lal 2010). The buffalo cannot yet be considered exactly as having a *"lactiferous habitus"* and therefore a *"catabolicus habitus"* such as that found in the high milk producing bovine cow which uses its reserves to compensate energy and protein deficiency during early lactation. As a matter of fact, within reasonable limits, the buffalo uses its reserves in its aim to reproduce and to the detriment of her own milk production.

The effects of the tendency toward seasonal reproduction in the buffalo are particularly evident. Studies conducted in Italy may be useful for countries wishing to increase the consistency of their production of buffalo milk during the year. When primiparous buffaloes are excluded from the survey (heifers are less sensitive to photoperiod), a decrease in calving rate between March and June for farms that are adopting the OBMS technique is observed in Italy whether OBMS is applied or not (Fig. 3). This confirms that the increase in daylight hours (April to June) or number of daylight hours >12 h, negatively interfere with reproductive activity. The buffalo that undergo OBMS can show anoestrus and this phenomenon is worsened by unfavourable climatic conditions.

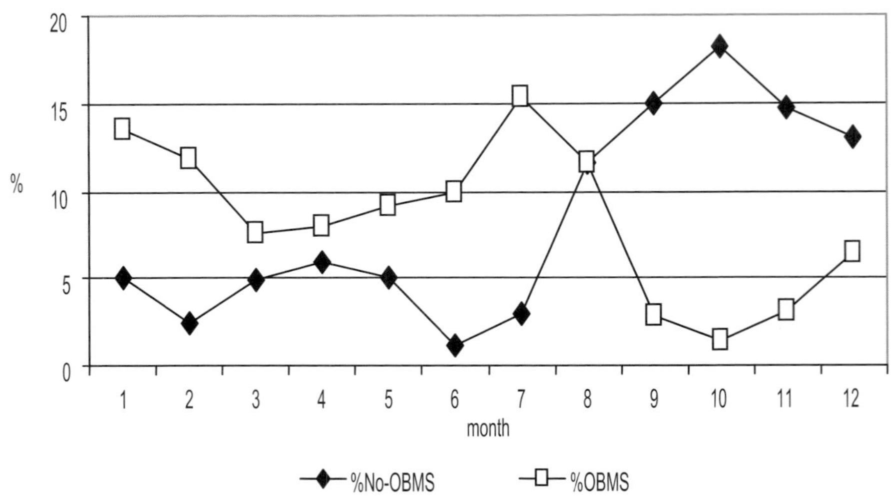

Fig. 3. Calving percentage in farms that use (%OBMS) or do not use (%No-OBMS) the out-of-breeding mating strategy (OBMS) technique.

It is possible to define a "temporary anoestrus" (<150 days) and a "deep anoestrus" (>150 days) based on the number of days open. It is also possible to distinguish between buffalo that come into oestrus within 70 days from calving, and conceive within or after 90 days, from those that come into oestrus after 70 days and conceive within or after 150 days (Zicarelli *et al.* 1994). Approximately 70% of buffaloes that deliver out of the breeding season showed RRC within 70 days from calving. Fifty-three percent of these buffalo were able to conceive within 3 months (around 75% of the animals that resumed the ovarian activity within 70 days) whereas 17.3% later than 3 months. The remaining 30% of animals had RRC after 70 days from calving and 10.6% and 18.8% conceived within and after 5 months, respectively.

Anoestrus can be identified as a non RRC after parturition or as an interruption of cyclic activity for varying reasons. Environmental conditions that are responsible for the anoestrus are accompanied by changes in blood hormones (Jain 1988) such as prolactin (Razdan *et al.* 1981), follicle stimulating hormone (Janakiraman *et al.* 1980), luteinizing hormone (Batra & Pandey 1982; Aboul-Ela *et al.* 1983), progesterone (Kaur *et al.* 1983; Qureshi *et al.* 2000), estradiol (Sheth *et al.* 1978; Heranjal *et al.* 1979; Razdan *et al.* 1981), thyroid hormones (Khurana & Madan 1985; Gupta & Dhoble 1988), and corticosteroids (Madan *et al.* 1983).

Some of these hormones represent the response to stressful factors rather than the cause of the arrest in reproductive activity. Buffalo that deliver out of the breeding season may need several months to conceive. During this period, they are not always acyclic, but are able to conceive and then undergo embryonic mortality, in particular between April and May, months characterized by progressively increasing day length. During the year, the embryonic mortality rate is 10% of the pregnanc es diagnosed at 40 days and is 22% for pregnancies that take place in the month of April (Zicarelli *et al.* 1994). The incidence of this event is affected by the "farm" factor and ranges between 10 and 45% if calculated on the pregnancies after AI diagnosed by ultrasonography at day 26 (Campanile *et al.* 2005).

A pregnancy is not always detected after the observation of a corpus luteum. It can be assumed that an early embryonic mortality or an anoestrus condition has occurred. The anoestrus condition may have been preceded by an ovarian cycle which forms a corpus luteum with inadequate function because of a short luteal phase or normal luteal phase with low progesterone (Zicarelli 1997; Zicarelli *et al.* 1997). This phenomenon has been found at the onset of anoestrus season in sheep, after first ovulation postpartum in bovine and during the prepubertal phase in both species (Garverick *et al.* 1992).

Some recent papers report an incidence of double ovulations of 15.5% in dairy cows (Lopez-Gautius *et al.* 2005). A similar value has been previously reported in buffalo (Zicarelli *et al.* 1988). In the latter, however, only 0.06% of double ovulation led to a twin pregnancy. The double ovulations reduce the efficiency of AI in the case of spontaneous oestruses, but not in the case of induced oestruses (Zicarelli *et al.* 1997).

In Italy, the OBMS technique leads to lesser fertility. In fact, when the OBMS technique was not applied, calving intervals of 400 to 445 days were recorded (Zicarelli *et al.* 2007). Recently, a mean inter-calving interval of 487±133 days was reported for 6,052 inter-calving intervals over a period of 5 to 10 years on 5 farms with an annual culling rate lower than 10% (Zicarelli *et al.* 2007). The OBMS technique was adopted and a constant rationing was given throughout the year. It was demonstrated that the shortest inter-calving periods were recorded in buffaloes that deliver between April and June, and that, consequently, conceived in the warmest months (between June and August). Short inter-calving intervals were also found in buffalo that delivered between July and September; the period of the year during which the highest temperatures are recorded in Italy. The longest inter-calving periods were recorded for buffaloes calving between October and December, because of the OBMS technique, which delays mating until February. Long inter-calving intervals were also found in buffaloes that calved between January and March, the coldest period of the year (Zicarelli *et al.* 1994; 1997; 2007). These buffalo would conceive in spring, the mildest period of the year, characterized by temperatures between 15 and 22°C. Conception is typically delayed until September, however, except for the 40% of animals that conceive within 90 days from calving. We can conclude, therefore, that in Italy nutrition and the warmest months, especially if a swimming-pool is present on the farm (Di Palo *et al.* 2009; Neglia *et al.* 2009), do not affect the inter-calving period. The main factor that has to be taken into account in Italy is the light stimulus. Buffaloes that deliver between January and March delay their conception until August to September, after three months of decreasing day length. Similarly, buffaloes that deliver in the period April to September show the shortest inter-calving period because after 58 days decreasing day length begins.

The majority of Indian and Egyptian authors assert that the lower concentration of calving observed between January and May depends on the reduced conception rate between March and July. This phenomenon is influenced by the hot and dry climate of this period of the year. In Italy, in farms that do not use the OBMS, a drop of calving is also observed between January and June (Fig. 1); a period of the year in which, unlike India, the climate is either cold or mild and moderately rainy. The fertility markedly improves between July and September; a period that in Italy coincides with the highest temperature (Fig. 4) and temperature humidity index of the year. This observation makes buffalo very different from cattle, that in the hottest months of the year (July to September), show a marked decrease in fertility.

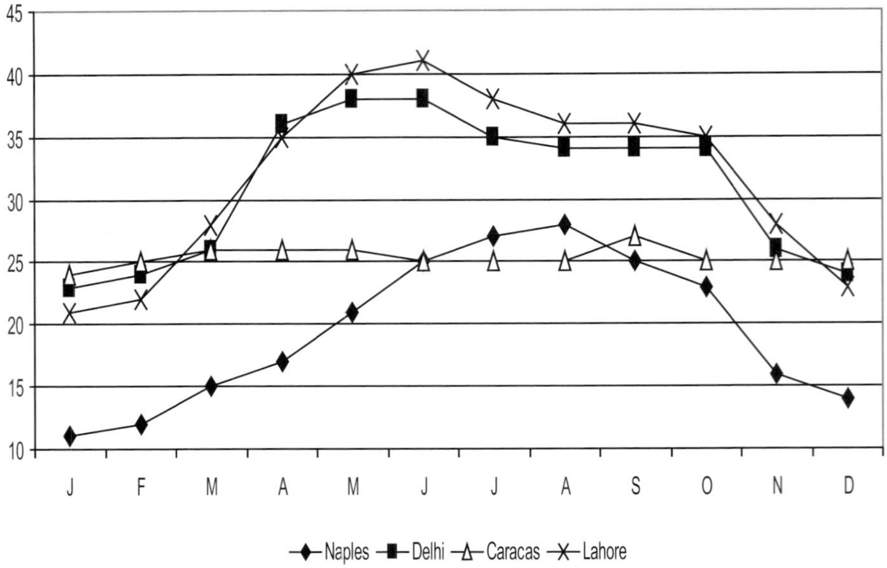

Fig. 4. Monthly maximum temperature (°C) in Naples, Delhi, Caracas, and Lahore. Calendar months (single letter abbreviations) are indicated on the x-axis.

We have already highlighted that in the areas located north of the equator a drop in the number of calvings is observed between January and June. The authors from countries located north of the equator attribute the anoestrus of buffalo to heat stress (India, Pakistan) or to the low environmental humidity (Venezuela). In our opinion, the decrease in calving rate between January and June (Fig. 1) depends on the reduced reproductive activity between March and September. In the latter period, the maximum daily temperature (Fig. 4) ranges between 15°C (March) and 27°C (August) in Naples, Italy; between 25°C and 38°C in Delhi, India; between 27°C (March) and 41°C (June) in Lahore, Pakistan; and between 25°C (March) and 26°C (August) in Caracas, Venezuela. The maximum daily temperatures that are recorded in Italy and in Venezuela rule out a direct action of environmental temperature on anoestrus. If only India and Pakistan are considered, it is not possible to exclude that heat stress, even if it is not the main factor, contributes to summer anoestrus. Furthermore, the RRC (August to September) coincides with a monthly maximum temperature of 28°C (August) and 25°C (September) in Italy, 25°C (August) and 27°C (September) in Venezuela, 34°C (September) in India and 36°C in Pakistan.

The monthly rainfall recorded in Italy and Venezuela between September and October is not different from that observed between March and May (Italy) and between June and August (Venezuela) when the lower conception rate is observed (Fig. 5). On the contrary, in India and in Pakistan the rainy season takes place between July and September. The cessation of reproductive activity in Italy and Venezuela, therefore, cannot be attributed to the rainfall. In India and Pakistan, the reproductive activity is good in October and November (calving August and September), when the temperature is lower and the rainfall is already minimal. The trend of daylight hours, although with different daily values, is shared by all the areas of breeding situated north of the equator (Fig. 6). Interestingly, a 4-year retrospective analysis of data (B Gasparrini,

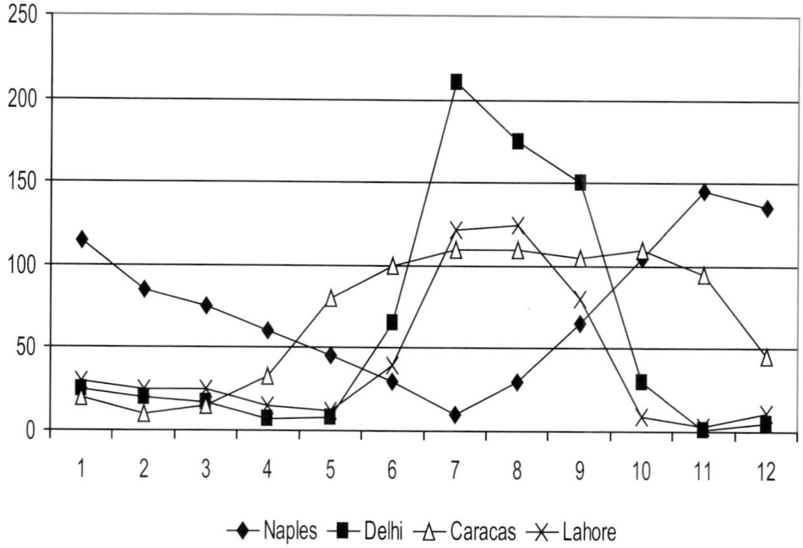

Fig. 5. Monthly rainfall (mm) in Naples, Delhi, Caracas, and Lahore.

unpublished observations) obtained in an in vitro embryo production laboratory showed that a significant decrease in blastocyst rate was observed between April to June compared with October to December. Intermediate values were recorded between July and September and between January and March. The drop in oocyte developmental competence coincides with the spring months that at our latitudes are characterized by mild environmental temperatures. This pattern confirms that the light stimulus plays the most critical role in determining seasonality.

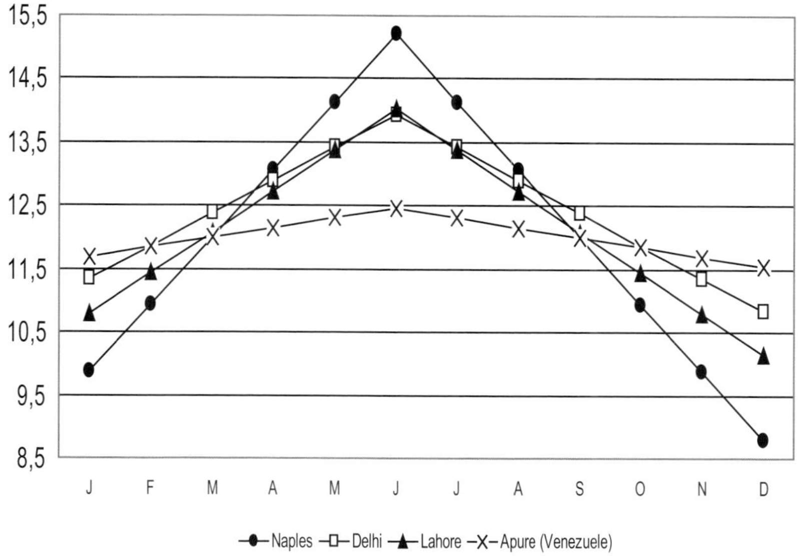

Fig. 6. Daylight hours (h) in Naples, Delhi, Appure (Venezuela), and Lahore. Calendar months (single letter abbreviations) are indicated on the x-axis.

South of the equator, Baruselli *et al.* (2001) demonstrated that the concentration of calving increases proportionally with increasing distance from the equator (Fig. 2). It is not possible to show any relationship between daily maximum temperature, rainfall and the calving calendar (Fig. 2) whereas an evident relationship exists between the calving calendar and the daylight hours at different latitudes (Fig. 7).

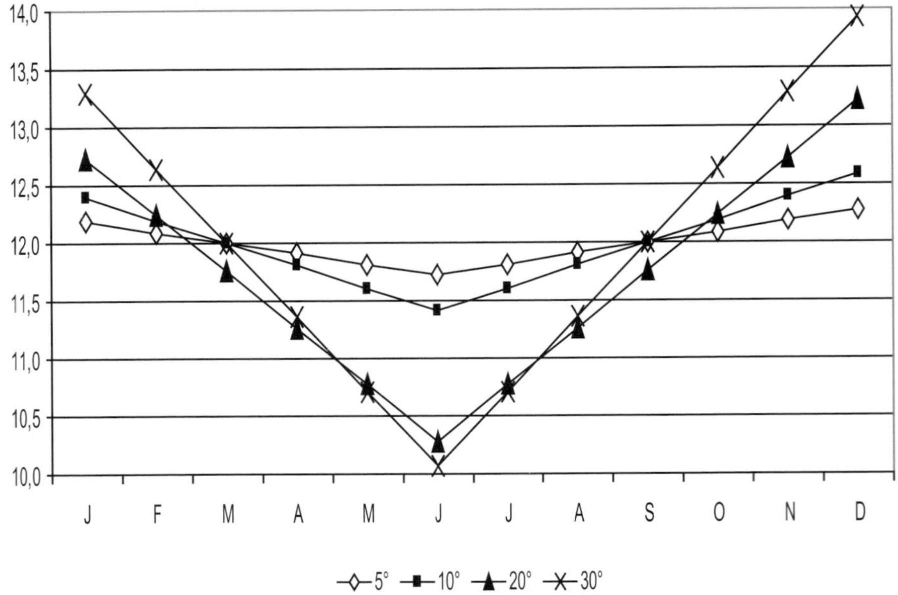

Fig. 7. Daylight hours (h) in Brazil as a function of latitude (°S). Calendar months (single letter abbreviations) are indicated on the x-axis.

Throughout this paper, the seasonality of the females has been considered. The phenomenon may affect the males as well. The effects are clear when the animals are maintained in free mounting condition. Recently, we observed in the same farm a higher pregnancy rate between January and April in buffaloes inseminated by AI compared with buffalo that were bred by using the bull. This perhaps occurred because the AI avoided the negative effect of the bull. We have recently verified that in April, only 23%, 31% and 29% of the bulls showed values higher than the average value for testosterone, diihydrotestosterone and androstenedione, respectively (Pelagalli *et al.* 2009).

Strategies to enhance reproductive performance

The delayed puberty and the consequent older age at first calving depend on both inappropriate weaning techniques and inadequate feeding during growth. The age at first calving was 28 to 32 months when feeding a diet characterized by an energy density of 0.8 MUF (MUF = Milk unit forages = 1700 kcal NE_l) and 12.5 to 13% protein content on a dry matter basis and a forage to concentrate ratio of 50 to 60%, (Zicarelli 2007). Embryonic mortality in buffalo is primarily due to a reduced secretion of progesterone by the corpus luteum. The importance of progesterone concentration during the first weeks of pregnancy for reducing embryonic mortality has been demonstrated in both cattle (Mann 2002) and buffalo (Campanile *et al.* 2005; 2007; 2008; 2009). In cattle, several treatments have been used typically within 5 days after conception to increase progesterone secretion by the existing corpus luteum or to induce ovulation and formation of an accessory corpus luteum (Mann 2002). Treatments on day 5 after insemination do not have any effect on reducing embryonic mortality in buffalo (Campanile *et al.* 2007). Treatment of buffaloes with a GnRH agonist, hCG or progesterone on day 25 after AI reduced embryonic mortality (Campanile *et al.* 2008).

Although the light/dark ratio is the main factor affecting reproductive efficiency, another important factor is the satisfaction of the buffalo's physiological need of water for bathing. The presence of a swimming-pool reduced the not pregnant buffaloes per corpora lutea ratio (NP/CL) found at rectal examination in buffaloes that calved between April and August (Di Palo *et al.* 2009; Neglia *et al.* 2009). The swimming pool apparently acted to reduce heat stress. The NP/CL ratio, as an indicator of an anomalous oestrous cycle or embryonic mortality, may be proposed as a specific tool for evaluating buffalo welfare (Di Palo *et al.* 2009).

The treatments for anoestrus are based on the use of progesterone devices combined with PMSG. The response is influenced by the effects of year and farm and are, therefore, variable. The above treatments in natural mating conditions do not have an immediate impact but in primiparous females they have a beneficial effect on the RRC. Unsatisfactory responses are perhaps more useful because they lead to the assessment of the environmental causes that underlie the reproductive failures (Zicarelli *et al.* 1994). For instance, we demonstrated that more space and better welfare conditions improved fertility in Italy. On 21 farms in which the OBMS is performed we observed that 38.1%, 52.4% and 4.8% of the farms increased fertility rate respectively in June, July to August and September (L. Zicarelli, unpublished observations). Out of the 8 farms that resumed fertility in June, 6 (75%) had at their disposal either covered sheds, that shorten the day length on average by 2 h during the year, or wide open spaces in which buffalo cows can move for at least 6 h/day or swimming pools. Out of the 11 farms that resumed fertility in July only 2 (18.2%) had swimming pools available (6/8 versus 2/11). In a farm with a variable number of breedings over 10 years, an increase in reproductive activity in June and July was recorded. Between January and June 77% and 68% of calving were observed, respectively, for 352 and 451 buffaloes. These finding suggest that the effects of season can in part be attenuated by improving the welfare status of the animals.

Conclusions

The seasonality in buffalo is influenced by the light/dark ratio throughout the year. In some countries the seasonality is influenced by nutritional factors. Furthermore, an improvement in the welfare of buffalo (swimming pool, space, brightness of the stalls, etc.) can increase the percentage of calvings between March and June. Delayed treatment of buffaloes with GnRH agonist, hCG or progesterone on day 25 after AI can reduce embryonic mortality in the months in which daylight hours increase. A significant improvement in reproductive efficiency can be achieved by increasing the culling rate from 10-14% to 25-30%, and hence eliminating older buffalo and those with reproductive problems.

References

Aboul-Ela MB, El-Keraby FE & Chesworth JM 1983 Seasonal variation in the LH release in response to GnRH in the buffalo. *Anim. Reprod. Sci.* **6** 229–232.

Avallone L, Parmeggiani A, Esposito L & Campanile G 1994 Correlation between prolactin, T3 and T4 levels in buffalo heifers during the whole year. Proceedings of the Fourth World Buffalo Congress, São Paulo, p. 477-479.

Baruselli PS, Bernardes O, Braga DPAF, Araujo DC & Tonhati H 2001 Calving distribution throughout the year in buffalo raised all over Brazil. Proceedings of the Sixth World Buffalo Congress, Maracaibo, Venezuela, p. 234-239.

Batra SK & Pandey RS 1982 Luteinizing hormone and oestradiol-17B in blood plasma and milk during the estrous cycle and early pregnancy in Murrah buffaloes.

Anim. Reprod. Sci. **5** 247-257.

Borghese A, Barile VL, Terzano GM, Pilla AM & Parmeggiani A 1995 Melatonin trend during season in heifers and buffalo cow. *Bubalus bubalis* **1** 61-64.

Campanile G, Shehu D, Esposito L, Di Palo R, Montemurro N, Zicarelli L, Terzano GM & Borghese A 1991 Onset of ovarian activity in Italian buffalo heifers. Proceedings of the Third World Buffalo Congress, Varna, p. 666-671.

Campanile G, Avallone L, d'Angelo A, Di Palo R & Di Meo C 1994 Influence of the season and of the number of days after calving on the pattern of thyroid hormones in buffalo cows. Proceedings of the Fourth World Buffalo Congress, São Paulo, p. 564-566.

Campanile G, Neglia G, Gasparrini B, Galiero G, Prandi A, Di Palo R, D'Occhio MJ & Zicarelli L 2005 Embryonic mortality in buffaloes synchronized and mated by AI during the seasonal decline in reproductive function. *Theriogenology* **63** 2334-2340.

Campanile G, Di Palo R, Neglia G, Vecchio D, Gasparrini B, Prandi A, Galiero G & D'Occhio MJ 2007 Corpus luteum function and embryonic mortality in buffaloes treated with a GnRH agonist, hCG and progesterone. *Theriogenology* **67** 1393-1398.

Campanile G, Vecchio D, Di Palo R, Neglia G, Gasparrini B, Prandi A, Zicarelli L & D'Occhio MJ 2008 Delayed treatment with GnRH agonist, hCG and progesterone and reduced embryonic mortality in buffaloes. *Theriogenology* **70** 1544-1549.

Campanile G, Neglia G, Vecchio D, Russo M & Zicarelli L 2009 Pregnancy in buffalo cows. In: *Pregnancy Protein Research*, p. 31-91, M. O'Leary and J. Arnett (Eds), Nova Science Publishers, Inc., New York.

Da Silva MET & Grodzki L 1991 Study of correlations between climatic factors and seasonal fertility of female buffaloes in the Northeast of the state of Parana. Brazil. Proceedings of the Third World Buffalo Congress, Varna, p. 689-700.

Di Palo R, Parmeggiani A, Campanile G & Zicarelli L 1993 Repeatability of melatonin plasma levels in buffaloes bred in Italy. *Atti della Societa Italiana delle Scienze Veterinarie*, **47** 331-335.

Di Palo R, Parmeggiani A, Spadetta M, Campanile G, Esposito L, Seren E & Zicarelli L 1997 Influence of changing farm on the repeatability of melatonin plasma level in Italian Mediterranean buffalo. Proceedings of the Fifth World Buffalo Congress, Caserta, p. 758-761.

Di Palo R, Ariota B, Zicarelli F, De Blasi M, Zicarelli G & Gasparrini B 2009 Incidence of pregnancy failures in buffaloes with different rearing system. *Ital. J. Anim. Sci.* **8** (Suppl. 2) 619-621.

Ferrara B 1957. Ricerche su alcune statistiche vitali nella popolazione bufalina dell'Italia Meridionale. Nota II: intervallo interparto e distribuzione dei parti. *Acta Med. Vet.* **3** 225-233.

Garverick HA, Zollers VG & Smith MF 1992 Mechanisms associated with corpus luteum lifespan in animals having normal or subnormal luteal function. *Anim. Reprod. Sci.* **28** 111-124.

Gasparrini B 2002 In vitro embryo production in buffalo species: state of the art. *Theriogenology* **57** 237-256.

Gupta SK & Dhoble RL 1988 Response of suboestrus rural buffaloes to PGF2α analogue in relation to levels of triiodothyronine (T3), tetraiodothyronine/ thyroxine (T4) and progesterone. Proceedings of the Second World Buffalo Congress, New Delhi, India.

Hassan F, Khan MS, Rehman MS, Sarwar M & Bhatti SA 2007 Seasonality of calving in Nili-Ravi Buffaloes, purebred Sahiwal and cross-bred cattle in Pakistan. *Ital. J. Anim. Sci.* **6** (Suppl. 2) 1298-1301.

Heranjal DD, Sheth AR, Wadadekar KB, Desai R & Rao SS 1979 Serum gonadotrophins and prolactin in anoestrus buffaloes. *Indian J. Dairy Sci.* **32** 383-385.

Jain GC 1988 Hormonal profiles in anoestrus rural buffaloes. Proceeding of the SecondWorld Buffalo Congress, New Delhi, India, p. 39.

Janakiraman K, Desai MC, Anim DR, Sheth AR, Moodbird SB & Wadadekar KB 1980 Serum gonadotropin levels in buffaloes in relation to phases of oestrous cycle and breeding periods. *Indian J. Anim. Sci.* **50** 601-606.

Kaur H, Arora SP & Sawhney A 1983 Progesterone and estradiol–17ß concentrations in blood plasma of buffaloes during different reproductive disorders. *Indian J. Anim. Reprod.* **3** 62.

Khurana ML & Madan ML 1985 Thyroxin secretion rate in buffaloes during hot dry, hot humid and cold season. Proceedings of the First World Buffalo Congress, Cairo, Egypt, p. 1165.

Le Van TY, Chupin D & Driancurt MA 1989 Ovarian follicular populations in buffaloes and cows. *Anim. Reprod. Sci.* **19** 171-178.

Lincoln GA 1992 Photoperiod-pineal-hypothalamic relay in sheep. *Anim. Reprod. Sci.* **28** 203-217.

Lopez-Gautius F, Lopez Bejar M, Fenech M & Hunter RH 2005 Ovulation failure and double ovulation in dairy cattle; risk factors and effects. *Theriogenology* **63** 1298-1307.

Madan ML 1988 Status of reproduction in female buffalo. Proceedings of the Second World Buffalo Congress, New Delhi, p. 89-100.

Madan ML, Naqvi SMK, Triu CV, Suri AK & Prakash BS 1983 Plasma estradiol - 17ß, progesterone and cortisol among anestrus rural animals. *Indian J. Anim. Reprod.* **3** 60

Mann GE 2002 Corpus luteum function and early embryonic death in the bovine. Proceedings of XXII World Buiatrics Congress, Hannover, Germany, p. 300-306.

Misra AK & Tyagi S 2007 In vivo embryo production in buffalo: present and perspectives. *Italian J. Anim. Sci.* **6** (Suppl. 2) 74-91.

Montiel U 2000 Aspectos reproductivos de la búfala. Comportamiento reproductivo en bufalas en un ambiente de bosque muy seco tropical. I Simposium Internacional de Búfalos de Venezuela, Maracaibo, p. 5-20.

Neglia G, Rendina M, Balestrieri A, Grasso FL, Potena A, Russo I & Zicarelli L 2009 Influence of a swimming-pool on fertility in buffalo species. *Ital. J. Anim. Sci.* **8** (Suppl. 2) 637-639.

Paul SS & Lal D 2010 Nutrient requirement of buffaloes,

Satish Serial Publishing House.

Parmeggiani A & Di Palo R 1994 Melatonina e stagionalità riproduttiva della bufala. Atti Conv. su "Miglioramento dell'efficienza produttiva e riproduttiva della specie bufalina" *Agricolture e Ricerca* **153** 41-48.

Pelagalli A, d'Angelo D, Mastellone V, Lombardi P, Avallone L, Zicarelli G, Sattar A, & Zicarelli L 2009 Influence of buffalo dams reproductive status on sexual hormone activity in bulls, *Pakistan Journal Zoology*, Supplementary Series, No **9**, p. 61-63.

Qureshi MS, Samad HA, Habib, Usman RH & Siddiqui MM 1999a Study on factors leading to seasonality of reproduction in dairy buffaloes. I. Nutritional factors. *Asian-Aust. J. Anim. Sci.* **12** 1019-1024.

Qureshi MS, Habib RH, Samad HA, Lodhi LA & Usman RH 1999b Study on factors leading to seasonality of reproduction in dairy buffaloes. II. Non-nutritional factors. *Asian-Aust. J. Anim. Sci.* **12** 1025-1030.

Qureshi MS, Habib G, Nawab G, Siddiqui MM, Ahmad N & Samad HA 2000 Milk progesterone profiles in various reproductive states in dairy buffaloes under field conditions. *Proc. Natl. Sci. Council Taipei Taiwan* **24** 70-75.

Razdan MN, Kakar ML & Galhotra MM 1981 Serum luteinizing hormone levels of non cycling buffaloes (Bubalus bubalis). *Indian J. Anim. Sci.* **51** 286-288.

Roy A, Raizada BC, Pandey MD, Yadav PC & Sengupta BP 1968 Effect of management on the fertility of buffalo cows bred during summer. *Ind. J. Vet. Sci.* **38** 554.

Seren E, Parmeggiani A, Mongiorgi S, Zicarelli L, Montemurro N, Pacelli C, Campanile G, Esposito L, Di Palo R, Borghese A, Barile VL, Terzano GM, Annicchiarico G, & Allegrini S 1994 Modificazioni endocrine durante il ciclo ovarico nella bufala. *Agricoltura e Ricerca* **153** 17-24.

Shah SNH 1990 Prolonged calving intervals in the Nili Ravi buffalo. PhD Thesis, Utrecht University.

Sheth AR, Wadadekar KB, Moodbidri SB, Janakiraman K & Paramesh M 1978 Seasonal alteration in the serum prolactin and LH levels in the water buffaloes. *Curr. Sci.* **47** 75-77.

Singh G 1988 Seasonal trend of calving and subsequent service-period in rural buffaloes in Punjab (India). *Acta Vet.Scand.* **83** 80-84.

Singh M, Chavdhary KC & Takkar OP 1988 Increasing the reproduction performance of buffaloes. Proceedings of the Second World Buffalo Congress, New Delhi, p. 271-282.

Singh B & Lal K 1992 Effect of season and breed on certain reproductive traits in buffaloes under village condition. *Indian J. Anim. Res.* **26** 15-19.

Vale WG, Ohashi OM, Sousa JS & Ribeiro HFL 1990 Studies on the reproduction of water buffalo in the Amazon Valley, Brazil. Livestock Reproduction in Latin America. International Atomic Energy Agency, Vienna, p. 201-210.

Vale WG, Ribeiro HFL, Silva AOA, Sousa JS, Ohashi OM & Souza HEM 1996 Buffalo a non-seasonal breeder in the Amazon Valley, Brazil. Proceedings of the 13th International Congress on Animal Reproduction, Vol. 3, Sydney, p. 19-33.

Vittoria A 1997 Third course on biotechnology of reproduction in buffaloes, Supplement, *Bubalus bubalis*, **4** 15-20.

Zicarelli L 1994 Management in different environmental conditions. *Buf. J. Suppl.* **2** 17-38.

Zicarelli L 1997 Reproductive seasonality in buffalo. Proceedings of the 3th International Course of Biotechnology in Buffalo Reproduction, Napoli, Suppl. *Bubalus bubalis*, p. 29-52.

Zicarelli L 1999 Nutrition in dairy buffaloes. *Perspectives of buffalo husbandry in Brazil and Latin America.* Tonhati H, Barnabe VH, Baruselli PS (Eds), Funep, Jabuticabal. p. 157-178.

Zicarelli L 2000 Considerations about the prophylaxis of the uterine and vaginal prolapse in Italian Mediterranean buffalo cows. *Bubalus bubalis* **3** p. 71-90.

Zicarelli L 2007 Can we consider buffalo a non precocious and hypofertile species? *Italian J. Anim. Sci.* **6** (Suppl. 2) 143-154.

Zicarelli L, Di Lella T & de Franciscis G 1977 Osservazioni e rilievi sui parametri riproduttivi e produttivi di bufale in allevamento presso un'azienda della piana del Sele. *Acta Med. Vet.* **23** 183-206.

Zicarelli L, Campanile G, Infascelli F, Esposito L & Ferrari G 1988 Incidence and fertility of heats with double ovulations in the Mediterranean buffalo cows of Italy. Proceedings of the Second World Buffalo Congress, New Delhi, India, p. 57-62.

Zicarelli L, Campanile G, Esposito L, Di Palo R, Boni R, Spadetta M, Montemurro N, Pacelli C, Borghese A, Barile VL, Terzano GM, Annicchiarico G, Allegrini S, De Benedetti A, Malfatti A, Lucaroni A & Todini L 1994 Anaestro e induzione dell'estro in bufale acicliche, (Anoestrus and oestrus induction in acyclic buffaloes), *Agric. Ric.* 153 25–40.

Zicarelli L, Esposito L, Campanile G, Di Palo R & Armstrong DT 1997 Effect of using vasectomized bulls in A.I. practice on the reproductive efficiency of Italian buffalo cows. *Anim. Reprod. Sci.* **47** 171-180.

Zicarelli L, Di Palo R, Neglia G, Ariota B, Varricchio E & Campanile G 2007 Estimation of the intercalving period in Italian Mediterranean buffalo. *Ital. J. Anim. Sci.* **6** (Suppl. 2) 709-712.

Zoheir KMA, Abdoon AS, Mahrous KF, Amer MA, Zaher MM, LiGuo Y & El-Nahass EM 2007 Effects of season on the quality and in vitro maturation rate of Egyptian buffalo (Bubalus bubalis) oocytes. *J. Cell. Anim. Biol.* **1** 29-33.

Gestation length in farmed reindeer

MP Shipka[1,2] and JE Rowell[1]

[1]*Department of High Latitude Agriculture, School of Natural Resources and Agricultural Sciences, University of Alaska Fairbanks, Fairbanks, Alaska;* [2]*Center of Reproductive Biology, Washington State University, Pullman, Washington*

Reindeer *(Rangifer tarandus tarundus)* are the only cervids indigenous to the arctic environment. In Alaska, reindeer are a recognized agricultural species and an economic mainstay for many native populations. Traditionally raised in extensive free-ranging systems, a recent trend toward intensive farming requires a more in-depth knowledge of reproductive management. Reported gestation length in reindeer varies, ranging from 198 to 229 d in studies performed at the University of Alaska Fairbanks. A switchback study that manipulated only breeding date demonstrated a mean increase in gestation length of 8.5 d among females bred early in the season. The negative correlation between conception date and gestation length is consistent with reindeer research at other locations and reports of variable gestation length in a growing number of domestic and non-domestic species. This paper reviews the phenomenon in reindeer and discusses some of the factors known to affect gestation length as well as possible areas for future research.

Introduction

Reindeer and caribou *(Rangifer tarandus)* are the only cervids indigenous to the arctic environment. With a circumpolar range extending from 45^0 to 80^0 N (Leader-Williams 1988) these animals have adapted to extremes in light, temperature, and nutrient availability and exhibit a number of characteristics that sets them apart from other deer species. Notably, they are the only deer in which both the male and female grow antlers; their highly gregarious nature contributes to the formation of massive herds that migrate greater distances in the spring and fall than any other deer; and they have been subjected to widespread domestication (Goss 1983). Caribou and reindeer are considered members of the same species even though they exhibit morphological and behavioral differences. Reindeer are considered the longest domesticated cervid, with a history of domestication going back thousands of years (Diamond 1999). It was because of their predisposition to agricultural practices that reindeer from Siberia were introduced to Alaska slightly more than 100 years ago. Over the ensuing century reindeer producers maintained their herds under free-range conditions utilizing grazing allotments of more than 400,000 hectares per herd. Such a system of extensive ranching was very successful and well suited to the northern ecosystem.

Intensive farming of reindeer, using traditional agricultural practices, is relatively new in Alaska and currently represents only a small fraction of the state's reindeer industry. However, this approach to reindeer farming occurs in at least 17 of the 48 contiguous states. The University of Alaska Fairbanks (UAF, 65^{0}N latitude) has established a program in Reindeer Reproductive Biology to support this emerging industry.

Corresponding author E-mail: mpshipka@alaska.edu

Reindeer reproductive biology

The initial goal of the program was to document the basic reproductive biology of reindeer and to provide a better understanding of the endocrinology of the estrous cycle and pregnancy in farmed Alaskan reindeer. Reindeer are similar to other cervids and domestic livestock in general. They have a mean estrous cycle length of 24 ± 1 d (range 18-29 d) (Shipka *et al.* 2007a). Reindeer females, under good husbandry conditions, will continue to cycle over the winter into March and April, (Bubenik *et al.* 1997, Blake *et al.* 2007, Shipka *et al.* 2007a). The endocrinology of pregnancy is also unremarkable and characteristic of a species dependent on luteal progesterone throughout gestation (Blake *et al.* 2007,Shipka *et al.* 2007a). Although the corpus luteum (CL) of pregnancy decreases in weight over the course of gestation, a functional CL is still present as late as 5.5 months (Roine 1974) and remains an important source of progesterone throughout gestation (Flood *et al.* 2005). Earlier studies in reindeer reproduction reported gestation lengths ranging from 208-240 d (McEwan & Whitehead 1972, Dott & Utsi 1973, Roine 1974, Bergerud 1975, Blom *et al.* 1983, Leader-Williams 1988, Reimers 2002), collectively providing a range in gestation length equivalent to almost two estrous cycles. In one study at UAF, the mean gestation length for 10 yearling females was 211 ± 2.2 d but the range was 198 to 221 d (Shipka *et al.* 2007a) while a contemporary study of 13 multiparous reindeer provided a mean gestation length of 216 d with a range of 212 to 220 d (Ropstad *et al.* 2005). The wide range in gestation length has generally been accepted within the context of how the data were collected: field observations of free-ranging animals compared to reindeer maintained in fenced settings under very different management regimens at very different latitudes. In addition, across the aforementioned studies, the means of establishing the time of breeding were equally variable and sample sizes generally small.

In an early study at UAF, 14 female reindeer were divided into 2 groups that remained well separated from any bulls. One group was introduced to the bull on Aug 23 while the other group was introduced to the bull on Sept 25. Although the study was designed to investigate the seasonal onset of ovarian activity, progesterone profiles established the time of breeding in 8 females and produced a variable gestation length ranging from 203 - 229 d. Breeding dates were spread over 26 days (Aug 31 – Sept 25) yet calving occurred over 7 days and there was a significant ($P < 0.001$) negative correlation between conception date and gestation length (Shipka *et al.* 2002). A retrospective examination of records from two reindeer herds at UAF where breeding dates (confirmed by systemic progesterone concentrations) and calving dates were known ($n = 39$) further strengthened this relationship. Females bred early in the season had a longer gestation than females bred later in the season (Shipka & Rowell 2006). The hypothesis that manipulating breeding date can alter gestation length was tested using a switchback design and, again, produced a significant ($P < 0.001$) negative relationship between conception date and gestation length (Rowell & Shipka 2009). The model generated by the switchback study has good predictive ability for female reindeer in good condition mated between late August and early October. Late bred animals consistently shorten gestation by 8-10 d. Despite small sample sizes, the results are strengthened by the documentation of a similar, highly significant, negative correlation between conception date and gestation length in Finnish reindeer (Ropstad *et al.* 2005, Holand *et al.* 2006, Mysterud *et al.* 2009) while anecdotal observations of this association in reindeer go back over 70 years (Schmit 1936, cited in Roine 1974). Across all these studies is the remarkably consistent, highly significant negative relationship between gestation length and breeding date.

Variable gestation length is not a unique observation. In the wild ruminant literature Berger (1992) introduced the concept of gestation plasticity in well conditioned bison and stressed the positive effect this had on maintaining calving synchrony. Recent documentation of a negative relationship between gestation length and conception date has been reported in a number of other species, most notably red deer (Asher 2006, Scott *et al.* 2008), Iberian red deer (Garcia *et al.* 2006), pronghorn antelope and bighorn sheep (Byers & Hogg 1995), Alaskan moose (Schwartz & Hundertmark 1993), alpacas (Davis *et al.* 1997), and dromedary camels (Elias *et al.* 1991). Although less apparent, the phenomenon has also been documented in domestic species. Howell and Rollins (1951) found season of breeding to be the single most important source of variation in gestation length of mares, independent of level of nutrition, with breeding in Sept – Nov producing the shortest gestation lengths. Even among non-seasonally breeding dairy cattle, analysis of data from 11 million parturitions found a moderate effect of month of conception on gestation length, with October conceptions producing a gestation length 2 d shorter than conceptions in January and February (Norman *et al.* 2009).

Factors affecting gestation length

Gestation length, defined as the period of time from conception to parturition, has historically been recognized as a species-specific, genetically determined event. However, it has also been equally recognized that gestation length can be modified by a number of factors such as

i. fetal influences (fetal genetics, fetal sex, pituitary/adrenal axis)
ii. maternal conditions (age, body size, and condition)
iii. environment (season, temperature, and nutrition).

Species and breed differences in gestation length have been well documented in domestic animals (sheep, goats, horses, and cattle) and between the various cervid species. Because of highly variable gestation lengths among cervid hybrids, Asher (2007) suggested that species specific gestation length is likely governed by relatively few genes. Red deer carrying cross-bred calves (wapiti X red deer) experience a 2.5% increase in mean gestation length (Moore & Littlejohn 1989). Although caribou and reindeer are considered the same species they differ in seasonal timing of reproductive events, with reindeer initiating estrous cycles 2-6 wk earlier than caribou even when both are raised under identical conditions (Leader-Williams 1988, Rowell & Shipka 2009). Information on hybrid gestation length is not available, however, reported mean gestation lengths of 216.7 (range 206-231) for captive and 227 (range 219-238) for wild caribou (McEwan & Whitehead 1972) are consistent with gestation lengths in reindeer (Shipka *et al.* 2007a). Hybridization between reindeer and caribou has occurred deliberately in an effort to increase carcass weight and may also occur where the ranges of the two subspecies overlap (Klein 1980), though gene flow between reindeer and caribou has been limited (Cronin *et al.* 2003). In our studies on gestation length the animals were all reindeer from the same genetic stock and thus genetics cannot account for the variable gestation length produced by manipulating breeding date.

Fetal influence through sex differences has been documented for a number of cervids including reindeer, with male reindeer calves reported to have slightly longer gestations (3-5 d) (Roine 1974, Mysterud *et al.* 2009) and greater birth weights than females calves (Eloranta & Nieminen 1986, Blake *et al.* 1998, Holand *et al.* 2006). Not all studies document a difference between male and female birth weight (Eloranta & Nieminen 1988). In the switchback study there was no difference in birth weight between male and female calves, although there was a tendency for birth weight of males to increase with gestation length. This relationship was not evident for females and the sex of the calf was independent of gestation length (Rowell & Shipka 2009). In both years of the switchback study the same sire was used to reduce any impact of the sire (through fetal genetics) on gestation length. Among red deer, no effect of calf sire was identified in a study of conception date and gestation length (Scott *et al.* 2008).

Age of the female at breeding can also affect gestation length. Maternal age and body weight are closely correlated; yearlings and primaparous reindeer are lighter, tend to breed later in the season, and have lighter offspring (Rognmo *et al.* 1983, Skogland, 1984, Eloranta & Nieminen 1988, Lenvik *et al.* 1988, Ronnegard *et al.* 2002, Reimers 2002). Mysterud *et al.* (2009) documented increasing gestation length with maternal age. This was partly due to the fact that older, heavier females bred earlier in the season and, thus, had longer gestation lengths. In the switchback study the sample size was too small to examine the effects of age although there was a tendency for older females to have longer gestation lengths. Nonetheless, they still exhibited an 8-10 d difference between early and late conceptions (Rowell & Shipka 2009).

Of the environmental impacts that can affect gestating females, the greatest body of information in semi domestic reindeer has examined the role of nutrition (reflected in maternal live weight and body condition) on gestation length, calf birth weight, and calf survival. It has been recognized for a long time that gestation length is extended in severely undernourished females (Bergerud 1975, Skogland 1984, Skogland 1990, Flydal & Reimers 2002) and the incidence of stillbirths increased when pregnancy occurred in females on a low plane of nutrition (Tveraa *et al.* 2003). The correlation between calf birth weight and survival is the same in reindeer as it is in many temperate region ungulates, low birth weight and late born calves experience higher mortality rates than do calves ≥ mean birth weight, born during the primary calving pulse (Bergerud 1975, Rognmo *et al.* 1983, Skogland 1984, Tveraa *et al.* 2003, Fauchald *et al.* 2004). Birth weight of calves is significantly correlated with dam body weight just prior to calving (Rognmo *et al.* 1983, Ronnegard *et al.* 2002, Tveraa *et al.* 2003). In a study of fetal growth characteristics among reindeer in Norway, fetal growth was reduced by 42% in females on poor quality ranges (Flydal & Reimers 2002, Reimers 2002). Fetal growth is apparently independent of female body condition for approximately the first two thirds of pregnancy, becoming susceptible to female condition only during the last third of gestation (Flydal & Reimers 2002). Among red deer, experimentally restricting food intake during the last third of pregnancy extended mean gestation length (8 d) and resulted in calves with the same birth weight as controls (Asher *et al.* 2005a). Conversely, when red deer were gestating hybrid calves (wapiti X red deer) dietary restriction resulted in lighter birth weight calves but no significant difference in gestation length, leading the authors to suggest that fetal genotype overrode mechanisms for extending gestation length (Asher *et al.* 2005b). Among reindeer, feed restriction during the last 120 days of pregnancy extended gestation by 13 days in the feed restricted group (lichen diet) but also reduced calf birth weight by 36.5% with 2 neonatal deaths (Fauchald *et al.* 2004).The impact of nutrition on gestation length in cervids has produced variable results making it difficult to extrapolate beyond the restrictions imposed by individual studies.

Seasonal fluctuations in weight and fat reserves are a typical feature of ungulates in temperate zones and have been well described in reindeer (characterized by increasing weight gain peaking in late summer followed by a gradual weight decrease that reaches a nadir around the time of parturition and initiation of lactation) (Leader-Williams 1988). Captive, well fed reindeer maintain a less dramatic but similar cyclic pattern of growth and will voluntarily reduce food intake over the winter, regardless of available forage. In the switchback study the reindeer were fed ad libitum, and while body weight fluctuated throughout the winter, they all followed the same relative pattern of body weight change over the course of pregnancy with no significant differences in weight loss identified among animals across the two year study. Reindeer in suboptimal body condition are quite capable of taking advantage of available food and gaining weight during winter months (Shipka *et al.* 2007a). Pregnant females provided *ad libitum* feed in late pregnancy gained 18% of body weight in one study (Sakkinen *et al.* 1999) and 12% of initial body weight in another (Fauchald *et al.* 2004). Given this information, it is important to realize that the variable gestation length identified in the switchback study cannot be linked to a late winter nutritional deficit. The females in that study did not lose appreciable weight during the last trimester, always had access to *ad libitum* feed, and, with the exception of the six wk that encompassed the two harem periods, they were managed as a single group throughout gestation and calving. The only manipulation was conception date.

Other than nutrition, relatively little is known about environmental impacts on gestation. Severe winter weather has been implicated in prolonging gestation in dall's sheep (Rachlow & Bowyer 1991). Alternatively, parturition and calving synchrony in Alaskan moose were not correlated with predation, snow depth or plant phenology (Bowyer *et al.* 1998). Evidence for direct effects of proximate environmental conditions on gestation length is inconsistent and difficult to demonstrate.

All of the above variables are known to affect gestation length, and all of them interact at different levels in reindeer populations. Yet none adequately explains the phenomenon of variable gestation length identified in captive reindeer here in Alaska or in the Scandinavian studies. Reindeer bred late in the season shorten gestation by 8.5 d (Rowell & Shipka 2009) or 10 d (Holand *et al.* 2006) A similar interval was identified in Iberian red deer (Garcia *et al.* 2006) and in red deer in New Zealand (Scott *et al.* 2008) While variable gestation enhances calving synchrony it doesn't necessarily produce highly synchronous calving. Early bred females, despite their longer gestation, still calved early, 18-20 d before the late bred females. This phenomenon is emphasized by the work of Mysterud *et al.*, (2009) who found gestation length to increase with maternal age; i.e. mature, heavier reindeer bred earlier and had longer gestation lengths. If gestation is being lengthened as a result of nutritional constraints on fetal growth during late pregnancy, then multiparous, well-conditioned females are the last group one would expect to extend gestation.

What is being described here appears to be a seasonal affect on gestation length (Berger 1992, Garcia *et al.* 2006, Holand *et al.* 2006, Mysterud *et al.* 2009), the earlier in the season a female is bred, the longer her gestation. These disparate gestation lengths produce calves of equivalent weight and viability (Shipka *et al.* 2007b), and are independent of nutrition. The possibility that gestation adjustment may be occurring early in pregnancy is worth investigating.

Embryonic diapause

Embryonic diapause or delayed implantation has been described as the 'uncoupling of mating and fertilization from birth' (Lopes *et al.* 2004) and is a very rare phenomenon in cervids. It has only been documented unequivocally in the roe deer (Short & Hay 1966) and suggested in Père David's deer (Brinklow & Loudon 1993). Key prerequisites for delayed implantation are an uncharacteristically long gestation length (as a function of maternal body weight) and a mechanism to prevent luteolysis during the period of blastocyst delay. Roe deer are monestrus, undergoing pseudopregnancy in the absence of conception (Short & Hay 1966, Aitken 1974, Lambert *et al.* 2001), have the longest gestation length among Cervidae ($\geq$ 285 d) (Brinklow & Loudon 1993) and are obligate delayed implanters (Short & Hay 1966). Père David's deer also have a long gestation (283-84 d) (Brinklow & Loudon 1993). Although Père David's deer are polyestrus, the first cycle of the season can range from 45-60 d in length (Curlewis *et al.* 1988) and Brinklow and Loudon (1993) have speculated that the extended cycles may be comparable to 'pseudopregnancy'. They concluded that Père David's deer most likely have a brief obligate delay of implantation or slower post implantation development compared to other cervids.

References

Abecia JA, Forcada F, Casao A & Palacin I 2008 Effect of exogenous melatonin on the ovary, the embryo and the establishment of pregnancy in sheep. *Animal* **2**, 399-404.

Abecia JA, Forcada F & Zuniga O 2002 Effect of melatonin on secretion of progesterone in sheep and on the development of ovine embryos in vitro. *Veterinary Research Communications* **26** 151-158.

Aitken RJ 1974 Delayed implantation in roe deer (*Capreolus capreolus*). *Journal of Reproduction & Fertility* **39** 225-233.

Asher GW 2007 Reproductive cycles in female cervids. In *Large Animal Theriogenology 2*, pp 921-936. Eds RS Youngquist & WR Threlfall. St Louis: Saunders, Elsevier.

Asher, GW 2006 Gestation length in red deer: genetically determined or environmentally controlled? In *Reproduction in Domestic Ruminants VI* pp 255-260 Eds JI Juengel, JF Murray & MF Smith. United Kingdom: Nottingham University Press.

Asher GW, Mulley RC, O'Neill KT, Scott IC, Jopson NB & Littlejohn RP 2005a Influence of level of nutrition during late pregnancy on reproductive productivity of red deerl. Adult and primiparous hinds gestating red deer calves. *Animal Reproduction Science* **86** 261-283.

Asher GW, Scott IC, O'Neill KT & Littlejohn RP 2005b Influence of level of nutrition during late pregnancy on reproductive productivity of red deer: (2) Adult hinds gestating wapiti x red deer crossbred calves. *Animal Reproduction Science* **86** 285-296.

Bazer FW, Spencer TE, Johnson GA & Burghardt RC 2009 Comparative aspects of implantation. *Reproduction* **138** 195-209.

Berger J 1992. Facilitation of reproductive synchrony by gestation adjustment in gregarious mammals: a new hypothesis. *Ecology* **73** 323-329.

Bergerud AT 1975 The reproductive season of Newfoundland caribou. *Canadian Journal of Zoology* **53** 1213-1221.

Berlinguer F, Leoni GG, Spezzigu A, Madeddu M, Satta V, Bebbere D, Contreras-Solis I, Gonzalez-Bulnes A & Naitana S 2009 Exogenous melatonin positively influences follicular dynamics, oocyte developmental competence and blastocyst output in a goat model. *Journal of Pineal Research* **46** 383-391.

Blake JE, Rowell JE & Shipka MP 2007 Reindeer Reproductive Management. In *Large Animal Theriogenology*, pp. 970-974. Eds RS Youngquist & WR Threlfall. St Louis, MI: Saunders, Elsevier.

Blake JE, Rowell JE & Suttie JM 1998 Characteristics of first-antler growth in reindeer and their association with seasonal fluctuations in steriod and insulin-like growth factor 1 levels. *Canadian Journal of Zoology* **76** 2096-2102.

Blom AK, Sjaastad OV & Jacobsen E 1983 Plasma levels of progesterone and oestradiol-17ß in reindeer (*Rangifer tarandus tarandus*) during pregnancy. *Acta Veterinaria Scandinavica* **24** 287-294.

Bowyer RT, Van Ballenberghe V & Kie JG 1998 Timing and synchrony of parturition in Alaskan moose: Long-term versus proximal effects of climate. *Journal of Mammalogy* **79** 1332-1344.

Brinklow BR & Loudon ASI 1993 Gestation period in the Père David›s Deer: evidence for embryonic diapause or delayed development. *Reproduction Fertility and Development* **5** 567-575.

Bubenik GA, Schams D, White RG, Rowell JE, Blake JE & Bartos L 1997 Seasonal levels of reproductive hormones and their relationship to the antler cycle of male and female reindeer. *Comparative Biochemistry and Physiology* **116B** 269-277.

Byers JA & Hogg JT 1995 Environmental effects on prenatal growth rate in pronghorn and bighorn: further evidence for energy constraint on sex-biased maternal energy expenditure. *Behavioral Ecology* **6** 451-457.

Cronin MA, Patton JC, Balmysheva N & MacNeil MD 2003 Genetic variation in caribou and reindeer (*Rangifer tarandus*). *Animal Genetics* **34** 33-41.

Curlewis JD, Loudon ASI & Coleman APM 1988 Oestrous cycles and the breeding season of the Père Davids's deer hind (*Elaphurus davidianus*). *Journal of Reproduction and Fertility* **82** 119-126.

Davis GH, Dodds KG, Moore GH & Bruce GD 1997 Seasonal effects on gestation length and birth weight in alpacas. *Animal Reproduction Science* **46** 297-303.

Diamond J 1999 Zebras, unhappy marriages and the Anna Kerenina principle. In *Guns, Germs, and Steel; the Fate of Human Societies*. Pp 157-175. New York: WW Norton and Company.

Dott HM & Utsi, MNP 1973 Artificial insemination of reindeer. *Journal of Zoology (London)* **170** 505-508.

Durotoye LA, Webley GE & Rodway RG 1997 Stimulation of the production of progesterone by the corpus luteum of the ewe by the perfusion of melatonin in vivo and by treatment of granulosa cells with melatonin in vitro. *Research in Veterinary Science* **62** 87-91.

Elias E, Degen AA & Kam M 1991 Effect of conception date on length of gestation in the dromedary camel (*Camelus dromedarius*) in the Negev Desert. *Animal Reproduction Science* **25** 173-177.

Eloranta E & Nieminen M 1986 The effects of maternal age and body weight on reindeer calf birth-weight and survival. *Rangifer* **1** 105.

Eloranta E & Nieminen M 1988 Calving and maternal body weight change in the reindeer. *Rangifer* **2***(special issue)* 64-65.

Fauchald P, Tveraa T, Henaug C & Yoccoz NG 2004 Adaptive regulation of body reserves in reindeer, *Rangifer tarandus*: A feeding experiment. *Oikos* **107** 583-591.

Flood PF, Tyler NJC, Read EK, Rodway MJ & Chedrese PJ 2005 Ovarian and placental production of progesterone and oestradiol during pregnancy in reindeer. *Animal Reproduction Science* **85** 147-162.

Flydal K & Reimers E 2002 Relationship between calving time and physical condition in three wild reindeer (*Rangifer tarandus*) populations in southern Norway.

Wildlife Biology **8** 145-152.

Garcia AJ, Landete-Castillejos T, Carrion D, Gaspar-Lopez E & Gallego L 2006 Compensatory extension of gestation length with advance of conception in red deer (*Cervus elaphus*). *Journal of Expermental Biology* **305A**, 55-61.

Garrett JE, Geisert RD, Zavy MT & Morgan GL 1988 Evidence for maternal regulation of early conceptus growth and development in beef cattle. *Journal of Reproduction and Fertility* **84** 437-466.

Goss RJ 1983 Deer Antlers. New York: Academic Press.

Holand O, Mysterud A, Roed KH, Coulson T, Gjostein H, Weladji RB & Nieminen M 2006 Adaptive adjustment of offspring sex ratio and maternal reproductive effort in an iteroparous mammal. *Proceedings of the Royal Society B* **273** 293-299.

Howell, CE & Rollins, WC 1951 Environmental sources of variation in gestation length of the horse. *Journal of Animal Science* **10** 789-796.

Hugentobler SA, Sreenan JM, Humpherson PG, Leese HJ, Diskin MG & Morris DG 2010 Effects of changes in the concentration of systemic progesterone on ions, amino acids and energy substrates in cattle oviduct and uterine fluid and blood. *Reproduction Fertility and Development* **22** 684-694.

Kleemann DO, Walker SK & Seamark RF 1994 Enhanced fetal growth in sheep administered progesterone during the first three days of pregnancy. *Journal of Reproduction and Fertility* **102** 411-417.

Klein DR 1980 Conflicts between domestic reindeer and their wild counterparts: A review of Eurasian and North American experience. *Arctic* **33** 739-756.

Lambert RT, Ashworth CJ, Beattie L, Gebbie FE, Hutchinson JSM, Kyle DJ & Racey PA 2001 Temporal changes in reproductive hormones and conceptus-endometrial interactions during embryonic diapause and reactivation of the blastocyst in European roe deer (*Capreolus capreolus*). *Reproduction* **121** 863-871.

Leader-Williams N 1988 Reindeer on South Georgia: The ecology of an introduced population. pp 1-319 Great Briton: Cambridge University Press.

Lenvik D, Ebsen B & Fjellheim A 1988 Relationship between the weight of reindeer calves in autumn and their mother's age and weight in the previous spring. *Rangifer* **8** 20-24.

Lincoln GA 1998 Photoperiod-melatonin relay in deer. *Acta Veterinaria Hungarica* **46** 341-356.

Lopes FL, Desmarais JA & Murphy BD 2004 Embryonic diapause and its regulation. *Reproduction* **128** 669-678.

Manjunatha BM, Devaraj M, Gupta PSP, Ravindra JP & Nandi S 2009 Effect of taurine and melatonin in the culture medium on buffalo in vitro embryo development. *Reproduction in Domestic Animals* **44** 12-16.

Mann GE, Fray MD & Lamming GE 2006 Effects of time of progesterone supplementation on embryo development and interferon-t production in the cow. *The Veterinary Journal* **171** 500-503.

McEwan EH & Whitehead PE 1972 Reproduction in female reindeer and caribou. *Canadian Journal of Zoology* **50** 43-46.

Mitchell LM, Dingwall WS, Mylne MJA, Hunton J, Matthews K, Gebbie FE, McCallum GJ & McEvoy TG 2002 Season affects characteristics of the pre-ovulatory LH surge and embryo viability in superovulated ewes. *Animal Reproduction Science* **74** 163-174.

Moore GH & Littlejohn RP 1989 Hybridisation of farmed wapiti (*Cervus elaphus manatobensis*) and red deer (*Cervus elaphus*). *New Zealand Journal of Zoology* **16** 191-198.

Mysterud A, Roed KH, Holand O, Yoccoz NG & Nieminen M 2009 Age-related gestation length adjustment in a large iteroparous mammal at northern latitude. *Journal of Animal Ecology* **79** 1002-1006.

Noel B, Mandiki SM & Paquay R 1999 Terminal follicular growth, ovulation rate and hormonal secretion after melatonin pretreatment prior to FGA-PMSG synchronisation in Suffolk ewes at the onset of the breeding season. *Small Ruminant Research* **32** 269-277.

Norman HD, Wright JR, Kuhn MT, Hubbard SM, Cole JB & VanRaden PM 2009 Genetic and environmental factors that affect gestation length in dairy cattle. *Journal of Dairy Science* **92** 2259-2269.

Pandi-Perumal SR, Srinivasan V, Maestroni GJM, Cardinali DP, Poeggeler B & Hardeland R 2006 Melatonin Nature's most versatile biological signal? *FEBS* **273** 2813-2838.

Rachlow JL & Bowyer RT 1991 Interannual variation in timing and synchrony of parturition in Dall's sheep. *Journal of Mammalogy* **72** 487-492.

Reimers E 2002 Calving time and foetus growth among wild reindeer in Norway. *Rangifer* **22** 61-66.

Renfree MB & Shaw G 2000 Diapause. *Annual Review of Physiology* **62** 353-375.

Rognmo A, Markussen KA, Jacobsen E, Grav HJ & Blix AS 1983 The effects of improved nutrition in pregnant reindeer on milk quality, calf birth weight, growth and mortality. *Rangifer* **3** 10-18.

Roine K 1974 Studies on reproduction in female reindeer. Helsinki: Helsingin Liikekirjapaino.Helsinki College of Veterinary Medicine.

Ronnegard L, Forslund P & Danell O 2002 Lifetime patterns in adult female mass, reproduction, and offspring mass in semidomestic reindeer (*Rangifer tarandus tarandus*). *Canadian Journal of Zoology* **80** 2047-2055.

Ropstad E, Veiberg V, Sakkinen H, Dahl E, Kindahl H, Holand O, Beckers JF & Eloranta E 2005 Endocrinology of pregnancy and early pregnancy detection by reproductive hormones in reindeer (*Rangifer tarandus tarandus*). *Theriogenology* **63** 1775-1788.

Rowell JE & Shipka MP 2009 Variation in gestation length among captive reindeer (*Rangifer tarandus tarandus*). *Theriogenology* **72** 190-197.

Sakkinen H, Timisjarvi J & Puukka M 1999 Nutrition-induced changes in blood chemical parameters of pregnant reindeer hinds (*Rangifer tarandus tarandus*).

Small Ruminant Research **32** 211.

Schwartz CC & Hundertmark KJ 1993 Reproductive characteristics of Alaskan moose. *Journal of Wildlife Management* **57** 454-468.

Scott IC, Asher GW, Archer JA & Littlejohn RP 2008 The effect of conception date on gestation length of red deer (*Cervus elaphus*). *Anim Reprod Sci* **109** 206-217.

Shipka MP & Rowell JE 2006 Gestation length in Alaskan reindeer. *Journal of Animal Science* **84** *(Suppl* 1).

Shipka MP, Rowell JE & Ford SP 2002 Reindeer bull introduction affects the onset of the breeding season. *Animal Reproduction Science* **72** 27-35.

Shipka MP, Rowell JE & Sousa MC 2007a Steroid hormone secretion during the ovulatory cycle and pregnancy in farmed Alaskan reindeer. *Journal of Animal Science* **85** 944-951

Shipka MP, Rowell JE & Young A J 2007b Relationship of Dam's body weight, milk components, and milk energy density to reindeer calf growth rate. *Journal of Animal Science* **58** 126-130.

Short RV & Hay MF 1966 Delayed implantation in the Roe deer (*Capreolus capreolus*) In *Comparative Biology of Reproduction in Mammals*, pp. 173-194. Ed IW Rowlands. New York: Academic Press.

Skogland T 1984 The effects of food and maternal conditions on fetal growth and size in wild reindeer. *Rangifer* **4** 39-46.

Skogland T 1990 Density dependence in a fluctuating wild reindeer herd; maternal vs offspring effects. *Oecologia* **84** 442-450.

Spencer TE, Olivier S & Eckhard W 2008 Genes involved in conceptus-endometrial interactions in ruminants: insights from reductionism and thoughts on holistic approaches. *Reproduction* **135** 165-179.

Tamura H, Nakamura Y, Korkmaz A, Manchester LC, Tan D-X, Sugino N & Reiter RJ 2009 Melatonin and the ovary: physiological and pathophysiological implications. *Fertility and Sterility* **92** 328-343.

Tarin JJ & Cano A 1999 Do human concepti have the potential to enter into diapause? *Human Reproduction* **14** 2434-2436.

Tveraa T, Fauchald P, Henaug C & Yoccoz NG 2003 An examination of a compensatory relationship between food limitation and predation in semi-domestic reindeer. *Oecologia* **137** 370-376.

Wallace JM, Robinson JJ, Wigzell S & Aitken RP 1988 Effect of melatonin on the peripheral concentrations of LH and progesterone after oestrus and on conception rate in ewes. *Journal of Endocrinology* **119** 523-530.

Unique strategies to control reproduction in camels

JA Skidmore, KM Morton and M Billah

Camel Reproduction Centre, P.O. Box 79914, Dubai, United Arab Emirates.

The reproductive efficiency of camels is low under natural pastural conditions and so the use of artifical insemination and embryo transfer are becoming increasingly important to improve their breeding potential. Methods to control their reproductive cycle are therefore essential. This review describes characteristics of the ovarian follicular wave pattern in camels and exogenous hormonal control of ovulation. It also summarizes the difficulties involved with artifical insemination and analyzing the highly gelatinous semen, and reports on the latest methods used to try and reduce the viscosity and liquefy camel semen. In addition an account is given of different hormonal and physical methods used to synchronise follicular waves, and various hormone treatments used to broaden the availability of ovulated, asynchronous and non-ovulated recipients are discussed.

Introduction

The family Camelidae originated in North America and split into three genera, *Camelus, Lama* and *Vicuña* approximately 11 million years ago (Stanley *et al.* 1994). Today there remains two species of large Old World Camelids indigenous to Africa and Asia namely, *Camelus bactrianus* (the Bactrian or two-humped camel) and *Camelus dromedarius* (the dromedary or one humped camel) and four species of New World Camelids, the domesticated llama (*Lama glama*) and alpaca (*Vicugna pacos*), and the wild guanaco (*Lama guanacoe*) and vicuña (*Vicugna vicugna*).

Both dromedary and Bactrian camels exhibit some unique aspects of reproductive physiology compared with other large domestic animals. For example, camels have a short breeding season during the cooler winter months (Wilson 1984), induced ovulation in response to coitus (Marie & Anouassi 1986), a very slow rise in peripheral serum progesterone concentrations after ovulation and a short luteal phase of only 8 – 10 days in the non – pregnant animal (Marie & Anouassi 1987; Skidmore *et al.* 1995) and a long gestation period of 13 months (Mehta *et al.* 1962). In addition they exhibit a long (8 – 10 month) period of lactation-related anoestrus which leads to a long inter-calving interval (Nawito *et al.* 1967). This low reproductive efficiency could be increased by various strategies to control the reproductive cycle and increased use of assisted reproduction techniques such as artificial insemination and embryo transfer. This paper briefly describes ovarian follicular dynamics in camels and outlines methods that can be used to control their reproductive cycle and increase breeding efficiency.

Corresponding author E-mail: luluskidmore@yahoo.com

Ovarian follicular dynamics

All camelids are induced ovulators. Therefore, during the breeding season follicles pass through periods of growth, maturity and regression if ovulation is not induced by mating (Musa & Abusineina 1978; El Wishy 1987). The use of serial real-time ultrasonographic examinations has shown that although the follicular wave pattern varies considerably between camels it can be divided into 3 phases: i) the growth phase which lasts 6 – 10 (±0.5) days; ii) a mature phase of approximately 7 – 8 (± 0.8) days, and (iii) a regression phase of 11 –12 (± 0.8) days (Skidmore *et al.* 1996). In all instances the new follicles become visible and start to grow before the mature follicle has completely regressed to give an interwave interval of 18.2 (± 1.0) days in dromedary camels (Skidmore *et al.* 1996) and 19 days in Bactrian camels (Niasari-Naslaji 2008).

In approximately 50% of follicular waves exhibited by domesticated female camels left separate from male camels the dominant follicle reaches a mature size of 1.3 –1.9 cm diameter, at which time it still responds to an ovulatory stimulus. In the remaining 50% of follicular waves however, the dominant follicle continues to grow to as large as 3.0 – 6.5 cm diameter when it will not ovulate. These large follicles take as long as 18.4 ± 0.8 days (range = 11–33 days) to reach their maximum diameter, they remain at the same size for 4.6 ± 0.5 days and take 15.3 ± 1.1 days to regress (Skidmore *et al.* 1996), although others have reported they can take anything from 8 – 45 days to regress (Tibary & Anouassi 1996). The speed of regression depends on the morphological characteristics of the anovulatory follicle as some follicles have a thin and richly – vascularized wall whilst others have an opaque and thick wall. In addition the contents are usually serous in the early stages but soon become haemorrhagic and show clotted blood and organized fibrin in the later stages (El Wishy 1988; Tibary & Anouassi 1997). Clearly, these overlarge follicles derive from the modern management practice of keeping male and female camels apart during the breeding season but the hormonal mechanisms that drive the development of such structures, and the reasons why they occur in only a proportion of unmated camels, have yet to be elucidated. As their occurrence can cause significant wastage in embryo transfer or artificial insemination programmes various methods have been applied to try and hasten the regression, or prevent development of these overlarge non-ovulated follicles. For example, Skidmore (1994) treated camels with a post-mature follicle of >3.0 cm diameter with either a single injection of 20 μg buserelin (Receptal) or daily injections of 150 mg of progesterone-in-oil for 14 days. Whereas it took 22 (± 1.5) days for the large follicle to regress in the untreated control group, regression occurred in 14.6 (± 1.3) days in animals injected with buserelin and 12.7 (± 1.5) days in those that received daily injections of progesterone. It is possible that the progesterone therapy suppressed the basal secretion rate of LH from the pituitary gland, thereby preventing any further growth or maintenance of the follicle. However since waiting for overlarge follicles to regress is very time consuming when trying to synchronize groups of donor and recipient animals for embryo transfer, it is preferable to prevent the occurrence of oversized, non-ovulatory follicles by inducing ovulation with an injection of GnRH when the follicle reaches 1.3 – 1.7cm diameter.

Control of ovulation

Previous studies have shown that ovulation can be induced in camelids by mating to an intact or vasectomized male (Marie & Anouassi 1987) or by a single intramuscular (i.m.) injection of seminal plasma (Pan *et al.* 1992; Adams *et al.* 2005). Ovulation must be controlled and synchronized when preparing animals for embryo transfer and artificial insemination. Mating to a vasectomized male, however, or inseminating or injecting seminal plasma is impractical due both to the difficulty of collecting camel semen and the risk of spreading veneral disease. Therefore, treatment with an LH-like gonadotrophic hormone preparation or a GnRH analogue at the optimal time in the follicular growth cycle is the most practical alternative. Ovulation rates of 80-85 % can be achieved by injecting either 20 μg of the GnRH analogue, buserelin, or 3000 i.u. human Chorionic Gonadotropin (hCG) when the dominant follicle measures 1.0 – 1.9 cm in diameter. This ovulation rate is reduced to < 20% if the follicle measures between 2.0 – 2.9 cm at the time of treatment and to zero if it measures > 3.0 cm (Skidmore *et al.* 1996).

Synchronisation of follicular waves

Previous embryo transfer studies in camels have indicated that optimal pregnancy rates are achieved when the degree of synchrony between donor and recipient camels is 0 – 2 days (McKinnon *et al.* 1994; Skidmore *et al.* 2002). Synchronisation of donor and recipient camels is best achieved either by selecting recipients from a random group of cycling animals or by treating them with a combination of progesterone-in-oil and eCG. Random selection involves serial ultrasonographic examination of the ovaries and administration of GnRH to all females presenting a mature "ovulable" follicle 24 h after the donor is mated (Skidmore *et al.* 2002). This method works well but it is labour intensive and is only feasible when a large number of recipient camels are available. McKinnon *et al.* (1994) synchronised groups of recipient and donor camels by treating them with progesterone-in-oil (100 mg/day) for 10 – 15 days followed by a single administration of 1500 i.u. eCG. Progesterone treatment stopped on the day of treatment with eCG in the donor camels and the recipients received a single dose of eCG 24 h later. This treatment of the recipients with eCG was given to ensure the presence of a mature follicle 24 – 48 h after the donor. However, although the progesterone treatment reduced the rate of follicular growth it did not inhibit it completely, so response to the eCG and time taken for the next follicle to reach a mature size was variable. This method involved daily handling and injection of the camels so it was time consuming, impractical and expensive. More recently Skidmore *et al.* (2009) compared the efficacy of various treatments intended to synchronise follicle wave cycles in dromedary camels by removing the existing follicle of unknown size, by either physical or hormonal means, and replacing it with a follicle capable of ovulating at a known time interval after treatment . Camels were randomly assigned to one of 5 groups and treated with i) 5mg oestradiol benzoate (i.m.) and 100mg progesterone; ii) 20μg GnRH analogue, (buserelin) i.m., iii) 20μg buserelin i.m. on day 0 and 500 μg prostaglandin analogue (estrumate; PG) on day 7, iv) all follicles ≥0.5cm were ablated using transvaginal guided ultrasound or v) 5 ml of saline given i.m. (controls). All the camels were subsequently injected with 20μg buserelin 14 days after the first treatment was given (i.e. on day T+14), and the intervals from treatment to new follicular wave emergence and the day on which the new dominant follicle reached 1.3cm were recorded. The mean interval from treatment to the time taken for new follicular wave emergence and for the new dominant follicle to reach a diameter of 1.3cm was shortest in the ablation group and longest in the oestradiol/progesterone treated group whereas the GnRH and GnRH/PG groups were intermediate (see Table 1). In both the GnRH and the GnRH/PG groups the majority of camels (11/15 in each group) had dominant follicles of 1.3 – 1.9cm in diameter by 14 days after the start of treatment and 21 of the 22 ovulated after GnRH injection given on day T+14. The ablation, oestradiol/progesterone and control groups however, showed greater variability in follicle size so that fewer of them ovulated after the GnRH injection. The results allowed the conclusion that two GnRH injections given 14 days apart or two GnRH injections 14 days apart plus PG given 7 days after the first GnRH treatment were the most effective methods to synchronise ovulation in dromedary camels at a fixed interval of 14 days after treatment. Similar results were obtained by Nikjou *et al.* (2008) in their attempts to synchronise follicular wave emergence in Bactrian camel. They compared treating one group of camels with two consecutive treatments of three norgestomet implants and 200mg progesterone i.m. given 7 days apart, with another group of camels that received two injections of GnRH given 14 days apart. The Bactrian camels treated with norgestamet implants did not respond consistently to progestogen treatment and therefore wave emergence was not synchronised, whereas in the group of camels that received two GnRH injections 14 days apart, four of five animals ovulated after the second GnRH indicating that this method was more successful at synchronising follicle wave emergence in Bactrian camels.

Table 1. Mean (±sem) time intervals (days) for new follicular wave emergence and the day on which the dominant follicle reached ≥1.3cm in diameter after oestradiol – 17β + progesterone, GnRH, GnRH + prostaglandin or follicle ablation treatments for the purposes of ovarian synchronization in camels.

	Treatment received				
	E/P	GnRH	GnRH/PG	ABL	Saline
Follicle emergence	6.36 ± 0.83^{a}	3.00 ± 0.48	4.47 ± 0.47	2.33 ± 0.48^{b}	4.3 ± 0.72^{b}
Follicle dominance	12.22 ± 1.01	11.14 ± 0.83	10.73 ± 0.72	8.83 ± 1.08^{c}	12.50 ± 0.57^{d}

E/P 5mg oestradiol benzoate and 100mg progesterone im.
GnRH 20 μg buserelin i.v.
GnRH/PG 20 μg buserelin i.v on T+0 + 500μg prostaglandin (cloprostenol) i.m. on T+7.
ABL follicle ablation
Saline 5ml saline i.m.
Those with different superscripts within rows are significantly different $^{ab}p<0.001$; $^{cd}p=0.044$
(From Skidmore *et al.* 2009)

Methods to broaden recipient availability for embryo transfer

To date embryo transfer experiments in camels have reported pregnancy rates of 60 – 70% when transferring Day 7 embryos to recipients that are negatively synchronized with the donor by 1 – 2 days (McKinnon *et al.*1994; Skidmore *et al.* 2002). However, as discussed above it can be difficult and time consuming to accurately synchronise donors and recipients. It would therefore be of great value to be able to establish pregnancies using non-ovulated or non-synchronised camels as recipients. A number of experimental approaches have been tested.

Treatment of recipients with Progesterone and eCG

Skidmore *et al.* (1992, 2002) showed it is possible to achieve and maintain pregnancies in non-ovulated progesterone-treated recipients by giving them daily i.m. injections of 150 mg of progesterone-in–oil starting 2 days before embryo transfer. This suggested that the degree of synchrony between embryo age and that of the recipient's uterus is perhaps not so important so long as serum progesterone concentrations remain elevated. However, since no CL was present in the ovaries of the recipient camels they required daily injections for the entire 13 month gestation period. This is because the placenta does not contribute to progesterone secretion, and all camelids depend entirely on progesterone from the CL to maintain their pregnancy. As daily injections are not practical for large numbers of recipients, a small number of recipients were each injected subcutaneously with Norgestamet (progestagen) implants at 10 day intervals. However 2 of 4 such treated recipients aborted 10 – 12 days after the start of treatment with the implants, so use of such implants is not recommended (Skidmore *et al.* 1992).

As daily injections are not practical another study investigated the possibility of stimulating the development of follicles in non-ovulated, progesterone-treated pregnant camels by injecting them i.m. with 2000 i.u. eCG on day 25 of gestation, and then inducing the follicles that subsequently mature to 1.3 cm diameter to ovulate with GnRH approximately 10 days later. The CL's that develop maintain the pregnancy for the remainder of gestation. Fourteen of 18 (77%) recipients that had received daily i.m. injections of 75 mg of progesterone-in-oil from 3 days before embryo transfer became pregnant and 7 (50%) remained pregnant after injections of eCG and GnRH. These results show that follicles can develop and subsequently ovulate in progesterone-treated animals and that the fetal maternal recognition of pregnancy signal produced by the conceptus can maintain the CLs that develop, thus eliminating the need for continuous exogenous progesterone therapy throughout pregnancy (J. Skidmore, unpublished data).

A further study investigated the possibility of establishing pregnancies in ovulated asynchronous, progesterone-treated animals. Embryos were transferred on Day 3 or 4 after ovulation into recipients receiving a daily i.m. injection of 75 mg progesterone-in-oil from 2 days before embryo transfer to 6 days after ovulation when it is reduced to 50 mg (day 7) and 25 mg (days 8 and 9). Nine of 16 (56%) recipients became pregnant (ov + 3 n = 4; ov + 4 n = 5) compared with 0/8 controls where the embryos were transferred into non-progesterone treated recipients on Day 4 after ovulation. These results again indicate that the degree of synchrony between embryo age and that of the recipient's uterus is perhaps less important so long as there is a sufficient level of progesterone in the blood. Once more this relieves the need for tight synchrony between the donor and recipient as recipients that ovulate 2 – 3 days after the donor can be maintained on progesterone until the embryo is established and secretes sufficient "maternal recognition of pregnancy signal" to maintain the CL itself (J. Skidmore, unpublished data)

Meclofenamic acid (Arquel)

A previous study has indicated firm evidence for the involvement of prostaglandins in luteolysis in camels as the oral administration of the prostaglandin synthetase inhibitor, meclofenamic acid, prevented both the luteolytic action of exogenous PGF2α and the normal increase in periphereal plasma PGFM concentrations in late dioestrus, thereby prolonging the luteal phase (Skidmore *et al*. 1998). A further study then investigated whether camels treated with meclofenamic acid during the luteal phase could be used as asynchronous recipients for embryo transfer. Meclofenamic acid was administered orally to camels from Day 7 after ovulation until 7 days after embryo transfer, and embryos transferred into these treated recipients on Days 8, 10, or 12 after ovulation. Pregnancy rates of 80%, 60%, or 70%, respectively, were achieved as compared to 10% in the control animals where embryos were transferred into non-treated recipients on Day 8 after ovulation (Skidmore & Billah 2005). This treatment again reduces the need for tight synchrony between donors and recipients as recipients that ovulate 4–5 days before the donor could be maintained on meclofenamic acid until the donor is flushed. This method has the added advantage that the CL is maintained by the conceptus once it is established, and further daily administration of exogenous progesterone or progestagens throughout gestation is unnecessary.

Artificial insemination

AI is an important technique in several species not only to ensure rapid genetic progress but also to enable more efficient use of superior males, eliminate need of transportation of live animals and reduce the spread of venereal diseases. Working with camel semen however produces many challenges due mainly to the difficulty of collecting and subsequent analysis and handling of the semen.

The preferred method for collection of camel semen is with an artificial vagina but not all males will accept one. It is easier to train young males to use an AV but mating times are not as long as with natural mating and therefore ejaculates may not be complete. Camel semen has a very viscous consistency immediately after collection and as the spermatozoa are entrapped in this viscous seminal plasma they do not display forward progressive motility. This makes spermatozoal motility very difficult to assess and highly variable. It has been reported that semen will liquefy if left on the lab bench for 20 – 30 min, although this does vary between ejaculates (Deen *et al.* 2003). Various other mechanical and enzymatic methods have therefore also been evaluated in an attempt to fully liquefy camel semen. Mechanical methods include gentle pipetting, vortexing, centrifugation and density gradient centrifugation. Only gentle pipetting of semen in a diluent, however, was effective in reducing semen viscosity without compromising sperm motility or viability (Morton *et al.* 2008), but it still does not completely liquefy the semen. There has been comparatively little research on the liquefaction of camel semen with enzymes although Deen *et al.* (2003) examined the effects of α-chymotrypsin (1% α-chymotrypsin in Tris buffer) and caffeine (0.2 mM caffeine supplemented in Tris extender) on spermatozoal motility and found that the addition of caffeine but not of α-chymotrypsin improved motility of individual sperm. In another study, treatment of camel semen with 0.05 mg/mL papain was successful in liquefying semen without detrimental effects to sperm acrosomal membranes (K. Morton, unpublished data). Moreover, the fertility after AI of fresh papain-treated sperm (30 % pregnancy rate) did not differ to fresh non-treated sperm (30 % pregnancy rate; K. Morton, unpublished data) demonstrating the beneficial nature of papain treatment to liquefy camel semen. A number of extenders have been used for fresh and liquid storage of semen but the best results to date have been achieved when the semen is diluted in either i) Green Buffer (I.M.V. Technologies, L'Aigle, France) ® plus 20% egg yolk (v:v; 50% pregnancy rate; Bravo *et al.* 2000; Skidmore & Billah, 2006) ii) an extender containing 11% lactose and 20% egg yolk (v:v; 50% pregnancy rate; Anouassi *et al.* 1992) or iii) INRA – 96 plus (I.M.V.; 36% pregnancy rate; Morton *et al.* 2010).

Artificial insemination also requires induction of ovulation in camels and because ovulation occurs 28 – 36 h after GnRH injection the optimum time for insemination would be 24 h after treatment. Initial studies have shown that pregnancy rates of 50% can be achieved when 300 x 10^6 motile spermatozoa are inseminated (Bravo *et al.* 2000) although more recently insemination of 150 x 10^6 live spermatozoa into the uterine body or just 80 x 10^6 into the tip of the uterine horn ipsilateral to the ovary containing the dominant follicle have both yielded pregnancy rates of 40 – 50% (Skidmore & Billah, 2006). Diluted semen can also be stored in a refrigerator or Equitainer (Hamilton Thorn) at 4°C for 24 h and providing at least 35 – 40% are motile after 24 h it can be inseminated (Bravo *et al.* 2000). However pregnancy rates are dramatically reduced to 20% in camels inseminated with cooled semen diluted in INRA compared with 0% when semen was diluted and cooled in Green Buffer (Morton *et al.* 2010) although previous studies by Bravo *et al.* (2000) did report pregnancy rates of 25% when inseminating semen cooled in Green Buffer for 24 h. Further studies have been carried out by Niasari-Naslaji *et al.* (2005) comparing the use of Green Buffer with their novel extender, SHOTOR diluent (2.6 g Tris, 1.35 g citric acid, 1.2 g glucose and 0.9 g fructose in 100 ml of water) for preserving Bactrian camel semen and it was concluded that the SHOTOR diluent was the better extender for chilling Bactrian semen for up to 12 h but no fertility results were recorded.

Conclusions

The increasing necessity to improve camel production has led to a more scientific approach to management of these animals. Ovulation can be controlled by using GnRH or gonadotrophic hormones if administered at the correct stage of the cycle and pregnancies can be achieved if camels are inseminated with semen diluted in Green Buffer, an extender containing 11 % lactose or INRA – 96 24 h after GnRH injection. The gelatinous nature of the semen makes it difficult to handle but the use of gentle pipetting or treatment with caffeine or papain has been successful in liquefying the semen and thus improves spermatozoal motility.

Hormonal methods using GnRH or a combination of GnRH and PG will successfully synchronise follicular waves in camels which has always been considered a necessary pre-requisite for embryo transfer. It is also possible, however, to achieve pregnancies in non-ovulated progesterone-treated recipients and to induce follicle growth and subsequent ovulation if they are treated with eCG and GnRH. The CLs that develop secrete sufficient progesterone to eliminate the need for continuous exogenous progesterone therapy throughout pregnancy. In addition, recipient availability has been broadened by treatment of ovulated, asynchronous recipients with progesterone or meclofenamic acid so that pregnancies can be successfully achieved in recipients that have ovulated up to 5 days before or 4 days after the donor.

These results show that controlled breeding and strategic use of hormone treatments should increase the efficiency of embryo transfer and AI programmes in camels and therefore improve their reproductive potential.

References

Adams GP, Ratto MH, Huanca W & Singh J 2005 Ovulation inducing factor in the seminal plasma of alpacas and llamas. *Biology of Reproduction* **73** 452 – 457.

Anouassi A, Adnani M, Raed EL 1992 Artificial insemination in the camel requires induction of ovulation to achieve pregnancy. *Proceedings of 1st International Camel Conference* pp 175 – 178. Eds WR Allen, AJ Higgins, IG Mayhew, DH Snow & JF Wade. R &W Publications (Newmarket) Ltd UK.

Bravo PW, Skidmore JA, Zhao XX 2000 Reproductive aspects and storage of semen in Camelidae. *Animal Reproduction Science* **62** 173 – 193.

Deen A, Sumant V, Shani MS 2003 Semen collection, cryopreservation and artificial insemination in the dromedary camel. *Animal Reproduction Science* **77** 223-233

El Wishy AB 1987 Reproduction in the female dromedary *(Camelus dromedarius)*. A Review. *Animal Reproduction Science* **82** 587 – 593

El Wishy AB 1988 A Study of the genital organs of the female dromedary (*Camelus dromedarius*). *Journal of Reproduction and Fertility* **82** 587 – 593.

Marie M & Anouassi A 1986 Mating induced luteinizing hormone surge and ovulation in the female camel (Camelus dromedarius). *Biology of Reproduction* **35** 792-798.

Marie M & Anouassi A 1987 Induction of luteal activity and progesterone secretion in the non-pregnant one-humped camel (*Camelus dromedarius*). *Journal of Reproduction and Fertility* **80** 183 – 192.

McKinnon AO, Tinson AH & Nation G 1994 Embryo transfer in dromedary camels. *Theriogenology* **41** 145-150.

Mehta VS, Prakash A & Singh M 1962 Gestation period in camels. *Indian Veterinary Journal* **39** 387-395.

Morton, K.M. Vaughan JL & Maxwell, WMC 2008 The continued development of artificial insemination technology in Alpacas. Rural Industries Research and Development Corporation, Kingston, ACT, Australia.

Morton KM, Thomson PC, Bailey KJ, Evans G & Maxwell WMC 2010 Artificial insemination in dromedary camels with fresh and chilled semen: preliminary results. Proceedings of the Ruminant Reproduction Symposium (submitted).

Musa BE & Abusineina ME 1978 The oestrous cycle of the camel (*Camelus dromedarius*). *Veterinary Record* 102 556-557.

Nawito MF, Shalash MR, Hoppe R & Rakha AM 1967 Reproduction in the female camel. *Bulletin of Animal Science Research Institute (Cairo)* No. 2 pp. 82.

Niasari-Naslaji A 2008 An update on Bactrian camel reproduction. *Journal of Camel Practice and Research* **15** No.1; 1-6.

Niasari-Naslaji A, Mosaferi S, Gharahdaghi AA, Abarghani A, Ghanbari A, Gerami A 2005 A novel extender for preservation of Bactrian camel (*Camelus bacterianus*) semen. *Reproduction Fertility and Development* **17** 198 – 199.

Nikjou D, Niasari-Naslaji A, Skidmore JA, Mogheiseh A

& Razavi K 2008 Synchronization of follicular wave emergence prior to superovulation in Bactrian camel (*Camelus bactrianus*). *Theriogenology* **69** 491-500.

Pan GW, Zhao XX, Chen BX, Jiang S, Huang YM, Zu YS & Wang HY 1992 The ovulation-inducing effect of seminal plasma in the Bactrian camel *Proceedings of 1st International Camel Conference* pp 159–162 Eds WR Allen, AJ Higgins, IG Mayhew, DH Snow & JF Wade. R &W Publications (Newmarket) Ltd UK

Skidmore JA 1994 Reproduction in the dromedary camel. PhD Thesis, University of Cambridge.

Skidmore JA & Billah M 2005 Embryo transfer in the dromedary camel (*Camelus dromedarius*) using asynchronous, meclofenamic acid-treated recipients. *Reproduction, Fertility and Development* **17** 417 - 421.

Skidmore JA & Billah M 2006 Comparison of pregnancy rates in dromedary camels (*Camelus dromedarius*) after deep intra-uterine versus cervical insemination. Theriogenology 66 292 – 296.

Skidmore JA, Allen WR, Cooper MJ, Ali Chaudhry M, Billah M & Billah AM 1992 The recovery and transfer of embryos in the dromedary camel: Results of preliminary experiments. *Proceedings of 1st International Camel Conference*. pp. 137-142. Eds. WR Allen, AJ Higgins, IG Mayhew, DH Snow & JF Wade. R & W Publications (Newmarket) Ltd. UK

Skidmore JA, Billah M & Allen WR 1995 The ovarian follicular wave pattern in the mated and non-mated dromedary camel (*Camelus dromedarius*) Journal of Reproduction and Fertility Supplement **49**: 545-548.

Skidmore JA, Billah M & Allen WR 1996 The ovarian follicular wave pattern and induction of ovulation in the mated and non-mated one - humped camel (*Camelus dromedarius*) . *Journal of Reproduction and Fertility* **106** 185 - 192.

Skidmore JA, Starbuck GR, Lamming GE & Allen WR 1998 Control of luteolysis in the one-humped camel (*Camelus dromedarius*). *Journal of Reproduction and Fertility* **114** 201 - 209.

Skidmore JA, Billah M. & Allen WR 2002 Investigation of factors affecting pregnancy rate after embryo transfer in the dromedary camel. *Reproduction, Fertility and Development* **14** 109 –116.

Skidmore JA, Adams GP & Billah M 2009 Synchronization of ovarian follicular waves in dromedary camels (*Camelus dromedarius*). Animal Reproduction Science **114** 249 -255.

Stanley HF, Kadwell M & Wheeler JC 1994 Molecular evolution of the family Camelidae: a mitochondrial DNA study. *Proceedings of the Royal Society. Lond. B* **256** 1 – 6.

Tibary A & Anouassi A 1996 Ultrasonographic changes of the reproductive tract in the female camel (*Camelus dromedarius*) during the follicular cycle and pregnancy. Journal of Camel Practice and Research **3** 71 – 90.

Tibary A. & Anouassi A 1997 Reproductive physiology in female camelidae. In: Institut Agronomique et Veterinarie Hassan II, Rabat, Maroc. (Eds) Theriogenology in camelidae. Abu Dhabi Printing and Publishing Company. pp 169-241

Wilson RT 1984 'The Camel." pp 53-102. Longmans (London), UK.

Abstract author index

A proposal for categorization of scrotum length and its relationship with andrological classification in extensively managed bulls

J Chacón, A Jiménez and B Vargas

Section of Andrology, Research Program on Applied Animal Andrology, School of Veterinary Medicine, Universidad Nacional (UNA), Heredia-Costa Rica

The bull´s breeding soundness evaluation (BSE) protocol comprises the assessment of many clinical attributes correlated with a sire's potential fertility under field conditions. Since the 1990's, the andrology section at UNA has given particular importance to the scrotal conformation during BSE in tropical bulls. This report proposes a simple categorization for the scrotum length (SL) and its relationship with andrological classification and semen quality in Costa Rican breeding sires.

The SL was classified on 4231 *Bos indicus* (BI, n=2888), *Bos taurus* (BT, n=802) and crossbred (BI x BT, n=541) bulls submitted to a single BSE during 1991 to 2009. It was categorized according to the distance between its distal part and the hock joint as: "Short", a scrotum clearly close to the body, with a non distinguishable neck; "Normal", an evident scrotal neck is present and the lower part of the sac does not extend beyond the limit of the hock; and "Long", the distal part of the scrotum is below the hock joint. After the BSE, bulls were classified according to the standards of the Society for Theriogenology. Means (%) for sperm abnormalities according to SL were compared by Duncan's test. The relationship between SL and BSE classification was analyzed by a Chi square test.

The overall prevalence (%) for short (S), normal (N) and long (L) scrotum was 4.2, 84.6 and 11.2 respectively. The frequency of sires with (L) was greater ($P<0.0001$) in BT (14.6%) compared with BI (10.8%) and BI x BT (8.2%). No differences were seen between species for (S). Relative prevalence (%) of (L) for most common breeds was: Indubrasil (23.4), Simmental (19.4), Holstein (16.4), Brown Swiss (16.1), Gyr (13.7), Indubrasil x Brahman (13.4), St. Gertrudis (12.6), Brahman (7.8), Simmental x Brahman (4.2), Nelore x Brahman (2.2) and Nelore (2.0). The overall prevalence of unsound breeding bulls was 36.2%. This percentage was lower for BI (30.7%) compared with both BT (43.9%) and BI x BT sires (46.1%). Regardless of the species, the occurrence of unsound bulls was greater in sires with (L) compared with (N) (72.4% vs. 34.1%; $P<0.0001$). The same pattern was seen for the frequency of pathologies (i.e., orchitis, hydrocele, sperm granuloma, and testicular atrophy) diagnosed during examination of the scrotal contents (7.2% vs. 1.1%; respectively). Differences concerning semen quality were also found in relation to scrotum length regardless of the species studied. Sperm motility was lower in bulls with (L) compared with (N) (53.8% vs. 63.8%, $P<0.0001$). Sires having (L) had higher levels of abnormal acrosomes, nucleus and head defects as well as proximal droplets compared with (N) (29.2% vs. 17.4%, $P<0.0001$). Although bulls with (L) had higher levels of tail defects and distal cytoplasmic droplets compared with (N) (10.4% vs. 6.9%), this was not significant. No statistical differences were found for spermiogramme variables when comparing (S) and (N).

Testicular function was impaired in bulls having a long scrotum since abnormalities in the sperm nucleus and head, as well as proximal cytoplasmic droplets were more frequently seen in these bulls compared with (N). Bulls having (L) are more exposed to testicular trauma. In addition, a long scrotum might, in some way, disturb the thermoregulation in this organ[1]. However, the mechanism of this impairment is not yet determined and the pathogenesis of this relationship deserves to be fully studied.

[1]Setchell, 1970. Testicular fluids, In: The Testis. NY Academic Press 1:46-147.

Functional and oxidative status of cryopreserved semen, collected from *Bos taurus* and *Bos indicus* raised under tropical conditions

MP Rodrigues[a], RP Bertolla[b], M Nichi[a], PAA Goes[a], EGA Perez[a], RC Barnabe[a] and VH Barnabe[a]

[a]*University of São Paulo, Faculty of Veterinary Medicine and Animal Science, São Paulo, Brazil;* [b]*São Paulo Federal University, Division of Urology, São Paulo, Brazil*

One of the main causes for impaired reproductive performance in bulls raised under tropical conditions is heat stress. In such conditions, European breeds (*Bos taurus* - Simmental) are much more sensitive to heat stress than Indian breeds (*Bos indicus*- Nelore). A hypothesis to explain greater vulnerability to heat stress is a higher susceptibility to oxidative stress which would induce structural and functional damage[1]. This influence could be even more deleterious when cryopreserving semen samples, which would increase the potential destructive influence of oxidative stress.

In order to test this hypothesis, semen samples of twenty Nelore (*Bos indicus*) and twenty Simmental (*Bos taurus*) bulls, raised under tropical conditions, were collected and cryopreserved. Ten sperm samples from each breed were collected during summer and ten during winter by electroejaculation. After thawing, semen samples were submitted to conventional (motility, vigor and sperm motility index) and functional analysis (plasmatic membrane integrity – Eosin/Nigrosin; acrosomal membrane integrity – Fast green / Bengal Rose; DNA fragmentation - Comet Assay, and mitochondrial activity - 3'3 diaminobenzidine -DAB). The sperm susceptibility to induced lipid peroxidation followed by measurement of thiobarbituric acid reactive substances (TBARS) was used to quantify sperm susceptibility against the oxidative stress. Statistical analyses were performed by using the SAS System for Windows.

Nelore bulls showed greater sperm quality during winter for the following parameters: motility (26.5% winter and 13.3% summer; P=0.02) and percentage of sperm showing high mitochondrial potential (DAB I; 22.3% winter and 13.3% summer; P=0.04). A breed effect was observed only during the winter, when Simmental bulls showed a lower percentage of sperm showing high mitochondrial activity (Simmental: 11.6% and Nelore: 22.3%; P=0.02). No differences were found on the susceptibility of sperm against the oxidative stress for neither breed nor season (P>0.05). Negative correlations were observed between DNA fragmentation and sperm quality, as evaluated by most of the tests performed (i.e., plasmatic membrane integrity, mitochondrial activity and motility).

These results indicate that *Bos indicus* bulls (compared with *Bos taurus*) showed greater cryopreserved sperm quality probably because of their resistance to tropical environments and good adaptability to extreme conditions. Furthermore, a hypothesis to explain the correlations found between DNA fragmentation and sperm quality may be explained by the damage caused to the plasma membrane by the cryopreservation which would increase the vulnerability of the mitochondria to damage. This, in turn, would lead to the release of pro-oxidative factors that would induce the DNA fragmentation. Additional studies are necessary to test this hypothesis.

[1]Nichi *et al.*, 2006. Theriogenology 66:822-828.

The effect of season on semen quality in *Bos indicus* and *Bos taurus* bulls raised under tropical conditions

GC Romitto, RF Gonçalves and VH Barnabe

Department of Animal Reproduction, College of Veterinary Medicine and Animal Science, São Paulo University, Cidade Universitária, SP, Brazil

Bull fertility is extremely important for efficient production of beef cattle bred by natural service under extensive production systems. Seasonal variations in the semen characteristics of bulls have been described in earlier studies concerning ejaculate volume and sperm concentration as well as morphologically altered spermatozoa. Under tropical conditions, cattle of the genotype *Bos indicus* are known to be more thermotolerant, and have higher fertility in response to heat stress than breeds of European origin (*Bos taurus*). In the present study, we tested the hypothesis that *Bos taurus* bulls have lower activity of antioxidant enzymes in their semen than *Bos indicus* bulls. Thirty Simmental (*Bos taurus*) and twenty five Nelore (*Bos indicus*) bulls, from 3 to 4 yr of age, were used for this study. These bulls were kept under an extensive management system, on pasture composed of brachiaria (*Brachiaria sp*), on a farm near Dourados, Mato Grosso do Sul, Brazil. Semen was collected twice annually (summer and winter) for 2 consecutive years. Semen was evaluated according to standard procedures for ejaculate volume, sperm concentration, gross motility, progressive motility and sperm morphology. To evaluate oxidative damage, malondialdehyde (lipid-peroxidation metabolite) concentrations were indirectly measured by semen concentrations of thiobarbituric acid reactive substances (TBARS). Simmental bulls had significantly greater percentages of major sperm defects during the summer than the winter ($20.3 \pm 3.1\%$ vs. $12.2 \pm 2.4\%$, respectively; mean $\pm$ S.E.M.). There was an interaction of breed and season for minor sperm defects ($P = 0.037$; highest in Nelore bulls in the summer) and an effect of season on total defects ($P = 0.066$; higher in summer). TBARS were higher in summer than in winter (728.1 ± 79.3 ng/mL vs. 423.8 ± 72.6 ng/mL, respectively; $P = 0.01$) for Simmental bulls, and no differences in Nelore bulls. The results support the hypothesis that heat stress not only interferes in spermatogenesis by increasing the rate of malformations, but also increasing the occurrence of lipid in the testicle and / or reducing the levels of antioxidants in semen.

Bovine subspecies influence in sperm chromatin susceptibility to fragmentation

R Simões, JM Baldrighi, WB Feitosa, CM Mendes, MA Peres, JA Visintin and MEOA Assumpção

Department of Animal Reproduction, University of São Paulo, São Paulo, Brazil

Particularities between bovine subspecies (*Bos taurus* vs. *Bos indicus*) must be considered before planning a reproductive management program. Various factors can influence reproductive efficiency such as the direct effects of climate on each bovine subspecies. For instance, fertility of *Bos taurus* bulls used for artificial insemination is depressed during summer months. This effect is observed to a lesser extent in *Bos indicus* bulls[1], mostly due to their adaptation to tropical regions. These facts could indicate that each bovine subspecies has different capacities to protect their spermatozoa from environmental damage. Studies in humans, mice and bulls indicate that increased fragmentation of chromatin is associated with disturbances in spermatogenesis, morphological abnormalities and infertility. The Sperm Chromatin Structure Assay (SCSA), a flow cytometric assay, provided evidence for a relationship between sperm chromatin structure and function[2]. The objective of the present study was to evaluate differences in DNA fragmentation index (DFI, likelihood of sperm contributing to infertility problems) between *Bos taurus* and *Bos indicus* bulls using the SCSA.

One-hundred and ninety-seven frozen semen samples from bulls of two different subspecies (*Bos taurus* n = 57; *Bos indicus* n = 140) were evaluated by flow cytometric analysis. The method described previously[2] was used as follows: samples were thawed at 37°C for 30 s and placed in 15 ml centrifuge tubes. The semen was then diluted in a buffer containing 0.01 M Tris-HCl, 0.15 M NaCl, and 1 mM and EDTA. An aliquot of 0.2 ml containing 2×10^6 cells was mixed with 0.4 ml of an acid-detergent solution (0.08 M HCl, 0.15 M NaCl, 0.1% Triton-X 100 v/v, pH 1.2) and after 30 s spermatozoa were stained by adding 0.6 ml of acridine orange (AO) staining solution (0.2 M Na_2HPO_4, 1 mM EDTA, 0.15 M NaCl, 0.1 M citric acid, 60 μM AO). Samples were examined 3 min after adding the acidified detergent in a flow cytometer; 5000 spermatozoa were evaluated in each sample.

The SCSA showed that DFI was greater for *Bos indicus* (2.71±0.13) than for *Bos taurus* (1.84±0.15; $P<0.0001$), indicating that *Bos indicus* bulls are more susceptible to DNA denaturation after low pH treatment. A previous study[1] had shown that *Bos taurus* bulls were more sensitive to heat stress thus leading to decreased pregnancy rates when compared with *Bos indicus*. However, sperm DNA fragmentation was not evaluated. It was speculated that *Bos taurus* sperm would be more sensitive to DNA fragmentation. Unexpectedly, the present data showed the opposite. A question raised is why *Bos indicus* bulls were more susceptible to a low pH challenge, considering that this subspecies is more adaptable to stress conditions. Some hypotheses are: *Bos indicus* bulls are more sensitive to the SCSA protocol or other pathways might be involved in controlling sperm DNA fragmentation. Further studies are being conducted in order to determine the effects of sperm DNA damage on fertilization in bovine.

[1]Pegorer *et al.*, 2007.Theriogenology 67:692-697.
[2]Evenson and Wixon, 2006.Theriogenology 65:979-991.

Automated evaluation of bull sperm quality using a novel, easy to operate flow cytometric platform – Guava EasyCyte Plus

JF Odhiambo, M Sutovsky and P Sutovsky

Division of Animal Sciences, University of Missouri-Columbia, Columbia, USA

The purpose of semen quality evaluation is to predict the fertility of the sample in an objective, rapid and inexpensive manner. This requirement often cannot be met, however, with traditional methods that rely on assessment of sperm motility, abnormal morphology and concentration. The use of the biomarkers of sperm quality such as ubiquitin (UBB) and lectin PNA (*Arachis hypogaea*/peanut agglutinin) for bull semen evaluation by flow cytometry, therefore, may eliminate the need for visual assessment by microscopy, especially in busy artificial insemination (AI) operations. Conventional flow cytometers are expensive, however, and difficult to operate in the industry settings. Herein, we adapt the easy to operate 'bench-top' micro-capillary flow cytometer platform, Guava EasyCyte Plus (IMV Technologies), to demonstrate a robust semen evaluation and purification technique based on ubiquitin (surface marker of defective spermatozoa) and PNA-lectin (surface marker of damaged sperm acrosomes).

Two trials were conducted. Semen samples for the first trial were obtained from two dairy bulls that had been subjected to temporary scrotal insults to induce variable semen quality, and collected periodically in a span of 3 or 7 months. Samples were fixed in formaldehyde and labeled with fluorescently-conjugated antibodies and lectin PNA. Fluorescent properties of the samples were evaluated by a conventional flow cytometer (Becton-Dickinson Facs Scan) and re-measured by the Guava EasyCyte Plus system. In the second trial, the sperm viability test, factory pre-set on Guava, was used to evaluate sperm viability after the depletion of defective spermatozoa using magnetic nanoparticles coated with anti-UBB antibody and PNA. Semen samples from 10 Holstein bulls were divided into 4 treatment groups: PNA particles, PSA particles (*Pisum sativum* lectin), anti-UBB antibody (MK-12-3) particles, and control (no particle pull-down). Sample volumes of 375 μL were mixed with 25 μL magnetic particles and 1 mL of warm PBS, incubated for 15 min at RT on a Dynal rotator set at the lowest speed, and depleted for 15 min using a magnet (Clemente Associates).

In the scrotal insulation trial, data from the two flow cytometers were highly and positively correlated ($P<0.001$) for total sperm PNA ($r=0.47$), total UBB ($r=0.68$) and intensity of ubiquitin ($r=0.90$) immunofluorescence. Proportion of sperm with abnormal morphology was negatively correlated with PNA fluorescence ($P<0.01$) but positively and highly correlated with UBB fluorescence obtained from the Guava EasyCyte Plus system ($r=0.63$, $P<0.001$). In the sperm depletion trial, samples depleted with anti-UBB or PNA particles, but not the control samples or samples depleted with PSA-particles, had greater viability. In a follow up experiment, the post-depletion viability was further improved by using a 50:50 mixture of anti-UBI and PNA particles.

Altogether these observations provide a rationale for the adaptation of ubiquitin and lectin PNA probes to sperm quality evaluation on the Guava EasyCyte Plus platform, the acquisition and operation cost of which is substantially lower than that of conventional flow cytometers.

Supported by USDA-NRI, Missouri Life Sciences Trust Fund and the Food for the 21st Century (F21C) Program of the University of Missouri.

Evaluation of membrane, acrosome, mitochondrial potential and chromatin integrity of bull semen using egg yolk-based and soybean lecithin-based extenders for cryopreservation

MB Koivisto[a], RB Prado[b], JT Carreira[a], LH Rodrigues[c] and SHV Perri[a]

[a]*UNESP - Univ Estadual Paulista, FOA, School of Veterinary Medicine, Araçatuba, São Paulo, Brazi;* [b]*Fertvitro, São José do Rio Preto, São Paulo, Brazil;* [c]*Lagoa da Serra, Sertãozinho, São Paulo, Brazil*

Artificial insemination has been widely used for genetic improvement in cattle. Although fertility with frozen–thawed bull semen is generally acceptable for AI, the cryopreservation techniques still result in the loss of 40–50% of viable sperm during the freezing–thawing process[1]. Semen diluents containing egg yolk as a cryoprotectant may pose hygienic risks and are difficult to standardize. Although a new generation of semen diluents free of animal ingredients is available, egg yolk-containing extenders are still widely used for cryopreserving semen[2]. The goal of this study was to evaluate the effects of egg yolk and soybean lecithin-based extenders for cryopreservation of bovine semen on sperm motility, plasma membrane, acrosomal membrane, mitochondrial function and chromatin integrity.

The ejaculate of four bulls was divided into two equal parts, one diluted with egg-yolk-Tris extender (A) and the other with a soy-lecithin based extender (Andromed®; Minitube, Verona, WI) (B). After dilution, semen was frozen and stored in liquid nitrogen according to pre-established patterns of the artificial insemination center. Semen samples with extender A and B of each bull were thawed and assessed regarding motility, concentration, membrane integrity through association of propidium iodide probes (PI), fluorescein isothiocianate - Pisum sativum (FITC-PSA) and lipophilic cationic carbocyanine (JC-1) and evaluation of chromatin integrity was performed by the acridine orange staining procedure. The statistical analysis was performed by using Analysis of Variance (ANOVA) and Wilcoxon test.

Sperm motility showed no statistical differences between extenders A and B (63.8 ±7.5%; 55.0±5.8%, respectively). The percentage of major, minor and total defects were similar for both extenders. The membrane, acrosome, mitochondrial and chromatin evaluations showed no statistical differences. The values for acrosome integrity for extender A and B were 36.2±5.2%; 40.7±19.6%, respectively; for membrane integrity 25.0±22.8%; 20.2±20.4%, respectively and for high mitochondrial potential 24.2± 29.4%; 20.0± 24.3%, respectively. For chromatin integrity the results were identical for group A and B.

Since no statistical difference between the extenders was identified, soybean lecithin may substitute the egg-yolk-Tris for cryopreservation of bull semen.

[1]Prathalingam *et al.*, 2006. Theriogenology 66:1894-1900.
[2]Aires *et al.*, 2003. Theriogenology 60:269-279.

Effect of adding taurine to a TRIS-based egg yolk extender on the viability of bull semen cooled at 5 °C

AM Crespilho[a], FO Papa[a], M Nichi[b], MF Sá Filho[b], FS Zahn[a] and JA Dell'Aqua[a]

[a]*São Paulo State University, Botucatu, Brazil;* [b]*University of São Paulo, Brazil*

Several reports have demonstrated the effectiveness of taurine, a sulfonic amino acid that acts as an antioxidant inhibiting lipid peroxidation, protecting bull sperm against the accumulation of ROS during cryopreservation. However, few studies have been conducted to determine the effect of taurine supplementation on the viability of liquid storage of bull semen under cooled conditions. The aim of the present study was to test the hypothesis that the addition of 50 mM of taurine in a TRIS-based egg yolk extender improves the quality of bull semen cooled at 5 °C for 96 h.

One ejaculate from each of ten Nelore bulls obtained by electroejaculation was used. Each ejaculate was fractioned into two aliquots, diluted in either TRIS egg yolk fructose extender (TRIS-Control) or TRIS with 50 mM taurine added (TAU), at the concentration of 30×10^6 total sperm per 0.5 mL straw. After packing, all the samples were submitted to passive cooling to 5°C in an isothermic box (Botutainer®, Brazil) and remained there for 96 h. The percentage of sperm total motility (MOT), progressive motility (PRO), average (um/s) path sperm velocity (VAP), and percentage of rapid sperm (RAP) as well as viable sperm and oxidative stress were determined in samples during the storage at 5 °C for 6, 24, 48, 72 and 96 h, respectively by computer-assisted sperm analysis, fluorescent probes propidium iodine and FITC-PSA, and using the quantification of Thiobarbituric acid reactive substances (TBARS). Data were analyzed by repeated measures of ANOVA and Tukey's test ($P < 0.05$).

Results of MOT were 86.30 ± 4.32^a; 73.10 ± 9.71^{ab}; 66.20 ± 12.25^b; 64.70 ± 15.51^b; 59.70 ± 14.98^b and 86.60 ± 4.48^a; 71.60 ± 11.28^{ab}; 68.70 ± 12.92^b; 67.70 ± 14.76^b; 60 ± 23.76^b% for TRIS and TAU treatments, respectively, at time 6, 24, 48, 72 and 96 h. The percentage of PRO, RAP and intact cells decreased after cooling for both treatments, but there were no significant differences on these parameters when TRIS or TAU groups were compared at each time. The VAP did not vary during the storage period on both groups. The total amount of TBARS was lesser ($P = 0.036$) for the TAU group than the TRIS group (921.84 ± 738.35^a vs. 698.63 ± 677.22^b ng/mL, respectively), but there was no significant effect of taurine addition on TBARS concentration during cooling. Sperm quality parameters for both groups decreased similarly during storage.

The conclusion is that the amino acid taurine indeed decreases the total amount of ROS production in the TRIS-based egg yolk extender diluted semen. Additional studies are necessary to verify the effect of taurine association with other antioxidants on ROS production during storage of bull semen at 5 °C in order to determine an effective protocol to protect against long term cellular damage during storage.

Effect of alpha tocopheryl acetate on cryopreserved semen quality of *Bos taurus* bulls raised under tropical environments

PAA Góes[a], M Nichi[a], EGA Perez[a], ROC Silva[a], MP Rodrigues[a], A Dalmazzo[a], CC Rocha[a], RC Barnabe[a], RP Bertolla[b] and VH Barnabe[a]

[a]*University of São Paulo, São Paulo, Brazil;* [b]*Sao Paulo Federal University, São Paulo, Brazil*

Oxidative stress is caused by reactive oxygen species (ROS) that may cause structural damage to biomolecules, DNA, lipids, carbohydrates and proteins, as well as other cellular components. Spermatozoa are particularly susceptible to oxidative stress, mainly due to reduced cytoplasm and high content of polyunsaturated fatty acids in its cellular membranes. Furthermore, previous studies indicate that oxidative stress is involved in damage caused by the cryopreservation of sperm. This effect could be even more pronounced in *Bos taurus* bulls raised under tropical environments. Treatments aiming to avoid the deleterious effects of the ROS are extremely important.

To test the effect of vitamin E supplementation in the extender, semen from four *Bos taurus* bulls were collected by artificial vagina and cryopreserved with Tris egg yolk with 0, 0.5, 2.5 and 5 mM of alpha tocopheryl acetate (Vitamin E). After thawing, samples were evaluated for motility characteristics using computer assisted sperm analysis (CASA, IVOS), membrane and acrosome integrities (eosin/nigrosin and fast green/bengal rose stain, respectively), mitochondrial activity (diaminobenzidine stain; DABI: full mitochondrial potential, DABIV: no mitochondrial potential) and, sperm susceptibility to the oxidative stress following challenge with ferrous sulphate and ascorbate (TBARS).

No effect of vitamin E treatment was found on motility characteristics evaluated by CASA. On the other hand, treatment with 5 mM of vitamin E showed higher percentage of sperm with intact membrane when compared with the control and those treated with 0.5 mM (46.7±9.6, 26.0±3.5, and 21.0±6.3%, respectively). Samples treated with 5 mM showed a higher percentage of sperm with impaired mitochondrial activity when compared with the same groups mentioned previously (DABII; 22.7±5.4, 44.0±3.5, and 36.2±4.4%, respectively). Furthermore, susceptibility to oxidative stress was greater in control samples when compared with groups treated with 5 mM of alpha tocopherol (7318.9±329.4 vs. 5822.7±452.5 ng of TBARS/10^6 sperm, respectively).

Results of this study indicate that treatment with vitamin E may protect the spermatozoa against the damage caused by cryopreservation. Vitamin E, due to its lipophilic characteristics, is an important antioxidant with action on cellular membranes. A hypothesis from these results is that vitamin E would play a protective effect on the plasma membrane, which in turn, would avoid damage to the mitochondria. Previous studies indicate that sperm mitochondria disruption plays an important role in the damage caused by oxidative stress due to the release of pro-oxidative factors. Therefore, the membrane and consequent mitochondrial protection of vitamin E would avoid the deleterious effects caused by oxidative stress on cryopreserved semen samples of bulls raised under tropical conditions.

The influence of epidermal growth factor on functions of ram cooling-stored spermatozoa

A Makarevich[a,c], E Spalekova[b], N Lukac[b], L Olexikova[a], Z Hegedusova[c] and J Pivko[a]

[a]Animal Production Research Centre Nitra, Slovak Republic; [b]Slovak Agricultural University, Nitra, Slovak Republic; [c]Research Institute for Cattle Breeding Ltd, Rapotin, Vikyrovice, Czech Republic

Epidermal growth factor (EGF) plays an important role in the control of reproductive functions. Although the presence of EGF receptors in spermatozoa of several mammalian species has been established[1], the role of EGF in sperm function is not known[2]. The aim of the study was to examine the effects of EGF on ram sperm characteristics following hypothermic storage.

Fresh ejaculates collected from three Lacoune rams were diluted in Triladyl extender and transported to the laboratory where the sperm samples were pooled and divided into groups according to EGF doses added (0, 100, 200 or 400 ng/ml of sperm suspension). Following 72 h of sperm storage at 4°C, the sperm samples were fluorescently stained for a plasma membrane integrity (peanut agglutinin, PNA-FITC), plasma membrane fluidity (annexin V-labeled membrane phosphatidylserine translocation) and apoptotic (Yo-Pro-1) markers and analyzed under a Leica fluorescent microscope. Sperm motility was measured using a CASA system and sperm fertilization rate was determined using an in vitro fertilization test on bovine prematured oocytes.

The 200 ng/ml dose of EGF decreased the proportion of spermatozoa with damaged plasma membranes (32.3% vs. 41.3% in control, $P<0.05$), and EGF doses of 200 and 400 ng/ml decreased the proportion of apoptotic cells (5.9% and 5.1% respectively vs. 12.7% in control, $P<0.05$), whilst the lower dose (100 ng/ml) was not effective. The proportion of spermatozoa with membrane phospholipid disorders (annexin V-labeled) in the control sample was approximately 8.5% of the whole sperm population. This value was not affected by any of the EGF concentrations tested.

A stimulatory effect of EGF on sperm motility was exhibited at all concentrations tested (96.1 ± 0.6%; 95.7 ± 0.6% and 96.0 ± 0.5% for 100, 200 and 400 ng/ml, respectively) compared with control (91.3 ± 0.7%). For the in vitro fertilization tests, the EGF concentration of 200 ng/ml was chosen. At this dose no differences in the oocyte fertilization rate between EGF (55.5%) and control (53.3%) groups were detected.

In summary, the EGF effect on ram sperm is dependent on concentration, with higher concentrations being more effective. EGF improved ram sperm viability and motility but their effects were not reflected in fertilizing ability of the sperm in vitro.

The study was supported from the SRDA grant – APVV-0514-07 and LA330 travel grant.

[1]Naz and Minhas, 1995. J Andrology 16:384-388.
[2]Oliva-Hernandez and Perez-Gutierrez, 2008. Theriogenology 70:1159-1169.

Effect of extenders on viability of sperm and pregnancy rate in ewes after intracervical insemination

Z Hegedusova[a,b], A Makarevich[a] and J Vejnar[c]

[a]Research Institute for Cattle Breeding, Ltd., Rapotin, Czech Republic; [b]Agriresearch Rapotin, Vikyrovice, Czech Republic; [c]Federation of sheep and goat breeders in the Czech Republic

The aims of our study were to evaluate pregnancy rate in ewes after artificial insemination and to test extenders for ram semen for short-term and long-term preservation. Data were obtained from 94 intracervical inseminations in Suffolk, Wallachian, Merinolandschaf and Texel ewes in reproductive and non-reproductive seasons (2008 and June 2009). Estrous cycles was synchronized in the ewes by using of intravaginal sponges Chronogest CR (Intervet/Schering-Plough Animal Health) for 14 d. On the day of sponge removal ewes were treated with PMSG – Sergon inj. (Bioveta, Czech Republic) at a dose of 500 to 600 IU. Intracervical insemination was performed from 50 to 58 h after the end of the synchronization process. For the intracervical insemination and the examination of extenders we used fresh semen or semen diluted with commercial products [Triladyl® (Minitüb, Tiefenbach, Germany), AndroMed® (Minitüb), Ovipro (Minitüb), Biladyl® (Minitüb), Biociphos® (IMV, L'Aigle, France)] or milk diluent.

Dilution of semen with the selected extender was carried out at the ratio 1:4. The treated ejaculate was transported to the laboratory in a climatic box at 16 to 18 °C and was placed in a stationary incubator at the same temperature. Then, 4 evaluations of sperm viability were done at the following times: 24, 48, 72 and 96 h of preservation.

Pregnancy rate ranged from 17.6% to 71.4%. Insemination carried out in the non-reproductive season (May, June) yielded a low pregnancy rate (17.6% in May; the pregnancy rate in June was higher, 55%). The pregnancy rate after the intracervical insemination in the reproductive season ranged from 52.6% to 71.4%.

Statistically significant differences were found between the extenders [Triadyl vs. Ovipro ($P<0.01$), Triadyl vs. Biladyl ($P<0.01$) and Triadyl vs. Biociphos ($P<0.05$)]. The extender Triladyl showed a high percentage of long-term viability. It was selected as a control for the overall evaluation. Other preservative extenders did not improve or deteriorate the sperm. A high percentage of sperm viability was found for the Ovipro extender but only for the first 48 h. For this reason, Ovipro appeared to be the best for short-term storage of semen.

Supported by projects MSM 2678846201 and LA 330 of the MEYS of the CR.

Cooled storage of ram semen extended in SHOTOR diluent and low-density lipoproteins (LDL)

S Gharibi, D Nikjou and A Niasari-Naslaji

Dept. Clinical Sciences, Faculty of Veterinary Medicine, University of Tehran, Tehran, Iran

Low-density lipoproteins (LDL) are the major component of egg yolk (EY) that protects sperm during the cooling process[1]. The present study investigated the possibility of replacing EY with LDL for cooled storage of ram semen.

LDL was extracted according to the method described previously[2]. Semen was collected using an artificial vagina from three fertile rams. Semen of good quality (>80% progressive motile sperm) were pooled and divided into two parts. Each part of semen was then extended at the ratio of 1:1 in SHOTOR diluent (Tris-based extender consisting of Tris: 2.36 g; citric acid: 1.3 g; glucose: 1.2 g and fructose 1.2 g in 100 ml of deionized water[3]; supplemented with either 12% EY (v/v) or 5% LDL (w/v). The diluted semen was then cooled within 1.5 to 2 h to 4°C, and stored at this temperature for 32 h. Assessment of progressive forward motility of sperm (PFM) was conducted immediately after collection, after reaching at 4°C and at 8, 24, and 32 h after incubation at 4°C. The experiment was replicated 6 times. Data were analyzed using GLM procedure in SAS including repeated measures in the model.

At the time of dilution, PFM did not differ between EY and LDL groups (88.8% vs. 89.8%; $P>0.05$). There was a significant reduction over time in PMF of both groups, from the time of collection till 32 h after incubation at 4°C ($P<0.001$); however, this reduction was significantly greater in EY (57.1%) compared with LDL (67.0%) at 32 h ($P<0.01$). There were also significant differences ($P<0.05$) between EY and LDL groups at 4 h (76.7 vs. 83.2), 8 h (69.7 vs. 79.5) and 24 h (63.0 vs. 71.8).

In conclusion, SHOTOR diluent supplemented with 5% LDL is a suitable extender for short-term preservation of ram semen.

[1]Bergeron and Manjunath. 2006. Mol Reprod Devel 73:1338–1344.
[2]Moussa *et al.*, 2002. Theriogenology 57:1695-1706.
[3]Niasari-Naslaji *et al.*, 2006. Cryobiology 53:12-21.

Effect of glutathione on ovine cryopreserved sperm function and oxidative status

EGA Perez[a], M Nichi[a], CHC Viana[b], RP Bertolla[c], CC Rocha[a], A Dalmazzo[a], MP Rodrigues[a], VH Barnabe[a] and RC Barnabe[a]

[a] *University of São Paulo, São Paulo, Brazil;* [b] *Pontifícia Universidade Católica de Minas Gerais, Poços de Caldas, Brazil;* [c] *São Paulo Federal University, São Paulo, Brazil*

The high susceptibility of ovine sperm to the oxidative stress occurs especially due to high content of polyunsaturated fatty acids (PUFAs) in its plasma membrane. The PUFAs provide the necessary fluidity to the plasma membrane. However, double bonds in the fatty acids are more susceptible to oxidative stress. In ovine sperm, the PUFA percentage in the membrane is higher than in others species such as humans and rabbits. Studies in humans indicate that cryopreservation may lead to damage to the sperm from oxidative stress. Previous studies from our group suggested that ovine sperm was particularly affected by hydrogen peroxide[1].

This study aimed to verify if the antioxidant reduced glutathione (GSH) may protect ovine cryopreserved sperm against damages caused by oxidative stress. Semen samples of four rams were cryopreserved using Tris-egg yolk extender supplemented with different concentrations of GSH (control, 1, 5 and 10 mM). After thawing, samples were evaluated using conventional (motility and vigor) and functional tests (for acrosome integrity, fast-green/ bengal rose staining, for membrane integrity, eosin-nigrosin staining, for mitochondrial activity, the 3-3´diaminobenzidine-DAB- staining). Susceptibility to chromatin denaturation was accessed by SCSA assay[2]. Aliquots of each thawed sample were submitted to a protocol of induced lipid peroxidation using ascorbate (20 mM) and ferrous sulphate (4 mM), with further measurement of tiobarbituric acid reactive substances (TBARS), an index of oxidative stress.

Treatment with GSH decreased the proportion of intact acrosomes. Samples treated with 5 mM GSH showed lower percentage of intact membrane (9.22 ± 1.32) cells when compared with control samples (15.06 ± 2.35) and those treated with 10 mM (18.31 ± 2.15). However, an increase on the percentage of sperm showing high mitochondrial activity was observed on samples treated with GSH (1 mM, 5 mM, and 10 mM) when compared with the control group (64.12 ± 3.75). No effect on the susceptibility of sperm against the oxidative stress (TBARS) was observed with the GSH treatment. Samples from the control group were more susceptible to chromatin denaturation when compared with the GSH treated groups (control: 12.32 ± 1.54, 1 mM, 5 mM, and 10 mM).

In conclusion, the addition of reduced glutathione (GSH) offers protection to DNA and mitochondrial activity of ovine sperm. The protection provided by the GSH may be limited to the internal cellular structures. Previous studies indicate that the GSH and glutathione peroxidase activities are compounds present mainly in cytoplasm. Therefore, the combination of GSH with an extracellular antioxidant would provide an increased protection of ovine cells against the damages caused by the oxidative stress during the cryopreservation.

[1] Perez *et al.,* 2010. Reprod Fertil Devel 22:175.
[2] Evenson *et al.,* 1999. Hum Reprod 14:1039.

Artificial insemination of dromedary camels with fresh and chilled semen: Effect of diluent and sperm dose, preliminary results

KM Morton, M Billah and JA Skidmore

Camel Reproduction Centre, Dubai, UAE

Artificial insemination (AI) is one of the most widely used reproductive technologies and there is considerable scope for its use in camel breeding programmes. The efficiency of AI in dromedary camels is low as the optimal diluent and sperm dose for AI with fresh and chilled semen have yet to be elucidated[1].

The objective of this study was to compare the fertility of fresh and chilled (24 h, 4°C) dromedary camel semen after AI. Semen was collected from four males (n = 5 ejaculates per male), split into two aliquots and diluted 1:1 with Green Buffer (GB, IMV Technologies, USA) or INRA-96 (IMV, France). Diluted semen was assessed for motility, acrosome integrity (FITC-PNA), sperm concentration, membrane integrity (HOS) and viability (Eosin/nigrosin)[1]. Diluted semen was then inseminated within 2 h of collection (fresh), or further diluted (1:2) and stored for 24 h in an equitainer (Hamilton-Thorne, USA) at 4°C before insemination (chilled). A total of 150, 300 or 600 (chilled only) x 10^6 motile sperm were inseminated into female camels (n = 79) 24 h after ovulation induction[2]. Pregnancy was diagnosed by ultrasound between 18 to 25 d after insemination[2]. Statistical analysis was performed by ANOVA after arc-sin transformation (sperm data) or Chi-square (pregnancy data) using GenStat with $P<0.05$ considered significant.

For fresh sperm, motility was greater after dilution in GB (67.4±1.7%) than INRA-96 (59.4±2.1%; $P<0.05$) while membrane integrity was greater after dilution in INRA-96 (64.9±2.5%) than GB (55.9±5.0%; $P<0.05$), but sperm viability (GB: 66.7±2.1%; INRA: 66.7±1.9%) and acrosome integrity (GB: 84.9±1.7%; INRA: 88.5±1.4%) were similar ($P>0.05$). For chilled sperm, motility (GB: 47.6±2.9%; INRA: 48.3±2.5%), membrane integrity (GB: 54.9±3.5%; INRA: 56.7±2.5%) and acrosome integrity (GB: 84.8±1.9%; INRA: 84.6±2.1%) were similar but sperm viability was greater after chilling in INRA (62.2±1.5%) than GB (58.9±1.0% $P<0.05$). For fresh semen, pregnancy rate was not affected by sperm diluent (GB: 8/23, 34%; INRA: 8/23, 34%; $P>0.05$) but was increased by AI of 300 x10^6 sperm (10/24; 41.6%) compared with 150 x10^6 (6/22; 27.2%; $P<0.05$). For chilled semen, pregnancy rate was greater after AI with semen chilled in INRA (3/17, 17.6%) compared with GB (0/16, 0.0%; $P<0.05$), and was increased by AI with 600 (2/8, 25 %) and 300 (2/19, 10.5%) compared with 150 x 10^6 motile sperm (0/10, 0.0%; $P<0.05$).

These results demonstrate that INRA-96 and GB are suitable diluents for fresh camel semen, but only INRA-96 is suitable for chilled preservation of dromedary camel semen. Pregnancies were achieved with chilled semen in dromedary camels, although the results were well below commercially acceptable levels. Further research is required to improve the pregnancy rates of dromedary camels using AI with fresh and chilled semen.

This research was kindly supported by His Highness General Shaik Mohammed bin Rashid Al Maktoum. The authors with to thank Aijaz Hussain and Abdul Rahman for their technical assistance.

[1]Morton *et al.*, 2008. Kingston, ACT, Australia.
[2]Skidmore and Billah, 2006. Theriogenology 66:292-296.

Preservation of pampas deer (Ozotoceros bezoarticus) semen I. Changes after the addition of a commercial extenders with 10 or 20% of egg yolk

A Sestelo[a], J Gil-Laureiro[b], N Citón[a], S González-Pensado[c] and R Ungerfeld[c]

[a]*Fundación Bioandina Argentina-Proyecto ARCA, Jardín Zoológico de la Ciudad de Buenos Aires, Argentina,*
[b]*Departamento de Reproducción, and* [c]*Departamento de Fisiología, Facultad de Veterinaria, Uruguay*

The pampas deer was originally distributed widely in the open grasslands in eastern South America, from 5° to 41° S, but now is an endangered species from which few isolated populations remain. As part of a program in which pampas deer reproductive biology is being studied, semen extraction and preservation is the first biotechnology to be applied. The objective of the experiment was to compare the use of a commercial semen extender with the addition of 10 or 20% egg yolk. Semen was obtained from 7 adult males by electroejaculation under general anesthesia during the breeding season (March to April). Quality of motility (QM, range 0 to 5, where 0 is no movement and 5 represents rapid, linear forward movement), percentage of motile spermatozoa (MS), progressive motility (PM), and abnormal spermatozoa (AS) were measured. Acrosomal integrity was classified as intact (IA), damaged (DA) or missing acrosome (MA). Split samples from each male were extended in a commercial diluent (red extender, IMV, France) with the two egg yolk concentrations, step wise cooled to 5°C, and assessed when the extender was added and at 5°. Before extention, general parameters were QM: 4.07 ± 0.25, MS: $79.3 \pm 1.7\%$; PM: $72.1 \pm 2.1\%$; AS: $64.0 \pm 4.0\%$; IA: 73.7 ± 4.8; DA: 23.2 ± 4.8; and MA: 3.2 ± 0.8. After the addition of the extenders, the only difference was a greater QM with the addition of 20% of egg yolk (3.5 ± 0.2 vs. 3.2 ± 0.3, $P=0.05$). When semen was cooled at 5°, the samples with the extender containing 20% of egg yolk had greater PM (69.3 ± 2.3 vs. $65.0 \pm 1.9\%$, $P=0.04$). On the other hand, IA was greater with 10% egg yolk (78.8 ± 4.8 vs. $75.5 \pm 5.4\%$, $P=0.02$). At this time, while QM tended to be better with 20% egg yolk (2.8 ± 0.2 vs. 2.7 ± 0.2, $P=0.09$), DA tended to be greater with 20% egg yolk (21.5 ± 5.2 vs. $18.7 \pm 4.8\%$, $P=0.06$). We concluded that differences between the diluents were not conclusive, making it necessary to test the use of other diluents to improve the results.

Preservation of pampas deer (*Ozotoceros bezoarticus*) semen II: thawed semen

F Beracochea[a], B Ceballos[b], A Sestelo[b], S González-Pensado[a], P Dos Santos-Neto[c] and R Ungerfeld[a]

[a]*Departamento de Fisiología, Facultad de Veterinaria, Montevideo, Uruguay,* [b]*Fundación Bioandina-Proyecto ARCA, Jardín Zoológico de la Ciudad de Buenos Aires, Argentina,* [c]*Laboratorio de Reprodução Animal, Universidade do Estado de Santa Catarina, UDESCCAV, Brasil*

The objective of this work was to evaluate the semen during post-thawing to determine if 10 or 20% of egg yolk is more efficient to optimize the cryopreservation of seminal material of the pampas deer (*Ozotoceros bezoarticus*) using the Red IMV extender. We used semen straws from 7 males, collected and cryopreserved during the breeding season (March to April), which were extended with a commercial extender (red extender, IMV, France) with 10% or 20% egg yolk before freezing. After thawing, we determined quality of motility (QM, range 0 to 5), percentage of motile spermatozoa (MS), progressive motility (PM), percentage of live spermatozoa [determined by Hypo Osmotic Swelling test (HOS)], and abnormal spermatozoa (AS). Acrosomal integrity was classified as intact (IA), damaged (DA) or missing acrosome (MA). Each sample was assessed at 0, 60 and 120 min after thawing, morphology and acrosomal integrity were determined at 0 and 120 min after thawing. The results of the HOS test were assessed after an incubation of 15 or 30 min. Quality of motility at 0 (2.5 ± 0.4) and 120 min (0.7 ± 0.7) was similar for both extenders, but 60 min after thawing tended to be better with the addition of 10% egg yolk (1.6 ± 0.6 vs. 1.5 ± 0.5, $P = 0.078$). There were no differences in MS (50.0 ± 9.4; 25.1 ± 12.9; and 10.4 ± 13.4% at 0, 60 and 120 min respectively) or PM (23.7 ± 11.7; 2.5 ± 3.6; 0.1 ± 0.5%). The decrease in QM from 60 to 120 min tended to be lower with the extender that contained 10% than that with 20% egg yolk (1.0 ± 0.64 vs. 0.9 ± 0.6, $P = 0.1$). There were no significant differences in the HOS test at 15 min (56.0 ± 3.5%), although less spermatozoa remained intact after 30 min in the samples that were extended with 20% of egg yolk (51.4 ± 3.5 vs. 53.1 ± 3.2, $P = 0.08$). In the samples extended with 20% egg yolk, less spermatozoa tended to have acrosome damage at 0 min than in the 10% egg yolk (49.0 ± 4.6 vs. 46.2 ± 4.0, $P = 0.07$), without differences at 120 min (48.2 ± 5.9). There were no differences at 0 and 120 min in spermatozoa with regard to intact acrosomes (44.1 ± 4.5%), and spermatozoa without acrosomes (MA) (7.9 ± 3.1%). There were not differences at 60 or 120 min in the percentage of AS (78.0 ± 4.7%). We concluded that there are no clear differences between the extenders. When the red extender is used it seems to be equal to extend pampas deer semen with 10 or 20% egg yolk.

Effect of antioxidant and polyunsaturated fatty acids on epididymal sperm in bulls

M Nichi[a], R Simões[a], PAA Góes[a], EGA Perez[a], ROC Silva[a], MP Rodrigues[a], A Dalmazzo[a], RC Barnabe[a], PEJ Bols[b] and VH Barnabe[a]

[a]*University of São Paulo, São Paulo, Brazil;* [b]*University of Antwerp, Antwerp, Belgium*

Sperm recovery from the caudae epididymides can be advantageous in case of the unexpected death of a genetically valuable animal, for propagating endangered species, and especially as an experimental model for research on semen. A key factor to be studied concerning the use of epididymal sperm is the cryopreservation technique. One of the main reasons for the negative impact of cryopreservation on sperm is oxidative stress, which may cause structural damage to biomolecules including, DNA, lipids, carbohydrates and proteins, as well as other cellular components. Spermatozoa are particularly susceptible to oxidative stress, mainly due to the reduced cytoplasm and the high content of polyunsaturated fatty acids (PUFA) in their membrane. This allows spermatozoa to be motile and confers a higher resistance against the damage caused by cryopreservation, but makes the sperm more susceptible to the attack of the reactive oxygen species (ROS).

The objective was to test the effect of adding decosaexaenoic acid (DHA), an important PUFA that is associated with antioxidants (e.g., vitamins E and C, reduced glutathione - GSH, superoxide dismutase - SOD, calatalase, glutathione peroxidase - GPx), to the semen extender with the aim of improving post-thaw semen quality. Sperm samples were collected from 30 caudae epididymides of bull testicles collected from abattoirs and were then cryopreserved. To test the effect of DHA and antioxidant treatments (in different concentrations and combinations) to the semen extender, spermatozoa were evaluated for membrane and acrosomal integrity (eosin/nigrosin and fast green/bengal rose stain, respectively), mitochondrial activity (diaminobenzidine stain), DNA integrity (sperm chromatin structure assay – SCSA) and, sperm susceptibility to oxidative stress (TBARS).

Results indicate that due to the treatment with DHA, epididymal sperm became more susceptible to oxidative stress (control: 178.3 ± 9.5^a, 5μM: 298.1 ± 53.2^b, and 10μM: 514.28 ± 43.34^c). On the other hand, when DHA (5μM) was associated with SOD (20 IU/mL), an improvement was found on progressive motility (control: 24.28 ± 4.82 vs. DHA+SOD: 34.43 ± 4.12%; $P<0.05$). Furthermore, the association between DHA and GSH (5 mM) induced an improvement in membrane and DNA integrity compared with the control group (57.83 ± 5.51 and 6.56 ± 0.64 vs. 38.62 ± 7.15 and 4.79 ± 0.41, respectively; $P<0.05$). However, when associated with Vitamin E, DHA had a detrimental effect on mitochondrial activity.

Our results indicate that the efficiency of the antioxidant treatment to epididymal sperm samples may depend on the concentration of the antioxidant used, the location of the deleterious influence of the oxidative stress and which ROS are causing damage. Furthermore, the treatment of DHA in combination with an antioxidant treatment, especially SOD and GSH, may be an alternative to improve post-thaw quality of semen samples.

Cryopreservation of goat epididymal sperm

ROC Silva[a], M Nichi[a], PAA Góes[a], EGA Perez[a], MP Rodrigues[a], A Dalmazzo[a], CC Rocha[a], RC Barnabe[a], RP Bertolla[b] and VH Barnabe[a]

[a]University of São Paulo, São Paulo, Brazil; [b]Sao Paulo Federal University, São Paulo, Brazil

Cryopreservation of epididymal sperm can be an important tool for research on semen. In goats, post thaw semen quality is one of the main limiting factors for the success of artificial insemination. It is well known that reactive oxygen species (ROS) lead to structural and functional damage to sperm, impairing or preventing fecundation. Spermatozoa are particularly susceptible to oxidative stress, mainly due to the reduced cytoplasm and high content of poly-unsaturated fatty acids in their membrane. This is even more relevant when considering cryopreservation, in which a deleterious influence of oxidative stress is known to impair post-thaw semen quality.

The aim of the present study was to examine the influence of cryopreservation on goat epididymal sperm. Semen was collected from epididymides of five goats by carefully dissecting the caudae. Samples were cryopreserved by using a commercial extender. After thawing, samples were submitted to motility evaluation by computer assisted sperm analysis (CASA, Ivos), examination of membrane and acrosomal integrity (eosin/nigrosin and fast green/bengal rose stain, respectively), mitochondrial activity (diaminobenzidine stain; DABI: full mitochondrial activity, DABIV: no mitochondrial activity) and, sperm susceptibility to oxidative stress (TBARS).

Cryopreservation had a deleterious effect on membrane integrity (pre-freeze: 84.1 ± 1.9 vs. post-thaw: $60.25 \pm 2.3\%$; $P<0.0001$) and on the susceptibility of sperm to oxidative stress (pre-freeze: 620.8 ± 107.8 vs. post-thaw: 3901.6 ± 186.7; $P<0.0001$). Post-thaw motility as evaluated by CASA showed that $59.4 \pm 5.5\%$ of cells were motile. Strong correlations were found between the higher susceptibility of sperm to oxidative stress (TBARS) and the percentage of cells having an intact membrane ($r=-0.95$, $P<0.0001$). On the other hand, the percentage of sperm showing no mitochondrial activity (DABIV) correlated significantly with VSL ($r=-0.91$, $P=0.03$) and progressive motility ($r=-0.89$, $P=0.04$).

Despite the significant loss of membrane integrity, the results found in the present study indicate that sperm collected from the caudae epididymides from goats could be used for artificial insemination. Further study using these samples for artificial insemination are in progress. The increased susceptibility of sperm to oxidative stress after thawing, and the strong negative correlation between TBARS and membrane integrity, indicate that oxidative stress may have an important deleterious influence on post-thaw semen quality. Therefore, an alternative to overcome such an effect on epididymal sperm in goats would be the use of antioxidants. In fact, previous studies by our group indicate that goat ejaculated sperm is particularly susceptible to hydrogen peroxide[1]. Therefore, the use of hydrogen peroxide scavengers such as glutathione peroxidase, reduced glutathione, and catalase may prove to be suitable antioxidants. However, further studies are necessary to prove such hypothesis for both ejaculated and epididymal sperm.

[1]Silva *et al.*, 2010. Reprod Fertil and Devel 22:316.

Preliminary surgical technique in the Sarda ram in preparation for stem cell transplantation

G Meloni[a], A Lai[a], L Mara[b], F Chessa[b], S Schmoelzl[c], V Farina[a], G Bomboi[a] and M Dattena[b]

[a]*Department of Animal Biology, Sassari University, Italy;* [b]*AGRIS-Sardegna, DIRPA (Agricultural Research Agency of Sardinia), Reproduction Division, Olmedo, Italy;* [c]*CSIRO, Armidale, Australia*

Transplantation of stem cells by microinjection into the testes of recipient males leads to establishment of donor-derived spermatogenesis. This system provides a model for the study of spermatogenesis, restoration of fertility, manipulation of different stem cell sources, and genetic modification of farm animals. The aim of this paper is to present a preliminary surgical technique for cell transplantation into ram testes.

Five adult rams were used for the injection of 4 ml of MitoTracker-green fluorescent label (Invitrogen; Carlsbad, CA USA) by surgical access into the extra-testicular rete. Each animal received acepromazine as a pre-anaesthetic. The scrotal and inguinal regions were prepared for surgery and the animal was positioned on its back and anaesthetised. Two 8 cm incisions were made in the middle-cranial part 4 cm lateral and parallel to the median raphe of the scrotum for each testes. The testis enclosed in the vaginal tunic was exposed by 8 cm incision performed in the middle-cranial position of the testis. The head of the epididymis was blunt dissected free of the tunica albuginea and reflected to expose the extratesticular rete. An intravenous 24-ga catheter was introduced 5 to 7 mm into the extra-testicular rete guided to the site by ultrasound using a 7.5 MHz probe. An insulin syringe was connected to the intravenous catheter and by gentle pressure 500 μl of air was injected to expand the mediastin. Soon after, 4 ml of fluorescent label was injected by using gentle pressure into the mediastin with ultrasound guide. The testis was placed back into the vaginal tunic with a correctly positioned epididymis and the tunic was stitched. The scrotum was closed with absorbable stitches. Five ml of Rapidexon (2 mg/ml; Cevavetem) was injected i.m. together with standard antibiotic therapy.

Fifteen days after the surgery, a single testis from two out of the five injected rams was removed and samples from different testis portions were sectioned with a cryostat and observed under a confocal microscope to evaluate the fluorescence in the mithocondria to confirm that the surgical technique was able to reach the seminiferous tubules. All tissue samples examined were fluorescent. Forty-five d after injection, all the rams were able to ejaculate by using an artificial vagina. Sperm was observed under a confocal microscope to evaluate spermatozoa fluorescence. All the sperm samples appeared to be fluorescent.

In conclusion, according to these preliminary results, this technique enabled: 1) complete and normal reproduction activity 45 d after surgery and; 2) a complete distribution of the label into the seminiferous tubules. This technique, therefore, provides a reliable surgical method for cell transplantation.

This work was supported by the Regione Autonoma della Sardegna (Grant numbers Cardiostam 2006, Biodiversita` APQ5/200).

Differential remodeling of oocyte, sperm and somatic chromatins in bovine oocytes

G Wee[a], S-T Shin[b] and Y-M Han[a]

[a]*Department of Biological Sciences, KAIST;* [b]*College of Veterinary Medicine, Chungnam National University, Korea*

ATP-dependent chromatin remodeling factors (ACRFs) modulate changes of chromatin structure such as condensation or decondensation through regulating histone-DNA interaction. In this study, behaviors of ACRFs and epigenetic modifiers were monitored during pronuclear formation to understand how maternal, paternal and somatic chromatin is respectively reprogrammed in the oocyte cytoplasm. Bovine oocytes fertilized by sperm insemination or reconstructed with somatic cells were recovered by time course (6 h to 24 h after sperm insemination; 1 h or 20 h after electrofusion). These samples were immunostained using various antibodies against Brg-1, BAF-170, Mi-2, hSNF2H, 5-MeC, AcH3K9, AcH4K5, mono-, di- and tri-methyl H3K9. After fertilization, Brg-1 and BAF-170 were observed in maternal chromatin during condensation earlier than sperm chromatin and then Brg-1 remained continuously until decondensation stage, whereas BAF-170 disappeared in condensed chromatin and reappeared during decondensation. Brg-1 and BAF-170 in sperm chromatin were reset during decondensation and then observed continuously during pronuclear formation. Only Mi-2 appeared at late pronuclear stage. Interestingly, hSNF2H appeared immediately in sperm chromatin after sperm penetration whereas remodeled later in maternal chromatin during decondensation, and then hSNF2H existed continuously in parental chromatin during pronuclear formation. These results indicate that Brg-1 regulate maternal chromatin remodeling whereas sperm chromatin is remodeled by hSNF2H. After somatic cell nuclear transfer, ACRFs of somatic chromatin seemed to be reprogrammed by oocyte cytoplasm, which was similar to reprogramming patterns of maternal chromatin in fertilized oocytes. Our findings suggest that remodeling of maternal and paternal chromatin by ACRFs may have a different mechanism, and that somatic chromatin behaves like a remodeling pattern similar to the maternal genome during pronuclear formation.

Sperm effect in the expression of genes related to cell cycle during early embryonic development in cattle

MP Milazzotto[a], WB Feitosa[b], FF Paula-Lopes[c], J Buratini Jr[d], JA Visintin[b] and MEOA Assumpção[b]

[a]Federal University of ABC, Santo Andre, SP–Brazil; [b]University of Sao Paulo, SP-Brazil; [c]UNIFESP-Diadema, Brazil; [d]UNESP, Botucatu, Brazil

Pre-implantation development in mammals is characterized by the transition of the genomic control from the oocyte to the embryo. After fertilization, during the first cleavages, embryonic development is supported by mRNA and proteins synthesized and stored during oogenesis. Thus, mRNA molecules of maternal origin decrease and embryogenesis gradually becomes dependent on the expression of genetic information derived from embryonic genome. It is known that sperm penetration initiates a cascade of events mediated by the release of intracellular calcium and other signaling proteins. It is unclear whether the absence of the sperm cell or artificial oocyte activation affects subsequent embryonic development. A key event in the transition of genomic control from the oocyte to the embryo is the beginning of mitotic cell cycle, which requires cyclin-dependent kinases (CDKs) and cyclins.

The objective of this study was to assess changes in levels of transcripts related to cell cycle (cyclin A, B and E, cdc2, CDK2 and CDK4) in the presence of the sperm cell and after artificial induction of oocyte activation during early embryonic development. Transcripts from bovine oocytes, in vitro produced (IVP) embryos (2 to 4 cells, 8 to 16 cells activated embryos and blastocysts) and parthenogenetic activated (PA) embryos (2 to 4 cells, 8 to 16 cells activated embryos and blastocysts) were evaluated. Transcripts were measured by Real Time PCR and data were analyzed using REST MCS beta software by Pair Wise Fixed Reallocation Randomization Test. Reactions were normalized by using the beta-actin housekeeping gene. All transcripts from oocytes were increased in relation to cleaved embryos in both IVP and PA groups. There was no difference between cleavage and blastocyst rates (68.7 and 28.2; 71.7 and 19.5; respectively, for IVP and PA). Comparing the expression of target genes, the PA group showed a greater expression of cyclins A, B, CDK2 and cdc2 compared with the IVP group. Upon activation, all genes studied, with the exception of CDK4 were expressed at a higher level in the PA group. After the initial activation of the embryonic genome in the PA group, all genes were more expressed in activated embryos compared with the 2 to 4 cell embryo. However, in the IVF group only cyclin A, E and CDK4 were increased in activated embryos compared with those in the initial mitotic division. At the blastocyst stage, only the transcripts related to cyclin A, B, cdc2, and CDK4 were more expressed in PA.

These results suggest that in both groups, there is an initial consumption of these transcripts in the early stages of embryonic development. However, in PA embryos, activation of the cell cycle genes seems to occur prior to the 8 to 16 cell stage, which can be harmful in terms of the control of other cellular functions.

Financial Support: FAPESP 07/58456-7.

Effects of spermatozoa containing abaxial tail attachment during *in vitro* embryo production (IVP) – preliminary results

MB Koivisto[a], DL Pavão[b], MM Piccolomini[b], MF Alves[b], AH Souza[c], JT Carreira[a] and M D'Angelo[b]

[a]*UNESP - Univ Estadual Paulista, FOA, School of Veterinary Medicine, Araçatuba, São Paulo, Brazil;* [b]*Animal Health Research Center, São Paulo Biological Institute, Brazil;* [c]*Accelerated Genetics, Baraboo,Wisconsin, USA*

Studies involving both laboratory tests and breeding trials are essential to develop further knowledge about the potential fertility of morphologically abnormal sperm. An in vitro fertilization and culture system was used to determine the effect of abaxial sperm tail attachment of bovine spermatozoa on fertilization and early embryonic development. Oocytes were aspirated from ovaries of slaughtered cows and those having an intact zona pellucida were selected and matured. After 20 to 24 h, the oocytes were fertilized with control semen [pool of semen from three Angus bulls – total defects <30%; abaxial attachment < 4.0%; post-thaw motility > 40%; percentage of intact acrosome (PIA) >51%] and semen containing a high percentage of abaxial attachment (pool of semen of one Angus bull – total defects: 65%; abaxial attachment 45.3%; post-thaw motility 47%; percentage of PIA >69%). Semen samples were treated with the discontinuous Percoll gradient technique and sperm concentration was adjusted to approximately 1×10^5 sperm for each oocyte. After the period of fertilization, the embryos were evaluated for their viability and morphology by light microscopy. A binomial distribution was assumed for cleavage and blastocyst rate. Data were analyzed with Proc GLIMMIX of SAS.

Cleavage rate was not different between Control (67.2%, n=201) and Pathology (67.3%, n=297; P>0.10) groups. Similarly, blastocyst production also did not differ between Control 43.0% and Pathology 44.8% (P>0.10), respectively.

In conclusion, our preliminary findings suggest that spermatozoa with abaxial attachment do not seem to have detrimental effects on embryo production during IVF procedures.

Developmental changes in the morphology and viability of in vitro-produced (IVP) bovine embryos experimentally contaminated with semen containing Stx2 Shiga-toxin-producing *Escherichia coli* (STEC)

M D'Angelo[a], MM Piccolomini[a], AC Goes[a], DL Pavão[a], MF Alves[a], AFC Nassar[a], S Miyashiro[a] and MB Koivisto[b]

[a]*Instituto Biológico de São Paulo, Centro de P&D de Sanidade Animal, Brazil;* [b]*UNESP - Univ Estadual Paulista - FOA – School of Veterinary Medicine, Brazil*

The assisted reproduction techniques, although increasingly used, still need research to assess health risks of oocytes, embryos and sperm, as embryonic and fetal mortality have a major impact on the efficiency of any livestock production system. The aim of this study was to evaluate by light microscopy, developmental changes in the morphology and viability of bovine embryos, fertilized experimentally with semen contaminated with Stx2 Shiga-toxin-producing Escherichia coli (STEC).

Oocytes were aspirated from ovaries of slaughtered cows and those showing intact zona pellucida were selected and matured. After 20 to 24 h, the oocytes were fertilized with control semen (control group, n = 418) and contaminated semen (infected group, n = 415) containing 200UFC STEC. Semen samples were treated by the technique of discontinuous Percoll gradient and sperm concentration was adjusted to approximately 1×10^5 sperm for each oocyte. After the period of fertilization, the embryos were evaluated for their viability and morphology by light microscopy. Statistical analysis was performed using the Chi-square test with Yates correction.

Morphological evaluation of the fertilized oocytes with contaminated semen showed cytoplasmic shrinkage, gaps in the division, blastomere asymmetry, granular ooplasm with dark brown color, vacuole formation and degeneration and disruption of the zona pellucida. These changes were not observed in the control group. Cleavage rate was 70.3% and 52.8%, respectively, for control and infected embryos, showing a significant difference ($P < 0.001$). A statistically significant difference was also observed after the 7th d of embryonic development, where 44.7% of morulae were noted in the control group and only 22.4% in the infected group ($P < 0.001$). STEC presence interferes with the cleavage rate and also inhibits and/or reduces embryonic development to the morula stage, besides inducing morphological changes during development.

For the IVP biotechnique, the rules for collection, processing and semen storage should be revised, to ensure that it is free of microorganisms. Appropriate disinfectants are extremely important for a good preputial hygiene of the bull and of the materials used during the collection. Likewise, the use of effective antibiotics in semen extenders also provide semen free from contamination, since the procedure used during *in vitro* fertilization (percoll) was not effective in reducing or eliminating STEC in our study.

Effects of an exogenous antioxidant on the in vitro bovine embryo production

E Dovolou[a,b], M Clemente[c], GS Amiridis[b] and I Messinis[a]

A. Gutierrez-Adan[c], and D. Rizos[c], [a]Clinic of Obstetrics & Gynaecology, Faculty of Medicine; [b]Clinic of Obstetrics & Reproduction, Vet. Faculty, Univ. of Thessaly, Greece; [c]Dept de Reproduction Animal, INIA, Spain

Reactive Oxygen Species (ROS) are the major contributors for the reduced rate of in vitro bovine embryo production. It is believed that they can cause meiotic arrest of oocytes, embryonic block and cell death. Here we report the effects of guaiazulene (G) -an exogenous antioxidant- in embryo development and in the quality of the produced blastocysts.

Bovine cumulus oocyte complexes (COC's) were aspirated from abattoir ovaries and COC's were matured in TCM199 with FCS and EGF at 39°C under an atmosphere of 5% CO_2 in air with maximum humidity. After 24 h, oocytes were inseminated with frozen/thawed semen and co-incubated for an additional 24 h. Zygotes were cultured in groups of 25 in 25 μl of SOF with 5% FCS at 39°C under an atmosphere of 5% CO_2, 5% O_2 in air with maximum humidity. In the first experiment the maturation medium was modified with addition of 0.1 mM of G (n=497), or 0.01 mM G (n=468), 0.05% DMSO-the G diluent (control$^+$ n=467), and 459 oocytes were used as control (control$^-$). In the second experiment, the culture medium was modified with the addition of 0.01 mM of G (n=344), 0.1 mM of G (n=345), 0.05% DMSO (Control$^+$, n=347) and 355 were the control$^-$. Blastocyst yield was recorded on d 6, 7, 8 and 9. All d 7 blastocysts from each experiment and group were snap frozen and stored for mRNA extraction. Quantification of transcripts for mRNA of genes related to metabolism (AKRIBI, PGHS-2 – COX-2, GADPH, GLUT-5) and to implantation (GPX1, G6PD, PLAC8) and to oxidation (MnSOD) was carried out by real time quantitative RT-PCR. Data for embryo development and on transcript abundance were analyzed by Chi-square and ANOVA, respectively.

In the first experiment, no differences were found between groups in terms of cleavage rate (Control$^-$: 74.20%; Control$^+$:74.58%; 0.1 mM: 71.63%; 0.01 mM: 71.61%) or d 9 blastocyst yield (Control$^-$: 28.26%; Control$^+$:25.80%; 0.1 mM: 25.25%; 0.01 mM: 25.86%). In the second experiment, cleavage rate tended to be greater in 0.01 mM group than in Control$^-$ (77.87% vs. 71.41% P=0.07). No other differences were detected in cleavage rate (Control$^+$:71.32%; 0.1 mM: 72.75%) or in the overall blastocyst yield on d 9 (Control$^-$: 25.50%; Control$^+$:26.71%; 0.1 mM: 25.75%; 0.01 mM: 29.58%).

In both experiments the relative abundance of genes studied varied between groups but these differences were not statistically significant. From our results it appears that under low oxygen incubation conditions, oxidation is not a major hurdle for the in vitro embryo production.

Cooperative communication between bovine in vitro embryos in group and WOW culture

L Vandaele[a], E Wydooghe[a], JL Leroy[b] and A Van Soom[a]

[a]*Department of Reproduction, Obstetrics and Herd Health, Faculty of Veterinary Medicine, Ghent University, Belgium;* [b]*Department of Veterinary Sciences, Faculty of Biomedical Pharmaceutical & Veterinary Sciences, Antwerp University, Belgium*

In vitro bovine embryo culture is traditionally done in groups of 25 because cooperative communication between embryos has shown to improve embryo development and quality. However, it is not known if the strength of cooperative communication is depending on embryo quality. Previous research demonstrated that developmental kinetics at 45 h post insemination (hpi) (fast: 5 to 8 cell stage or slow: 2 to 4 cell stage) can be used as a predictive embryo quality parameter[1]. The aim of the present study was to compare potential cooperative communication between fast and slow embryos in different culture systems based on blastocyst development, total cell number and apoptotic cell number.

A total of 1590 immature bovine oocytes were matured in serum free conditions (TCM199 supplemented with 20 ng/ml EGF and 0.1% gentamycin) and fertilized in vitro. Presumed zygotes (n=1494) were denuded 24 hpi and cultured in 50 μL droplets of modified synthetic oviduct fluid (SOF) medium with 2% bovine serum albumin (BSA) at 39.0°C in 5% CO_2, 5% O_2 and 90% N_2. At 45 hpi cleavage rate was recorded and embryos having 5 or more cells were classified as fast developing embryos, while embryos with only 2 to 4 cells were classified as slow developers. Slow and fast embryos were randomly divided over 3 different culture systems: Classical culture system (50 μl droplets) with fast (ClasF) or slow developers (ClasS); Individual culture in 20 μl droplets with fast (IndF) or slow developers (IndS) and culture in Well-of-the-Well (WOW)[2] of fast (WowF) and slow developers (WowS). At 7 d post insemination (dpi), blastocyst development was assessed and in all blastocysts total cell number (TCN) and apoptotic cell ratio (ACR) were determined using TUNEL-staining.

Blastocyst percentage of fast cleaving embryos was not different between culture conditions and varied between 27.8±4.57% for ClasF, 30.1±5.41% for IndF and 35.4±4.91% for WowF. For slow cleaving embryos, blastocyst percentage in ClasS (12.6±3.06%) and WowS (9.2±2.67%) was greater than in IndS (2.4±1.40%). Furthermore, TCN (between 82.2 and 118.5) was not different between the different culture conditions of fast developing embryos and slow developing embryos, respectively. For both fast and slow developing embryos ACR was lower in traditional group culture (5.7±0.41% in ClasF and 5.2±0.56% in ClasS) in comparison with WowF (7.1±0.4%) and IndF (8.7±0.60%) or WowS (8.1±0.76%) and IndS (8.7±1.43%), respectively.

Cooperative effect between embryos is more important for slow cleaving embryos, since development competence of individually cultured fast cleavers was not hampered. The higher ACR in WowF and WowS in comparison with ClasF and ClasS might indicate that the cooperative effect may be hampered by the relative large distance between embryos in the WOW-system (670μm). Other researchers have claimed that 165μm is the optimal distance between embryos in a group[3].

[1]Vandaele *et al.*, 2007. Reproduction 133:709-718.
[2]Vajta *et al.*, 2000. Mol Reprod Dev 55:256-264.
[3]Gopichandran and Leese 2006. Reproduction 131:269-277.

Heat stress affects on in vitro embryo production of Holstein heifers, high-producing cows in peak lactation and repeat-breeder cows

RM Ferreira[a], H Ayres[a], MR Chiaratti[a], ML Ferraz[b], CA Rodrigues[c], YF Watanabe[d] and PS Baruselli[a]

[a]*University of São Paulo, São Paulo, Brazil;* [b]*Vida Reprodutiva, São Paulo, Brazil;* [c]*SAMVET, São Paulo, Brazil;* [d]*VITROGEN, São Paulo, Brazil*

Previous reports have indicated the occurrence of low fertility associated with summer heat stress (HS) in Holstein cattle. In the present work, we hypothesized that 1) Holstein cattle under HS would have compromised in vitro embryo production (IVP) compared with cattle in fresh season; 2) heifers (H) would have greater IVP than peak lactation (PL) and repeat-breeders (RB; >3 services) cows; 3) RB would have compromised IVP compared to non-RB cows.

This experiment was conducted on 2 commercial dairy farms in southeast Brazil in summer and winter 2009. Cattle started a protocol to synchronize follicular wave emergence: 2 mg estradiol benzoate (Sincrodiol®, OuroFino, Brazil) + 50 mg progesterone (OuroFino, Brazil) + 150μg D-cloprostenol (Sincrocio®, OuroFino, Brazil) i.m. + a norgestomet ear implant (Crestar®, Intervet, Brazil) on d 0, implant removal and OPU on d 5. Respiration rate (RR), rectal temperature (RT), and cutaneous temperature (CT) were recorded on d 0. Semen from a single Holstein bull previously tested was used in IVP. Statistical analyses were done using PROC GLIMMIX of SAS (SAS Institute, Cary, NC, USA). Heifers were on average 16.8 ± 0.3 mo old; PL and RB cows had 110.4 ± 3.8 vs. 425.3 ± 17.5 d in milk, milk production of 34.3 ± 0.7 vs. 23.2 ± 0.9 kg, and number of insemination of 0.7 ± 0.1 vs. 7.1 ± 0.3; mean $\pm$ SE; $P<0.0001$. Heifers and cows had similar RR during the fresh month, but cows had their RR increased during the hot months [fresh vs. HS: H=40.59 ± 1.04 (n=34) vs. 44.78 ± 1.30 (n=36), PL=43.74 ± 1.49^b (n=32) vs. 72.86 ± 2.25^a (n=37), RB=43.10 ± 1.23^b (n=31) vs. 73.83 ± 1.41^a (n=36); $P<0.0001$]. Heifers kept similar RT in fresh months and HS (38.65 ± 0.07 vs. 38.61 ± 0.06, $P>0.05$), while PL and RB cows had their RT raised during HS (PL=39.21 ± 0.07^b vs. 39.76 ± 0.12^a, RB=38.81 ± 0.07^b vs. 39.51 ± 0.11^a; $P<0.0001$). The CT was lower in heifers than cows [H=31.37 ± 0.14^b (n=70), PL=32.73 ± 0.22^a (n=69), RB=32.40 ± 0.22^a (n=67); $P<0.0001$] and during the fresh month compared to HS [fresh=31.09 ± 0.09 (n=97), HS=33.10 ± 0.17 (n=109); $P<0.0001$]. At IVP, the cleavage rate was similar among categories [H=51.7% (194/375), PL=37.9% (148/390), RB=41.9% (279/666); $P<0.18$] and periods [fresh=42.3% (414/979), hot=45.8% (207/452); $P=0.45$]. However, the blastocyst rate was greater ($P<0.0001$) in heifers during both, the fresh month [H=30.3%^{a} (74/244); PL=22.0%^{b} (42/191); RB=22.5%^{b} (93/413)] and HS [H=23.3%^{a} (35/150); PL=14.6%^{b} (15/103); RB=7.9%^{c} (14/177)]. Also, within each category, blastocyst rate was reduced during the HS ($P<0.0001$).

In conclusion, the HS negatively affected the IVP in Holstein cattle, regardless of the category. Heifers were capable of keeping similar RR and RT during the fresh month and HS. Also, heifers were superior to cows in the IVP during both periods. RB cows were severely compromised by HS and poorer in IVP than non-RB cows during this period.

Acknowledgements: Farms Santa Rita and Campestre, Vida Reprodutiva, LMMD, SAMVET, VITROGEN, OuroFino Saúde Animal, CAPES, and FAPESP (proc2009/0938-3).

Bovine viral diarrhea virus in fetal bovine serum batches

E De Stefano, NTC Galleti, CP Ribeiro, LH Okuda, AHC Nogueira, and EM Pituco

Instituto Biológico, Centro de Pesquisa e Desenvolvimento de Sanidade Animal, Laboratório de Viroses de Bovídeos, São Paulo, SP, Brazil

Bovine viral diarrhea virus (BVDV) is a widespread and costly cattle pathogen. Infections with BVDV are either acute or persistent. Persistently infected animals are affected in early fetal life, before onset of immunological competence. Fetal bovine serum (FBS), which has long been used as a supplement for tissue culture media supplying growth factors and attachment factors essential for cell culture, has been incriminated as the source of noncytopathic BVDV. This is a problem because it is used in the manufacture of veterinary and human immunological products. Cell culture established from infected fetuses is often contaminated with BVDV and remains so indefinitely[1]. Because noncytopathic BVDV does not induce a cytopathic effect, infection of cell cultures may not be detected unless the samples are tested by immunocytochemical, ELISA and/or molecular procedures. It is necessary, therefore. to use BVDV-free FBS batches in order to avoid viral dissemination, by applying contaminated vaccine, and interference in the diagnostic of any virological diseases.

From 2005 to 2009 samples were analyzed at the Biological Institute of São Paulo Brazil. There were 277 FBS batches coming from commercial suppliers. RT-PCR, ELISA and isolation in MDBK cell culture with immunoperoxidase staining was used to determine the presence of BVDV.

The number of batches found positive was 14.8% (41/277) by at least one method. From the total, 13.8% (38/277) were positive for RT-PCR, 5.8% (16/277) for ELISA and 5.4% (15/277) were positive for both ELISA and PCR. Noncytopathic BVDV was isolated from 1.4% (4/277) of the batches of FBS. Although there was detected viral nucleic acid and/or viral protein in 14.8% of the batches, in only 1.4% was the virus isolated, and this may be due to the viral inactivation during the industrialization process.

Finally, these findings indicate that BVDV is an endemic infection in Brazil and must be a matter of concern in control programs of reproduction diseases of ruminants. Furthermore, there is a significant risk that adventitious BVDV from FBS may lead to contamination in the veterinary biologics industry. We concluded that detection of BVDV in batches of FBS is important for several reasons. It is recommended to avoid the use of FBS in diagnostic procedures without preliminary tests for pestivirus infections.

[1]Bolin *et al.,* 1991. J Vet Diagn Invest 3: 199-203.

Evaluation of ovarian follicular production in ewes submitted to follicular aspirations at a one week interval: pilot study

PPM Teixeira, MEF Oliveira, LC Padilha, ASL da Silva, TF Motheo, MB Bandarra and WRR Vicente

Department of Preventive Medicine and Animal Reproduction, São Paulo State University (UNESP), Jaboticabal, Brazil

The production of embryos from oocytes in vitro is one way to expand the gene pool derived from superior female animals[1,2]. Follicular aspiration is an important technique that needs to be studied so that oocytes can be collected efficiently with minimal damage to the ovary[3]. The aim of the present study was to quantify ovarian follicles in ewes that underwent two follicular aspirations in one week and to verify if this procedure and interval influenced the efficiency of the aspiration technique. Six Santa Inês ewes had estrus synchronized with 60 mg MAP sponges (d 0) for 6 d. At d 5, 37.5μg of D-cloprostenol and 300 I.U. eCG were injected intramuscularly. After synchronization, ewes were stimulated with 80 mg of FSHp and 300 I.U. eCG in a single injection, 36 h before surgery.

Ovarian follicles were counted and aspirated by using a video-laparoscopic procedure under general anesthesia. Video-assisted ovariectomies were performed seven d later, and harvested ovaries were grossly evaluated and then processed for histological analysis (hematoxylin and eosin - HH and Masson´s Trichrome MT). Inflammatory content and fibrous tissue formation were scored as absent (0), mild (1), moderate (2), or severe (3). One–way ANOVA and Tukey tests were performed to evaluate number of oocytes and to compare results between each aspiration. Histological data were compared by the Wilcoxon Signed Rank test ($P<0.05$). Mean $\pm$ standard error (SEM) of the number of aspirated oocytes in the first session was 8 ± 1.3 (right ovary) and 8 ± 2.3 (left ovary) and in the second aspiration was 7.5 ± 0.8 (right ovary) and 8 ± 1.3 (left ovary). No statistical difference was detected for the number of oocytes collected at the first and the second aspirations. In addition, ovaries did not show significant gross and histological abnormalities after follicular aspirations ($P=0.12$) with average $\pm$ SEM score of 0.7 ± 0.5 (HH and MT) which corresponds to focal regions of fibrous tissue and mononuclear infiltrate probably caused by previous trauma induced by the procedures. In conclusion, this pilot study showed that sequential follicular aspirations at a one week interval were harmless to the ovaries. The procedure as well as the chosen interval did not interfere with the efficiency of the aspiration technique.

[1]Morton *et al.*, 2005. Reprod Dom Anim 40:422-428.
[2]Basso *et al.*, 2008. O Embrião 38:9-13.
[3]Viana *et al.*, 2003. Preq Vet Bras 23:119-124.

Follicular differentiation and oocyte quality in the cow

AL Nivet[a], C Vigneault[b], P Blondin[b], and MA Sirard[a]

[a]Centre de Recherche en Biologie de la Reproduction, Animal Sciences Department; [b]Laval University, Québec, Canada and L'Alliance Boviteq, St-Hyacinthe, Canada

Dairy cow fertility has decreased over the past 20 years. Combinations of genetic and environmental factors are suspected to explain the loss in fertilty. In some cases *in vitro* fertilization (IVF) must/may be used. The success rate has been relatively weak when compared with *in vivo* fertilization until the process of FSH coasting, or FSH withdrawl, was introduced in 2002. FSH coasting is the duration between the last FSH injection and transvaginal aspiration. Although FSH withdrawal is associated with increased competence when aspirated oocytes are processed for *in vitro* maturation and IVF, this has not been optimized nor explained. The goal of the project is firstly to define the oocyte competence window during the coasting process and secondly to better understand *in vivo* mechanisms underlying the oocyte developmental competence acquisition during follicular differentiation

Cycling cows (n = 6) were stimulated with 3 d of FSH (6 X 40 mg NIH Folltropin-V given at 12 h intervals), followed by a coasting (no FSH) period of four different durations (20, 44, 68 or 92 h). Each animal was exposed to the 4 conditions and served as its own control. Each animal was treated during the luteal phase to prevent spontaneous ovulation. At the scheduled time, transvaginal aspirations of immature oocytes were performed, followed by IVF of half the oocytes and RNA extraction of the other half. Follicular cells were aspirated at all the selected times and were snap-frozen to study their gene expression with a global approach (microarray) in correlation with time and blastocyst rate obtained. Statistical analyses were performed with SAS software (rsreg procedure,).

Developmental results indicated that the best coasting duration is approximately 55 h and the oocyte competence window is between 44 h and 68 h of coasting. The best statistical blastocyst rate estimations, with quadratic regression model, are within these conditions and the blastocyst rate is more than 75%.

An optimal duration between the FSH surge and transvaginal aspiration seems to be crucial for optimal oocyte quality. The next step is to better understand what happens in the follicle during that period to understand the signaling pathway leading to developmental competence.

Supported by NSERC and FQRNT.

Changes in metabolic hormone profiles of donor and recipient ewes and their connection to the outcome of superovulation and embryo transfer

N Vass[a], P Balogh[a], A Jávor[a], M Kulcsár[b], V Faigl[b], G Huszenicza[b] and S Cseh[b]

[a]*University of Debrecen, Institute of Animal Sciences, Debrecen, Hungary;* [b]*SZIE, Faculty of Veterinary Sciences, Budapest, Hungary*

Assisted reproductive technologies have been introduced to overcome reproductive inefficiencies in sheep and to accelerate genetic gain. Superovulation and embryo transfer can be applied to correctly choose females to allow extra genetic gain through the production of males with positive indexes used for artificial insemination. Sheep embryo transfer technology has improved and it has become used worldwide in sheep breeding. Little progress, however, has been achieved in superovulation/ovarian stimulation during the last decade. The variability of the superovulatory response still remains to be improved. It has been well documented that several factors (breed, season, treatment protocol) influence the efficacy of superovulation and embryo transfer. There is limited data (mainly obtained in bovine) available on the role of metabolic hormones (IGF-1, insulin, T4) in superovulation and the pregnancy rate of recipient animals after embryo transfer. The effects of IGF-I on steroidogenesis, cell proliferation, aromatase activity, folliculogenesis, ovulation, fertilization, implantation and embryonic development have, however, been well documented. In this study, the possible role of metabolic hormones on the efficiency of superovulation and embryo transfer were studied in sheep.

Donor and recipient ewes were treated with intravaginal sponges (40 mg; Chronogest, Intervet, France) for 12 d in breeding season and out of breeding season. Superovulatory treatment (6 x 0.8 mL; Stimufol, France) was started on d 10. Laparoscopic insemination of donors was applied 36 h after sponge removal. Recipient ewes were treated with PMSG (i.m.) (400 IU per ewe, Folligon, Intervet, France) at the time of sponge removal. Rams, fitted with harnesses and crayons were introduced to the flock 24 h after PMSG administration. Blood samples were taken 3 times from the donor (n = 12) and recipient (n = 20) ewes (d 0: at the time of artificial insemination of donors/heat observation of recipients, d 2: at the beginning of fasting before surgery, d 4: at the time of embryo flushing/embryo transfer). The blood concentrations of IGF-1, insulin, and T4 were determined.

There were significant differences between blood IGF-1 and insulin for the breeding compared with the non-breeding season. We found a relationship between the number of corpora lutea ($P < 0.005$), the number of embryos flushed ($P < 0.001$), the number of transferable embryos obtained ($P < 0.001$) and the blood concentrations of IGF-1. Lower T4 concentrations were found in the breeding season and in pregnant recipients ($P < 0.001$).

In conclusion, our results indicate that metabolic hormones (IGF-1, insulin, T4) may play an important role in folliculogenesis, steroidogenesis, oocyte maturation, and embryonic development in sheep. Further investigations are needed to determine their exact mechanism of action, especially the role of T4 in embryo transfer programs.

Successful pregnancies of vitrified *in vitro* produced (IVP) Holstein blastocysts derived from sorted and unsorted semen after a fixed-time embryo transfer – A field trial in Thailand

S Sangsritavong[a], R Parnpai[b], C Laowtammathron[b], C Lorthongpanich[b], P Ittiworapong[a] and RL Monson[c]

[a]*Biotec Central Research Unit, Thailand Science Park;* [b]*Embryo Technology and Stem Cell Research Center, Suranaree University of Technology, Thailand;* [c]*Department of Animal Science, University of Wisconsin-Madison, USA*

Dairy producers have desired a methodology to manipulate the sex of offspring in order to generate more heifer calves. Flow cytometer sorted X-and Y- chromosome-bearing sperm have been used for *in vitro* production of blastocysts in several species including bovine. The widespread implementation of IVP embryo transfer in the bovine has been limited by cost, efficiency and conception rate. Using sex-sorted semen to skew gender ratio in favor of females could enhance the application of IVP embryos. The objective of this study was to evaluate conception rates of vitrified IVP blastocysts derived from sex-sorted or unsorted semen in bovine. Ovaries from Holstein cows were obtained from abattoirs and cumulus oocyte complexes were aspirated for *in vitro* maturation. After maturation, oocytes were inseminated with percoll separated X-sorted or unsorted sperm and cultured in modified CR1aa medium for 8.5 d at 38.5°C, and 5% CO_2 in humidified air. A three-step pre-equilibration procedure was used for the rapid cooling vitrification of good and excellent quality d 7 to 8.5 IVP Holstein blastocysts. All embryos were kept in liquid nitrogen prior to transfer into synchronized recipients. Recipient heifers were prepared for timed embryo transfer using a steroid-based synchronization of ovulation protocol. Intravaginal progesterone-releasing devices (CIDR) were inserted into the vagina of 320 cross-bred Holstein heifers. Simultaneously, heifers were treated with progesterone (50 mg) and estradiol-17ß (2 mg) via i.m. injection (d 0). On d 6 of the protocol, heifers were treated with 25 mg $PGF_{2\alpha}$ followed by removal of the CIDR on d 7. On d 8 all animals were treated with 1 mg estradiol benzoate. Corpus luteum (CL) size was confirmed by ultrasonography on d 15 (i.e., 8 d after CIDR removal). Heifers that carried at least one CL were selected as suitable recipients. Vitrified IVP blastocysts derived from both sex-sorted and unsorted sperm were warmed and assessed for quality. Only good and excellent quality blastocysts were transferred to recipients. Vitrified IVP blastocysts derived from unsorted semen yielded greater conception rates than blastocysts derived from sex-sorted semen (31.0%; 36/116 vs. 19.4%; 24/124; P=0.10). Conception rates in recipient heifers with larger CL were greater (conception rates for CL diamater of 11 to 14 mm, 15 to 19 mm, and > 19 mm were 28% (4/14), 32% (16/50) and 42% (6/14), respectively). These results suggest that a methodology combining *in vitro* produced bovine embryos using sex sorted sperm and cryopreservation via rapid cooling vitrification could be an effective tool for dairy producers to enhance the production of heifer calves for replacements, but only if conception rates can be improved.

Acknowledgement: This study was financially supported by National Center for Genetic Engineering and Biotechnology (BIOTEC), Thailand.

Successful cryopreservation of embryos produced from superovulated ewes inseminated with sex-sorted ram spermatozoa

SP de Graaf, KH Beilby, WMC Maxwell and G Evans

Faculty of Veterinary Science, The University of Sydney, Australia

Pre-selection of sex of offspring has been realised through the use of flow cytometrically sorted spermatozoa within artificial insemination and *in vitro* fertilisation programs. In the sheep industry, considerable interest exists in the successful use of this technology when combined with multiple ovulation and embryo transfer (MOET)[1]. The present study was conducted to determine the feasibility of utilising sex-sorted ram spermatozoa to produce pre-sexed embryos from superovulated ewes for cryopreservation and transfer.

Semen was collected from two Merino rams, and split into two parts for sex-sorting and freezing (S) or standard freezing (non-sorted Control) using previously established techniques[2]. Intrauterine inseminations were conducted using commercial laparoscopic techniques on superovulated mature Merino ewes ($n = 18$) in synchronised estrus utilising either 15×10^6 or 30×10^6 motile sex-sorted (S_{15} or S_{30}, respectively) or Control spermatozoa (C_{15} or C_{30}, respectively). Resultant embryos and unfertilised ova were recovered by retrograde flush (via surgical-median laparotomy) 6 d after insemination and morulae to blastocysts frozen using a modified slow-freeze technique. Thawed embryos were cultured for 6 h prior to transfer into synchronised recipients ($n = 15$) or kept for sex-determination by PCR analysis. Pregnancy was diagnosed at d 54 by real-time cutaneous ultrasound.

The fertilisation rate with spermatozoa from all groups was similar (S_{15}: 45/51, 88.2%; S_{30}: 36/50, 76.6%; C_{15}: 17/27, 65.4%; C_{30}: 2/3, 66.7%; $P > 0.05$) as was the percentage of embryos designated as transferable ($P > 0.05$). Five of the 29 (17.2%) embryos transferred (derived from sex-sorted treatments) resulted in a fetus at ultrasound and all resultant lambs were of the predicted sex. Fifteen of 16 (93.8%) embryos produced with sex-sorted spermatozoa were found to be of the predicted sex after PCR analysis.

To our knowledge, these are the first recorded births of lambs produced following the transfer of cryopreserved embryos derived from artificial insemination of superovulated sheep with sex-sorted, frozen-thawed ram spermatozoa. The similar levels of fertilisation and embryo survival obtained for sex-sorted and control groups, albeit with low replication, supports the established hypothesis that sex-sorted ram spermatozoa are not functionally compromised[1,3].

Supported by XY Inc. and Bioniche Animal Health Australasia.

[1]de Graaf *et al.* 2007. Theriogenology 67:550-555.
[2]Beilby *et al.* 2009. Theriogenology 71:829-835.
[3]de Graaf *et al.* 2009. Theriogenology 71:89-97.

Comparison of superovulatory response and reproductive performance after flushing with and without CIDR in early postpartum suckling Japanese Black cows

K Oshima, Y Ochiai, T Kojima and N Yamamoto
National Agricultural Research Center for Western Region, Oda, Japan

Embryos can be recovered after superovulation during the voluntary waiting period in postpartum suckled beef cows. We are attempting to improve reproductive efficiency in Japanese Black cows by means of embryo recovery following superovulation within 60 d postpartum during the voluntary period. The aim of this study was to investigate the effect of a CIDR used in superovulation on superovulatory responses and reproductive performance after flushing.

Seventy-one postpartum suckling cows were used. At 40 d postpartum, the cows were classified into two groups: (1) timed superovulation using CIDR (CIDR+; n = 36) and (2) superovulation without CIDR following natural ovulation (CIDR−; n = 35). In the CIDR+ group, cows received CIDR at 40 d postpartum (d 0) and were subsequently superovulated with a total dose of 20 Armour units of FSH twice daily with gradually decreasing doses from d 5 to 7. On d 7, the CIDR was withdrawn and 0.75 mg cloprostenol was injected. In the CIDR− group, cows were superovulated during the second postpartum estrous cycle with the same medication schedule but without a CIDR. The superovulation treatment in the CIDR− group was initiated 7 d after estrus. Cows were artificially inseminated twice at estrus. Embryos were recovered non-surgically 7 or 8 d after estrus. The ovaries were examined by ultrasonography and the number of CL and remaining follicles were counted. After uterine flushing, the cows were re-employed for reproductive purposes. The intervals to first estrus and conception after flushing and days open were examined. Data were analyzed by using a Student's *t*-test.

The interval from caving to flushing in the CIDR− group (60.5 ± 5.6 d, mean ± SD) was longer ($P < 0.05$) than that in the CIDR+ group (56.9 ± 1.5 d). There were no differences between the CIDR+ and CIDR− groups in the number of CL (16.1 ± 7.5 vs. 17.9 ± 8.1), recovered ova or embryos (12.6 ± 8.1 vs. 11.9 ± 9.1), and transferable and freezable embryos (8.3 ± 7.3 and 6.8 ± 5.7, respectively vs. 9.1 ± 8.6 and 7.7 ± 7.3, respectively). The number of remaining follicles in the CIDR+ group (7.0 ± 7.5) was greater ($P < 0.05$) than that in the CIDR− group (2.5 ± 2.6). The CIDR+ and CIDR− groups showed no differences in the intervals of first estrus after flushing and conception and days open (11.4 ± 9.2, 38.9 ± 21.3 and 95.9 ± 21.3 d, respectively vs. 8.6 ± 4.5, 33.1 ± 30.3 and 93.7 ± 30.9 d, respectively).

Using a CIDR in a superovulation treatment in early postpartum suckling Japanese Black cows neither affects the recovered embryo quality nor the reproductive performance after flushing.

Efficiency of the P-36 protocol, associated with eCG or LH administration on the last day of superovulation treatment, in Angus (Bos taurus) donors

FS Rosa, ALM Bonotto, LA Trinca, MFG Nogueira and CM Barros

IB - University of Sao Paulo State, Brazil

Recent studies with a superovulatory protocol called P-36 have shown that replacement of the last two doses of FSH by eCG improves embryo yield in *Bos indicus* cattle, presumably due to the LH like activity of eCG. The objective of the present study was to verify the efficiency of protocol P-36/eCG in Angus cattle and to test the replacement of eCG by LH in the last day of superovulatory treatment. In Exp.1, 22 Angus cows were allotted to 4 groups: LH60 (Control), LH60/eCG, LH60/LH and LH60/FSH+LH. Each donor was superovulated 3 times, such that each animal received 3 of 4 treatments, totaling 17 cows in the first two groups and 16 in the others (incomplete block design). At a random stage of the estrous cycle the donors received an intravaginal device (IVD) containing 1.0 g of progesterone and estradiol benzoate (3.0 mg, i.m, d 0). In the control group, the animals were superovulated with decreasing doses of pFSH; whereas, in groups LH60/eCG and LH60/LH the last two doses of pFSH were replaced by eCG (i.m, each dose=200 IU) or pLH (i.m., each dose= 1.0 mg), respectively. Finally, the cows from group LH60/FSH+LH received two doses of 1.0 mg of LH simultaneously with the last two doses of pFSH. All animals were treated with a $PGF_{2\alpha}$ analog on D6, and the IVD was removed 36 h afterwards. Ovulation was induced with 12.5 mg of pLH (i.m.), on D8, and the animals were FTAI 12 and 24 h after pLH. In Exp.2, 17 cows were allocated in 3 groups: LH48, LH60 and LH48/FSH+LH. The difference between the first and the second experiment is that in groups LH48 and LH48/FSH+LH, the hormone used to induce ovulation was administered 48 h after $PGF_{2\alpha}$, instead of 60 h. Each donor was superovulated 3 times and received all treatments (cross-over design). Embryo flushing was performed on D15-16, in both experiments, and data were analyzed by ANOVA (Proc Mixed, SAS). In Exp.1, replacement of eCG by LH (group LH60/LH), resulted in a decline ($P<0.05$) in the number of total embryos and transferable embryos, when compared with the other groups. However, addition of pLH to the last two doses of pFSH (LH60/FSH+LH) improved embryo quality and numerically increased the total embryo yield (87) compared with LH60 (43) and LH60/LH group(13). In Exp. 2, there was no significant difference among treatments in embryo yield. Nevertheless, group LH48/FSH+LH had a greater number of excellent and good embryos than the others ($P<0.05$). It is concluded that eCG can be replaced by FSH and LH, in the last day of superovulatory treatment of the P-36 protocol, without affecting viable embryos yield.

Supported by FAPESP and fellowship (Rosa FS) from CAPES (Brazil).

Prediction of superovulatory responses in the cow: effects of the estrous cycle and breeding conditions on anti-Müllerian hormone endocrine concentrations

C Rico[a], C Médigue[c], F Clément[c], E Briant[b], M Dupont[b], S Fabre[a] and D Monniaux[a]

[a]*Physiologie de la Reproduction et des Comportements;* [b]*Unité Expérimentale de l'Orfrasière, INRA Nouzilly, France;* [c]*INRIA Paris-Rocquencourt, Le Chesnay, France*

In cattle, ovarian responsiveness to FSH stimulation is highly variable between individuals and difficult to predict. We have established that anti-Müllerian hormone (AMH), secreted by granulosa cells of growing follicles, is a possible endocrine predictor of the ovarian response to superovulation in the cow[1]. For an accurate test of high prognostic value, the optimal time at which to perform this blood test has to be assessed. This study aimed to establish: 1) whether AMH should be measured at a given day of the estrous cycle of cows or anytime and 2) whether breeding conditions could affect AMH levels.

Twenty-seven Holstein dairy cows were superovulated and their ovarian response was assessed by counting large follicles >7 mm in diameter at estrus and corpora lutea (CL) after ovulation by ovarian ultrasonography. Then cows were assigned to 2 groups, according to their high (H, number of CL>10) or low (L, number of CL<10) ovarian response. Afterwards, daily changes in plasma AMH concentrations were studied throughout a natural estrous cycle in groups H (n=6) and L (n=5). The effects of breeding conditions on plasma AMH concentrations were studied on 16 other cows (8 in groups H and L) between January and May through monthly blood sampling. They received food supplementation with a cereal-based concentrate from February and were put out to grazing from April onwards.

During the studied estrous cycle, plasma AMH concentrations decreased between estrus (d 0) and d 6 and increased thereafter, and were consistently greater in group H compared with group L. The numbers of large follicles and CL observed in response to the superovulatory treatment were highly correlated with plasma AMH concentrations measured at d 0 ($r=0.87$, $P<0.001$; $r=0.74$, $P<0.01$, respectively) and after d 11 until the end of the estrous cycle ($r>0.84$; $r>0.65$, respectively). In contrast, AMH concentrations between d 4 and d 7 were not correlated with the number of CL. For the 16 cows studied between January and May, plasma AMH concentrations remained low in the L group and were not affected by changes in breeding conditions. In contrast, in group H, plasma AMH concentrations dropped significantly in February ($P<0.001$) after food supplementation, then returned to initial values in March and dropped again in May ($P<0.001$) after putting out the cows for grazing.

For an accurate prediction of superovulatory responses, AMH concentrations should be measured in plasma either at estrus or after d 11 of an estrous cycle. Moreover, changes in diet can affect plasma AMH concentrations in cows with a high capacity for ovarian response to superovulation, and consequently the prognostic value of the AMH blood test may be affected.

[1]Rico *et al.,* 2009. Biol Reprod 80:50-59.

Production of bovine chimeric embryos, by aggregation of post-compaction developmental stage half-embryos

IP Emanuelli[a,b], BCS Campanha[a], DM de Souza[a], CP Godoi[a], MPM Mancini[a] and MFG Nogueira[a]

[a]*Laboratory of Embryo Micromanipulation, Dept. of Biological Sciences, São Paulo State University, Assis, São Paulo, Brazil;* [b]*Animal Breeding Biotechnology Center, Maringá Univ. Center, Maringá, Paraná, Brazil*

To aggregate mammalian embryos (*i.e.*, embryonic chimeras) pre-compaction developmental stages are well reported as more efficacious than morulae or blastocysts. However, when MOET is used to recover farm animal embryos, they could be in more advanced developmental stages (post-compaction).

The aim of this work was, primarily, to evaluate the feasibility of demi-morulae (DM) and demi-blastocysts (DB) to produce bovine embryonic chimeras and the effect of the treatment with phyto-hemaglutinin-L (PHA) during bovine embryo aggregation and, secondarily, to perform a pilot test with mouse embryos to obtain previous data about post-compaction developmental stage embryo aggregation effectiveness.

Transgenic (C57/BL6/EGFP; GFP) or non-transgenic (Swiss Webster; SW) mice were superovulated and the embryos were recovered. Embryos were manipulated in M2 medium (room temperature), and aggregation groups consisted of GM1 (two DB, n=28), GM2 (DB and DM, n=20) and GM3 (two whole zona free 8 to 16 cells embryos, n=25). After 24 h incubation (KSOMaa under oil, at 37°C, 5% CO_2 in maximum humidity), the presence of chimera was verified, and, in a subset of chimeras, the percentage of area occupied by GFP strain (GM2, n=3 and GM3, n=3) was measured. Bovine ovaries were used to obtain 270 COC that were matured in drops (90 μL) of TCM-199 bicarbonate medium, supplemented with 10% FCS, and incubated *in vitro* for 22 to 24 h. After *in vitro* fertilization, the presumptive zygotes were transferred to SOF culture medium to *in vitro* culture. IVM, IVF and IVC were performed under 38.5°C, 5% CO_2 in air and saturated humidity. The aggregation was tested between two whole zona free 8 to 16 cells embryos in the presence (GB1, n=16) or absence of PHA (GB2, n=14); and between one DM and one DB with (GB3, n=15) or without PHA (GB4, n=12). Groups GB1 and GB3 were treated with 500 μg of PHA/mL for 3 min. After PHA treatment, the pairs of embryos were allocated in WOW, under same previous culture conditions, until expansion (d 7). At 24 h of culture, embryonic aggregation pairs were first evaluated to detect a unique and cohesive cell mass.

Chimerism rates results were (3.6, 15.0 and 60.0% for GM1, GM2 and GM3, respectively; $P<0.001$ with GM3 differing from others; $P\leq0.003$) or were not different (62.5, 42.9, 40.0 and 25.0%; GB1, GB2, GB3 and GB4, respectively; $P=0.252$). The mean percentage ($\pm$sd) of GFP cells in the resultant mouse chimera were 51.3$\pm$4.1 (GM2) and 50.6$\pm$10.0% (GM3; $P=0.91$). It was concluded that in those conditions, the embryonic chimerism by aggregation of bovine half-embryos is a feasible procedure and that PHA treatment did not increase the rate of embryo chimerism.

Funding and fellowships from FAPESP (Sao Paulo, Brazil).

Serial nuclear transfer using pre-activated oocyte cytoplasm increases *in vitro* but not *in vivo* development in cattle

NT Standley[a], RSF Lee[a], LW Chamley[b] and DN Wells[a]

[a]*AgResearch Ruakura, Hamilton, New Zealand;* [b]*Department of Obstetrics and Gynaecology, University of Auckland, New Zealand*

The nuclei of differentiated cells can be reprogrammed to a totipotent state following nuclear transfer (NT) using cytoplasm from metaphase II-arrested oocytes. However, few reconstructed embryos develop into viable cloned offspring. The objective of this study was to determine the potentially beneficial effects of alternative sources of cytoplasm in a bovine serial (or double) NT (SNT) procedure. For the second NT reconstruction step, cytoplasm was obtained from either 2-cell *in vitro* produced (IVP) embryos or pre-activated oocyte cytoplasts (PAC) and development directly compared to NT and IVP controls.

NT embryos were produced with serum-starved male fibroblasts and oocyte cytoplasts, using established zona-free procedures[1]. Reconstructs were artificially activated 3 to 4 h post-fusion using ionomycin and 6-dimethylaminopurine. *In vitro* fertilisation was used to generate IVP embryos from the same batch of oocytes. In addition, PACs were generated by activating zona-free oocyte cytoplasts concomitantly with NT. The following day, 2-cell NT and zona-free IVP embryos (both in early S-phase) were separated into individual blastomeres. Single NT donor blastomeres were fused either to a 1-cell PAC or two enucleated recipient IVP blastomeres, generating PAC-SNT or IVP-SNT reconstructs, respectively. Both had approximately 50% greater cytoplasmic volume compared with IVP and NT 1-cells. Zona-free embryos were cultured individually for 7 d in 5 μL drops of AgResearch synthetic oviduct fluid medium. Embryos from each treatment were transferred in pairs to synchronised recipient heifers. Concepti were recovered on d 26 of gestation, following slaughter. Data were analysed by ANOVA.

A greater proportion of 2-cell embryos developed to transferable quality compacted morula and blastocyst stages on d 7 following NT compared with IVP (108/284 = 38% vs. 71/500 = 14%, respectively; $P < 0.001$). For SNT embryos, a greater proportion developed to transferable quality stages following PAC-SNT compared to IVP-SNT (38/73 = 52% vs. 15/98 = 15%, respectively; $P < 0.001$). Moreover, *in vitro* development with PAC-SNT was greater than NT ($P < 0.05$), whereas IVP-SNT was less than NT ($P < 0.001$) and not different to IVP controls. The proportion of transferred blastocysts resulting in apparently normal, viable concepti on d 26 was similar for IVP (8/16 = 50%), NT (7/16 = 44%) and IVP-SNT groups (7/15 = 47%), while PAC-SNT appeared less (4/16 = 25%; $P < 0.27$). There were no differences in morphometric measurements amongst potentially viable embryos.

PAC-SNT reconstructs had significantly greater *in vitro* development than other treatments, but this was not evident *in vivo* at d 26 of gestation. The zona-free cloning method was very advantageous for the otherwise technically demanding SNT procedure and allows the volume of cytoplasm to be greatly increased. Additionally, the use of cytoplasts from more advanced IVP embryos, just after the time of embryonic genome activation, may provide cytoplasm rich in reprogramming factors and mRNA transcripts critical for normal development of clones.

Supported by the NZ Foundation for Research, Science and Technology.

[1]Oback and Wells, 2003. Cloning Stem Cells 5:243-256.

Bovine sperm cell DNA fragmentation is not induced by high exogenous DNA concentration

E Lopes, WB Feitosa, CM Mendes, MP Milazzotto, FF Paula-Lopes, JA Visintin and MEOA Assumpção

Department of Animal Reproduction, College of Veterinary Medicine, University of São Paulo, Brazil

Sperm mediated gene transfer (SMGT) has been described as a promising approach for transgenic animal production. Although SMGT is a simple, fast and low-cost method of gene transfer, it has not been used widely. The low rate of stable DNA integration into the recipient genome and the low repeatability have limited the widespread use of this technology. An increase in exogenous DNA concentration may be an alternative to enhance DNA uptake into sperm cells and consequently increase SMGT efficiency. A high concentration of exogenous DNA may trigger, however, sperm endonuclease activation, leading to an apoptosis-like process. The aim of the present work was to evaluate the effect of a high exogenous DNA (plasmid) concentration on sperm cell transfection and its effect on endogenous DNA integrity.

10^6 sperm/mL were incubated for 90 min with 100, 300 or 500 ng of plasmid. In order to verify the transfection rate after incubation, sperm cells were treated with DNase I for 30 min to degrade non-associated plasmid, followed by DNA extraction with phenol-chloroform. The transfection rate was quantified by real-time PCR. The DNA integrity of sperm cells was evaluated by flow cytometry using the TUNEL protocol and Sperm Chromatin Structure Assay (SCSA). Data were analyzed by ANOVA and Tukey's Test for multiple comparisons at the 5% ($P<0.05$) significance level.

An increase in plasmid concentration (100, 300 and 500 ng) did not increase plasmid uptake by sperm cells (0.02 ± 0.01, 0.06 ± 0.07 and 0.09 ± 0.1 ng, respectively), possibly due to the increase in endonuclease activity which resulted in degradation. Endonuclease activity can result, however, in both exogenous (plasmid) and endogenous DNA degradation. Interestingly, in the present work, no effect of plasmid concentration (0, 100, 300 and 500 ng) on sperm cell DNA integrity was observed by TUNEL assay (96.7 ± 0.9, 96.1 ± 1.4, 96.4 ± 1.2 and 95.8 ± 1.2%; respectively) or by SCSA (93.5 ± 3, 90.4 ± 2.7, 93.2 ± 3.6 and 94.2 ± 2.5%, respectively).

In conclusion, plasmid uptake by sperm cells was not affected by the plasmid concentration during 90 min of incubation. Additionally, the increase in plasmid concentration was not able to trigger an apoptosis – like process in bovine sperm leading to DNA fragmentation.

Financial support was provided by FAPESP 03/10234-7 and 03/07456-8.

Aberrant prostaglandin metabolism in the uterus of early pregnant cattle following somatic cell nuclear transfer

SE Ulbrich[a], V Zakhartchenko[b], E Wolf[b], HD Reichenbach[c], M Büttner[d], C Angioni[e], G Geisslinger[e] and HHD Meyer[a]

[a]*Physiology-Weihenstephan, Technical University of Munich, Freising, Germany;* [b]*Institute of Animal Breeding and Biotechnology, Gene Center, Ludwig-Maximilians-University of Munich, Munich, Germany;* [c]*Institute of Animal Breeding, Bavarian State Institute for Agriculture, Grub, Germany;* [d]*Bavarian Health and Food Safety Authority, Oberschleißheim, Germany;* [e]*Institute of Clinical Pharmacology/ZAFES, Johann Wolfgang Goethe-University Frankfurt, Frankfurt a.M., Germany*

The uterine histotroph comprises signalling molecules which critically account for an intact embryo-maternal communication. Prostaglandins (PG) are important mediators of female reproductive events. We recently showed that during early pregnancy in cattle, PGI_2 was the predominant PG in the uterine lumen followed by $PGF_{2\alpha}$ > PGE_2 > PGD_2 ≈ TXB_2[1]. An unbalanced production and action of PG may cause reproductive disorders. Bovine somatic cell nuclear transfer (SCNT) pregnancies are frequently characterized by placental failure initiated at the onset of pregnancy prior to implantation[2] and thus provide an interesting *in vivo* model for studying early embryo-maternal communication.

We quantitatively analyzed PG present in uteri of SCNT pregnancies (n = 8) in comparison to normal IVF pregnancies (n = 10). Additionally, endometrium and trophoblast tissue were examined regarding specific enzymes and receptors involved in PG generation and function. SCNT and IVF embryos were cultured under identical conditions to the blastocyst stage (d 7) until being transferred to synchronized recipients, which were slaughtered at d 18 of pregnancy. Uterine flushings were analyzed for PG using LC-MS/MS as well as for interferon-τ (IFNT) using a bioassay. Endometrial and trophoblast RNA was extracted for qRT-PCR analysis.

The uterine concentration of IFNT did not differ with respect to origin of embryo (P = 0.5). However, uterine flushings from pregnancies obtained with SCNT embryos had lower levels of PGI_2 (4423 ± 1286 vs. 9709 ± 907 pg/mL, P = 0.006, measured as 6-keto $PGF_{1\alpha}$) and PGE_2 (978 ± 232 vs. 1656 ± 212 pg/mL, P = 0.03) than pregnancies obtained with IVF embryos. $PGF_{2\alpha}$ was also slightly lower in SCNT pregnancies, while the 15-keto metabolites of $PGF_{2\alpha}$ and PGE_2 were elevated (270 ± 60 vs. 102 ± 23 pg/mL, P = 0.03, and 117 ± 20 vs. 26 ± 4 pg/mL, P < 0.001, respectively). Day 18 trophoblasts normally synthesize high amounts of PG with marginal PG catabolism, whereas the endometrium has a higher PG metabolic turnover than the trophoblast. Interestingly, transcripts of PG synthases I and E were both lower in the endometrium of SCNT as compared with IVF pregnancies (1.7-fold, P < 0.001 and 1.4-fold, P = 0.05, respectively), while the mRNA of 15-hydroxyprostaglandin dehydrogenase forming 15-ketoprostaglandin metabolites was neither changed in trophoblast nor endometrial tissue. The mRNA of endometrial target receptors of PGI_2 (PPARγ) and PGE_2 (PTGER4) had lesser expression in SCNT pregnancies (1.9-fold, P = 0.02 and 1.5-fold, P = 0.001, respectively) as well.

A reciprocal embryonic and maternal contribution to an aberrant prostaglandin metabolism with possible adverse fertility consequences seems feasible. Protein verification will further disentangle the causes of unbalanced PG levels in the uterine lumen and verify whether inadequate signaling transfer may be causing detrimental downstream target effects.

[1]Ulbrich *et al.*, 2009. Reproduction 138:371-382.
[2]Bauersachs *et al.*, 2009. Proc Natl Acad Sci 106:5681-5686.

Atypical expression of steroidogenic genes in somatic cell nuclear transfer-derived bovine placentae at d 40 of pregnancy

M Binelli[a], A Verduzco[b], HR Kohan-Ghadr[b], DR Arnold[c], R Lefebvre[b], LC Smith[b] and BD Murphy[b]

[a]*College of Veterinary Medicine and Animal Science, Pirassununga, University of São Paulo, Brazil;* [b]*CRRA, Faculté de Médecine Vétérinaire, Université de Montréal, Saint Hycinthe, Canada;* [c]*College of Agrarian and Veterinary Sciences, São Paulo State University, Jaboticabal, Brazil*

In cattle, there is a 5 to 7% pregnancy success rate for embryos obtained by somatic cell nuclear transfer (SCNT). The SCNT-derived placentae at term show gross morphological abnormalities, such as large and fused placentomes. Recently, we detected global transcriptome changes at the window of placentome formation between SCNT- and artificial insemination (AI)-derived placentae. Differentially expressed genes included genes associated with placental steroidogenesis. The bovine placenta synthesizes steroids that are expected to regulate placental function and fetal development. Our objective was to compare expression of a series of genes coding for steroidogenic enzymes between SCNT and AI placentae.

Cotyledons were collected from cows slaughtered at d 40 of pregnancy (AI, N=8; SCNT, N=8) and subjected to total RNA extraction followed by cDNA synthesis. Differential expression of Scarb1, StAR, Hsd3b Cyp17, Cyp11A1, SULT1E1 and STS between AI and SCNT cotyledons was measured by quantitative real time PCR. Tissue localization of steroidogenic enzymes was evaluated by fluorescent immunohistochemistry and confocal microscopy.

There was a reduction in the abundance of transcripts of Scarb1 ($P<0.1$) and StAR, Hsd3b, Cyp17 and Cyp11A1 ($P<0.01$) in placentae from SCNT compared with AI gestations. Protein localization of Scarb1, Cyp11A1 and Cyp17 was restricted to mononuclear trophoblastic cells, indicating that these are the main cell type responsible for steroid synthesis in d 40 placentae. The reduced expression of Scarb1 and StAR transcripts suggests deficient uptake and cellular transfer of cholesterol across the mitochondrial membrane. Altered levels of the Hsd3b, Cyp11A1 and Cyp17 in cloned gestations are expected to lead to a reduction in progesterone and estrogen synthesis by the placenta. Altered levels of the aforementioned gene transcripts in cloned pregnancies could contribute to the abnormal placental and fetal development associated with losses in SCNT pregnancies.

Supported by NSERC Strategic Grant funds and by FAPESP, CAPES, CNPq and CONACYT scholarships.

Atlas of expression of candidate genes at the utero-conceptus interface during early pregnancy in the cow: A comparative analysis between normal and cloned pregnancies

M Guillomot[a], O Sandra[a], E Campion[a], G Taghouti[a], F Biase[a], C Rabel[b], I Hue[a], L Gall[a], C Richard[a], H Jammes[a], JP Renard[a], R Oliveira[b], R Wallace[b] and H Lewin[b]

[a]Institut National de la Recherche Agronomique, Jouy-en-Josas, France; [b]University Illinois, Urbana-Champaign, USA

It is now well established that embryo manipulations associated with reproductive technologies impact the embryonic viability and maintenance of pregnancy to term. In cattle, the rates of pregnancy and birth of viable offspring are very low after somatic cloning by nuclear transfer (SCNT) and most of the pregnancy losses after SCNT are associated with placental defects. Transcriptomic analyses show that both uterine and extra-embryonic tissues present differential expression patterns of several families of genes during early pregnancy in inseminated or SCNT embryos carrying females[1,2,3]. Although abnormal gene expression highlighted involvement of these factors during pregnancy, little is known about their function during the peri-implantation period in cattle. To bridge a gap between molecular analyses and cellular interactions between the bovine endometrial and extra-embryonic tissues during early pregnancy, we initiated a program aiming to construct an atlas of localized expression of candidate gene networks by in situ hybridization (ISH). Selection of genes was based on their differential expression levels in AI versus SCNT extra-embryonic tissues and cyclic versus AI or SCNT endometrium. Seven families of genes will be considered: 1) cell adhesion molecules and extra-cellular matrix, 2) trophoblast differentiation, 3) imprinted genes, 4) VEGF system, 5) IGF system 6) cell signalling pathways and 7) cell differentiation and apoptosis. Endometrial tissues and conceptuses were collected from slaughtered cows at D18 and D34 of pregnancy after artificial insemination (AI) or transfer of SCNT blastocysts. In AI pregnancies, our preliminary observations on 22 genes indicated that 11 genes had a specific localization in the trophoblast (*Fizzled4, Peg3 ,adfp, cpa3, cited ,hand1, fabp5,tkdp4, dkk1*) or in the endometrium (*fabp3,Angpt2*) and 11 were distributed in both the conceptus and the uterine compartments (*decorin, H19, Igf2, Fn1, col1a2, calmodulin, claudin4, coupTfII, c11orf34, VEGF, Hif1α*). Studies are in progress to compare the patterns of expression of these genes during SCNT pregnancy.

The authors wish to thank D. Le Bourhis and Y. Heyman for cloning embryos and embryo transfers, respectively.

[1]Degrelle *et al.*, 2005. Dev Biol 288:448-460
[2]Everts *et al.*, 2008. Physiol Genomics 33:65-77.
[3]Mansouri-Attia *et al.*, 2009. Proc Natl Acad Sci 106:5687-5692.

Myogenesis of bovine fœtal clones: genomic profiling across pregnancy

I Hue[a], D Valour[a], E Liszewska[a], A de la Foye[b], B Meunier[b], B Picard[b], O Sandra[a], Y Heyman[a] and I Cassar-Malek[b]

[a]*UMR1198, INRA, Jouy, France;* [b]*UR1213, INRA, Theix, France*

Somatic cloning (NT) has often been studied with regard to placental defects and large offspring syndrome (LOS) occurrence but scarcely with regard to foetal muscle defects. We recently showed that disturbances in both primary and secondary myogenesis occur in bovine cloned foetuses using somatic cells from Holstein and Charolais breeds[1]. This may impact the meat quality derived from clones and their offspring, but may also reveal early discrepancies in the mesodermal lineage since myotubes and myoblasts originate from somites.

To further identify molecular pathways that may underly early disturbances in myogenesis, we analysed the transcriptome of cloned and control bovine muscle (NT: n=4, AI: n=4) at 30 d of gestation (dg). Using a bovine oligo-array (22K, INRA-AGENAE), 340 oligonucleotides corresponding to 215 genes were found to be differentially expressed between clones and controls ($P<0.015$). We also performed a comparative proteomic analysis (using 2D-gel electrophoresis) of the Semitendinosus muscle at 60 and 260 dg and found changes in the muscle proteome in clones vs. controls (60 dg: n=8 per group, 260 dg: n=4 per group).

As indicated by data mining of the transcriptomic and proteomic data, few functions were affected, mainly lipid metabolism and angiogenesis at 30 dg, regulation of cell cycle/apoptosis at 60 dg, and energy metabolism and chaperone activity at 260 dg. At 30 dg, using the Ingenuity Pathway software we identified 4 interconnected networks related to lipids. Moreover, a differential expression of homeobox transcription factors and their target genes was also detected, as well as several genes involved in myogenesis and angiogenesis.

The authors wish to thank G. Gentes, C. Barboiron, A. Delavaud and N. Hafsia for genomic analyses; D. Le Bourhis and C. Richard for cloning and transfer of the embryos, respectively.

[1]Cassar-Malek *et al.*, 2010. Cloning and Stem Cells 12 (in press).

Effects of the endocrine disrupting compounds, phthalates, on developmental competence of bovine oocytes

Z Roth and D Grossman

Department of Animal Sciences, Robert H. Smith Faculty of Agriculture, Food and Environment, the Hebrew University, Rehovot, Israel

The possible exposure of humans and animals to industrial chemicals and pesticides has been a growing concern over the last decade. Phthalate esters are a class of water-insoluble, synthetic organic chemicals used widely in a variety of industrial applications (e.g., perfumes, lotions, cosmetic, toys and medical devices). As plasticizers, phthalates are not chemically bound to the plastic product, but leak out from PVC items into the environment. Dibutyl phthalate (DBP), Di-(2-ethylhexyl) phthalate (DEHP) and its primary metabolite mono-(2-ethylhexyl) phthalate (MEHP) are the most abundant phthalates in the environment. The objective was to use phthalates and bovine oocytes as a model to extend our knowledge about endocrine-disrupting compounds and the risk associated with early embryonic losses.

A system for in vitro production of embryos was used to examine the effects of phthalates on oocyte developmental competence. Cumulus-oocyte complexes (COCs) were matured (22 h, 38.5°C, 5% CO_2), fertilized (18 h, 38.5°C, 5% CO_2) and the resultant embryos were cultured for 8 d (KSOM; 38.5°C, 5% $CO_{2,}$ 5% O_2). Groups of COCs were exposed to 50 μM DEHP or 50 μM MEHP (n = 340 and 420, respectively) during maturation; cleavage rate and blastocyst rates were noted on d 2 and d 7 to 8, respectively. mRNA was isolated from 2-cell stage embryos for sqPCR in order to examine the expression of candidate genes (Cyclin A, ZAR1, ASAH1, OCT4) involved in early embryonic development. A TUNEL procedure was employed on 8-d blastocysts to determine apoptotic index.

Exposure of COCs to DEHP or MEHP during maturation reduced the cleavage rate ($P < 0.05$) and the proportion of embryos that developed to the blastocyst stage ($P < 0.05$). The total cell count for blastocysts that developed from MEHP-treated oocytes was lower than blastocysts that developed from control oocytes ($P < 0.05$). This decrease in cell number was not associated with an increased proportion of TUNEL positive cells, suggesting that a mechanism other than apoptosis is responsible for the decrease in cell number.

Exposure of oocytes to MEHP during maturation reduced the expression of the OCT4 gene. OCT4 is responsible for the pluripotency of the developing blastocyst, therefore, alterations in its expression could underlie at least some of the reduced embryonic development noted for MEHP-treated oocytes. ASAH1 is a pro-apoptotic factor involved in ceramide metabolism. Nevertheless, the increase in ASAH-1 noted for MEHP-treated embryos was not accompanied by an increased proportion of TUNEL-positive cells. MEHP did not affect the expression of genes at the 2-cell stage for ZAR1, involved in oocyte arrest, nor did it affect cyclin A, involved in cell cycle.

These results demonstrate the actions of phthalalates on the oocyte that lead to embryos with deviated patterns of gene expression and developmental competence.

Elevated nonesterified fatty acid concentrations during bovine oocyte maturation and the consequences on embryo development and viability

V Van Hoeck[a], RG Sturmey[b], PEJ Bols[a] and JL Leroy[a]

[a]*Laboratory of Veterinary Physiology, University of Antwerp, Belgium;*
[b]*Hull-York Medical School, United Kingdom*

Negative energy balance (NEB) in dairy cows leads to elevated nonesterified fatty acid (NEFA) concentrations in follicular fluid which is associated with impaired oocyte development and reduced fertility[1]. Previous research has showed that exposure to saturated long chain fatty acids during final maturation contributes to aberrant oocyte development, a finding recently associated with a reduction in embryo quality in terms of cell number and apoptotic cell ratio[2]. The present study wanted to expand this knowledge and focused on the effect of elevated NEFA exposure during oocyte maturation on amino acid turnover of the resulting embryo; an important metabolic marker of early embryo viability.

During serum-free maturation, 734 bovine COCs were exposed in three replicates to 1) physiological NEFA concentrations = CONTROL (150 μM total NEFA, i.e., oleic, stearic and palmitic acid), 2) elevated (75 μM) stearic acid concentrations = HIGH SA and 3) elevated (425 μM total) NEFA concentrations = HIGH COMBI NEFA. After serum-free in vitro maturation (24 h) and fertilization (22 h), zygotes were cultured in SOF + 5% FCS medium. d 7 embryos were graded for developmental stage and cultured singly in 5 μL droplets for 24 h. The amino acid composition in spent and blank medium was measured non-invasively by HPLC. Data were analysed with binary logistic regression (embryo development) and mixed model ANOVA after logistic transformation for normality reasons (amino acid turnover).

No significant effect of maturation condition on cleavage rates was observed. However, maturation in HIGH COMBI and HIGH SA resulted in reduced blastocyst rates (14.9 and 18.3%, respectively) compared with CONTROL (25.2%) ($P<0.05$). Zygotes had a significantly lower chance to form a blastocyst when the oocyte was matured in HIGH COMBI conditions (23.6% compared with 45.3 and 36.9% in the CONTROL and SA group, respectively). HIGH COMBI embryos showed an elevated amino acid consumption (factor 1.8) ($P<0.01$), production (factor 1.7) ($P=0.02$) and total turnover (factor 1.7) ($P<0.01$) compared with CONTROL embryos. HIGH SA embryos displayed a significant higher amino acid consumption (factor 1.9) ($P<0.01$) and turnover (factor 1.6) ($P<0.03$) compared with CONTROL embryos.

This study demonstrated that embryos arising from oocytes matured under NEB conditions with elevated NEFA concentrations have a reduced developmental competence and are metabolically more active than CONTROL embryos. Up-regulated embryo metabolism has previously been associated with elevated DNA damage and low embryo viability[3]. This may ultimately lead to embryonic mortality and thus contribute to declining fertility in high yielding dairy cows.

This study is funded by the Flemish Research Fund (FWO grant 1106910N: Veerle Van Hoeck).

[1]Leroy *et al.*, 2005. Reproduction 130:485-495.
[2]Van Hoeck *et al.*, 2010. Reprod Fertil Devel 22:335.
[3]Sturmey *et al.*, 2009. Hum Reprod 24:81-91.

Saturated free fatty acid during maturation of bovine oocytes impairs early embryonic development

H Aardema, PLAM Vos, BAJ Roelen, JB Helms and BM Gadella

Faculty of Veterinary Medicine, Utrecht University, The Netherlands

Fertility in high producing dairy cows has declined over the last decades. An increased serum and follicular fluid concentration of free fatty acids (FFA), due to body fat mobilization in the early post-partum period, is believed to cause this fertility decline. FFA concentration and composition changes in the environment of the oocyte might affect oocyte quality and lipid storage depots.

To investigate this, cumulus oocyte complexes (COCs) from 3 to 8 mm follicles of slaughterhouse ovaries were exposed to saturated (palmitic acid) or unsaturated (oleic acid) FFA during maturation. COCs were matured in medium (TCM-199) containing 0, 100, 250 or 500 μM palmitic or oleic acid or a combination of 250 μM palmitic and 250 μM oleic acid (10 mM fatty acid was pre-bound to 10% fatty acid-free BSA). Concentrations were based on *in vivo* measured FFA concentrations in follicular fluid in the early post partum period. After 23 h of maturation, COCs were fertilized (4 runs, 450 per group) and cultured until the blastocyst stage, or fixed (3 runs, 80 per group) for nuclear (TOPRO-®-3) and lipid droplet staining (C1-BODIPY®-500/510-C12). Confocal microscopy was performed to determine lipid droplet size in μm (mean) and the number of lipid droplets per oocyte. Lipid droplet number and log of size were analyzed by linear modeling with Bonferroni with condition as a fixed factor (mean $\pm$ SEM, $P<0.05$).

Palmitic and oleic acid had an opposite effect on the size of lipid droplets in oocytes, with smaller lipid droplets after exposure to 250 or 500 μM palmitic acid ($1.59\pm0.15\ \mu m^2$ and $1.59\pm0.17\ \mu m^2$) compared to the control group ($2.50\pm0.17 \mu m^2$). The number of lipid droplets decreased in oocytes exposed to 500 μM palmitic acid (224 ± 23) and increased after exposure to 500 μM oleic acid (610 ± 17), compared with oocytes from control medium (477 ± 16). Lipid droplet features of oocytes exposed to a combination of 250 μM palmitic and 250 μM oleic acid (414 ± 31 and $2.02\pm0.17 \mu m^2$) were not different from control oocytes. Exposure of COCs to FFA during maturation did not affect the percentage of oocytes in metaphase-II of meiosis, but exposure to palmitic acid resulted in impaired embryonic development in a dose-dependent manner. The percentage of blastocysts was lower after exposure to 250 or 500 μM palmitic acid (13 ± 2.4% and 2.8 ± 1.3%), compared with control oocytes (20 ± 1.6%) or oocytes exposed to 100, 250 or 500 μM oleic acid (23 ± 1.3%, 23 ± 3.3% and 28 ± 3.3%, $P<0.05$). The negative effects of palmitic acid were completely diminished by simultaneous exposure with oleic acid during maturation (26 ± 5.5%).

We conclude that palmitic acid elicited negative effects on early embryonic development, possibly induced by palmitate-induced lipid depletion which may end in embryo starvation. Remarkably, negative effects of palmitic acid were neutralized by simultaneous exposure to oleic acid during maturation. The adverse effect of FFA on lipid droplet features in oocytes and early embryonic development is under current investigation.

Project is sponsored by Pfizer Animal Health.

Silencing the progesterone receptor gene in bovine zygotes: effects on subsequent embryonic development

CM O'Meara[a], JD Murray[b], JF Roche[a] and P Lonergan[a]

[a]*University College Dublin, Belfield, Dublin 4, Ireland;* [b]*University of California, Davis, USA*

Elevated progesterone (P4) post-conception is associated with an increase in embryonic growth rate and pregnancy rate in cattle. A large body of evidence exists to demonstrate P4-induced effects on endometrial gene expression. The detection of progesterone receptor mRNA (PGR) in bovine embryos, however, suggests a potential direct effect of P4 on the embryo. The aim of this study was to use small interfering RNAs (siRNAs) to silence the PGR in bovine zygotes to determine a functional role, if any, for PGR in early embryo development.

In vitro produced bovine zygotes (16 h post insemination) were randomly assigned to one of 3 groups over 2 experiments. Zygotes were microinjected with siRNA targeting either PGR (n = 383) or luciferase (n = 409, LUCI), or left as non-injected controls (n = 392). In Experiment 1, cleavage rate at 24 h post insemination (pi) and blastocyst development on d 8 (day of IVF = d 0) was recorded. In Experiment 2, developmental competence at 48 h (≥ 4-cell rate) and at 72 h (≥ 8-cell rate) pi was recorded. Eight-cell embryos and d 7 blastocysts (Exp 2) were snap frozen for qPCR determination of mRNA relative abundance. Data were analysed using ANOVA.

Microinjection of PGR siRNA resulted in a lower cleavage rate and fewer embryos reaching the 4-cell, 8-cell and blastocyst stages compared with non-injected controls ($P < 0.05$). Cleavage rate was reduced in zygotes injected with PGR siRNA compared with both LUCI and non-injected controls (76.1% vs. 87.5% and 85.4%, respectively; $P < 0.05$). Fewer zygotes developed to the 8-cell stage following injection with PGR siRNA compared with both negative (LUCI) and positive (non-injected) controls (22.7% vs. 39.7% and 40.1%, respectively; $P < 0.05$). While blastocyst yield was lower in zygotes microinjected with PGR siRNA (31.1%) compared with LUCI siRNA (37.9%), the difference was not significant. Microinjection of zygotes with PGR siRNA lead to a 30% and 70% reduction in progesterone receptor mRNA relative abundance in 8-cell embryos and d 7 blastocysts, respectively ($P < 0.05$).

In conclusion, microinjection of zygotes with PGR siRNA resulted in a lower cleavage rate and fewer embryos developing to the 8-cell stage and blastocyst stage, suggesting a potential functional role for this receptor in early development.

Supported by Science Foundation Ireland (07/SRC/B1156).

Embryonic effect on uterine blood flow in cows during early pregnancy

A Honnens, M Steufmehl, K Bruening, C Wrenzycki and H Bollwein

Clinic for Cattle, University of Veterinary Medicine, Hanover, Germany

Successful establishment of pregnancy requires complex interactions between the embryo and its maternal environment. Previous investigations indicate that changes in uterine blood flow are part of the early embryo-maternal communication. In that regard, uterine perfusion showed a marked rise seven d after insemination in cows undergoing a superovulation program, but it had not been clarified if the rise was due to maternal or embryonic effects.

The objective was to test the hypothesis that uterine blood flow in superovulated cows is stimulated by the presence of embryos. Eight cows were treated and investigated in three different models following a latin-square model. In models A and B, cows underwent a superovulatory treatment following a standard protocol using FSH and $PGF_{2\alpha}$, and were artificially inseminated three times every 12 h, beginning 48 h after $PGF_{2\alpha}$, with the semen of a fertile bull in model A and using seminal plasma without sperm in model B, respectively. As a non-superovulated control, cows were artificially inseminated twice, 12 h apart, during spontaneous oestrus without a preceding hormonal treatment, in model C. In all models, the time of the first insemination was defined as d 0. Blood flow measurements were conducted using colour Doppler sonography of the uterine arteries on d 1, 3, 5 and 7. On d 7, the number of corpora lutea was counted and embryos were recovered and classified according to IETS. Cows successfully passed models A and C, if at least four and one, respectively, transferable embryos were recovered.

After maximum three passages per model, seven cows successfully passed model A, and five cows successfully passed model C. So for statistical analyses including models A and B, seven cows, and including models A, B and C, only five cows, respectively, were used. In model A, 6.9 (min: 4, max: 11) transferable embryos were found. The number of corpora lutea did not differ ($P>0.05$) between models A (12.7 ± 1.1) and B (12.1 ± 1.8). Between d 1 and 7, uterine blood flow volume (BFV) increased ($P<0.05$) by 51% in model A, but no rise ($P>0.05$) was observed in models B and C. On d 3, 5 and 7, BFV was higher ($P<0.05$) in model A compared with model B; on d 1 of both models, values did not differ ($P>0.05$). Only on d 7, BFV was greater ($P<0.05$) in models A and B compared with model C. No further differences ($P>0.05$) were observed between models A and B on the one hand and model C on the other hand.

In conclusion, the presence of embryos positively affected BFV in superovulated cows. This effect was present within 3 d after insemination. This indicates that uterine perfusion plays a role in embryo-maternal communication during the first week of pregnancy.

Measurement of interferon-tau (IFN-τ) stimulated gene expression in blood leukocytes for pregnancy diagnosis within 18 to 20 d after insemination in dairy cattle

JC Green[a], CS Okamura[a], SE Poock[b] and MC Lucy[a]

[a]Division of Animal Sciences and [b]College of Veterinary Medicine, University of Missouri, Columbia, USA

The objective was to diagnose pregnancy within 18 d after insemination by measuring interferon-stimulated gene (ISG) expression in circulatory leukocytes. We identified candidate ISG in a microarray experiment and then performed a series of in vivo experiments to determine the utility of ISG for early pregnancy detection in lactating dairy cows and nonlactating dairy heifers. Based on the microarray results, three genes were selected [2′-5′ oligoadenylate synthetase 1(Oas1), myxovirus resistance gene 2 (Mx2), and interferon stimulated gene 15 kDa protein (Isg15)] because they were known to be interferon-stimulated genes (ISG) and were also differentially expressed in the samples. Primers were synthesized for the respective genes and used for real time reverse transcriptase polymerase chain reaction (RTPCR). Three in vivo experiments were conducted. In the first experiment, blood samples were collected and RNA was isolated from leukocytes of pregnant ($n=5$) and nonpregnant ($n=15$) dairy cows on each of d 14, 16, 18, and 20 after insemination. There was an interaction between status and day ($P<0.01$) for ISG expression (Mx2 and Isg15) because ISG expression was greater in pregnant compared with nonpregnant cows on d 18 and d 20. In the second experiment, we attempted to define the shortest interval to pregnancy detection with ISG by collecting blood samples on d 17 (Exp. 2A) or d 18 (Exp. 2B). For Exp. 2A, blood was collected from pregnant ($n=16$) and nonpregnant ($n=16$) cows on d 17 after insemination. There was an effect of status for Mx2 ($P<0.056$) and Oas1 expression ($P<0.018$). On d 17, therefore, pregnant cows had greater Mx2 and Oas1 but Receiver Operator Characteristic (ROC) curves showed that the increase was too small to develop a suitable cut-off for a reliable pregnancy test. For Exp. 2B, blood samples were collected from pregnant ($n=21$) and nonpregnant ($n=21$) cows on d 18 after insemination. For both Mx2 and Oas1, there was an interaction between status and parity ($P<0.021$ and $P<0.083$, respectively). Primiparous pregnant cows had greater ISG expression than primiparous nonpregnant cows on d 18. For multiparous cows, however, pregnant and nonpregnant cows were similar for ISG expression on d 18. Regardless of parity, ROC curves showed that the increase in ISG on d 18 was too small to develop a suitable cut-off for a reliable pregnancy test. The possibility of correcting for pre-insemination ISG expression was examined in a final series of experiments. Blood samples were collected from cows ($n=54$) and heifers ($n=24$) during the luteal phase preceding insemination. A second sample was collected from the same cows [pregnant ($n=13$) and nonpregnant ($n=41$)] and heifers [pregnant ($n=17$) and nonpregnant ($n=7$)] 18 d after insemination. The ratio of the second sample (after insemination) to the first sample (before insemination) minimally increased the sensitivity of the ISG test for pregnancy detection. As before, there was an effect of parity for cows (greater expression in primiparous cows; $P<0.05$). There was a large increase in ISG expression on d 18 of pregnancy in heifers that could be measured for a reliable pregnancy test. The conclusion from the studies is that a reliable ISG-based method for pregnancy detection could be applied as early as d 18 but only in heifers. Older cows have a lesser response that reduces the sensitivity of the ISG test on or before d 18.

Maternal circulating C-type natriuretic peptide (CNP) is produced by trophoblast binucleate cells during ovine pregnancy

BA McNeill[a], GK Barrell[a], TCR Prickett[b] and EA Espiner[b,]

[a]*Lincoln University, Lincoln, New Zealand;* [b]*University of Otago, Christchurch School of Medicine, Christchurch, New Zealand*

C-type natriuretic peptide (CNP) is a paracrine/autocrine factor with important roles in vascular health and skeletal growth. Recent studies in pregnant sheep and red deer have identified extremely high maternal concentrations of plasma CNP and a related amino-terminal fragment (NTproCNP) which show distinctive temporal patterns associated with fetal and placental maturation[1]. Although the concentrations of CNP and NTproCNP are higher in maternal compared with fetal plasma, CNP protein forms are more abundant in the fetal cotyledon and greatly exceed concentrations in the maternal caruncle[1]. However the cellular site of placental CNP production is unknown.

To identify the cellular source of CNP within the placenta, whole placentomes were collected from twin-bearing ewes at d 124 of pregnancy and processed for immunohistochemical staining for CNP, NTproCNP and pregnancy-associated glycoprotein (PAG) - a positive marker of the trophoblast binucleate cell (BNC). Immunohistochemistry revealed strong staining of NTproCNP, CNP and PAG in the cytoplasm and perinuclear regions of the BNC. Intense CNP and NTproCNP staining was also evident surrounding the placental blood vessels. The similarity of the staining pattern of both CNP forms and co-localisation with PAG provide strong evidence that CNP is synthesised in the BNC and is the primary source of the peptide in maternal circulation during pregnancy. The immunopositive localisation of CNP around placental blood vessels supports previous findings in the mouse[2] and is consistent with the hormone's known vasodilator actions and probable role in placental angiogenesis.

Although CNP has traditionally been regarded as a paracrine/autocrine factor, its localisation to the BNC suggests a novel endocrine role during pregnancy, in addition to important paracrine actions within the placenta itself. BNCs are formed within the fetal trophoblast and migrate to the maternal-fetal interface to release contents of their granules into the maternal circulation, thus enabling the fetus to manipulate the maternal endocrine environment while evading detection by the maternal immune system. Although the function of CNP in the maternal circulation remains to be determined, likely actions include redirection of nutrients to favour fetal growth, as has been proposed for other products of the BNC such as ovine placental lactogen, and sustaining high rates of uterine blood flow[3]. Monitoring CNP levels during pregnancy may provide a novel index of maternal and fetal well-being in ruminants.

[1]McNeill et al., 2009. Endocrinology 150:4777-4783.
[2]Cameron et al., 1996. Endocrinology 137:817-824.
[3]Itoh et al., 1998. Endocrinology 139:3329-3341.

Embedding phenotypic information to a microarray study. Case: endometrial receptivity in lactating dairy cows

T Tiirikka[a], V Ahola[a], M Räty[a], T Hurme[a], C Grosse-Brinkhaus[b], D Salilew-Wondim[b], P Sørensen[c], D Valour[d], B Grimard[e], JP Renard[d], D Tesfaye[b], J Vilkki[a] and J Peippo[a]

[a]*MTT Agrifood Research Finland, Jokioinen, Finland;* [b]*University of Bonn, Bonn, Germany;* [c]*University of Aarhus, Tjele, Denmark;* [d]*INRA, Jouy-en-Josas, France;* [e]*ENVA, Maisons-Alfort France*

Good fertility is very important for the dairy industry. We have conducted *in silico* modeling of pathways related to success of embryo transfer. The data were obtained from an Affymetrix microarray study concerning endometrial receptivity of lactating Finnish Ayrshire dairy cows. The cows were subjected to endometrial biopsy on d 0, 7 and 14 of the first detectable estrous cycle after calving followed by embryo transfer during the subsequent cycle. Phenotypic data for fertility and milk production were gathered from the recipients.

The data were analyzed using R and Bioconductor packages. LIMMA (Linear Model for Microarray Analysis) package was used to find gene expression differences. The effect of incrementing phenotypic information to genotype results was studied using GSEA (Gene Set Enrichment Analysis), CCA (Canonical Correlation Analysis) and standard hyper geometric test. We analyzed genes for significantly enriched time points by using fold change (FC>2) and error-corrected P-values. This information was mapped to corresponding KEGG and GO categories to elucidate active metabolic routes and processes. The initial number of differentially expressed genes linked to pathways was 6152.

Without adding phenotypic data, there were 10 KEGG pathways with $P<0.05$. With phenotypic data, the differentially expressed genes created 11 enriched pathways at time point 0. Instead of adding many new pathways, the phenotype data provided valuable gene-gene interaction data as was later observed on the other time points. Due to the similarities of immunological processes and the ones in reproductive systems, there was a significant amount of immunology-related gene ontologies. In terms of top enriched genes, however, the sorted lists created by CCA and GSEA varied only a little. This could be because of the annotation status of the Affymetrix GeneChip array.

More thorough gene expression information was extracted by creating signaling pathways of the significant genes. In addition, SNPs located close to or in the gene region of the enriched genes were collected from dbSNP (build 130). The signaling pathways were created with Genomatix BiblioSphere Pathway Edition (Genomatix, Munich, Germany). We found several interesting candidate genes in few biological pathways, the most promising pathway being the peroxisome proliferator-activated receptor pathway (PPAR). Genes ACOX2, PLTP and FABP7 contained 577 SNPs that created 219 new transcription factor (TF) binding sites and lost 187 sites, but only 6 SNPs were found in coding exons. The PPAR pathway was finally narrowed down to a delta subunit component. Currently we are finding additional TF binding sites that are affected by SNPs and locating orthologous regions in other species. The biological verification of candidate genes is under way.

Acknowledgments: These results are obtained through the EC-funded FP6 Project "SABRE".

The immune response to pregnancy may be a key driver of reproductive performance

CG Walker[a,b], S Meier[b], MD Littlejohn[b], JR Roche[b] and MD Mitchell[b,c]

[a]*DairyNZ Ltd, Hamilton, New Zealand;* [b]*The Liggins institute, University of Auckland, New Zealand;* [c]*UQ Centre for Clinical Research, RBWH campus, Herston, Brisbane, Queensland, Australia*

Over the past three decades, there has been a significant decline in dairy cattle fertility. A large proportion of pregnancy losses are believed to occur during the pre-implantation period, when the developing embryo is elongating rapidly and signaling its presence to the maternal system. The objective of this study was to elucidate potential mechanisms involved in successful pregnancy establishment through transcriptional profiling of both pregnant and non-pregnant cows. Both caruncular and intercaruncular endometrial tissues were analyzed, with samples taken at d 17 (immediately pre-implantation) after estrous synchronization. Within this study two diverse genetic strains were used that exhibit differential reproductive performance - animals with predominately North American ancestry (NA), and those with New Zealand ancestry (NZ). Agilent 44k bovine specific microarrays were employed in a reference design, followed by investigation with Genespring GX software and Ingenuity pathway analysis.

Microarray analysis revealed 1,657 differentially expressed transcripts with more than a 1.5 fold change in expression ($P<0.05$) between pregnant and cycling animals in both caruncular and intercaruncular tissue. Ingenuity pathway analysis of these genes revealed enrichment for molecules relating to the immune response to pregnancy, including; OAS1 (13 fold), OAS2 (7 fold), TAP1 (2.4 fold), TAP2 (1.5 fold), PSMB8 (1.7 fold), PSMB9 (1.9 fold), B2M (1.9 fold), HLA-G (1.5 fold), MUC-1 (1.6 fold), IDO (5.7 fold), TTS (2.4 fold), CCL11 (13 fold),CCL2 (2 fold), IL15 (1.5 fold), IL7 (2.1 fold), IL1α (2 fold), IL1RN (2.2 fold), C1q (2 fold), C1r (2.2 fold), C1s (2.4 fold), C4 (2.6 fold), C2 (3.6 fold), C3 (1.7 fold), PTX3 (2.6 fold). Further, several of these immune response genes were also differentially expressed between the two strains of cattle.

This analysis supports the idea that the immune response to the embryo is tightly regulated during early pregnancy. Expression of genes that confer immunological protection to the embryo, along with those important for maintaining the immunological integrity of the uterus from potential invading pathogens appear to be of particular importance. Further evidence for the importance of this response comes from differential expression of these genes in the two cattle strains used in the study, implying that altered expression of these genes may contribute to the differential fertility seen between the two strains.

A role for activin and follistatin during embryo implantation in the ewe

A O'Connell[a], JJ Holdgate[a], KP McNatty[b], PR Hurst[c], GH Davis[a], FW Bazer[d], TE Spencer[d] and J Juengel[a]

[a]AgResearch Invermay, Mosgiel, New Zealand; [b]Victoria University, Wellington, New Zealand; [c]University of Otago, Dunedin, New Zealand; [d]Texas A&M University, College Station, USA

For the developing conceptus (embryo and its extra-embryonic membranes) to successfully implant and survive, it needs to achieve immunotolerance within the uterine environment of the mother. Activin, together with its bio-neutralizing agent, follistatin (FST) are known to modulate the immune response[1]. Previously, we found higher levels of activin, but not FST, in the plasma and uterine fluid of ewes that repeatedly exhibited low conceptus survival. In the current study, *in situ* hybridisation was used to assess expression of the inhibin beta A (*INHBA*) subunit (of which two combine to form activin) and FST genes in uterine tissues during the luteal phase (non-pregnant) of the oestrous cycle and during gestation in ewes.

Following oestrous synchronisation, uterine tissues from ewes considered to have normal rates of embryonic survival were collected on d 10, 12, 14 and 16 of the oestrous cycle and d 10, 12, 14, 16, 18 and 20 of gestation and fixed in 4% paraformaldehye and processed into paraffin blocks (n = 4 per time point). *In situ* hybridisation was used to detect the presence and cellular localizations of *INHBA* and *FST* mRNAs in $\sim 5\ \mu m$ sections of uterine tissue.

During the oestrous cycle, *INHBA* mRNA expression was observed in the stromal cells but not the ductal glands of the endometrium. Uterine stromal cells showed weak expression on d 12 and more intense expression by d 16 of the oestrous cycle. In contrast, during gestation *INHBA* mRNA expression was observed primarily in the endometrial ductal glands. Expression of *INHBA* mRNA was weak on d 14 but strong expression was observed by d 18 of gestation. Conversely, moderate expression of *FST* mRNA was limited to the luminal epithelium for all days in non-pregnant animals and d 10 to 16 of pregnant animals. However, *FST* mRNA was most abundant in the trophoblast giant binucleate cells and interacting luminal epithelium on d 18 and 20 of gestation.

Uterine derived activin is synthesised in the glandular epithelium of the ewe at a time when *FST* is expressed by the interacting trophoblast. Activin is known to stimulate macrophages in the uterus of the mouse[2] and elevated levels of activin, but not *FST*, have been observed in the uterine fluid of ewes with low embryonic survival. Therefore the possibility exists that activin and follistatin have a role in modulating immunotolerance within the maternal uterine environment for successful implantation warrants further investigation.

[1]Phillips *et al.*, 2001. Mol cell Endocrinol 180:155-162.
[2]Wang *et al.*, 2009. Cell Mol Immunol 6:387-392.

Differential effects of arginine, leucine, glutamine and glucose on expression of interferon tau, orinithine decarboxylase and nitric oxide synthase by ovine conceptuses

J Kim[a], RC Burghardt[b], G Wu[a], GA Johnson[b], TE Spencer[a] and FW Bazer[a]

[a]*Departments of Animal Science and* [b]*Veterinary Integrative Biosciences, Texas A&M University, College Station, USA*

Arginine (Arg), leucine (Leu), and glucose, but not glutamine (Gln), stimulate protein synthesis through the phosphorylation of mTOR signaling molecules to increase proliferation of an established ovine trophectoderm cell line[1]. Therefore, this study examined effects of Arg, Leu, Gln and glucose (select nutrients) on gene expression and protein synthesis in explant cultures of d 16 ovine conceptuses recovered from ewes by flushing each uterine horn with 20 ml customized DMEM F12 medium containing one-tenth the amount of each amino acid and glucose in fully supplemented DMEM F12 medium. Conceptuses were starved for 6 h in each respective nutrient-free customized DMEM F12 medium (e.g., Arg-free medium for Arg treatment) and then cultured in either 0.2 mM Arg, 0.2 mM Leu, 0.5 mM Gln or 4 mM glucose for 18 h at 37°C with rocking under an atmosphere of 50% O_2, 45% N_2, 5% CO_2. After incubation, conceptuses were homogenized and the homogenate stored at -80°C until analyzed. The mRNAs and proteins for MTOR (mammalian target of rapamycin), RPS6 (ribosomal protein S6), RPS6K (RPS6 kinase), and eukaryotic translation initiation factor 4E-binding protein 1 (EIF4EBP1), as well as nitric oxide synthases (NOS) 2 and 3, ornithine decarboyxlase (ODC1), GTP cyclohydrolase I (GCH1) and interferon tau (IFNT) were analyzed using RT-PCR and immunoblotting. MTOR, RPS6K, EIF4EBP1, RPS6, ODC1, NOS, and IFNT mRNA levels were not affected by any of the select nutrients, but GCH1 mRNA increased ($P<0.05$) in response to Arg. In contrast, the select nutrients increased ($P<0.05$) translation of mRNAs for MTOR, RPS6, RPS6K, and EIF4EBP1 proteins. Arg and glucose increased ($P<0.01$) the abundance of ODC1, NOS2 and GCH1 proteins, whereas Leu and Gln failed to increase ODC1 and NOS proteins. Only Arg increased ($P<0.01$) the abundance of IFNT. These results indicate that Arg, Leu, Gln and glucose differentially increase the abundance of NOS2, NOS3, ODC1, GCH1 and IFNT proteins in ovine conceptuses. Those effects were associated with increased abundance of both total and phosphorylated forms of MTOR, RPS6, RPS6K and EIF4EBP1 which results in dissociation of 4EBP1 to allow EIF4E to stimulate mRNA translation. The increase in GCH1 mRNA and protein is significant as GCH1 is a rate-limiting enzyme for synthesis of tetrahydrobiopterin, an essential cofactor for all isoforms of NOS to generate nitric oxide. The results of this study provide important insights into mechanisms whereby select nutrients act differentially to increase transcription (GCH1), but primarily translation of mRNAs for cell signaling molecules that affect conceptus growth, development, and survival during the peri-implantation period of pregnancy.

This research was supported by USDA CSREES National Research Initiative Grant 2006-35203-17283.

[1]Kim *et al.*, 2009. Proc Soc Study Reprod, Page 158.

Systems biology of mammalian embryo implantation and early placental development

R Oliveira[a], G Taghouti[b], Y Heyman[b], I Hue[b], O Sandra[b], JP Renard[b], M Guillomot[b] and H Lewin[a,c]

[a]*Department of Animal Sciences, University of Illinois, Urbana, USA;* [b]*Institut National de la Recherche Agronomique, Unité Mixte de Recherche, Biologie du Développement et Reproduction, Jouy-en-Josas Cedex, France;* [c]*Institute for Genomic Biology, University of Illinois, Urbana, USA*

Embryo implantation is a critical event that has three distinct stages: apposition, adhesion, and in some species, trophoblast invasion of the uterus. For the process to occur there has to be synchronized cross-talk between the embryonic trophoblast and the endometrium. We have employed a systems approach to understanding the interacting gene networks in trophoblast and endometrium in ruminants during the early post-implantation period[1], with somatic cell nuclear transfer (SCNT) being used as a perturbation system of the process. Ruminants are a valuable model for such studies because they are efficiently cloned by SCNT, have a similar gestation period to humans and, unlike mice, ruminant embryos undergo gastrulation prior to implantation, thus permitting *ex vivo* studies of this critical developmental process. In the present study, thirteen genes considered to be involved in the communication between conceptus and endometrium on the basis of our earlier transcriptome analyses were assayed for gene expression using quantitative PCR (qPCR) among endometrial and trophoblast tissue samples biopsied at d 30 and 60 of gestation. The 13 genes were: *BCL2L1*, *CSH1*, *CTSB*, *ESRRA*, *HDAC7A*, *HIF1A*, *IGF2BP2*, *KPNA1*, *MGAT1*, *PNPLA6*, *SIVA*, *STAT1*, and *TLR4*. The tissues tested were trophoblast and endometrium (caruncles and intercaruncular areas) derived from artificial insemination (AI), *in vitro* fertilization (IVF) and SCNT conceptuses. We collected a total of 67 samples from d 30 and d 60 AI, IVF and SCNT pregnancies. Significant effects were found for tissue source (trophoblast, caruncle or intercaruncular areas) for 11/13 genes ($P<0.01$), while treatment (AI, IVF or SCNT) affected expression of 6/13 genes ($P<0.05$). Day of sampling (d 30 or d 60) had significant effects on the expression of 9/13 genes ($P<0.01$), thus indicating the importance of development on gene expression patterns. Two genes, *STAT1* and *BCL2L1* showed a significant tissue by treatment by day interaction. These two genes were preferentially expressed in maternal tissues, with over expression in SCNT and IVF pregnancies at d 30 relative to AI. These results suggest signaling abnormalities through *STAT1* and increased apoptosis in the maternal component of the developing placenta of IVF and SCNT embryos. We propose that SCNT and IVF perturb the cross-talk between the trophoblast and endometrium, thus contributing to abnormalities in implantation and early placental development. In surviving conceptuses, these abnormalities may lead to fetal pathologies, such as Large Offspring Syndrome and hydropsy frequently observed in clones during later stages of pregnancy.

[1]Mansouri-Attia *et al.*, 2009. Proc Natl Acad Sci 106:5687-5692.

Expression of reproductive genes during fetal development in cattle

JH Hernandez-Medrano[a], K Derecka[a], A Peters[a], BK Campbell[b] and R Webb[a]

[a]*School of Biosciences, The University of Nottingham, Loughborough, LE12 5RD, UK;* [b]*Division of Human Development, The University of Nottingham, Queen's Medical Centre, Nottingham, NG7 2UH, UK*

In humans and rodents, α-gonadotrophin (α-SU) is the earliest subunit expressed in the fetal pituitary gland[1], while in sheep fetuses, pituitary mRNA for oestradiol receptors (ERα and ERβ) was reported at 80 d of gestation[2]. Conversely, in cattle information regarding expression of reproductive genes is scarce. The aim of the present study was to describe gene expression of gonadotrophin subunits (α-SU, LHβ and FSHβ), GnRH receptor (GnRHR), ER-α, ER-β and inhibin/activin subunits (α, βA and βB) in the fetal pituitary gland at different stages of development in cattle using a multiplexed PCR system, which allowed evaluation of up to 30 genes in a single PCR reaction.

Bovine fetal pituitary glands were dissected, frozen in liquid nitrogen and gestational age (GA) estimated using crown-rump length measurements. Fetuses were grouped into first (1st, <90 d; n=4); early (91 to 150 d; n=6) and late (151 to 180 d; n=3) second (2nd); and third (3rd; >210 d; n=3) trimesters of gestation. Pituitary gland RNA was extracted and DNase treated before multigene expression assays were carried out (GenomeLab GeXP Genetic Analysis System; Beckman-Coulter Inc.). Gene specific primers (F and R) attached to common universal tag sequences were designed and individually evaluated using a positive RNA control (adult pituitary RNA), before fetal samples were analysed. Controls included reactions in which template RNA and reverse transcriptase were not added and an internal quality control of the system (Kanamycin resistance RNA). Individual gene expression was normalised using three housekeeping genes (Actin B, GAPDH and Histone 2A) and resulting values were compared using one-way ANOVA.

Expression of α-SU and FSHβ subunits was observed at 65 d and LHβ at 75 d of GA. Expression of all gonadotrophin subunits increased from 1st to 2nd trimester ($P<0.05$). Despite an increase in LHβ and α-SU gene expression during 3rd trimester ($P<0.05$), FSHβ expression did not change ($P>0.05$). At 65 d of GA, expression of GnRHR and ER-β was observed, while ER-α expression occurred during the early 2nd trimester (GA=91 to 150 d). GnRHR expression tended ($P=0.063$) to increase with age, whereas expression of ERs did not change ($P>0.05$) throughout gestation. Inhibin/activin subunit gene expression was detected during the 1st trimester (GA<90d), and did not change during pregnancy ($P>0.05$).

In conclusion, the reproductive genes studied were expressed in fetal pituitary glands between 65 and 150 d of gestation. A differential pattern of gene expression according to age was observed, with some genes showing higher expression with increasing GA (i.e., α-gonadotrophin and LHβ), while others did not change throughout pregnancy. Whether this differential pattern of expression is linked to developmental changes observed during fetal life requires further research.

Study funded by The University of Nottingham/Pfizer and CONACYT-Mexico.

[1]Simmons *et al.*, 1990. Genes and Development 4:695-711.
[2]Shaub *et al.*, 2008. Gene Expression Patterns 8:457-463.

Identification of gene expression indicative of pregnancy in the pre-attachment period in bovine peripheral blood leukocytes

A Hammerle-Fickinger[a], S Bauersachs[b], E Wolf[b], HHD Meyer[a], MW Pfaffl[a] and SE Ulbrich[a]

[a]*Physiology-Weihenstephan, Technical University of Munich, Freising, Germany;* [b]*Institute of Animal Breeding and Biotechnology, Gene Center, Ludwig-Maximilians-University of Munich, Munich, Germany*

The establishment of pregnancy comprises the regulation of a number of functional complexes necessary to modulate the local paracrine and peripheral endocrine environment of the mother. In ruminants, the pregnancy recognition factor interferon-τ (IFNT) mainly exerts its effect in the uterus by inhibiting luteolytic $PGF_{2\alpha}$ secretion. However, recent studies[1] have shown that an induction of interferon-regulated genes may be observed in bovine peripheral blood leukocytes as early as d 15. Moreover, ovine uterine venous blood contains bioactive IFNT during early pregnancy, thus demonstrating that IFNT exerts an endocrine mode of action[2]. As the uterus may locally perceive IFNT or another secreted factor from the hatching blastocyst, maternal recognition of pregnancy might even occur earlier.

Blood samples were collected from healthy control and pregnant Brown Swiss heifers on d 4, 8, 12, 16, 18 and 20 following estrus and insemination, respectively. Total RNA was extracted from white blood cells (PBL). Microarray hybridization (one color) analyses were conducted using a custom designed 4x44k array (Agilent) for the analysis of d 4, 8 and 12 of pregnancy versus control (n = 3 animals per group). Quantitative RT-PCR was performed to validate differentially expressed genes (DEG) obtained from microarray results and to evaluate further candidate genes of interest (interferon-related genes, components of the complement system, cytokines) for all time points (n = 7 animals per group).

Expression ratios calculated by significance analysis of microarray (SAM) did not reveal differentially expressed genes at any of the time points under analysis. A paired local pooled error test (PLPE) analysis (FDR < 0.05, P < 0.05 and at least 1.5-fold signal difference between control and pregnant animals) revealed 73, 36, and 38 DEG at d 4, 8 and 12, respectively. A successful validation of DEGs by RT-qPCR analysis was achieved only infrequently probably due to the low number of biological replicates (n = 3) used for array analysis. However, out of 19 specific qRT-PCR assays using n = 7 animals per group, analyses revealed 12 genes as differentially expressed at d 8 (P < 0.03), one single gene each for d 8 and 12, and 6, 9 and 14 genes for d 16, 18 and 20, respectively, which were regulated up to 3.3-fold between pregnant and control animals. Advanced statistical analysis by Principal Components Analysis (PCA) of DEGs and the respective peripheral progesterone concentration indicated that the gene signatures at d 8, 18 and 20 are clearly separating controls from pregnant animals at each respective day. Thus the analyzed genes may represent groups of biomarkers which taken together may be indicative of early pregnancy. Whether these genes are showing a response due to local IFNT, to cell surface antigens exposed to the maternal immune system or to a combination of both remains to be shown.

Peripheral PBL may be holding valuable information of local uterine events taking place during early pregnancy. The specific read-out of informative gene expression may be a promising analytical approach for early pregnancy detection. The molecular mechanisms underlying the observed differential gene expression in PBL during the pre-attachment period remain to be unraveled.

[1]Yankey *et al.*, 2001. J Endocrinol 170:R7-11.
[2]Oliveria *et al.*, 2008. Endocrinology 149:1252-1259.

Effects of maternal uterine environment on embryonic development, birth weight and post-natal growth rate in breeds of sheep of dissimilar mature bodyweight

RK Sharma, TJ Parkinson, PR Kenyon and HT Blair

Massey University, Palmerston North, New Zealand

Human[1] and animal[2] studies have shown that post-natal growth, development and health are affected by both genotype and the maternal environment that an individual experiences *in utero*. Two experiments were undertaken to examine the effects of uterine environment upon early embryonic development, birth weight and post natal growth rates of lambs.

Purebred embryos were transferred within and reciprocally between two breeds of sheep of markedly different body weight and size (Cheviot: 58 kg; Suffolk: 74.0 kg) to establish four groups of pregnancies: Suffolk in Suffolk (SinS; large control), Suffolk in Cheviot (SinC; restricted uterine environment) Cheviot in Suffolk (CinS; luxurious uterine environment) and Cheviot in Cheviot (CinC; small control). Embryos were thereafter removed on d 19 of gestation (post-slaughter flushing: Experiment 1, n = 10/group), or pregnancies were allowed to go to term (Experiment 2) and the lambs were then reared to 6 months of age.

On d 19, SinC embryos were smaller (11.04 $\pm$ 0.57 mm) than SinS (13.42 $\pm$ 0.53 mm: $P<0.05$), but CinS embryos (15.23 $\pm$ 0.68 mm) were bigger ($P<0.05$) than CinC (12.84 $\pm$ 0.53 mm). There were fewer ($P<0.05$) binucleate cells in SinC than SinS trophoblasts, but tended ($P=0.07$) to be more in CinS than CinC. At full term, birthweight of SinC lambs (5.0 $\pm$ 0.2 kg; n = 29) was lower ($P<0.05$) than SinS lambs (5.9 $\pm$ 0.2 kg; n = 31), but CinS (5.5 $\pm$ 0.2 kg; n = 21) and CinC (5.2 $\pm$ 0.2 kg; n = 22) lambs did not differ significantly from each other. Body dimensions (head width/length, crown-rump length, limb lengths) were also significantly ($P<0.05$) smaller in SinC than SinS lambs, but did not differ ($P>0.50$) between CinC and CinS lambs. There were fewer cotyledons ($P<0.05$) in CinS (56 $\pm$ 6.) than SinS (74 $\pm$ 6) placentas, whereas cotyledons were heavier ($P<0.05$) in CinS (2.4 $\pm$ 0.2 g) than SinS (1.7 $\pm$ 0.2 g) placentas.

Liveweight, body dimensions and growth rates were measured 3, 6, 9, 12 and 24 weeks after birth. There were no differences ($P>0.05$) in growth rates between SinC and SinS or between CinS and CinC lambs. Liveweight and body dimensions of SinC lambs remained lower ($P<0.05$) than those of SinS lambs, but there were no differences ($P>0.05$) in liveweight or body dimensions between CinS and CinC lambs.

In conclusion, by d 19, a restricted uterine environment had resulted in development of smaller embryos, whereas a luxurious uterine environment had accelerated development. By full term, however, lambs born from a restricted environment remained smaller, but those from a luxurious environment were not larger than controls. Because post natal growth rates were similar between groups, the differences between groups that were present at birth were perpetuated thereafter.

[1] Barker, 1995. British Medical Journal 311:171-174.
[2] Allen *et al.*, 2004. Reproduction 127:67-77.

Bovine luteal prolactin receptor expression: Potential involvement in regulation of progesterone during the estrous cycle and pregnancy

IM Thompson, J Bubolz, M Ozawa, QE Yang and GE Dahl

University of Florida, Gainesville, USA

Prolactin is a multifunctional hormone synthesized and secreted by the anterior pituitary gland and numerous other tissues including the ovary. In rodents, prolactin has long been identified as a luteotropic factor, characterized by enhanced progesterone secretion. A decrease in prolactin receptor expression in the corpus luteum (CL) of rodents leads to an increased expression of 20α-hydroxysteroid dehydrogenase (20α-HSD) and a subsequent decrease of serum progesterone concentrations. Thus, prolactin receptors are key components in regulation of progesterone secretion and maintenance of the CL. We performed quantitative RT-PCR (qRT) to examine changes in gene expression of prolactin receptors (long form: *l-PRLR*; short form: *s-PRLR*) and 20α-HSD in bovine CL throughout the estrous cycle and during pregnancy. In addition, western blotting was used to determine protein abundance. Ovaries with CL were collected at a local abattoir and luteal stages were classified by macroscopic observation as early (d 1 to 4 after ovulation; n=6), mid- (d 5 to 10; n=6), late (d 11 to 17; n=6) and regressing (d 18 to 20; n=6). Pregnant CL (n=6) was determined by the presence of conceptus (d 28 to term). Quantitative RT-PCR revealed that the mRNAs for both forms of prolactin receptor were expressed at all the luteal stages. Expression of *s-PRLR* and *l-PRLR* mRNA was less during the early and regressing luteal stages compared with mid- and late stages. Expression of the *s-PRLR* in CL of pregnant animals was greater than early, mid- and regressing CL and did not differ from late luteal stage expression. Expression of *l-PRLR* did not differ among pregnant and mid and late luteal CL stages. A greater expression of *l-PRLR* was observed, however, in pregnant versus early and regressing CL. In addition, qRT results showed the presence of 20α-HSD mRNA during all luteal stages of the estrous cycle, with the greatest expression observed during the regressing luteal stage. Interestingly, expression of 20α-HSD mRNA was greater than either form of prolactin receptor during the regressing luteal stage. Moreover, relative to prolactin receptor, 20α-HSD mRNA expression was the lowest during pregnancy and the late luteal stage. Western blotting revealed transcripts of both prolactin receptors during all luteal stages and pregnancy, with a prevalence of the *s-PRLR* protein. Densitometry analysis indicated a significant decrease in both prolactin receptor protein levels during the regressing luteal stage. Protein levels of *s-PRLR* were greater than *l-PRLR* during early, mid and late luteal stages and did not differ during the regressing luteal stage. In addition, 20α-HSD protein levels were lowest during early and greatest during regressing luteal stages. Moreover, protein levels of both prolactin receptors were lower than 20α-HSD during the regressing luteal stage. In conclusion, results of the current study suggest a possible involvement of prolactin receptors, especially *s-PRLR*, in regulation of progesterone levels during bovine estrous cycle and pregnancy.

Expression of local angiogenic and anti-angiogenic factors in the bovine corpus luteum

B Berisha, S Schilffarth, HHD Meyer and D Schams

Physiologie Weihenstephan, Technische Universität München, Freising, Germany

The ovary offers an excellent system for studying and understanding molecular mechanisms of angiogenesis and angiolysis under physiological conditions. The aim of this study was to characterize mRNA and protein expression patterns of some angiogenic and anti-angiogenic factors in the bovine corpus luteum (CL) during the estrous cycle and pregnancy as well as during induced luteolysis in the cow. The mRNA expression was analyzed by a quantitative real-time PCR, and the protein concentration was evaluated by enzyme immunoassay (EIA) or radioimmunoassay (RIA). In experiment 1, CL were collected at the following stages of an estrous cycle (d 0 = estrus); d 1 to 2, 3 to 4, 5 to 7, 8 to 12, 13 to 16, > 18 (after regression) and of pregnancy (month 1 to 2, 3 to 4, 6 to 7, > 8). In experiment 2 (induced luteolysis), cows on d 8 to 12 of an estrous cycle were injected with a prostaglandin (PG)$F_{2\alpha}$ analogue and CL were collected by transvaginal ovariectomy before and 0.5, 2, 4, 12, 24, 48 and 64 h after $PGF_{2\alpha}$ injection. The following angiogenic factors were examined: VEGF-A_{121}, VEGF-A_{165}, VEGF-A_{189}, and hypoxia inducible factor-1α. Anti-angiogenic factors that were characterized included: vasohibin-1, vasohibin-2, thrombospondin-1, thrombospondin-2, CD36 and CD47. In addition VEGF-A and thrombospondin-2 were examined in protein level. The results obtained showed a remarkable inverse and significantly regulated expression pattern between examined angiogenic and anti-angiogenic factors during estrous cycle and induced luteolysis in bovine CL. The expression levels of angiogenesis stimulating factors were high during early luteal phase and decreased significantly from d 8 to 12 to d > 18 and after luteal regression. In contrast, inhibiting local anti-angiogenic factors increased or remained up regulated in CL tissue at the end of estrous cycle and after induced luteolysis. In conclusion, angiogenic and anti-angiogenic factors are involved in the local mechanisms regulating angiogenesis and angiolysis in CL. The interaction between pro- and anti-angiogenic factors impacts CL formation, function and regression in the cow.

Temporal regulation of bovine luteal angiogenesis by PDGF and VEGFA *in vitro*

RS Robinson[a], AJ Hammond[b], GE Mann[b], MG Hunter[b] and KJ Woad[b]

[a]*School of Veterinary Medicine and Science &* [b]*School of Biosciences, University of Nottingham, Sutton Bonington Campus, Loughborough, UK*

The growth and development of the corpus luteum (CL) is dependent on angiogenesis. The principle pro-angiogenic factors include vascular endothelial growth factor A (VEGFA), fibroblast growth factor 2 (FGF2), and platelet-derived growth factor (PDGF). Recently, we have developed a culture model of luteal angiogenesis that incorporates luteal steroidogenic and vascular cell types. In this model, endothelial cells proliferate and form intricate networks which are stimulated by both VEGFA and FGF2[1] Previously, we have shown that continuous blockade of PDGF and VEGFA signalling by specific tyrosine kinase inhibitors markedly reduced the formation of endothelial networks[2]. The objective of this study was to determine whether there were specific windows of sensitivity to PDGF and/or VEGFA inhibition that represent major periods of endothelial cell cluster formation (d 0 to 3), tubule initiation (d 3 to 6) and network establishment (d 6 to 9).

Cells were enzymatically dispersed from early bovine CL and then plated onto fibronectin-coated coverslips in culture wells. The cells were grown in the presence of luteinising hormone, FGF2 and VEGFA. Cells were treated in triplicate wells with either 2 μM SU1498 (VEGF receptor inhibitor) or 2 μM AG1295 (PDGF receptor inhibitor) or neither (control) on d 0 to 3, d 3 to 6, or d 6 to 9 of culture (n=4 cultures). At the end of culture (d 9) endothelial cells were immunolocalised by von willebrand factor and development of networks assessed by image analysis. In the control wells, endothelial cells formed networks with tubule-like structures. The total area of endothelial networks was markedly reduced with AG1295 treatment on d 0 to 3 ($P<0.01$; $47\pm17\%$ of control), which was comparable to blanket inhibition (d 0 to 9; 21% of control)[2]. Treatment with AG1295 on d 0 to 3 reduced the number of endothelial clusters ($P<0.05$) rather than mean size of each cluster ($P>0.15$). There was no effect of the other treatment windows on any of the endothelial network parameters (e.g. for total endothelial cell area: d 3 to 6: $75\pm10\%$ of control; d 6 to 9 $120\pm20\%$ of control; $P>0.05$). While the total area of endothelial staining was lower in each of the treatment windows with the VEGF receptor inhibitor, SU1498, this was not significant ($P>0.05$). In contrast, blanket inhibition with SU1498 from d 0 to 9 reduced total endothelial cell area by 55% ($P<0.05$).

In conclusion, there was no specific window of sensitivity to VEGFA inhibition, suggesting that VEGFA signaling plays a modulatory role throughout luteal angiogenesis. In contrast, the formation of the endothelial cell clusters was sensitive to PDGF signaling inhibition. Since PDGF receptors are predominantly found on pericytes, this indicates a role for pericytes in the early stages of luteal angiogenesis.

This work was supported by BBSRC (grant BB/F002998) and Pfizer Ltd

[1]Robinson *et al.*, 2007. Reproduction 135:405-13.
[2]Woad *et al.*, 2009. Reproduction 138:581-8.

Neutrophils and chemokine interleukin-8 rapidly increase in the corpus luteum after $PGF_{2\alpha}$ administration in the mid-cycle cow

K Shirasuna[a], S Raddatz[b], J Sineenavd[a], HJ Schuberth[c], H Bollwein[b], T Shimizu[a] and A Miyamoto[a]

[a]*Graduate School of Animal and Food Hygiene, Obihiro University of Agriculture and Veterinary Medicine, Obihiro, Japan;* [b]*Clinic for Cattle and* [c]*Institute of Immunology, University of Veterinary Medicine Hannover, Hannover, Germany*

The corpus luteum (CL) undergoes dynamic changes in its function and structure during the estrous cycle. Active angiogenesis and progesterone (P) synthesis occur during development, while the drastic decrease of P secretion (functional luteolysis) and disruption of vascular vessels and luteal cells (structural luteolysis) are induced by luteolytic action of prostaglandin $F_{2\alpha}$ ($PGF_{2\alpha}$). It is well known that various types of immune cells such as CD4-positive T-cells, CD8-positive T-cells, gd-T cells, macrophages and eosinophils exist in the bovine CL and have an essential role in luteal function, but there is little information about neutrophils and their major chemokines interleukin-8 (IL8) and chemokine (C-X-C motif) ligand 1 (CXCL1). In addition, many studies have examined the time course of molecular and cellular responses of the CL to $PGF_{2\alpha}$ from 0.5 or 2 h after administration. However, $PGF_{2\alpha}$ can reach the CL much earlier because in vivo administration of $PGF_{2\alpha}$ stimulates oxytocin release from the CL within 5 min. The aim of the present study was, therefore, to investigate the change in the number of neutrophils as well as mRNA expression of IL8 and CXCL1 immediately after the onset of PGF-induced luteolysis in the cow. Cows (n = 5 for each time point) at the mid luteal phase (d 10 to 12; d 0 = estrus) were injected with $PGF_{2\alpha}$ (0 min) and ovaries were collected by ovariectomy at 0 min, 5 min, 15 min, 30 min, 2 h and 12 h. Number of neutrophils within the CL were analyzed by Periodic acid-Schiff staining. To investigate the function of IL8 as a luteal chemotactic mediator, we tested the migration of neutrophils using a transmigration assay with bovine IL8 and the CL culture supernatants from the mid-cycle CL. The mRNA expression of IL8 and CXCL1 increased at 30 min and 15 min after $PGF_{2\alpha}$ administration, respectively, and were maintained at high levels during luteolysis. Interestingly, the number of neutrophils significantly increased at 5 min after $PGF_{2\alpha}$ administration, when the level of neutrophilic chemoattractant had not yet started to increase. These neutrophils did not express $PGF_{2\alpha}$ receptor mRNA, indicating that $PGF_{2\alpha}$ can not directly attract neutrophils into the CL. In the transmigration assay, the CL supernatants as well as IL8 (10 to 100 ng/ml) stimulated neutrophil migration. These findings indicate that $PGF_{2\alpha}$ rapidly activates neutrophil migration without stimulation of neutrophilic chemoattractant within 5 min after $PGF_{2\alpha}$ administration. Taken together, neutrophils and their chemoattractants IL8 and CXCL1 may be involved in the bovine luteolytic cascade, but some unknown mechanisms appear to exist to attract neutrophils rapidly into the CL.

eCG treatment increases the progesterone in subsequent diestrus in lactating buffaloes

NAT Carvalho[a], LU Gimenes[b], H Ayres[b], DC Souza[b], K Neves[b] and PS Baruselli[b]

[a]*Unidade de Pesquisa e Desenvolvimento de Registro/Pólo Regional do Vale do Ribeira/APTA, Registro–SP, Brazil;* [b]*Departamento de Reprodução Animal, FMVZ-USP, São Paulo-SP, Brazil*

Protocols for fixed-time artificial insemination in anoestrous buffaloes (*Bubalus bubalis*) are based on the use of progesterone devices. Equine chorionic gonadotropin (eCG) is known for stimulating follicular growth and for luteotrophic effects. For these reasons, eCG is frequently used in hormonal treatments of anoestrous cattle. The aim of this study was to evaluate the effect of eCG treatment on follicular response, diameter of CL and progesterone (P4) concentration during diestrus following synchronized ovulation in buffaloes treated with intravaginal progesterone devices.

Forty lactating buffaloes (>40 d after parturition) were assigned into two groups (no-eCG: n=20 and eCG: n=20) according to parity, days postpartum, body condition score, presence of a dominant follicle and a CL on d -12 (D-12), D0 and D9. All buffaloes received an intravaginal progesterone device (DIB®; Syntex SA, Argentina) plus 2.0 mg of estradiol benzoate IM (D0; RicBE®; Syntex). On D9, DIB® was removed and a dose of $PGF_{2\alpha}$ (0.15 mg d-cloprostenol, Preloban®, Intervet/Schering-Plough) was administered. On this day, buffalo in Group eCG received 400 IU of eCG (Folligon®, Intervet/Schering-Plough). After two d (D11), each buffalo was treated with 10μg of GnRH (Conceptal®, Intervet/Schering-Plough). Buffaloes were examined by ultrasonography (Mindray DP2200Vet, 7.5MHz) on D-12, D0, D9, D11 to D14 (12 h apart), D16, D20 and D24. Serum samples were collected in all animals in order to measure P4 concentration on D16, D20 and D24. Data were analyzed in SAS for Windows by using PROC GLM (diameter of ovulatory follicle, interval device removal to ovulation, and ovulation rate) and PROC MIXED (diameter of CL from D16 to D24, and P4 concentration from D16 to D24).

There were no significant differences between no-eCG and eCG Groups on diameter of ovulatory follicle (12.3±0.9 vs. 13.7±0.6 mm), interval between device removal and ovulation (67.3±4.2 vs. 70.6±2.6 h), and ovulation rate (45.0±0.1 vs. 65.5±0.1%). Concerning CL diameter, there was no effect of treatment (P=0.14) or interaction treatment by time (P=0.11). However, there was a time effect (D16=14.5 ± 0.7^c vs. D20=17.0 ± 0.9^b vs. D24=18.9 ± 0.9^a mm; P<0.01). For P4 concentrations, there was no interaction treatment by time (P=0.16), although there was an effect of treatment (no-eCG=1.98 ± 0.34^b vs. eCG= 2.92 ± 0.44^a ng/mL; P=0.02) and time (D16=0.46 ± 0.06^c vs. D20=2.56 ± 0.29^b vs. D24=4.59 ± 0.58^a ng/mL; P<0.01).

These results indicate that treatment with eCG can increase P4 concentrations during diestrus following synchronized ovulation in lactating buffaloes treated with an intravaginal progesterone device.

Effects of nutritional status on corpus luteum function in non-lactating cyclic cows

T van Haeften[a], KJ Oosterhuis[a], JJ Hölzenspies[a], HM Knijn[b] and PLAM Vos[a]

[a]*Faculty of Veterinary Medicine, University of Utrecht, the Netherlands;* [b]*CRV, Arnhem, the Netherlands*

Negative energy balance (NEB) in dairy cows negatively affects fertility by influencing oocyte quality and ovarian, as well as corpus luteum (CL) function. NEB is supposed to interfere with normal lipid metabolism in CL and as such may alter progesterone production. In this study, we have analyzed changes in lipid content and progesterone (P4) production in CL of cyclic cows that were kept under restricted feeding (fasting) conditions, as a standardized model for NEB.

Two groups of synchronized cows were used in a cross-over study, which consisted of two experimental periods in which cows were fed a control diet of concentrates for 33 d or with a transition diet (hay 7 d), followed by feed withdrawal for 4 d, after which they returned to the control diet. During the experimental period, NEFA and ß-hydroxy butyrate blood levels, as indicators for NEB were measured daily. After estrus (d = 0), small samples of CL tissue were obtained using a transvaginal ultrasound-guided biopsy technique at d 8, 12 and 15. Paraformaldehyde-fixed tissue samples were processed for biochemical triacylglycerol (TAG) quantification. Lipid droplet distribution and quantification analysis was performed on sections using the neutral lipid stain Bodipy® and image analysis. CL function was measured by determining P4 blood levels during the entire estrous cycle.

Plasma NEFA and ß-hydroxybutyrate levels in the fasting group were greater on d 12 (1.1 ± 0.10 mmol/L; 0.78 ± 0.20 mmol/L, respectively) when compared with the control group (0.27 ± 0.02 mmol/L; 0.36 ± 0.003mmol/L, respectively). TAG concentrations of the CL of the fasting group increased from 10.24 ± 3.67 nmol/mg tissue at the start of the fasting period (d 8) to 15.01 ± 5.22 nmol/mg tissue (d 12). In the control group, TAG concentrations ranged from 11.01 ± 3.64 nmol/mg on d 8 to 8.07 ± 3.89 nmol/mg on d 12. After fasting, TAG levels in the fasting group returned to control values again. Lipid droplet analysis using Bodipy® revealed a similar increase in lipid content. In the control group, a constant number of lipid droplets/cell was observed on d 12 and 15 (3.87 ± 1.25 and 3.55 ± 1.91, respectively). In the fasting group, the number of lipid droplets averaged from 8.45 ± 1.17 on d 12 to 5.50 ± 1.50 on d 15. Surprisingly, blood P4 concentrations in the fasting group increased during fasting when compared with the control group (11.40 ± 2.40 ng/ml and 7.68 ± 4.45 ng/ml on d 12, respectively).

A brief period of food deprivation seems to induce NEB-like conditions in cyclic dairy cows as demonstrated by increased NEFA and ß-hydroxybutyrate blood levels. These elevated NEFA levels probably cause the observed lipid accumulation as demonstrated by increased TAG concentrations and increased lipid droplet numbers in CL samples. Whether these increased lipid levels underlie altering CL function as indicated by elevated P4 levels is a subject of current research.

Effect of ovulatory follicle size on luteal weight and steriodogenic enzyme expression

GA Perry, KL Gebhart, BL Perry, MG Gonda, CL Wright and RC Bott

Department of Animal and Range Sciences, South Dakota State University, Brookings, USA

Secretion of progesterone by the corpus luteum is necessary for the establishment and maintenance of pregnancy. It has been reported that corpora lutea from small follicles secrete decreased concentrations of progesterone and have decreased pregnancy success following GnRH-induced ovulation in fixed-time AI protocols. The objective of this study was to correlate ovulatory follicle size at time of GnRH-induced ovulation with d 10 luteal weight and to determine the effect of follicle size and luteal weight on expression of LH receptor (LHr), StAR, CYP11A1, and 3ß-HSD. Cows were synchronized with the CO-Synch protocol (d -9, 100 μg GnRH; d -2, 25 mg $PGF_{2\alpha}$; d 0, 100 μg GnRH; n=21). Estrus was detected with the HeatWatch System. Location and size of the ovulatory follicle was determined on d 0 at the time of GnRH by transrectal ultrasonography. Blood samples were collected on d 3, 4, 5, 7, and 9 for determination of concentrations of progesterone. Luteal tissue was collected on d 10 (n=5 estrus and n=16 no estrus). Total cellular RNA was extracted and relative mRNA expression was determined by real-time RT-PCR and corrected for GAPDH expression. Cows that exhibited estrus tended (P=0.09) to have larger follicles than cows that did not exhibit estrus (15.3±0.8 mm and 13.7±0.4 mm), but there was no difference (P=0.99) in d 10 luteal weight (5.0±0.7 g and 5.0±0.4 g). Ovulatory follicle size tended (P=0.056) to have a positive correlation with luteal weight on d 10 (R-squared=0.18). For every one mm increase in ovulatory follicle size, d 10 luteal weight increased by 0.33 g. When ovulatory follicle size was grouped into small (<12 mm), medium (12 to 15.5 mm), and large (>15.5 mm) follicles, follicle size (P=0.04) and time (P<0.01) influenced concentrations of progesterone, and there tended to be a follicle size by time interaction (P=0.08). However, there was no effect of estrus (P=0.16), luteal weight (P=0.47), estrus by time (P=0.21), or luteal weight by time (P=0.50) interaction on circulating concentrations of progesterone. In addition, there was no effect of estrus, follicle size, or luteal weight on LHr expression (P=0.99, 0.87, and 0.85, respectively), StAR expression (P=0.35, 0.70, and 0.16, respectively), CYP11A1 expression (P=0.64, 0.74, and 0.69, respectively), or 3ß-HSD expression (P=0.39, 0.11, and 0.69, respectively). In summary, as ovulatory follicle size increased, d 10 luteal weights tended to increase, and cows that exhibited estrus tended to have larger follicles than cows not in estrus. When larger follicles were induced to ovulate, greater concentrations of progesterone were observed, but estrus, follicle size, and luteal weight did not influence expression of steriodogenic enzymes. Therefore, the increased concentrations of progesterone among cows that ovulated larger follicles are likely the result of increased luteal weight and not changes in steroidogenic enzyme expression.

Impact of reduced progesterone during the follicular wave on ovulatory follicle diameter and progesterone concentrations in the subsequent estrous cycle

GA Bridges, BL Sparks, PJ Gunn and KS Fisher

Department of Animal Sciences, Purdue University, West Lafayette, USA

For optimal fertility, estrous synchronization protocols must enable the ovulation of a follicle that elevates blood estradiol concentrations before ovulation, contains a viable oocyte, and subsequently develops into a CL that produces adequate progesterone. Reduced peripheral progesterone concentrations during a follicular wave should provide increased gonadotropin support to the ovulatory follicle. Such a manipulation may promote increased estradiol production by the dominant follicle, the ovulation of a more viable oocyte, and enhance the secretion of progesterone by the subsequent CL, all of which have the potential to increase fertility in cattle.

The objective of this experiment was to evaluate the effect of reduced progesterone concentrations during the follicular wave on dominant follicle growth, ovulatory follicle diameter and luteal function in beef heifers. On d -7 (d 5 of the estrous cycle), heifers assigned to the reduced progesterone treatment (LoP4; n = 10) received a CIDR and were administered two doses of $PGF_{2\alpha}$ (25 mg;) given 8 h apart. On d -5, the remaining heifers received a CIDR (n = 11; Con treatment), and heifers in both treatments received GnRH (100 μg). On d 0, CIDR inserts were removed and all heifers received 25 mg of $PGF_{2\alpha}$, with a second dose of $PGF_{2\alpha}$ (25 mg) given 8 h later. Ovarian ultrasonography was performed on d -5, -3 and then daily following CIDR removal for 5 d or until ovulation was confirmed. Blood samples were collected on d 0, 6, 10, 14, and 18 to evaluate circulating concentrations of progesterone.

All (11/11) heifers in the Con treatment and 8/10 heifers in the LoP4 treatment ovulated to GnRH. At CIDR removal, circulating concentrations of progesterone were greater ($P < 0.05$) in the Con (8.41 ± 0.54 ng/mL) than LoP4 (4.61 ± 0.25 ng/mL) treatment. Dominant follicle diameter from d 0 (LoP4; 11.2 ± 0.4 mm, Con; 10.1 ± 0.3 mm) to d 3 (LoP4; 14.6 ± 0.4 mm, Con; 14.0 ± 0.4 mm) was greater (treatment; $P < 0.05$, treatment x d; $P > 0.10$) in the LoP4 than Con treatment. By d 4, 14 heifers had ovulated and the remaining heifers, with the exception of one heifer in the Con treatment who failed to ovulate, ovulated by d 5. On the day preceding ovulation, the diameter of the dominant follicle did not differ between treatments (Con; 14.2 ± 0.4 mm, LoP4; 14.7 ± 0.4 mm). Circulating concentrations of progesterone in the subsequent luteal phase tended ($P = 0.10$) to be greater in the LoP4 than Con treatment. In summary, reducing circulating concentrations of progesterone during the development of the follicular wave accelerated follicular growth and resulted in a marginal increase in progesterone concentrations in the subsequent estrous cycle.

Characteristics of bovine follicular growth and follicular function under low plasma progesterone concentrations induced by using the "corpus luteum absent" model

M Matsui[a], K Yamane[a], H Lee[a], S Haneda[a], A Miyamoto[b] and Y-I Miyake[a]

[a]*Department of Applied Veterinary Medicine;* [b]*Graduate School of Animal and Food Hygiene, Obihiro University of Agriculture and Veterinary Medicine, Obihiro, Japan*

Failure of a positive feedback response to estradiol (E_2) may cause follicular cysts in lactating dairy cows[1]. Progesterone (P_4) exposure of the hypothalamus may prevent cyst formation by maintaining this positive E_2 feedback mechanism[2]. We recently demonstrated that repeated follicular aspirations could prevent CL formation, maintain low plasma P_4 concentrations and induce a persistent follicle (CL absent model). Follicular growth may be altered under low plasma P_4 concentrations. The effects of continuous low plasma P_4 concentrations on the growth and function of follicles destined to become persistent were examined using the CL absent model in the present study.

Eleven cows received $PGF_{2\alpha}$ at 10 d after spontaneous ovulation. At 36 h after $PGF_{2\alpha}$ injection, the follicular fluid (FF) of all follicles with a diameter > 6 mm was aspirated using an ultrasound-guided technique. Follicular aspirations were repeated at 3, 6 and 9 d after first aspiration. Five cows showed no CL formation and maintained low plasma P_4 concentrations continuously from the time of first follicle aspiration. Measurement of diameter and collection of FF from the largest follicle were performed at 5 (d5NCL), 7 (d7NCL) or 9 d (d9NCL) after the last aspiration (CL absent model). The day of FF collection was set up as d 0 again and then the measurement of follicle diameter and collection of FF were repeated. In the control group, the dominant follicle at 6 d after ovulation was aspirated to induce new follicular recruitment. The diameter of the largest follicle was examined and its FF was collected at 5 (d5C), 7 (d7C) or 9 d (d9C) after the start of follicle recruitment in the control group. Concentration of E_2, total insulin-like growth factor-I (IGF-I) and free IGF-I in FF were analyzed. Blood samples for hormonal analysis (E_2 and total IGF-I) were also collected at the same time as follicular aspiration.

The diameter of d9NCL was greater than that of d9C. Concentration of E_2 in plasma and FF were greater in d5NCL, d7NCL and d9NCL compared with d5C, d7C and d9C, respectively. Total IGF-I concentrations in FF of CL absent model were greater than that of control. In the CL absent model, free IGF-I concentrations in FF tended to be greater compared with the control group. Free IGF-I in FF of d9NCL was greater than that of d9C.

Follicular growth and E_2 synthesis within the dominant follicle were stimulated during follicular growth in the CL absent model. Increased LH pulse frequency under continuous low plasma P_4 levels induced by the CL absent model may alter follicular growth and function and then induce a persistent follicle.

[1]Dobson and Alam, 1987. J Endocrinol 113:167-171.
[2]Gümen and Wiltbank, 2002. Biol Reprod 66:1689-1695.

Contributions of follicle size to establishment and maintenance of pregnancy in suckled beef cows using reciprocal embryo transfer

JA Atkins[a], MF Smith[a], MD MacNeil[b], EM Jinks[a] and TW Geary[b]

[a]*Division of Animal Sciences, University of Missouri, Columbia, USA;* [b]*USDA ARS Fort Keogh, Miles City, Montana, USA*

GnRH-induced ovulation of a small dominant follicle reduced pregnancy success in cattle. A reciprocal embryo transfer study was conducted at Fort Keogh from 2007 to 2009 in order to differentiate between follicular effects on pregnancy mediated through oocyte quality or uterine environment. Suckled beef cows (n = 1,166) were administered GnRH on d -9 (GnRH1), $PGF_{2\alpha}$ on d -2, and GnRH (GnRH2) either with (donor cows; n = 810) or without (recipient cows; n = 354) artificial insemination on d 0. Single embryos (n = 394) or oocytes (n = 45) were recovered from the donor cows (d 7; ET) and all live embryos were transferred into recipients the same day. Embryos from cows that ovulated a small (< 12.5 mm) or large follicle (≥ 12.5 mm) were transferred into cows that ovulated either a small or large follicle to remove co-linearity of follicle sizes pre- and post- d 7 of pregnancy; small to small (S-S; n = 71), small to large (S-L; n = 111), large to small (L-S; n = 122) and large to large (L-L; n = 50). Probability of successful fertilization increased with increasing diameter of the ovulatory follicle (P = 0.08) and serum concentrations of estradiol at GnRH2 (P = 0.006). The probability of embryo survival up to d 7 increased with increasing serum concentrations of progesterone at $PGF_{2\alpha}$ (P = 0.008) and follicle diameter at GnRH2 (P = 0.02). The stage of the embryo development was positively associated with serum concentrations of progesterone at ET (P = 0.05) but negatively associated with ovulatory follicle diameter at GnRH2 (P = 0.06). No direct effect of follicle size in either donor or recipient cows was detected for maintenance of pregnancy to d 27 or d 72 (P > 0.10). Probability of pregnancy at d 27 increased with increasing concentrations of estradiol at GnRH2 (P = 0.09) and progesterone at ET (P = 0.0005) in the recipients cows. There was no direct effect of donor serum concentrations of estradiol (GnRH2) or progesterone (ET) on pregnancy at d 27 (P > 0.10). In summary, increased ovulatory follicle diameter influenced the probability of pregnancy through increased serum concentrations of estradiol on d 0, increased fertilization rate, increased incidence of a live embryo on d 7, and increased progesterone production from the resulting corpus luteum.

Supported by NRI grant 2006-35203-17284 from USDA-CSREES.

Factors affecting preovulatory concentrations of estradiol and its role in establishment and maintenance of pregnancy in suckled beef cows using reciprocal embryo transfer

EM Jinks[a], JA Atkins[a], KG Pohler[a], MF Smith[a], GA Perry[b], MD MacNeil[c] and TW Geary[c]

[a]*University of Missouri, USA;* [b]*South Dakota State University, USA;* [c]*USDA ARS Fort Keogh, Miles City, Montana, USA*

In postpartum beef cows, GnRH-induced ovulation of small dominant follicles decreased pregnancy rates and increased late embryonic/fetal mortality; however, ovulatory follicle size had no apparent effect on the establishment or maintenance of pregnancy when ovulation occurred spontaneously[1]. To differentiate between effects of ovulatory follicle size on oocyte quality and uterine environment, a reciprocal embryo transfer study was conducted at Fort Keogh from 2007 to 2009. One objective was to examine the relationship between preovulatory serum concentrations of estradiol in donor and recipient cows and establishment and maintenance of pregnancy. Suckled beef cows (n=1,166) were administered GnRH1 on d -9, $PGF_{2\alpha}$ on d -2, and GnRH2 on d 0 either with (donor cows; n=810) or without artificial insemination (recipient cows; n=354). Single embryos (n=394) or oocytes (n=45) were recovered from the donor cows (d 7; ET) and all live embryos were transferred into recipients the same day. Embryos from cows that ovulated a small (<12.5 mm) or large follicle (≥12.5 mm) were transferred into cows that ovulated either a small or large follicle to remove co-linearity of follicle sizes pre- and post- d 7 of pregnancy. Ovulatory follicle size in both donors and recipients was positively correlated with serum concentration of estradiol at GnRH2 ($r=0.45$, $P<0.0001$) and estradiol at GnRH2 was greater ($P<0.01$) in cows that ovulated in response to GnRH1. Serum concentration of estradiol at GnRH2 was positively correlated with progesterone at ET ($r=0.34$, $P<0.0001$) and donors with greater estradiol were more likely to yield a fertilized embryo than an unfertilized oocyte ($P<0.0001$). There was no effect of donor estradiol at GnRH2 on embryo stage ($P=0.49$) or quality ($P=0.14$). Using data from the Perry et al. (2005) study[1], we determined pregnancy rate was significantly decreased when estradiol at GnRH2 was <8.4 pg/ml. Therefore, we retrospectively divided donor and recipient cows into four groups [low estradiol (<8.4 pg/ml) or high estradiol (≥8.4 pg/ml)] based on serum concentration of estradiol at GnRH2. Pregnancy rate at d 27 for low-low (n=78), low-high (n=80), high-low (n=91), and high-high (n=101) groups (donor-recipient) was 45[a], 65[b], 43[a], and 61[b]% respectively ([ab]$P<0.02$). Estradiol at GnRH2 had no effect on pregnancy maintenance to d 72 in the preceding groups. In summary, serum concentration of estradiol at GnRH2 was positively correlated with ovulatory follicle size, fertilization, and the establishment but not maintenance of pregnancy and its effects were likely mediated through improved uterine environment.

Supported by NRI grant 2006-35203-17284 from USDA-CSREES.

[1]Perry et *al.*, 2005. Proc Natl Acad Sci 102:5268-5273.

Circulating concentrations of pregnancy associated glycoproteins (PAGs) are associated with embryo/fetal survival but not ovulatory follicle size in suckled beef cows

KG Pohler[a], JA Atkins[a], EM Jinks[a], CL Johnson[a], MF Smith[a], JA Green[a], MD MacNeil[b] and TW Geary[b]

[a]*University of Missouri, USA;* [b]*USDA ARS Fort Keogh, Miles City, Montana, USA*

GnRH-induced ovulation of small dominant follicles resulted in increased late embryonic/fetal mortality around the time of embryo-uterine attachment. Pregnancy associated glycoproteins (PAGs) are secreted by binucleated trophoblast cells into the maternal circulation and have been used to monitor the presence of an embryo/fetus and placental function. The objective was to examine the relationship between ovulatory follicle size, embryo/fetal survival, and circulating concentrations of PAGs. In experiment 1, postpartum beef cows (n=69) were treated with the CO-Synch protocol (GnRH1 on d -9, $PGF_{2\alpha}$ on d -2, and GnRH2 and artificial insemination [AI] 48 h later [d 0]) and classified into one of four ovulatory follicle size groups: 1) small follicle (≤ 12 mm; n=9), 2) small-medium follicle (12 to 13 mm; n=20), 3) medium-large follicle (14 to 15 mm; n=28) or 4) large follicle (≥ 16 mm; n=12). The first increase ($P<0.0001$) in serum PAG concentration after insemination occurred on d 24 and PAG concentration decreased before a decrease in progesterone in cows that lost an embryo/fetus. The PAG secretion pattern from d 24 to 60 after insemination (d 0) was affected by day ($P<0.0001$), but not ovulatory follicle size or the interaction of ovulatory follicle size by day. In experiment 2, suckled beef cows (n=1,166) were administered the CO-Synch protocol either with (donor cows; n=810) or without (recipient cows; n=354) AI on d 0. Single embryos (n=394) or oocytes (n=45) were recovered from the donor cows (d 7; ET) and all live embryos were transferred into recipients the same day. Embryos from cows that ovulated a small (< 12.5 mm) or large follicle (≥ 12.5 mm) were transferred into cows that ovulated either a small or large follicle to remove co-linearity of follicle sizes pre- and post- d 7 of pregnancy; small to small (S-S; n=71), small to large (S-L; n=111), large to small (L-S; n=122) and large to large (L-L; n=50). The following results only include cows that established pregnancy at d 27 (n=195). Compared with cows that maintained pregnancy, cows that exhibited late embryonic/fetal mortality after d 27 had decreased ($P<0.05$) concentrations of PAGs on d 27. Serum concentrations of PAGs at d 27 were not affected by ovulatory follicle size ($P=0.85$), embryo stage at ET ($P=0.75$), embryo quality at ET ($P=0.64$), or estradiol at GnRH2 ($P=0.62$). In summary, there was no relationship between PAGs and ovulatory follicle size or serum concentrations of estradiol at GnRH2, embryo stage or quality on d 7; however, cows that lost an embryo after d 27 had lower concentrations of PAGs on d 27 compared with cows that maintained pregnancy.

Supported by USDA NRI grant 2006-35203-17284 from USDA-CSREES.

Follicle diameter at timed insemination influences the pregnancy in suckled *Bos indicus* cows inseminated with gender selected semen

MF Sá Filho[a], JM Baldrighi[a], L Penteado[b], EP Campos Filho[c], and PS Baruselli[a]

[a]*Departamento de Reprodução Animal, FMVZ-USP, São Paulo-SP, Brazil;* [b]*FIRMASA-IATF, Campo Grande-MS, Brazil;* [c]*SEXING-Technologies Brasil, Sertãozinho-SP, Brazil*

Follicular diameter at fixed time artificial insemination (FTAI) in suckled *Bos indicus* cows can influence ovulation rate, occurrence of estrus following progesterone source removal in a FTAI protocol, and pregnancy per artificial insemination (P/AI) using conventional semen. However, few investigations have been performed to identify the importance of dominant follicle diameter at insemination with gender-selected semen.

The aim of this study was to evaluate the effect of largest follicle (LF) diameter at FTAI on P/AI in suckled *Bos indicus* cows to FTAI with conventional (CON) or gender-selected semen (SEX). A total of 853 suckled Nelore *Bos indicus* cows between 30 and 60 d postpartum from two commercial farms were used. Information about parity, body condition score (BCS) at the beginning of FTAI protocol and type of semen were recorded for every cow. Estrus was synchronized by using an intravaginal device containing 1.0 g of progesterone plus an i.m. injection of 2.0 mg of estradiol benzoate (EB). Females received prostaglandin $F_{2\alpha}$ (0.5 mg of sodium cloprostenol) plus an injection of equine chorionic gonadotropin (300IU) at progesterone device removal (eight d after insertion) and 1 mg of EB 24 h afterwards. Cows were inseminated 60 to 64 h after progesterone withdrawal. The ovaries were examined by transrectal ultrasonography (7.5MHz, CTS-3300V, SIUI, China) at FTAI. During the exam the LF was measured and classified as <11 mm or ≥11 mm. At FTAI, cows were randomly assigned into four groups according to the LF diameter present (<11 mm or ≥11 mm) and the type of semen used (CON or SEX), in a 2x2 factorial design. To reduce variation between SEX and CON semen that might affect P/AI, the gender selected or conventional semen was obtained from the same ejaculate from each sire (two sires were used). All cows were examined for pregnancy by transrectal ultrasonography on d 30 after FTAI.

No effects of parity (P=0.24) or BCS (P=0.28) at the beginning of the synchronization protocol on P/AI were observed. There was a tendency (P=0.08) for an interaction between type of semen and the LF at FTAI on P/AI [CON≥11mm=59.1% (101/171); CON<11mm=51.0% (131/257); SEX≥11mm=56.8% (104/183); and SEX<11mm=36.8% (89/242)]. Effects of the type of semen [CON=54.2% (232/428) vs. SEX=45.4% (193/425), P=0.02] and the LF at FTAI [≥11mm=57.9% (205/354) vs. <11mm=44.1% (220/499), P<0.001] on the P/AI were observed.

The presence of a larger follicle at FTAI was associated with greater P/AI following FTAI in *Bos indicus* cows. The use of gender selected semen resulted in lower P/AI than the use of the non-gender selected semen. Additionally, identification of LF at FTAI may be an interesting tool to optimize the use of gender selected semen in FTAI programs.

Acknowledgements: Fazenda Boa Vista and the Herbran Agropecuária staff and the financial support provided by Sexing Technologies Brasil and Intervet Shering Plough.

Transcriptome differences between oocytes recovered from cows of high and low progesterone level

X Cao[a], D Salilew-Wondim[a], AAC de Wit[b], H Woelders[b], F Rings[a], M Hoelker[a], K Schellander[a] and D Tesfaye[a]

[a]*Institute of Animal Science, Animal Breeding and Husbandry Group, University of Bonn, Germany;* [b]*Animal Breeding and Genomics Centre, Wageningen UR Livestock Research, The Netherlands*

Progesterone is believed to be one of the ovarian hormones affecting the developmental competence of oocytes in vivo by inducing or switching off some molecular pathways. However, the molecular signatures and pathways influenced by the level of progesterone or its mechanism in oocyte development is poorly understood. The present study was aimed at investigating differences in molecular signatures in oocytes derived from Holstein-Friesian heifers with high or low progesterone level, euthanized on d 0 or d 12 of the estrous cycle. Total RNA was isolated from three pools of 30 oocytes for each heifer group, in triplicate using the PicoPure™ RNA isolation kit (ARCTURS, München, Germany). The gene expression patterns were analyzed using cDNA array. The microarray data analysis was performed using linear model for microarray data (LIMMA), R software (www.r-project.org) and bioconductor packages (www.bioconductor.org). The result revealed that 42 genes were differentially expressed (DE) ($P \leq 0.05$, fold change ≥ 1.4) comparing oocytes from heifers with high versus low progesterone level on d 0 of the estrous cycle. Gene ontology showed that genes that were up-regulated in oocytes from high progesterone heifers included genes related to signal transduction (STAT3, CHL1), zinc ion binding (ZFP91), mitotic cell cycle (AURKA) and NADH dehydrogenase activity (FL405). But, genes that were down-regulated in oocytes of high progesterone group comprised genes involved in transcription (PWP1, ZNF519, and MSX1), cell cycle (PTTG1, PRC1, CCNB1), polyamine biosynthesis (ODC1) and microtubule cytoskeleton organization (TUBA1B, TUBA1C). Similarly, a total of 57 DEGs were found comparing oocytes from high versus low progesterone heifers on d 12 of the estrous cycle. Genes expressed higher in the high progesterone group included genes involved in signal transduction (STAT3, FEZ2), transcription (CASK, MSX1), cell cycle (PTTG1, PRC1) and polyamine biosynthesis (ODC1). Genes expressed lower in the high progesterone group included genes involved in transcription (PAPOLG, LMO3, SOX4, MAML1, MYF5), signal transduction (CHL1, GOLT1B) and steroid biosynthesis (HSD17B11). Comparing oocytes from high versus low progesterone heifers of d 0 and d 12 combined, 9 DEGs were found. From those, STAT3 was found to be increased in high progesterone level both in d 0 and 12. However, TPM3, CHL1 and FL405 was found to be abundant in high progesterone level at d 0 but became lower during d 12. Similarly, the expression of PTTG1, PRC1, MSX1, TUBA1C and ODC1 were decreased in high progesterone level at d 0 of the estrous cycle but increased at d 12 of the estrous cycle. Therefore, this data showed that the effect of progesterone on the expression of developmentally related genes is dependent on the day of the estrous cycle.

Comparisons of mRNA expression for insulin-like growth factor (IGF) type 2 receptor (IGF2R) and IGF-1 in small ovarian follicles between cattle selected and not selected for twin ovulations

SE Echternkamp[a], PA Aad[b] and LJ Spicer[b]

[a]*USDA, ARS, U.S. Meat Animal Research Center, Clay Center, Nebraska, USA;*
[b]*Oklahoma State University, Stillwater, USA*

Both IGF-1 and -2 stimulate ovarian follicular cell proliferation and antral follicle development. Actions of IGF-1 and -2 are mediated through the IGF type 1 receptor, whereas binding of IGF-2 to the IGF2R results in its degradation. Information on the role of IGF2R in regulating bovine follicular development is limited, but IGF-1 reduced IGF2R in bovine follicular cells in vitro[1]. Because cattle selected for twin ovulations (Twinner) have greater blood and follicular fluid IGF-1,[2] increased antral follicle numbers may result from IGF-1-mediated reduction in IGF2R.

Experimental objectives were to assess relationships among IGF2R, aromatase, and IGF-1 mRNA expression in small (<5 mm) antral follicles and to determine their association with increased follicular development in Twinner cattle. Ovaries were collected from cyclic (d 5 or 6) Twinner (n=11) and non-Twinner (n=12) cows; pieces of cortex were fixed in 4% formaldehyde, dehydrated in ethanol and then xylene, and embedded in paraffin. Expression of mRNA was evaluated by in situ hybridization using ^{35}S-UTP-labelled antisense and sense probes published for IGF2R, aromatase, and IGF-1. Slides were exposed to Kodak NTB-2 emulsion for 4 wk. Silver grain density was quantified in four areas of the granulosa and thecal layers of each antral follicle (2 to 7 follicles/cow) by Bioquant Nova Prime image analysis. Antisense minus sense density measurements were averaged for four replicates per follicle and specific expression data were analyzed for effect of genetic line using Proc Mixed of SAS.

Antral follicles from Twinners were smaller in diameter than non-Twinner follicles (1.9±0.1 vs. 2.3±0.1 mm; P=0.08), but thickness of granulosa layer did not differ (76.8±19.2 vs. 75.0±16.0 microns, respectively). Abundance of IGF2R mRNA was less within granulosa (3.4±0.8 vs. 6.3±0.8% specific grains; P<0.01) and thecal cells (3.1±0.7 vs. 4.9±0.6%; P<0.05) of Twinner vs. non-Twinner follicles, whereas abundance of aromatase mRNA was greater in granulosa of Twinner vs. non-Twinner follicles (17.5±1.6 vs. 7.8±1.4%; P<0.01). Expression of aromatase and IGF2R mRNA was correlated negatively in granulosa (r=0.42; P≤0.01) and thecal (r=0.24; P=0.05) layers. IGF-1 mRNA was primarily in the granulosa layer, including cumulus, and its expression did not differ between Twinners vs. non-Twinners (14.6±2.8 vs. 13.7±2.3% specific grains); granulosa IGF-1 and IGF2R mRNA were correlated negatively (r=0.25; P=0.05).

Decreased abundance of IGF2R mRNA and increased aromatase mRNA in small antral follicles of Twinner cows are likely the consequence of increased extra-ovarian IGF-1 within Twinners. The inverse relationship between abundance of aromatase and IGF2R mRNA is consistent with increased IGF-2 stimulation of steroidogenesis as a result of decreased IGF2R. We hypothesize that decreased expression of IGF2R mRNA in Twinner ovarian follicles contributes to increased follicular development by increasing free IGF-2.

[1]Spicer and Aad, 2007. Biol Reprod 77:18-27.
[2]Echternkamp *et al.*, 2004. J Anim Sci 82:459-471.

Associations of the bovine follicular health, mitotic activity and intrafollicular amounts of IGFBP-4 on d 5 or 6 of the first follicular wave

T Moonmanee[a], C Navanukraw[a] and S Guntaprom[b]

[a]*Department of Animal Science, Faculty of Agriculture, Khon Kaen University, Khon Kaen, Thailand;*
[b]*Rajamangala University of Technology Isan Kalasin Campus, Thailand*

Insulin-like growth factor (IGF)-I and IGF binding proteins (IGFBPs) have been found to play a crucial role in the selection of bovine dominant follicles. Dominant follicles are characterized by greater mitotic activity and lower amounts of IGFBP-4 whereas atretic follicles are characterized by apoptosis of granulosa cells. No associations have yet been made, however, between mitotic activity, follicular health and intrafollicular amounts of IGFBP-4. The aim of the study, therefore, was to investigate the interactions of mitotic activity, follicular health and intrafollicular of IGFBP-4. Eight mature Thai native crossbred beef cows (60 ± 7 mo of age; 461 ± 14 kg BW) received two injections (11 d apart) of a $PGF_{2\alpha}$ analogue (Estrumate®) to synchronize estrus. Ovaries were collected from a slaughterhouse on d 5 or 6 of the subsequent estrous cycle. Surface diameter of all follicles ≥ 3 mm was determined. Follicular fluid was gently aspirated and stored at -20°C until determination of protein and IGFBP-4 by Bradford and Western blot analysis as previously described[1]. Follicular health was determined morphologically and classified as previously described[2]. Mitotic activity of granulosa and theca cells was evaluated by immmunohistochemistry using a monoclonal PCNA antibody (Cell Signaling Technology, CA, USA). The labeling index was calculated as the number of PCNA labeled nuclei expressed as percentage of total nuclei[3]. A total of 19 healthy and 10 unhealthy follicles were analyzed. Follicular diameters in healthy follicles were smaller than unhealthy follicles (6.9 ± 0.7 vs. 9.6 ± 1.5 mm; $P < 0.01$). Regardless of follicular health, labeling index (%) of granulosa and theca cells were greatest (34.0 ± 3.5 and 29.2 ± 2.3; $P < 0.05$) in small follicles (3 to 6 mm) compared with large follicles (>10 mm; 22.1 ± 2.9 and 19.4 ± 3.3) but were not different when compared with medium size follicles (7 to 10 mm; 31.7 ± 3.9 and 26.4 ± 3.0). Intrafollicular amounts of IGFBP-4 quantitated by densitometry were expressed arbitrarily in units. Follicular fluid amounts of IGFBP-4 were less ($P < 0.05$) in healthy follicles regardless of follicular size. The interaction of mitotic activity and intrafollicular amounts of IGFBP-4 may play significant roles in follicular growth and atresia.

This study was supported by Strategic Scholarships Fellowships Frontier Research Networks, Office of the Higher Education Commission, Thailand Research Fund, and Agricultural Biotechnology Research Center for Sustainable Economy, Khon Kaen Univeristy.

[1]Mihm *et al.*, 2000. Biol Reprod 63:811-819.
[2]Hendriksen *et al.*, 2003. Biol Reprod 69:2036-2044.
[3]Grazul-Bilska *et al.*, 2007. J Anim Sci 85:1914-1922.

Temporal patterns of circadian clock gene expression differ between stroma and dominant follicles in periovulatory ovine ovaries

BA Murphy, C Blake, A-M Martin, N Forde, JA Browne and ACO Evans

School of Agriculture, Food Science and Veterinary Medicine, University College Dublin, Ireland

The precise timing from follicular cyclooxygenase (COX2) induction to ovulation in rats, cows and mares is highly conserved[1], suggesting similar temporal regulation. The mammalian circadian (24 h) system responds to changes in environmental photoperiod by communicating time-of-day information from the suprachiasmatic nucleus to each organ. Cellular rhythms are thereby synchronized via highly conserved molecular clockwork mechanisms that in turn regulate tissue-specific transcriptional activity. Recent discoveries of: 1) an LH-regulated rodent ovarian circadian clock[2], 2) clock gene regulation of ovarian steroidogenesis[3], and 3) clock gene oscillation in granulosa cells; highlight a potentially important link between circadian regulation and the process of ovulation. This prompted an investigation of the role played by photoperiod and core clock gene expression patterns in the ovine pre-ovulatory ovary.

72 Suffolk-cross cull ewes were presynchronized using intravaginal progestagen sponges and administration of eCG. Sponge removal was staggered by 12 h (n=36 per group) for anticipated ovulation either midway during daylight or darkness h. 36 h after sponge removal, animals were culled and ovaries harvested at 6 h intervals for 24 h (n=4 per time point), encompassing a 24 h pre-and post-ovulatory period. Ovarian stroma and follicle wall preparations (theca interna with attached granulosa cells) were dissected, snap frozen and stored at -80°C before isolation of total RNA. Blood samples were collected every 3 h by jugular venipuncture for the period 24 to 48 h after sponge removal to detect the LH surge. Quantitative (q) PCR assays were designed to detect mRNA expression levels using SYBR® Green (Applied Biosystems) for the core clock genes (*Per2, Arntl* and *Cry1*), in addition to other transcripts important in the ovulatory cascade (*3ß-HSD* and *StAR*).

Serum LH analysis revealed that photoperiod had no effect on the timing of the LH surge after sponge removal (~36 h). Expression data were aligned relative to the time of sponge removal (SR) and circadian time (CT) to differentiate between circadian and prevailing hormonal regulation of transcription. One-way ANOVA for CT revealed significant variation in the temporal pattern of *Arntl, Cry1* and *3ß-HSD* expression in ovarian stroma ($P=0.0346$, $P=0.0124$, $P<0.0001$; respectively), while in follicular tissue there were no significant patterns identified. One-way ANOVA for SR revealed that *3ß-HSD* expression rose sharply in stroma at expected ovulation time ($P=0.0003$) whereas in follicular tissue significant temporal expression patterns were demonstrated for *Per2, Star* and *3ß-HSD* ($P=0.0087$, $P=0.0289$, $P=0.0445$; respectively). Except for *3ß-HSD,* each of these genes demonstrated a 24 h cyclic expression pattern in the tissue examined. Our findings strongly suggest that stroma tissue function is regulated by time-of-day signals while follicular steroidogenesis likely involves the clock gene *Per2* temporally regulating *Star* and *3ß-HSD.*

[1]Sirois *et al.*, 2004. Hum Reprod Update 10:373-385.
[2]Karman and Tischkau, 2006. Biol Reprod 75:624-632.
[3]Nakao *et al.*, 2007. Endocrinology 148:3031-3038.

Comparison of intrafollicular levels of different isoforms of follistatin and activin during follicular wave growth in cattle

C Glister[a], SJ Sunderland[b], MP Boland[b], JF Roche[b], JJ Ireland[c] and PG Knight[a]

[a]School of Biological Sciences, University of Reading, Reading RG6 6UB, UK; [b]Faculty of Veterinary Medicine, University College Dublin, Ireland; [c]Dept. Animal Science, Michigan State University, East Lansing, USA

We investigated whether post-emergence antral follicle growth is associated with changing intrafollicular concentrations of different isoforms of follistatin (FS) and activin. Heifers (n = 28) were ovariectomized at five times during an estrous cycle[1]: d 0 (follicular phase, pre-LH surge), d 1 (post-LH surge, pre-ovulation), d 3 (selection phase), d 6 (dominance phase) and d 12 (atretic phase). Daily ovarian ultrasonography was performed and blood samples were collected every 4 to 6 h to determine gonadotrophin and steroid profiles. Follicular fluid (FF) was aspirated from follicles > 5 mm and total FS, activin-A, activin-AB, inhibin-A, estradiol (E) and progesterone (P) concentrations were measured. Six different FS isoforms were quantified by immunoblotting[2]. At each time-point, the largest and second largest follicle were classified as the morphologically dominant (DF) or largest subordinate (SF1) follicle, respectively. FF from the remaining follicles > 5mm was pooled for analysis (SF2p).

Serum FSH concentrations were transiently increased during d 0.5 to 1.5 and 8 to10.5 in association with emergence of the first and second wave of follicular growth. Follicular diameter was positively correlated with E/P ratio (r = 0.56) and negatively correlated with activin-A (r = -0.34), activin-AB (r = -0.80) and 'total' FS (r = -0.70). Six different FS isoforms were detected in bFF (apparent *Mr*: 65, 41, 37, 35, 31 and 29 kDa) representing, on average, 6, 13, 24, 26, 13 and 17%, respectively of total FS. Follicular diameter was positively correlated with % abundance of the 41 kDa FS isoform (r = 0.59) but negatively correlated with % abundance of 31 and 29 kDa FS isoforms (r = -0.56, -0.41).

During growth of the first follicular wave (d 3 to 6) FS, activin-A, activin-AB and inhibin-A decreased in DF but were maintained or increased in SF1 and SF2p. During subsequent atresia of DF (d 6 to 12), FS and activin-AB remained lower in DF than in SF1 and SF2p while inhibin-A increased in DF to a level higher than in SF1 or SF2p. Activin/inhibin ratio fell 4-fold through d 3, 6 and 12 in DF but did not vary in SF1 or SF2p. There was an effect of follicle status (i.e., DF, SF1, SF2p) on % abundance of the 41, 37, 31 and 29kDa FS isoforms and an effect of cycle d (i.e., d 3, 6, 12) on % abundance of the 65kDa isoform.

In 'follicular phase' follicles, there was an effect of follicle status on E, FS and activin-AB concentrations and on activin/FS ratio and E/P ratio. There was also an effect of cycle day (i.e. pre- versus post-LH surge) on activin-A, activin-AB, FS levels and activin/inhibin ratio. FS concentration was much lower in DF than in SF1 or SF2p. There was also an effect of follicle status, but not cycle day, on the % abundance of the 41, 31 and 29kDa FS isoforms.

In conclusion (1) six *Mr* isoforms of FS and two isoforms of activin were detected in FF of follicular- and luteal-phase dominant and subordinate follicles, and (2) there were follicle status-dependent changes in the relative amounts and proportions of the above proteins that supports their involvement in the follicle selection/dominance mechanism.

[1]Sunderland *et al.*, 1996. Biol Reprod 54:453-462.
[2]Glister *et al.*, 2006. J Endocrinol 188:215-225.

Fibroblast growth factor and bone morphogenetic protein regulation of Sprouty gene expression in bovine granulosa cells

CA Price[a], J Juengel[b], J Buratini Jr[c] and ZL Jiang[a,d]

[a]Université de Montréal, St-Hyacinthe, QC, Canada; [b]AgResearch Invermay, Mosgiel, New Zealand; [c]Universidade Estadual Paulista, Botucatu, SP Brazil; [d]Northwest A&F University, Yangling, ShaanXi, China

Fibroblast growth factors (FGF) form a large family of proteins mainly involved in tissue patterning and organ development. FGFs also affect reproductive function. Convincing evidence has been presented for a role for FGFs in oocyte–cumulus signaling in mice, specifically the ability of FGF8 to stimulate cumulus glycolysis in cooperation with bone morphogenetic protein (BMP)-15. FGF8 belongs to a FGF subfamily that also contains the structurally related proteins, FGF17 and FGF18. All three activate the same FGF receptors, although the pattern of expression (in cattle) differs: FGF8 and FGF17 are expressed in the oocyte, whereas FGF18 is restricted to the theca. FGF signaling involves the Ras/MEK/extracellular signal-regulated kinase (ERK), phospholipase-C (PLC) and phosphatidylinositol-3-kinase (PI3K) and Akt pathways depending on cell type, but this has not been explored in the follicle. Similarly, downstream target genes of FGF signaling in the follicle have not been identified, with the notable exception of the MEK inhibitor, Sprouty2, which is expressed in mouse cumulus in response to FGF8. The objectives of the present study were to identify the main pathways and target genes of FGF8 and FGF18 in bovine granulosa cells.

Bovine ovaries were obtained from a local abattoir, and granulosa cells from small follicles (2 to 5 mm diameter) were placed in serum-free medium containing FSH. Medium was changed on d 2 and 4, and on d 5 the cells were stimulated with 10 ng/ml of FGF8 or FGF18. FGF8-treated cells were co-treated with or without ovine BMP15 (6 ng/ml) or GDF9 (25 ng/ml). Total RNA was extracted and target gene expression was measured with real-time RT-PCR. In separate experiments, signaling pathways were explored by measuring relative levels of phospho-ERK and phospho-Akt by Western blotting.

The addition of FGF8 but not FGF18 resulted in a robust increase in phospho-ERK, and a rapid increase in Sprouty2 mRNA levels. Abundance of mRNA encoding Sprouty1 and 4 were also stimulated by FGF8, but more slowly. Inhibitors demonstrated that PI3K and PKC pathways were also involved in FGF8 stimulation of Sprouty2. FGF8 increased abundance of mRNA encoding NR4A transcription factors, but FGF18 did not. FGF8 increased levels of mRNA encoding the cell cycle regulator GADD45B, whereas FGF18 decreased GADD45B mRNA levels. Co-treatment with FGF8 and BMP15 abolished the stimulatory effect of FGF8 on Sprouty and GADD45B mRNA levels but did not alter the effect on NR4A mRNA. Co-culture with GDF9 had a similar effect.

In conclusion, these data demonstrate that members of the FGF8 subfamily employ quite different signaling pathways in granulosa cells, and illustrate how BMP and GDF modulate FGF signaling/action.

This research was supported by Chinese Scholarship Council and NSERC (Canada).

Expression of mRNA encoding FGF22 and FGFR1B around follicle deviation in Nelore (*Bos indicus*) heifers

J Buratini Jr.[c], ACS Castilho[a], MF Machado[a], R Ereno[a], CM Barros[a] and CA Price[b]

[a]Department of Pharmacology, Institute of Biosciences, UNESP, SP, Brazil; [b]Centre de Recherché en Reproducion Animale, University of Montreal, Canada; [c]Department of Physiology, Institute of Biosciences, UNESP, SP, Brazil

Fibroblast growth factors (FGF) are grouped into several FGF subfamilies according to structural and functional properties. FGF play a number of different physiological roles including regulation of folliculogenesis. The FGF7 subfamily includes FGF7, FGF10 and FGF22, which activate FGFR2B and FGFR1B. Both FGF7 and FGF10 have been shown to inhibit oestradiol secretion from granulosa cells. Recently we showed that FGF22 and FGFR1B are expressed in theca cells of bovine antral follicles, and mRNA abundance for both genes was lower in oestrogenic compared with non-oestrogenic follicles. This suggests that these FGFs may be involved in follicle regression.

The objective of the present study was to determine if FGF22 and its receptor are involved in the control of follicular selection. We assessed mRNA expression of FGF22 and FGFR1B in theca cells from dominant and subordinate follicles around the time of deviation in Nelore heifers. In this sub-species, morphological divergence occurs on average 2.5 d after ovulation when the diameter of the dominant follicle is around 6.0 mm. Oestrous cycles of thirteen heifers were synchronized and ovulation was detected by ultrasound monitoring every 12 h. Heifers were slaughtered 2 ($n=4$), 2.5 ($n=5$) and 3 ($n=4$) days after ovulation. Theca cells were isolated from the two largest follicles and submitted to total RNA extraction. For each heifer, we classified the follicles as 'Dominant' and 'Subordinate' based on abundance of CYP19 mRNA in granulosa cells of the same follicle. FGF22 and FGFR1B mRNA abundance was measured by real time RT-PCR and expressed as ddCt values with cyclophilin A as housekeeping gene. Effects of follicle status and day on FGF22 and FGFR1B mRNA abundance were tested with paired t-tests.

Follicular diameter did not differ between the dominant and subordinate follicles on d 2 or 2.5, but approached significance on d 3 (8.4 ± 0.3 vs. 6.6 ± 0.4 mm; $P=0.05$). FGF22 mRNA abundance did not change with day or between dominant and subordinate follicles. FGFR1B mRNA abundance was greater in theca cells from subordinate follicles compared with dominant follicles on d 2 ($P=0.002$) but not on d 2.5 or 3 ($P>0.05$). In conclusion, expression of FGFR1B was decreased in dominant, oestrogenic follicles before morphological divergence. This suggests that FGF signaling through this receptor plays a role in determining the fate of the future dominant follicle.

Supported by FAPESP.

Differences of follicular growth and blood flow in the follicular wall between the first and second wave dominant follicles in cows

R Miura, M Matsui, S Haneda and Y-I Miyake

Obihiro University of Agriculture and Veterinary Medicine, Japan

In recent years, several estrus synchronization protocols were developed to increase insemination rate but conception rate per insemination has not improved. The characteristics of the dominant follicle when the estrus synchronization protocol is started may be important for sucessful synchronizaton because follicles grow under different endocrine conditions during the estrous cycle in cows[1]. The influence of endocrine status on follicular growth was characterized by comparing the dominant follicle (DF) from the first and second follicular wave.

Follicular growth and blood flow in the follicular wall of the DF during the first wave (W1; n = 8) and second wave (W2; n = 8) were examined in multiparous Holstein dry cows. In W1, the DF diameter was measured on d 4, 5 and 6 of the estrous cycle (d 0 = estrus) using transrectal ultrasonography. To induce follicular maturation, $PGF_{2\alpha}$ and GnRH were given on d 7 and 9, respectively. A diameter and blood flow area (BFA) of DF on d 7, 9 and 10 were measured by using transrectal color Doppler ultrasonography. In W2, ovulation of the DF was induced by GnRH injection on d 6 to induce a new follicular wave, then ovulation was confirmed on d 8. A diameter of DF was measured on d 11, 12 and 13, and then $PGF_{2\alpha}$ and GnRH were given on d 14 and 16, respectively. A diameter and BFA of DF were also measured on d 14, 16 and 17. In both groups, the DF was examined from 4 d (D4) to 10 d (D10) after follicle wave emergence (D1 = day of spontaneous ovulation in W1, or day of induced ovulation by GnRH in W2).

Diameter of W1 DF was greater than W2 DF at D9 and D10 ($P < 0.05$). From D7 to D9, the diameter of the DF increased in W1 ($P < 0.05$), but no significant changes were observed in W2. BFA was greater ($P < 0.05$) for W1 DF versus W2 DF at D10. BFA of DF in W1 at D10 was greater than at D7 and D9 ($P < 0.001$). In W2, although BFA of DF was greater for D10 versus D7 ($P < 0.001$), there is no significant difference between D9 and D10. Blood flow area/follicle circumference (BFA/FC) of DF was greater ($P < 0.05$) for W1 versus W2 DF at D10. BFA/FC of DF at D10 were greater than at D7 and D9 in W1 ($P < 0.001$). But there was no significant change from D7 to D10 in W2.

The increase in diameter and blood flow of the DF was greater in W1 than in W2 during the period of follicular maturation. Since characteristics of DF were different between W1 and W2, follicular growth and function may be affected on by endocrine condition, such as progesterone profile.

[1]Wolfenson *et al.*, 1999. J Reprod Fertil 117:241-247.

Number of follicles during follicular waves is positively associated with fertility in dairy cows

F Mossa[a], ST Butler[b], DP Berry[b], F Jimenez-Krassel[c], P Lonergan[a], GW Smith[c], JJ Ireland[c] and ACO Evans[a]

[a]Agriculture Food Science and Veterinary Medicine, University College Dublin, Ireland; [b]Teagasc, Moorepark Dairy Research Centre, Fermoy, Co. Cork, Ireland; [c]Department of Animal Science, Michigan State University, USA

Our previous results documented that the total number of ovarian follicles ≥3 mm in diameter (antral follicle count, AFC) during follicular waves varies among animals of similar age, but is highly repeatable within individuals and indicative of total number of healthy follicles and oocytes in ovaries of cattle.

To address the hypothesis that AFC is positively associated with fertility in cows, AFC was assessed using transrectal ultrasonography for two consecutive days during the first wave of follicular growth in 306 Holstein–Friesian dairy cows (aged 3.5 ± 1.7 years) 1 to 4 months postpartum. Based on AFC, cows were classified into three groups: low ≤15 follicles (n = 126), intermediate 16 to 24 follicles (n = 122) or high ≥25 follicles (n = 58). During the breeding season, cows were artificially inseminated following estrus detection. Ultrasonographic examinations were conducted 30 to 36 and 60 to 66 d post-AI and at 150 d after the beginning of the breeding season to determine pregnancy status. The following reproductive parameters were analyzed: calving to first service interval, calving to conception interval, services per cow during the breeding season, conception rate to first service and overall pregnancy rate. Fixed effects models, logistic regression, survival analysis and ordinal regression were used. The predicted probability of a successful pregnancy at first service for animals with high, intermediate and low AFC was 42%, 50% and 36%, respectively and the respective values for overall pregnancy rate at the end of the breeding period were 90%, 80% and 73%. The odds of a successful pregnancy to first service were greater ($P < 0.05$) for animals with intermediate AFC compared to animals with low AFC, while no difference existed between animals with high AFC compared to low AFC. However, animals with high AFC had a 3.34 times greater odds of conceiving at the end of the breeding season compared with those with low AFC. Fifty per cent of the cows in the high and intermediate groups had conceived by d 103 after calving, while it took until d 112 ($P < 0.05$) after calving for 50% of the cows in the low group to conceive. No difference in 21-d submission rate was evident among groups, but animals with a high AFC received fewer ($P < 0.05$) services during the overall breeding season compared with animals with a low AFC.

In summary, cows with a high AFC had higher pregnancy rates, shorter calving to conception intervals and received fewer services during the breeding season compared with cows with a low AFC. We conclude that cows with high compared with low numbers of follicles growing during follicular waves have an enhanced reproductive performance.

Funded by the Irish Department of Agriculture, Fisheries and Food (RSF 06 328).

Using growth traits and adipose function to identify indicators of heifer fertility

RA Cushman, MF Allan, TG McDaneld, LA Kuehn, LA Rempel, AK Lindholm-Perry, WM Snelling and HC Freetly

USDA-ARS U.S. Meat Animal Research Center, Clay Center, Nebraska, USA

The identification of early indicators of fertility would increase profitability by improving the quality of heifers chosen to enter the breeding herd. Growth traits are closely linked to age at puberty and could be predictors of initiation of reproductive cycles and heifer fertility. Adipose has been classically thought of as a tissue that stores excess energy; however, during the last decade it has been recognized as an endocrine organ that secretes hormones, growth factors, and adipokines. Therefore, adipose represents an easily accessible tissue that could produce biomarkers of fertility that also could be linked to growth traits or feed efficiency.

Crossbred beef heifers (n=422) were observed for behavioral estrus with the aid of Estrotect patches starting at 6 mo of age. At 363.7±0.7 d of age, a subcutaneous adipose biopsy was collected from the tail head under epidural anesthesia; and at 416.3±0.6 d of age heifers were pastured with fertile bulls for a 63-d breeding season. Heifers were examined by ultrasonography to determine pregnancy status 45 d after the end of the breeding season; pregnancy status was confirmed at calving. Random adipose samples from 22% of the heifers that were pre-pubertal (n=15) or pubertal (n=77) at the time of biopsy were analyzed by real-time RT-PCR to determine relative levels of peroxisome proliferator-activated receptor-γ (PPAR-γ) mRNA because PPAR-γ has been linked to adiposity, fertility, and ovarian function.

Heifers that were pre-pubertal at biopsy were 10.2±3.5 kg lighter at weaning (P=0.004) and 6.3±2.0 d younger at biopsy (P=0.002) but did not differ in weight at breeding (P=0.41) or in pregnancy rate (P=0.42). Pre-pubertal heifers were 6.9±3.0 d younger at calving (P=0.02), but calving day did not differ between the groups (P=0.64). Age at puberty did not differ between heifers that were diagnosed pregnant (n=373) and heifers that were diagnosed open (n=49; P=0.83). Messenger RNA levels of PPAR-γ did not differ between pre-pubertal and pubertal heifers (P=0.88); however, PPAR-γ mRNA levels tended to increase in a linear manner as age at puberty increased (P=0.1). Heifers that were diagnosed pregnant (n=84) and heifers that were diagnosed open (n=8) did not differ in PPAR-γ mRNA levels (P=0.34).

Messenger RNA levels of PPAR-γ in the adipose were not a predictor of fertility. In future studies, biopsies will be collected at weaning because this is an ideal management point for making decisions on replacement heifers and because weaning weights were lower in heifers that reached puberty at a later age.

Biochemical and topographical changes in glycoconjugates of the cervical epithelium associated with the onset of oestrus in cattle

K Pluta, C Dolphin, ACO Evans and SD Carrington

School of Agriculture, Food Science and Veterinary Medicine, University College Dublin, Belfield, Dublin 4, Ireland

The cervix and its secretions undergo biochemical and physical changes under the differential influences of oestrogen and progesterone. At oestrus, the cervical epithelium is soft and thickened and cervical mucus is thin and watery, facilitating sperm transit. During the rest of the cycle and pregnancy the cervical epithelium is firm and mucus viscoelasticity increases, enhancing cervical barrier function. The molecular scaffolding of mucus gels is formed by mucins, which are heavily O-glycosylated glycoproteins. Thus, changes in the cervix barrier, and the physicochemical behaviour of its secretions, may be correlated with changes in the glycosylation of mucins and other cervical glycoconjugates. The glycosylation profile of bovine cervical tissues in the perioestrus period has not yet been fully described. Therefore, we investigated them histochemically and biochemically.

Cervical tissue samples were collected from synchronized beef heifers that were slaughtered at (i) 12 h after CIDR removal, (ii) 24 h after CIDR removal, (iii) at the onset of oestrus, (iv) 12 h after the onset of oestrus, (v) 48 h after the onset of oestrus, and (vi) 7 d after the onset of oestrus (luteal phase). A range of histological techniques were used to map overall patterns of mucin glycosylation (Periodic Acid Schiff's, Alcian Blue, High Iron Diamine). Biotinylated lectins (DBA, PNA, UEAI, WGA, SNA, MALII) were also used to detect the presence and distribution of a range of sugar structures coupled with image analysis.

Epithelial stores of neutral and acidic mucins rise significantly from before the onset of oestrus and remain high up to 48 h afterwards. Sialylated mucins predominate at the bases of cervical folds, whereas sulphated mucins are more abundant at their apices and were not significantly different among time points. Similar differences between apical and basal staining were also noted in staining by DBA and SNA. Sialic acid (α2-6 linked) was detected by SNA binding, but MAL binding of α2-3 linkages was not observed.

The different glycosylation microenvironment at the bases of the cervical folds may explain previous literature showing that this location is a favoured conduit for sperm transit. While there are major changes in the overall quantity of stored mucins in the perioestus period, and minor qualitative differences in lectin staining at different timepoints, quantitative analysis did not suggest that any of the techniques used would be useful in predicting oestrus on the basis of changes in the lectin staining profile of cervical tissues or secretions.

Funded by Science Foundation Ireland (07/SRC/B1156).

Sexual attractiveness of estrous ewes synchronized with intravaginal sponges impregnated with medroxiprogesterone

M Gatti and R Ungerfeld

Departamento de Fisiología, Facultad de Veterinaria, Montevideo, Uruguay

Chemical signals released to the environment by an animal may stimulate physiological changes in others animals of the same species. Sexual attractiveness is a factor that determines whether a female is preferred by males. Vaginal secretions are an important source of signals that determine attractiveness in ewes[1]. These authors reported that alterations of vaginal flora negatively affect sexual attractiveness of estrous ewes. As the use of intravaginal sponges for estrous synchronization alters vaginal flora[2], our hypothesis was that estrus expression of ewes previously synchronized with intravaginal sponges will be less attractive than spontaneous natural estrus. The experiment was performed during the breeding season with two groups of 36 Corriedale x Milchschaf ewes (37.9 ± 0.7 kg). Estrus of 18 ewes was synchronized with intravaginal sponges impregnated with medroxiprogesterone acetate (50 mg, Sincrovin, Lab. Santa Elena, Montevideo, Uruguay) (group MAP), and the other 18 were in natural spontaneous estrus (group SE). Sexual attractiveness was determined with Tilbrook's attractiveness tests[3] in 12 groups of six estrous ewes (3 MAP and 3 SE) located in a small pen (4 m x 4 m). The courting and mating time that the ram spent with each ewe was recorded. After 5 min, the ewe with which the ram spent more time (most attractive ewe, ranked 1, scale 1 to 6) was taken out from the pen. The procedure was repeated until the ram ranked the 6 ewes. Sexual rank was compared with Friedman test for randomized block design. SE ewes were more attractive than MAP ewes: 2.9 ± 0.3 vs. 4.1 ± 0.3 respectively ($P < 0.002$). We concluded that ewes with spontaneous estrus are more attractive than ewes treated with intravaginal sponges. The lower sexual attractiveness of MAP ewes was probably related to alterations in vaginal flora.

[1]Ungerfeld and Silva, 2005. Appl Anim Behav Sci 93:245-250.
[2]Suárez *et al.*, 2005. Small Rum Res 63:39-43.
[3]Tilbrook and Lindsay, 1987. Appl Anim Behav Sci 17:129-138.

Uterine expression of Na^+/H^+ antiporters 1, 2, and 4 in beef cows following CIDR removal

JK Grant and GA Perry

Department of Animal and Range Sciences, South Dakota State University, Brookings, USA

Research has shown that uterine pH decreases at the onset of estrus in cows. When synchronized with a fixed-time AI protocol, cows that exhibited estrus around the time of AI had decreased uterine pH at insemination and greater pregnancy rates than cows that did not exhibit estrus. Additionally, research has reported the presence of Na^+/H^+ exchanger isoform 1, 2, and 4 in mouse uterine epithelium and their ability to extrude H^+ from the uterus to regulate uterine pH. Therefore, the objective of this study was to determine changes in uterine expression of Na^+/H^+ antiporter 1, 2, and 4 in cows from CIDR removal through 60 h following CIDR removal. Angus-cross beef cows (n = 40) were synchronized with a PG-CIDR protocol. Cows received $PGF_{2\alpha}$ on d -9, GnRH and insertion of a CIDR on d -6, and $PGF_{2\alpha}$ and CIDR removal on d 0. At CIDR removal, transrectal ultrasonography was performed to determine dominant follicle size. Cows were blocked by follicle size at time of CIDR removal, and uterine biopsies were collected every 12 h from CIDR removal (h 0) to h 60. Total cellular RNA was extracted from all biopsies, and relative mRNA levels were determined by real-time RT-PCR and corrected for GAPDH expression. Onset of estrus was determined by the HeatWatch Estrous Detection System from d 0 to d 5, and mean interval to estrus was 70.5 ± 1.7 h. There was no effect of estrus on expression of Na^+/H^+ antiporter 1, 2, or 4 ($P = 0.43$, $P = 0.33$, and $P = 0.88$, respectively). In addition there was no effect of time on expression of antiporter 4 ($P > 0.25$). Alternatively, there was an effect of time ($P < 0.05$ and $P = 0.04$) on antiporter 1 and 2 expression and an estrus by time interaction ($P = 0.05$, $P < 0.01$, and $P < 0.04$, respectively) on expression of antiporter 1, 2, and 4. Among cows that exhibited standing estrus, expression of antiporter 1 was decreased at 48 h compared to h 0 ($P = 0.05$), antiporter 2 expression was decreased at 12, 24, 36, 48, and 60 h compared to h 0 ($P < 0.01$), and antiporter 4 expression was decreased at 36, 48, and 60 h compared to h 0 ($P < 0.02$). Among cows that did not exhibit estrus, expression of antiporter 1, 2, and 4 did not change ($P > 0.14$, $P > 0.35$, and $P > 0.06$; respectively). In summary, expression of Na^+/H^+ antiporter 1, 2 and 4 decreased following CIDR removal among cows that exhibited standing estrus, but did not change among cows that did not exhibit estrus.

Underfeeding affects IGF-1 and gene expression in genital tract tissues in high producing dairy cows

D Valour[a], SA Degrelle[a], G Marot[b], S Dejean[c], O Dubois[a], I Hue[a], G Germain[a], P Humblot[d], A Ponter[a], G Charpigny[a] and B Grimard[a]

[a]*Biologie du Développement et de la Reproduction, Institut National de la Recherche Agronomique, Jouy en Josas, France;* [b]*INRA, UR337 Station de Génétique Quantitative et Appliquée, Jouy en Josas, France;* [c]*Institut de Mathématiques, Université Paul Sabatier, Toulouse, France;* [d]*Union Nationale des Coopératives d'Elevage et d'Insémination Animale, Cedex Maisons Alfort, France*

A decline in fertility in high producing dairy cows has been observed in France since the 1980s and is a cause of huge economic losses for dairy farmers. The decrease in fertility is linked to genetic (milk production potential) and environmental factors (alimentation). The negative energy balance observed during the postpartum period results from interactions between these factors. Previous studies have shown that this physiological state leads to modifications in gene expression profiles, particularly in the liver. The purpose of this project was to evaluate the influence of negative energy balance during the postpartum period on the gene expression profiles in the somatic tissues of the genital tract (oviduct, endometrium and corpus luteum). Holstein cows were randomly assigned to one of two treatment groups at calving: control (100% requirements, n=4) and underfed (40% requirements, n=4). There was no difference between the groups at calving for: age, body condition score, previous milk yield, sire fertility index and milk index. Blood samples were taken regularly postpartum and plasma analysed for selected metabolites and hormones. Oestrus was synchronised 80 d postpartum and tissue samples were taken from each pair of cows (control and underfed) 4, 8, 12 and 15 d later. Metabolic and transcriptomic data were generated. Principal canonical pathways altered in the different tissues were highlighted and statistical correlations between gene expression and blood metabolites were calculated. The main modifications in gene expression were found in the oviduct and in the endometrium whereas; the corpus luteum was not affected. The biological pathways which were modified differentially by energy balance were involved in lipid metabolism (Fatty Acid Binding Protein 5: *FABP5*), but also in other biological pathways potentially linked to fertility (Lipase H *LIPH*). Using statistical correlation analysis the data were integrated into a model which highlighted the central role of insulin-like growth factor-1 (*IGF-1*). In addition, IGF-1 appears to be a good predictor of energy balance in dairy cows.

Acknowledgments: This work received the financial support of the ANR GENANIMAL.

Immunohistochemical detection of estrogen and progesterone receptors in endometrial glands and stroma during the postpartum anestrus of Nelore (*Bos indicus*) cows

RS Lima[a], I Martin[a], WC Marques Filho[a], MMP Rodrigues[b], R Laufer-Amorim[b] and JCP Ferreira[a]

[a]*Department of Animal Reproduction and Veterinary Radiology, School of Veterinary Medicine and Animal Science (FMVZ) UNESP – Univ Estadual Paulista, Brazil;* [b]*Departament of Veterinary Clinic, (FMVZ) UNESP – Univ Estadual Paulista, Brazil*

During the estrous cycle, expression of estrogen (ERα) and progesterone (PR) receptor in the bovine reproductive tract is controlled by plasma concentrations of estrogens and progesterone. Estrogen is responsible for the stimulation of not only its own receptor expression, but PR as well. While progesterone can stimulate a decrease in uterine ERa after estrus; it also down-regulates uterine epithelial PR after several days of stimulation during the estrous cycle[1,2]. Little is known concerning the role ovarian follicular development may have on expression of uterine steroid receptors during the puerperal anestrous period in cattle. The objective of the present study was to determine if uterine expression of ERα and PR were affected by follicular growth and development during the postpartum anestrus period.

Fourteen postpartum, anestrous Nelore purebred cows were used in the study. Anestrus was determined based on the reproductive history which was confirmed in each cow by plasma progesterone concentration (<1 ng/ml) and on the absence of corpus luteum assessed by transrectal ultrasonography. During the ultrasonographic examination, the maximum follicle diameter was recorded and animals were separated into two groups - Group 1: cows with follicles <6 mm (n=7) and Group 2: cows with follicles ≥ 6 mm (n=7). Endometrial biopsies were collected and immunohistochemically stained for evaluation of ERα and PR in the uterine glandular epithelium and stroma. The number of positive nuclei and staining intensity of the nuclei (score 1 to 4) was evaluated for both ERα and PR.

High counts of positive nuclei (>80%) and high intensity of immunostaining (>2.7) for ERα and PR in the glandular epithelium and stroma were observed in the two groups. The score of immunostaining for the PR in the glandular epithelium, however, was higher in Group 2 (3.6) compared with Group 1 (2.7; $P<0.05$). When glandular epithelium and stroma were compared within each group, the relative number of ERα positive nuclei in the Group 1 was higher in the glandular epithelium (88.1) compared with stroma (80.5; $P<0.05$) and the score of immunostaining for the PR in Group 2 was higher in the glandular epithelium (3.6) compared with stroma (3.0; $P<0.05$).

Despite the fact that the follicular growth occurs during the anestrous period but has lower steroidogenic capability[3], steriod production appears to be sufficient for steroid receptor expression similar to that of animals during a regular estrous cycle[1]. However, the immunostainning intensity of PR in the glandular epithelium increased as the follicular diameter enlarged. Our results suggest that the mechanisms that control the expression of receptors during anestrus are similar to that observed during the estrous cycle.

This study was supported by FAPESP and FUNDUNESP, Brazil.

[1]Martin *et al.*, 2008. Reprod Domest Anim 43:415-421.
[2]Robinson *et al.*, 2001. J Reprod Fertil 122:965-979.
[3]Garverick *et al.*, 1988. J Anim Sci 66:104-111.

Morphometric evaluation of endometrial glands and progesterone serum levels in three different breeds of cattle in the Colombian tropics

AM Gonella[a], HA Grajales[a], R Martínez[b], Y Abuabara[b] and A Hernández[a]

[a]*Universidad Nacional de Colombia, Bogotá, Colombia;* [b]*Centro de Investigaciones Turipaná- Corpoica, Montería, Colombia*

In the cow, endometrial gland secretion is essential for embryonic development and implantation. Romosinuano (Romo) and costeño con cuernos (CCC) are Colombian-adapted cattle breeds with high reproductive efficiency. These breeds also have very high serum progesterone concentrations during the luteal phase of the estrous cycle[1]. This study was undertaken to measure progesterone serum concentration and endometrial gland morphology of three different breeds located in low lands of the Colombian tropics to determine if there is a relationship between endometrial morphology and serum progesterone concentrations during the estrous cycle.

Serum and endometrial biopsy samples were taken from 42 animals [Romo=15, CCC=15 and Holstein X Cebu (F1)=12] on d 0, 5, 10, 15 and 20 of the estrous cycle (d 0=estrus). Animals were maintained under good management conditions in Montería, Colombia (20 m above sea level, temperature = 27°C and 83% humidity). Radioimmunoassay was performed with a commercial kit (Coat-A-Count Progesterone kit, Diagnostics Products Corporation, Los Angeles, CA, USA) and all biopsy samples were stained with hematoxylin and eosin for microscopic evaluation. Ten optical fields (40x) were randomly chosen to calculate number, perimeter and area of glandular ducts and deep glands using computerized software (LECO 2001, LECO Instruments Ltd., St. Joseph, MI, USA). All data were subjected to a two-way analysis of variance for repeated measurements (SAS 9.0). To normalize data, logarithm transformations were carried out for progesterone values. The latter were different on d 5 ($P<0.1$) and 15 ($P<0.05$) of the estrous cycle among breeds. On d 5, serum progesterone concentrations (mean$\pm$SD) were 2.9 ± 1.34 ng/ml for Romo, 3.1 ± 2.03 ng/ml for CCC and 4.9 ± 1.95 ng/ml for F1 cows. On d 15, serum progesterone concentrations were 12.4 ± 5.22 ng/ml, 10.8 ± 5.26 ng/ml and 8.1 ± 1.91 ng/ml, respectively. No differences were detected for perimeter of superficial and deep glands. However, there was a breed ($P<0.05$) and time ($P<0.001$) effect on endometrial gland area measured as the percentage of total endometrial area.

The endometrial gland area was related to the progesterone concentrations[3], being higher during the luteal phase, and higher for the Romo and CCC ($P<0.05$) as compared with the crossbred cattle. It is suggested that greater serum progesterone concentrations stimulate an increase in uterine histotroph, which might account for the previously reported high reproductive efficiency of adapted cattle breeds in the Colombian tropics.

[1]Baez *et al.*, 2007. Livestock Research for Rural Development 19:132.
[2]Boos *et al.*, 1996. Anim Reprod Sci 44:11-21.
[3]Wang *et al.*, 2007. Reproduction 134:365-371.

Cyclooxygenase-2 (COX-2) distribution in endometrium of cycling and anoestrous ewes treated with GnRH with or without progesterone priming

C Tasende, G D'Anatro, C López, S Acuña, and EG Garófalo

Biochemistry, Faculty of Veterinary, Uruguay

The aim of this study was to investigate the distribution of COX-2 in the caruncular (CLE) and intercaruncular (ICLE) uterine luminal epithelium of cycling and anoestrous Corriedale ewes treated with GnRH with or without progesterone (P) priming.

Uteri and blood samples were collected after slaughter by exsanguination from 19 cycling ewes during the breeding season on d 1 (n = 7), 6 (n = 6) or 13 (n = 6) after oestrus detection (d 0). Twenty-two ewes in seasonal anoestrus were assigned to two groups: GnRH (n = 11) and P + GnRH (n = 11). The GnRH ewes were treated every 2 h with GnRH (6.7 ng i.v.) for 16 h, followed by bolus injection of GnRH (4 μg, d 0) at 18 h. The P + GnRH ewes were treated with P (0.33 g, CIDR) for 10 d and immediately after CIDR removal they were treated according to the same protocol as the GnRH ewes. Ewes were slaughtered by exsanguination on d 1 (n = 6, for each treatment) and d 5 (n = 5, for each treatment) after bolus injection (d 0). Samples of uterus and blood for COX-2 and P determinations (respectively) were immediately collected. The COX-2 was studied in CLE and ICLE by immunohistochemistry. The immunostaining was scored as negative (0), faint (1), moderate (2) or intense (3) and the proportion (n) of cells per field were expressed in a scale 0 to 10. The average of immunostaining intensity was calculated as $1n_1 + 2n_2 + 3n_3$. The data were analysed by ANOVA. The P concentrations (nmol/L, mean $\pm$ pooled s.e.m.) were 0.7 ± 0.6, 7.1 ± 0.9 and 10.3 ± 0.9 for d 1, 6 and 13 respectively in cycling ewes during the breeding season. In anoestrous ewes, the P concentrations at d 5 were lower in GnRH than P + GnRH treated ewes (3.1 ± 0.61 vs. 6.5 ± 0.54, respectively, $P < 0.001$).

In cycling ewes, the COX-2 distribution was influenced by the day of the cycle ($P < 0.001$). The intensity was greater at d 13 than at d 1 and 6 ($P < 0.05$). No differences between CLE and ICLE were found. In anoestrous ewes, the COX-2 distribution was influenced by treatments and day and there was interaction between both ($P < 0.05$). The COX-2 intensity on d 1 was lower in CLE in GnRH than P + GnRH ewes and no variation were found in ICLE. On d 5 the intensity was greater in GnRH ewes than P + GnRH ewes in both CLE and ICLE. The intensity in P + GnRH ewes in CLE decreased from d 1 to 5. On the contrary, in the GnRH ewes the COX-2 intensity increased from d 1 to 5 in both CLE and ICLE.

The increment of endometrial COX-2 expression at d 13 of the oestrous cycle is consistent with its participation in the known mechanism of normal luteolysis. The higher COX-2 expression at d 5 in GnRH – when compared with the P + GnRH – ewes suggest that COX-2 could be involved in triggering premature luteolysis, as a mechanism causing a short luteal phase.

The countercurrent transfer of $PGF_{2\alpha}$ from the uterus to the ovary at the time of luteolysis in ruminants is controlled by a prostaglandin transporter-mediated mechanism

JA McCracken[a], J Lee[b], SK Banu[b], R Rodriguez[b], TK Nithy[b] and JA Arosh[b]

[a]Department of Animal Science, University of Connecticut, Storrs, USA; [b]Reproductive Endocrinology and Cell Signaling Laboratory, Department of Veterinary Integrative Biosciences, College of Veterinary Medicine and Biomedical Sciences, Texas A&M University, College Station, USA

In ruminants, prostaglandin $F_{2\alpha}$ ($PGF_{2\alpha}$) is the uterine luteolytic hormone. During luteolysis, $PGF_{2\alpha}$ is synthesized and released from the endometrium in a pulsatile pattern. The unique structure of the vascular utero-ovarian plexus (UOP) allows the countercurrent transport of luteolytic $PGF_{2\alpha}$ pulses from the uterus directly to the ovary thus bypassing the systemic circulation where otherwise $PGF_{2\alpha}$ would be metabolized in the pulmonary circulation before reaching the ovary. The underlying molecular basis for the countercurrent transport of $PGF_{2\alpha}$ from the utero-ovarian vein to the ovarian artery in the UOP is not known.

The objective of the present study was to determine the role of the prostaglandin transporter protein (PGT) in the compartmental transport of $PGF_{2\alpha}$ from uterus to ovary through the UOP at the time of luteolysis using the sheep as a ruminant model. First, the expression of the PGT protein was determined in the UOP throughout the estrous cycle (n = five sheep per day of cycle). Second, [3H]-$PGF_{2\alpha}$ with or without a PGT inhibitor was infused into a uterine vein on cycle day 15 and the amount of [3H]-$PGF_{2\alpha}$ transferred to the adjacent ovarian artery was determined with (n = four sheep) or without (n = four sheep) the co-infusion of a PGT inhibitor. The effect of the PGT inhibitor on the transfer of endogenous $PGF_{2\alpha}$ generated by exogenous oxytocin was also investigated (n = five sheep for both test and control animals).

Using immunohistochemistry with quantification by Image-pro Plus, it was found that the PGT protein was expressed in the tunica intima, tunica media, and tunica adventitia of the utero-ovarian vein and the ovarian artery of the UOP, and that the expression levels were significantly greater ($P < 0.05$) on d 10 to 15 compared with d 3 to 6 of the estrous cycle. Maximal expression of PGT protein was observed on d 15 ($P < 0.05$). No significant difference ($P > 0.05$) in the expression levels of PGT was found for UOPs ipsilateral and contralateral to the ovary containing the corpus luteum. Pharmacological inhibition of the PGT protein reduced ($P < 0.05$) the countercurrent transfer of both exogenous [3H]-$PGF_{2\alpha}$ and oxytocin-induced endogenous of $PGF_{2\alpha}$ from the utero-ovarian vein to the ovarian artery by > 80%.

Taken together, these results indicate that at the time of luteolysis in sheep, the countercurrent transfer of $PGF_{2\alpha}$ from the uterus to the adjacent ovary through the UOP is regulated by a PGT-mediated mechanism. These findings also suggest that impaired PGT-mediated transport of $PGF_{2\alpha}$ from the utero-ovarian vein to the ovarian artery could adversely influence luteolysis and thus affect reproductive efficiency in ruminants.

Supported by the National Research Initiative (NRI) Competitive Grants program, Cooperative State Research, Education, and Extension Service (CSREES) USDA award 2008-35203-19101 to Joe A. Arosh and in part by USDA award 2004-35203-14176 to John A. McCracken.

In vitro evidence that leptin can modulate melatonin-induced prolactin secretion from ovine pituitary

M Szczesna[a], DA Zieba[a], B Klocek-Gorka[a] and K Romanowicz[b]

[a]*Agricultural University, Laboratory of Genomics and Biotechnology, Krakow, Poland;* [b]*Polish Academy of Sciences, Jablonna, Poland*

In temperate latitudes, sheep are seasonal breeders whose reproductive activity is regulated mainly by photoperiod. In this species, photoperiod and variable concentrations of melatonin can modulate secretion of pituitary hormones. Leptin, a hormone produced primarily by adipocytes, exerts influence on energetic homeostasis. However, contradictory results have been obtained in studies that investigated the secretion of prolactin (PRL) in sheep in response to leptin, under non-lactating conditions. The aim of this study was to investigate interactions between leptin and melatonin in the regulation of PRL secretion in short-term cultures of ovine pituitary explants, and to test the hypothesis that the day length can modify this interaction. Anterior pituitary glands from 15 Polish Longwool ewes were collected during different times of the year (May, July, September, October, November). Tissues were cut into approximately 100-mg explants, placed on a stainless steel grid covered with lens paper, and incubated in a gas-liquid interface in 2.5 ml of Medium 199 with or without melatonin (100 ng/ml). Cultures were carried out under 95% humidified air and 5% CO_2 at 37°C. After equilibration, explants were treated with control medium or medium containing leptin (50 ng/ml or 100 ng/ml) in a 90-min experiment. Incubation was continued for an additional 3.5 h period. Samples of medium were harvested every 30 min and stored at -20°C until RIA for PRL. Effects of leptin treatment on PRL secretion changed in a seasonally-dependent manner. In May and July, exogenous leptin (50 ng/ml) tended to stimulate PRL release, but this effect was only significant ($P<0.01$) in July. In autumn, a larger dose of leptin had no influence on PRL secretion. In October, the 50 ng/ml dose of leptin stimulated PRL release ($P<0.01$). In May, PRL concentrations were greater in explant media after 50 ng/ml of leptin compared with 100 ng/ml; however, during October and November these results were reversed. Melatonin stimulated PRL release in every month and the melatonin-induced increase in PRL release was inhibited by leptin in May, July, October and November. Melatonin affected secretion of PRL from ovine pituitary explants and exogenous leptin modulated this process.

Leptin treatment changes expression of the SOCS-3 gene in ovine anterior pituitary and medial basal hypothalamus in a seasonally-dependent manner

M Szczesna, DA Zieba and B Klocek-Gorka

Agricultural University, Department of Swine and Small Ruminant Breeding, Laboratory of Genomics and Biotechnology, Krakow, Poland

Suppressor of cytokine signaling (SOCS) proteins negatively regulate cytokine-induced signaling pathways and may be involved in leptin resistance. Leptin specifically induces expression of those factors in the hypothalamus in rodents. The aim of this study was to investigate whether leptin can modify the expression of SOCS-3 mRNA in the mediobasal hypothalamus (MBH) and anterior pituitary in seasonally-breeding sheep and to test the hypothesis that this process may be involved in photoperiod-driven changes in leptin sensitivity. Polish Longwool ewes surgically-fitted with third ventricle cannulas (n = 12), were used during the long-day season (LD, May) and an additional 12 ewes were used during the short-day season (SD, November). Animals were 2 to 3 yr of age and were fed *ad libitum*. During LD, ewes were anovulatory and during SD estrous cycles were synchronized. Treatments consisted of intracerebroventricular injection of: Ringer-Locke buffer (Control), or leptin at rates of 0.5 μg/kg (L1) and 1.0 μg/kg BW (L2), respectively. One h after injection, ewes were slaughtered and explants of MBH and anterior pituitaries were collected and snap frozen in liquid nitrogen. Total RNA from tissues was prepared and semiquantitative expression of SOCS-3 mRNA was performed using RT-PCR. The PCR products were separated on a 3% agarose gel, stained with ethidium bromide and analyzed using the Dscan Ex. v.3.1.0. program. In the MBH, leptin increased ($P < 0.001$) SOCS-3 mRNA expression during LD compared with controls. Concentrations of SOCS-3 mRNA in MBH during LD were almost twice in L2 compared with L1 ($P < 0.05$). There was no effect of leptin treatment on hypothalamic SOCS-3 expression during SD. In the anterior pituitary, leptin action was reversed compared with MBH. There were no changes in SOCS-3 mRNA after leptin infusion in LD, but during SD, exogenous leptin stimulated transcription of the SOCS-3 gene in a dose-dependent manner. These results provide evidence that in seasonal breeding sheep, the pattern of leptin action on expression of SOCS-3 mRNA differs between MBH and anterior pituitary in a seasonally-dependent manner. Results also indicate that, despite the occurrence of leptin resistance in the hypothalamus during LD, sensitivity of the anterior pituitary may be preserved.

Effect of energy supplementation on ovarian follicle profile in pre-pubertal Nelore heifers

GP Nogueira, LM Pavanello and RS Cipriano

UNESP-Universidade Estadual Paulista, Veterinary Medicine, Clovis Pestana 793, Araçatuba-SP, Brazil

Nelore is the main Brazilian beef breed. The breed is well adapted for tropical weather and extensive management but heifers reach puberty at 24 months of age. The major research aim is to decrease Nelore heifer age at puberty to 12 months. This will increase herd productivity up to 16%. Fat plays a crucial role in a heifer's age at puberty. The objective was to evaluate the ovarian follicle profile and age at first ovulation in pre-pubertal Nelore heifers supplemented with protected fat and high energy.

After weaning (8 months of age) 31 heifers from a commercial herd were tamed and adapted during 3 months to animal ration (R), protected-fat (F, Megalac®), corn (C) and sugar-cane bagasse (B) ingestion. Heifers were sorted according biotype (precocious and non-precocious) and equally distributed into 3 groups: Control (n=10; 2.2 kg R, 0.5 kg C, 5 kg B); Fat (n=11; 2.2 kg R, 0.2 kg F, 5 kg B); or Excess (n=10; 2.2 kg R, 0.2 kg F, 0.5 kg C, 5 kg B). The treatment duration was 82 d during the breeding season (from 358 to 440 d of age). Heifers had free access to pasture during the trial. Ovarian ultrasound was performed every 4 d and also daily for 17 d every other month either before (240 to 356 d of age) or during treatment. Body weight was measured every 15 d.

Only one heifer ovulated at 420 d of age and 246 kg body weight (Fat group). Live body weight did not vary between groups either before ($P=0.92$) or during treatment ($P=0.32$, Cont=267±29 kg, Fat=254±33 kg and Exc=254±25 kg). There was no difference in the largest follicle diameter either before ($P=0.58$; Cont=6.9±1.9 mm, Fat=7.2±1.6 mm and Exc=6.8±1.7 mm) or during treatment ($P=0.32$; Cont=9.0±1.1 mm, Fat=9.4±1.3 mm and Exc=9.0±1.6 mm). The total number of follicles did not vary before treatment ($P=0.46$; Cont= 6.2±1.4, Fat= 5.8±1.2 and Exc= 5.7±1.5). After nutritional treatment at 373 to 389 d of age, groups receiving fat had lesser numbers of follicles than control heifers ($P=0.019$, Cont= 8.1±1.7, Fat=6.9±1.6 and Exc= 6.6±1.7). At all the other daily evaluated intervals (246 to 274, 277 to 293, 323 to 338 and 418 to 434 d of age), there were no differences either in follicle numbers or largest follicle diameter.

In *Bos indicus* pre-pubertal heifers, energy excess had limited beneficial effect on age at first ovulation. During one period (373 to 389 d of age) fat supplementation decreased the number of follicles.

Acknowledgements: Fapesp for founding 08/57486-4 and scholarship 08/57492-4.

Effect of flushing and temporary calf removal on follicular development in primiparous Hereford cows

C Viñoles[a], L Veloz[b], MA Trobo[b], C García-Pintos[b] and M Carriquiry[c]

[a]National Research Institute for Agriculture, Tacuarembó, Uruguay; [b]Undergraduate students School of Veterinary Medicine, Montevideo, Uruguay; [c]School of Agronomy, Montevideo, Uruguay

Long periods of anoestrus (>120 d) in primiparous cows limit their reproductive efficiency[1]. Short-periods of improved nutrition and temporary weaning increase early pregnancy rate[2], but the underlying mechanisms involved in this response remain unknown.

To evaluate the effects of improved nutrition (flushing) and temporary weaning on follicular development and the quality of the cumulus oocyte complex (COC), 30 primiparous Hereford cows [388±7 kg body weight (BW) and 3.6±0.2 units of body condition score (BCS), scale 1 to 9] and their calves (120±2 kg BW) were selected at 103±1 d postpartum. The 2x2 factorial trial design included the effect of supplementation (n=15) and temporary weaning (n=15). The supplement (2.5 kg/cow of whole rice middlings; 90.3% DM, 10% CP, 9% EE, 14% NDF) was fed daily for 23 d and calves were temporary weaned by applying nose plates for 14 d. All cows grazed native pasture. Cows were injected three times with prostaglandin $F_{2\alpha}$ ($PGF_{2\alpha}$) 11 d apart. Thirty-six h after the last $PGF_{2\alpha}$ injection, cows were ovariectomized and all follicles >5 mm were dissected. Follicles were classified as healthy if they were pink or red, had blood vessels and the oocyte was found in the follicular fluid. The COC was classified using a scale from 1 (best quality) to 3 (worst quality) depending on the number and characteristics of the granulosa cell layers and the aspect of the cytoplasm. Means from a mixed model analyses were considered to differ when $P<0.05$.

The supplement did not affect cow BW or BCS but increased calf BW (130±2 kg vs. 124±2 kg). Temporary weaned calves were lighter (125±2 kg vs. 130±2 kg; $P<0.05$) but their mothers were heavier (405±7 kg vs. 396±2 kg) compared to those that suckled *ad libitum*. The supplement alone reduced the frequency of cyclic cows (4/7) that was increased by temporary weaning (7/8; $P<0.05$). The total numbers of follicles (67±10), the number of follicles >5 mm (4±1) and the number of healthy follicles (2±0.4) did not differ among groups. Supplementation increased the frequency of COC classified as class 1 (10/25 vs. 2/19). The mean size (7±1 mm) and the maximum diameter of healthy follicles (8±1 mm) were similar among groups. The size of healthy follicles and the quality of the COC were not correlated.

We conclude that supplementation decreases the frequency of primiparous cows that ovulate if it is not associated with temporary weaning. Nutrition had no effect on the number, health or size of follicles, but improved the quality of the COC. These results may explain the higher fertility observed in supplemented and temporarily weaned cows in previous studies.

[1]Quintans *et al.*, 2009. Ann Mtg Eur Assoc Anim Prod, Barcelona, Spain, 241.
[2]Pérez-Clariget *et al.*, 2007. Archivos Latinoamericanos de Producción Animal 15:114.

Effect of flushing on follicular health and quality of the cumulus oocyte complex in cyclic Hereford cows grazing native pastures

C Viñoles[a], L Veloz[b], MA Trobo[b], C García-Pintos[b] and M Carriquiry[c]

[a]National Research Institute for Agriculture, Tacuarembó, Uruguay; [b]Undergraduate students School of Veterinary Medicine, Montevideo, Uruguay; [c]School of Agronomy, Montevideo, Uruguay

A positive energy balance increases the size and the steroidogenic capacity of the dominant follicle[1]. The steroidogenic capacity of a follicle correlates positively with the quality of the cumulus oocyte complex (COC), thus with its developmental capacity[2]. The information linking the effect of a nutritional supplementation on the health of follicles and the quality of the COC, however, is lacking.

Thirteen cyclic multiparous Hereford cows (492 ± 6 kg body weight and 5.6 ± 0.1 units of body condition, scale 1 to 9) were randomly allocated to two groups: control, non-supplemented (n = 7) and supplemented (n = 7). The supplement (2.5 kg/cow of whole rice middlings, 90.3% DM, 10% CP, 9% EE, 14% NDF) was offered daily for 23 d. All cows grazed native pastures. Cows were injected three times with prostaglandin $F_{2\alpha}$ ($PGF_{2\alpha}$) 11 d apart to synchronize follicular growth. Feeding started the day after the first $PGF_{2\alpha}$. Thirty-six h after the last $PGF_{2\alpha}$ injection, cows were ovariectomized and all follicles > 5 mm were dissected and the oocytes were recovered. Follicles were classified as healthy if they were pink or red, had blood vessels and the oocyte was found in the follicular fluid. The COC was classified using a scale from 1 (best quality) to 3 (worst quality), depending on the number and characteristics of the granulosa cell layers and the aspect of the cytoplasm. Means from a mixed models analyses were considered to differ when $P < 0.05$.

Supplementation did not affect cow body weight or body condition score. The total number of follicles was similar between control (42 ± 10) and supplemented cows (30 ± 12). The total number of follicles > 5mm (3 ± 1 vs. 4 ± 1) and the number of healthy follicles > 5 mm (3 ± 0.4 vs. 3 ± 0.4), were not different between control and supplemented cows, respectively. Supplementation increased the frequency of COC classified as class 1 (4/13 vs. 0/18; $P < 0.05$) and decreased the frequency of COC classified as class 3 (3/13 vs. 10/18; $P < 0.05$). Supplementation did not affect the mean size of 5 to 10 mm follicles (7 ± 0.4 vs. 6 ± 0.4 mm for control and supplemented cows, respectively) or the maximum size (13 ± 0.8 for control and supplemented cows) of healthy follicles. The size of healthy follicles and the quality of the COC were not correlated.

We conclude that supplementation has no effect on the number, health or size of follicles but improves the quality of the COC that may have important implications for cow fertility. The effect on COC quality may be caused by a better endocrine milieu promoted by glucose and metabolic hormones, independent of the size (e.g. steroidogenic capacity) of the follicles.

[1]Butler, 2003. Livestock Prod Sci 83:211-218.
[2]Araki *et al.*, 1998. J Reprod Devel 44:359-365.

Effect of short-prepartum supplementation on reproductive and productive performance in primiparous beef cows under grazing conditions

A Scarsi[a], A Astessiano[b], G Banchero[a], M Carriquiry[b] and G Quintans[a]

[a]*Instituto Nacional de Investigación Agropecuaria, INIA, Treinta y Tres, Uruguay;* [b]*Facultad de Agronomía, Montevideo, Uruguay*

Multiparous dairy cows increased their reproductive performance after a short-term prepartum supplementation[1]. Grazing conditions improved supply of nutrients in the last month of gestation in multiparous beef cows and enhanced reproductive performace, possibly due to a modification in the partitioning of nutrients between body reserves and milk production[2]. The aim of this experiment was to evaluate the effect of a short-term prepartum supplementation on reproductive and productive parameters in cow performance. Twenty-five Aberdeen Angus x Hereford crossbred cows were grouped into two blocks according expected calving date. Sixty d before the expected calving date, cows were assigned randomly to two treatments: i) cows grazed native pastures (CON; n=14); ii) cows grazed native pasture and were supplemented (SUP; n=11) with 1 kg/100kg body weight (BW) of a mix (67:33% as-fed basis; 16% CP, 11% ADF) of sorghum grain and protein concentrated from 36±2.8 d prepartum until calving (d=0). Cows of both treatments grazed together during the whole experimental period and were offered on average 14 kg DM/100 kg BW of native pasture (8.5% CP, 69.9% NDF, 37.6% ADF, 59.8% OMD). Body weight and body condition score (BCS) were recorded from -42 to 170 d postpartum (DPP) every 28 d. All cows were bled by jugular venipunture from d -42 to 112 for progesterone analysis. Resumption of ovarian activity was defined as the first of two consecutive samples with progesterone concentration greater than 1 ng/ml. Data were analyzed using linear models with repeated measures and the model included effects of treatment, BW, BCS, interaction of treatment by day postpartum (DPP) and covariance correction. Analyses were carried out using the PROC MIXED procedure (SAS v 9.1). The proportions of cows cycling or getting pregnant were analyzed with a generalized linear model (PROC GENMOD, SAS v 9.1).

Cows in the SUP treatment weighed more ($P<0.05$) than CON cows (422±6.78 vs. 413±6.78 kg). Also BW changed significantly ($P<0.001$) along the experimental period. Cows lost BW from -28 to 28 d and then gained BW until d 112 when they started losing BW again. Body condition score was similar between SUP and CON cows (4.25±0.08 units). Moreover there was a trend ($P=0.06$) for the interaction between treatments and time for BCS, which reflected a greater decline in BCS in CON compared with SUP cows (0.85±0.08 vs. 0.69±0.08 units for CON and SUP cows, respectively). The average milk production of cows was similar in CON and SUP cows (4.22±0.57 kg/d). Milk production decreased over time ($P<0.001$) from 5.6 kg/d at d 30 to 3.3 ± 0.6 kg/d at d 180. The proportion of cycling cows was similar between SUP and CON cows (55 vs. 43% for SUP and CON, respectively). Similarly, no differences were found in pregnancy rate (36% for CON and SUP cows). In the conditions of the present experiment primiparous cows did not increase their reproductive performance with a short-term prepartum supplementation. We can speculate that younger cows are partitioning nutrients in a different manner with respect to multiparous cows and are prioritizing nutrients for growth. Further research is needed in this area.

[1]Chagas *et al.*, 2006. J Dairy Sci 89:1981-1989.
[2]Carriquiry *et al.*, 2009. J Anim Sci 87(E-Suppl 2):M238.

Short-prepartum supplementation effect on productive and reproductive parameters in multiparous beef cows under grazing conditions I

A Scarsi[a], A Astessiano[b], G Banchero[a], M Carriquiry[b] and G Quintans[a]

[a]*Instituto Nacional de Investigación Agropecuaria, INIA, Treinta y Tres, Uruguay;* [b]*Facultad de Agronomía, Montevideo, Uruguay*

Under extensive spring calving conditions, the last third of gestation takes place in winter, when native pastures are-low producing. Pregnant cows, therefore, mobilize a high quantity of body reserves[1]. The objective of this study was to evaluate the effects of a prepartum short-term supplementation in beef cows grazing native pastures on body weight (BW), body condition score (BCS, 1 = thin 8 = fat), plasma insulin, ovarian activity and pregnancy rate. The experiment involved 26 multiparous Aberdeen Angus x Hereford crossbred cows. Sixty days before the expected calving date, cows were assigned randomly to two treatments: i) cows grazed native pastures (CON; n = 13): ii) cows grazed native pasture and were supplemented (SUP; n = 13) with 1 kg/100 kg BW of whole-rice bran (14.9% CP, 20.7% NDF, 8.2% ADF). In the early morning SUP cows were separated from CON cows and were supplemented in feeding troughs during the last 40 ± 0.6 d of gestation (calving = d 0). Cows of both treatments grazed together during the entire experimental period and were offered on average 9 kg DM/100 kg BW of native pasture (9.5% CP, 69.4% NDF, 41.1% ADF, 55% OMD). Body weight and BCS were recorded every 28 d. Blood samples were collected in all cows weekly by jugular venipunture from d -42 to 112 for insulin and progesterone analyses. Resumption of ovarian activity was defined as the first of 2 consecutive samples with progesterone concentration greater than 1 ng/ml. The breeding season started at d 60 and lasted 60 d. Data of BW, BCS and plasma insulin were analyzed using linear models with repeated measures and the model included effects of treatment, interaction of treatment by day postpartum (DPP) and covariance correction using the PROC MIXED procedure. The probabilities of cows cycling or getting pregnant were analyzed with a generalized linear model (PROC GENMOD, SAS).

Cow BW and BCS did not differ between treatments (453 ± 3 kg, 4.0 ± 0.1), however, there was a trend for the interaction between treatment and DPP for BCS ($P = 0.06$). The nadir of BCS was reached at 60 DPP in both groups of cows, but SUP tended ($P = 0.069$) to lose less BCS than CON (0.5 vs. 0.7 units for SUP and CON cows, respectively). Plasma insulin concentrations did not differ between treatments (4.07 ± 0.22 μU/ml). The probability of cows cycling during the first 120 DPP was greater ($P = 0.002$) in SUP than in CON cows (92 vs. 69%). Also, the probability of pregnancy was greater ($P = 0.002$) in SUP than CON cows (84% vs. 61 for SUP and CON, respectively). A short prepartum supplementation increased reproductive performance although the real underlying mechanisms involved in this response remain unclear. Further research is needed.

[1]Quintans *et al.*, 2009. EAAP 60th 21:241.

Short-prepartum supplementation effect on productive and reproductive parameters in multiparous beef cows under grazing conditions II

A Scarsi[a], A Astessiano[b], G Banchero[a], M Carriquiry[b] and G Quintans[a]

[a]*Instituto Nacional de Investigación Agropecuaria, INIA, Treinta y Tres, Uruguay;* [b]*Facultad de Agronomía, Montevideo, Uruguay*

During the last trimester of gestation, pregnant cows present high nutrient demands and generally mobilize body reserves when they are managed on native pastures during the winter. The objective of this study was to evaluate the effects of a prepartum short-term supplementation in beef cows grazing native pastures on milk production and calves performance. Twenty six multiparous Aberdeen Angus x Hereford crossbred cows were used in this experiment. Sixty days before the expected calving date, cows were assigned randomly to two treatments: i) cows grazed native pastures alone (CON; n=13); ii) cows grazed native pasture and were supplemented (SUP; n=13) with 1 kg/100 kg body weight (BW) of whole-rice bran (14.9% CP, 20.7% NDF, 8.2% ADF) during the last 40 ± 0.6 d of gestation (calving=d 0). Milk production (MP) was assessed by milking procedure at 30 d postpartum (pp) and every 30 d thereafter until weaning (d 180). All cows were bled weekly by jugular venipuncture from d -42 to 112 for non-esterified fatty acid (NEFA) analysis. Calf BW was recorded at birth and every 28 d until weaning. Data were analyzed using linear models with repeated measures analyses using the PROC MIXED procedure (SAS v9.1).

Average MP did not differ between treatments (4.7 ± 0.21 kg/d). There was an effect of time on MP, because there was a decrease ($P<0.001$) in MP during the postpartum period. Moreover, MP at d 30 was 6.4±0.4 kg/d whereas at d 180 it was 4.4±0.4 kg/d. A treatment by time interaction on NEFA concentrations was found ($P<0.001$). At d -28, SUP cows had lesser ($P<0.05$) NEFA concentrations than CON cows (0.44±0.05 vs. 0.58±0.05 mmol/L for SUP and CON, respectively). However, during the postpartum period SUP cows had greater ($P<0.0001$) NEFA concentrations than CON cows (0.52±0.02 vs. 0.37±0.02 mmol/L for SUP and CON, respectively). Calf BW did not differ between treatment at birth (40.3±1.4 kg) or at weaning (188.0±3.0 kg). Under the conditions of the present experiment, a short-term prepartum supplementation did not affect milk production or calf weight.

Nutritional regulation of body condition score at the initiation of the transition period in dairy cows on grazing conditions: hepatic expression of the somatotropic axis genes

M Carriquiry[a], ML Adrien[b], V Artegoitia[b], D Mattiauda[a] and A Meikle[b]

[a]*School of Agronomy, UDELAR, Montevideo, Uruguay;* [b]*School of Veterinary Medicine, UDELAR, Montevideo, Uruguay*

The somatotropic axis varies with nutritional status and lactation of cows, and has been associated with reproductive performance. Reduced insulin-like growth factor (IGF)-I concentrations during the transition period have been related to prolonged postpartum anestrus on confined and grazing production systems1,2 and hepatic growth hormone receptor (GHR) and IGF binding protein (BP)-2 mRNA expression have been positively associated with pregnancy establishment 3.

Multiparous Holstein cows (n = 10), blocked by body weight and expected calving date, were used to investigate the effect of different body condition score (BCS, scale 1 to 5) at 30 d before calving, induced by a differential nutritional management from -100 until -30 d, on hepatic expression of somatotropic axis genes during the transition period. From -100 to -30 d, cows were offered different planes of nutrition with approximately 7, 14 or 20 kg DM/cow of a long-term pasture to achieve a desired BCS at –30 d. Body condition score was determined every 15 d, and cows had to gain 0.5 points (HI) or to maintain (LO) BCS at least in two subsequent observations to be included in the study. From -30 to +45 d cows were managed together. Liver biopsies were collected at -15, +15, and +45 d and GHR, IGF-I, BP-2, and BP-3 mRNA were determined by real time PCR using hypoxanthine phosphoribosyltransferase as a control gene. Means from mixed model analyses differed when $P < 0.05$.

Cows had similar BCS at -100 d and differed after the nutritional treatment, but all groups presented similar BCS at +21 d. Circulating IGF-I concentrations were greater in HI than LO cows (98.9 vs. 79.6 ± 5.7 ng/mL) and decreased from pre to postpartum. Expression of GHR mRNA was greater in HI than LO cows (1.51 vs. 0.67 ± 0.55) and decreased at +45 d for HI cows while remained constant for LO cows. Expression of IGF-I and BP3 mRNA were not affected by BCS at -30 d, days or their interaction. In contrast, BP2 mRNA was reduced in HI than LO cows (4.2 vs. 11 ± 1.8) and peaked at +15 d. The ratio BP3/BP2 tended to be greater ($P = 0.09$) in HI than LO cows and to decrease ($P = 0.07$) from pre to postpartum (0.17, 0.09, 0.08 ± 0.03 for -15, +15, and +45 d, respectively). Circulating IGF-I was correlated ($r = 0.44$, $P = 0.03$) with BP3/BP2 ratio. Days to first ovulation were reduced for HI than LO cows (39.1 vs. 22.1 ± 2 d).

The plane of nutrition that resulted in different BCS at the initiation of the transition period affected the liver expression of the somatotropic axis genes that can be reflected in the endocrine/metabolic milieu which in turn may be associated with a differential length of the anestrous period.

[1]Meikle et al., 2004. Reproduction 127:727-737.
[2]Taylor et al., 2004. Vet Rec 155:583-588.
[3]Rhoads et al., 2008. J Dairy Sci 91:140-150.

Effects of polyunsaturated fatty acids (PUFA) supplementation on serum concentrations of progesterone and insulin of dairy cows

BI Cappellozza[a], P Moriel[a], LF Ferraretto[a], A Aboin[a], FVR Vieira[a], RF Cooke[b] and JLM Vasconcelos[a]

[a]*FMVZ/UNESP, Botucatu, Brazil;* [b]*Oregon State University, Eastern Oregon Agricultural Research Center, Burns, USA*

Supplementation with PUFA for 28 d beginning at AI increased pregnancy rates in beef cows, and this outcome was attributed, in part, to the beneficial effects of PUFA on serum progesterone (P4) concentrations[1]. To determine if PUFA also increases serum P4 concentrations in dairy cows, and potentially benefits their reproductive function, two experiments were conducted.

In experiment 1, 11 non-lactating, non-pregnant, ovariectomized Gir x Holstein cows were assigned to one of three treatments, arranged in a 3 × 3 Latin square design with experimental periods of 7 d each: 1) control (4.5 kg/cow daily of a grain-based concentrate), 2) SF (control with the inclusion of 220 g/cow daily of a saturated fatty acid source; Megalac®, Church and Dwight, Princeton, NJ, USA), and 3) PF (control with the inclusion of 220 g/cow daily of a PUFA source; Megalac-E®, QGN Carbonor, Rio de Janeiro, Brazil). Blood samples were collected at d 7 of each experimental period, immediately prior to and at 3, 6, 9 and 12 h relative to treatment feeding for determination of serum P4 and insulin concentrations. In Exp. 2, 45 non-lactating, pregnant, multiparous and primiparous Holstein cows were randomly assigned to receive a corn silage-based diet added with one of the following treatments for a 14-day period: 1) control (500 g/cow daily of ground corn + 220 g/cow daily of kaolin), 2) SF (500 g/cow daily of ground corn + 220 g/cow daily of a saturated fatty acid source; Megalac®, Church and Dwight), and 3) PF (500 g/cow daily of ground corn + 220 g/cow daily of a PUFA source; Megalac-E®, QGN Carbonor). Blood samples were collected on d 7 and d 14, immediately prior to and at 3, 6, 9 and 12 h relative to treatment feeding for determination of serum P4 concentrations.

In experiment 1, control cows had greater ($P=0.02$) serum concentrations of P4 compared with PF cows (1.34 vs. 1.20 ng/mL of P4, respectively), but similar ($P=0.29$) compared with cows fed SF (1.28 ng/mL of P4). Serum concentrations of P4 were also similar ($P=0.23$) between SF and PF cows. Dietary treatment did not affect ($P=0.47$) serum concentrations of insulin. In experiment 2, dietary treatments did not affect ($P=0.65$) serum P4 concentrations in multiparous cows. However, PF heifers had greater ($P=0.03$) serum P4 concentrations compared with control cohorts (7.58 vs. 6.43 ng/mL of P4, respectively), but similar ($P=0.77$) compared with SF heifers (7.43 ng/mL of P4).

In conclusion, fatty acid supplementation increased serum P4 concentrations in non-lactating dairy heifers, but the same effect was not observed in multiparous cohorts.

[1]Lopes *et al.*, 2009. J Anim Sci 87:3935-3943.

Effects of polyunsaturated fatty acids (PUFA) supplementation on progesterone production and time of luteolysis in non-pregnant Nelore cows

CN Lopes[a,b], RFG Peres[a], M Reis[a], T Araújo[b], RF Cooke[c] and JLM Vasconcelos[a]

[a]FMVZ/UNESP, Botucatu, Brazil; [b]QGN Carbonor, Rio de Janeiro, Brazil; [c]Oregon State University, Eastern Oregon Agricultural Research Center, Burns, USA

Three experiments were conducted to further understand the mechanisms through which PUFA supplementation after AI enhances reproductive performance in beef cows[1]. In experiment 1, 51 multiparous non-lactating Nelore cows with synchronized ovulation were used to determine if PUFA influences progesterone (P4) production during the estrous cycle and timing of luteolysis. In experiment 2, 43 multiparous non-lactating Nelore cows with synchronized ovulation were used to evaluate if PUFA changes the responsiveness of a 6-d old corpus luteum to exogenous prostaglandin $F_{2\alpha}$ (12.5 mg of dinoprost tromethamine, i.m.). In experiment 3, 27 multiparous lactating Nelore cows with synchronized ovulation and approximately 30 to 40 d postpartum were used to determine if PUFA alters the incidence of short cycles. For all experiments, cows were randomly assigned to one of the three dietary treatments offered daily during the experimental period: 1) Control (100 g of mineral mix + 100 g of ground corn + 100 g of kaolin), 2) SF (100 g of mineral mix + 100 g of ground corn + 100 g of a saturated fatty acid source; Megalac®, Church and Dwight, Princeton, NJ, USA), and 3) PF (100 g of mineral mix + 100 g of ground corn + 100 g of PUFA source; Megalac-E®, QGN Carbonor, Rio de Janeiro, Brazil).

In experiments 1, 2, and 3, no treatment effects were detected ($P > 0.10$), respectively, in serum P4 concentrations, time and rate of luteolysis, and in the incidence of short cycles. When data from experiments 1 and 2 were combined, serum P4 concentrations were greater ($P=0.01$) on d 6 following ovulation in PF cows compared with SF and control cohorts (4.45, 3.25 and 3.48 ng/mL of P4, respectively, SEM=0.28).

These results indicate that although PUFA supplementation did not influence overall P4 concentrations during the estrous cycle, time of luteolysis, corpus luteum responsiveness to prostaglandin $F_{2\alpha}$, and incidence of short cycles, it increased serum P4 concentrations on d 6 following ovulation, which can be one of the mechanisms through which PUFA supplementation enhances reproductive performance in beef cows.

[1]Lopes *et al.*, 2009. J Anim Sci 87:3935-3943.

Effects of polyunsaturated fatty acids (PUFA) supplementation during different periods on pregnancy rates of Nelore beef cows

CN Lopes[a,b], RFG Peres[a], I Claro Jr.[a], T Martins[a], M Tavares[a], T Araújo[b], RF Cooke[c] and JLM Vasconcelos[a]

[a]*FMVZ/UNESP, Botucatu, Brazil;* [b]*QGN Carbonor, Rio de Janeiro, Brazil;* [c]*Oregon State University, Eastern Oregon Agricultural Research Center, Burns, USA*

Supplementation with PUFA for 28 d, but not for 16 d, beginning at AI increased pregnancy rates in Nelore beef cows[1]. To further explore these outcomes, two experiments evaluating different lengths in post-AI PUFA supplementation were conducted. The supplemental treatments offered during both experiments were: 1) control (100 g of mineral mix + 100g of ground corn + 100 g of kaolin), 2) SF (100 g of mineral mix + 100 g of ground corn + 100 g of a saturated fatty acid source; Megalac®, Church and Dwight, Princeton, NJ, USA), and 3) PF (100 g of mineral mix + 100 g of ground corn + 100 g of PUFA source; Megalac-E®, QGN Carbonor, Rio de Janeiro, Brazil).

In experiment 1, 1457 multiparous lactating Nelore cows, averaging 40 to 60 d postpartum, were randomly allocated to 28 *Brachiaria humidicula* pastures. Pastures were assigned to one of the following supplementation schemes for 28 d beginning at fixed-time AI (d 0): 1) control from d 0 to 28, 2) SF from d 0 to 14 and control from d 15 to 28, 3) PF from d 0 to 14 and control from d 15 to 28, 4) SF from d 0 to 21 and control from d 22 to 28, 5) PF from d 0 to 21 and control from d 22 to 28, 6) SF from d 0 to 28, 7) PF from d 0 to d 28. In experiment 2, 502 multiparous lactating Nelore cows, averaging 40 to 60 d postpartum, were randomly allocated to 12 *B. humidicula* pastures. Pastures were assigned to one of the following supplementation schemes for 21 d beginning at fixed-time AI (d 0): 1) PF from d 0 to 14 and control from d 15 to 21, 2) control from d 0 to 6 and PF from d 7 to 21, 3) control from d 0 to d 13, and PF from d 14 and 21, 4) PF from d 0 to 21.

In experiment 1, cows fed PF for 21 and 28 d after AI had greater ($P<0.05$) pregnancy rates compared with all other treatments combined (50.4 vs. 42.4%, respectively). No differences were detected in pregnancy rates between cows receiving PF for 21 or 28 d (50.9 vs. 49.8 %, respectively). In experiment 2, cows receiving PF for 21 d after AI had greater ($P<0.05$) pregnancy rates compared with cows receiving PF for 14 d after AI (46.8 vs. 33.6 %, respectively). No further effects were detected.

These results indicate that PUFA increases pregnancy rates if supplemented for at least 21 d following AI.

[1]Lopes *et al.,* 2009. J Anim Sci 87:3935-3943.

Effects of polyunsaturated fatty acids (PUFA) supplementation on pregnancy rates to fixed-time AI in crossbred dairy cows

RFG Peres[a], CN Lopes[a,b], I Claro Jr.[a], T Araújo[b], RF Cooke[c] and JLM Vasconcelos[a]

[a]*FMVZ/UNESP, Botucatu, Brazil;* [b]*QGN Carbonor, Rio de Janeiro, Brazil;* [c]*Oregon State University, Eastern Oregon Agricultural Research Center, Burns, USA*

Supplementation with PUFA for 28 d beginning at AI increased pregnancy rates in Nelore beef cows[1]. The objective was to determine if PUFA supplementation during the same time frame would also increase pregnancy rates to a fixed-time AI protocol in *Bos indicus*-influenced dairy cows.

Multiparous lactating Gir x Holstein dairy cows (n=374), maintained on pasture and averaging 40 to 150 d postpartum, were assigned to receive a 2 mg treatment of estradiol benzoate (Estrogin®; Farmavet, São Paulo, Brazil) and an intravaginal progesterone releasing device (CIDR®; containing 1.9 g of progesterone; Pfizer Animal Health, Sao Paulo, Brazil) on d -11 of the study, a 12.5 mg prostaglandin $F_{2\alpha}$ treatment (Lutalyse®; Pfizer Animal Health) on d -4, a 0.5 mg treatment of estradiol cypionate (ECP®; Pfizer Animal Health) and CIDR® removal on d -2, followed by TAI on d 0. In addition to the pasture consumption and a common concentrate offered daily, cows were randomly assigned to receive one of the two supplement treatments offered daily for 28 d following AI: 1) control (500 g/cow of ground corn), 2) PF (230 g/cow of PUFA source; Megalac-E®, QGN Carbonor, Rio de Janeiro, Brazil). Pregnancy status was verified by detecting a fetus with transrectal ultrasonography on d 28. Pregnancy rates were analyzed with the LOGISTIC procedure of SAS, and the model included the effects of treatment, parity, days postpartum, BCS, and appropriate interactions. No significant interactions containing the treatment variable were detected. Pregnancy rates were greater ($P<0.05$) in PF-fed cows compared with control cohorts (46.5 vs. 37.2 %, respectively).

These results indicate that, similarly to our previous research effort with beef cows[1], PUFA supplementation after AI increased pregnancy rates in *Bos indicus*-influenced lactating dairy cows.

[1]Lopes *et al.*, 2009. J Anim Sci 87:3935-3943.

The effect of microalgae supplementation on the mRNA expression for gluconeogenic enzymes in liver of transition dairy cows

M Hostens[a], L Peelman[b], V Fievez[c] and G Opsomer[a]

[a]*Department of Obstetrics, Reproduction and Herd Health, Faculty of Veterinary Medicine;* [b]*Department of Animal Nutrition, Genetics, Breeding and Ethology, Faculty of Veterinary Medicine;* [c]*Laboratory for Animal Nutrition and Animal Product Quality, Faculty of Bioscience Engineering, Ghent University, Ghent, Belgium*

Many efforts have been made to alleviate the negative energy balance (NEBAL) of high yielding dairy cows early postpartum. One of the proposed means is the induction of milk fat depression (MFD) in order to substantially decrease the 'loss' of energy as the production of fat is associated with the highest demand for energy[1]. When fed to dairy cows during transition, docosahexaenoic acid (DHA) enriched microalgae (Schizochytrium spp.) are able to induce a MFD as described recently by our research group[2]. In contrast to the proposed mechanism to diminish the NEBAL in dairy cows, the MFD was accompanied by an increase in milk production leading to an even more severe NEBAL as measured in the serum as well as in the follicular fluid. The objective of the present experiment was to investigate the mRNA expression in the liver of 9 candidate genes known to be involved in the adaptation of the intermediary metabolism of the dairy cows in the transition period and to determine changes in abundance of these mRNA in response to MFD in the postpartum period. The expression of these genes might partially explain the increase in milk production and worsened NEBAL.

Holstein Friesian cows were fed either a control diet (C; n=8), or a diet in which 2 kg of concentrates was replaced by an iso-energetic concentrate containing microalgae (ALG; n=8) from wk -3 to 9 relative to calving. Liver biopsies were taken on d 2 and d 30 postpartum. Milk production parameters were monitored until wk 9 postpartum. The mRNA expression was assessed by means of RT–qPCR. Data analysis was performed using the PROC MIXED procedure of SAS. ALG increased milk yield ($P=0.057$) whereas milk fat yield ($P=0.005$) and milk fat content ($P=0.011$) decreased. Protein yield ($P=0.465$) was not affected but a tendency for reduced milk protein content ($P=0.094$) was observed.

The relative mRNA abundance was significantly higher at d 2 as compared to d 30 for pyruvate carboxylase ($P=0.0052$) and lower for growth hormone receptor 1A ($P=0.0027$) and insulin like growth factor-I ($P=0.046$). Similar time dependent changes in early lactation have been reported by Greenfield et al. (2000)[3] and Lucy et al. (2008)[4]. Neither the diet nor the interaction between time of sampling and the diet significantly affected the mRNA abundance.

Further studies should focus on the role of the liver in the regulation of EBAL in response to MFD as induced by ALG in postpartum dairy cows.

[1]Jensen, 2002. J Dairy Sci 85:295-350.
[2]Hostens *et al.*, 2009. Rum Phys 2009:712-713.
[3]Greenfield *et al.*, 2000. J Dairy Sci 83:1228-1236.
[4]Lucy, 2008. Reprod Dom Anim 43(Suppl.2):31-39.

Nutritional supplements, metabolic and reproductive hormones, and ovarian activity in Australian Cashmere goats

M Shikh Maidin, JTB Milton, PA Hawken and GB Martin

UWA Institute of Agriculture, The University of Western Australia, Crawley, Australia

In sheep, short-term supplements increase ovulation rate, perhaps due to actions of leptin and insulin on the follicles, but decrease the circulating concentrations of progesterone due to an increase in the catabolism and clearance of progesterone by the liver. Generally, goats are more fecund than sheep so the processes that determine reproductive outcomes may differ, including their responses to nutritional supplements. We therefore studied the effect of a short-term supplement of high-protein lupin grain in Cashmere goats.

We allocated 28 females into two equal groups: the control group received a daily allowance that ensured maintenance of body mass (90% chaff, 10% lupins per head per d); the treated group was fed a diet that supplied twice the daily requirements for maintenance. The cycles of all females were synchronized via an 18 d treatment with intravaginal progestagen pessaries (CIDR). The nutritional treatments lasted for 21 d, commencing 10 d before CIDR withdrawal (i.e., 11 d prior to introduction of bucks; d 1). The bucks were removed on d 5. Blood was sampled every 2 d, from d 1 of nutritional treatment until d 12 after CIDR removal (d 0). Plasma was separated and later assayed for progesterone, insulin and leptin. During the period of supplementary feeding, the concentrations of insulin and leptin were greater ($P<0.001$) in the treatment group than in the control group. This difference disappeared immediately after the end of supplementation. During the preovulatory period (d -10 to d 0), the concentration of progesterone was greater ($P<0.05$) in control than in treated females but, during the early post-ovulatory period (d 1 to 12), this effect was reversed. Ovulation rate was determined by laparoscopy on d 12 after CIDR removal, and there was no significant difference between groups (2.14 ± 2.73 treated vs. 1.79 ± 1.45 controls; $P>0.05$).

In conclusion, female goats fed with high-protein lupin grain showed an elevation in the concentration of insulin and leptin, as seen in female sheep. This was not associated with a significant increase in ovulation rate. Furthermore, does supplemented with lupins had higher post-ovulatory concentration of progesterone than does in the control group. It therefore seems that, in contrast to sheep, nutrition does not accelerate the catabolism and clearance of progesterone by the liver.

Thank you to Ministry of Higher Education Malaysia (MOHE) to providing the scholarship and to Rural Industries Research & Development Corporation (RIRDC) for research funding.

Unrecognized variation in gestation length and birth weight of Droughtmaster calves produced through fixed-time AI

BM Burns[a], AD Herring[b], A Laing[a], G Fordyce[a], J Bertram[a], T Grant and S Hiendleder[c]

[a]*Agri-Science Queensland, Department of Employment, Economic Development and Innovation;* [b]*Texas A&M University, College Station, USA;* [c]*University of Adelaide, Roseworthy, South Australia*

Large variation in gestation length and birth weight has been widely documented among reciprocal crosses of *Bos indicus* and *Bos taurus* cattle. Historically, this was thought to be a function of maternal uterine influence such as blood flow. This phenomenon, however, also exists in embryo transfer calves where all surrogate dams are of the same genotype. In 2007, a collaborative project was initiated to investigate epigenetic influence on growth and size traits in several defined *Bos indicus-Bos taurus* populations in Australia and the United States.

This report describes variability for gestation length (GL) and birth weight (BWT) in 33 Droughtmaster calves produced through fixed-time AI in northern Queensland. Droughtmaster is a stabilized *Bos indicus* (50%), *Bos taurus* (50%) composite breed established in Australia. Maiden 2-yr-old heifers (n = 133) were bred on 8 January, 2009 to two Droughtmaster sires (one high growth and one average growth based on BREEDPLAN EBV). Placental (amnion length and width, placentome width and thickness; 2 measurements per time point) and fetal (crown-rump length, foreleg length) characteristics were evaluated by ultrasound on d 49, 56 and 63 of gestation. Birth date and BWT were recorded for resulting calves (n = 33). Traits were evaluated through ANOVA for effects of AI bull, sex of calf and potential AI bull x sex of calf interaction. Correlations among all traits were also evaluated. The range in GL was from 267 to 300 d, and the range in BWT was 21 to 37 kg. There were no significant differences for AI bull, calf sex, or the interaction for any trait. Average placentome width (APW) or thickness (APT) was not correlated to GL; however, BWT was correlated to APW at d 56 ($r = 0.46$, $P < 0.01$) and at d 63 ($r = 0.35$, $P < 0.05$). Average placentome thickness and APT were not related to crown-rump or foreleg length; crown-rump and foreleg length were not correlated to GL or BWT. The correlation between GL and BWT was 0.63 ($P < 0.001$). The amount of variation, based on CV%, appeared similar for APW (11.0, 9.1, 13.4) and APT (23.3, 15.8, 14.9) for d 49, 56, 63, respectively, as BWT (14.4); however, CV appeared lower for crown-rump length at d 49 (7.8%) and d 56 (4.7%) and for foreleg length at d 63 (6.4%).

Potential interactions between maternal and fetal genotypes are likely to be important predictors of birth weight and gestation length in *Bos indicus-Bos taurus* composite calves, and placental traits may be more useful to predict birth weight than early fetal measurements. We hypothesize that epigenetic influences may contribute to previously unexplained variation in many production traits where *Bos indicus-Bos taurus* crosses are used and should continue to be investigated.

Obstetrical assistance and neonatal vitality in dairy Holstein cows

CI Vannucchi, LCG Silva, RA Silva Jr., BS Mesquita, RD Mingoti, BG Freitas, TAF Vechiato and PH Risolia

Faculty of Veterinary Medicine, University of São Paulo, Brazil

Prolonged parturition may lead to neonatal asphyxia and unfavorable consequences to the dam. Premature obstetrical assistance, however, is known to cause neonatal problems and retained placenta. The aims of the present study were to compare neonatal vitality and the incidence of retained placenta in Holstein dairy cows submitted to obstetrical assistance or presenting spontaneous calving.

Twelve Holstein cows and their calves were grouped into: Spontaneous Group (SPOG; n = 7) and Assistance Group (ASSG; n = 5). Spontaneous calving was considered to be a normal parturition with no obstetrical intervention and the time passing from the second stage of parturition (rupture of the allantois) and calf delivery below 2 h. Cows of the ASSG were submitted to extraction of the calf within the same time passing as the SPOG but still presenting normal parturition. Calves were subjected to clinical assessment through the Apgar score[1] every 10 min during the first hour of birth. Arterial blood gas and blood glucose concentration (mg dL^{-1}) were analyzed at birth, 2 and 4 h after calving. Arterial pH, oxygen tension (pO2; mmHg), carbon dioxide tension (pCO2; mmHg), total carbon dioxide (TCO2; mM), bicarbonate concentration (mM), base excess (BE; mM), oxygen saturation (SO2; %), sodium and potassium concentration (mMol L^{-1}) were measured as a manner to verify acid-basic balance. Placenta retention was diagnosed within 12 h after fetal expulsion. Values were compared using ANOVA and Tukey's Test for multiple comparisons with a significance level of 5%.

No statistical differences were found between SPOG and ASSG regarding acid-base changes, Apgar score, body temperature and blood glucose during the 4 h of birth. Regardless of the obstetrical intervention, all calves presented hypoxemia (low arterial pO_2 concentration) during the initial 4 h of birth. On the other hand, normal blood pH and bicarbonate concentration were verified, indicating no metabolic disorders and adequate tissue oxygenation. In addition, pCO2 was within the normal range, suggesting proper pulmonary gas exchange. Hence, the high oxygen consumption at tissue level lead to a decrease in blood oxygen tension in order to maintain a tissue acid-base balance. No retained placenta was observed in both SPOG and ASSG.

In conclusion, a calving period of less than 2 h can favor neonatal adaptation to extra-uterine life. Obstetrical intervention in less than 2 h of calving does not cause any neonatal injury or predisposition to retention of fetal membranes and proved to be a safe medical assistance at this time point.

[1]Silva *et al.*, 2009. Reprod Domest Anim 44:160-163.

Monitoring endocrine profiles for prediction of stillbirth in Holstein-Friesian dairy cattle

O Szenci[a], ÁC Bajcsy[a], E Bryd[a], I Mádl[b], J Tibold[b], N Melo de Sousa[c], A Bella[c], JF Beckers[c], M Keresztes[a], V Faigl[a], M Kulcsár[a] and G Huszenicza[a]

[a]*Szent István University, Budapest, Hungary;* [b]*Agroprodukt Co., Pápa, Hungary;* [c]*University of Liege, Liege, Belgium*

During the last decades, there is a declining trend in conception and calving rates in high yielding Holstein dairy cows. At the same time, the gradual increase in stillbirth rates, especially in Holstein heifers, has until recently received relatively little attention. Birth weight and gender of the calf, parity and age of the dam and season of calving are all factors associated with calving difficulties and stillbirths. Other causes of stillbirths not related to calving difficulties are, for example, infections (e.g., BVD), insufficient placenta development and/or function, metabolic disorders of the cow, and congenital malformations of the calf. The objective of the present study was to investigate the possible effect of hormonal disturbances on the incidence of stillbirth in dairy cattle on a Holstein-Friesian dairy farm in Hungary.

In the first experiment (A), 94 dairy cattle were sampled three times during the periparturient period (at drying-off, 3 wk prior to expected calving, and within 1 h after calving). In the second experiment (B), 86 cattle were sampled at the two last occasions. Dairy cattle were grouped according to the incidence of stillbirth: Group 1 (control) and Group 2 (stillbirth). Hormone and pregnancy protein parameters measured by RIA were as follows: progesterone, estradiol, cortisol, thyroxin, triiodothyronine, insulin, insulin-like growth factor-1 and pregnancy associated glycoprotein (PAG). Differences between the two groups (control vs. stillbirth) were evaluated by Student-t test (at individual time points) and ANOVA (considering time and group effect together).

Comparing the groups with normal calving and stillbirth, concentrations of each of the measured hormones and PAGs changed significantly during the sampling period (time effects, $P<0.001$) in both experiments. At the same time, Group (control vs. stillbirth) did not influence the hormone or PAG concentrations with the only exception being estradiol concentrations in experiment B ($P=0.028$). The Group by time interactions were not significant. When the Student t-test was used to detect group differences at each sampling time, progesterone concentrations immediately after calving in both experiments were greater ($P<0.001$) in the cattle with stillbirths. Similarly, significant differences between the estradiol concentrations could be detected immediately after calving in experiment A ($P<0.01$), however, in these cases estradiol concentrations were lower in cattle with stillbirths than in the controls. Changes in the progesterone and estradiol may be one of the reasons for stillbirth in dairy cattle however more examinations are needed to confirm this hypothesis. Other hormones measured did not explain the incidence of stillbirth in dairy cattle.

This study was supported by OMFB 0173-177/2006.

Plasma pregnancy associated glycoproteins and insulin-like growth factor I five days prior to calving are inappropriate to predict viability of calves

M Piechotta, I Tapken, M Kaske and H Bollwein

Clinic for Cattle, University of Veterinary Medicine, Hannover, Germany

Growth and development of the placenta are critical for fetal development and thereby neonatal viability[1]. Insulin like growth factor I (IGF-I) affects cell growth, differentiation and proliferation of the placenta and may, therefore, also be crucial for calf viability. Plasma concentrations of pregnancy associated glycoproteins (PAG) produced by trophoblast giant cells were already suspected to be lower during late pregnancy and at time of parturition in cases of stillbirth and low calf viability[2].

The objective was to investigate whether IGF-I and PAG plasma concentrations may be predictive for calf viability in primiparous (prp) and pluriparous (plp) cows. Plasma samples were taken daily between d 270 after AI until spontaneous calving from 47 prp (body weight 571 ± 52 kg) and 87 plp (body weight 685 ± 81 kg) Holstein Friesian cows which calved without complications (i.e., excluding dystocia, twins and stillbirths). Plasma IGF-I (immunoradiometric assay; Beckman Coulter, USA) and PAG concentrations were evaluated from all samples taken at the fifth day before calving. Immediately after calving, calf body weight, neck-rump-length (NRL) and APGAR-score (vital: 7-8 points; endangered: 6-4; non-vital: 3-1 points) were recorded.

No differences ($P > 0.05$) were found between prp and plp cows for IGF-I (136 ± 49 vs. 139 ± 49 ng/ml; mean ± SD) and PAG concentrations (1638 ± 757 vs. 1714 ± 1106 ng/ml). The coefficients of variations were 35.4% (IGF-I) and 68.1% (PAG). Body weights (39.7 ± 4.6 kg vs. 45.6 ± 5.0 kg; $P < 0.001$) and NRL of calves (86.7 ± 7.0 vs. 90.5 ± 5.9 cm; $P = 0.001$) were lesser in prp compared with plp cows. No correlations ($P > 0.05$) were found between IGF-I or PAG and birth weight / NRL. No differences ($P > 0.05$) in the number of vital or less vital calves were found between prp (vital n = 39; endangered n = 7; non-vital n = 1) and plp cows (vital n = 68; endangered n = 15; non vital n = 4). Neither IGF-I nor PAG concentrations differed ($P > 0.05$) between cows with vital, endangered or non-vital calves.

Although the birth weight and size of the calves from prp cows were significantly less compared with plp cows, IGF-I and PAG concentrations five d before calving were comparable. IGF-I was reported as an important factor regulating placental development, but did not differ between cows with vital and non vital calves. In contrast to other studies, PAG levels five d prior to calving were not lower in cases of less vital calves. Moreover, the inter-individual variance of PAG was high. In conclusion, neither PAG nor IGF-I seemed to be suitable parameters to predict viability of calves in dairy cattle shortly before calving.

[1]Reynolds and Redmer, 1995. J Anim Sci 73:1839-1851.
[2]Kornmatitsuk *et al.*, 2004. Acta Vet Scand 45:47-68.

Steroid sulfatase expression pattern in the ovine fetal brain during late gestation

MB Rabaglino, J Winikor, M Sutherland and CE Wood

University of Florida, Gainesville, USA

Parturition is a highly regulated endocrine process. In ruminants, estrogen produced by the placenta plays an essential role in stimulating the hypothalamus-pituitary-adrenal axis in the fetal brain. In fetal circulation, estrogen is presented mostly as sulfoconjugated estrogen that needs to be deconjugated by the enzyme steroid sulfatase (STS) in order to bind the estrogen receptor, targeting biological active estrogen to specific tissues. We hypothesized that an induction of STS expression occurs toward the end of gestation in the ovine fetal brain, probably in response to high levels of circulating estradiol sulfate. The objectives were: to measure the gene and protein expression for STS in different regions of the fetal brain at different late gestational ages (Exp. 1); and to compare the gene and protein expression of STS in different brain regions in fetuses treated with estradiol sulfate (Exp. 2).

In Exp. 1, mRNA was extracted from different brain regions (i.e., brainstem, hypothalamus, hippocampus, pituitary, cerebellum and cortex) of ovine fetuses at the following developmental ages: 80, 100, 120, 130 and 145 d of gestation (4 to 5 per group). cDNA was synthesized by reverse transcription of mRNA and quantified by Taqman PCR. Primers and probe were designed from the ovine STS mRNA, purified from placenta and sequenced using the Sanger method. STS expression for each sample was normalized to β-actin. Data were expressed as cycle time (Ct) values and relative quantifications of each gene were determined by the difference in Ct, calculating fold changes in gene expression for each sample. Protein expression for each sample was measured by Western blot using rabbit anti-STS previously made in this laboratory. STS gene and protein expression varied significantly throughout the latter half of gestation in all brain regions except hypothalamus. In general, the pattern was a tendency to increase toward the end of gestation, for both gene and protein expression, with higher concentration at 145 d of gestational age compared with 80 d ($P<0.05$).

For Exp. 2, a total of 4 sets of chronically-catheterized ovine twin fetuses were studied with one infused with estradiol-3-sulfate intracerebroventricularly (1 mg/day) and the other untreated (control fetus). After euthanasia, mRNA and protein were extracted from the following brain regions: brainstem, cerebellum, cortex, hippocampus and hypothalamus. mRNA and protein were measured as described in Exp. 1. No significant difference in mRNA abundance was found in the estradiol sulfate-treated fetus compared with the control fetus. Nonetheless, protein abundance was significantly increased in cortex and hippocampus in the treated fetuses ($P<0.05$).

In conclusion, there is an increased deconjugation of sulfoconjugated estrogens in the fetal brain at the end of gestation. The results suggest that increased exposure of the fetal brain to estradiol-3-sulfate reduces the turnover of the STS protein but does not alter STS gene transcription. The cause of increased STS gene transcription in the fetal brain in the latter half of gestation is unclear.

Supported by HD57561 to CEW.

Effects of a protracted induction of parturition on placental maturation in cattle

H Bollwein[a], D Hartmann[a], A Honnens[a], D Rath[b], H Niemann[b] and C Pfarrer[c]

[a]Clinic for Cattle, University of Veterinary Medicine Hannover, Germany; [b]Institute of Farm Animal Genetics, Friedrich-Loeffler-Institute, Mariensee, Germany; [c]Department of Anatomy, University of Veterinary Medicine, Hannover, Germany

As the etiopathology of retained placenta is still not resolved in cattle, we compared the effects of a protracted and a conventional induction of parturition on placental maturation and the occurrence of retained placenta. Furthermore, we tested the usefulness of color Doppler ultrasonography of the uterine arteries as a non-invasive method for the assessment of placental maturation. This technique has been successfully used to monitor changes in uterine perfusion throughout the entire pregnancy.

Protracted induction of labor (PIL) was precipitated in 13 cows by administration of 1.3 mg dexamethasone i.m. between d 268 and 273 of gestation twice daily, and 40 mg dexamethasone i.m. on d 274 of gestation. For conventional induction of labor (CIL), 10 cows received 40 mg dexamethasone on d 274 of gestation. A third group (CON, n=11) served as a non treated control group. Within two h after birth, 2 placentomes were extracted from the uterus and used for assessment of placental maturation by histology and immunohistochemistry. Blood flow volume (BFV) and pulsatility index (PI) in both uterine arteries were measured daily in groups PIL and CIL and every second day in group CON from d 268 of gestation until labor by transrectal Doppler ultrasonography. After each examination blood was collected for the measurement of estrone (E) in plasma.

The incidence of retained placenta was lower ($P<0.05$) in the PIL group (54 %) compared with the CIL group (70 %), but in both groups higher ($P<0.05$) than in CON (9%). Until 4 d before parturition, no differences ($P>0.05$) in E were detected between groups, but from this time onwards the PIL group increased and showed greater E concentrations compared with the cows of the CON- and CIL-groups. Staining with Masson-Goldner and pan-cytokeratin indicated an increased degree of atrophy and flatness of the maternal crypt epithelium in cows without retained placenta compared wiht cows with retained placenta. Staining with anti-caspase-3 verified the observations as more apoptotic cells were detected in the CON and PIL group compared with CIL. Uterine BFV and PI neither differed ($P>0.05$) between the three groups nor between cows with or without retained placenta.

In conclusion, a protracted induction of labor resulted in a lower incidence of placental retention, which seems to be due to a better placental maturation. Differences in placental maturation cannot be detected by color Doppler ultrasonography of the main uterine arteries.

Concentration of progesterone in the blood serum in cows with and without retained fetal membranes

S Skuja and V Antāne

University of Agriculture, Latvia

Retained fetal membranes (RFM) in cows postpartum (PP) can cause inflammation of the uterus, inhibit the ovarian function and uterine involution and negatively affect other aspects of reproduction. The blood progesterone (P_4) concentration decreases shortly before parturition and remains at a low level during the PP period until the ovarian activity becomes renewed. The aim of the research was assess ovary activity in cows with and without RFM using blood P_4 concentrations.

Sixty Holstein Friesian cows, 45 with RFM and 15 without RFM (NRFM), were analyzed for serum P_4 concentration every two d for six weeks. RFM cows were divided into three groups: group 1 – cows with RFM, removed manually and treated; group 2 – cows with RFM, not removed manually and treated; and group 3 – cows with RFM, not removed manually and not treated. Progesterone was established with a fully automated sample selective analyzer Elecsys 2010 (Roche Diagnostics).

The serum P_4 concentration on the second day PP was greater in RFM cows (1.38±0.36 ng/ml) than in NRFM cows (0.80±0.11 ng/ml). Such a tendency remained during the enitre study. During the first 18 d PP in cows with RFM, the mean P_4 concentration exceeded 1 ng/ml whereas in NRFM cows it remained lower. Subsequently (d 18 to 32), P_4 concentration increased from 1.24±0.14 ng/ml to 6.43±0.76 ng/ml in RFM cows but in NRFM the P_4 increased from 0.74±0.11 ng/ml to 3.40±1.15 ng/ml. The differences between the groups were significant ($P<0.05$). The next time P_4 was established (d 42 PP), the P_4 level was decreased in both groups of cows: in RFM group to 3.34±0.32 ng/ml, in the NRFM group to 1.97±0.68 ng/ml ($P<0.05$). When analysing the P_4 concentration in blood in individual animals during six weeks PP, it was found out that the P_4 level was constantly low (<1 ng/ml) in 32% of RFM cows and 20% of NRFM cows; thus a conclusion can be drawn that in the examined animals that ovulation did not take place.

In conclusion, in cows with RFM, the PP serum P_4 concentrations were greater and decreased slower in comparison with NRFM. This could be a factor for a delayed folliculogenesis and ovulation.

Uterine infection is associated with decreased mRNA for IGF-I in liver and increased negative energy balance in post partum cows

EJ Williams[a], RA Law[b], HS Gilmore[b], F Carter[a], FJ Young[b], CP Ferris[b], CS Mayne[b], MG Diskin[c], S Cody[a], P Lonergan[a], JF Roche[a], MA Crowe[a] and ACO Evans[a]

[a]*School of Agriculture, Food Science and Veterinary Medicine, University College Dublin, Dublin, Ireland;* [b]*Agri-Food & Biosciences Institute, Hillsborough, Northern Ireland;* [c]*Teagasc, Athenry, Co Galway, Ireland*

Uterine infection is prevalent in postpartum dairy cows and persists in up to 50% of animals. Furthermore, it has been suggested that severe negative energy balance is a risk factor for uterine infection, which is associated with changes in the growth hormone–insulin-like growth factor (GH-IGF) axis. Therefore, the aim of the present study was to test the hypothesis that animals with more severe energy deficit would suffer more uterine infection and decreased liver expression of gene transcripts for IGF-I and GH receptor postpartum compared with animals that did not have infection.

Fifty-three Holstein-Friesian cows were monitored from calving until d 35 postpartum. Energy status was calculated using the equations described previously[1]. Uterine health was assessed by vaginal mucus character score (range 0 to 3) on d 14 and 21 postpartum. Animals with a vaginal mucus score of 2 or 3 on d 14 and/or d 21 postpartum were classed as 'infected' (n = 23) and animals with a vaginal mucus character score of 0 or 1 on both d 14 and 21 postpartum were classed as 'clean' (n = 30). Liver tissue was biopsied from all cows on d 35 ± 5 postpartum, total RNA was isolated and reverse transcribed to cDNA. Real-time reverse-transcription PCR assays previously validated in bovine liver were then used to detect transcripts of the key hepatic genes IGF-I, GH Receptor 1a (GHR1a) and Total GH Receptor (GHRt). Gene expression was determined following normalisation to the reference gene GAPDH using the relative standard curve method and was expressed in arbitrary expression units.

Infected animals had more severe cumulative energy deficit between calving and d 35 postpartum compared with clean animals (-1306 ± 241 vs. -646 ± 153 MJ; P = 0.022). Furthermore, expression of IGF-I mRNA in the liver was lower in infected animals when compared with clean animals (118 ± 12 vs. 172 ± 16 units; P = 0.01). However, liver GHR1a and liver GHRt mRNA expression were not different between the groups (122 ± 16 vs. 115 ± 20 units, P = 0.41 for GHR1a and 134 ± 9 vs. 131 ± 17 units, P = 0.44 for GHRt).

We conclude that cows with postpartum uterine infection were associated with having more severe energy deficit and reduced liver IGF-1 expression in the early postpartum period compared with clean cows. It is unclear if uterine infection in the early postpartum period increased the severity of metabolic disorders or if uncoupling of the GH-IGF axis contributed to uterine infection in post partum dairy cattle.

Funded by SFI (07/SRC/B1156).

[1]Thomas, 2004. Feed into milk: An Advisory Manual. Nottingham University Press.

Detection of uterine miRNA and related molecular networks and pathways underlying bovine subclinical endometritis

DW Hailemariam[a], M Hoelker[a], F Rings[a], M Drillich[b], W Heuwieser[b], K Schellander[a] and D Tesfaye[a]

[a]*Institute of Animal Science, Animal Breeding and Husbandry Group, University of Bonn, Germany;* [b]*Clinic for Reproduction, Section of Production Medicine and Quality Management, Free University of Berlin, Berlin, Germany*

The aberrant expression of microRNAs (miRNAs) has been associated with establishment and progression of various disorders in the mammalian uterus. Subclinical endometritis is the presence of polymorphonuclear leukocytes (PMN) in uterine cytology samples after 21 d postpartum in clinically normal dairy cows and has a negative impact on reproductive performance. With the objective of detecting uterine miRNAs and related molecular networks and pathways, we collected endometrial cytology samples from dairy cows at flushing using cytobrush technique and categorized cows on the basis of PMN proportions as healthy (PMN = 0) and with subclinical endometritis (PMN > 5%). After isolating total RNA from both healthy (n = 6) and subclinical (n = 6) groups using miRNeasy mini kit (Qiagen, Hilden, Germany) following manufacturers protocol, cDNA was synthesised using RT^2 miRNA frist Strand kit (SABiosciences, Frederick, MD USA) from equal amounts of RNA in both groups. We then used 96-well Genome RT^2 miRNA qPCR assay (SABioscience) and identified the differentially expressed miRNAs in subclinical endometritis as compared with their healthy counterparts. Furthermore, we filtered high ranking target genes (predicted using microcosem algorithm and available at http//microrna.sanger.ac.uk/) and uploaded into the web-based pathways analysis tool, Ingenuity Pathway Analysis (IPA), to identify molecular networks and biological functions underlying bovine endometritis. Here, we report that out of 352 miRNAs in which their expression was assessed, 23 were found to be differentially expressed (15 up and 8 were down-regulated in sub-clinical endometritis). The expression profiling of six selected miRNAs (miR-24, miR-215, miR-27a, miR-223, miR-619, miR-423) at different stages of the estrous cycle and pregnant group (d 0, d 3, d 14, pregnant) showed a variable expression level. The expression pattern of miR-619 and miR-423 conform to the expression of estrogen while the expression of miR-24 and miR-215 follows the pattern of progesterone expression during the estrous cycle. The Ingenuity Pathway Analysis (IPA) of the predicted target genes (680) of the 23 miRNAs revealed biological functions and molecular pathways that potentially relate to subclinical endometritis in bovine. The IPA identified 28 significant molecular networks underlying the biological functions from which we identified the top five networks, such as; gene expression, hematological system development and function, cellular development (score = 42), cell death, cardiovascular disease (score = 33), Connective tissue development and function, nervous system development and function, skeletal and muscular system development and function (score = 32), cell signaling, amino acid metabolism, post translational modification (score = 31), cell cycle, connective tissue development and function, cancer (score = 31). Besides, 39 significant canonical pathways have been identified in which most of them are related to reproductive diseases and disorders and cellular proliferation. Taken together, we identified aberrantly expressed miRNAs in bovine subclinical endometritis and subsequently traced the biological functions and molecular pathways. The role of these aberrantly expressed miRNAs may be important for the establishment of pregnancy in cattle.

Gene expression profiling reveals the potential role of antimicrobial calcium-binding proteins of the S100 family as biomarkers in bacterial lipopolysaccharide (LPS)-induced inflammation in bovine endometrium

T Swangchan-Uthai, CRM Lavender, Z Cheng, AA Fouladi-Nashta and DC Wathes

Royal Veterinary College, London, United Kingdom

Bovine postpartum uteri are susceptible to contamination with bacteria: this leads to infection causing endometritis, associated with poor fertility. The endometrial cell plays an important role in the immune response against bacterial endotoxin LPS through the Toll-like receptor4/CD14/MD2 complex signalling pathway[1]. Recently, microarray analysis of the endometrium obtained from postpartum cows in mild or severe negative energy balance (SNEB) showed that SNEB cows had up-regulated many genes involved in inflammatory responses including several antimicrobial peptides[2].

The objective was to study the role of LPS on mRNA expression of the calcium binding protein family (*S100A8, S100A9, S100A12*), other potentially relevant genes and *18S rRNA* as the reference gene in bovine endometrium. An in vitro model of bovine endometrium was developed. Cultures of mixed epithelial and stromal cells were grown to confluence in 24 well plates and half were incubated with LPS (100 ng/ml). Total RNA samples were collected at 0, 1, 6, 12, 24 and 48 h post-treatment and analysed by 2-step RT-qPCR. Treatments were replicated 6 times and experiments conducted on three separate occasions. LPS versus control treatment and time courses were compared using mixed model analysis.

At 24 h, the proportionately greatest increase following LPS stimulation was in *S100A8* mRNA, which increased 10-fold ($P<0.001$). Levels of mRNA for the pro-inflammatory cytokine *IL1B* and the chemokine *IL8* increased 7-fold ($P<0.001$). Gene expression of *S100A12* and the chemokine *CXCL5* increased 5-fold ($P<0.001$ and $P<0.005$, respectively). Relatively smaller increases were observed in *TNFα, MMP1* and *MMP13* which increased 2-fold ($P<0.05$ to $P<0.001$). Three antimicrobial peptides *DEFB5, LAP* and *SLP1* were significantly up-regulated in uteri of SNEB cows[2] but their expression was not altered by LPS in vitro. Time course in the S100 family expression showed that LPS treatment increased *S100A8* levels up to 18-fold ($P<0.001$) at 6 h, peaking at 12 h (19-fold, $P<0.001$) before decreasing over 48 h. Similarly, increased expression of *S100A12* mRNA was evident at 6 h (4-fold, $P<0.001$), peaking approximately 5-fold ($P<0.001$) after 12 h, with sustained expression at 48 h. The *S100A9* mRNA was maximal at 6 h (2-fold, $P<0.01$) post stimulation and had returned to the control level by 24 h.

These results provide evidence that endometrial cells respond to LPS by increased expression of known target genes. It is predicted that these gene changes are involved in triggering an inflammatory response, mediating synthesis of antimicrobial proteins and altering connective tissue remodelling in the postpartum bovine uterus. The S100 family genes have both antimicrobial and chemotactic activity. Our data indicate that they may play a major role in the innate immune system of the postpartum uterus, providing surface defense against the exposure to bacterial endotoxin experienced during involution.

This study was funded by The Royal Thai Government and The Royal Veterinary College.

[1]Herath *et al.*, 2009. Endocrinology 150:1912-1920.
[2]Wathes *et al.*, 2009. Physiological Genomics 39:1-13.

The effect of postpartum uterine infection on subsequent preovulatory follicle gene expression during the breeding season in postpartum cows

SW Walsh, EJ Williams, PA McGettigan, JP Mehta, JA Browne and ACO Evans

School of Agriculture Food Science and Veterinary Medicine, and the Conway Institute, University College Dublin, Ireland

Approximately 90% of dairy cows have uterine bacterial contamination within 2 wk postpartum. This is associated with decreased follicular growth and function and can have a negative effect on fertility even after clinical resolution of the infection. The objective of this experiment was to investigate if uterine infection early postpartum has long-term effects on preovulatory follicle function in Holstein-Friesian lactating cows.

Uterine bacterial infection was determined in Holstein-Friesian cows (n = 12; average lactation 3.8) by characterisation of vaginal mucus between d 21 and 27 postpartum and by cytological examination of uterine flushings between d 38 and 45 postpartum. Animals with evidence of uterine pathology (INF; n = 5) had a mucus score 3 and/or >10% neutrophils present on cytological examination. Estrous cycles of INF cows and non-infected cows (CONT; n = 7) were synchronized. On d 8 (d 0 = estrus) a previously used CIDR was inserted intravaginally. Animals received a luteolytic dose of $PGF_{2\alpha}$ on d 13 and the CIDR was removed 2 d later. They were slaughtered between 24 and 30 h after CIDR removal, i.e., preovulatory follicle before estrus (average 82.6 d in milk). At slaughter the ovaries were recovered, the follicles were dissected and measured, follicular fluid was aspirated and the granulosa and theca cells were separated and isolated. The preovulatory follicle was identified based on diameter and follicular fluid estradiol concentrations. Total RNA was extracted from granulosa and theca cells and gene expression was assessed using RNAseq technology (Illumina Genome Analyzer).

Both INF and CONT animals had no signs of uterine infection at slaughter. Preovulatory follicle diameters (18.1 vs. 17.6 mm) and follicular fluid estradiol concentrations (307 vs. 560 ng/ml) were not different ($P>0.05$) between CONT and INF groups, respectively. The expressions of 19,956 transcripts were detected. We found 255 transcripts representing 251 genes to be differentially expressed ($P<0.05$) in CONT compared with INF cows across both theca and granulosa cells. Of the 255 transcripts, 78 were specific to granulosa tissue, whereas 173 were specific to theca tissue (no common transcripts). Across both tissue types, 86 transcripts had greater and 23 transcripts had lesser expression ($P<0.05$) in INF compared with CONT cows. We found 28 over-represented GO (Gene Ontology) terms which included hormone activity, calcium channel activity and lipid catabolic process. Of particular note was the lesser expression of genes involved in hormone activity (IGFBP2, CYP17A1, FOXG1) and greater expression of genes involved in immune function (IL6R) in INF animals compared with CONT animals.

In conclusion, there were a small number of differentially expressed genes between INF and CONT animals that may be important for follicle function. However, the persistent effect of uterine infection on fertility may be mediated through an altered uterine rather than follicle environment.

Funded by Science Foundation Ireland (07/SRC/B1156).

Dairy cattle reproductive viral diseases in the South-eastern region of Brazil

BA Rodrigues, LC Torres, JB Barreto Filho, MVC Ferraz Júnior, RL Previdelli and TF Silva

Department of Veterinary Medicine, Federal University of Lavras, Lavras, Minas Gerais, Brazil

Minas Gerais State is the major dairying area in Brazil, which has the sixth largest milk production in the world. Two regions in this state, the Triangle and the Southern, are responsible for 41.25% of milk production with 1,767 and 1,234 millions of liters per year[1], respectively. These regions have experienced an increase in dairy industry of 20% (Southern) and 35% (Triangle) in the last decade. Cattle density is about 16.1 cows/km^2 in the Southern and 14.5 cows/km^2 in the Triangle regions. Some reproductive diseases, such as infectious bovine rinotracheitis (BoHV-1) and bovine viral diarrhea (BVDV) can cause great economic losses, and its diagnosis is important to animal health and herd management. The insidious nature of BVDV, which uses the reproductive system to maintain and spread itself, has led to important reproductive failures and abortions in both dairy and beef cattle on a worldwide level. BoHV-1 is primarily associated with rinotracheitis, pustular vulvovaginitis, balanopostitis and abortion. The objective of this work was to evaluate the prevalence of these viruses in the Triangle and Southern regions of Minas Gerais.

At the beginning of this study, 319 cows (not immunized against BoHV-1 or BVDV with clinical history of abortion) were examined (BoHV-1: 105 in the Triangle and 77 in the Southern; BVDV: 137 in the Southern). For the diagnosis, virus neutralization technique was used (samples BoHV-1 Nebraska and BVDV 1 - SINGER) in Madin Darby bovine kidney (MDBK) cells.

All the herds studied were positive to BVDV (18 farms in Triangle) or BoHV-1 (28 farms, 18 from the Southern region and 10 from the Triangle). BVDV seroprevalence in the Southern region was 54%. For BoHV-1, seroprevalence of 79% and 84% were observed in the Triangle and Southern regions, respectively. No significant differences were detected among virus titration, except in two farms that have experienced recent BVDV outbreaks in the Southern region ($P<0.05$). The IBR seroprevalence between regions did not differ ($P > 0.05$).

In conclusion, these reproductive diseases are endemic in both regions, and their prevalence is high. Factors influencing the spread and behavior of these viruses are under investigation.

Financial support: CNPq, FAPEMIG and VALLÉE S.A.

[1]IBGE, 2007. Produção da Pecuária Municipal 35:30-56.

Vaccination against reproductive diseases associated with timed artificial insemination affects pregnancy outcome and its subsequent losses in lactating dairy cows

MHC Pereira[a], M Meneghetti[b] and JLM Vasconcelos[a]

[a]FMVZ – UNESP/Botucatu, São Paulo, Brazil; [b]Laboratórios Pfizer LTDA, São Paulo, Brazil

Reproductive diseases may have a considerable economic impact on bovine production. Many infectious agents have been identified as potential causes of bovine pregnancy losses, being the most common ones: infectious bovine rhinotracheitis (IBR), bovine viral diarrhea virus (BVDV) and Leptospirosis[1,2] The objective was to evaluate the prevention against these agents on reproductive performance of dairy cows. This study was conducted with 1,889 lactating purebred (Holstein) and crossbred (Holstein x Gir) dairy cows from 35 dairy farms. Average milk production was 22.8±8.2 kg per day. Two experiments were performed. Exp. 1 used cows (n = 793) that had been vaccinated against IBR/BVD/Leptospirosis every 12 mo and Exp. 2 used cows (n = 1096) that had never received the vaccine before. In both experiments all cows were timed artificially inseminated (TAI) and randomly divided into two groups to receive or not receive the first injection of vaccine against IBR/BVDV/Leptospirosis (5.0 mL, i.m., Cattle Master® 4 + L5, Pfizer Animal Health, Lincoln, USA) at the beginning of an eleven-day TAI protocol and a second dose when the first pregnancy diagnosis was performed by ultrasound scan (Aloka SSD-500, 5.0 mHz) to define the conception rate to TAI protocol. The second ultrasound scan was done 41 d later to determine the pregnancy rate on d 71 and pregnancy loss between 30 and 71 d of gestation. All the cows were synchronized with the same TAI protocol. Data was analyzed by a logistic Regression Procedure from SAS. In Exp. 1, the cows were already vaccinated with Cattle Master® 4 + L5. The additional immunization program did not improve conception rate to the TAI protocol on d 30 ($P>0.10$) the pregnancy rate on d 71 ($P>0.10$) or the pregnancy loss between the two diagnoses. In Exp. 2, in which cows received the vaccine program for the first time, animals that received Cattle Master® 4 + L5, compared with control cows had greater ($P=0.038$) conception rate [44.3% (247/558) vs. 38.1% (205/538)] on d 30; greater ($P=0.003$) pregnancy rates [40.9% (228/558) vs. 32.2% (173/538)] on d 71 and lower ($P=0.009$) pregnancy loss [7.7% (19/247) vs. 15.6% (32/205)] between 30 and 71 d of gestation. In dairy farms that already have Cattle Master® 4 + L5 in their annual sanitary program, the additional use of it in association with the TAI protocol is not necessary. However, in the group of cows that had never been vaccinated before, the use of Cattle Master® 4 + L5 had a positive impact on the pregnancy rate on d 71, due to the higher conception rate and lower pregnancy loss. This data shows that the prevention against reproductive diseases (IBR/BVDV/Leptospirosis) can be an important tool to improve reproductive performance of lactating dairy cows.

Acknowledgments: Pfizer Animal Health – Brazil.

[1]Kirkbride, 1992. J Vet Diagn Invest 4:374-379.
[2]Murray, 1990. Vet Rec 127:543-547.

Changes in cerebrospinal fluid concentration of melanin-concentrating hormone in anoestrous ewes in response to the ram effect

HG Quintela[a], P Lagos[c], S Alzugaray[b], P Torterolo[c] and R Ungerfeld[a]

[a]*Departamento de Fisiología,* [b]*Departamento de Morfología y Desarrollo Área de Histología y Embriología, Facultad de Veterinaria, Montevideo, Uruguay;* [c]*Departamento de Fisiología, Facultad de Medicina, Montevideo, Uruguay*

Melanin-concentrating hormone (MCH) is a neuropeptide whose expression and synthesis in the hypothalamus is stimulated by estrogen in monkeys[1] and rats[2]. The introduction of rams to anoestrous ewes that were isolated from males (the ram effect) stimulates an increase in LH pulsatility followed by a follicular phase, an LH peak and ovulation. Our aim was to measure the changes in MCH concentration in cerebrospinal fluid (CSF) of anoestrous ewes stimulated by the ram effect. Sixteen acyclic Corriedale ewes were isolated from rams (minimum distance = 1 km) during 30 d before the experiment began (non-breeding season). Cerebrospinal fluid was obtained by using lumbosacral puncture before the introduction of the rams (n = 5) and then 12 h (n = 6), and 24 h (n = 5) after the introduction of the rams. The MCH concentration was measured with a commercial ELISA kit. The MCH concentration increased (P = 0.01) from 1.58 ± 0.06 (before) to 1.69 ± 0.07 and 1.72 ± 0.09 ng/mL at 12 and 24 h after the introduction of the rams, respectively. The MCH concentrations at 12 and 24 h were similar. We concluded that the MCH release into the CSF increased after the introduction of rams to anestrous ewes. Our working hypothesis is that the increase in oestradiol during the induced follicular phase stimulates the MCH synthesis and release within the hypothalamus.

[1]Murray *et al.*, 2006. J Neuroendocrinol 18:157-167.
[2]Viale *et al.*, 1999. Peptides 20:553-559.

Undernourished photoperiod-treated male goats are able to stimulate the reproductive activity in does by the male effect

JA Delgadillo, JA Flores, A Lemiere, S Secundino, H Hernández, G Duarte and J Vielma

Centro de Investigación en Reproducción Caprina, Departamento de Ciencias Médico Veterinarias, Universidad Autónoma Agrria Antonio Narro, Torreón, Coahuila, Mexico

Estrous behavior and ovulatory activity in female goats during the anestrous season can be stimulated when they are suddenly exposed to a male. This technique of biostimulation is called "the male effect". Some factors, such as nutritional level, can modify the ability of males to stimulate the sexual activity in does exposed to "the male effect". Indeed, undernourished male goats induced less anestrous does to ovulate than do the well-nourished ones. The aim of this study was to determine if undernourished goat bucks sexually stimulated by a photoperiodic treatment are able to stimulate the reproductive activity of does as do the well-nourished ones.

Two groups of male goats (n = 7 each) were exposed to 2.5 mo of long days (16 h of light/d) from November 1 to stimulate their sexual activity during the non-breeding season. The undernourished bucks were fed 0.5 maintenance requirements and had a body condition score (BCS) of 1.5 ± 0.1, while the well-nourished bucks were fed 1.5 maintenance requirements and had a BCS of 3.0 ± 0.1. Two groups of multiparous anovulatory does (n = 26 each) were exposed to undernourished and well-nourished bucks during 18 d (n = 2 males by group). Estrous behavior was recorded twice daily (0800 and 1700 h). Ovulations and pregnancy rates were determined 20 and 45 d after male introduction by transrectal and abdominal ultrasonography, respectively. Chi-square and independent t-student test were used as appropriate.

The percentages of does detected in estrus were similar in females in contact with undernourished and well-nourished bucks (23/26; 89% in both groups; $P > 0.05$). However, the interval between male introduction and onset of the estrous behavior was greater in does exposed to undernourished (9.5 ± 0.6 d) than in those exposed to well-nourished bucks (2.5 ± 0.6 d; $P < 0.05$). The proportion of does that ovulated did not differ between females exposed to undernourished (25/26; 96%) or well-nourished bucks (26/26; 100%; $P > 0.05$). The pregnancy rates did not differ between does in contact with undernourished (20/26; 77%) and well-nourished bucks (22/26, 83%; $P > 0.05$).

These results demonstrate that the undernourished photoperiod treated male goats are able to stimulate the reproductive activity of anovulatory goats. However, the estrous latency was greater in females in contact with undernourished than in those exposed to well-nourished males. This difference could be attributed to the low sexual behavior displayed by undernourished males when introduced into female groups to stimulate estrous behavior, or to their inability to detect estrous behavior.

Follicular status does not modify the ovarian responding pattern of female goats exposed to the sexually active males

R Ungerfeld[a], JA Flores[b], H Hernandez[b] and JA Delgadillo[b]

[a]*Departamento de Fisiología, Facultad de Veterinaria, Montevideo, Uruguay;* [b]*Centro de Investigación en Reproducción Caprina, Universidad Autónoma Agraria, Antonio Narro, Torreón, Coahuila, México*

The introduction of sexually active bucks stimulates an increase in LH pulse frequency that ends with an LH surge similar to that observed during the follicular phase of a normal oestrous cycle in anestrous goats, followed by an ovulation. After the first male-induced ovulation, most goats display a short luteal phase, that ends 5 to 6 d later, but in others a luteal phase of normal length is observed. The aim of the current study was to determine if the follicular size at the introduction of the bucks influences the probability of its ovulation in anestrous does exposed to sexually active bucks.

The experiment was conducted in Torreón, Coahuila México (26° N) during the non-breeding season (March to April) with 13 anoestrous goats (no CL observed in 3 consecutive weekly ultrasound observations). Four bucks were subjected to a long-day treatment (16 h of light/day) from November 1 to January 15 followed by natural photoperiod to stimulate their sexual activity during the non-breeding season. On March 29 (d 0) at 0900 h, one of the four treated males was introduced in the pen (5 m x 5 m) where the females were placed and remained with them during 6 d. Estrous behavior was recorded twice daily by direct visual observation throughout the study. Ultrasound examinations were performed once daily from d -7 to -1, and twice daily from d 0 to 6 with an Aloka 500 ultrasound equipped with a 7.5 MHz linear probe. Follicles that ovulated were categorized according to the diameter at the moment when females were exposed to males as small (<3.9 mm), medium (4.0 to 5.9 mm) or large (>6.0 mm).

All females ovulated (13/13) and 12 came into estrus during the first 5 d after exposure to males. The growth rate of the ovulatory follicles increased after the introduction of the bucks (before: 1.1 ± 0.1 mm/d vs. after: 1.5 ± 0.1 mm/d; $P<0.05$). The percentage of follicles from each category that finally ovulated did not differ ($P>0.05$; small 47.8%, medium 34.8%, and large 17.4%). From those follicles that ovulated, the growth rate of those that were small at the moment of the introduction of the bucks was greater (2.1 ± 0.1; $P<0.05$) than that observed in those that were medium (1.3 ± 0.1) and large follicles (1.1 ± 0.1).

The size of the follicles present when bucks were introduced did not affect the probability of ovulation, or the time length needed to ovulate. All follicles increased their growth rate but the growth rate was greater when the follicles were smaller at the time of male exposure.

Ovarian response in prepubertal beef heifers exposed to androgenised steers

C Fiol, N Curbelo, G Larraz and R Ungerfeld

Facultad de Veterinaria, Montevideo, Uruguay

Biostimulation is an effective method to induce estrous cyclicity. Cyclicity is induced through the genital stimulation by the male, pheromones or other less defined external cues. Biostimulation may be used to reduce age of puberty in heifers[1]. The physiological mechanisms through which females respond to stimulation by the male remains unknown. Greater numbers of small and large follicles were observed in biostimulated than in isolated prepuberal beef heifers[2]. Postpartum beef cows exposed to bulls had shorter inter-wave intervals and greater maximum dominant follicle (DF) diameter than isolated ones[3].

The objective of this experiment was to determine if the introduction of androgenized steers (AS) to prepubertal heifers stimulates ovarian follicular growth. Thirty prepubertal Hereford heifers (24 mo of age, 257.5±32.5 kg) and 3 AS were used. From d -10 to d 0 (joining with AS) all heifers were grazed together. On d 0 animals were assigned to two groups: 1) exposed to AS from d 0 to 80 (Exposed, EH, n=15), or 2) isolated from males (Control, CH, n=15). Both groups grazed low quality native pastures in two paddocks separated by 600 m, so CH females could not see or smell the males. Daily ovarian ultrasonographic evaluations were done in all the heifers during 40 d (d -10 to 30) to determine the diameter of the largest follicle. During the same period, estrous behavior was recorded in both groups twice daily. Thereafter, ovarian ultrasonographic determinations were done every week (d 32 to 60) and every 10 d (d 60 to 80) to determine the presence of the corpus luteum indicating that an ovulation has occurred.

Cumulative proportion of cyclic heifers was greater for EH than CH on d 60 (33.3 vs. 0%, $P=0.01$), 70 (47 vs. 0%, $P<0.005$) and 80 (53 vs. 0%, $P<0.001$). Maximum DF diameter was greater in EH than in CH by d 5 (6.2±0.8 vs. 5.2±0.6 mm; $P=0.001$), 7 and 8 (6.7±0.5 vs. 5.7±0.5 mm; $P<0.05$) and from d 11 to 17 (7.7±0.6 and 6.9±0.5 mm, EH and CH, respectively; $P<0.05$). When analyzed in a 5 d interval, EH had greater DF than CH by d 15 (6.5±0.8 vs. 5.9±0.6 mm; $P<0.05$) and d 25 (8.1±0.5 vs. 7.4±0.4 mm; $P<0.01$).

Exposure of prepubertal beef heifers to AS was effective to advance the onset of cyclic activity. Follicular development during the first 20 d of exposure was greater for exposed heifers, but none of those follicles ovulated during that period. Although ovulation was delayed, the presence of AS increased the cyclic activity.

Financial support: Fondo Clemente Estable, ANII, Uruguay.

[1]Fiol *et al.*, 2010. Theriogenology *in press*.
[2]Bastidas *et al.*, 1997. Arch Latinoam Prod Anim 5:390-392.
[3]Berardinelli *et al.*, 2009. Biol Reprod 81:544.

The male effect improves reproductive performance in ewes maintained under extensive conditions in arid central Mexico

AL Ramos-Rojas[b], L Gijón-Palafox[a], AA Trejo-González[c], JA Delgadillo[d], R Soriano-Robles[a], C Murcia-Mejía[e], MS Retana-Márquez[a], RJ Scaramuzzi[f], GB Martin[g] and M Muñoz-Gutiérrez[a]

[a]*UAMI, Mexico;* [b]*UAMX, Mexico;* [c]*FESC, UNAM, Mexico;* [d]*CIRCA, UAAAN, AP México;* [e]*FMVZ, UNAM, Mexico;* [f]*Marie Curie Professor, INRA, UMR Physiologie de la Reproduction et des Comportements, France;* [g]*School of Animal Biology, UWA, Australia*

In the arid regions of Central Mexico (Hidalgo), the fertility of sheep is low. A simple, inexpensive management technique that improves the reproductive performance of these flocks would result in significant economic benefits to the subsistence farmers in the region. One option is the 'male effect', a simple way to induce synchronized ovulations in anoestrous ewes. The present trial was carried out to test whether the male effect could improve the fertility of anoestrous ewes maintained under the arid conditions in central Mexico.

From April 10 to June 22, 162 mixed breed (Corriedale x Ramboillet x Suffolk) adult anoestrous ewes (BCS: median range 1.5 to 2.5) were kept for 60 d with 14 sexually-active rams (treated with 16 h light from January 25 to April 9). The control group ($n=52$) was maintained in isolation from rams. On June 21, after mating had been confirmed in ewes exposed to the male effect, the control females were treated with progestagen sponges for 12 d. To monitor the characteristics of the oestrous cycles induced by the male effect, progesterone was assayed in plasma from jugular blood that had been sampled daily from 50 ewes (25 treated and 25 controls), from 2 d before until 47 d after ram introduction.

89/162 (55%) of the ewes exposed to the male effect had an induced oestrous cycle. This was followed by a second oestrous cycle in 51/162 ewes (31%) and by a third oestrous cycle in 23/162 ewes (14%). In the control group, none of the ewes had an oestrous cycle over the same period ($P<0.05$). In the ewes exposed to males, the delay from the introduction of males to the first detected oestrous cycle was 15 ± 1.5 d (mean$\pm$SE). There were no differences ($P=0.101$) among the lengths of the first, second and third detected cycles induced by the males (17 ± 1.0 d; 17 ± 1.0 d and 20 ± 1.3 d). The progesterone concentration was greater in the ewes exposed to rams (1.41 ± 0.20 ng/mL) compared with controls (0.46 ± 0.03 ng/mL; $P<0.001$). The percentage of pregnant ewes was greater in the male effect group (65%) than in the control group (45%; $P=0.007$) after progestagen sponge treatment.

In conclusion, the male effect improved the induction of oestrous cyclicity and pregnancy rate in ewes maintained under extensive conditions in an arid environment.

Supported by Universidad Autónoma Metropolitana Iztapalapa 1440902 and PROMEP-SEP 14410747 Mexico.

Effects of transport stress and kisspeptin on blood prolactin concentrations in Japanese Black beef

H Kadokawa[a], K Noguchi[a], Y Hajiri[a], D Fujisaki[a], K Takeshita[b] and Y Fujii[b,]

[a]*Yamaguchi University, Yamaguchi, Japan;* [b]*Yamaguchi Prefectural Agriculture and Forestry General Engineering Center, Yamaguchi, Japan*

It is now well established that kisspeptin, the signals through the kisspeptin receptor (GPR54), provides a direct and robust stimulus to the hypothalamic network of gonadotropin realeasing hormone (GnRH) neurons that govern gonadotropin secretion from the anterior pituitary. Kisspeptin may have other important roles in brain or pituitary, including controlling secretions of prolactin[1,2]. The nature of the roles remains to be defined, however, especially in males under various environmental conditions. In this study, we evaluated the effects of transport stress and kisspeptin on blood concentrations of luteinizing hormone (LH), and prolactin.

Intact male Japanese Black beef calves (5 months old) were used in this study. On the day preceding the injection with kisspeptin-10 or saline, all animals were fitted with an indwelling jugular vein catheter. On the day of trial, males were given transport stress by trucking for 2 h, from 930 to 1130 h, or remained in the house. Blood samples were collected to obtain plasma at 15-min intervals from the males from 1200 to 1700 h, for analysis of the concentrations of cortisol, LH and prolactin. Males received an injection of saline only or 1 mg of human kisspeptin-10 dissolved in saline at 1200 h. After assays for cortisol, LH and prolactin, we calculated the maximum concentration observed among serial samples during the 300 min (maximum concentration) and the timing of samples containing them for comparison by ANOVA. Also, we evaluated the effect of transport stress and the injectate on blood hormone concentration using repeated-measure ANOVA.

Transport stress increased blood cortisol concentrations. As expected, injection with kisspeptin-10, but not saline only, increased blood LH concentrations. Transport stress had no significant effect on the maximum LH concentration, its timing, and other parameters. Transport stress decreased blood prolactin concentrations in the first hour after the injection. Kisspeptin-10 injection did not increase prolactin concentration as surge-shape immediately after the injection. However, the kisspeptin-10 group had significant ($P<0.01$) higher prolactin concentration than the saline group in the period from 1500 to 1700 h, only after the transport stress.

Kisspeptin-10, therefore, had no significant rapid effect on prolactin, however, further studies are required to evaluate its delayed effect on prolactin under various environmental condition.

[1]Kadokawa *et al.*, 2008. J Endocrinol 196:331–334.
[2]Kadokawa *et al.*, 2008. Anim Reprod Sci 105:404–408.

Effects of temperament on reproductive and physiological responses of beef cows

RF Cooke[a], AB Scarpa[a], C Mueller[b], T DelCurto[b] and DW Bohnert[a]

[a]*Oregon State University – Eastern Oregon Agricultural Research Center, Burns, USA;* [b]*Oregon State University – Eastern Oregon Agricultural Research Center, Union, USA*

Recent research demonstrated that excitable temperament altered physiological parameters and impaired reproductive performance of beef cows[1]. However, this evaluation was only performed in *Bos indicus*-influenced cows. Therefore, the objective of this study was to evaluate the effects of excitable temperament on plasma concentrations of cortisol and acute-phase proteins, and pregnancy rates of *B. taurus* cows.

A total of 435 multiparous lactating Angus × Hereford cows, located at two different research stations (Burns, n = 241; Union, n = 192) were sampled for blood and evaluated for body condition score (BCS) and temperament before the beginning of the breeding season. Temperament was assessed by chute score and chute exit velocity score, which were combined into a final temperament score (1 to 5 scale; 1 = calm temperament, 5 = excitable temperament). Cows were classified according to the final temperament score (≤ 3 = adequate temperament, > 3 = excitable temperament). Blood samples were analyzed for plasma concentrations of cortisol, haptoglobin, and ceruloplasmin. During the breeding season, cows were exposed to mature Angus bulls for a 50-d breeding season (1:18 bull to cow ratio). However, cows located at the Union station were also assigned to a estrus synchronization + timed-AI protocol before bull exposure. Pregnancy status was verified by detecting a fetus with rectal palpation approximately 180 d after the end of the breeding season.

Plasma cortisol concentrations were greater ($P < 0.01$) in cows with excitable temperament compared with cohort with adequate temperament (19.7 vs. 15.1 ng/mL, respectively). No effects were detected ($P > 0.26$) for BCS and plasma concentrations of haptoglobin and ceruloplasmin. Pregnancy rates tended to be reduced ($P = 0.10$) in cows with excitable temperament compared with the cohort with adequate temperament (89.3 vs. 94.0 % as pregnant cows divided by total exposed cows, respectively). Further, the probability of cows to become pregnant during the breeding season was affected quadratically ($P = 0.05$) by temperament score (91.4, 95.0, 94.3, 87.6, and 59.3% of pregnancy probability for temperament scores of 1 through 5, respectively).

Results from this study indicated that excitable temperament is also detrimental to reproductive performance of *B. taurus* beef cows, independently of BCS and breeding system. Further, this effect can be associated, at least in part, with increased plasma cortisol concentrations of cows with excitable temperament.

[1]Cooke *et al.*, 2009. J Anim Sci 87:4125-4132.

Effects of acclimation to handling on performance, reproductive, and physiological responses of replacement beef heifers

RF Cooke[a], H Montilla[b], AB Scarpa[a], FM Nery[a], FNT Cooke[a], CT Estill[b] and DW Bohnert[a]

[a]*Oregon State University – Eastern Oregon Agricultural Research Center, Burns, USA;* [b]*Oregon State University – Veterinary Teaching Hospital, Corvallis, USA*

Acclimation to human handling improved temperament and decreased age at puberty and interval to pregnancy in replacement beef heifers[1]. However, this strategy was evaluated in *Bos indicus*-influenced heifers. The objective of this study, therefore, was to evaluate the effects of acclimation to human handling on growth, temperament, plasma concentrations of cortisol and acute-phase proteins, and puberty attainment of *Bos taurus* heifers.

Thirty-eight Angus heifers were initially evaluated, within 30 d after weaning, for body weight (BW) and puberty status via transrectal ultrasonography and plasma progesterone concentrations (d 0 and 10), and for temperament by measurements of chute score and exit velocity (d 10 only). On d 11, heifers were stratified by puberty status, temperament, BW and age, and randomly assigned to receive or not receive (control) the acclimation treatment. Acclimated heifers were exposed to a handling process 3 times weekly (Mondays, Wednesdays, and Fridays) for 4 weeks (d 11 to 39 of the experiment). The acclimation treatment was applied individually to heifers by processing them through a handling facility, whereas control heifers remained undisturbed on pasture. Heifer puberty status, evaluated by plasma progesterone concentrations and BW were assessed again on d 40 and 50, d 70 and 80, d 110 and 120, and d 140 and 150 of the study. Blood samples collected before (d 10) and at the end of the acclimation period (d 40) were also analyzed for plasma concentrations of cortisol, haptoglobin, and ceruloplasmin. Heifer temperament was assessed again on d 40 of the study.

No treatment effects were detected for BW gain ($P=0.89$). Acclimated heifers had greater exit velocity ($P=0.04$) but reduced plasma concentrations of cortisol ($P=0.04$) and haptoglobin compared with control heifers after the acclimation period (2.09 vs. 1.53 m/s for chute score; 25.7 vs. 34.11 ng/mL for cortisol; 5.27 vs. 5.90 absorbance at 450 nm $\times$ 100 for haptoglobin). No treatment effects were detected for puberty attainment ($P=0.50$).

Results from this study indicated that acclimation to human handling after weaning reduced circulating concentrations of substances associated with behavioral stress but did not improve temperament or hasten puberty in *Bos taurus* replacement beef heifers.

[1]Cooke *et al.*, 2009. J Anim Sci 87:3043-3412.

Monitoring estrus expression and behavioral irregularities with a pedometric system in grazing beef herds

R Gabrieli[a] and A Antman[b]

[a]Extension Service, Ministry of Agriculture, Israel; [b]SAE Afikim, Israel

In many countries beef herds are raised in grazing plots. There is no data available regarding daily observations of reproductive activity of the cows because there is no operating system for daily estrus detection in extensive grazing plots. Cows are diagnosed for pregnancy by a veterinarian 45 d after the breeding season is ended and none of the pregnant cows are culled. There is no available data to indicate whether a cow failed to conceive because: 1) she was not cycling, 2) she was in estrus but not mated, or 3) she conceived but then aborted.

The objectives of this field trial were to test the feasibility of operating an estrus detection pedometric system by SAE Afikim in a typical grazing beef herd, to obtain daily observations of estrus activity for the majority of the herd, maintain stable activity graphs, and identify deviations from base line activity as expression of estrus or something else. Successful accomplishment of the preceding objectives would allow the breeder to accept online data-based decisions pertaining to treating an individual cow, improving management, or culling.

A typical Israeli beef herd was selected. The herd had 129 Simmental cows from 3 to 5 years of age, and at their 2nd or 3rd calving. The area of the grazing plot was approximately 250 acres. Pedometers were put on 60 cows and daily data were captured on 47 cows. Visual detection of estrus was conducted to compare with the results of the pedometric system. We encountered some technical problems with identification in the field that were solved by proper grounding of the antenas. Opening the detection system for time periods longer than 4 hours, resulted in irregular activity graphs. Individual manual inspection revealed an irregular daily pattern of visiting the water trough (location of the antenas). Shortening the detection period to 4 h daily resulted in detection of 95% of the cows and stable activity graphs on which deviations could be seen clearly.

The system detected 46 of 47 cows that were cyclic and had pedometric data. Three cows did not express estrus during the period, were not pregnant at pregnancy check, and did not calve. Three cows showed estrus, were not pregnant at pregnancy check, and did not calve. Another cow was in estrus, was pregnant on the pregnancy check and aborted. The system also showed depression in activity of a cow that was limping. This implies a possibility for earlier detection of health problems using the system. Another cow showed an activity deviation that could not be explained as an estrus. The observation discovered that the cow's calf was sick, and the higher activity was due to the cow going back and forth to the calf that did not follow her. This implies the possibility for the use of the system for detecting early health problems with the calves as well. Deviations in the graphs of the whole group occurred upon weaning of the calves. Some deviations in individual cow graphs could not be explained. These require further research.

An integrated approach to development and application of precise methods of estrous cycle control for beef heifers and cows: A project retrospective

DJ Patterson, DA Mallory, JM Nash and MF Smith

University of Missouri, Columbia USA

Improvements in methods to control the estrous cycle of beef cattle have outpaced progress in the publics' understanding of how best to implement new technologies. Despite the recent development of estrous synchronization protocols that facilitated the use of fixed-time AI in postpartum beef cows, the same degree of success in beef heifers has not been realized. The objectives of this project were based on the economic need to improve the competitive position of the U.S. beef industry through an integrated effort designed to increase adoption of reproductive procedures. These objectives included: 1) Research in development of new reproductive management strategies for replacement beef heifers to synchronize estrus and facilitate successful use of fixed-time AI; 2) Implementation of a comprehensive Extension education program focused on transfer of technology that would facilitate and expand the use of fixed-time AI in postpartum beef cows; and 3) Development of a comprehensive education program for veterinarians and extension field staff, and veterinary and animal science undergraduate and graduate students focused on the use of estrous synchronization and AI. Outcomes stemming from Objective 1 included the development of two long-term progestin-based protocols to synchronize estrus before fixed-time AI in beef heifers (CIDR Select and 14-d CIDR-PG protocols). Outcomes resulting from Objective 2 included comprehensive field demonstrations across Missouri involving 73 farms and 7,028 cows. All cows were synchronized using the CO-Synch + CIDR protocol with fixed-time AI performed 66 h after CIDR removal and PG. Pregnancy rates resulting from fixed-time AI averaged 62%. Outcomes stemming from Objective 3 were focused on the development of a new web based curriculum entitled "Fundamentals of Beef Reproduction and Management: Focus on Estrous Synchronization". The curriculum consists of three courses including an overview of physiological principles that underlie estrous synchronization, and a review of commercially available estrous synchronization products; a review of specific estrous synchronization protocols recommended for beef heifers and cows; and an overview of management considerations for implementing an estrous synchronization program, including a description of the impact of estrous synchronization on reproductive management. The curriculum is now available through the University of Missouri Division of Animal Sciences website at http://animalsciences.missouri.edu/, and the NCBA Cattle Learning Center. The project, in addition, supported an internship in reproductive management of beef cattle, which over the past 14 years provided opportunities for 140 students in breeding programs involving over 175,000 heifers and cows on farms and ranches in twelve states. Collectively, the development of new estrous synchronization protocols for beef heifers, on-farm field demonstrations with beef cows, course curricula, and student internships support strategies that will enhance the successful use of estrous synchronization and AI among beef producers in the U.S.

This project was supported by National Research Initiative Competitive Grant no. 2005-55203-15750 from the USDA Cooperative State Research, Education, and Extension Service.

Impact of gender-selected semen on AI pregnancy rates, gender ratios, and calf performance in crossbred postpartum beef cows

JB Hall[a], A Ahmadzadeh[a], RH Stokes[a], C Stephenson[a] and J Ahola[b]

[a]*University of Idaho, Moscow, USA;* [b]*Colorado State University, Fort Collins, USA*

Gender-selected semen (GSS) is widely used in the dairy industry to produce replacement females. Pregnancy rates (PR) to GSS in dairy heifers range from 30 to 50%, but PR in lactating dairy cows are poor. Gender-selected semen from beef bulls is increasingly commercially available. The potential impact of GSS use in the beef industry is great, but limited information is available on the effect of GSS on PR or gender ratios in beef cattle, especially postpartum beef cows.

The objectives of the experiment were: 1) compare PR of cows inseminated with GSS or conventional semen (CON), 2) examine gender ratios in GSS and CON cows when a single AI service is followed with natural service for 45 d, and 3) compare the performance of calves produced from GSS and CON. In year 1, all cows (n=216) were estrous synchronized using a controlled intervaginal drug releasing (CIDR) device-based protocol. Thirty-seven estrual cows were selected for insemination with GSS (1 sire). All remaining cows were bred to one of 6 sires on estrus or fixed-time AI (FTAI). In year 2, all cows (n=100 GSS; n=223 CON) were estrous synchronized with the CO-Synch + 5-d CIDR protocol[1] and inseminated by FTAI. There were 2 GSS and 8 CON sires. In both years, cows were a minimum of 40 d postpartum and body condition score of 4. Pregnancy detection was performed via ultrasound on d 50 to 60 after AI and via palpation on d 90 after AI. Pregnancy and calving data were recorded for both years and weaning data were available for year 1.

In both years, there was no difference ($P>0.5$) in PR between GSS and CON cows. Pregnancy rates in year 1 averaged 67.5% (25/37; GS) and 57.5% (103/179: CON). For CON cows in year 1 that displaed estrus before AI, PR was 64.7%. In year 2, PR was 50.5% (46/97; GSS) and 53.8% (120/223; CON). There was no interaction ($P>0.2$) among estrus status at AI and semen type on PR. However, more cows ($P<0.05$) observed in estrus became pregnant to AI regardless of semen type (56.3% vs. 44.7% for estrus and no estrus, respectively). Female to male ratios after natural service were 78:22 (GSS) and 47:53 (CON). Calf survivability and weaning weights were not different ($P>0.2$) between GSS and CON sired calves.

In this study, PR to GSS were not significantly different than CON. In addition, PR to GSS in postpartum beef cows averaged 53%. The results from this experiment should not be over-interpreted due to relatively limited number of cows and bulls used. However, we conclude that gender-selected semen is a viable option for altering gender ratios in beef cattle.

[1]Beef Reproductive Task Force, 2009.

Effect of PRID or PRID alpha on the interval to the LH peak and ovulation

W Kanitz[a], I Mücke[a], F Schneider[a], G Nürnberg[a] , C Leiding[b] and F Becker[a]

[a]*Leibniz Institute for Farm Animal Biology, Dummerstorf, Germany,* [b]*BVN Neustadt-Aisch, Germany*

An optimal interval between artificial insemination (AI) and ovulation is very important for fertilization and pregnancy rates. Artificial insemination at a fixed time requires an optimal interval; one where physiological processes and ovarian function are considered. The aim of this study was to investigate the interval from PRID or PRID alpha (PRID without estradiol) removal to the LH-Peak and ovulation. The specific aim was to decrease the variance of this interval to facilitate fixed-time AI.

Experiment 1: Eighteen (n=6 per treatment group) Simmental heifers received a PRID for 9 d. Treatment started on d 3/4 or d 11/12 or d 18/19 of the oestrous cycle. All animals received a luteolytic dose of PGF_{2a} directly after PRID removal. Frequent blood sampling was performed via jugular catheter for 60 h at 2 h intervals starting 44 h after PRID removal. Ultrasound scanning of the ovaries was performed for 42 h at 6 h intervals starting 66 h after PRID removal. LH concentrations were determined by using an enhanced chemiluminescence immunoassay system (ECLIA; sensivity <0.03 ng/ml, intra-assay CV=6.4 %, inter-assay CV=8.9 %).

Experiment 2: The same heifers as in Exp. 1 received PRID alpha after one additional natural cycle. Treatment, blood sampling, LH determination and ultrasound scanning were done as in Exp. 1.

Experiment 3: Based on the results from Exp. 1 and 2 the same heifers received PRID alpha independent of stage of oestrous cycle for 9 d after one natural cycle. All heifers received 10 μg Buserelin (Receptal®, Intervet) 50 h after PRID removal and PGF_{2a} administration. Samples for LH determination were recovered for 10 h at 2 h intervals starting 40 h after PRID removal and additionally 1 and 2 h after GnRH application.

Data were analyzed by an one-way ANOVA model, with a fixed factor 'group', using proc GLM of SAS® (SAS Systems, Release 8.2, SAS Institute Inc., Cary, NC USA). All post-hoc tests were adjusted by Tukey correction to ensure a multiple error rate of 0.05. Additionally confidence intervals (1-alpha=0.95) were calculated.

In Exp. 1 and 2, 31 animals (86.1 %) showed signs of oestrus and this result was independent of estradiol administration. The mean interval from PRID removal to LH peak ranged from 55.3±7.8 to 56.5±5.5 h in Exp. 1. It was not influenced by start of treatment. The confidence interval for the parameter was 39 to 71 h. The mean interval from PRID removal to ovulation was 79.4 h with a confidence interval of 65 to 93 h.

The mean interval from PRID alpha removal to LH peak ranged from 50.7±5.5 to 61.0±5.5 h in Exp. 2. It was not significantly influenced by start of treatment. The confidence interval for the parameter was 39 to 72 h. The mean interval from PRID removal to ovulation was 78.7 h with a confidence interval from 64 to 92 h.

GnRH application synchronized the LH peak in treated animals. The mean interval from PRID alpha removal to LH peak was 53.0 h with a confidence interval of 52.4 to 53.6 h. The mean interval from PRID removal to ovulation was 77.7 h after GnRH treatment. The confidence interval was 75.2 to 80.0 h. The interval from LH peak to ovulation was not influenced by GnRH (mean: 24.3 h, confidence interval 21.9 to 26.8 h).

In conclusion PRID alpha is as efficient as PRID in synchronizing the interval to LH peak and ovulation. Ovulations can be synchronized efficiently, if physiological processes are considered.

Gonadotropin secretion stimulated by whitefish GnRH in ruminants

H Kadokawa[a], Y Joh[b], H Kamada[c] and Y Yamada[b]

[a]*Yamaguchi University, Yamaguchi, Japan;* [b]*National Agricultural Research Center for Hokkaido Region, Sapporo, Japan;* [c]*National Institute of Livestock and Grassland Science, Tsukuba, Japan*

Gonadotropin-releasing hormone (GnRH) is the primary hypothalamic peptide that controls reproductive function by regulating the secretion of LH and FSH. The traditional view was that eutherian mammals express only a single form of GnRH, known as mammalian GnRH. However, more than 60 novel decapeptides have now been identified as GnRH structural variants in different species and more than one form of GnRH is expressed in most species, including human. We previously reported that sheep brains have the undefined peptide detected by antisrerum to GnRH-II[1] and MALDI/TOFF mass spectrometry, although ruminants have no active gene for GnRH-II. Whitefish GnRH (pGlu-His-Trp-Ser-Tyr-Gly-Met-Asn-Pro-Gly-NH_2) is a novel form of GnRH observed in basal salmonid which belong to one of most important places in the evolutionary tree. We evaluated whether whitefish GnRH has an effect on gonadotropin release in ruminants.

In first experiment, Holstein heifers were used on 3 d after ovulation. The 1 mg of synthetic whitefish GnRH was injected into the jugular vein of the heifers at time 0 and blood samples were collected at -30, -15, 0, 1, 2, 3, 4, 5, 10, 15, 20, 30, 45, 60, 75, 90, 105, 120, 150, 180, 240, and 300 min for radioimmunoassay (RIA) for LH and FSH. In the second experiment, prepubertal female lambs were used in an active immunization trial and treated with KLH carrier protein only or 1 mg/head of synthetic whitefish GnRH conjugated to the KLH. After booster immunizations and confirming the existence of desired antibodies in the blood of all lambs, the blood samples were collected at 10 min intervals for 6 h for the gonadotropin RIA. In the third experiment, three Holstein dry cows were implanted with third ventricular cannula. On 3 d after the induced ovulation, the blood samples were collected at 15 min intervals for an hour to determine basal levels, then, 1 mg/ml of whitefish GnRH dissolved in saline were injected through the catheter at time 0. After the injection, further peripheral blood samples were collected at 15 min intervals for 6 h for the gonadotropin RIA.

In the first experiment, we observed a significant surge in the levels of both LH and FSH after the intravenous injection in all heifers. In the second experiment, the LH pulse frequency was suppressed in sheep immunized with the synthetic whitefish GnRH, but not in sheep immunized with the KLH only. In third experiment, we observed the significant surge-shape increases in the levels of both LH and FSH after the intravenous injection in 1 of 3 cows.

Whitefish GnRH, therefore, can stimulate gonadotropin release in ruminants. Further studies are required to evaluate the existence of GnRH variants in ruminant brains.

[1]Kadokawa *et al.,* 2008. Biol Reprod Special Issue 307.

Effects of long-term subcutaneous implant of deslorelin (GnRHa-Suprelorin®) in Nelore cows

WC Marques Filho[a], JCP Ferreira[a], R Sartori[b], E Trevisol[a] and I Martin[a]

[a]*Department of Animal Reproduction and Veterinary Radiology, School of Veterinary Medicine and Animal Science, Univ Estadual Paulista, São Paulo, Brazil;* [b]*Department of Animal Science, ESALQ, USP, São Paulo, Brazil*

Long-term treatments with GnRH agonists (deslorelin) have been used in a variety of species to control reproductive activity. The main reported effect of deslorelin implant in cattle is the down-regulation of GnRH receptors on gonadotrophs that desensitizes the anterior pituitary gland to GnRH and abolishes the pulsatile release of FSH and LH[1]. Such effects lead to suppression of follicular growth and an arrest of follicles at 2 or 3 mm in diameter after continuous treatment for 28 d[1,2]. However, deslorelin implants have not been tested in *Bos indicus* cattle which is the objective of this experiment.

Fifteen cycling adult Nelore cows (body condition score ≥ 3; 1 to 5 scale) were used. Estrous cycles were synchronized by the follow protocol: D-11: 2 mg of estradiol benzoate i.m. (Estrogin®; Farmavet, Brazil) + intravaginal progesterone device 1 g (DIB®; Intervet Schering-Plough, Brazil); D-3: 12.5 mg tromethamine Dinoprost i.m. (Lutalyse®, Pfizer Saúde Animal, Brazil) + removal of intravaginal progesterone device; D-2: 1 mg estradiol benzoate IM (Estrogin®) and D0: transrectal ultrasound ovary examination.

All animals had ovulated on d 11 of the protocol and 10 cows were chosen randomly to receive the subcutaneous deslorelin bioimplant in the outer side of the right ear where it remained for 70 d. During this period there were no ovulations. Two patterns of follicular development were observed. In the first 35 d after implantation the follicular waves emerged sequentially at regular intervals of 10-11 (7-16) d and the follicular diameter reached values similar to those observed during the normal estrous cycle (from 1.1 to 1.4 cm)[3]. Occasionally larger follicles were observed with diameters ranging from 1.5 to 1.6 cm, and in two animals the follicles reached a diameter of only 0.8 to 1 cm. After d 35, the waves occurred at regular intervals of about 10 d. However, the follicular diameter remained lesser than 0.6 cm in 5 animals, and between 0.6 and 0.9 cm in 3 animals.

The patterns of follicular development observed in the first half of implantation period were similar to that observed in pregnant cows and suggested that gonadotropin release occurred in a manner sufficient to allow follicular wave emergence, selection and deviation of dominant follicles. However, as no ovulations were seen, the ovulatory surge of LH appeared to be abolished. Conversely, after d 35 the follicular development model suggested that the secretion patterns of gonadotropins changed with the decrease of LH pulsatility as the follicular diameter remained near deviation

Long-term treatments with GnRH agonists (deslorelin subcutaneous implants) affected the follicular development of Nelore cows. The extent of suppression of follicular growth, however, was lesser than that observed in *Bos taurus* cows.

This study was supported by FAPESP, FUNDUNESP/Brazil and Peptech Animal Health/Australia.

[1]D'Occhio *et al.*, 2000. Anim Reprod Sci 61:433–442.
[2]Silvestre *et al.*, 2009. Anim Reprod Sci 110:79-95
[3]Martin *et al.*, 2004. Acta Scientiae Veterinariae 32:234.

Follicular and ovulatory response following a pLH challenge in pre-pubertal Nelore heifers

RS Cipriano, JC Freitas and GP Nogueira

UNESP- Universidade Estadual Paulista – Veterinary Medicine, Araçatuba-SP, Brazil

Puberty in beef heifers is an important event that is regulated by gonadostatic mechanisms that control the frequency of LH pulses from the hypothalamic-pituitary axis. Reduced LH pulse frequency results in reduced follicular growth and less ovulation. Nelore cattle, although well adapted to tropical weather, first ovulate at 24 mo of age. Consequently, decreasing the age at puberty in the Nelore breed is crucial for the Brazilian beef industry and may increase a breeder's revenue by 16%.

This research evaluated the effect of an injection of 5 mg of pLH on folicular growth and ovulatory follicular capacity in pre-pubertal Nelore heifers. Ovaries from 30 pre-pubertal Nelore heifers that were approximately 540 d of age were evaluated daily and 20 heifers with growing follicles (>9mm) were divided into 2 groups of 10 animals each. Heifers had the same weight (P=0.37) in each group: Control group 310±28 kg (275 to 365 kg) and Treated 320±21 kg (294 to 354 kg). Treated heifers received a single injection of 5 mg of pLH (i.m.) and heifers in the Control group received 2 ml of saline. Ovaries of heifers in each group were subsequently evaluated by ultrasound (Aloka Prosound-2, 7.5 MHz probe) every 12 h for the first 24 h and every 6 h until 36 h and the largest follicle diameter was measured. Ovulation was defined as the disappearance of the largest follicle at the subsequent ultrasound evaluation. Data were analyzed by repeated measures ANOVA.

pLH treatment induced ovulation in one treated heifer between 28 and 36 h. The heifer weighed 308 kg and had a 10 mm follicle at the moment of pLH injection. Follicle diameter increased from 0 to 28 h in Treated heifers (P=0.001, from 10.2±1 mm to 11.6±1.6 mm) but decreased from 0 h to 36 h in Control heifers (P=0.025, from 10.6±1.5 mm to 9.5±1.4 mm). After 24 h of pLH injection the largest follicle diameter was greater (P=0.05) in treated (11.6±1.6mm) than Control (10.2±1.4mm) heifers.

After a pLH challenge the percentage of ovulation was low (10%) as a consequence of the animal status or the dose that was used. The ovulated follicle became a CL and 5 d later was producing 1.9 ng/ml of serum progesterone. Although conservative, the utilized dose was sufficient to stimulate follicular growth as treated animals had larger dominant follicles than control animals. It was possible to conclude that a growing follicle is responsive to pLH in prepubertal Nelore heifers but efficiency of the ovulatory response needs further investigation.

Acknowledgements: Fapesp for founding 08/57486-4 and scholarship 08/57492-4.

Induction of first postpartum LH surge with GnRH or estradiol benzoate administration, in Nelore cows with or without nutritional supplementation

VG Pinheiro[a], RA Satrapa[b], JRLM Cury[b], GP Nogueira[c] and CM Barros[c]

[a]*Department of Animal Reproduction – FMVZ;* [b]*Department of Pharmacology – IBB, University of São Paulo State (UNESP), Botucatu, São Paulo, Brazil;* [c]*FOA-UNESP*

The presence of calf, body condition score, number of births (multiparous vs. primiparous) and breed are factors that influence the duration of postpartum anoestrus in beef cows. The objective of the present study was to evaluate, during early postpartum, the time of re-establishment of pituitary LH stores, measured by the hypothalamic-pituitary axis responsiveness to exogenous administration of GnRH or EB. Primiparous lactating Nelore cows (*Bos indicus,* n = 38) were randomly allocated into four groups, according to the hormonal treatment: EB Group (1 mg EB, i.m., Estrogin®, Farmavet, Sao Paulo, Brazil; n = 11), GnRH Group (100μg, licerelina, i.m, Gestran Plus□, ARSA S.L.R., Buenos Aires, Argentina; n = 9), EB-SUP (n = 9) and GnRH-SUP (n = 9). The supplemented (SUP) groups were supplemented with a balanced diet, based on cotton meal and ground corn. The drugs were administered from 7 d postpartum (±4 d), at intervals of 7 d, until 140 d postpartum or the occurrence of the first ovulation that was observed by weekly ultrasonography (US, Aloka 900, Tokyo, Japan, transrectal probe 7.5 MHz). Blood samples were collected just before and 4 h (GnRH groups) or 18 h (EB groups) after hormone administration in order to determine LH concentrations by RIA. The data were analysed by regression analysis (PROC PHREG) and Fisher exact test. The occurrence of an LH surge until 140 d postpartum was significantly less frequent in the EB group (2/11 cows) when compared with the other groups [EB-SUP (6/9); GnRH (7/9), and GnRH-SUP (7/9), $P<0.01$]. Excluding the EB group, since only 2 cows had increased LH concentrations, an LH surge was observed earlier (days postpartum ± SEM) in animals that were supplemented (GnRH-SUP, 30.4 ± 0.9) compared with non supplemented cows (GnRH, 41.6 ± 1.3, $P<0.09$), and in cows that were treated with GnRH (GnRH-SUP, 30.4 ± 0.9) vs. EB-SUP (73.5 ± 0.9, $P<0.001$). In conclusion, nutritional supplementation advanced the first postpartum LH surge induced by GnRH or EB. Additionally, EB administration did not induce the LH surge in most Nelore cows in the EB group, possibly due to the sensitivity of the hypothalamus to negative feedback of estrogens, inhibiting the pre-ovulatory LH surge.

Supported and fellowship (Pinheiro VG and Satrapa RA) from FAPESP (Sao Paulo, Brazil).

Ovarian function in Nelore beef cows (*Bos indicus*) after different hormonal treatments to induce ovulation

R Machado[a], MA Bergamaschi[a], CA Oliveira[b] and M Binelli[b]

[a]*Embrapa Pecuária Sudeste, São Carlos, Brazil;* [b]*Universidade de São Paulo, São Paulo, Brazil*

Synchronization of ovulation is a tool to carry out timed artificial insemination. However, available protocols to induce ovulation provide variable results. This study evaluated different treatments to induce ovulation in Nelore (*Bos indicus*) cows.

Group GnRH/$PGF_{2\alpha}$ (n = 40) received the Ovsynch protocol[1] based on the administration of two injections of GnRH agonist (Buserelin acetate; 8 μg i.m.) given 9 d apart and a $PGF_{2\alpha}$ analogue (d-Cloprostenol; 0.15 mg i.m.) given 48 h before the 2nd GnRH injection; Group Norg (n = 30): animals received 3 mg Norgestomet and 5 mg Estradiol valerate i.m. with an auricular implant containing 3 mg Norgestomet at an unknown stage of the oestrous cycle (d 0). On d 9, the implant was withdrawn; and group NorgeCG (n = 30): same treatment as Norg plus Equine Chorionic Gonadotrophin (eCG; 400 IU, i.m.) at implant removal[2]. Ovulation rate was determined by ultrasound and cows that ovulated were submitted daily to transrectal ultrasound assessment of follicular and luteal dynamics, as well as determination of plasma progesterone concentration (P_4) up to the subsequent natural ovulation.

All treatments induced synchronized ovulation in most cows (62.5%, 70.0% and 70.0% respectively to GnRH/$PGF_{2\alpha}$, Norg and NorgeCG; P > 0.05). Inter-ovulatory interval (22.5±0.7 d) as well as diameter of the dominant follicle at luteolysis (9.6±1.1 mm) and preovulatory follicle diameter at the induced (12.73±0.69 mm) and subsequent natural (13.17±0.52 mm) cycle were not affected (P > 0.05) by treatments. Overall function of the corpus luteum (CL) generated after induced ovulation was affected by treatments (P < 0.05), except the luteal phase length, which was similar among cows (17.6±0.5 d). Respectively for GnRH/$PGF_{2\alpha}$, Norg, and NorgeCG, the maximum volume of CL (mm^3) was: 7117.3±125.7[a], 5437.8±405.9[b] and 6927.5±405.9[a]; the day of CL maximum volume was: 14.4±0.6[a], 7.7±0.5[c] and 9.2±0.5[b]; the plasma P_4 concentration (ng/mL) at that day was: 6.2±1.7[a], 4.5±0.5[b] and 6.1±0.5[a]; the highest plasma P_4 (ng/mL) in the estrous cycle subsequent to induction of ovulation was 6.8±1.7[b], 6.4±0.6[b] and 8.2±0.6[a] and the day in the estrous cycle of highest plasma P_4 was 13.4±0.6[a], 11.4±0.6[b] and 11.3±0.6[b].

In conclusion, GnRH/$PGF_{2\alpha}$ based protocol delays the increase in progesterone concentration after synchronized ovulation, which can be potentially hazardous to embryo transport, maternal recognition of pregnancy and maintenance of early gestation[3]. eCG may be added to the Norg protocol when luteal function is to be optimized because it increased the dimensions of the CL and concentration of progesterone over the subsequent estrous cycle compared to Norg alone.

[1]Pursley *et al.*, 1995. Theriogenology 44:915-923.
[2]Baruselli *et al.*, 2004. Anim Reprod Sci 82-83:479-486.
[3]Mann and Lamming, 2001. Reproduction 121:175-80.

Influence of dose of $PGF_{2\alpha}$ and length of CIDR treatment on reproductive performance of non-lactating Nelore beef cows

MV Biehl[a], AV Pires[a], JLM Vasconcelos[b], R Sartori[a], JRS Gonçalves[c], LG Lima[c], DD Nepomuceno[a], I Susin[a], GB Mourão[a] and ML Day[d]

[a]*Escola Superior de Agricultura Luiz de Queiroz, Piracicaba - SP, Brazil;* [b]*FMVZ/UNESP, Botucatu-SP, Brazil;* [c]*Estação Experimental Georgina Hildegard Von Pritzelwitz, Londrina-PR, Brazil;* [d]*Ohio State University, Columbus, USA*

The objective was to compare reproductive performance of non-lactating Nelore cows (n=286) in which estrus was synchronized using either a 5 or 7 d estradiol benzoate (EB) + CIDR-based protocol and 3 doses of $PGF_{2\alpha}$. Cows were blocked according to body weight (mean 364±39 kg) and BCS (2.55±0.16, scale of 1 to 5) in a 2x3 factorial arrangement. Cows received 2 mg EB at the time of CIDR insertion, which was offset by 2 d to achieve either 5 (5 d) or 7 (7 d) d of CIDR treatment. On the day of CIDR removal, cows received either 12.5, 25 or 50 mg $PGF_{2\alpha}$ i.m. The treatments were 5d12.5 (n=50; e.g., 5 d CIDR treatment and 12.5 mg $PGF_{2\alpha}$), 5d25 (n=46), 5d50 (n=48), 7d12.5 (n=48), 7d25 (n=48), and 7d50 (n=46).

Estrus detection was performed for 120 h after CIDR removal and artificial insemination (AI) was performed according to the AM/PM protocol. Beginning 16 d after CIDR removal, estrus detection was again performed for 144 h and cows that showed estrus were AI. Pregnancy diagnosis was performed by ultrasonography 60 d after the first AI. Overall, estrus was detected in 238/286 cows (83.2%). A main effect of duration of CIDR treatment indicated that more ($P<0.05$) cows were detected in estrus across the 7d (overall mean and SE for 7d) than 5 d (mean across 5 d treatments) treatments.

Mean time of onset of estrus did not differ among treatments and was 70.1±17.3 h after CIDR removal. Conception rate was also greater ($P<0.05$) across doses of $PGF_{2\alpha}$ in the 7d (mean for 7d) than the 5d (mean for 5 d) treatments. Accordingly, pregnancy rate during the synchronization period was greater ($P<0.05$) in the 7 d (mean) than 5 d (mean) treatments. A CIDR x $PGF_{2\alpha}$ dose interaction was detected for total AI pregnancy rate with the greatest ($P<0.05$) pregnancy rates detected in the 7d12.5 and 5d50 treatments and the lowest detected in the 5d12.5 and 7d50 treatments. In an EB+CIDR synchronization protocol that included 2 mg EB at the time of CIDR insertion, reproductive performance was greater with a 7 d than 5 d CIDR treatment.

Acknowledgement: This study was supported by Fundação de Amparo à Pesquisa do Estado de São Paulo - FAPESP, Brazil. A.V.Pires and G.B. Mourão are recipients of research productivity scholarship from CNPq.

Effects of GnRH at initiation of the 5-d timed AI program and timing of induction of ovulation relative to AI on ovarian dynamics and fertility of dairy heifers

FS Lima, H Ayres, M Favoreto, RS Bisinotto, LF Greco, ES Souza, RS Marsola, CA Risco, WW Thatcher and JEP Santos

Department of Animal Sciences, University of Florida, Gainesville, USA

Pregnancy per insemination (P/AI) in dairy heifers is low in timed AI protocols based on GnRH and $PGF_{2\alpha}$; however, a recent program[1] resulted in 52 to 61% pregnancy in heifers inseminated at a fixed time. The protocol is comprised of an injection of GnRH and insertion of an intravaginal progesterone device (CIDR) followed 5 d later by CIDR removal and an injection of $PGF_{2\alpha}$, and AI concurrent with a second GnRH injection 72 h after $PGF_{2\alpha}$.

Two experiments were conducted. Objectives of experiment 1 and 2 were, respectively: to evaluate the need for the first GnRH injection on ovarian responses and P/AI of dairy heifers and to determine the effects of timing of induced ovulation relative to AI on fertility of dairy heifers.

In experiment 1, 602 heifers were assigned randomly to receive GnRH or to remain as untreated Control on study d 0. Ovaries were scanned on study d 0 and 5. All heifers received a CIDR on d 0, an injection of $PGF_{2\alpha}$ and removal of the CIDR on d 5, and GnRH and timed AI on d 8. Blood was sampled and analyzed for progesterone (P4) on d 5 and 8. Pregnancy was diagnosed on d 32 and 67 after AI. Ovulation to the first GnRH was greater (P=0.001) for GnRH (35.4%) than Control (10.6%). Presence of new CL at $PGF_{2\alpha}$ injection was greater (P=0.001) for GnRH (43.1%) than Control (20.8%), although the proportion of heifers with a CL at $PGF_{2\alpha}$ did not differ (P=0.35) between treatments (GnRH=88.2% vs. Control=86.0%). P4 on the day of AI was greater (P=0.01) for GnRH than Control (0.52±0.06 vs. 0.31±0.06 ng/mL). Luteal regression (P4 <1 ng/mL) did not differ (P=0.16) between treatments (GnRH=90.2% vs. Control=94.9%) but a lesser (P<0.01) proportion of GnRH than Control heifers had P4 <0.5 ng/mL on the day of AI (73.8 vs. 88.2%). P/AI was not affected by treatment either on d 32 or 67 (GnRH=52.7 and 51.9% vs. Control=53.3 and 50.4%), and pregnancy loss did not differ (P=0.11) between treatments (GnRH=1.5% vs. Control=5.6%).

In experiment 2, 1,316 heifers were assigned randomly to receive a CIDR on d 0, $PGF_{2\alpha}$ and removal of the CIDR on d 5, and either GnRH 56 h after $PGF_{2\alpha}$ and AI 16 h after GnRH (OVS56) or GnRH and AI 72 h after $PGF_{2\alpha}$ (COS72). P/AI on d 32 did not differ (P=0.43) and they were 58.6 and 63.0 for OVS56 and COS72, respectively.

Use of GnRH on the first day of the 5-d CIDR synchronization program resulted in low ovulation rate and no improvement in P/AI. Also, timing of induction of ovulation relative to AI did not influence P/AI in dairy heifers.

[1]Rabaglino *et al.,* 2010. J Dairy Sci 93:1050-1058.

The effect of eCG given as part of an Ovsynch whole herd synchrony program on a seasonal calving herd in Victoria

DS Beggs[a], JC Kelly[a] and JF Hasler[b]

[a]*Warrnambool Veterinary Clinic, Warrnambool, Victoria, Australia;* [b]*Bioniche, Belleville, Ontario, Canada*

A pilot trial was conducted on a seasonal calving dairy herd in western Victoria to assess the effect of eCG given at the time of $PGF_{2\alpha}$ injection in a standard Ovsynch whole herd synchrony program. All cows that calved more than 30 d before the planned start of AI in the current season and which had reliable records of age and calving date were included in the trial (n = 508). Cows were divided into control (n = 255) and treatment (n = 253) groups on the basis of having an odd or even ear tag number in an attempt to stratify the groups by age. All cows received 100 μg gonadorelin (Gonabreed®, Parnell) on d 0, 500 mg cloprostenol (Estromil®, Troy) on d 7, 100 μg gonadorelin on d 9 and fixed time insemination approximately 16 h later, on d 10. In addition to this, the treatment group received 400 i.u. eCG (Pregnecol®, Bioniche) at the time of $PGF_{2\alpha}$ injection on d 7. All cows were tail painted 21 d prior to the commencement of the synchrony. At the time of the first GnRH injection cows were recorded as either cycling or non-cycling on the basis of the tail paint having been rubbed. It was hypothesised that eCG might increase fertility in an OvSynch program by hastening the development of follicles that take longer to emerge after the first GnRH injection so that they are capable of ovulation at the time of the second GnRH, as well as increasing the size of follicles at this time generally. Cows were pregnancy tested and the pregnancy was staged using ultrasound at both 7 and 14 wk after the fixed time AI.

An overall statistically significant increase in 25 d in-calf rate of 28% (41.2 to 52.6) and an increased 6 wk in calf-rate of nearly 25% (47.5 to 58.9). Much of the previous work involving Ovsynch programs and their derivatives in recent times has been directed at non-cycling cows. This trial demonstrated a statistically significant increase in 6 wk in calf rate for cows that were previously observed cycling at the time of treatment of 19% (55.1% to 65.8%, n = 233).

Acknowledgements: The Authors would like to acknowledge the assistance of Bioniche, and the farmers who helped so much.

Strategy to improve conception rate and reduce incidence of ovarian cysts in lactating postpartum dairy cows under a tropical environment

C Navanukraw[a], T Moonmanee[a], S Guntaprom[b] and K Kaewprom[c]

[a]*Department of Animal Science, Faculty of Agriculture, Khon Kaen University, Khon Kaen, Thailand;* [b]*Rajamangala University of Technology Isan Kalasin Campus, Thailand;* [c]*Faculty of Agriculture Technology, Rajabhat Mahasarakham University, Maha Sarakham, Thailand*

A tropical environment (hot and humid conditions) has been shown to alter the duration of estrus, conception rate, uterine function, endocrine status, follicular growth and development, and early embryonic development[1]. Two experiments were conducted to determine the effect of TAI protocols on progesterone (P4) concentrations, corpus luteum (CL) development, and conception rates and to reduce the incidence of ovarian cysts in lactating postpartum dairy cows. Experiment 1, Holstein crossbred dairy cows (n = 54) were assigned by parity to one of three TAI protocols (control = Ovsynch, Ovsynch + 3,000 IU hCG on d 5 after TAI, and Ovsynch + 100 µg GnRH on d 5 after TAI). Cows received TAI in the morning (6 am) to avoid heat stress or approximately 16 h after the second GnRH. Cows treated with 3,000 IU hCG or 100 µg GnRH had a greater number of CL than control cows (1.8±0.1, 1.8±0.2, and 0.8±0.1, respectively) and had greater P4 concentrations on d 12 after TAI than the control group (6.4±0.3, 5.1±0.4, and 3.8±0.5 ng/ml, respectively). However, conception rates were not different (55.5, 55.5, and 38.9%, respectively; $P > 0.05$). Experiment 2, Holstein crossbred dairy cows (n = 20) were identified as having follicular or luteal cysts by using transrectal ultrasonography as previously described[2]. Cows with follicular cysts (n = 12) were intramuscularly treated with 100 µg GnRH; whereas, cows with luteal cysts (n = 8) were intramuscularly treated with 25 mg $PGF_{2\alpha}$. Responsiveness of cows with luteal cysts to $PGF_{2\alpha}$ treatment was 100% (8/8) and greater ($P < 0.05$) than cows with the follicular cysts to GnRH treatment which was 33.3% (4/12). The P4 concentration of the luteal cysts was significantly decreased from 4.1±0.8 ng/ml at 0 h to 0.3±0.8 ng/ml by 48 h. However, the P4 concentration of the follicular cysts was not significantly increased from 0.3±0.2 ng/ml at 0 h to 1.3±0.2 ng/ml by 48 h. Thus, these strategies could be applied to improve the conception rate and reduce incidence of ovarian cysts in lactating postpartum dairy cows under heat stress.

This study was supported by Thailand Research Fund (TRF) and Agricultural Biotechnology Research Center for Sustainable Economy (ABRCSE), Khon Kaen University.

[1]Jordan, 2003. J Dairy Sci 86:E104-E114.
[2]Ambrose *et al.*, 2004. Can Vet J 45:931-937.

Ovine fixed time artificial insemination using a short term oestrous synchronization protocol with eCG and EB

C Castilho[a], MZ Costa[b], MF Almeida[a] and IC Giometti[a]

[a]*Universidade do Oeste Paulista (UNOESTE), Presidente Prudente (SP), Brazil;* [b]*Fundação Educacional de Andradina (FEA), Andradina (SP), Brazil*

Many advantages can be obtained by using estrous synchronization protocols in sheep reproduction. In intensive production systems that attempt to concentrate births or obtain 3 births every 2 years, estrous synchronization is required, especially in breeds with established reproductive seasonality. The aim of the study was to test short term hormonal protocols for fixed time artificial insemination (FTAI) using progesterone for 6 d and equine chorionic gonadotropin (eCG) or estradiol benzoate (EB) as ovulation inducers.

The experiment was conducted in São Paulo State, Brazil and included 31crossbred ewes, ranging in age from 3 to 5 years, in good body condition, grazing Tifton 85 grass (*Cynodon dactylon*) and Aruana grass (*Panicum Maximum cv.*) with free access to water and minerals. Each ewe was implanted with a 0.33 g progesterone releasing intravaginal device (CIDR, Pfizer, Brazil) and randomly divided into 3 groups. In the control group (G-C) 10 ewes had the progesterone devices for 9 d and at progesterone withdraw they received an injection of 12 mg of dinoprost (Lutalyse, Pfizer) and 300 units of eCG (Folligon, Intervet, Brazil). The groups G-eCG (12 ewes) and G-EB (9 ewes) had the progesterone device removed after 6 d and all animals were treated with 12 mg of dinoprost (Lutalyse). Twenty-four h after withdraw of the device, the animals in the G-eCG group were treated with 300 units of eCG (Folligon), and the animals in the G-EB group were treated with 1 mg of estradiol benzoate (Estrogin, Farmavet, Brazil). Intra-uterine artificial insemination was conducted by laparoscopy at fixed time (FTAI) 50 h after withdraw. Pregnancy detection was performed 30 d after insemination by trans-abdominal ultrasonography (Aloka SSD500 with a 5MHz probe). The results were statistically analyzed by Fisher's exact test test. There was a significant difference ($P<0.05$) in pregnancy rate between the G-eCG (66.6%) and G-EB (11%) groups, and these groups did not differ statistically from the G-C (30%).

In conclusion, it was possible to use a short time (6 d) progesterone treatment in an estrous synchronization protocol for ewes when combined with eCG to induce ovulation instead of EB.

[1]Killen and Caffery, 1982. Australian Veterinary Journal 59:95.

Influence of seasonality on long estrus synchronization protocols in Santa Inês sheep

MEF Oliveira[a], H Ayres[b], LG Oliveira[a], PPM Teixeira[a], SD Bicudo[c], JF Fonseca[d] and WRR Vicente[a]

[a]UNESP, Jaboticabal-SP, Brazil; [b]USP, São Paulo-SP, Brazil; [c]UNESP, Botucatu-SP, Brazil; [d]EMBRAPA, Sobral-CE, Brazil

Low levels of progesterone (P4) during long estrous synchronization protocols in ewes can promote excessive growth of the follicles, resulting in large persistent and aged ovulatory follicles. Timing of ovulation or the LH surge in relation to the onset of estrus is also more variable with lower progesterone[1]. These findings as well as an effect of seasonality may contribute to a reduction in fertility in ewes[2]. In southeastern Brazil, seasonality is not very marked, however, three seasons can be identified (anoestrus, transition and breeding).

This study was designed to investigate the influence of seasonality on ovulation in long synchronization protocols, with or without a P4 device, in Santa Inês sheep. Seventy adult ewes were treated with one of two synchronization protocols during three seasons (2 x 3 factorial; Anoestrus: $G\text{-}1_{CIDR}$, n=12 and $G\text{-}2_{CIDR}$, n=11; Transition: $G\text{-}1_{CIDR}$, n=12 and $G\text{-}2_{CIDR}$, n=12; Breeding: $G\text{-}1_{CIDR}$, n=11 and $G\text{-}2_{CIDR}$, n=12). Estrus was synchronized with a P4 device (CIDR) for 14 d. However, in $G\text{-}2_{CIDR}$, the CIDR was replaced by a new one on d 7 (d 0=P4 administration). Doses of 2.5 mg of dinoprost prostaglandin $F_{2\alpha}$, i.m. were administered on d 0 and 14. All ewes received 300 I.U. of eCG on d 14. Ultrasonographic examination of ovaries was performed every 8 h for 5 d after the end of treatment to determine the moment of ovulation and the diameter of the ovulatory follicle. Data were analyzed by GLIMMIX by using SAS. There was no group by season interaction; therefore, the main effects of the variables are presented.

All ewes ovulated at the end of the synchronization protocols. There was no effect of treatment on time of ovulation ($G\text{-}1_{CIDR}$ 74.4±2.3, vs. $G\text{-}2_{CIDR}$ 77.0±2.5 h after the end of the protocols; P=0.31), number of ovulations ($G\text{-}1_{CIDR}$ 1.3±0.1 vs. $G\text{-}2_{CIDR}$ 1.2±0.1; P=0.39) or diameter of the first ovulatory follicle ($G\text{-}1_{CIDR}$ 6.3±0.2 vs. $G\text{-}2_{CIDR}$ 7.5±0.2 mm; P=0.46). However, there was an effect of season on time of ovulation (anoestrus: 64.7±1.1[c] vs. transition: 88.7±1.9[a] vs. breeding: 73.2±2.7[b] h after the end of the protocols; [abc]P<0.0001), number of ovulations (anoestrus: 1.31±0.12[ab] vs. transition: 1.04±0.04[b] vs. breeding: 1.43±0.16[a]; [ab]P<0.06), and diameter of the first ovulatory follicle (anoestrus: 7.8±0.2[a] vs. transition: 7.1±0.1[b] vs. breeding: 7.3±0.2[ab] mm; [ab]P<0.04).

These results showed that the effect of the two synchronization protocols on ovulation was similar. However, season influenced the ovulation time and the diameter of the first ovulatory follicle. Finally, both protocols were effective during each season.

Financial support: FAPESP

[1]Viñoles *et al.*, 2001. Theriogenology 55:993-1004.
[2]Rosa and Bryant, 2003. Small Ruminant Research 48:155-171.

Reproductive performance in goats following estrus and ovulation synchronization with different progesterone time exposure, gonadotropins (eCG, hCG) and fixed-time intrauterine or transcervical insemination or natural service

E Loetz[a], L Dawson[a,b], J Hayes[a], I Portugal[a], T Sahlu[a] and J Malayer[b]

[a]*E. (Kika) de la Garza American Institute for Goat Research, Langston University, Oklahoma,*
[b]*Oklahoma State University, Stillwater, USA*

Reproductive performance (RP) is the largest determinant of income in a livestock enterprise[1]. Maintaining genetic selective pressure and decreasing costs to breed females require hormonal estrus/ovulation synchronization and fixed-time breeding. Synchronization protocols focusing on ovarian follicular dynamics have been validated on the basis of 5 to 6 d progesterone use and eCG or estradiol benzoate[2,3]. The use of eCG in combination with hCG in lieu of eCG alone has not been addressed.

The RP of cyclic dairy, meat and fiber goats (n = 879) was evaluated along with meat × fiber crossbreds using ultrasonography at 46 ± 4 d after breeding. All goats ranged from 1.5 to 11 yr of age with an average herd age of 4.1 ± 1.6 yr. The effect of gonadotropins on reproductive efficiency traits (RET) was evaluated from first-time breeding goats (n = 533). Data were fitted to logistic regression models. Independent variables were: a) estrus/ovulation synchronization protocols: Extra-long (XL) progesterone (P4) exposure (24 d CIDR-G), long (L; 12 to 14 d CIDR-G or Synchromate-B ear implant), short (S; 5 to 6 d CIDR-G) and two control cohorts (N) non-synchronized and NNT (non-synchronized and not fixed-time bred). b) type of breeding: Natural service (NS); laparoscopically-aided intrauterine (LAI) and transcervical AI, (TrAI) and c) use of eCG/hCG at 0, 140IU/70IU and 400IU/200IU. Secondary blocking variables were goat phenotype, breeding yr, age, parity, sire, AI and technician. RP was evaluated with RET: conception rate (CR), pregnancy rate (PR), fertility (F), prolificacy (P), fecundity (Fc), kidding rate (KR), litter size of fertile goats (LS/F) and LS at kidding (LS/K).

RET for synchronized, fixed-time bred goats were: CR = 57%, PR = 50%, F = 61%, P = 1.8, Fc = 1.09, KR = 61%, LS/F = 1.8 and LS/K = 1.8, compared with NNT goats which had: CR = 79% ($P<0.001$), PR = 67% ($P<0.001$), F = 53% ($P<0.02$), P = 1.7 ($P<0.008$), Fc = 0.89% ($P<0.0001$), KR = 52% ($P=0.07$), LS/F = 1.95 ($P<0.02$) and LS/K = 2.0 ($P<0.008$). Fixed-time NS resulted in the greatest PR with 66% compared with the 46% PR for fixed-timed LAI ($P<0.0001$) or the latter compared to the 27% PR attained with fixed-time TrAI ($P<0.02$).

We conclude that synchronization protocols with 5 to 6 d use of P4 and a combination of eCG/hCG reduce RET's. The use of eCG/hCG in P4-based synchronization protocols has a different effect on CR and LS depending on gonadotropin dose level. As expected, breeding type has a significant effect on all 6 RET's (odds ratios) studied with ($P<0.044$) for CR, ($P<0.025$) for P and ($P<0.001$) for the remaining RET's. Fixed-time breeding decreased RP when goats not-synchronized were compared with goats not-synchronized and not fix-timed bred.

[1]Luther, *et al.*, 2007. Small Rum Res 72:227-231.
[2]Menchaca and Rubianes, 2007. Reprod Domest Anim 42:590-593.
[3]Menchaca *et al.*, 2007. Anim Reprod Sci 102:76-87.

Lack of evidence for a gonadotrophic effect of royal jelly on progesterone-treated goats

L Alvarez, A Sánchez, D Gamboa and B De Luna

Facultad de Medicina Veterinaria y Zootecnia, Universidad Nacional Autónoma de México, Mexico

In progesterone-treated goats and sheep, an injection of eCG is necessary in order to promote a greater estrus and ovulatory response. eCG is too expensive and induces some negative consequences when used repeatedly.[1] Royal Jelly (RJ) is a natural substance produced in the pharyngeal glands of the bee (*Apis mellifera*) and used to feed young larvae and the queen bee. In several investigations carried out in sheep, injected or orally administered RJ during the 12 d of CIDR use induced the same estrus and ovulatory response as eCG.[2,3]

The objective of this study was to determine whether RJ can substitute for eCG in CIDR-based treatments without adversely affecting the results in adult dairy goats during the non-breeding season (April). Thirty-five goats received the CIDR device during 12 c. The eCG group (n = 12) was injected with 200 I.U. of the gonadotropin at CIDR withdrawal; the RJ group (n = 12) received a daily intramuscular injection of 1 g of RJ during the period of CIDR treatment; the CIDR group (n = 11) did not receive any additional treatment. A fourth group (Con, n = 12) was included as a control and received no treatment whatsoever. Estrus was detected every 4 h after CIDR removal using an aproned male. The estrus response, fertility (measured at kidding after 148 to 158 d) and number of kids per group were recorded.

Expression of estrus was greater in the eCG group (100%) than in the remaining groups (RJ, 33%; CIDR, 0% and Con, 0%) and occurred at shorter intervals (eCG, 34.2 ± 2.6; RJ, 61.5 ± 4.6; h $\pm$ SE; $P < 0.05$). Fertility was greater in the eCG group (91%) than in the others (RJ, 16%; CIDR, 0% and Con, 0%), the response was not different between RJ, CIDR and Con groups ($P > 0.05$). The number of kids was not different between groups ($P > 0.05$).

There was no evidence of a gonadotropic effect of RJ in progesterone-treated goats. It is concluded that administering 1 g of RJ during the time of CIDR treatment does not increase the reproductive results expressed in percentages of estrus and fertility.

[1]Roy *et al.*, 1999. Biol Reprod 60:805-813.
[2]Husein and Haddad, 2006. Anim Reprod Sci 93:24-33.
[3]Husein and Kridli, 2002. Anim Reprod Sci 74:45-53.

Subject index